Dietary Reference Intakes: RDA, AI*

Elements

Life Stage Group	Calcium (mg/d)	Chromium (µg/d)	Copper (µg/d)	Fluoride (mg/d)	Iodine (µg/d)	Iron (mg/d)	Magnesium (mg/d)	Manganese (mg/d)	Molybdenum (µg/d)	Phosphorus (mg/d)	Selenium (µg/d)	Zinc (mg/d)	Potassium (g/d)	Sodium (g/d)	Chloride (g/d)
Infants															
0–6 mo	200*	0.2*	200*	0.01*	110*	0.27*	30*	0.003*	2*	100*	15*	2*	0.4*	0.12*	0.18*
6–12 mo	260*	5.5*	220*	0.5*	130*	11	75*	0.6*	3*	275*	20*	3	0.7*	0.37*	0.57*
Children															
1–3 y	700	11*	340	0.7*	90	7	80	1.2*	17	460	20	3	3.0*	1.0*	1.5*
4–8 y	1,000	15*	440	1*	90	10	130	1.5*	22	500	30	5	3.8*	1.2*	1.9*
Males															
9–13 y	1,300	25*	700	2*	120	8	240	1.9*	34	1,250	40	8	4.5*	1.5*	2.3*
14–18 y	1,300	35*	890	3*	150	11	410	2.2*	43	1,250	55	11	4.7*	1.5*	2.3*
19–30 y	1,000	35*	900	4*	150	8	400	2.3*	45	700	55	11	4.7*	1.5*	2.3*
31–50 y	1,000	35*	900	4*	150	8	420	2.3*	45	700	55	11	4.7*	1.5*	2.3*
51–70 y	1,000	30*	900	4*	150	8	420	2.3*	45	700	55	11	4.7*	1.3*	2.0*
>70 y	1,200	30*	900	4*	150	8	420	2.3*	45	700	55	11	4.7*	1.2*	1.8*
Females															
9–13 y	1,300	21*	700	2*	120	8	240	1.6*	34	1,250	40	8	4.5*	1.5*	2.3*
14–18 y	1,300	24*	890	3*	150	15	360	1.6*	43	1,250	55	9	4.7*	1.5*	2.3*
19–30 y	1,000	25*	900	3*	150	18	310	1.8*	45	700	55	8	4.7*	1.5*	2.3*
31–50 y	1,000	25*	900	3*	150	18	320	1.8*	45	700	55	8	4.7*	1.5*	2.3*
51–70 y	1,200	20*	900	3*	150	8	320	1.8*	45	700	55	8	4.7*	1.3*	2.0*
>70 y	1,200	20*	900	3*	150	8	320	1.8*	45	700	55	8	4.7*	1.2*	1.8*
Pregnancy															
14–18 y	1,300	29*	1,000	3*	220	27	400	2.0*	50	1,250	60	12	4.7*	1.5*	2.3*
19–30 y	1,000	30*	1,000	3*	220	27	350	2.0*	50	700	60	11	4.7*	1.5*	2.3*
31–50 y	1,000	30*	1,000	3*	220	27	360	2.0*	50	700	60	11	4.7*	1.5*	2.3*
Lactation															
14–18 y	1,300	44*	1,300	3*	290	10	360	2.6*	50	1,250	70	13	5.1*	1.5*	2.3*
19–30 y	1,000	45*	1,300	3*	290	9	310	2.6*	50	700	70	12	5.1*	1.5*	2.3*
31–50 y	1,000	45*	1,300	3*	290	9	320	2.6*	50	700	70	12	5.1*	1.5*	2.3*

Note: This table (taken from the DRI reports, see www.nap.edu) presents Recommended Dietary Allowances (RDAs) in bold type and Adequate Intakes (AIs) in ordinary type followed by an asterisk (*). An RDA is the average daily dietary intake level sufficient to meet the nutrient requirements of nearly all (97–98 percent) healthy individuals in a group. It is calculated from an Estimated Average Requirement (EAR). If sufficient scientific evidence is not available to establish an EAR, and thus calculate an RDA, an AI is usually developed. For healthy breast-fed infants, an AI is the mean intake. The AI for other life stage and gender groups is believed to cover the needs of all healthy individuals in the groups, but lack of data or uncertainty in the data prevent being able to specify with confidence the percentage of individuals covered by this intake.

Data from: DIETARY REFERENCE INTAKES series, National Academies Press. Copyright ©1997, 1998, 2000, 2001, 2005, and 2011, by the National Academy of Sciences. These reports may be accessed via www.nap.edu. Courtesy of the National Academies Press, Washington, DC. Reprinted with permission.

Dietary Reference Intakes: RDA, AI*

Vitamins

Life Stage Group	Vitamin A (µg/d)[a]	Vitamin C (mg/d)	Vitamin D (µg/d)[b,c]	Vitamin E (mg/d)[d]	Vitamin K (µg/d)	Thiamin (mg/d)	Riboflavin (mg/d)	Niacin (mg/d)[e]	Vitamin B6 (mg/d)	Folate (µg/d)[f]	Vitamin B12 (µg/d)	Pantothenic Acid (mg/d)	Biotin (µg/d)	Choline (mg/d)[g]
Infants														
0–6 mo	400*	40*	10*	4*	2.0*	0.2*	0.3*	2*	0.1*	65*	0.4*	1.7*	5*	125*
6–12 mo	500*	50*	10*	5*	2.5*	0.3*	0.4*	4*	0.3*	80*	0.5*	1.8*	6*	150*
Children														
1–3 y	300	15	15	6	30*	0.5	0.5	6	0.5	150	0.9	2*	8*	200*
4–8 y	400	25	15	7	55*	0.6	0.6	8	0.6	200	1.2	3*	12*	250*
Males														
9–13 y	600	45	15	11	60*	0.9	0.9	12	1.0	300	1.8	4*	20*	375*
14–18 y	900	75	15	15	75*	1.2	1.3	16	1.3	400	2.4	5*	25*	550*
19–30 y	900	90	15	15	120*	1.2	1.3	16	1.3	400	2.4	5*	30*	550*
31–50 y	900	90	15	15	120*	1.2	1.3	16	1.3	400	2.4	5*	30*	550*
51–70 y	900	90	15	15	120*	1.2	1.3	16	1.7	400	2.4[h]	5*	30*	550*
>70 y	900	90	20	15	120*	1.2	1.3	16	1.7	400	2.4[h]	5*	30*	550*
Females														
9–13 y	600	45	15	11	60*	0.9	0.9	12	1.0	300	1.8	4*	20*	375*
14–18 y	700	65	15	15	75*	1.0	1.0	14	1.2	400[i]	2.4	5*	25*	400*
19–30 y	700	75	15	15	90*	1.1	1.1	14	1.3	400[i]	2.4	5*	30*	425*
31–50 y	700	75	15	15	90*	1.1	1.1	14	1.3	400[i]	2.4	5*	30*	425*
51–70 y	700	75	15	15	90*	1.1	1.1	14	1.5	400	2.4[h]	5*	30*	425*
>70 y	700	75	20	15	90*	1.1	1.1	14	1.5	400	2.4[h]	5*	30*	425*
Pregnancy														
14–18 y	750	80	15	15	75*	1.4	1.4	18	1.9	600[j]	2.6	6*	30*	450*
19–30 y	770	85	15	15	90*	1.4	1.4	18	1.9	600[j]	2.6	6*	30*	450*
31–50 y	770	85	15	15	90*	1.4	1.4	18	1.9	600[j]	2.6	6*	30*	450*
Lactation														
14–18 y	1,200	115	15	19	75*	1.4	1.6	17	2.0	500	2.8	7*	35*	550*
19–30 y	1,300	120	15	19	90*	1.4	1.6	17	2.0	500	2.8	7*	35*	550*
31–50 y	1,300	120	15	19	90*	1.4	1.6	17	2.0	500	2.8	7*	35*	550*

Note: This table (taken from the DRI reports, see www.nap.edu) presents Recommended Dietary Allowances (RDAs) in **bold type** and Adequate Intakes (AIs) in ordinary type followed by an asterisk (*). An RDA is the average daily dietary intake level sufficient to meet the nutrient requirements of nearly all (97–98 percent) healthy individuals in a group. It is calculated from an Estimated Average Requirement (EAR). If sufficient scientific evidence is not available to establish an EAR, and thus calculate an RDA, an AI is usually developed. For healthy breast-fed infants, an AI is the mean intake. The AI for other life stage and gender groups is believed to cover the needs of all healthy individuals in the groups, but lack of data or uncertainty in the data prevent being able to specify with confidence the percentage of individuals covered by this intake.

[a] As retinol activity equivalents (RAEs). 1 RAE = 1 µg retinol, 12 µg β-carotene, 24 µg α-carotene, or 24 µg β-cryptoxanthin. The RAE for dietary provitamin A carotenoids is two-fold greater than retinol equivalents (RE), whereas the RAE for preformed vitamin A is the same as RE.

[b] As cholecalciferol. 1 µg cholecalciferol = 40 IU. vitamin D.

[c] Under the assumption of minimal sunlight.

[d] As α-tocopherol. α-Tocopherol includes *RRR*-α-tocopherol, the only form of α-tocopherol that occurs naturally in foods, and the *2R*-stereoisomeric forms of α-tocopherol (*RRR*-, *RSR*-, *RRS*-, and *RSS*-α-tocopherol) that occur in fortified foods and supplements. It does not include the *2S*-stereoisomeric forms of α-tocopherol (*SRR*-, *SSR*-, *SRS*-, and *SSS*-α-tocopherol), also found in fortified foods and supplements.

[e] As niacin equivalents (NE). 1 mg of niacin = 60 mg of tryptophan; 0–6 months = preformed niacin (not NE).

[f] As dietary folate equivalents (DFE). 1 DFE = 1 µg food folate = 0.6 µg of folic acid from fortified food or as a supplement consumed with food = 0.5 µg of a supplement taken on an empty stomach.

[g] Although AIs have been set for choline, there are few data to assess whether a dietary supply of choline is needed at all stages of the life cycle, and it may be that the choline requirement can be met by endogenous synthesis at some of these stages.

[h] Because 10 to 30 percent of older people may malabsorb food-bound B_{12}, it is advisable for those older than 50 years to meet their RDA mainly by consuming foods fortified with B_{12} or a supplement containing B_{12}.

[i] In view of evidence linking folate intake with neural tube defects in the fetus, it is recommended that all women capable of becoming pregnant consume 400 µg from supplements or fortified foods in addition to intake of food folate from a varied diet.

[j] It is assumed that women will continue consuming 400 µg from supplements or fortified food until their pregnancy is confirmed and they enter prenatal care, which ordinarily occurs after the end of the periconceptional period—the critical time for formation of the neural tube.

Data from: DIETARY REFERENCE INTAKES series, National Academies Press. Copyright ©1997, 1998, 2000, 2001, 2005, and 2011, by the National Academy of Sciences. These reports may be accessed via www.nap.edu. Courtesy of the National Academies Press, Washington, DC. Reprinted with permission.

A Modern and Personal Approach to Nutrition

Nutrition: From Science to You helps students understand the science of nutrition and how to successfully apply it to their personal lives fute careers. Thoroughly updated to better meet the needs of tomorrow's nutrition and allied health professionals, the **4th Edition** provides students with more inter-professional applications, increased coverage of emerging and high interest topics such as the microbiome and Leaky Gut syndrome, and new dietary and nutrition guidelines.

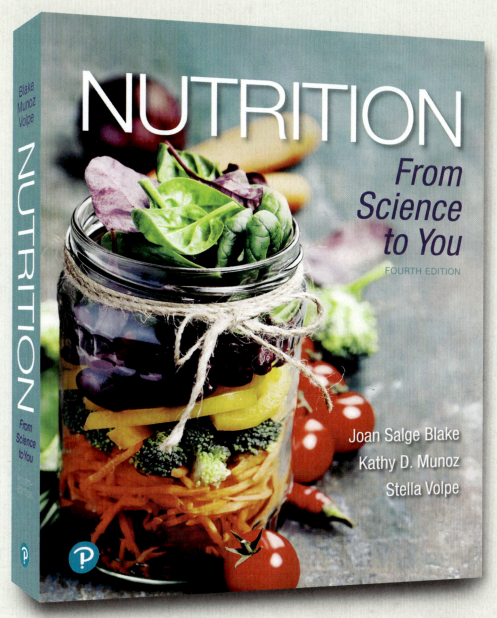

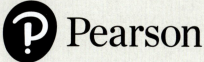

Helping Students Make
Connections Between

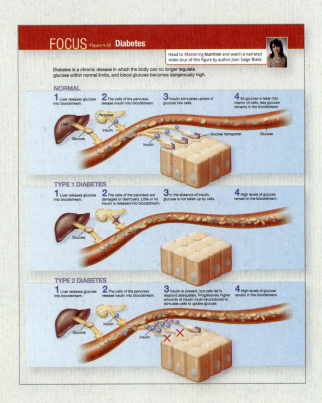

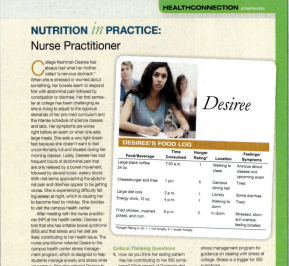

Nutrition, Themselves, and Their Future Careers

Health Connections appear in each chapter directly before the Visual Chapter Summary. Tied to learning outcomes, these figures highlight diseases and disorders in which nutrition plays a major role, as well as nutritional practices that offer unique health benefits.

NEW! and EXPANDED! Coverage of important topics, including:

- Prediabetes
- Non-celiac gluten sensitivity
- FODMAP diet
- FITT and HIIT
- Prebiotics and synbiotics
- And more!

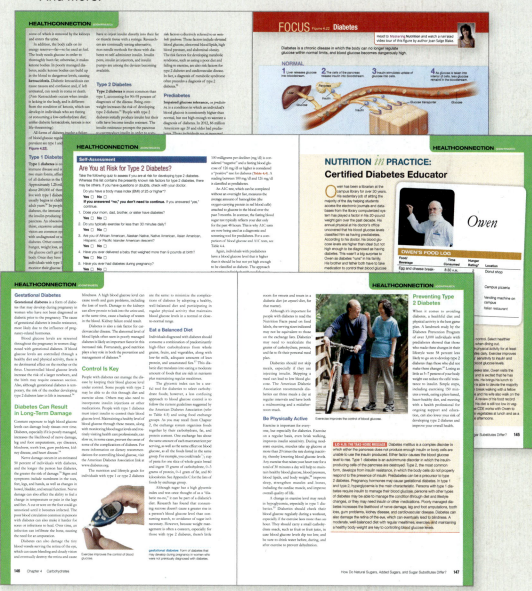

BEFORE CLASS

Mobile Media and Reading Assignments Ensure Students Come to Class Prepared

UPDATED! Dynamic Study Modules help students study effectively on their own by continuously assessing their activity and performance in real time. These are available as graded assignments prior to class, and accessible on smartphones, tablets, and computers.

NEW! Instructors can now remove questions from Dynamic Study Modules to better fit their course.

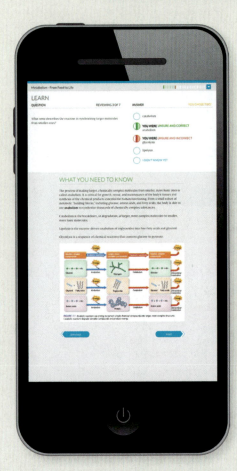

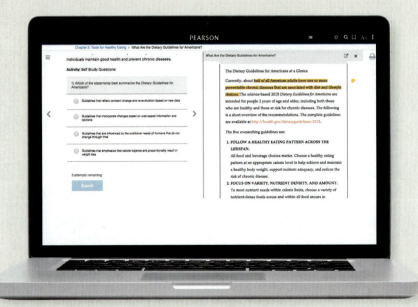

UPDATED! Pearson eText now optimized for mobile:

- Pearson eText mobile app offers offline access
- Seamlessly integrated videos and other rich media
- Accessible (screen-reader ready)
- Configurable reading settings, including resizable type and night reading mode
- Instructor and student note-taking, highlighting, bookmarking, and search

During & After Class with
MasteringNutrition™

DURING CLASS

Engage students with Learning Catalytics

Learning Catalytics, a "bring your own device" student engagement, assessment, and classroom intelligence system, allows students to use their smartphone, tablet, or laptop to respond to questions in class.

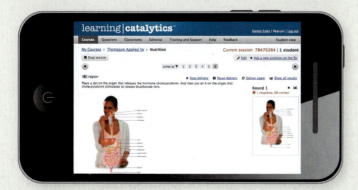

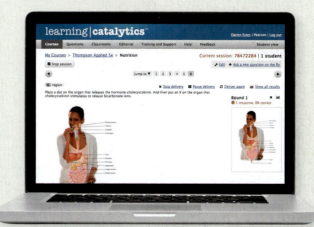

AFTER CLASS

Mastering Nutrition Delivers Diet Analysis Tools and Activities to students

Mastering Nutrition includes Access to MyDietAnalysis
MyDietAnalysis is available as a single sign on to Mastering Nutrition. For smartphone users, a mobile website version of MyDietAnalysis is available. Students can track their diet and activity intake accurately, anytime and anywhere, from their mobile device.

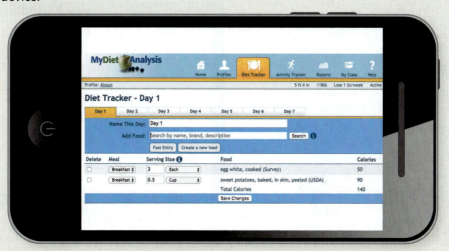

AFTER CLASS

Easy to Assign, Customize, Media-Rich, and Automatically Graded Assignments.

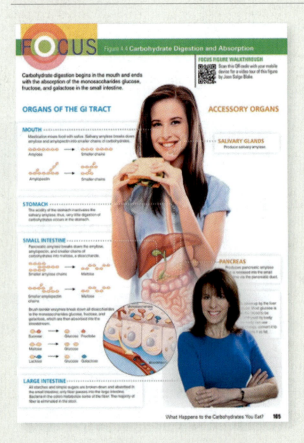

NEW! Focus Figure Coaching activities are interactive, mini-lessons narrated by author Joan Salge Blake. These video walkthroughs, and associated coaching activities, help students understand key concepts.'

NEW! MDA Personalized Dietary Analysis activities guide students in a thorough investigation of their dietary intake and are focused on the most commonly assigned topics in diet analysis projects. Follow-up feedback and a reflection question help students understand how to improve their diets. **Activities can also be automatically graded,** saving instructors valuable time from grading their students' lengthy diet analysis projects

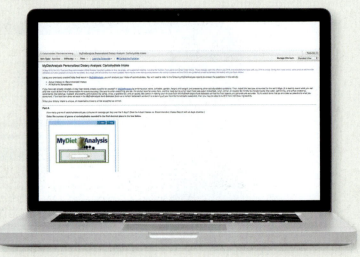

During & After Class with
MasteringNutrition

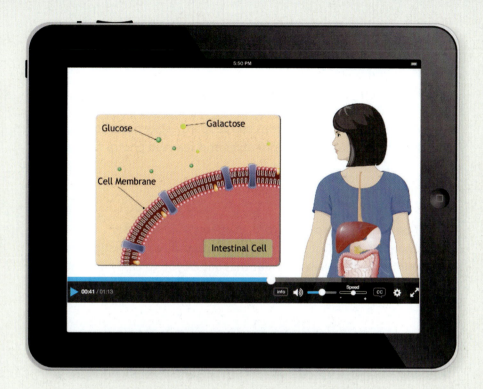

Nutrition Animations help students master tough topics with associated auto-graded coaching activities that contain hints and wrong-answer feedback.

NutriTools Coaching Activities allow students to combine and experiment with different food options and learn firsthand how to build healthier meals.

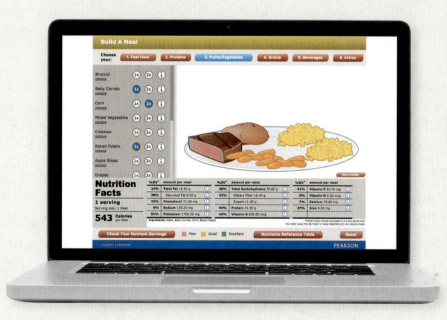

Additional videos in Mastering Nutrition include Math Videos, ABC News Videos, and Joan Salge Blake's Practical Nutrition Tips!

Resources for YOU, the Instructor

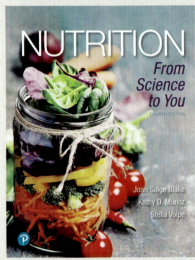

Mastering Nutrition

Mastering Nutrition provides you with everything you need to prep for your course and deliver a dynamic lecture, in one convenient place. Resources include:

MEDIA ASSETS FOR EACH CHAPTER

- *ABC News* Lecture Launcher videos
- Nutrition Animations
- Practical Nutrition Tip videos
- PowerPoint Lecture Outlines
- PowerPoint clicker questions and Jeopardy-style quiz show questions
- Files for all illustrations and tables and selected photos from the text

TEST BANK

- Test Bank in Microsoft, Word, PDF, and RTF formats
- Computerized Test Bank, which includes all the questions from the printed test bank in a format that allows you to easily and intuitively build exams a quizzes.

TEACHING RESOURCES

- Instructor Resource and Support Manual in Microsoft Word and PDF formats
- Learning Catalytics: Getting Started
- Getting Started with Mastering Nutrition

STUDENT SUPPLEMENTS

- Eat Right! Healthy Eating in College and Beyond
- Food Composition Table

Measuring Student Learning Outcomes?

All of the Mastering Nutrition assignable content is tagged to book content and to Bloom's Taxonomy. You also have the ability to add your own learning outcomes, helping you track student performance against your learning outcomes. You can view class performance against the specified learning outcomes and share those results quickly and easily by exporting to a spreadsheet.

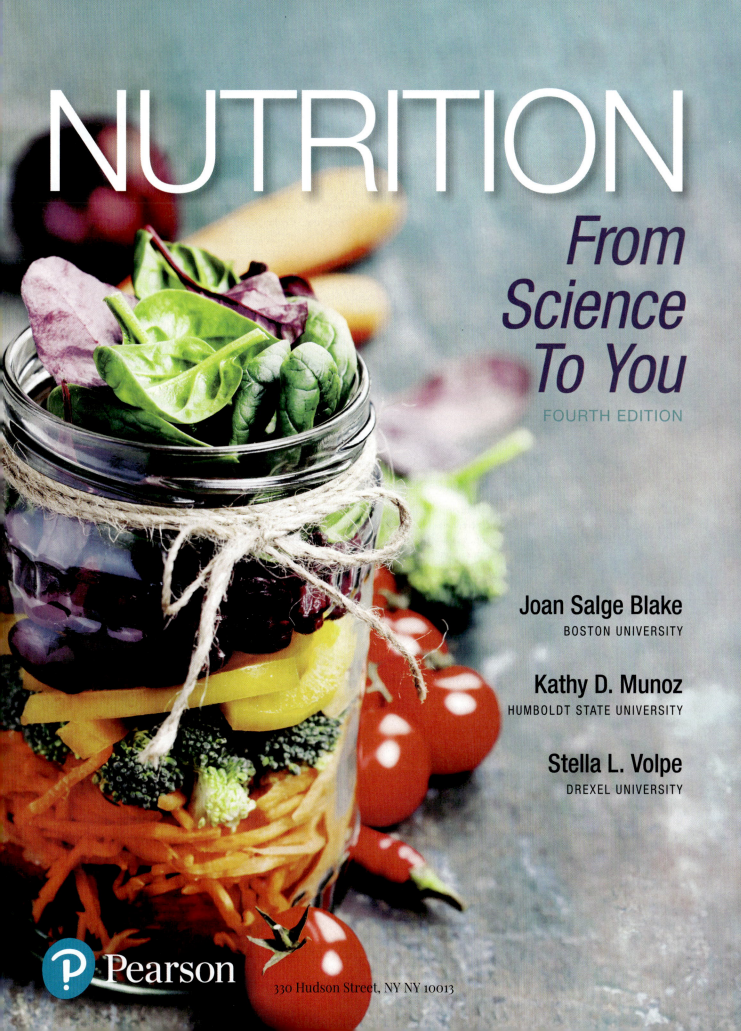

NUTRITION

From Science To You

FOURTH EDITION

Joan Salge Blake
BOSTON UNIVERSITY

Kathy D. Munoz
HUMBOLDT STATE UNIVERSITY

Stella L. Volpe
DREXEL UNIVERSITY

Pearson

330 Hudson Street, NY NY 10013

Courseware Portfolio Manager: Michelle Yglecias
Content Producer: Lizette Faraji
Managing Producer: Nancy Tabor
Courseware Director, Content Development: Barbara Yien
Development Editor: Laura Bonazzoli
Courseware Editorial Assistant: Nicole Constantine, Crystal Trigueros
Rich Media Content Producer: Lucinda Bingham
Full-Service Vendor: SPi Global
Copyeditor: Laura Patchkovsky
Compositor: SPi Global
Art Coordinator: Morgan Ewald, Lachina Publishing Services
Design Manager: Mark Ong

Interior Designer: Gary Hespenheide
Cover Designer: Gary Hespenheide
Rights & Permissions Project Manager: Linda DeMasi, Cenveo Publishing Services
Rights & Permissions Management: Ben Ferrini
Photo Researcher: Clare Maxwell
Manufacturing Buyer: Stacey Weinberger, LSC Communications
Executive Product Marketing Manager: Neena Bali, Alysun Burns
Field Marketing Manager: Mary Salzman
Printer/Binder: LSC Communications, Inc.
Cover Printer: Phoenix Color/Hagerstown
Cover Photo Credit: Natalia Klenova/Shutterstock

Cataloging-in-Publishing data is on file with the Library of Congress
Names: Blake, Joan Salge, author. | Munoz, Kathy D., 1951- author. | Volpe, Stella, 1963- author.
Title: Nutrition : from science to you / Joan Salge Blake (Boston University), Kathy D. Munoz (Humboldt State University), Stella L. Volpe (Drexel University).
Description: Fourth edition. | New York : Pearson, [2019]
Identifiers: LCCN 2017056138
Subjects: LCSH: Nutrition–Textbooks.
Classification: LCC RA784 .B553 2019 | DDC 613.2–dc23
LC record available at https://lccn.loc.gov/2017056138

ISBN 10: **0-13-466826-X;** ISBN 13: **978-0-134-66826-0** (Student edition)
ISBN 10: **0-134-79645-4;** ISBN 13: **978-0-134-79645-1** (Instructor's Review Copy)

1 18

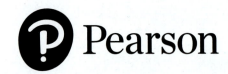

www.pearson.com

Brief Contents

Contents

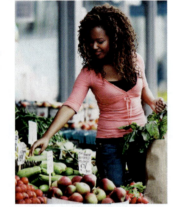
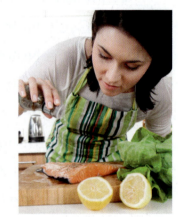

3
Digestion, Absorption, and Transport   75

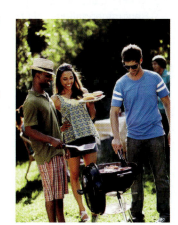

4
Carbohydrates   111

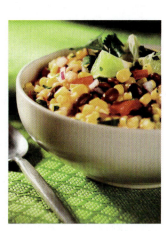

5

Lipids 157

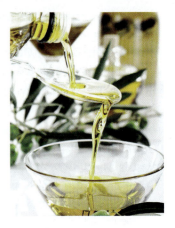

6

Proteins   205

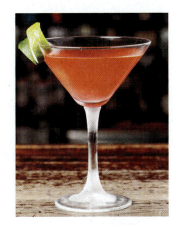

7

Alcohol   247

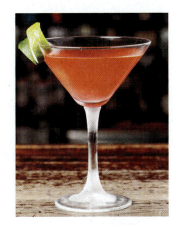

8
Energy Metabolism 281

9
Fat-Soluble Vitamins 317

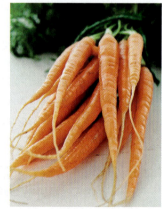

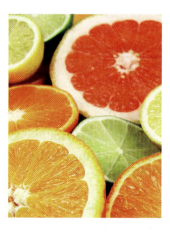

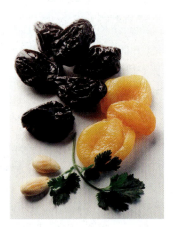

13
Trace Minerals   469

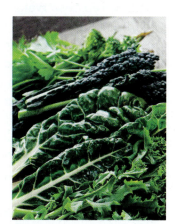

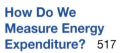
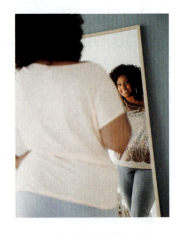

16
Nutrition and Fitness 577

17
Life Cycle Nutrition: Pregnancy through Infancy 619

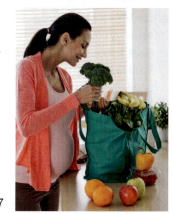

18
Life Cycle Nutrition: Toddlers through Adolescents 665

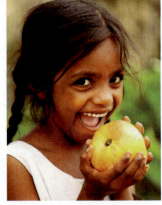

21

Global Nutrition and Malnutrition   779

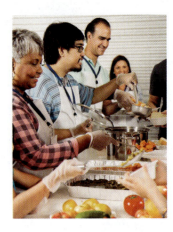

Appendices

Special Features

Scan this QR code to access all Focus Figure Narrated Walkthroughs videos, Calculation Corner videos, and MP3 Tutor Sessions for this edition.

FOCUS FIGURE

HEALTH CONNECTION

Calculation Corner

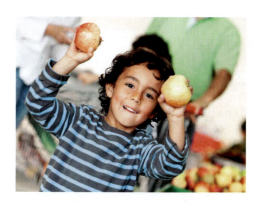

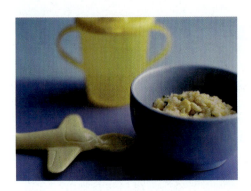

Chemistry Boost

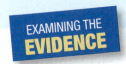

EXAMINING THE EVIDENCE

NUTRITION *in* PRACTICE

Self-Assessment

About the Authors

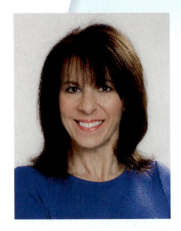

Joan Salge Blake, MS, RD, LDN
Boston University

Dr. Joan Salge Blake is a Clinical Associate Professor and Dietetics Internship Director at Boston University's Sargent College of Health and Rehabilitation Sciences. She teaches both graduate and undergraduate nutrition courses. She received her MS and EdD from Boston University.

Joan is a member of the Academy of Nutrition and Dietetics (formerly the American Dietetic Association) and the Massachusetts Dietetic Association (MAND). She has been a presenter and Presiding Officer at both the AND Annual Meeting and the MAND Annual Convention and is a guest lecturer at both the Boston University Goldman School of Dental Medicine and the Boston University School of Medicine. She was previously named MDA's "Young Dietitian of the Year" and is the past Director of Education and Nominating Committee Chairperson for the MDA. She currently serves on the MDA board. Joan has received the Whitney Powers Excellence in Teaching award from Boston University and the Annie Galbraith Outstanding Dietitian award from the Massachusetts Dietetic Association.

In addition to teaching and writing, Joan has a private practice specializing in weight management and lifestyle changes. Joan is often asked to translate complex nutritional issues in popular terms in the media. She has conducted over 1,000 media interviews and is a contributor of nutrition articles in a variety of news outlets. Joan was an AND National Media Spokesperson for nine years.

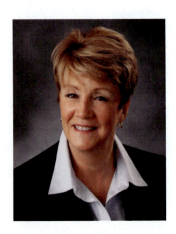

Kathy D. Munoz, EdD, RDN
Humboldt State University

Kathy D. Munoz is a professor emerita and professor of nutrition in the Department of Kinesiology and Recreation Administration at Humboldt State University. She teaches undergraduate introductory nutrition, exercise nutrition, and weight management courses, and teaching preparation in higher education courses in the Extended Education, College of eLearning. She received her EdD from the University of Southern California in curriculum design and an MS in Foods and Nutrition with a minor in exercise physiology from Oregon State University.

Kathy is a member of the Academy of Nutrition and Dietetics and the California Dietetic Association. Her professional memberships include Dietitians in Integrative and Functional Medicine (DIFM), Sports, Cardiovascular, and Wellness Nutrition (SCAN), and Weight Management (WM).

Kathy has published articles in *Research Quarterly for Exercise and Sport, Children's Health Care,* the *Journal of Nutrition Education,* and the *International Journal of Sport Nutrition and Exercise,* and has co-authored a series of nutrition and physical activity curriculum guides for elementary teachers. Kathy has also been recognized for her research in, and development of curriculum for, asynchronous learning.

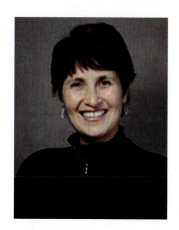

Stella L. Volpe, PhD, RD, LDN, FACSM
Drexel University

Dr. Stella Lucia Volpe is Professor and Chair of the Department of Nutrition Sciences at Drexel University. Stella is a nutritionist and exercise physiologist who has built a program of research focusing on three interrelated areas that traverse the lifespan: (1) obesity and diabetes prevention via mineral supplementation, (2) weight management through diet, exercise, and educational programs, and (3) environmental change leading to weight management. She is conducting a cross-sectional, long-term study assessing body composition, resting metabolic rate, maximal oxygen consumption and diet in athletes. In addition, she has recently completed a three-year, school-based obesity prevention trial.

Stella received her BS in Exercise Science from the University of Pittsburgh, her MS in Exercise Physiology from Virginia Tech, and her PhD in Nutrition, also from Virginia Tech.

Prior to beginning her faculty appointment at Drexel University, Stella was on the faculty of the University of Pennsylvania, and previous to that, she was on the faculty at the University of Massachusetts, Amherst. Stella is both a Certified Clinical Exercise Physiologist (American College of Sports Medicine [ACSM]), and a Registered Dietitian Nutritionist. She is a Fellow of the ACSM. Stella is a competitive athlete in field hockey, rowing, ice hockey. She enjoys being active with her husband and their German Shepherd dogs, Sasha and Bear.

Preface

Why We Wrote *Nutrition: From Science to You*

We wrote *Nutrition: From Science to You* to provide you with a solid foundation about nutrition and how it affects *you* and your nutritional needs, concerns, and questions.

Between the three of us, we have more than 60 years of experience teaching college-level nutrition. We've conducted and published research, studied the literature, and listened to and watched our students learn the science. We've taken copious notes regarding students' questions, interests, concerns, and misunderstandings, both in and outside the classroom. These years of experience have culminated in a textbook that we believe translates the latest nutrition science into a readable format to provide you with information that you can easily incorporate into your life and the lives of others.

As a college student, you are exposed to a steady stream of nutrition and health information from the media, your family and friends, and the Internet. Although you may think Google has the answer to your nutrition questions, we have seen students frequently fall victim to misinformation found on the Web. We designed *Nutrition: From Science to You* to be as user friendly as possible, and packed exclusively with sound nutrition information. The text goes beyond basic nutrition science and provides realistic advice and strategies to help you apply what you learn in your own life. The text is written to meet *your* nutritional concerns and answer *your* questions.

Remember, nutrition matters to *you!* What you eat today and tomorrow will affect you and your body for years to come. Just as important, what you learn about nutrition today will enable you to make a positive effect on the lives of others from now on.

New to This Edition

- **The 2015 Dietary Guidelines of America and Nutrition Facts Panel** are fully integrated into the fourth edition.
- **Focus Figure Video Walkthroughs** narrated by author Joan Salge Blake provide a video tour of the full-page Focus Figure, where each part is broken down and further explained by Joan Salge Blake, just as she would do in the classroom. Students can access these videos in—and instructors can assign them from—Mastering Nutrition.
- **Inter-professional Nutrition in Practice case studies** encourage critical thinking and emphasize the applicability of the content to your own life and future career. Some case studies draw upon Joan Salge Blake's experience as a dietitian working with actual clients, while others have been created with a new focus for those students interested in pursuing other allied health professions such as nursing, physical therapy, etc.
- **New and expanded topics such as:** prediabetes, non-celiac gluten sensitivity, FODMAP diet, FITT and high intensity interval training, prebiotics and synbiotics, and more. In addition, Chapter 8, including metabolism and energy metabolism pathways, has been significantly restructured for clarity.

Other Key Features

- **Learning Outcomes** are used to structure the chapter: each main heading is accompanied by its own learning outcome; **The Take-Home Message** at the end of each main section repeats the learning outcome number before a brief summation of the key points; and the **Visual Chapter Summary** is organized by learning outcome number and contains key images and concepts. This strong pedagogical structure throughout the chapter promotes comprehension and facilitates study and review.
- **Health Connections** appear in each chapter directly before the Visual Chapter Summary. These sections, which are tied to learning outcomes, highlight diseases and disorders in which nutrition plays a major role, as well as nutritional practices that offer unique health benefits.
- **Content has been updated throughout** to be consistent with new guidelines, data, research, and trends.
- **Mastering™ Nutrition,** the online homework, tutorial, and assessment system, delivers self-paced tutorials and activities that provide individualized coaching, focus on your course objectives, and are responsive to your personal progress. The Mastering system is the most effective and widely used online homework, tutorial, and assessment system for the sciences. It helps instructors maximize class time with customizable, easy-to-assign, and automatically graded assessments that motivate students to learn outside of class and arrive prepared for lectures. Mastering Nutrition for the fourth edition includes new Focus Figure Coaching Activities, updated NutriTools Coaching Activities, and much more. Learn more at www.masteringhealthandnutrition.com.
- **MyDietAnalysis mobile website** is available, so you can track your diet and activity intake accurately, anytime, and anywhere from your mobile device. Learn more at www.mydietanalysis.com. Access to MyDietAnalysis is included in Mastering Nutrition at no additional cost.
- **Examining the Evidence** features look at the latest research on hot topics in nutrition today. These features guide you to making better, informed choices in your personal nutrition, while also demonstrating the ways nutrition professionals are constantly expanding and refining our understanding of nutritional science.
- **Exploring Micronutrients** within Chapters 9, 10, 12, and 13 are self-contained sections that incorporate photos, illustrations, and text to present each vitamin and mineral. Each micronutrient is discussed using the same categories (forms, absorption and transport, functions, daily needs, food sources, and toxicity and deficiency symptoms) for a consistent and easy-to-study format.
- **Chemistry Boosts** review chemistry concepts within the context in which you need to know them.
- **Calculation Corners** walk through mathematical equations used in the chapter and give you practice working the equations themselves. These features also have corresponding math video activities in Mastering Nutrition.
- **True or False?** pretests open each chapter with 10 true/false statements that help you realize that the things you think you know about nutrition aren't always accurate. Answers are given at the end of the chapter.
- **Table Tips** give practical ideas for incorporating adequate amounts of each nutrient into your diet using widely available foods.
- **Self-Assessments** throughout the book ask you to think about your own diet and behaviors and how well you are meeting your various nutrient needs.

Chapter-by-Chapter Updates

Nutrition research and applications continue to expand our understanding of this advancing and dynamic science. To keep pace, we've reorganized the content, and visually improved the figures and tables to enrich student learning in each chapter in the 4th edition of *Nutrition: From Science to You.*

Chapter 1: What Is Nutrition?

- Learning Outcomes tie into major headings, The Take-Home Messages, and Visual Chapter Summaries.
- Updated statistics on such key topics as the obesity epidemic, consumption trends, the quality of the American diet, leading causes of death in the United States.
- Moved content on meeting nutrition needs into its own section with Learning Outcome and The Take-Home Message.
- Created a new Health Connection on *Finding Credible Nutrition Information.*

Chapter 2: Tools for Healthy Eating

- Learning outcomes are highlighted to match the major headings, the Take-Home Message, and visual chapter summaries.
- Added a new Focus Figure 2.3, *Dietary Reference Intakes.*
- Created a new Focus Figure 2.10, *The Nutrition Facts Panel,* to describe the newest proposed food label changes.
- Developed a new Health Connection, with accompanying Learning Outcome and The Take-Home Message, on *Portion Distortion* to provide guidance on how to recognize healthy portion sizes to reduce the risk of weight gain.

Chapter 3: Digestion, Absorption, and Transport

- Learning Outcomes tie into major headings, The Take-Home Messages, and Visual Chapter Summary sections.
- Added a new Figure 3.12 summarizing the actions of digestive hormones.
- Added a new Figure 3.13 on how the cardiovascular and lymphatic systems transport nutrients.
- Added a new Figure 3.16 on the effects celiac disease has on the wall of the small intestine.
- Consolidated coverage of celiac disease and other digestive disorders into a new Health Connection with accompanying Learning Outcome and The Take-Home Message.

Chapter 4: Carbohydrates

- Learning Outcomes tie into major headings, The Take-Home Messages, and Visual Chapter Summaries.
- Created a new Figure 4.9 on absorption and storage of monosaccharides.
- Added a discussion of hypoglycemia to the section on regulating blood glucose.
- Added a new Focus Figure 4.23, *Diabetes,* showing the mechanisms involved in both type 1 and type 2 diabetes.
- Revised all carbohydrate food source diagrams to feature new foods.
- Added a discussion of glycemic index and glycemic load to the section on best food sources of carbohydrates.
- Created a new Examining the Evidence feature, *Do Sugar-Sweetened Beverages Cause Obesity?*
- Updated coverage of sugar substitutes.
- Relocated Health Connection on diabetes and included Learning Outcome and The Take-Home Message.

Chapter 5: Lipids

- Learning Outcomes tie into major headings, The Take-Home Messages, and Visual Chapter Summaries.
- Revised headings to clarify when the discussion covers lipids in general or triglycerides specifically.
- Revised the Focus Figure 5.16, *Lipid Digestion and Absorption*.
- Created a new Figure 5.15, *Lipoproteins*, to illustrate the both the size and compositions differences between the lipoproteins.
- Created a new Figure 5.18 on the metabolism of linoleic acid and alpha-linolenic acid.
- Moved both Figure 5.19 on the production of bile from cholesterol and Figure 5.20 on the phospholipid bilayer to the section discussing the roles of phospholipids and cholesterol in the body.
- Revised all lipid food source diagrams to feature new foods.
- Updated the research on the Mediterranean Diet in a new Spotlight box and added a new figure of the latest Healthy Mediterranean Diet Pyramid.
- Added a new Examining the Evidence feature, *Is Coconut Oil the Next Superfood?*
- Updated the Health Connection on heart disease and added a Learning Outcome and The Take-Home Message.
- Created a new Focus Figure 5.25, *Atherosclerosis*.

Chapter 6: Proteins

- Learning Outcomes tie into major headings, The Take-Home Messages, and Visual Chapter Summaries.
- Revised Figure 6.1 on the structural differences between carbohydrates, proteins, and fats.
- Revised Figure 6.2 on the organization and shape of proteins.
- Modified Focus Figure 6.6 on the digestion and absorption of protein.
- Revised Focus Figure 6.7 on protein synthesis.
- Modified Figure 6.9 on deamination and transamination.
- Moved coverage of amino acid score, PDCAAS, biological value, protein quality to the section discussing food sources of protein.
- Updated the statistics and references in the Examining the Evidence feature, *Does Soy Reduce the Risk of Disease?*
- Revised all protein food source diagrams to feature new foods.
- Expanded the Health Connection on vegetarian diets, with accompanying Learning Outcome and The Take-Home Message, to include benefits and potential risks of vegetarian diets.
- Added Figure 6.20, *MyVeganPlate*.

Chapter 7: Alcohol

- Learning Outcomes tie into major headings, The Take-Home Messages, and Visual Chapter Summaries.
- Reorganized the order of the topics presented and updated latest statistics and research.
- Moved content on reasons for drinking into its own section with Learning Outcome and The Take-Home Message.
- Moved content on short-term effects of alcohol into its own section with Learning Outcome and The Take-Home Message.
- Expanded the coverage of the negative impact of alcohol consumption, including the statistics on depression.

- Moved *Figure 1, How Red Wine May Affect the Risk of Cardiovascular Disease* to the Examining the Evidence, *Does Moderate Alcohol Consumption Provide Health Benefits?*
- Expanded the information on the moderate consumption of alcohol to emphasize the age-related benefits not seen in younger adults.
- Expanded the content on alcohol abuse and alcoholism in the Health Connection, with accompanying Learning Outcome and The Take-Home Message, and updated statistics on the prevalence of different types of alcohol abuse.

Chapter 8: Energy Metabolism

- Learning Outcomes tie into major headings, The Take-Home Messages, and Visual Chapter Summaries.
- Modified references to high-energy electrons and hydrogen ions throughout the chapter.
- Created a new figure for the Chemistry Boost box that illustrates oxidation-reduction reactions.
- Revised Figure 8.5, *The Metabolic Fate of Food*.
- Created a new Table 8.2, *Glucogenic and Ketogenic Amino Acids*
- Revised Figure 8.11, *Fatty Acids Are Oxidized for Energy*.
- Revised Figure 8.13, *The Electron Transport Chain*.
- Revised explanation of electron transport chain and oxidative phosphorylation.
- Revised Figure 8.18, *The Metabolism of Alcohol*.
- Created a new Figure 8.19 to illustrate galactosemia.
- Expanded the Health Connection, with accompanying Learning Outcome and The Take-Home Message, on inborn errors of metabolism.

Chapter 9: Fat-Soluble Vitamins

- Learning Outcomes tie into major headings, The Take-Home Messages, and Visual Chapter Summaries.
- For each fat-soluble vitamin, included the Learning Outcome at the beginning of the section, and added a new The Take-Home Message at the end.
- Revised all fat-soluble vitamin food source diagrams to feature new foods.
- Created a new Focus Figure 9.8, *Retinal and Its Role in Vision*.
- Revised Table 9.4 on the function, daily needs, food sources, toxicity, and deficiency of each fat-soluble vitamin.
- Moved the Nutrition in Practice on vitamin D deficiency to fall within the vitamin D section.
- Created a new Health Connection, with accompanying Learning Outcome and The Take-Home Message, on the role of vitamin supplements in good health.
- Added a new Figure 9.27 on dietary supplement labels.

Chapter 10: Water-Soluble Vitamins

- Learning Outcomes tie into major headings, The Take-Home Messages, and Visual Chapter Summaries.
- Revised Figure 10.1, *Digesting and Absorbing Water-Soluble Vitamins*.
- Moved Figure 10.3 on the functions of B vitamins in energy metabolism to the section discussing the primary functions of water-soluble vitamins.
- Revised Table 10.1 on the function, daily needs, food sources, toxicity, deficiency, and active form of each water-soluble vitamin.
- For each water-soluble vitamin, included the Learning Outcome at the beginning of the section, and added a new The Take-Home Message at the end.

- Revised all water-soluble vitamin food source diagrams to feature new foods.
- Revised Figure 10.16, *Pantothenic Acid and Energy Metabolism.*
- Revised Figure 10.20, *Vitamin B₆ Assists in Transamination.*
- Revised Figure 10.23, *The Digestion of Folate*
- Added new Figure 10.28 on the absorption of vitamin B_{12}, including the reactions of vitamin B_{12} with the R protein and intrinsic factor in the gastrointestinal tract.
- Revised discussion of how folate deficiency may mask vitamin B_{12} deficiency.
- Updated the information in the Examining the Evidence feature on vitamin C and the common cold.
- Added a new Health Connection, with accompanying Learning Outcome and The Take-Home Message, on the role of a healthy diet and lifestyle in cancer risk.

Chapter 11: Water

- Learning Outcomes tie into major headings, The Take-Home Messages, and Visual Chapter Summaries.
- Revised Figure 11.1, *The Composition of the Body.*
- Revised Figure 11.5, *Sources of Body Water and Routes of Excretion.*
- Updated the Examining the Evidence feature on bottled water to include the most recent research.
- Updated coverage of the health effects of too much or too little water with the latest research and moved into a new Health Connection, with accompanying Learning Outcome and The Take-Home Message,
- Added a new Focus Figure 11.12, *Fluid Balance during Exercise.*

Chapter 12: Major Minerals

- Learning Outcomes tie into major headings, The Take-Home Messages, and Visual Chapter Summaries.
- Revised Table 12.2 on the function, daily needs, food sources, toxicity, and deficiency, of each major mineral.
- For each major mineral, included the Learning Outcome at the beginning of the section, and added a new The Take-Home Message at the end.
- Revised all major mineral food source diagrams to feature new foods.
- Revised Figure 12.4, *Sodium Helps Transport Some Nutrients.*
- Revised Figure 12.8 to illustrate the size of a kidney stone.
- Created a new Focus Figure 12.11 on the hormonal regulation of blood calcium levels.
- Revised and updated the content on bone mass and osteoporosis in the Health Connection, with accompanying Learning Outcome and The Take-Home Message.

Chapter 13: Trace Minerals

- Learning Outcomes tie into major headings, The Take-Home Messages, and Visual Chapter Summaries.
- Revised Table 13.1 on the function, daily needs, food sources, toxicity, deficiency, and interaction of each trace mineral.
- For each trace mineral, included the Learning Outcome at the beginning of the section, and added a new The Take-Home Message at the end.
- Revised all trace mineral food source diagrams to feature new foods.
- Expanded the Health Connection, with accompanying Learning Outcome and The Take-Home Message, to include the causes, symptoms, testing, and treatment for both microcytic and macrocytic anemia.

- Revised Figure 13.18 compares healthy red blood cells to microcytic and macrocytic red blood cells affected by anemia.

Chapter 14: Energy Balance and Body Composition

- Learning Outcomes tie into major headings, The Take-Home Messages, and Visual Chapter Summaries.
- Added a new Focus Figure 14.1 describing energy balance, negative energy balance, and positive energy balance.
- Expanded discussion of the health risks associated with underweight and overweight.
- Added Table 14.6 defining the terms underweight, overweight, and obesity classified by BMI.
- Added Table 14.7 listing different methods of classifying obesity in adults.
- Created a new Health Connection, with accompanying Learning Outcome and The Take-Home Message, on disordered eating using updated content previously located in Chapter 15.
- Added Table 14.8 presenting the diagnostic criteria for classifying eating disorders.
- Added Table 14.9 explaining the warning signs associated with eating disorders.
- Added a Self-Assessment feature, *Are You At Risk for an Eating Disorder?*

Chapter 15: Weight Management

- Learning Outcomes tie into major headings, The Take-Home Messages, and Visual Chapter Summaries.
- Updated all statistics about the prevalence of overweight and obesity.
- Added new information on weight bias and discrimination and the classification of obesity as a disease by the AMA.
- Created a new Figure 15.1 describing the cost of treating obesity in America.
- Created a new Focus Figure 15.2 on hormonal regulation of hunger and satiety.
- Created a new Figure 14.4 illustrating lipoprotein lipase activity in lean, overweight, and obese adults.
- Included a new section on the role of nutrigenomics and epigenetics in obesity and weight management.
- Created a new Figure 15.5 on the structure of an epigenome.
- Added a discussion of decreased physical activity due to the prevalence of the automobile.
- Added a new Examining the Evidence feature on carbohydrates and their role in obesity.
- Expanded the discussion on low-energy-density foods as they relate to weight management.
- Added a new Examining the Evidence feature on microbiomes and their possible link to obesity.
- Added a new Examining the Evidence feature on whether anaerobic or aerobic exercise is the most effective for weight loss.
- Revised and updated the content on obesity medications and bariatric surgery in the Health Connection feature, with accompanying Learning Outcome and The Take-Home Message.

Chapter 16: Nutrition and Fitness

- Learning Outcomes tie into major headings, The Take-Home Messages, and Visual Chapter Summaries.
- Added a new Focus Figure 16.5 on energy sources that fuel different levels of activity.

- Added a new Table 16.3 on the timing of foods and amount of macronutrients needed to improve exercise performance.
- Added a new Nutrition in Practice on an athlete, which introduces the student to the process of nutrition counseling and dietetics in a real-world setting.
- Revised the Spotlight feature on the female athlete triad with the latest diagnostic terminology.
- Created a new Health Connection, with accompanying Learning Outcome and The Take-Home Message, on the role of various dietary supplements in exercise performance and fitness.
- Added discussion of the potential risks and benefits of bicarbonate loading and amino acid supplementation.

Chapter 17: Life Cycle Nutrition: Pregnancy through Infancy

- Learning Outcomes tie into major headings, The Take-Home Messages, and Visual Chapter Summaries.
- Revised coverage of fetal health risks associated with pregnancy in overweight or underweight women with latest research.
- Revised coverage of fetal health risks associated with drug use during pregnancy.
- Revised discussion of goals for weight gain during pregnancy.
- Revised discussions of iron and vitamin D needs during pregnancy to emphasize the value of supplementation for most women.
- Revised Figure 17.8, *The Letdown Response.*
- Revised coverage of the relationship between breast-feeding and risk of developing food allergies with latest research.
- Updated discussion of feeding infants juice with the latest recommendations from the AAP.
- Updated the Health Connection on food allergies and added a Learning Outcome and The Take-Home Message.

Chapter 18: Life Cycle Nutrition: Toddlers through Adolescence

- Learning Outcomes tie into major headings, The Take-Home Messages, and Visual Chapter Summaries.
- Updated discussion of young children's iron needs.
- Revised Figure 18.3 on the USDA's SuperTracker website.
- Revised coverage of the National School Lunch Program.
- Added discussion of the School Breakfast Program.
- Added a section on determining childhood overweight and obesity.
- Updated Figure 18.4, *Increase in Overweight among U.S. Children and Adolescents.*
- Updated and expanded section on the factors contributing to overweight and obesity in children to include discussions of sugary beverages, genetics, family environment, targeting marketing, and peer influence.
- Updated the Examining the Evidence feature, *Does Sugar Cause Behavior Problems in Children?*
- Updated coverage of eating disorders in adolescents with latest research.
- Updated and expanded Health Connection, with accompanying Learning Outcome and The Take-Home Message, on health effects of childhood obesity to include risks of CVD and psychological problems, as well as approaches to obesity reduction and management.

Chapter 19: Life Cycle Nutrition: Older Adults

- Learning Outcomes tie into major headings, The Take-Home Messages, and Visual Chapter Summaries.
- Updated discussion of lifestyle factors that contribute to the leading causes of death in older Americans.
- Revised discussion of changes in body composition during aging.
- Created a new Table 19.1 on the recommended dietary changes for older adults.
- Updated the Examining the Evidence feature, *Does Kilocalorie Restriction Extend Life?*.
- Updated discussion of older adults' potential benefit from supplements with latest research.
- Revised coverage of Alzheimer's disease.
- Added a new Health Connection, with accompanying Learning Outcome and The Take-Home Message, on hypertension.

Chapter 20: Food Safety, Technology, and Availability

- Learning Outcomes tie into major headings, The Take-Home Messages, and Visual Chapter Summaries.
- Revised chapter opening section.
- Updated statistics throughout chapter.
- Revised Figure 20.1, *Bioaccumulation of Toxins*.
- Revised Figure 20.3 on cross-contamination.
- Updated Table 20.2, *Safe Food Temperatures*.
- Revised Table 20.3, *Agencies that Oversee the Food Supply*.
- Revised Figure 20.7, *The Farm-to-Table Continuum*.
- Moved coverage of label terms for animal foods to the section on the use of hormones and antibiotics.
- Updated and relocated discussion of organic food production.
- New Figure 20.13 of a sustainable systems framework.
- Updated coverage of genetically engineered food in a new Health Connection, with accompanying Learning Outcome and The Take-Home Message.

Chapter 21: Global Nutrition and Malnutrition

- Learning Outcomes tie into major headings, The Take-Home Messages, and Visual Chapter Summaries.
- Revised focus of chapter to address hunger as well as other forms of malnutrition, including overnutrition.
- Added a new section defining hunger, malnutrition, undernutrition, and overnutrition.
- Updated statistics about the prevalence of hunger and food insecurity in the United States and worldwide.
- Updated Figure 21.1, *Hunger in the United States*.
- Created new Figure 21.2 on world population growth.
- Added a new section on food deserts in the United States.
- Created a new Figure 21.3 showing food insecurity worldwide.
- Added new sections on food waste and nutrition transition to the discussion of malnutrition worldwide.
- Added new section on malnutrition in overweight and obese individuals.
- Created new Table 21.2, *Food Assistance Programs in the United States*.

- Added a new section on global programs addressing issues related to food and water supply.
- Revised discussion of health effects of chronic hunger in a new Health Connection, with accompanying Learning Outcome and The Take-Home Message.

Supplements

Mastering Nutrition with MyDietAnalysis with Pearson eText

www.masteringnutrition.pearson.com

The Mastering Nutrition with MyDietAnalysis online homework, tutorial, and assessment system delivers self-paced tutorials that provide individualized coaching, focus on your course objectives, and are responsive to each student's progress. Set up your course in 15 minutes with proven, assignable, and automatically graded nutrition activities that reinforce your course's learning outcomes.

- **Visual Chapter Summary Coaching Activities** review the main ideas of the chapter while incorporating engaging assessments.
- **NEW Focus Figure Narrated Walkthrough Coaching Activities** guide students through key nutrition concepts with interactive mini-lessons.
- **NEW MyDietAnalysis Personalized Diet Analysis Activities** provide students with hands-on diet analysis practice that can also be automatically graded.
- **Reading Quizzes** (20 questions per chapter) ensure that students have completed the assigned reading before class.
- **Dynamic Study Modules** help students study effectively by continuously assessing student performance and providing practice in areas where students struggle the most.
- 25 *ABC News* **Videos** with quizzing bring nutrition to life and spark discussion on current hot topics in the nutrition field. They include multiple-choice questions that provide wrong-answer feedback to redirect students to the correct answer.
- **40 Nutrition Animations Activities** explain big-picture concepts that help students learn the hardest topics in nutrition. These animations have questions that provide wrong-answer feedback that address students' common misconceptions.
- **Math Video Coaching Activities,** accessible through Mastering, provide hands-on practice of important nutrition-related calculations.
- **Mobile-ready NutriTools Coaching Activities** allow students to combine and experiment with different food options and learn firsthand how to build healthier meals.
- **MP3 Chapter Summary** relate to chapter content and come with multiple-choice questions that provide wrong-answer feedback.
- **Access to *Get Ready for Nutrition*** gives students extra math and chemistry study assistance.
- **The Study Area** is broken down into learning areas and includes videos, animations, MP3s, and much more.

MyDietAnalysis Premium Website

www.mydietanalysis.com

MyDietAnalysis was developed by the nutrition database experts at ESHA Research, Inc. and is tailored for use in college nutrition courses. MyDietAnalysis is available as a single sign-on to Mastering Nutrition.

- View a classwide nutritional average. MyDietAnalysis will allow you to see a nutritional profile of your entire class, enabling you to base your lecture on your students' needs.
- Video help with associated quizzes covers the topics students struggle with most.
- A mobile website version of MyDietAnalysis is also available for mobile devices.

Learning Catalytics

Learning Catalytics is a "bring your own device" student engagement, assessment, and classroom intelligence system that allows students to use their smartphones, tablets, or laptops to respond to questions in class. With Learning Catalytics, you can assess students in real-time using open ended question formats to uncover student misconceptions and adjust lecture accordingly and automatically create groups for peer instruction based on student response patterns, to improve discussion productivity.

Digital Instructional Resources

These valuable teaching resources include everything you need to create lecture presentations and course materials, including JPEG and PowerPoint® files of all the art, tables, and selected photos from the text, and "stepped-out" art for selected figures from the text, as well as animations, all available for download from within Mastering Nutrition or www.pearson.com.

The Digital Instructional Resources includes:
- PowerPoint lecture outlines with links to Nutrition Animations and *ABC News* Lecture Launcher Videos
- Media Link PowerPoint slides for easy importing of videos and animations
- PowerPoint slides with a Jeopardy-type quiz show
- Questions for Classroom Response Systems (CRS) in PowerPoint format, allowing you to import the questions into your own CRS
- Instructor's Resource and Support Manual
- Test Bank (Microsoft® Word, RTF, and PDF files) and Computerized Test Bank
- Introduction to Mastering Nutrition
- Introductory video for Learning Catalytics
- *East Right! Healthy Eating in College and Beyond*
- *Food Composition Table*

Acknowledgments

It takes a village, and then some, when it comes to writing a dynamic textbook. *Nutrition: From Science to You* is no exception. We personally want to extend our gratitude to all of those who passionately shared their expertise and support to make *Nutrition: From Science to You* better than we could have envisioned.

Beginning with the energetic staff at Pearson, we would like to thank Michelle Yglecias, who helped make our vision for this textbook into a reality. Laura Bonazzoli's comprehensive developmental editing improved the clarity of *Nutrition: From Science to You* and made it more enjoyable to read. A special thank you to Barbara Yien, Director of Development, as well, for helping steer the ship while Michelle Yglecias was on maternity leave.

Crackerjack Rich Media Content Producer Lucinda Bingham and Mastering Nutrition Content Development Lead Lorna Perkins worked diligently to create the best media supplements for *Nutrition: From Science to You*. Thanks also to editorial assistant Nicole Constantine for all of her behind-the-scenes work.

A very special thanks to Lizette Faraji, Content Producer, and Nathaniel Jones, Project Manager at SPi Global, for all of their hard work shepherding this book through to publication. Our humble appreciation also goes to Gary Hespenheide, whose design made the text, art, and photos all come alive; and to design manager Mark Ong.

Marketing takes energy, and that's exactly what Executive Product Marketing Managers Neena Bali, Alysun Burns, and Field Marketing Manager, Mary Salzman, generate nonstop. The many instructors who reviewed the first, second, and third editions, as well as those who reviewed and class-tested early versions of this book, are listed on the following pages. We are grateful to all of them for helping in the development of *Nutrition: From Science to You*.

The village also included loyal contributors who lent their expertise to specific chapters. They are: Whitney Evans, PhD of Brown University Alpert Medical Schoolwho revised the three "life cycle" chapters; Kellene Isom, MS, RD, LDN of Brigham and Women's Hospital, who overhauled and expanded the food safety, technology, and sustainability chapter; and Claire Alexander, who updated the global nutrition and malnutrition chapter.

Lastly, an endless thanks to our colleagues, friends, and especially our families. Joan would like to "thank my family, Adam, Brendan, and Craig for their love and support when I was working more than I should have been." Kathy sends a special thanks to "my husband Rich and our children Heather, Wes, and Ryan for keeping me sane and grounded, and my sister Vicki for her steadfast support." Stella would like to acknowledge "my husband, Gary Snyder, for his constant support; and our wonderful dogs, Sasha and Bear, for always making me smile! And to my Mom and Dad, who both instilled in me a wonderful relationship with food, especially home grown and homemade food."

Reviewers

First Edition

Janet Anderson
Utah State University

Sandra Baker
University of Delaware

Gita Bangera
Bellevue College

Lisa Blackman
Tarrant County College, Northwest

Jeanne Boone
Palm Beach State College

John Capeheart
University of Houston-Downtown

Susan Chou
American River College

Nicole Clark
Indiana University of Pennsylvania

Susan Cooper
Montana State University-Great Falls College of Technology

Jessica Coppola
Sacramento City College

Lynn Monahan Couch
West Chester University of Pennsylvania

Wendy Cunningham
California State University, Sacramento

Jeannette Davidson
Bradley University

Holly Dieken
The University of Tennessee at Chattanooga

Johanna Donnenfield
Scottsdale Community College

Roberta Durschlag
Boston University

Brenda Eissenstat
The Pennsylvania State University

Sheryl L. Fuller-Espie
Cabrini College

Eugene J. Fenster
Metropolitan Community College, Longview

Alyce D. Fly
Indiana University

Sara Folta
Tufts University

Betty Forbes
West Virginia University

Sue Fredstrom
Minnesota State University, Mankato

Teresa Fung
Simmons College

Susan Gaumont
Chandler-Gilbert Community College

Jill Golden
Orange Coast College

Gloria Gonzalez
Pensacola State College

Donna Handley
The University of Rhode Island

William Helferich
University of Illinois at Urbana-Champaign

Catherine Howard
Texarkana College

Karen Israel
Anne Arundel Community College

Seema Jejurikar
Bellevue College

Jayanthi Kandiah
Ball State University

Vicki Kloosterhouse
Oakland Community College

Allen Knehans
The University of Oklahoma

Kathy Knight
The University of Mississippi

Shui-Ming Kuo
University at Buffalo

Robert D. Lee
Central Michigan University

Sharon Lemons
Tarrant County College, Northwest

Darlene Levinson
Oakland Community College

Rose Martin
Iowa State University

Mary Martinez
Central New Mexico Community College

George F. McNeil
Fort Hays State University

Monica Meadows
The University of Texas at Austin

Kathleen Melanson
The University of Rhode Island

Mithia Mukutmoni
Sierra College

Pat Munn
Metropolitan Community College, Longview

Megan Murphy
Southwest Tennessee Community College

Dan Neisner
Walla Walla Community College

Corin Nishimura
Leeward Community College

Anna Page
Johnson County Community College

Jill Patterson
The Pennsylvania State University

Janet Peterson
Linfield College

Gwendolyn Pla
Howard University

Roseanne Poole
Tallahassee Community College

Linda Pope
Southwest Tennessee Community College

Elizabeth Quintana
West Virginia University

Denise Russo
Cabrillo College

Kevin Schalinske
Iowa State University

Diana Spillman
Miami University

Sherry Stewart
Navarro College

Leeann Sticker
Northwestern State University

Susan Swadener
California Polytechnic State University, San Luis Obispo

Janelle Walter
Baylor University

Sandy Walz
West Chester University of Pennsylvania

Daryle Wane
Pasco-Hernando State College

Garrison Wilkes
University of Massachusetts-Boston

Jessie Yearwood
El Centro College

Gloria Young
Virginia State University

Maureen Zimmerman
Mesa Community College

Second Edition

Ellen Brennan
San Antonio College

Wendy Buchan
California State University, Sacramento

Nicole A. Clark
Indiana University of Pennsylvania

Mary Dean Coleman-Kelly
The Pennsylvania State University

Eugene J. Fenster
Metropolitan Community College, Longview

Karen Friedman-Kester
Harrisburg Area Community College

Amy Frith
Ithaca College

Susan Edgar Helm
Pepperdine University

Shanil Juma
Texas Woman's University

Allen Knehans
The University of Oklahoma Health Sciences Center

Julia L. Lapp
Ithaca College

John Radcliffe
Texas Woman's University

Nancy L. Shearer
Cape Cod Community College

Eric Vlahov
The University of Tampa

Heidi Wengreen
Utah State University

Third Edition

Julie Albrecht
University of Nebraska Lincoln

Sandra Brown
University of Delaware

Donna M. Cain
Collin County Community College

Jana Gonsalves
American River College

Cindy Hudson
Hinds Community College

Ruth Anne McGinley
Harrisburg Area Community College

Judith Myhand
Louisiana State University

Rebecca Orr
Collin County Community College

John Radcliffe
Texas Woman's University

Jacqueline Vernarelli
Fairfield University

Stanley Wilfong
Baylor University

Fourth Edition

Valerie Amend
Ball State University

Carol Barnes
Mississippi College

Christina Sullivan
City College of San Francisco

Alison Borkowska
Pennsylvania State University

Wendy Buchan
California State University, Sacramento

Kevin Cooper
Sierra College

Rebecca Creasy
Texas A&M University

Yanyan Li
Husson University

Rosanna Licht
Pasco-Hernando State College

Marcia Magnus
Florida State University

Adam Pennell
California State University, Bakersfield

Shelia Taylor
Ozarks Technical Community College

Yolanda Williams
Harrisburg Area Community College, Harrisburg

Class Testers

Janet Anderson
Utah State University

Jeanne Boone
Palm Beach State College

Jessica Coppola
Sacramento City College

Robert Cullen
Illinois State University

Gloria Gonzales
Pensacola State College

Jill Goode-Englett
University of North Alabama

Debra Head
University of Central Arkansas

Lenka Humenikova-Shriver
Oklahoma State University

Allen Knehans
The University of Oklahoma

Janet Levin
Pensacola State College

Darlene Levinson
Oakland Community College

Anna Miller
De Anza College

Vijaya Narayanan
Florida International University

Anna Page
Johnson County Community College

Nancy Parkinson
Miami University

Renee Romig
Western Iowa Tech Community College

Janet Sass
Northern Virginia Community College, Annandale

Susan Swadener
California Polytechnic State University, San Luis Obispo

Janelle Walter
Baylor University

Suzy Weems
Baylor University

Jennifer Zimmerman
Tallahassee Community College

I am nothing without my ABCs. Thanks.

—*Joan Salge Blake*

I dedicate this to my family for their love and support that sustained me through the development of this book. And to my students, both present and past, for whom this book was written.

—*Kathy D. Munoz*

I would like to dedicate this book to my Mom, Felicetta Volpe, and my Dad, Antonio Volpe (in memory). I would also like to dedicate this book to my husband, Gary Snyder, and our dogs, Sasha and Bear.

—*Stella Lucia Volpe*

NUTRITION

From Science To You

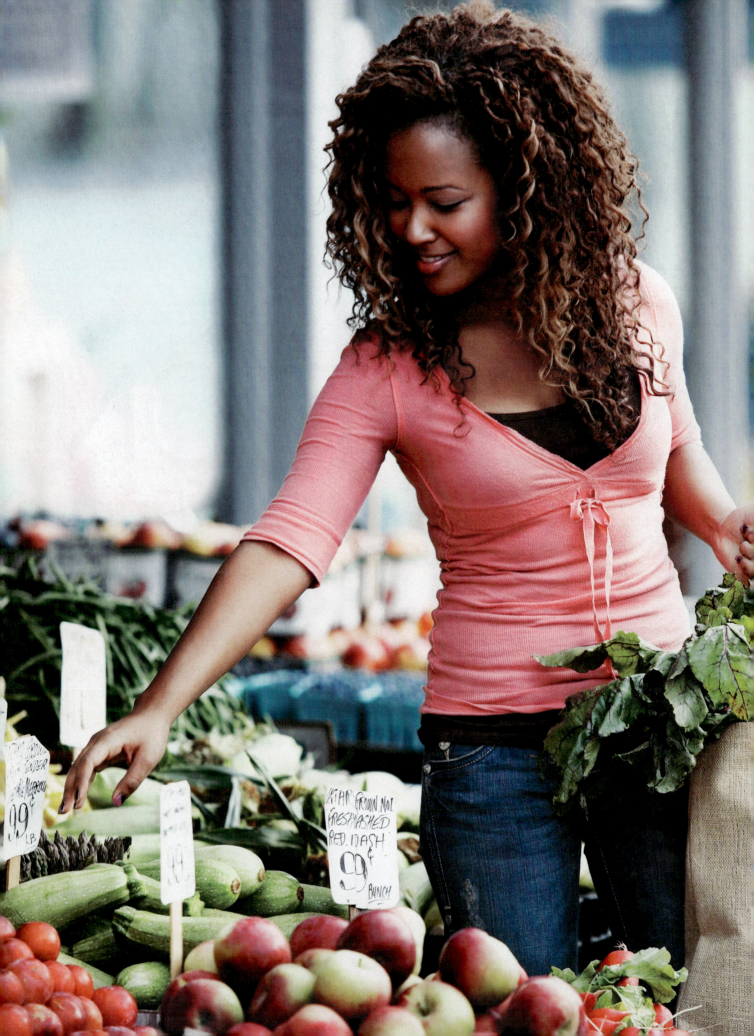

What Is Nutrition?

Learning Outcomes

After reading this chapter, you will be able to:

1.1 Discuss the factors that drive our food choices.

1.2 Define the term *nutrition* and characterize nutrients.

1.3 Explain the primary roles of the six classes of nutrients found in food.

1.4 Describe the best approach to meeting your nutritional needs.

1.5 Summarize three ways in which diet influences health.

1.6 Summarize the ABCD method used to assess the nutrient status of individuals and populations.

1.7 Discuss the current nutritional state of the average American diet.

1.8 Describe the scientific method that leads to reliable and accurate nutrition information.

1.9 Explain how to identify reliable nutrition information and how to recognize misinformation.

True or False?

1. Food choices are driven primarily by flavor. **T**/**F**
2. Nutrition is the study of dietary supplements. **T**/**F**
3. Carbohydrates provide our main source of energy. **T**/**F**
4. Alcohol is a nutrient. **T**/**F**
5. Taking a dietary supplement is the only way to meet your nutrient needs. **T**/**F**
6. The most effective method of nutritional assessment is to ask clients to write down what they've eaten in the last 24 hours. **T**/**F**
7. About 25 percent of all Americans are obese. **T**/**F**
8. Eliminating all fat from the diet will reduce your risk of developing heart disease. **T**/**F**
9. Cancer is the leading cause of death in the United States. **T**/**F**
10. You can get good nutrition advice from anyone who calls him- or herself a nutritionist. **T**/**F**

See page 36 for the answers.

During the course of a day, we make over 200 decisions about food, from when to eat, how much to eat, and what to eat, to how the food is prepared, and even what size plate to use.[1] You make these decisions for reasons you may not even be aware of. If your dietary advice comes from media sound bites, you may receive conflicting information. Last week's news flash announced that eating more protein would help you fight a bulging waist. Yesterday's headline boldly announced that limiting sugary drinks was the key. This morning, the TV news lead was a health report on the weight-loss benefits of consuming more dietary fiber.

It can be frustrating when nutrition news seems to change daily, but the research behind this barrage of news illustrates the progress nutrition scientists are making toward understanding what we eat and how it affects our health. Today's research validates what nutrition professionals have known for decades: Nutrition plays an invaluable role in your health.

In addition to exploring the factors that affect food choice, this chapter introduces you to the study of nutrition. Let's begin with the basic concepts of why and what you eat, why a healthy diet is important to your well-being, and how you can identify credible sources of nutrition information.

What Drives Our Food Choices?

LO 1.1 Discuss the factors that drive our food choices.

Have you ever considered what drives your food choices? Or are you on autopilot as you stand in line at the sub shop and squint at yet another menu board? Do you enjoy some foods and eat them often, while avoiding others with a vengeance? You obviously need food to survive, but beyond your basic instinct to eat are many other factors that affect your food choices. These factors include taste and enjoyment; culture and environment; social life and trends; nutrition knowledge; advertising; time, convenience, and cost; and habits and emotions (Figure 1.1).

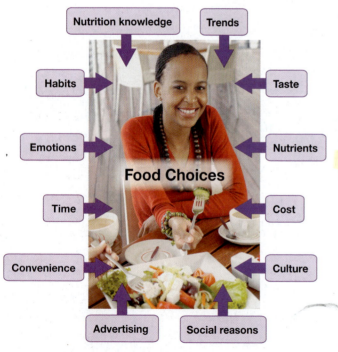

Nutrition knowledge · Trends · Habits · Taste · Emotions · Nutrients · Food Choices · Time · Cost · Convenience · Culture · Advertising · Social reasons

▲ Figure 1.1 Many Factors Influence Your Food Choices

Taste and Enjoyment

Research confirms that when it comes to making food choices, taste is the most important consideration.[2,3] This shouldn't be too much of a surprise, considering there are more than 10,000 taste buds in the mouth. These taste buds tell you that chocolate cheesecake is sweet, fresh lemon juice is sour, and a pretzel is salty. Our preferences for sweet, salty, or creamy foods may be influenced by our genes[4] and may change as we age.[5]

We have a taste for fat, which may also be genetically linked.[6] When fat is combined with sugar, such as in a sugar-laden doughnut, our preference for that food is even stronger.[7]

Texture also affects our likelihood of enjoying foods. We enjoy a flaky piecrust but dislike one that is tough; we prefer crunchy apples to mealy ones, and creamy rather than lumpy soups. Almost 30 percent of adults dislike slippery foods, such as oysters and okra.[8] Researchers have suggested that people's preferences for sweetness, high fat, and specific textures begin early in life and this makes them resistant to change.[9]

Culture and Environment

Enjoying food is not just a physiological sensation. Other factors, such as our culture and the environment, also play a role in which foods we eat.[10] If you were a student in Mexico, you may regularly feast on corn tortillas and tamales, as corn is a staple of Mexican cuisines. In India, meals commonly include lentils with rice and vegetables, whereas Native Americans often enjoy stews of mutton (sheep), corn, vegetables, and berries. And, in Asian countries, rice likely would be front and center on your plate.

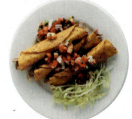
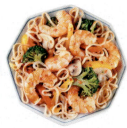

Roughly one in three Americans is of Hispanic, Native American, Asian, or African descent. Cultural food preferences often influence food choices.

The environment in which its people live significantly influences a culture's cuisine. This includes the climate and soil conditions as well as the native plants and animals and the distance people live from rivers, lakes, or the ocean. Foods that are available and accessible are more likely to be regularly consumed than foods that are scarce. For example, native Alaskans feast on fish because it is plentiful, but eat less fresh produce, which is difficult to grow locally. For most Americans today, global food distribution networks have made eating only locally available foods less of an issue than in the past; however, the tendency persists for some food items.

Our food environment—the variety of food choices available, the size and shape of plates and glassware, the packaging of foods, and the types and amounts of food that are visible—has a strong influence on what and how much we consume. We eat more food when the serving plates are larger and drink less when beverages are served in taller glasses. Environmental cues also affect eating patterns. You are more likely to linger over a meal when the light is dimmed,[11] or quickly finish your meal when you are standing rather than sitting. Physical cues, such as a friend's empty appetizer plate covered with disposed-of cocktail sticks, may signal you to eat more of your appetizer.

Social Life and Trends

Every year on the fourth Thursday in November, approximately 48 million turkeys are consumed when Americans gather with family and friends to celebrate Thanksgiving.[12] A person is likely to eat more on Thanksgiving than on any other Thursday, and this is partly because of the number of people eating with them. Eating dinner with others has been shown to increase the size of the meal by over 40 percent, and the more people present at the meal, the more you'll eat.[13]

Eating is an important way to bond with others. Sharing a meal with family or friends stimulates conversation, creates traditions, and expands our food experiences. Although eating a quick meal in the campus cafeteria may not provide you the most healthy food options, it will allow you to socialize with classmates.

For many people, activities such as watching a football game with fellow fans or going to a movie with friends often involve particular foods. More pizzas are sold on Super Bowl Sunday than on any other day of the year.[14] Movie theater owners bank on their patrons buying popcorn, candy, and beverages at the concession stand before heading in to watch the film.[15]

Food choices are also affected by popular trends. For instance, home cooks in the 1950s bought bags of "newfangled" frozen vegetables in order to provide healthy meals in less time. A few decades later, vegetables went upscale and consumers bought them as part of ready-to-heat stir-fry mixes. Today, shoppers pay a premium for bags of fresh veggies, like carrots, that have been prewashed and peeled, sliced, or diced, and they pay even more if the food is labeled "organic." In 2013 alone, Americans spent more than $35 billion on organic foods.[16] Millennials (people born between about 1980 and 2000) who are parents are the biggest group of consumers buying organic foods.

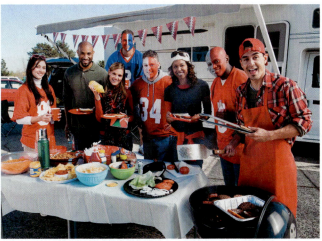

Eating junk food while watching sports or attending a sporting event sometimes seems like an American way of life.

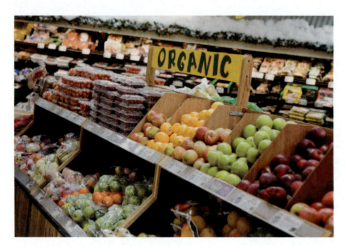

The USDA certifies that foods labeled "organic" are grown without the use of toxic and persistent pesticides or fertilizers.

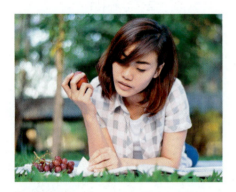

Rates of fruit and vegetable consumption increased among consumers exposed to the FNV advertising campaign.

Food sustainability and food waste are also topics that are on the radar of restaurant patrons and shoppers, who may choose vegetarian meals or smaller portions out of concerns for the environment. Supermarkets provide dozens of choices in flavored and enhanced bottled teas and waters, which are trendy beverages among college students. As food manufacturers pour more money into research and development, who knows what tomorrow's trendy foods will be?

Nutrition Knowledge

Individuals may choose certain foods they associate with good health or avoid other foods they associate with poor health. For example, many Americans consume vegetables, fruits, and whole grains because they perceive them as healthy choices that can help them control their blood pressure or reduce their risk of colon cancer.[17] At the same time, many Americans worry about fried foods causing heart disease.

When it comes to weight management, some consumers believe that specific dietary components are the culprits behind weight gain. While 3 in 10 consumers believe that overeating any type of food will cause weight gain, one in four believe that sugar is more likely to cause you to pack on the pounds.[18]

The more aware you are of the effects of food choices on health, the more likely you are to make an effort to improve those choices. If you believe that choosing low-sodium foods will decrease your blood pressure or that eating yogurt with active cultures will improve your digestion, you are more likely to choose these foods. Many consumers are label-reading in the supermarket, checking the expiration date, Nutrition Facts panel, and ingredients list before buying a food product.[19]

Advertising

The food and beverage industry spends over $136 million annually on advertising.[20] Food companies spend these large sums on advertising for one reason: It works, especially on young people. American children view an estimated 30 hours of food commercials on the television annually, and more than half of these advertisements are for unhealthy foods.[21]

In contrast, commercials for fruits and vegetables are rare, which is unfortunate because healthy foods can be successfully marketed. The Fruit and Vegetable (FNV) campaign, the brainchild of the Partnership for a Healthier America (PHA), a nonprofit organization working with public, private, and nonprofit leaders to develop strategies to end childhood obesity, knows that celebrity marketing to kids is powerful. They recruited influential actors and athletes, all pro bono, to get kids to chow down more produce. Their research showed that 70 percent of individuals who were aware of FNV stated that they purchased and ate more fruits and vegetables after seeing or hearing about the campaign.[22]

Time, Convenience, and Cost

When it comes to making a meal, time is often at a premium. A recent survey reported that close to 60 percent of Millennials spend as little as 15 minutes cooking dinner during the week.[23] Consequently, supermarkets are now offering more prepared and partially prepared foods. If chicken is on the menu tonight, you can buy it uncooked at the meat counter in the supermarket, or you can go to the deli and buy it hot off the rotisserie, cooked and stuffed with bread crumbs or grilled with teriyaki sauce. Rice or pasta side dishes and cooked vegetables are also available to complete the meal.

Convenience has also become more of a factor in food selection. Foods that are easily accessible to you are more likely to be eaten. Decades ago, the most convenient way to get a hot cup of coffee was to brew it at home. Today, Americans are more likely to get their latte or half-caff from one of the 29,000 coffee shops across the United States.[24]

For reasons related to both time and convenience, people eat out more often today than they did a few decades ago. In the 1970s, Americans spent less of their household budget on eating out, compared with today.[25] Because cost is often an issue when considering where to eat out, most meals consumed away from home are fast food, which is often cheaper and quicker than more nutritious meals. Though cheap fast food may be easy on the pocketbook, it is taking its toll on the health of Americans. Epidemiological research suggests that low-cost, high-calorie diets, such as those that incorporate lots of burgers, fries, tacos, and soft drinks, increase the risk of obesity, especially among those at lower socioeconomic levels.[26]

The good news is that cheaper food doesn't have to always mean fast food, and when healthy foods are offered at lower prices, people do buy them. More Americans, especially urban Millennials, are opting for boxes of fresh fruits and vegetables or meal kits delivered directly to their door. They may eat home-cooked meals more often because of these services.[27]

Researchers have found that lowering the cost of fresh fruits and vegetables improves the consumption of these nutritious foods.[28] This suggests that price reductions are an effective strategy to increase the purchase of more-healthful foods.

Habits and Emotions

Your daily routine and habits often affect both when you eat and what you eat. For example, if you routinely start your day with a bowl of cereal, you're not alone. Ready-to-eat cereals are the number-one breakfast food choice among Americans.[29] Many individuals habitually snack when watching television or sitting at the computer.[30]

For some individuals, emotions can sometimes drive food choice: feeling happy or sad can trigger eating. In some cases, appetite is suppressed during periods of sadness or depression; in others, food is used as an emotional crutch during times of stress, depression, or joy.

LO 1.1: THE TAKE-HOME MESSAGE Taste and enjoyment are the primary reasons people prefer certain foods. A food's availability makes it more easily become part of a culture, and many foods can be regularly eaten out of habit. Advertising, food trends, limited time, convenience, emotions, and the perception that foods are healthy or unhealthy also influence food choices.

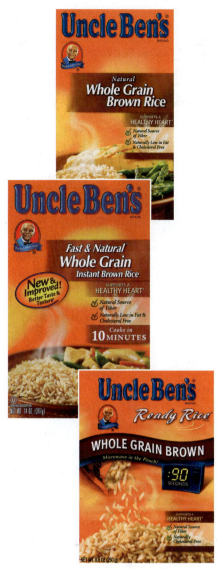

Although brown rice is a healthy whole-grain addition to any meal, it generally takes almost an hour to cook. For time-strapped consumers, food manufacturers have developed brown rice that cooks in 10 minutes and a precooked, microwavable variety that reheats in less than 2 minutes.

What Is Nutrition?

LO 1.2 Define the term *nutrition* and characterize nutrients.

The science of **nutrition** is the study of food and the nutrients we need to sustain life and reproduce. It examines the way food nourishes the body and affects health. Since its inception, the science of nutrition has explored how food is digested, absorbed, transported, metabolized, and used or stored in the body. Nutritional scientists study how much we need of each nutrient, the factors that influence our needs, and what happens if we don't consume enough. As with any science, nutrition is not stagnant. The more we discover about the relationship between nutrition and well-being, the greater the impact will be on long-term health.

nutrition Science that studies how nutrients and other components of foods nourish the body and affect body functions and overall health.

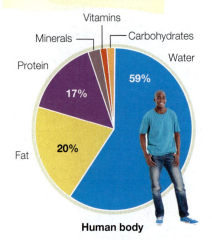

Human body

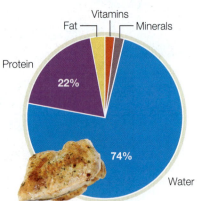

Chicken breast

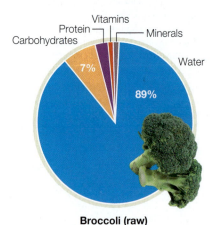

Broccoli (raw)

▲ **Figure 1.2 Nutrients in Foods and in the Body**
Water is the most abundant nutrient found in foods and in the body. Carbohydrates, fats, protein, vitamins, and minerals make up the rest. Note that foods also contain non-nutritive compounds, such as phytochemicals and fiber.

Nutrients Are Essential Compounds in Food

The body is one large organism made up of millions of cells that grow, age, reproduce, and die, all without your noticing. You slough off millions of skin cells when you towel off after a shower, yet your skin isn't noticeably thinner today than it was last week. Your body replaces skin cells at a rate fast enough to keep you covered, and it manufactures new cells using the same nutrients found in a variety of foods. As cells die, **nutrients** from food provide the building blocks to replace them. Nutrients also provide the energy we need to perform all body functions and processes, from maintaining heartbeat to playing tennis.

There are six categories of nutrients found in foods and in the body: carbohydrates, lipids (fats), protein, vitamins, minerals, and water. Foods also often contain beneficial non-nutrient compounds, such as phytochemicals or zoochemicals, and nondigestible fiber, as well as chemicals added by food manufacturers to enhance color, flavor, or texture or extend shelf-life.

Plant foods are made up of about 10 percent carbohydrates, fats, proteins, vitamins, and minerals (**Figure 1.2**). The rest is typically water, and plant foods contain more water (about 90 percent) than do animal foods (about 70 percent). Animal foods are composed of about 30 percent protein, lipids, vitamins, and minerals. One unique quality of animal foods, with the exception of dairy products, is that they do not contain any carbohydrates by the time we consume them.

A healthy human body is about 60 percent water. The other 40 percent is made up of protein and fat, as well as a small amount of stored carbohydrates, minerals in bone, and small amounts of vitamins. Thus, the old saying is true that *we are what we eat*, from the carbohydrates in broccoli to the proteins in meat. The six biochemical ingredients needed to sustain life are all provided by the foods in our diets.

In general, nutrients are **essential**—they must come from foods because either they cannot be made in the body at all, or they cannot be made in sufficient amounts to meet the body's needs. The body can make a few **nonessential nutrients** in sufficient quantities. An example is vitamin D, which is synthesized in the skin upon exposure to sunlight. Under some circumstances, *nonessential* nutrients can become *essential*. We refer to these nutrients as *conditionally essential*. If you are not exposed to enough sunlight, you will not be able to synthesize an adequate amount of vitamin D. You must then obtain vitamin D from foods and/or supplements.

Most Nutrients Are Organic

Carbohydrates, proteins, lipids, and vitamins are the most complex of the six classes of nutrients. These nutrients are **organic** because their chemical structures contain carbon. Organic nutrients also contain the elements hydrogen and oxygen, and in the case of proteins and some vitamins, nitrogen is also part of the molecule (**Figure 1.3**).

Minerals are the least complex of the nutrients. From calcium to zinc, each mineral is an individual element, and its atoms are exactly the same whether found in food or in the body. For instance, the structure of zinc found in lean meats and nuts is the same as that found in a cell membrane or a hair follicle. Minerals are **inorganic** because, as individual elements, they do not contain carbon. Water, a three-atom molecule composed of hydrogen and oxygen, is also inorganic. The Chemistry Boost will help you visualize elements and molecules.

Some Nutrients Provide Energy

All creatures need energy in order to function, and humans are no exception. **Energy is defined as the capacity to do work.** It also provides a source of heat. The body derives chemical energy from certain nutrients in foods, which store energy in their chemical

Each nutrient contains a unique combination of chemical elements.

		Carbon	Hydrogen	Oxygen	Nitrogen	Single elements
Organic	**Carbohydrates**	X	X	X		
	Lipids	X	X	X		
	Proteins	X	X	X	X	
	Vitamins	X	X	X	Some vitamins contain nitrogen	
Inorganic	**Minerals**					X
	Water		X	X		

bonds. During digestion and metabolism, the bonds are broken and the energy is released. This chemical energy released when the foods are digested can be converted into adenosine triphosphate (ATP), a form of energy the body can use. Carbohydrates, lipids (fats), and proteins are defined as the **energy-yielding nutrients** because they contribute energy to the body. Alcohol, although not a nutrient, also provides energy.

Scientists use the metric system to measure weight, volume, and distance. Grams are the fundamental units of measurement for weight; liters are the fundamental units for volume; and meters are the units used to measure distance. The metric system is a decimal system; that is, larger and smaller units are multiples or divisions of 100. For example, a kilogram is 1,000 grams (*kilo* = 1,000) and a centimeter is a hundredth of a meter (*cent* = 100). This uniform system of measurement allows scientists all over the world to share and compare data. Appendix B provides commonly used metric units.

Scientists measure the energy in foods in kilocalories. A **kilocalorie** is defined as the amount of energy needed to raise the temperature of one kilogram of water 1 degree

Chemistry Boost

Chemical Bonds

Most nutrients consist of carbon, hydrogen, and oxygen. These elements combine to form compounds through chemical reactions. An atom of each element can carry a positive or negative charge and can form a set number of bonds with other elements. For example, carbon can form bonds with four elements, hydrogen can form one bond, and oxygen can form two bonds, as illustrated below. Two or more atoms bonded together are called *molecules*. Molecular oxygen, for example, contains two oxygen atoms (O_2). Compounds are molecules containing two or more different elements. Water (H_2O) is a compound. Molecules tend to be more stable than atoms, and, like atoms, can carry a positive or negative charge. Charged atoms or molecules are called *ions*.

$$H-C-H \quad\quad H-O-H$$

Methane (CH_4)   Water (H_2O)

nonessential nutrients Nutrients that can be made in sufficient quantities in the body to meet the body's requirements and support health.

organic Describing compounds that contain carbon or carbon–carbon bonds.

inorganic Describing elements or compounds that do not contain carbon.

energy Capacity to do work.

energy-yielding nutrients Three nutrients that provide energy to the body to fuel physiological functions: carbohydrates, lipids, and protein.

kilocalorie Amount of energy required to raise the temperature of 1 kilogram of water 1 degree centigrade; used to express the measurement of energy in foods; 1 kilocalorie is equal to 1,000 calories.

Celsius. A kilocalorie is not the same as a *calorie* (with a lowercase *c*), which is a much smaller unit of measurement. (In fact, a "calorie" is so small that one slice of bread contains about 63,000 calories.) One kilocalorie is equal to 1,000 calories.

To add to the confusion, the term *Calorie* (with an uppercase *C*) is used on nutrition labels to express the energy content of foods and is often used in science textbooks to mean kilocalories. This text refers to the units of energy found in foods as kilocalories, abbreviated *kcalories* or *kcals*.

Each energy-yielding nutrient provides a set number of kilocalories per gram. Thus the number of kilocalories in one serving of a given food can be determined based on the amount (in grams) of carbohydrates, protein, and fat in the food. Carbohydrates and protein provide 4 kilocalories per gram; so, for example, a food that contains 5 grams of carbohydrate and 3 grams of protein would have 32 kilocalories ([5 × 4] + [3 × 4] = 32). Fats yield 9 kilocalories per gram, more than twice the number of kilocalories in either carbohydrates or protein. Alcohol contains 7 kilocalories per gram, which must be taken into account when calculating the energy of alcohol-containing foods and beverages (**Figure 1.4**).

Use the Calculation Corner to determine the number of kilocalories in a snack of potato chips and cola.

Energy in foods and in the body is trapped within the bonds that keep the molecules together. When the bonds are broken during the process of metabolism, a significant amount of energy, including some heat, is released. The energy can then be used to digest and absorb the meal, contract muscles, fuel the heartbeat, synthesize new cells, and perform other functions. The Chemistry Boost will help you visualize covalent bonds.

People's energy needs vary according to their age, gender, and activity level. Males generally need more energy because they weigh more and have more muscle mass (which

▶ **Figure 1.4 The Energy-Yielding Nutrients and Alcohol Provide Kilocalories**
Carbohydrates, fats, and protein provide energy, or kilocalories, to fuel the body. Alcohol also contains kilocalories.

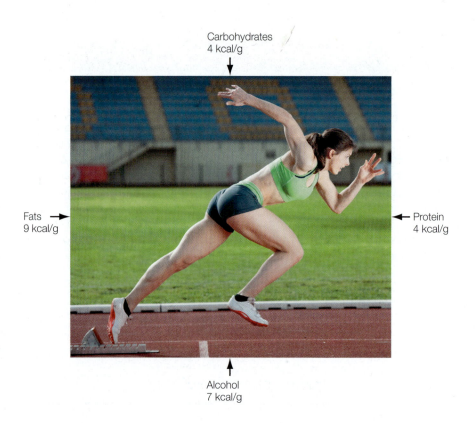

Carbohydrates
4 kcal/g

Fats →
9 kcal/g

← Protein
4 kcal/g

Alcohol
7 kcal/g

Calculating Kilocalories in a Snack of Chips and Soda

Suppose you ate an entire 8-ounce bag of potato chips and drank a 16-ounce cola while you studied for an exam. Together these two items contain 144 grams of carbohydrate (in the cola and chips), 12 grams of protein (from the chips), and 60 grams of fat (also in the chips). How many kilocalories did you consume?

(a) To calculate the total kilocalories in this snack, multiply the total grams of each energy nutrient times the number of kilocalories per gram of that nutrient. Remember, a gram of carbohydrate and protein each contain 4 kilocalories and a gram of fat contains 9 kilocalories.

$$(144 \text{ g} \times 4 \text{ kcals/g}) + (12 \text{ g} \times 4 \text{ kcals/g}) + (60 \text{ g} \times 9 \text{ kcals/g}) = 1{,}164 \text{ kcals}$$
$$576 \text{ kcals} + 48 \text{ kcals} + 540 \text{ kcals} = 1{,}164 \text{ kcals}$$

In one sitting, you consumed more than 1,100 kilocalories, which for some people may be more than half of the amount they need to meet their daily energy requirement. If behaviors like this become habits, they can quickly result in weight gain.

(b) Another useful measure for assessing the nutritional quality of the snack is the percentage of fat, protein, and/or carbohydrate found in the food (you learn in later chapters that there are ranges for each nutrient that are considered part of a healthy diet). For example, what percentage of kilocalories in the chips and soda is from fat? To answer this question, divide the fat kilocalories by the total kilocalories in the food and multiply by 100:

$$(540 \text{ kcals} \div 1{,}164 \text{ kcals}) \times 100 = 46\% \text{ fat}$$

Almost half of the kilocalories in this snack are from fat. Do you think this is likely to be a desirable proportion?

For practice, complete the same calculations for carbohydrate and protein.

Go to **Mastering** Nutrition and complete a Math Video activity similar to the problem in this Calculation Corner.

Covalent Bonds

A chemical reaction unites two atoms by creating a bond that forms a new molecule. A covalent bond is formed when atoms share their electrons, as in the case of water. The oxygen atoms require two additional electrons and the hydrogen atoms need one electron to be stable. When these three atoms combine, the oxygen shares one electron with each of the hydrogen atoms and the hydrogen atoms share one electron with the oxygen atom. The atoms are held together because of their affinity to share each other's electrons. The covalent bond that is formed is strong and difficult to break. Trapped within the bonds is stored energy that is released when the bonds are broken.

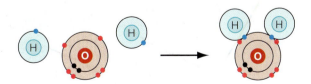

requires more kilocalories to function) and less body fat. Younger people require more energy than older adults because they are still growing and therefore synthesizing more new tissue. Physically active individuals require more energy than sedentary people to fuel their activities and meet their body's basic energy needs.

Energy that is not used to fuel the body will be stored, predominantly as fat, for later use. If you regularly consume more kilocalories than you expend, you will accumulate stored fat in adipose tissue and gain weight. The opposite is also true. Eating fewer kilocalories than the body needs will result in the breakdown of stored energy and weight loss.

LO 1.2: THE TAKE-HOME MESSAGE Nutrition is the science of how nutrients and other components of foods nourish the body, and how the body uses nutrients to manufacture and replace cells and produce energy. Most nutrients are essential; that is, they cannot be synthesized in adequate amounts to meet body needs. Carbohydrates, lipids, proteins, and vitamins are organic nutrients composed of the chemical elements carbon, hydrogen, oxygen, and sometimes nitrogen. Minerals and water are inorganic because they don't contain carbon. Energy in foods is measured in kilocalories. The energy-yielding nutrients—carbohydrates (4 kilocalories per gram), lipids (9 kilocalories per gram), and proteins (4 kilocalories per gram)—provide fuel to be used by the body or stored for future use. Alcohol (7 kilocalories per gram) is not a nutrient but does provide energy.

macronutrients Essential nutrients, including water and the energy-containing carbohydrates, lipids, and proteins that the body needs in large amounts.

micronutrients Essential nutrients the body needs in smaller amounts: vitamins and minerals.

What Are the Primary Roles of the Six Classes of Nutrients?

LO 1.3 Explain the primary roles of the six classes of nutrients found in food.

Individual nutrients supply energy, regulate metabolism, and provide structure (**Table 1.1**). Some nutrients, including carbohydrates, lipids, proteins, and water, are called **macronutrients** (*macro* means "large") because they are needed in much larger amounts to support normal functioning. Vitamins and minerals, though equally important to health, are considered **micronutrients** (*micro* means "small") because they are required in smaller amounts to perform their key roles. We introduce each of the six classifications of nutrients briefly in this chapter; they are discussed in much greater detail later in the textbook.

Carbohydrates Are the Primary Energy Source

All forms of carbohydrates are composed of carbon (*carbo-*), hydrogen, and oxygen (*hydrate* means "water"). Carbohydrates supply simple sugar, called glucose, which is the primary source of energy for most body cells.

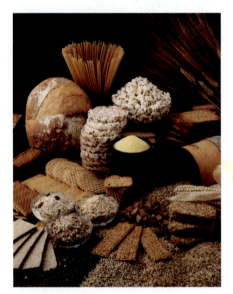
Carbohydrates are found in a variety of foods, including breads, grains, and pasta.

TABLE 1.1	Functions of the Major Nutrients by Type			
	Nutrient	**Provides Energy**	**Participates in Growth, Maintenance, Support, or Structure**	**Regulates Body Processes**
Macronutrients	Carbohydrates	Yes	No	No
	Protein	Yes	Yes	Yes
	Fats	Yes	Yes	Yes
	Water	No	Yes	Yes
Micronutrients	Vitamins	No	Yes	Yes
	Minerals	No	Yes	Yes

Carbohydrates are found in most foods. Breads, cereals, nuts, fruits, legumes (dry beans, peas, and lentils), other vegetables, and dairy products are all rich in carbohydrates. The only foods that do not provide significant amounts of carbohydrates are animal products other than dairy, such as eggs, meat, poultry, and fish. (Chapter 4 covers carbohydrates in detail.)

Lipids Also Provide Energy

The term *lipid* refers to a diverse group of organic compounds including fats (also called *triglycerides*), phospholipids, and sterols that are insoluble in water. These nutrients contain the same chemical elements as carbohydrates, including carbon, hydrogen, and oxygen. The difference is that lipids are much more concentrated than carbohydrates and contain less oxygen.

Triglycerides make up the majority of the lipids we eat and are found in margarine, butter, oils, and animal products. Triglycerides are an important energy source for the body, especially during rest and sleep. The body stores excess energy as triglycerides in the adipose tissue beneath the skin, which insulates the body and cushions the organs. (Chapter 5 presents more information on lipids.)

Proteins Provide the Building Blocks for Tissue Synthesis

Proteins contribute the basic building blocks, known as amino acids, to synthesize, grow, and maintain tissues in the body. The tissues in muscles, bones, and skin are primarily made up of protein. Proteins also participate as neurotransmitters in the complex communication network between the brain and the rest of the body, and they play a role in the immune system and as **enzymes** that catalyze chemical reactions.

Proteins are similar in composition to carbohydrates and lipids in that they contain carbon, hydrogen, and oxygen. But proteins are unique in that they all contain the element nitrogen, and some also contain sulfur. Proteins can be used for energy but are usually not a primary energy source.

Protein is found in a variety of foods, including meats, dairy products, nuts, and seeds. Legumes such as soy also provide significant protein, and certain other vegetables, whole grains, and some fruits provide small amounts. (Chapter 6 covers protein in detail.)

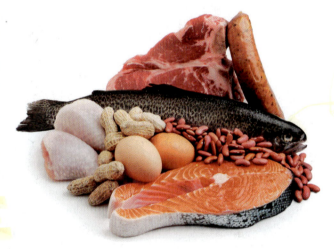

Meats and dairy products are excellent sources of protein. Plant products, such as nuts, seeds, and legumes, also provide protein to the diet.

Vitamins and Minerals Play Vital Roles in Metabolism

Vitamins and minerals do not provide energy, but they are involved in numerous key functions in the body. They are essential to help regulate metabolism, for example, and without them we would be unable to convert carbohydrates, fats, and proteins to energy or to sustain numerous other chemical reactions. A deficiency of vitamins and minerals can cause a cascade of ill health effects ranging from fatigue to stunted growth, weak bones, and organ damage. The metabolic fate of carbohydrates, protein, and fats in the body depends on consuming enough vitamins and minerals in the daily diet.

Vitamins

Many vitamins function as **coenzymes**; that is, they help enzymes catalyze reactions in the body. For example, the B vitamin thiamin attaches to and assists an enzyme involved in carbohydrate metabolism. Vitamins also activate enzymes that participate in building bone and muscle, energy production, fighting infections, and maintaining healthy nerves and vision.

There are 13 known vitamins, and each has a unique chemical structure. They are grouped into two classifications according to their **solubility**, which affects how they are

enzymes Proteins in living cells that act as catalysts and control chemical reactions.

coenzymes Substances, such as vitamins or minerals, that facilitate the activity of enzymes.

solubility Ability to dissolve into another substance.

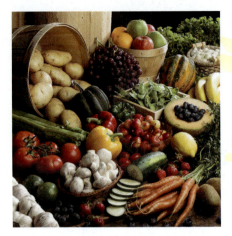

A wide variety of fruits and vegetables are abundant sources of water-soluble vitamins.

absorbed, stored, and excreted. **Water-soluble vitamins**, which include vitamin C and the eight B-complex vitamins, are easily absorbed and excreted by the body and need to be consumed daily. The **fat-soluble vitamins**—A, D, E, and K—are stored in the liver and fatty tissues and thus don't need to be consumed on a daily basis. (Vitamins are discussed in Chapters 9 and 10.)

Minerals

Minerals are inorganic elements that assist in body processes and are essential to the structure of hard tissues, such as bone, and soft tissues, such as the red blood cells. Minerals like calcium and phosphorus work with protein-containing hormones and enzymes to maintain and strengthen teeth and bones. A deficiency of any of the minerals can cause disease symptoms. Falling short of daily iron needs, for example, can cause fatigue and impair your immunity.

Minerals are classified by the amount needed in the diet and total content found in the body. **Major minerals** are needed in amounts of at least 100 milligrams per day and are found in amounts of at least 5 grams in the body. Calcium and magnesium are two examples of major minerals. In addition to contributing to the structure of bones and teeth, some major minerals help maintain fluid balance, participate in energy metabolism, or contribute to muscle contractions. (Each individual major mineral is described in Chapter 12.)

Trace minerals are needed in amounts of less than 100 milligrams per day and are found in amounts of less than 5 grams in the body. Iron and zinc are two examples of trace minerals. Among other functions, trace minerals transport oxygen and carbon dioxide, participate in cell growth and development, control the metabolic rate, and play a role in body defenses. (Chapter 13 provides more specific detail on the role of trace minerals.)

Water Is Critical for Numerous Functions

Some of the essential roles of water in the body probably seem obvious, as it makes up the majority of all body fluids, including digestive secretions, blood, urine, and perspiration. Less obvious is the fact that water is part of every cell in the body, from muscle and bone cells to brain and nerve cells. Water is also vital to several key body functions. It is essential during metabolism, for example, because it provides the medium in which metabolic reactions take place. Water functions in digestion and absorption and as a transport medium that delivers nutrients and oxygen to the cells through blood and lymph and excretes waste products through the urine and feces. Water helps maintain body temperature and acts as a lubricant for the joints, eyes, mouth, and intestinal tract. It surrounds vital organs and cushions them from injury. Because the body can't store water, it must be replenished every day to maintain hydration. (The role of water in the body is discussed in Chapter 11.)

water-soluble vitamins Vitamins that dissolve in water; they generally cannot be stored in the body and must be consumed daily.

fat-soluble vitamins Vitamins that dissolve in fat and can be stored in the body.

major minerals Minerals found in the body in amounts greater than 5 grams; also referred to as *macrominerals*.

trace minerals Minerals found in the body in amounts less than 5 grams; also referred to as *microminerals*.

LO 1.3: THE TAKE-HOME MESSAGE The six classes of essential nutrients—carbohydrates, lipids (fats), protein, vitamins, minerals, and water—each have specific roles in the body. Carbohydrates and lipids are the body's primary energy sources. Proteins can be used for energy, but their main role is to provide the building blocks for body structures and functional compounds. Vitamins, minerals, and water are needed to use the energy-producing nutrients and for various body processes.

How Can You Be Sure to Meet Your Nutritional Needs?

LO 1.4 Describe the best approach to meeting your nutritional needs.

There is no question that you need all six classes of nutrients to function properly. A chronic deficiency of even one nutrient will impact the body's ability to function in the short term. Over time, chronic deficiencies, excesses, and imbalances will affect long-term health.

Is there more to a healthy diet than just meeting your basic nutrient needs? And is there an advantage to consuming the essential nutrients through food rather than taking them as supplements?

The Best Approach Is to Consume a Balanced Diet

Most credible nutrition experts will tell you that the best way to maintain nutritional health is to eat a variety of foods, including whole grains, fruits, vegetables, lean meats, and low-fat dairy. Among the reasons for this recommendation is that foods provide a variety of nutrients. For example, low-fat milk is high in carbohydrates and protein and provides a small amount of fat. Milk is also a good source of the vitamins A, D, and riboflavin, as well as the minerals potassium and calcium, and is approximately 90 percent water by weight.

Furthermore, foods almost always contain a variety of non-nutrient compounds that enhance health. Foods that are thought to provide health benefits beyond basic nutrition are known as **functional foods**. Americans have been consuming functional foods to improve their health since the late 1920s, when iodine was first added to salt. Today's functional foods include foods such as oatmeal, genetically modified foods that are developed to have a higher nutrient content, and foods that contain or have been fortified with phytochemicals and zoochemicals.

Phytochemicals are non-nutritive chemicals that occur naturally in plants. Consuming a diet rich in phytochemicals is associated with a reduced risk of developing certain diseases. At least 900 different phytochemicals have been identified in foods and more are likely to be discovered. For example, lutein is found in spinach, lycopene is found in tomatoes, and anthocyanins are found in dark purple grapes. The disease-fighting properties of phytochemicals may be due to more than the compounds themselves. It is the interactions between the phytochemicals and nutrients, fiber, or other unknown substances in the food that provide the health benefits.[31] Phytochemicals extracted from foods and put in a pill do not produce the same positive health effects. In contrast, foods with added phytochemicals, such as margarine with added phytosterols, have the same appearance and taste as your favorites but provide added health benefits.

Zoochemicals are naturally occurring, health-enhancing chemicals found in animal-based foods. Examples include lutein and zeaxanthin found in egg yolks, which may protect against vision disorders such as macular degeneration and the formation of cataracts. Omega-3 fatty acids added to butter substitutes may improve heart health and reduce inflammation, protecting us against heart disease, cancer, and a decline in cognitive function. And the beneficial bacteria (called *probiotics*) present in yogurt support intestinal health and function.

Table 1.2 provides a guide to functional foods. These foods can be part of a healthy, well-balanced diet. Keep in mind that whole grains, fruits, vegetables, healthy vegetable oils, lean meat and dairy products, fish, poultry, and nuts and seeds all contain varying amounts of naturally occurring phytochemicals or zoochemicals and are the quintessential functional foods. Consumers who choose packaged functional foods, such as snack bars and juices, should take care not to overconsume any one compound.

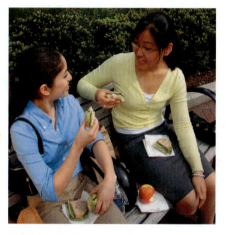

Healthy eating is a way of life.

functional foods Foods that may provide additional health benefits beyond their basic nutrient value.

phytochemicals Non-nutritive plant compounds, found in fruits and vegetables, that may play a role in fighting chronic diseases.

zoochemicals Non-nutritive animal compounds that play a role in fighting chronic diseases.

TABLE 1.2   Your Guide to Functional Foods

This Compound	Found in This/These Functional Food(s)	May Have This Health Benefit
Beta-carotene	Carrots, pumpkin, cantaloupe, broccoli	Functions as an antioxidant in the body
Lycopene	Tomatoes, tomato sauce	May lower risk of prostate cancer
Soy protein	Tofu, soy milk	Lowers risk of heart disease
Beta-glucan	Oatmeal, oats, oat bran	Lowers blood cholesterol
Plant sterol and stanol esters	Fortified margarines, like Benecol spreads	Lowers blood cholesterol
Omega-3 fatty acids	Salmon, sardines, tuna	May reduce the risk of heart disease
Whole grains	Whole-wheat bread, brown rice, popcorn	May reduce the risk of some cancers and heart disease
Flavanols	Dark chocolate, green apples	May contribute to heart health
Anthocyanins	Berries, red grapes, cherries	Act as antioxidants, may contribute to brain function
Probiotics	Active cultures in fermented dairy products such as yogurt	Support intestinal health

Some Nutrient Needs Can Be Met with Fortified Foods or a Supplement

Some individuals with dietary restrictions or higher nutrient needs may benefit from taking a supplement if they cannot meet their nutrient requirements through whole foods alone. For example, someone who is *lactose intolerant* (has difficulty digesting milk products) may have to meet his or her calcium needs from sources other than dairy products. Calcium-fortified orange juice or soymilk or a calcium supplement would be an option for such an individual. Pregnant women should take an iron supplement because their increased need for this mineral is unlikely to be met through a healthy diet alone.

Note that a balanced diet, fortified foods, and dietary supplements aren't mutually exclusive. Some or all of these sources of nutrients, phytochemicals, and zoochemicals can be combined as the best nutritional strategy for good health.

> **LO 1.4: THE TAKE-HOME MESSAGE** A balanced diet providing a variety of whole foods rich in nutrients, phytochemicals, and zoochemicals reduces the risk of developing certain diseases and is the best way to meet nutritional needs. People who cannot meet their nutrient needs through food alone may benefit from consuming fortified foods and/or taking a supplement.

How Does Diet Influence Your Health?

LO 1.5 Summarize three ways in which diet influences health.

Your diet can positively affect your health by reducing your risk of chronic diseases, preventing nutrient-deficiency diseases, and interacting in beneficial ways with your genes. Let's look a little further at each of these three key influences.

A Healthy Diet Reduces the Risk of Chronic Disease

A healthy diet reduces the risk of **chronic disease**. Of the top 10 leading causes of death in the United States, four are chronic diseases linked to poor nutrition. These include heart disease, cancer, stroke, and diabetes (**Table 1.3**). Eating well helps us achieve and maintain a healthy weight and reduce the risk for all four of these chronic diseases, which are significantly increased in people who are obese.

chronic disease Noncommunicable disease characterized by a slow onset, long duration, and gradual progression.

TABLE 1.3	Leading Causes of Death in the United States	
Disease/Cause of Death	**Nutrition Related**	
1. **Heart disease**	X	
2. **Cancer**	X	
3. Respiratory diseases		
4. Accidents		
5. **Stroke**	X	
6. Alzheimer's disease		
7. **Diabetes**	X	
8. Influenza and pneumonia		
9. Kidney disease		
10. Suicide		

Source: Centers for Disease Control. 2017. Leading Causes of Death. Available at www.cdc.gov.

Nutrition also plays an important role in preventing other chronic diseases and conditions that can reduce quality of life. A healthy diet, for example, can help keep bones strong and reduce the risk of developing osteoporosis. Evidence also suggests that a healthy diet can reduce the risk of *hypertension* (high blood pressure), age-related vision loss, and many other chronic conditions.

A Healthy Diet Prevents Nutrient-Deficiency Diseases

Our understanding of the link between nutrition and health began to develop several centuries ago with discoveries of the health effects of certain foods. For example, in the 1600s some seagoing merchants realized that providing their sailors with citrus fruits prevented scurvy, a disease characterized by tissue breakdown. By the year 1800, the British Navy began routinely supplying sailors with limes, and the term *limey* for a British sailor was born.

Although scientists had begun to recognize the value of certain foods in treating disease, it wasn't until the early 1900s that the concept of *essential nutrients* was widely accepted and many vitamins and minerals were identified. For example, vitamin C, the "anti-scurvy agent" in citrus fruits, was discovered in 1912. Throughout the early decades of the twentieth century, nutrition science became more quantitative, addressing the questions of how much of each nutrient is required and how individuals might vary in their nutrient needs. Nutrition research advanced further as dietary surveys conducted by the government gathered population data. As a result of these efforts, nutrient-deficiency diseases are now rare throughout the developed world.

In the twenty-first century, nutrition science has evolved to study the role of nutrients and functional foods not only in preventing chronic disease but also in promoting longevity. A key contribution to this evolution has been our increasing understanding of the relationship between our diet and our genes.

A Healthy Diet Can Positively Affect Gene Expression

Most chronic diseases stem from the interplay between our genetic makeup and environmental factors, which include our diet (**Figure 1.5**). Each one of us carries a unique combination of genes—segments of DNA—that we inherited from our parents. Because genes are chemical instructions for assembling body proteins, they are responsible for our appearance, our metabolism, and our susceptibility to disease. Some genes have variations in their codes (mutations) that increase susceptibility to diseases such as cancer, cardiovascular disease, and diabetes, whereas other gene variants enhance the body's ability to

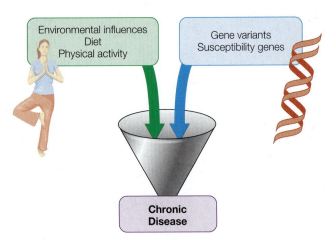

▲ **Figure 1.5 Chronic Disease Is a Mixture of Genetic Influences and Our Environment**

gene expression Processing of genetic information to create a specific protein.

epigenetics Study of the variety of environmental factors and other mechanisms influencing gene expression.

nutritional genomics Study of the relationship between genes, gene expression, and nutrition.

registered dietitian nutritionist (RDN) Health professional who is a food and nutrition expert; RDNs obtain a college degree in nutrition from an Academy of Nutrition and Dietetics–accredited program and pass a national exam.

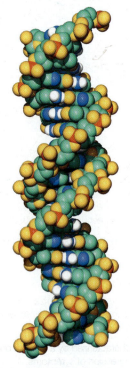

The study of nutritional genomics may one day allow individuals to tailor their diets to their DNA.

resist chronic disease. Variants alone rarely cause disease directly; usually, they increase the risk that the disease will develop given a conducive environment.

The interactions between genes and your environment are complex. Scientific advances point to a variety of mechanisms by which nutrition—a key aspect of the cellular environment—interacts with genes to influence your risk of disease. While you can't change the genetic cards you are dealt, by improving the quality of your diet, you can change the way you play the game.

The Human Genome Project (HGP) mapped the sequence of all of the genes (the genome) in humans. Completion of the HGP has enabled nutritionists, geneticists, and other researchers to actively examine the synergistic effects of nutrition and genetics. This reaction either increases or decreases **gene expression**, producing greater or smaller amounts of proteins, which in turn affects body function. The study of the mechanisms by which factors such as food intake alter gene expression without changing the DNA sequence is known as **epigenetics**. For example, folate, one of the B vitamins, may alter the expression of genes as the embryo develops during early pregnancy. A deficiency of folate during this critical time increases the risk of specific birth defects in the baby. We talk more about this in Chapter 10.

Until recently, nutrition research and genetic research contributed separately to our understanding of human health and disease. Studied together, these two fields help us understand how genetic variations influence an individual's response to his or her diet (*nutrigenetics*), and how nutrients and other components of foods influence genetic expression (**nutritional genomics**, or *nutrigenomics*).

Recent advances in nutritional genomics have already yielded potential clinical applications. For example, research has shown that chronic inflammation can be reduced with consumption of certain bioactive compounds found in food. These compounds include vitamin C in fruits and vegetables, vitamin E in wheat germ and vegetable oils,[32] and the omega-3 fatty acids in fish.[33] Increasing dietary intake of these compounds may regulate the expression of genes coding for proteins active in inflammation.

Nutritional genomics may have tremendous potential to provide personalized dietary recommendations based on an individual's genetic makeup. Ultimately, a future **registered dietitian nutritionist (RDN)** may be able to use this information to recommend dietary modifications specific to a patient's DNA.

LO 1.5: THE TAKE-HOME MESSAGE Eating a balanced diet that includes adequate but not excessive amounts of all nutrients is the best way to stay healthy and reduce the risk of developing four of the top 10 leading causes of death in the United States, including heart disease, cancer, stroke, and diabetes. A healthy diet also prevents nutrient-deficiency diseases such as scurvy. In addition, a healthy diet influences gene expression in ways that may increase or decrease your risk of disease.

How Do We Assess Nutritional Status?

LO 1.6 Summarize the ABCD method used to assess the nutrient status of individuals and populations.

How do you know if you are eating enough of the essential nutrients? If you suspect you may not be meeting all of your nutrient needs, or you have been diagnosed with a nutrition-related disease, turn to a nutrition professional, such as an RDN. The RDN will conduct a complete assessment to find out if you are getting too much, too little, or the right amount of all nutrients.

Nutrition professionals describe a person's *state of nutrition* as either healthy or **malnourished**. Someone who lacks a specific nutrient, or isn't consuming enough energy, is **undernourished**, which means that person is at risk of losing too much weight or developing a disease related to a nutrient deficiency. In contrast, an individual who overconsumes a particular nutrient, or eats too many kilocalories, is described as being **overnourished**. This person runs the risk of becoming overweight, developing diseases such as diabetes or heart disease, or potentially accumulating toxic amounts of a specific nutrient in the body.

The ABCD Method Is Used to Assess the Nutritional Status of Individuals

Evaluating a person's current nutrition status begins with a look at that person's health history, including any experiences with **acute** or chronic illness, and diagnostic procedures, therapies, or treatments that may increase nutrient needs or induce **malabsorption**. Does the patient have a family history of diabetes or heart disease? Has the patient been overweight or underweight in the past? To learn more about evaluating your own family history, see the Self-Assessment.

Self-Assessment

How Healthy Is Your Family Tree?

You inherited your DNA from your parents, so the extent to which DNA affects health is largely hereditary. Does your family have a history of heart disease, diabetes, or obesity? What about other chronic diseases or conditions? Before you learn about the role that healthy eating plays in preventing chronic diseases, ask your parents and grandparents about your family's health history. If there are certain diseases or conditions that run in your family, you'll want to pay particular attention to these as you learn more throughout this text.

An easy way to gather information about your family's health history is by visiting My Family Health Portrait at http://familyhistory.hhs.gov. The site generates a family tree report according to the medical history you enter. Save a copy of the report for future reference.

Along with the health history, nutrition professionals use a number of specialized methods to assess the nutritional status of individuals. You can use the mnemonic ABCD to help you remember these methods, which include collecting **a**nthropometric data, collecting **b**iochemical (laboratory) data, conducting a **c**linical exam, and performing **d**ietary intake assessments (**Table 1.4**). ABCD is more of a framework than a chronological guideline. Each portion builds off the other, but it is not necessary to conduct the method in any specific order.

Assessing Dietary Intake through Questionnaires and Interviews

Questioning an individual about his or her dietary intake and diet history is an important aspect of a nutrition assessment. A detailed diet history is conducted by a skilled interviewer who knows just what types of questions to ask to help a patient remember not only current food intake but food intake in the past.

Two tools used to collect dietary intake data are questionnaires and interviews. Food frequency questionnaires and food records can be used to gather information about how often a specific food or category of food is eaten. A nutrition interview can reveal data about lifestyle habits, such as how many meals are eaten daily, where they are eaten, and who prepares them.

malnourished Characterized by an inappropriate level of essential nutrients to maintain health; overnourishment and undernourishment are forms of malnutrition.

undernourished Characterized by an inadequate energy intake or a deficiency in quality or quantity of one or more individual nutrients.

overnourished Characterized by an excessive intake of energy or one or more individual nutrients.

acute Characterized by a sudden onset and rapid progression of symptoms.

malabsorption Condition characterized by impaired absorption of nutrients through the gastrointestinal tract.

TABLE 1.4	The ABCDs of Nutrition Assessment	
Type of Assessment	**Measurements**	**What They Determine**
Anthropometric	Height Weight Body mass index Waist-to-hip ratio Waist circumference	Growth, obesity, changes in weight, and risk of developing chronic diseases such as diabetes and heart disease
Biochemical	Blood, urine, and feces	Protein, mineral, and vitamin status and disease
Clinical	Observe hair, fingernails, skin, lips, mouth, muscles, joints, overall appearance	Signs of deficiencies and excesses of nutrients
Dietary Intake	Diet history Diet record Food frequency questionnaire 24-hour dietary recall	Usual nutrient intake and deficiencies or excesses of various nutrients

One of the easiest ways to determine an individual's intake of nutrients is to use the *food frequency questionnaire (FFQ)*. This form of assessment provides evidence of consumption patterns over time. For example, if you wanted to determine the usual calcium intake over time of an older woman with osteoporosis, an FFQ could be used to indicate the number of servings of dairy foods "per day, per week, and per month," as well as whether she "seldom" or "never" consumes milk, cheese, or yogurt. The FFQ is a reasonably reliable, accurate, and inexpensive method to assess usual intake.[34]

This assessment tool is not as helpful in assessing the actual amount consumed of a nutrient, nor does it always accurately reveal usual intake. For that information, a food record or 24-hour dietary recall usually provides a better picture.[35]

A *food record* is simply a diary of what foods and beverages are eaten, how much, and when they are eaten over a defined period of time. Food records are often kept for 3–7 days and are considered by some to be one of the best methods for collecting diet information. There are drawbacks to this method. The accuracy depends on the individual's skill and commitment to keeping a valid record. Many people start out strong and then lose interest or simply forget to record the food. Or, they might alter their usual food intake to avoid feeling embarrassed about what they eat.

Food records can be kept in written form, such as a journal, or with an electronic diet analysis program. There are also new digital and mobile devices that may help improve the accuracy, ease, and evaluation of recording dietary intake.[36]

The FFQ or a diet record should be selected based on the specific information the assessor needs to know, such as iron intake over time and how much iron the individual eats daily, as well as the assessor's ability to complete the instrument accurately. The information obtained from these tools is then compared with current dietary standards, which we discuss in the next chapter.

Whether a handwritten log or a smartphone app, food diaries can be useful tools for assessing nutritional status.

The *24-hour dietary recall* method is a quick assessment conducted by a trained interviewer who asks a patient to recall all the food and drinks, including snacks, eaten the previous day. This tool relies on the skills of the interviewer and the individual's ability to remember what he or she ate and drank the day before. Because dietary intake varies from one day to the next, one 24-hour period may not provide an accurate estimate of typical intake.

Collecting Anthropometric Data

body mass index (BMI) Measurement calculated using the metric formula of weight in kilograms divided by height in meters squared; used to determine whether an individual is underweight, at a healthy weight, overweight, or obese.

Data about body size or body composition is also called *anthropometric data*. In adults, this usually means height, weight, **body mass index (BMI)**, waist-to-hip ratios, and waist circumference. For children, growth charts have been developed that compare height to weight, as well as how a child's height and weight compare with others of the same age. All of these measurements are easily obtained with a scale and tape measure.

The BMI is a measure of weight relative to height, and waist circumference measures abdominal fat. Body composition measurements can provide data on an individual's lean body tissue and percentage of body fat. The measurements can be assessed with specialized equipment, such as skin calipers or the Bod Pod. (We discuss these measurements in greater detail in Chapter 14.)

Data collected from anthropometric measurements is then compared with reference standards. Patterns and trends become evident when more than one measurement is taken over time and compared with the initial values. By combining the results of the BMI and waist circumference with other information gathered during the nutrition assessment, an individual's risk of developing diseases associated with obesity, such as diabetes and heart disease, can be determined.

Conducting a Clinical Examination

A person who is malnourished will exhibit physical symptoms as the body adjusts to the lack or excess of nutrients. Therefore, several parts of the body can be inspected during a clinical exam for evidence of malnutrition. Observing the hair, skin, eyes, fingernails, tongue, and lips can provide clues that point to under- or overnutrition. For example, cracks at the corners of the mouth can be evidence of B-vitamin deficiencies, whereas small pinpoint hemorrhages on the skin may reflect a deficiency of vitamin C. Observations of physical symptoms should be followed up by more direct measurements, including laboratory assessments.

Collecting Biochemical Data

Laboratory tests based on body fluids, including blood and urine, can be important indicators of nutritional status, but they are also influenced by non-nutritional factors. Biochemical tests of urine assess nutritional status by measuring, for example, how fast a nutrient is excreted through the urine and the metabolic by-products of various nutrients found in urine. Blood tests may measure levels of albumin (a blood protein) to screen for protein deficiency; low hemoglobin levels in the blood indicate iron-deficiency anemia; and a high fasting blood sugar level may suggest diabetes.

Surveys Are Used to Assess the Nutritional Status of a Population Group

Assessing the nutritional status of an individual in a clinical setting is one thing, but how do we determine the nutritional status of a population? What percentage of Americans is meeting the dietary recommendations for healthy eating? To find out, researchers collect dietary intake information on a large scale. The information is used by researchers in many ways, such as to determine the adequacy of the current nutrient recommendations for different population groups, to evaluate and develop food assistance programs, and to assess risk of nutritional deficiencies.

Populations are typically assessed through the use of surveys. Numerous national surveys have been developed by a variety of federal agencies to assess the health and nutritional status of Americans. The National Health and Nutrition Examination Survey (NHANES) is one of the most prominent. Conducted annually, it is used to determine the nutritional status of Americans of all ages and to monitor their risk behaviors over time. The intake of carbohydrates, lipids, protein, vitamins, minerals, and fiber is collected using a 24-hour recall method and reported in the document *What We Eat in America*.

The Framingham Heart Study, which coined the term *risk factors*, had a major impact on the dietary intake of Americans. This study used surveys to collect longitudinal data on two generations and more than 10,000 participants to establish the current recommendations for the prevention of cardiovascular disease.

LO 1.6: THE TAKE-HOME MESSAGE An individual's nutritional status is assessed by gathering information from health history, dietary record, and anthropometric, clinical, and biochemical (laboratory) data. When the information from the ABCD methods is viewed together, a comprehensive picture of the individual's nutritional status can be determined. The National Health and Nutrition Examination Survey is used to determine the nutritional status of a large population. The Framingham Heart Study provided the foundation for the current dietary recommendations for heart health.

How Healthy Is the Average American Diet?

LO 1.7 Discuss the current nutritional state of the average American diet.

The food supply in the United States provides an array of nutritious choices to meet the dietary needs of Americans. Fresh fruits and vegetables, whole grains, lean meats, fish, and poultry are easily accessible and affordable through local grocery stores and farmers markets. With such an abundance of healthy foods to choose from, are Americans adopting healthy diets?

The Quality of the American Diet Needs Improvement

In general, the American diet is too high in added sugars, sodium, and saturated fat.[37] **Added sugars** account for 13 percent of America's daily kilocalories. This is largely due to Americans' love of soft drinks, other sugary beverages, and sweets and treats.[38] High sodium intake is a risk factor for hypertension, and Americans consume far more than is recommended. The American diet also contains too much saturated fat, the form of fat linked to cardiovascular disease. Whereas the recommended intake is to consume less than 10 percent of your total daily kilocalories from saturated fat, Americans, on average, are consuming over 11 percent. However, most Americans don't exceed the recommended dietary cholesterol intake limit of 300 milligrams per day.[39]

In contrast, our intake of fiber and certain vitamins and minerals is too low.[40] Our low fiber intake is partly due to inadequate consumption of fruits and vegetables and overconsumption of refined grains, which provide far less fiber than whole grains. (The role of dietary fiber in health is discussed in Chapter 4.) American women fail to meet their recommended intake for iron, and Americans in general don't consume enough vitamin D, potassium, and calcium.[41] In an attempt to balance their poor choice in foods, over 50 percent of Americans take at least one vitamin or mineral supplement per day.[42]

Our lack of a healthy diet may be due in part to where we eat and with whom we eat. Today, many Americans eat most of their meals away from home.[43] Some of us eat in the car or buy takeout meals or prepared foods from the supermarket. Research suggests that increasing the number of meals consumed as a family may improve the dietary quality of the entire family. Eating family meals together seven or more times per week has been associated with consuming an additional serving of both fruits and vegetables daily as compared with families who do not dine together.[44]

The majority of Americans understand the positive benefits of eating breakfast, yet nearly 25 percent of Americans skip this morning meal.[45] Breakfast, which often includes foods from the dairy, grains, and fruit groups, is an important meal that could provide Americans with fiber (whole-grain cereal), vitamin D and calcium (milk), and potassium

added sugars Sugars added to foods during processing and/or packaging.

(bananas, orange juice). Many Americans are falling short of fiber and these three nutrients in their daily diet.

Rates of Overweight and Obesity in Americans Are Too High

As Americans take in more kilocalories than they burn in their sedentary lives, they create a recipe for overweight and obesity. Overall, more than 35 percent of American adults are obese.[46] Rates within certain populations and geographical regions are even higher (**Figure 1.6**). Along with these increases in obesity have come higher rates of type 2 diabetes, particularly among children, and increased rates of heart disease, cancer, and stroke. Reducing America's obesity rate is therefore a top public health priority.

Healthy People 2020 Provides Health Objectives for Americans

The U.S. Surgeon General has issued calls for a nationwide health improvement program since 1979. The latest edition of this report, *Healthy People 2020*, contains a set of health objectives for the nation to achieve over the second decade of the twenty-first century.[47]

There are more than 35 topic areas in *Healthy People 2020*, ranging from ensuring that Americans have adequate access to health services to improvements in their diet and physical activity. Objectives are developed within each topic area. For example, research indicates that Americans' body weights are increasing rather than decreasing. Thus, "Nutrition and Weight Status" is one topic area. The numerous objectives developed within this topic area, if fulfilled, will help Americans improve their diet and reduce their weight and their risk for chronic disease. **Table 1.5** lists a few objectives in this topic area.

As you can see from the table, consuming adequate amounts of fruits and vegetables is beneficial to managing one's weight. Americans should increase their intake of both of these food sources to help them improve their nutrition and weight status.

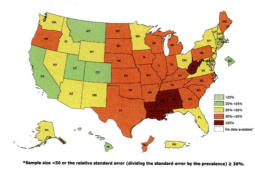

Prevalence¹ of Self-Reported Obesity Among U.S. Adults by State and Territory, BRFSS, 2015

¹ Prevalence estimates reflect BRFSS methodological changes started in 2011. These estimates should not be compared to prevalence estimates before 2011.

*Sample size <50 or the relative standard error (dividing the standard error by the prevalence) ≥ 30%.

a

Obesity Trends* Among U.S. Adults
BRFSS, 1985
(*BMI ≥30, or ~ 30 lbs. overweight for 5' 4" person)

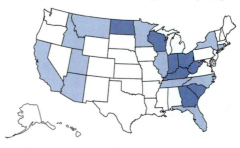

No Data | <10% | 10%–14%

Source: Behavioral Risk Factor Surveillance System, CDC.

b

▲ **Figure 1.6 Obesity Trends Among U.S. Adults**
Over the past few decades, rates of obesity have risen significantly in the United States.
Source: Centers for Disease Control. 2016. "Prevalence of Self-Reported Obesity among U.S. Adults." Available at www.cdc.gov.

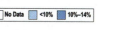

TABLE 1.5	*Healthy People 2020* Nutrition and Weight Status Objectives		
Objectives		**Target for Americans (%)**	**Status of Americans (%)**
Increase the proportion of adults who are at a healthy weight		33.9	30.8
Reduce the proportion of adults who are obese		30.5	33.9
Reduce the proportion of children and adolescents ages 2–19 who are considered obese		14.5	16.1
Increase the contribution of fruits to diets of the population age 2 years and older		0.9 cups/1,000 kcals	0.5 cups/1,000 kcals
Increase the variety and contribution of vegetables to the diets of the population age 2 years and older		1.1 cups/1,000 kcals	0.8 cups/1,000 kcals

Source: United States Department of Health and Human Services. Nutrition and Weight Status: Objectives. Updated January 12, 2017. *Healthy People 2020*. Available at www.HealthyPeople.gov. Accessed January 2017.

What Is Credible Nutrition Research?

LO 1.8 Describe the scientific method that leads to reliable and accurate nutrition information.

If you Google the word *nutrition*, you will get a list of about 14.5 million entries in 0.25 seconds. Obviously, the world is full of nutrition information at our fingertips. But is it credible?

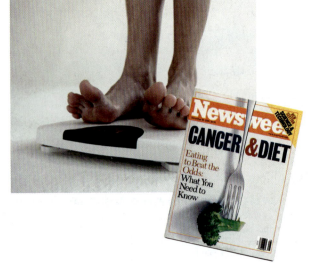

Nutrition-related stories often lead in newspapers and magazines and on websites.

Anyone who has attempted to lose weight can probably tell you how hard it is to keep up with the latest diet advice—because it seems to keep changing. In the 1970s, waist watchers were told that carbohydrates were the bane of their existence and that a protein-rich, low-carbohydrate diet was the key to shrinking their waistline. A decade later, avoiding fat was the way to win the battle of the bulge. By 2000, carbohydrates were being ousted again, and protein-rich diets were back in vogue. More recently, high-protein diets have been losing popularity and high-carbohydrate diets are once again being promoted for weight loss. So . . . are you frustrated yet?

Whereas diet trends and popular wisdom seem to change frequently, basic scientific knowledge about nutrition does not. Results from individual studies are often deemed newsworthy and publicized in the media, but the results of one report do not radically change expert opinion. Only when multiple, affirming research studies have been conducted is a **consensus** reached about nutrition advice. News of the results of one study is just that: news. In contrast, advice from an authoritative health organization or committee, such as the American Heart Association or the Dietary Guidelines Advisory Committee, which is based on a consensus of research information, is sound information that can be trusted for the long term.

Sound Nutrition Research Begins with the Scientific Method

Sound research studies begin with a process called the **scientific method**. Scientists observe something in the natural world, ask questions, and propose an explanation (or **hypothesis**) based on their observations. They then test their hypothesis by conducting an experiment. There are many steps in the scientific method and many adjustments are made along the way before a scientist has gained enough information to draw a conclusion about his or her hypothesis. In fact, the entire process can take years to complete.

Let's walk through a nutrition-related study in which scientists used the scientific method to study rickets (**Figure 1.7**). *Rickets* is a disease in children in which the leg bones are so weakened that they cannot hold up the child's body weight. The legs bow as a result. In the early 1800s, parents often used cod-liver oil to treat rickets because it seemed to provide a miraculous cure.

consensus Agreed-upon conclusion of a group of experts based on a collection of information.

scientific method Process used by scientists to gather and test information for the sake of generating sound research findings.

hypothesis Idea or explanation proposed by scientists based on observations or known facts.

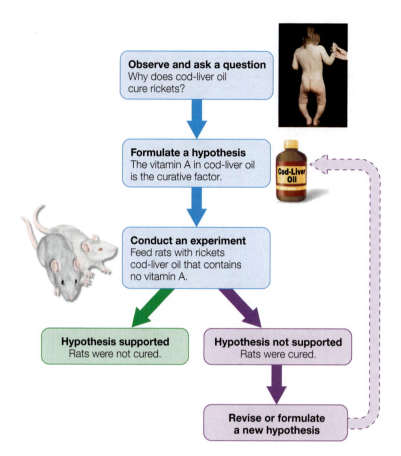

Observe and ask a question
Why does cod-liver oil cure rickets?

Formulate a hypothesis
The vitamin A in cod-liver oil is the curative factor.

Conduct an experiment
Feed rats with rickets cod-liver oil that contains no vitamin A.

Hypothesis supported
Rats were not cured.

Hypothesis not supported
Rats were cured.

Revise or formulate a new hypothesis

Scientists noticed the cod-liver oil curing phenomenon and asked themselves why cod-liver oil cured rickets. In doing so, these scientists were using the first step in the scientific method: observing and asking questions.

The second step of the scientific method is to formulate a hypothesis. Because cod-liver oil is very rich in vitamin A, scientists initially thought that this vitamin was the curative factor. To confirm this, scientists proceeded to the third step, which was to conduct an experiment.

The scientists altered the cod-liver oil to destroy its vitamin A. The altered oil was given to rats that had been fed a diet that caused rickets. Surprisingly, the rats were still cured of rickets. This disproved the scientists' original hypothesis that vitamin A was the curative factor. They then needed to modify their hypothesis, as it was obvious that there was something else in the cod-liver oil that cured rickets. They next hypothesized that it was the vitamin D in the oil that cured the rats. They conducted another experiment to confirm this hypothesis, which it did.

What good would it be to make such an important discovery if other scientists couldn't find out about it? Fortunately, scientists today share their findings by summarizing and submitting their research to a **peer-reviewed journal** (**Figure 1.8**). Other scientists (peers) review the researchers' findings to make sure that they are sound. If so, the research study is published in the journal. After that, it may be picked up by the popular press and reported. If the relationship between vitamin D and rickets were discovered today, it would probably be the lead story on CNN.

As more and more studies confirmed that vitamin D could cure and prevent rickets, a theory developed. By the 1920s, researchers knew with great certainty that vitamin D prevents rickets, and that a deficiency of vitamin D can cause deformed bones in children. Because of this, there is a consensus among health professionals as to the importance of vitamin D in the diets of children.

peer-reviewed journal Journal in which scientists publish research findings, after the findings have gone through a rigorous review process by other scientists.

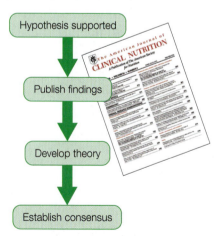

Hypothesis supported

Publish findings

Develop theory

Establish consensus

▲ **Figure 1.8 A Hypothesis Can Lead to a Scientific Consensus**
When a hypothesis is supported by research, the results are published in peer-reviewed journals. Once a theory has been developed and supported by subsequent experiments, a consensus is reached in the scientific community.

Scientists Use a Variety of Experiments to Test Hypotheses

laboratory experiment Scientific experiment conducted in a laboratory; some involve animals.

observational research Research that involves systematically observing subjects to see if there is a relationship to certain outcomes.

epidemiological research Research that studies the variables that influence health in a population; it is often observational.

experimental research Research involving at least two groups of subjects receiving different treatments.

experimental group In experimental research, the group of participants given a specific treatment, such as a drug, as part of the study.

control group In experimental research, the group that does not receive the treatment but may be given a placebo instead; used as a standard for comparison.

Scientists can use different types of experiments to test a hypothesis. A **laboratory experiment** is done within the confines of a lab setting, such as the rickets experiments with rats. Research conducted with humans is usually observational or experimental.

Observational research involves exploring factors in two or more groups of subjects to see if there is a relationship to a certain disease or health outcome. One type of observational research is **epidemiological research**, which looks at health and disease in populations of people. For example, scientists may notice that there is a higher incidence of rickets among children who live in Norway than among children who live in Australia. Through their observations, they may find a relationship between the lack of sun exposure in Norway and the high incidence of rickets there compared with sunny Australia. However, the scientists can't rule out that the difference in the incidence of rickets in these two populations may also be due to other factors in the subjects' diet or lifestyle. This type of research does not answer the question of whether one factor directly causes another.

Experimental research involves at least two groups of subjects. One group, the **experimental group**, is given a treatment, and another group, the **control group**, isn't. When scientists hypothesized that vitamin D cured rickets, they would have randomly assigned children with rickets to one of two groups (**Figure 1.9**). The scientists would have

▶ **Figure 1.9 Controlled Scientific Experiments**
Scientists use experimental research to test hypotheses.

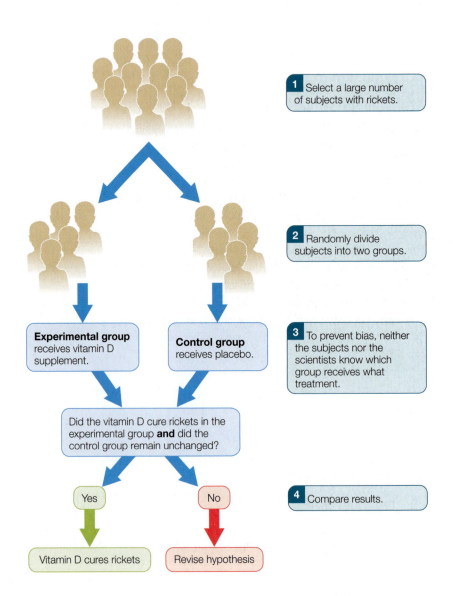

1 Select a large number of subjects with rickets.

2 Randomly divide subjects into two groups.

Experimental group receives vitamin D supplement.

Control group receives placebo.

3 To prevent bias, neither the subjects nor the scientists know which group receives what treatment.

Did the vitamin D cure rickets in the experimental group **and** did the control group remain unchanged?

Yes

No

4 Compare results.

Vitamin D cures rickets

Revise hypothesis

given the experimental group a vitamin D supplement but would have given the control group a **placebo**, which looked just like the vitamin D supplement but contained only sugar. If neither of the two groups of subjects knew which pill they received, then the subjects were "blind" to the treatment. If the scientists who gave the placebo and the vitamin D supplement also didn't know which group received which treatment, the experiment would be called a **double-blind placebo-controlled study**. The scientists would also have to make sure that the variables were the same or controlled for both groups during the experiment. For example, they couldn't let the control group go outside in the sunshine and at the same time keep the experimental group of subjects inside, since sunlight is known to allow humans to synthesize vitamin D. The exposure to the sunshine would change the outcome of the experiment.

A double-blind placebo-controlled study is considered the "gold standard" of research because all of the variables are the same and controlled for the groups of subjects and neither the subjects nor the researcher are biased toward one group.

In any scientific research, sample sizes must be large enough to ensure that differences found in the study are due to the treatment rather than to chance. Studying an entire population is usually impossible because the population is too large, the study would be too expensive or time-consuming, or all members of the population do not want to participate. This was the case with the vitamin D and rickets study mentioned earlier. It would be virtually impossible to measure all children with rickets. Instead, a sample of children with rickets was used and a statistical comparison was done to estimate the effects on the population. Generally, the larger the sample size, the more confident the researchers are that the data reflects reliable differences that would most likely be seen in the population.

The beauty of science is that one discovery builds on another. Though this may seem frustrating when the findings of one research study contradict the results of another from just a few months before, conflicting findings actually help scientists formulate new questions. Though many hypotheses fail along the way, a great many discoveries are also made.

LO 1.8: THE TAKE-HOME MESSAGE Sound nutrition advice is based on years of research using the scientific method. Several methods can be used to conduct nutrition research, including laboratory experiments on animals, experimental research on humans, and observational, particularly epidemiological, research. In double-blind placebo-controlled studies, neither the subjects nor the researchers are aware of who is receiving treatment, and such studies are therefore considered the gold standard of experimental research. Findings from observational and epidemiological research are only considered valid if the study was conducted with an adequate sample size of subjects.

placebo Inactive substance, such as a sugar pill, administered to a control group during an experiment.

double-blind placebo-controlled study Experimental study in which neither the researchers nor the subjects in the study are aware of who is receiving the treatment or the placebo.

How Can You Find and Recognize Credible Nutrition Information?

LO 1.9 Explain how to identify reliable nutrition information and how to recognize misinformation.

If you need legal advice, you seek the expertise of an attorney. If you need knee surgery, you go to an orthopedic surgeon. Where do you go for nutrition advice?

Seek Information from Nutrition Experts

Who is a credible expert with training in the field of nutrition? Different health professionals have varying levels of nutrition training, but by far the professional with the most nutrition training is the registered dietitian nutritionist (RDN). An RDN has completed at least a bachelor's degree from a university or college accredited by the Academy of Nutrition and Dietetics (AND) and has passed the national exam administered by the credentialing body of the AND. The Academy of Nutrition and Dietetics is the largest professional organization in the United States, with a membership of over 89,000 nutrition experts. RDNs must maintain registration with the national organization and participate in continuing professional education to remain current in the fast-changing world of nutrition, medicine, and health.

RDNs are trained to administer **medical nutrition therapy** and work with patients to make dietary changes that can help prevent diseases such as heart disease, diabetes, stroke, and obesity. Many physicians, based on the diagnoses of their patients, refer them to RDNs for nutrition advice and guidance. RDNs must participate in continuing professional education in order to remain current in the fast-changing world of nutrition, medicine, and health and to maintain their registration. RDNs work in

hospitals and other health care facilities, private practice, universities, medical schools, professional athletic teams, food companies, and other nutrition-related businesses.

Some individuals other than RDNs, including those with advanced degrees in nutrition, can also provide credible nutrition information. Some physicians and nurses have taken a nutrition course in school and gone on to get a master of science in public health (MPH), which involves some nutrition courses, or an MS in nutrition at an accredited university or college.

Some **public health nutritionists** may have an undergraduate degree in nutrition but didn't complete a supervised practice so are not eligible to take the AND exam. These individuals can work for state or local governments developing community outreach nutrition programs, such as programs for older adults.

In order to protect the health of the public, over 40 states currently license nutrition professionals. A person who meets these qualifications is a **licensed dietitian nutritionist (LDN)** and so will have the letters "LDN" after his or her name. Because RDNs have completed the rigorous standards set forth by the Academy of Nutrition and Dietetics, they automatically meet the criteria for LDN and often will have both "RDN" and "LDN" after their names.

Be careful when taking nutrition advice from a trainer at the gym or the person who works at the local health food store. Whereas some of these people may be credible, many are not, and thus less likely to give you information based on solid scientific evidence. Anyone who calls him- or herself a **nutritionist** may have taken few or no accredited courses in nutrition.

Beware of Quackery

Whereas credible nutrition experts can provide highly useful nutrition guidance, people of questionable credentials often dole out misinformation, usually for the sake of turning a profit. These skilled salespeople specialize in health **quackery**, or fraud, introducing health fears and then trying to sell services and products to allay these newly created fears. Part of their sales pitch is to make unrealistic promises and guarantees.

To avoid falling for one of their shady schemes, be leery of infomercials, magazine ads, mail-order catalogs, and websites that try to convince you that:

- There is a quick fix for what ails you.
- Their product is all natural and miraculously cures.
- One product does it all.

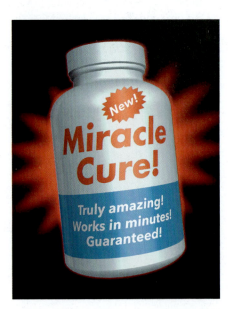

medical nutrition therapy Integration of nutrition counseling and dietary changes, based on individual medical and health needs, to treat a patient's medical condition.

public health nutritionists Individuals who may have an undergraduate degree in nutrition but who are not registered dietitian nutritionists.

licensed dietitian nutritionist (LDN) Individual who has met specified educational and experience criteria deemed by a state licensing board necessary to be considered an expert in the field of nutrition. An RDN would meet all the qualifications to be an LDN.

nutritionist Generic term with no recognized legal or professional meaning. Some people may call themselves a nutritionist without having any credible training in nutrition.

quackery Promotion and selling of health products and services of questionable validity. A quack is a person who promotes these products and services in order to make money.

- You can lose a lot of weight in a short amount of time and without dieting or exercising.
- The product contains a secret ingredient.
- The product shrinks tumors.
- There is no risk, as there is a money-back guarantee. (Good luck getting your money back!)

Evaluate Nutrition News with a Critical Eye

In your lifetime, you will read thousands of newspaper and website headlines, as well as watch and listen to countless television and radio reports announcing sensational headlines about nutrition. Dramatic headlines are designed to grab your attention, but they can be misleading. Whether they're delivered via a magazine or newspaper, TV, or online, these headlines should always be considered with a critical eye.

The media are routinely bombarded by press releases sent from medical journals, food companies, organizations, and universities about research being conducted and/or conferences being sponsored by these institutions. These releases are sent for one reason: to gain publicity. Reputable news organizations that report these findings will seek out independent experts in the field to weigh in on the research and, just as importantly, explain how these findings relate to the public. Even with this added context, there's often much detail that's left out of the story. Here are some questions to consider when hearing or reading about a new study, finding, or claim in the mainstream media:

- **Was the Research Finding Published in a Peer-Reviewed Journal?** You can be more confident that studies published in a peer-reviewed journal have been thoroughly reviewed by experts in this area of research. In most cases, if there are flaws in the study, the study does not get published. If the research isn't published in a peer-reviewed journal, you have no way of knowing

if the study was conducted in an appropriate manner and whether the findings are accurate. A study about the possible virtues of chocolate in fighting heart disease that is published in the *New England Journal of Medicine* has more credibility than a similar article published in a baking magazine.

- **Was the Study Done Using Animals or Humans?** Experiments with animals are often used to study how a particular substance affects a health outcome. But if the study is conducted in rats, it doesn't necessarily mean that the substance will have the same effect if consumed by humans. This doesn't mean that animal studies are frivolous; they are important stepping-stones to designing and conducting similar experiments involving humans.
- **Do the Study Participants Resemble Me?** When you read or hear about studies involving humans, you should always find out more information about the individuals who took part in the research. For example, were the people in the chocolate studies college-age subjects or older individuals with heart disease? If older adults were studied, then would these findings be of any benefit to young adults who don't have heart disease?
- **Is This the First Time I've Heard About This?** A single study in a specific area of research is a lonely entity in the scientific world. Is this the first study regarding the health benefits of

chocolate? If the media article doesn't confirm that other studies have also supported these findings, this one study may be the *only* study of its kind. Wait until you hear that these research findings have been confirmed by a reputable health organization, such as the American Heart Association, before considering making any changes in your diet. Reputable organizations will only change their advice based on a consensus of research findings.

Know How to Evaluate Nutrition Information on the Internet

Many people turn to various websites when they have a question about health or nutrition. In fact, approximately 60 percent of American adult Internet users have surfed millions of websites looking for health and medical information.[48] Remember that anyone with computer skills can put up a slick website, and many promote misleading or false information.

To help evaluate the validity of websites, the National Institutes of Health (NIH) has developed nine questions to consider:[49]

1. **Who Runs and Pays for the Site?** Credible websites are willing to show their credentials. For example, the National Center for Complementary and Integrative Health (www.nccih.nih.gov) provides information about its association

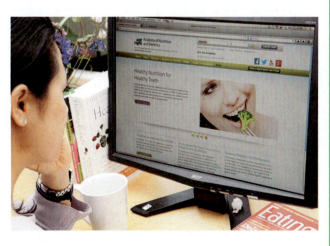

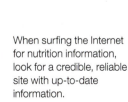
When surfing the Internet for nutrition information, look for a credible, reliable site with up-to-date information.

with the NIH and its extensive ongoing research and educational programs.

Also, running a website is expensive, and finding out who's paying for a particular site will tell you something about the reliability of its content. Websites sponsored by the government (with URLs ending in .gov), a nonprofit organization (ending in .org), or an academic institution (ending in .edu) are more reliable than many commercial websites (ending in .com or .net). Some commercial websites, such as WebMD, carry articles that can be reliable if credible health professionals write them, but other websites may be promoting information to suit a company's own purposes. For example, if the funding source for the website is a vitamin and mineral supplement company, are all the articles geared toward supporting the use of supplements? Does the website have advertisers and do their products influence the content of the website?

2. **What Is the Purpose of the Site?** Look for the "About This Site" link. This will help you understand the website's purpose. For example, at www.nutrition.gov, the purpose is to "provide easy access to the best food and nutrition information across the federal government." This website doesn't exist to sell anything, but to help you find reliable information.

3. **Where Does the Information Come From?** You should always know who wrote what you are reading. Is the author a qualified nutrition expert or did she or he interview

qualified individuals? If the site obtained information from another source, was that source cited?

4. **What Is the Basis of the Information?** Is the article's information based on medical facts and figures that have references? For example, any medical news items released on the American Heart Association website (www.heart.org) will include the medical journal from which the information came. In fact, the website will often include the opinion of experts regarding the news item.

5. **How Is the Information Reviewed?** Check to see if the website has an editorial board of medical and health experts and if qualified individuals review or write the content before it is released.

6. **How Current Is the Information?** Once a website is on the Internet, it will stay there until someone removes it. Consequently, the health information that you read may not be the most up to date. Check the date; if it is over a year old, check to see if it has been updated.

7. **What Is the Site's Policy on Linking to Other Sites?** Some medical sites don't like to link to other sites, as they don't have control over other sites' credibility and content. Others do link, if they are confident that these sites meet their criteria. Don't assume that the link is credible.

8. **How Does the Site Handle Personal Information?** Websites track the pages consumers visit to analyze popular topics. Sometimes they elicit personal information such as gender,

age, and health concerns, which can then be sold to interested companies. Credible sites should state their privacy policy and if they will or will not give or sell this information to other sources.

9. **How Does the Site Manage Interactions with Visitors?** Contact information of the website's owners should be listed in case readers have any concerns or questions that they want answered. If the site is associated with social media sites such as Twitter or Facebook, you should know how it is moderated. Read the postings before you jump in.

When obtaining information from the Internet, carefully peruse the site to make sure that it is credible and contains up-to-date information and that its content isn't influenced by those who fund and support the website.

LO 1.9: THE TAKE-HOME MESSAGE

Credible nutrition information is obtained from trained nutritional professionals including registered dietitian nutritionists or other valid experts. These professionals have the education and experience to provide reliable nutrition information to achieve an overall healthy diet. Use a critical eye when considering health and nutrition headlines in the media, and be careful when obtaining nutrition information from the Internet. Peruse the website to make sure it is credible, contains up-to-date information, and its content is not influenced by those that fund and support the website.

Visual Chapter Summary

LO 1.1 Many Factors Drive Your Food Choices

Food choices are influenced by personal taste, culture and environment, social life and trends, nutrition knowledge, advertising, time, convenience, and cost. People often eat out of habit, in response to emotions, and, of course, because food is delicious.

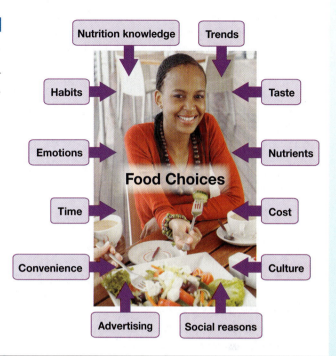

Nutrition knowledge · Trends · Habits · Taste · Emotions · Nutrients · Food Choices · Time · Cost · Convenience · Culture · Advertising · Social reasons

LO 1.2 Nutrition Is the Science of Food

Nutrition is the science that studies how the nutrients in food nourish the body, manufacture and replace cells, and produce energy. There are six categories of nutrients: carbohydrates, lipids, proteins, vitamins, minerals, and water. Carbohydrates, lipids, proteins, and vitamins contain carbon and are classified as organic. Minerals and water are inorganic because they do not contain carbon. Carbohydrates and proteins each contain 4 kilocalories per gram, while fats contain 9 kilocalories per gram. Alcohol, though not a nutrient, also contains energy at 7 kilocalories per gram.

		Carbon	Hydrogen	Oxygen	Nitrogen	Single elements
Organic	Carbohydrates	X	X	X		
	Lipids	X	X	X		
	Proteins	X	X	X	X	
	Vitamins	X	X	X	Some vitamins contain nitrogen	
Inorganic	Minerals					X
	Water		X	X		

LO 1.3 Six Nutrient Groups Have Primary Roles in the Body

Carbohydrates, fats (lipids), and proteins provide energy in the form of kilocalories. Carbohydrates are the body's preferred source of energy. Fats insulate the body and cushion internal organs. The primary role of dietary protein is to build and maintain body tissues. Proteins also act as enzymes that catalyze chemical reactions. Vitamins and minerals do not provide energy but are necessary to properly metabolize carbohydrates, fats, and protein. Many vitamins aid enzymes in the body. Water bathes the inside and outside of the cells, helps maintain body temperature, acts as a lubricant and protective cushion, and delivers nutrients and oxygen to the cells.

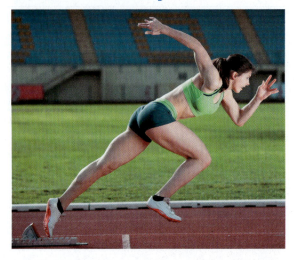

LO 1.4 Eating a Balanced Diet Is the Best Approach to Meeting Your Nutritional Needs

A balanced diet that helps prevent chronic diseases includes whole foods and functional foods providing phytochemicals, zoochemicals, and fiber. In some situations, consumption of whole foods and enriched and fortified foods can be combined with dietary supplements for good health.

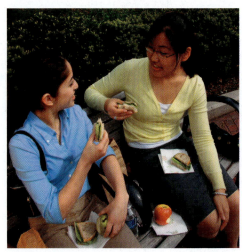

LO 1.5 A Healthy Diet Can Reduce the Risk of Chronic Disease, Prevent Deficiency Disease, and Enhance Gene Expression

A healthy diet plays an important role in reducing the risk for many of the leading causes of death in the United States, including heart disease, cancer, stroke, and type 2 diabetes. It also prevents nutrient-deficiency diseases such as scurvy and iron-deficiency anemia. Interactions between nutrition and disease are explored in the science of nutritional genomics, which studies the relationship between genes, gene expression, and nutrition.

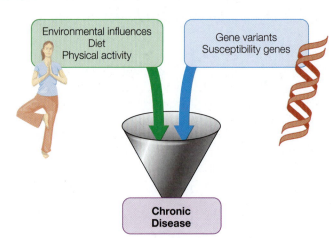

Environmental influences
Diet
Physical activity

Gene variants
Susceptibility genes

Chronic Disease

LO **1.6** We Assess Nutritional Status Using the ABCD Method

The ABCD methods for assessing an individual's nutritional status include—after taking the health history—collecting anthropometric and biochemical laboratory data, clinical observation, and conducting dietary intake surveys. The nutritional status of population groups is determined by national surveys and studies, including the National Health and Nutrition Examination Survey and the Framingham Heart Study.

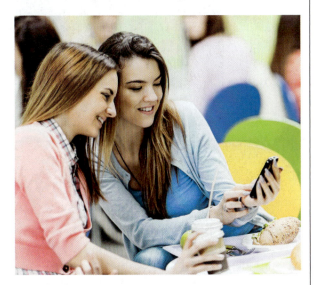

LO **1.7** The Average American Diet Needs Improvement

Most Americans are not meeting all their nutrient needs without exceeding their kilocalorie requirements. The average American diet is high in added sugars, sodium, and saturated fat, but low in vitamin D, calcium, potassium, and fiber. In addition, the rates of overweight and obesity among Americans are too high.

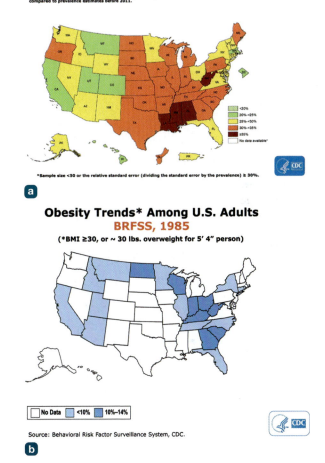

Prevalence¹ of Self-Reported Obesity Among U.S. Adults by State and Territory, BRFSS, 2015

¹ Prevalence estimates reflect BRFSS methodological changes started in 2011. These estimates should not be compared to prevalence estimates before 2011.

<20%
20%–<25%
25%–<30%
30%–<35%
≥35%
No data available*

*Sample size <50 or the relative standard error (dividing the standard error by the prevalence) ≥ 30%.

a

Obesity Trends* Among U.S. Adults
BRFSS, 1985
(*BMI ≥30, or ~ 30 lbs. overweight for 5' 4" person)

No Data   <10%   10%–14%

Source: Behavioral Risk Factor Surveillance System, CDC.

b

LO **1.8** The Scientific Method of Research Provides Credible Nutrition Information

Sound nutrition information is the result of numerous scientific studies conducted according to the scientific method, which includes observing, formulating a hypothesis, and conducting one or more experiments. Studies are reviewed by the medical and scientific community. Nutrition research is conducted through laboratory experiments, experimental research, and observational and epidemiological studies. Findings are presented in peer-reviewed journals.

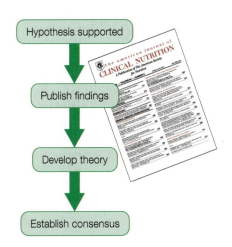

Hypothesis supported

Publish findings

Develop theory

Establish consensus

LO 1.9 Reliable Nutrition Information Comes from Authoritative Sources

Nutrition advice should come from credible sources including registered dietitian nutritionists who have the education and training to provide reliable and accurate information. Individuals who call themselves nutritionists may or may not have a credible nutrition education. Use critical thinking to evaluate media headlines and product claims relating to health and nutrition. When looking for nutrition and health information on the Internet, seek out the sites of credible organizations that provide up-to-date information from reliable sources.

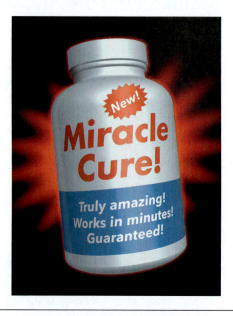

Terms to Know

- nutrition
- nutrients
- essential nutrients
- nonessential nutrients
- organic
- inorganic
- energy
- energy-yielding nutrients
- kilocalorie
- macronutrients
- micronutrients
- enzymes
- coenzymes
- solubility
- water-soluble vitamins
- fat-soluble vitamins

- major minerals
- trace minerals
- functional foods
- phytochemicals
- zoochemicals
- chronic disease
- gene expression
- epigenetics
- nutritional genomics
- registered dietitian nutritionist (RDN)
- malnourished
- undernourished
- overnourished
- acute
- malabsorption
- body mass index (BMI)
- added sugars

- consensus
- scientific method
- hypothesis
- peer-reviewed journal
- laboratory experiment
- observational research
- epidemiological research
- experimental research
- experimental group
- control group
- placebo
- double-blind placebo-controlled study
- medical nutrition therapy
- public health nutritionists
- licensed dietitian nutritionist (LDN)
- nutritionist
- quackery

Check Your Understanding

LO1.1 1. Megan picks up a sandwich at the campus food truck after class every day before dashing off to her part-time job. Which of the following most likely drives Megan's food choice?
   a. her ethnic background
   b. her busy schedule
   c. her emotions
   d. her limited budget

LO1.2 2. Nutrition is
   a. the study of genes, how they function in the body, and the environment.
   b. the study of how the body functions.
   c. the study of nutrients and other components of foods and their effect on body functions and health.
   d. the study of hormones and how they function in the body.

LO1.2 3. Minerals are considered an organic nutrient because they contain the element carbon.
   a. True
   b. False

LO1.2 4. A slice of whole-wheat bread contains 1 gram of fat, 18 grams of carbohydrate, and 4 grams of protein. How many kilocalories does it contain?
   a. 65 kilocalories
   b. 72 kilocalories
   c. 89 kilocalories
   d. 97 kilocalories

LO1.3 5. Which of the following roles do nutrients perform in the body?
   a. Nutrients provide energy.
   b. Nutrients provide structure for bone, muscle, and other tissues.
   c. Nutrients facilitate metabolism.
   d. Nutrients perform all of the above functions.

LO1.4 6. Dietary supplements are necessary to meet your nutrient needs.
   a. True
   b. False

LO1.5 7. Which of the following statements about diet and health is true?
   a. The top five causes of death in the United States are all related to nutrition.
   b. Nutritional genomics is the study of how the foods we eat alter the structure of our DNA.
   c. Components of the foods we eat can alter the expression of our genes as proteins.
   d. Cancer is an example of a nutrient-deficiency disease.

LO1.6 8. Which of the ABCD assessments yields data about body weight and body composition?
   a. Anthropometric
   b. Biochemical
   c. Clinical
   d. Dietary intake

LO1.7 9. The current state of the American diet is reflected in the fact that more than _____ percent of American adults are obese.
   a. 35
   b. 45
   c. 55
   d. 65

LO1.8 10. The first step in the scientific method is to
   a. make observations and ask questions.
   b. form a hypothesis.
   c. conduct an experiment.
   d. develop a theory.

Answers

1. (b) While food choices are influenced by many factors, including ethnic background, emotions, and costs, in Megan's case her limited time for food preparation and/or shopping most strongly influences her choice of this fast-food sandwich.

2. (c) Nutrition is the science related to how nutrients and other components in foods are used in the body and how they affect health. The study of genes is called genetics. Physiology is the study of how the body functions. The study of hormones is called endocrinology.

3. (b) Minerals are actually inorganic nutrients because they do not contain carbon. Nutrients that do contain carbon, including protein, carbohydrates, lipids, and vitamins, are classified as organic.

4. (d) A slice of bread contains 97 kilocalories: $(18\text{ g} \times 4\text{ kcal}) + (4\text{ g} \times 4\text{ kcal}) + (1\text{ g} \times 9\text{ kcal})$.

5. (d) Nutrients help perform numerous vital body functions. Carbohydrates, protein, and fats provide energy in the form of kilocalories; protein and some minerals help build body tissues; and several vitamins and minerals are essential during metabolic processes.

6. (b) False. Dietary supplements can be beneficial for individuals with diet restrictions or higher nutrient needs, but they are not essential. Consuming a diet rich in a variety of whole foods is the best way to achieve a healthy, balanced diet.

7. (c) Components of the foods we eat can alter the expression of our genes as proteins. Nutritional genomics studies these and other links between genetics and diet. The foods we eat do not, however, alter the structure of our DNA. Three of the top five causes of death in the United States—not all five—are related to nutrition. Cancer is a multifactorial disease in which nutrition may play a role, but cancer is not caused by a nutrient deficiency.

8. (a) Anthropometric measurements yield data about body weight and body composition. Biochemical measurements are tests of blood, urine, and feces, and clinical tools are observations of your hair, skin, muscles, and overall appearance to assess for signs of deficiencies or excess nutrients. Dietary intake records diet history or uses a survey, food frequency questionnaire, or diet record to assess nutrient intake.

9. (a) Over 35 percent of American adults are considered obese.
10. (a) The scientific method begins with scientists observing and asking questions. They then formulate a hypothesis and test it using an experiment to confirm their hypothesis. After many experiments that confirm their hypothesis, a theory is developed.

Answers to True or False?

1. **True.** Taste is the strongest motivating factor for choosing foods. However, numerous other factors—including culture, social setting, health, advertising, habit, emotion, time, cost, and convenience—also play a role in food choice.
2. **False.** Nutrition is the science related to how nutrients are used in the body and how they affect health.
3. **True.** Carbohydrates are the primary source of energy to the body.
4. **False.** Whereas alcohol does provide kilocalories, eliminating it from the diet would not result in malnutrition. Therefore, alcohol is not a nutrient.
5. **False.** There is no replacement for whole foods in a healthy diet. A supplement can augment a healthy diet, but it can't replace it to meet your nutritional needs.
6. **False.** The 24-hour diet record is one tool for gathering information about the quality of a client's diet, but it doesn't reveal a complete picture. Long-term food records, interviews, and anthropometric data are also needed.
7. **False.** In 2015, more than 35 percent of American adults were considered obese.
8. **False.** Eliminating all fat from the diet is incompatible with life. In the short term, it would result in nutrient deficiencies and do little to reduce your risk of heart disease. Chronic disease such as heart disease is often the result of a cluster of risk factors including an overall poor-quality diet, lack of exercise, and tobacco use, as well as heredity.

9. **False.** Heart disease is the leading cause of death among Americans. The good news is that your diet can play an important role in reducing your risk.
10. **False.** There is no standard for or legal definition of the word *nutritionist*, so it does not convey expert status. In fact, anyone can call him- or herself a nutritionist.

Web Resources

Examples of reliable nutrition and health websites include:

- Academy of Nutrition and Dietetics: www.eatright.org
- Agricultural Research Service: www.ars.usda.gov
- American Cancer Society: www.cancer.org
- American College of Sports Medicine: www.acsm.org
- American Medical Association: www.ama-assn.org
- Center for Science in the Public Interest: www.cspinet.org
- Centers for Disease Control and Prevention: www.cdc.gov
- Food and Drug Administration: www.fda.gov
- Food and Nutrition Information Center: www.nal.usda.gov/fnic
- National Institutes of Health: www.nih.gov
- NHANES Surveys: www.cdc.gov/nchs/nhanes.htm
- Nutrition.gov: www.nutrition.gov
- Shape Up America!: www.shapeup.org
- Vegetarian Resource Group: www.vrg.org

References

1. Van Meer, F., Charbonnier, L., and Smeets, P. 2016. Food Decision-Making: Effects of Weight Status and Age. *Current Diabetes Reports* 16:2–8.
2. Freeland-Graves, J., and S. Nitzke. 2013. Position Paper of the Academy of Nutrition and Dietetics: Total Diet Approach to Healthy Eating. *Journal of the Academy of Nutrition and Dietetics* 113:307–317.
3. Food Information Council Foundation. 2016. Food Decisions 2016. Available at http://www.foodinsight.org/articles/2016-food-and-health-survey-food-decision-2016-impact-growing-national-food-dialogue. Accessed January 2017.
4. Freeland-Graves, J. 2013.
5. Freeland-Graves, J. 2013.
6. Shen, Y., O. Kennedy, and L. Methven. 2017. The Effect of Genotypical and Phenotypical Variation In Taste Sensitivity on Liking of Ice Cream and Dietary Fat Intake. *Food Quality and Preference* 55:79–90.
7. Ambrosini, G., D. Johns, K. Northstone, P. Emmetee, and S. Jebb. 2016. Free Sugars and Total Fat Are Important Characteristics of a Dietary Pattern Associated with Adiposity Across Childhood and Adolescence. *Journal of Nutrition* 146:778–784.
8. Drewnowski, A. 1997. Taste Preferences and Food Intake. *Annual Review of Nutrition* 17:237–253.
9. Ambrosini, G., 2016.
10. Van Meer, F., 2016.
11. Wansink, B., C. R. Payne, and M. Shimizu. 2010. "Is This a Meal or Snack?": Situational Cues that Drive Perceptions. *Appetite* 54:214–216.
12. National Turkey Foundation. 2016. *Turkey Facts and Trivia*. Available at www.eatturkey.com. Accessed January 2017.
13. Freeland-Graves, J. 2013.
14. National Restaurant Association. 2011. *Pizza Is King of Super Bowl Takeout*. Available at www.restaurant.org. Accessed January 2017.
15. Udland, M. 2015. Here's How Movie Theaters are Still Making Money Even Though Ticket Sales are Down. *Business Insider*. Available at www.businessinsider.com/movie-concessions-drive-amc-earnings-2015-2. Accessed January 2017.
16. Organic Trade Association. 2015. Quick Stats. Available at www.ota.com. Accessed January 2017.
17. Food Information Council Foundation. 2016. Food Decisions 2016.
18. Ibid.
19. Ibid.
20. Statista. 2016. Statistics and Facts About Food Advertising. Available at https://www.statista.com/topics/2223/food-advertising/. Accessed January 2017.
21. Vilaro, M., T. Barnett, A. Watson, J. Merten, and A. Mathews. 2017. Weekday and Weekend Food Advertising Varies on Children's Television in the USA but Persuasive Techniques and Unhealthy Items Still Dominate. *Public Health* 142:22–30.
22. Blake, JS. 2016. Celebrity Watching in the Produce Aisle. Available at http://salge-blake.blogspot.com/2016/07/celebrity-watching-in-produce-aisle.html. Accessed January 2017.
23. International Food Information Council (IFIC) Foundation's *2015 Food and Health Survey*: the Millennials. 2015. Available at www.foodinsight.org/2015-food-health-survey-millennial-research. Accessed January 2017.
24. Specialty Coffee Association. 2015. *US Coffee Shops*. Available at www.scaa.org. Accessed January 2017.
25. U.S. Department of Agriculture. 2016. *Food Expenditures*. Available at www.ers.usda.gov. Accessed January 2017.

26. Burgoine, T., N. Forouhi, S. Griffin, S. Brage, N. Wareham, and P. Monsivatis. 2016. Does Neighborhood Fast-Food Outlet Exposure Amplify Inequalities in Diet and Obesity?: A Cross-Sectional Study. *American Journal of Clinical Nutrition* 103:1540–1547.

27. Mintel International Group. 2016. *Cooking Enthusiasts.* Available at www.mintel.com/. Accessed January 2017.

28. Sy, S., J. Penalvo, S. Abrahams-Gessel, S., Alam, A. Pandya, D. Mozaffarian, and T. Gaziano. 2016. Changes in Food Prices Improve Cardiovascular Disease (CVD) Outcomes. *Circulation* 133:AP280.

29. Mintel International Group. 2016. *What's for Breakfast?* Available at www.mintel.com. Accessed January 2017.

30. Maddison, R., L. Foley, C. N. Mhurchu, Y. Jiang, A. Jull, H. Prapavessis, M. Hohepa, and A. Rodgers. 2011. Effects of Active Video Games on Body Composition: A Randomized Controlled Trial. *American Journal of Clinical Nutrition* 94:156–163.

31. Crowe, K, and C. Francis. 2013. Position of the Academy of Nutrition and Dietetics: Functional Foods. *Journal of the Academy of Nutrition and Dietetics* 113:1096–1103.

32. Bolarin, D., E. Ekpe, K. Saidu, and E. Eyam. 2016. Overview of Foods with Antioxidant Effects-Clinical Relevance. *European Journal of Food Science and Technology* 4:1–9.

33. Crowe, K. 2013.

34. Forster, H, M. Walsh, M. Givney, L. Brennan, and E. Gibney. 2016. Personalised Nutrition: The Role of New Dietary Assessment Methods. *Proceedings of the Nutrition Society* 75:96–105.

35. Eaton, D. K., E. O. Olsen, N. D. Brener, K. S. Scanlon, S. A. Kim, Z. Demissie, and A. L. Yaroch. 2013. A Comparison of Fruit and Vegetable Intake Estimates from Three Survey Question Sets to Estimates from 24-Hour Dietary Recall Interviews. *Journal of the Academy of Nutrition and Dietetics* 113(9):1165–1174.

36. Illner, A-K., H. Freisling, H. Boeing, I. Huybrechts, S. P. Crispim, and N. Slimani. 2012. Review and Evaluation of Innovative Technologies for Measuring Diet in Nutritional Epidemiology. *International Journal of Epidemiology* 41(4):1187–1203.

37. U.S. Department of Agriculture, Agricultural Research Service. 2016. *What We Eat in America, NHANES 2013-2014.* Available at https://www.ars.usda.gov/northeast-area/beltsville-md/beltsville-human-nutrition -research-center/food-surveys-research -group/docs/wweianhanes-overview/. Accessed January 2017.

38. U.S. Department of Health and Human Services and U.S. Department of Agriculture. 2015. 2015–2020 *Dietary Guidelines for Americans.* 8th Edition. Available at http://health.gov/dietaryguidelines/2015/guidelines/.

39. U.S. Department of Agriculture, Agricultural Research Service. 2016.

40. U.S. Department of Agriculture, Agricultural Research Service. 2016. *What We Eat in America, NHANES 2013–2014.* Available at https://www.ars.usda.gov/northeast-area /beltsville-md/beltsville-human-nutrition -research-center/food-surveys-research -group/docs/wweianhanes-overview/. Accessed January 2017.

41. Ibid.

42. Kantor, E., C. Rehm, M. Du., E. White, and E. Giovannucci. 2016. Trends in Dietary Supplement Use Among US Adults from 1999–2012. *Journal of the American Medical Association* 316:1464–1471.

43. U.S. Department of Agriculture. 2016.

44. Golden, N., M. Schneider, and C. Wood. 2016. Preventing Obesity and Eating Disorders in Adolescents. *Pediatrics* 138(3):e20161649.

45. Buckner, S., P. Loprinzi, and J. Loenneke. 2016. Why Don't More People Eat Breakfast?: A Biological Perspective. *American Journal of Clinical Nutrition* 103:1555–1559.

46. Centers for Disease Control. 2016. *Adult Obesity Facts.* Available at www.cdc.gov. Accessed January 2017.

47. U.S. Department of Health and Preventative Services. Updated 2017. *Healthy People 2020.* Available at www.healthypeople.gov. Accessed January 2017.

48. Fox, S., and M. Duggan. 2013. *Health Online 2013. Pew Research Center's Internet and American Life Project.* Available at www.pewinternet .org. Accessed January 2017.

49. National Center for Complementary and Integrative Health Medicine. Updated 2014. Online Health Information: Can You Trust It? Available at https://nccih.nih.gov/health/webresources. Accessed January 2017.

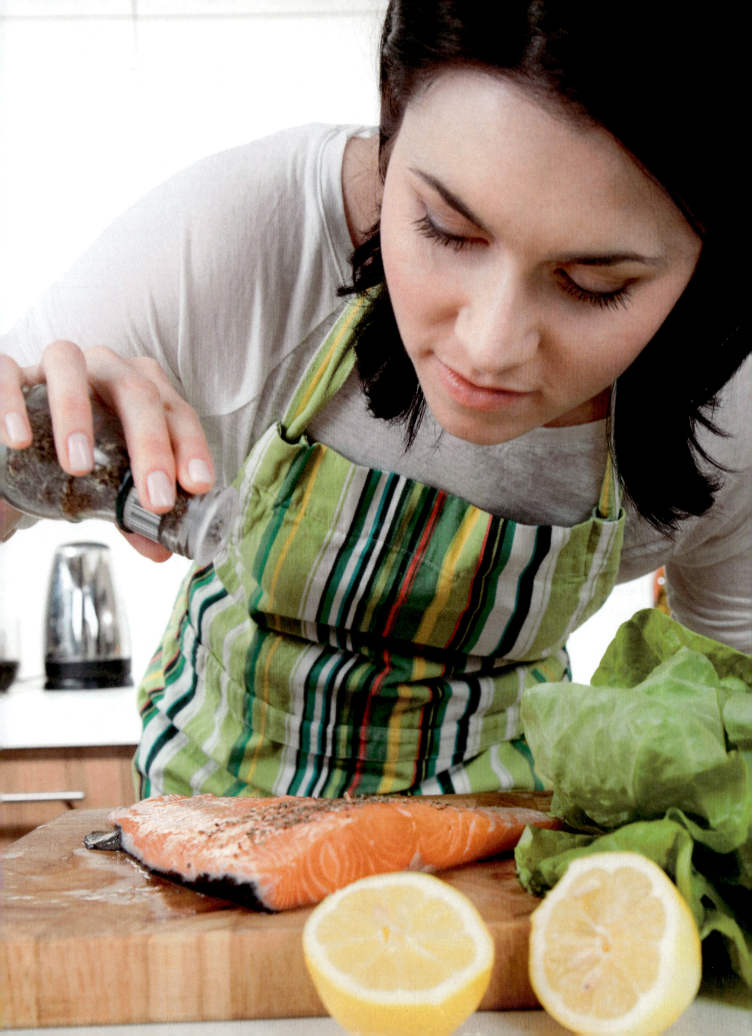

Tools for Healthy Eating

Learning Outcomes

After reading this chapter, you will be able to:

2.1 Describe the key principles of healthy eating.

2.2 Distinguish between the Dietary Reference Intake terms *EAR, AI, RDA, UL,* and *AMDR.*

2.3 Describe the recommendations included in the *Dietary Guidelines for Americans.*

2.4 Discuss the concept of MyPlate, including the food groups and typical foods represented.

2.5 Explain how the exchange system can be used as a guide to plan a balanced diet.

2.6 Identify the required components of a food label and Nutrition Facts panel.

2.7 Compare the terms *portion* and *serving size* and summarize the health benefits of controlling your portions.

True or False?

1. Having a balanced diet means eating the same number of servings from each food group. **T**/**F**

2. There isn't any risk in overconsuming the essential nutrients in your diet. **T**/**F**

3. The current Dietary Reference Intakes for vitamins and minerals are set at the amount you should consume daily to maintain good health. **T**/**F**

4. If you follow the advice in the *Dietary Guidelines for Americans,* you can reduce your risk of dying from chronic diseases such as heart disease and diabetes mellitus. **T**/**F**

5. According to the USDA MyPlate food guide, there are five basic food groups. **T**/**F**

6. Healthy oils are a food group in MyPlate. **T**/**F**

7. Exchange lists are similar to MyPlate except the foods are based on the carbohydrate, protein, fat, and kilocalorie contents. **T**/**F**

8. A nutrient content claim on a food label tells you why that nutrient is good for you. **T**/**F**

9. All packaged foods must contain a food label. **T**/**F**

10. A portion of food is defined as a standard serving size. **T**/**F**

See page 71 for the answers.

Many Americans believe that to eat a healthful diet means giving up their favorite foods. Nothing could be farther from the truth! With a little planning, you can still occasionally eat almost any food even if it contains added sugars and fat and is high in kilocalories. All it takes are the right tools to balance those higher kilocalorie foods with more nutritious choices each day.

The good news is that a number of tools are available to help you achieve a healthful, balanced eating plan. This chapter explains how to use these tools in a consistent manner that over time will lead to better eating habits. Let's begin with a discussion of what healthy eating is.

What Are the Key Principles of Healthy Eating?

LO 2.1 Describe the key principles of healthy eating.

Healthy eating means you need to **balance**, **vary**, and **moderate** your nutrient intake. In addition, a healthy diet includes foods that are high in **nutrient density** and low in **energy density**.

Healthy Eating Means Balance between Food Groups

A balanced diet includes healthy proportions of all nutrients and is adequate in energy. A diet that lacks balance can cause undernutrition. For instance, a student subsisting largely on bread, bagels, muffins, crackers, chips, and cookies might be eating too much carbohydrate and fat but too little protein, vitamins, and minerals. If the diet lacks a particular nutrient, such as protein, over time the body suffers from malnutrition. A meal that contains foods from the grain, vegetable, fruit, meat, and dairy groups, such as a lunch of a turkey-and-cheese wrap with lettuce and tomato plus an apple, provides the proper proportion of foods from each of the food groups. This balancing act prevents overnutrition of a specific nutrient, such as fat,[1] or too many kilocalories, which can lead to overweight and obesity. Consuming adequate amounts of all essential nutrients is key to avoiding nutrient deficiencies and, in many cases, chronic disease.

balance Diet principle of providing the correct proportion of nutrients to maintain health and prevent disease.

vary Diet principle of consuming a mixture of different food groups and foods within each group.

moderate Diet principle of providing reasonable but not excessive amounts of foods and nutrients.

nutrient density Measurement of the nutrients in a food compared with the kilocalorie content; nutrient-dense foods are high in nutrients and low in kilocalories.

energy density Measurement of the kilocalories in a food compared with the weight (grams) of the food.

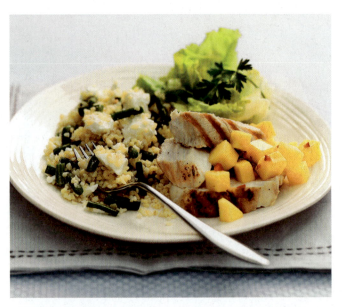

A meal that contains foods from every food group is part of a balanced, healthy diet.

Healthy Eating Means Consuming a Variety of Foods

Choosing a variety of foods improves the quality of the diet because the more varied the food choices, the better the chance of consuming adequate amounts of all the essential nutrients.[2] Even within one food group, the nutrient composition of foods can vary dramatically. For example, while broccoli is a good source of folate, it has less than half the vitamin A of a carrot. Similarly, if the only fruit you eat is bananas, your diet would include an excellent source of potassium, but could be low in vitamin C. Because no single food or food group contains everything you need to be healthy, you should choose a variety of foods from within each food group and among food groups each day. This is the basic principle of the *Fruits & Veggies—More Matters* campaign developed by the Produce for Better Health Foundation and the Centers for Disease Control and Prevention.[3] This campaign promotes eating a variety of colorful fruits and vegetables—which are rich in vitamins, minerals, fiber, and phytochemicals—each day to help reduce the risk of cancer and heart disease and slow the effects of aging.

Healthy Eating Means Moderate Intake of All Foods

According to many registered dietitian nutritionists (RDNs), "there are no good or bad foods, just good or bad habits." What they mean is that all foods—even less nutritious foods—can be part of a healthy diet, as long as they are consumed in moderation. Foods such as sweets and fried or packaged snack foods should be eaten only in small amounts to avoid consuming too much sugar and saturated fat, as well as too many kilocalories. Finally, these foods can displace more nutritious choices, resulting in a diet that lacks essential nutrients. Even some healthy foods, such as nutrient-dense nuts, can be high in kilocalories and should be consumed in moderation. Healthy eating doesn't mean you can't enjoy your favorite foods. It simply means eating those foods in moderation by limiting the **portion** size and number of servings you eat.

Many people overestimate the appropriate portion sizes of foods. An entire body of research is devoted to studying factors that affect how much we put on our plates. The important point is that, in general, we tend to consume portions larger than necessary to meet our kilocalorie needs. See the Health Connection on pages 65–67 for examples of visuals you can use to estimate portion sizes. For suggestions on eating a balanced, varied, and moderate diet, see the Table Tips.

Healthy Eating Includes Nutrient-Dense Foods

Healthy eating also means choosing foods that are nutrient dense. Nutrient-dense foods are high in nutrients, such as vitamins and minerals, but low in energy (kilocalories), providing more nutrients per kilocalorie (and in each bite) than less nutrient-dense foods.[4] Fresh fruits and vegetables, for example, are nutrient dense because they are high in B vitamins, vitamin C, and minerals such as calcium and magnesium, as well as dietary fiber, while usually providing fewer than 60 kilocalories per serving.

Nutrient-dense foods are also low in saturated fat and added sugars. To illustrate this concept, compare the nutrient density of two versions of the same food: a baked potato and potato chips (**Figure 2.1**). Although a medium baked potato and one ounce of potato chips have about the same number of kilocalories, the baked potato provides much higher amounts of vitamins and minerals than the deep-fried chips.

Though many foods, such as vegetables, are clearly nutrient dense, and other foods, such as candy, are clearly not, some foods do not fit neatly into these two categories. Items such as dried fruits, nuts, peanut butter, and avocados are higher in kilocalories, but they are also excellent sources of important nutrients, including polyunsaturated fatty acids, calcium, and iron. Other foods, such as whole milk or yogurt, are higher

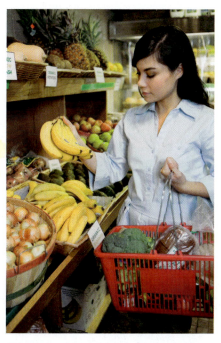

Choosing a variety of nutrient-dense foods you enjoy is a key to eating a healthy diet.

portion Quantity of a food usually eaten at one sitting.

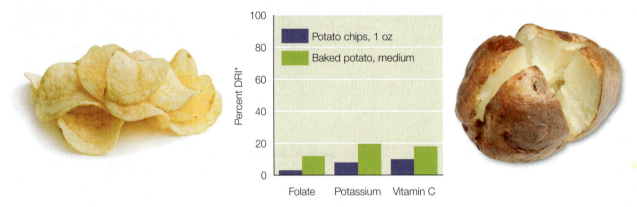

▲ Figure 2.1 Which Is the Healthier Way to Enjoy Potatoes?
Whereas one ounce of potato chips and one medium baked potato have similar kilocalories, their nutrient content is worlds apart. A baked potato contains more folate, potassium, and vitamin C, and fewer fat kilocalories, than its fried counterpart. The baked potato is therefore more nutrient dense than potato chips.
* Note: Based on the percentage of the DRI for 19- to -50-year-old males. All these percentages apply to females in the same age range, except for vitamin C. Females have lower vitamin C needs than males, so a baked potato provides over 20 percent of the DRI of this vitamin for women.

in saturated fat and kilocalories than their nonfat or low-fat counterparts, but still provide significant amounts of calcium, riboflavin, vitamins A and D, and protein. Some foods, such as fruit-flavored yogurt and some fortified cereals, contain added sugars in addition to several essential nutrients. Do you think these foods can be considered nutrient dense?

In all of these scenarios, the answer is yes. Whereas nutrient dense usually means high in nutrients and low in energy, foods that are high in nutrients and high in energy can also be considered nutrient dense. The key is to be aware of the extra kilocalories and make up for them elsewhere in the diet. If you don't like skim milk and won't drink it, but do enjoy the taste of whole milk, then drinking whole milk is a more healthy choice than drinking soda.

Healthy Eating Includes Low-Energy-Dense Foods

In contrast to nutrient density, energy density refers to foods that are high in energy but low in weight or volume, such as that potato chip. A serving of deep-fried chips weighs much less than a plain baked potato, but is considerably higher in kilocalories. Therefore, the chip contains more energy per gram. A big, leafy green salad, on the other hand, is large in volume but low in energy density, because of its high water content.

Most high-fat foods are considered energy dense.[5] This is because fat has 9 kilocalories per gram and is thus 2.25 times more energy dense than either carbohydrates or protein at 4 kilocalories per gram. Individuals who choose low-energy-dense foods will generally have diets that are lower in fat and higher in nutrient content.

Eating a low-energy-dense diet can sometimes be the key to weight loss. Recent studies have found that leaner individuals ate more low-energy-dense foods and fewer kilocalories, while consuming a greater volume of food, compared with their obese counterparts.[6] Even modest changes in dietary intake may promote and help maintain weight loss[7] over time.[8] One reason for this may be that eating higher-volume, lower-energy foods means larger portions for the same number of kilocalories. Other reasons may include improved **satiety** and appetite control.[9] In other words, low-energy foods will "fill you up before they fill you out."

If you are trying to maintain your current weight, or lose weight, you are probably on a limited energy budget and need to choose foods that are nutrient dense and low in kilocalories. Use the guide in **Table 2.1** to help stretch your energy budget while consuming the most nutrient-dense foods.

satiety Feeling of satiation, or "fullness," after a meal before hunger sets in again.

TABLE 2.1 — Bargain Shopping on an Energy Budget

Foods	Energy Density	Are They an Energy Bargain?
Soups Fruits Vegetables	0.0–0.6 kcal/g	**Great Energy Bargain:** Eat as much of these low-energy-density foods as you want; however, take care that soups don't contain too much sodium and are made with broth rather than cream.
Starchy fruits and vegetables Lean meats Beans and legumes	0.6–1.5 kcal/g	**Good Energy Bargain:** Consume healthy portions of these foods.
Cheese Salad dressings Snack foods	1.5–4.0 kcal/g	**More Expensive Choices:** These foods should be chosen carefully and consumed in moderation.
Chocolates Chips Candy Deep-fat fried foods Desserts	4.0–9.0 kcal/g	**Very Expensive Choices:** Eat less of these foods and be aware of the portion size to avoid overconsuming kilocalories.

Source: Adapted from B. Rolls. 2012. *The Ultimate Volumetrics Diet: Smart, Simple, Science-Based Strategies for Losing Weight and Keeping It Off.* New York: HarperCollins.

Many Resources Are Available for Planning a Healthy Diet

Do you think all this advice for planning a healthy diet is hard to keep straight? If so, you're not alone. Fortunately, several tools can help you avoid both under- and overnutrition, including:

- The Dietary Reference Intakes (DRIs), which provide recommendations regarding your nutrient needs
- The *Dietary Guidelines for Americans,* which provide broad dietary and lifestyle advice
- MyPlate, part of the ChooseMyPlate.gov Web-based initiative, which is designed to help you eat healthfully and implement the recommendations in the DRIs and the advice in the *Dietary Guidelines*
- The exchange system, which groups foods according to their macronutrient content, thus making it easier to plan meals
- The Nutrition Facts panel on food labels, which contains the percent Daily Values, and which can help you decide which foods to buy

Together, these tools help you plan a balanced, moderate, and varied diet that meets your nutrient and health needs. **Table 2.2** compares these tools, and the following text sections discuss each in more detail.

TABLE 2.2 — Putting It All Together: Tools for Healthy Eating

	DRIs	Dietary Guidelines for Americans	MyPlate	Nutrition Facts Panel	Exchange Lists for Healthy Eating
What Are They?	Specific reference values for each nutrient by age and gender.	Guidelines for nutrition and health that are informed by the most current scientific evidence, updated every 5 years.	A representational icon that depicts five food groups using the familiar mealtime visual of a place setting.	Contains important nutrition information to be used to compare food products.	Lists that are organized into food groups by their carbohydrate, protein, fat, and kilocalorie contents.
How Do They Guide You in Healthy Eating?	DRIs provide recommendations to prevent malnutrition and chronic diseases for each nutrient. The upper level is designed to prevent overnutrition or toxicity.	The *Dietary Guidelines* emphasize following a healthy, plant-based diet to maintain a healthy weight and reduce the risk for chronic disease.	MyPlate is the focal point for the Web-based ChooseMyPlate.gov initiative, which provides information to build a healthy diet based on the *Dietary Guidelines for Americans*.	You can use the Nutrition Facts panel to compare the nutrient density of foods.	It's easy to plan healthy menus with a variety of foods. The exchanges are based on specific food portion sizes plus various fat levels in foods.

(continued)

TABLE 2.2 Putting It All Together: Tools for Healthy Eating *(continued)*

	DRIs	*Dietary Guidelines for Americans*	MyPlate	Nutrition Facts Panel	Exchange Lists for Healthy Eating
What Are They Made Up Of?	EARs, RDAs, AIs, ULs, and AMDRs	Key messages emphasize healthy eating patterns, as well as limiting intake of added sugars, saturated fats, sodium, cholesterol, and caffeine.	Recommendations are made for physical activity as well as five food groups, plus oils: 1. Vegetables 2. Fruits 3. Grains 4. Protein 5. Dairy 6. Oils	Information is presented about: • Serving size, servings per package, and kilocalories per serving • Macronutrients • Dietary fiber • Vitamins and minerals • % Daily Values	Exchange lists consist of six food groups: 1. Starch 2. Meat 3. Vegetables 4. Fruit 5. Milk 6. Fat

LO 2.1: THE TAKE-HOME MESSAGE Healthy eating emphasizes consuming the right amount of food from a variety of food groups to provide an adequate intake of nutrients and a moderate level of energy. Choosing nutrient-dense and low-energy-dense foods ensures a diet high in nutrient content and low enough in energy to prevent weight gain. A variety of tools are available to help individuals make healthy choices.

What Are the Dietary Reference Intakes?

LO 2.2 Distinguish between the Dietary Reference Intake terms *EAR, AI, RDA, UL,* and *AMDR.*

The **Dietary Reference Intakes (DRIs)** are issued by the Food and Nutrition Board (FNB) of the National Academy of Medicine. They identify the amounts of each nutrient that people in a specific life stage need to consume to maintain good health, prevent chronic diseases, and avoid unhealthy excesses.[10] The recommendations are grouped according to life stage—such as childhood, older age, or pregnancy—because **nutrient requirements** differ according to these stages. A teenager may need more of a specific nutrient than a 55-year-old (and vice versa) and women need more of certain nutrients during pregnancy and lactation. Many of the recommendations also differ by gender. Males and females vary in some of their nutrient requirements because of differences in their anatomy and physiology.[11]

The National Academy of Medicine periodically organizes committees of U.S. and Canadian scientists and health experts to update the DRIs to reflect the latest scientific research. Since the 1940s, the DRIs have been updated 10 times. In the 1990s, nutrition researchers identified expanded roles for many nutrients. Though nutrient deficiencies were still an important issue, research suggested that higher amounts of some nutrients could play a role in disease prevention. Also, as consumers began using more dietary supplements and fortified foods, committee members grew concerned that excessive consumption of some nutrients might be as unhealthy as, or even more dangerous than, not consuming enough. Hence, the FNB convened a variety of committees between 1997 and 2004 to take on the enormous task of reviewing the research on vitamins, minerals, carbohydrates, fats, protein, water, and other substances such as fiber and developing the current DRI reference values. The DRIs are continually updated as research evolves.

Dietary Reference Intakes (DRIs) Reference values for nutrients developed by the Food and Nutrition Board of the National Academy of Medicine, used to plan and evaluate the diets of healthy people in the United States and Canada. It includes the Estimated Average Requirement (EAR), the Recommended Dietary Allowance (RDA), the Adequate Intake (AI), and the Tolerable Upper Intake Level (UL).

nutrient requirements Amounts of specific nutrients needed to prevent malnutrition or deficiency; reflected in the DRIs.

The DRIs Encompass Several Reference Values

The DRIs cover five reference values: the Estimated Average Requirement (EAR), the Recommended Dietary Allowance (RDA), the Adequate Intake (AI), the Tolerable Upper Intake Level (UL), and the Acceptable Macronutrient Distribution Range (AMDR) (**Focus Figure 2.2**). Each of these values is unique, and serves a different need in planning a healthy diet.

Estimated Average Requirements

The DRI committee members begin by reviewing a variety of research studies to determine the **Estimated Average Requirement (EAR)** for a nutrient. They may look at studies that investigate the consequences of eating a diet too low in the nutrient and the associated side effects or physical changes that develop, as well as how much of the nutrient should be consumed to correct the deficiency. They may also review studies that measure the amount a healthy individual absorbs, stores, and maintains daily. Additionally, they look at research studies that address the role the nutrient plays in reducing the risk of associated chronic diseases, such as heart disease. After a thorough review process, the EAR for the nutrient is determined.

The EAR is the average amount of a nutrient projected to meet the needs of 50 percent of healthy Americans by age and gender.[12] The EAR is a good starting point to determine the amount of a nutrient an individual should consume daily for good health. As you can see from Focus Figure 2.2, if a nutrient's requirements were set using the EAR, 50 percent of the individuals would need more and 50 percent would need less than this amount to meet their needs.

An EAR for each nutrient is established based on a measurement that indicates whether an individual is at risk of a deficiency. For example, to determine the EAR for iron for a 19-year-old female, scientists measure hemoglobin concentrations in the blood. The measurement differs from nutrient to nutrient. If there aren't enough studies or collected data to develop an appropriate measurement for a nutrient, an EAR or requirement for that nutrient is not established. Once the EAR has been set for each nutrient, the RDA can be calculated.

Recommended Dietary Allowances

The **Recommended Dietary Allowance (RDA)** is based on the EAR, but it is set higher. It represents the amount for each nutrient that should meet the needs of nearly all (97–98 percent) of the individuals in a specific gender and age group. Let's use iron to illustrate the relationship between the EAR and the RDA. After careful review of the latest research on iron metabolism, the EAR for iron was set at 6 milligrams per day for both men and women over all age groups.[13] The amount is increased to an RDA of 18 milligrams per day to cover the needs of 97 to 98 percent of females ages 19–30. For 19- to 30-year-old males, the RDA for iron is 8 milligrams daily. The RDA for each nutrient according to age and gender is presented in the front of the textbook.

If there is insufficient evidence to determine an EAR for a nutrient, the RDA can't be calculated. When this is the case, such as with fluoride, an Adequate Intake can provide an alternative guideline.

Adequate Intakes

Adequate Intake (AI) is a formal reference value that is estimated based on the judgment of the members of the FNB, according to the latest research. The AI is the next best scientific estimate of the amount of a nutrient that groups of similar individuals should consume to maintain good health.

There are several differences between the RDAs and the AIs. First, the RDAs are based on EARs, whereas the AIs are set without having established an EAR. If a nutrient

Estimated Average Requirement (EAR) Average daily amount of a nutrient needed by 50 percent of the individuals in a similar age and gender group.

Recommended Dietary Allowance (RDA) Recommended daily amount of a nutrient that meets the needs of nearly all individuals (97–98 percent) in a similar age and gender group. The RDA is set higher than the EAR.

Adequate Intake (AI) *Approximate* daily amount of a nutrient that is sufficient to meet the needs of similar individuals within a population group. The Food and Nutrition Board uses AIs for nutrients that do not have enough scientific evidence to calculate an RDA.

Head to Mastering Nutrition and watch a narrated video tour of this figure by author Joan Salge Blake.

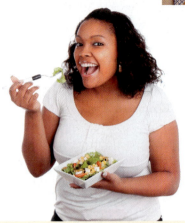

Dietary Reference Intakes (DRIs) are specific reference values for each nutrient issued by the Food and Nutrition Board of the National Academy of Medicine. They identify the amounts of each nutrient that one needs to consume to maintain good health.

DRIs FOR MOST NUTRIENTS

EAR The Estimated Average Requirement (EAR) is the average daily intake level estimated to meet the needs of half the people in a certain group. Scientists use it to calculate the RDA.

RDA The Recommended Dietary Allowance (RDA) is the average daily intake level estimated to meet the needs of nearly all people in a certain group. Aim for this amount!

AI The Adequate Intake (AI) is the average daily intake level assumed to be adequate. It is used when an EAR cannot be determined. Aim for this amount if there is no RDA!

UL The Tolerable Upper Intake Level (UL) is the highest average daily intake level likely to pose no health risks. Do not exceed this amount on a daily basis!

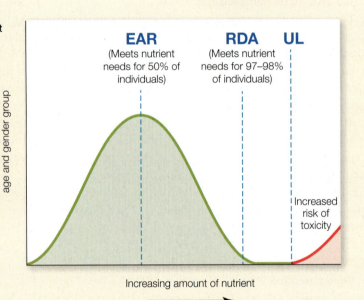

DRIs RELATED TO ENERGY

AMDR The Acceptable Macronutrient Distribution Range (AMDR) is the recommended range of carbohydrate, fat, and protein intake expressed as a percentage of total energy.

EER The Estimated Energy Requirement (EER) is the average daily energy intake predicted to meet the needs of healthy adults.

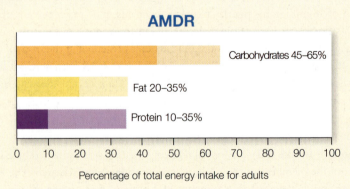

has an AI, then more research must be done to accurately set an RDA. Second, the RDAs should cover the needs of 97–98 percent of the population, but the AIs do not estimate how many people will be covered because the EAR is not available. Finally, for infants, AIs are the only estimations for nutrients to evaluate dietary adequacy. This is because conducting the types of studies necessary to determine an EAR would be unethical.

The nutrients with AIs are noted in the DRI tables in the front of your textbook and include some vitamins and minerals, such as biotin, pantothenic acid, vitamin K, fluoride, and potassium.

Tolerable Upper Intake Level

Because consuming too much of some nutrients can lead to harmful side effects, the FNB developed the **Tolerable Upper Intake Level (UL)**. The Tolerable Upper Intake Level is not a recommended intake. It refers to the highest amount of a nutrient that is unlikely to cause harm if consumed daily. The higher the consumption above the UL, the higher the risk of **toxicity**. These reference values became necessary because of individuals' increased interest in consuming dietary supplements and fortified foods in pursuit of their supposed health benefits. For example, the American Association of Poison Control Centers report approximately 60,000 annual cases of vitamin toxicity from dietary supplements.[14] Unfortunately, many Americans believe that vitamin supplements are safe in any dose but that consuming too much of other nutrients, such as fat or cholesterol, can have a deleterious effect.

Not all nutrients have UL values. This doesn't mean that high intakes of those nutrients are safe, however. The UL for selected nutrients according to age and gender is presented in the front of the textbook.

Acceptable Macronutrient Distribution Ranges

To ensure that intake of the energy nutrients is adequate and proportionate to physiological needs, recommended ranges of carbohydrate, fat, and protein intakes have been developed. These are called the **Acceptable Macronutrient Distribution Ranges (AMDRs)**. The AMDRs are as follows:

- Carbohydrates should comprise 45–65 percent of your daily kilocalories
- Fat should comprise 20–35 percent of your daily kilocalories
- Proteins should comprise 10–35 percent of your daily kilocalories

Consuming the energy-yielding nutrients in these ranges will ensure that kilocalorie and nutrient needs are met, while the risk of developing chronic diseases such as heart disease and obesity is reduced.[15] Practice calculating the AMDR using the Calculation Corner. (We cover this in greater detail in Chapter 14.)

Estimated Energy Requirements

No DRI has been established for energy (kilocalorie) intake. The method used to determine the amount of energy you need, or your **Estimated Energy Requirement (EER)**, uses a different approach than the RDAs or AIs. The EER is calculated based on age, gender, height, weight, and activity level and indicates the amount of energy needed to maintain energy balance. Individuals who consume more energy than they need will gain weight. Equations to provide a general estimate of energy needs are included in Chapter 14.

You Can Use the DRIs to Plan a Quality Diet

You can use the DRIs to make healthy food choices and plan a quality diet. To meet your needs, your goal should be to achieve the RDA or the AI of all nutrients, but not exceed the UL. **Table 2.3** summarizes how to use the DRIs to plan a quality diet. (You will also find the DRIs for all nutrients on the inside front cover of this textbook.)

Tolerable Upper Intake Level (UL) Maximum daily amount of a nutrient considered safe in a group of similar individuals.

toxicity Level of nutrient intake at which exposure to a substance becomes harmful.

Acceptable Macronutrient Distribution Ranges (AMDRs) Healthy range of intakes for the energy-containing nutrients—carbohydrates, proteins, and fats—expressed as a percentage of total daily energy. The AMDRs for adults are 45–65 percent carbohydrates, 10–35 percent protein, and 20–35 percent fat.

Estimated Energy Requirement (EER) Amount of daily energy to maintain a healthy body weight and meet energy needs based on age, gender, height, weight, and activity level.

Calculating AMDR

Use the following scenario to calculate the AMDR for carbohydrate and fat:

Suppose a woman needs 2,150 kcal per day to maintain her current healthy weight.

The AMDR for carbohydrates is 45–65 percent of total daily kilocalories. To determine the number of kilocalories she needs to obtain daily from carbohydrates, we run the following equations:

$$2,150 \text{ kcal} \times 45 \text{ percent carbohydrates} = 2,150 \times 0.45 = 968 \text{ kcal}$$
$$2,150 \text{ kcal} \times 65 \text{ percent carbohydrates} = 2,150 \times 0.65 = 1,398 \text{ kcal}$$

Thus, of the 2,150 kcal the woman eats each day, 968–1,398 kcal should be from carbohydrates.

The AMDR for fat is 20–35 percent of daily kilocalories. Therefore:

$$2,150 \text{ kcal} \times 20 \text{ percent fats} = 2,150 \times 0.20 = 430 \text{ kcal}$$
$$2,150 \text{ kcal} \times 35 \text{ percent fats} = 2,150 \times 0.35 = 753 \text{ kcal}$$

Of the 2,150 kcal the woman eats each day, 430–753 kcal should be from fat.

Can you calculate the AMDR for your daily intake of kilocalories?

Go to **Mastering** Nutrition and complete a Math Video activity similar to the problem in this Calculation Corner.

TABLE 2.3	The Do's and Don'ts of the DRIs
Reference Value	**When Planning Your Diet**
Estimated Average Requirement (EAR)	**Don't** use this amount.
Recommended Dietary Allowance (RDA)	**Do** aim for this amount!
Adequate Intake (AI)	**Do** aim for this amount if an RDA isn't available.
Tolerable Upper Intake Level (UL)	**Don't** exceed this amount on a daily basis.
Acceptable Macronutrient Distribution Range (AMDR)	**Do** follow these guidelines regarding the percentage of carbohydrates, protein, and fat in the diet.

Source: Adapted from the Subcommittee on Interpretation and Uses of Dietary Reference Intakes and the Standing Committee on the Scientific Evaluation of Dietary Reference Intakes, Institute of Medicine and Food and Nutrition Board. 2003. *Dietary Reference Intakes: Applications in Dietary Planning*. Washington, DC: National Academics Press. Reprinted with permission.

Each chapter in this textbook further explains what each nutrient is, why it is important, how much (based on the DRIs) you need to consume, and how to get enough, without consuming too much, in your diet.

LO 2.2: THE TAKE-HOME MESSAGE The Dietary Reference Intakes are specific reference values that help individuals determine daily nutrient needs to maintain good health, prevent chronic diseases, and avoid unhealthy excesses. The reference values include the EAR, RDA, AI, UL, and AMDR. The EER can help determine the appropriate amount of energy needed to maintain a healthy body weight given one's age, gender, height, weight, and activity levels. You should try to meet your RDA or AI and consume below the UL for each nutrient daily while maintaining sufficient energy intake.

What Are the *Dietary Guidelines for Americans*?

LO 2.3 Describe the recommendations included in the *Dietary Guidelines for Americans*.

Whereas the DRIs were released to prevent undernutrition, the **Dietary Guidelines for Americans** were developed out of concern over the incidence of overnutrition among Americans. By the 1970s, research had shown that Americans' overconsumption of foods rich in saturated fat, cholesterol, and sodium was increasing their risk for chronic diseases such as heart disease and stroke.[16] In 1977, the U.S. government released the *Dietary Goals for Americans*, which were designed to improve the nutritional quality of Americans' diets and to try to reduce the incidence of overnutrition and its associated health problems.[17]

Amid controversy over the scientific validity of the goals, the government asked scientists to participate in the next revision. Their work culminated in the 1980 *Dietary Guidelines for Americans*, which emphasized eating a variety of foods to obtain a nutritionally balanced diet. Since 1990, the U.S. Department of Agriculture (USDA) and the Department of Health and Human Services (HHS) have been mandated by law to update the guidelines every 5 years. The guidelines shape all federally funded nutrition programs in areas such as research and labeling and educate consumers about healthy diet and lifestyle choices.[18]

The *Dietary Guidelines for Americans* are designed to help individuals age 2 and over improve the quality and content of their diet and make other lifestyle choices to lower their risk of chronic diseases and conditions, such as diabetes mellitus, cardiovascular disease, certain cancers, osteoporosis, and obesity.

The most recent guidelines build on the previous reports and encourage Americans to follow healthy eating patterns. They also include updated guidance on added sugars, sodium, cholesterol, and caffeine.[19] The Spotlight on page 50 provides an overview of the current dietary guidelines.

> **LO 2.3: THE TAKE-HOME MESSAGE** The *Dietary Guidelines for Americans* reflect the most current nutrition and lifestyle advice for good health and reduced risk for chronic disease. They are updated by the USDA and HHS every 5 years.

What Is MyPlate?

LO 2.4 Discuss the concept of MyPlate, including the food groups and typical foods represented.

Released in 2011, **MyPlate** is an icon that serves as a reminder for healthy eating (**Figure 2.3**). Its online component, ChooseMyPlate.gov, is a Web-based communication and education initiative that provides information, tips, and tools to help people build a diet based on the DGAs and the DRIs. These include an interactive tool based on the USDA Food Patterns, which identify the amounts of food to consume from each of the basic food groups, as well as oils, at a range of kilocalorie levels, in order to provide a balanced diet. Together, the MyPlate icon and accompanying website promote proportionality, moderation, variety, and personalization.

Dietary Guidelines for Americans
Guidelines published every 5 years by the Department of Health and Human Services and the United States Department of Agriculture that provide dietary and lifestyle advice to healthy individuals age 2 and older to maintain good health and prevent chronic diseases. They are the basis for the federal food and nutrition education programs.

MyPlate Icon that serves as a reminder for healthy eating and a website providing nutritional information and educational tools based on the *Dietary Guidelines for Americans* and the Dietary Reference Intakes (DRIs).

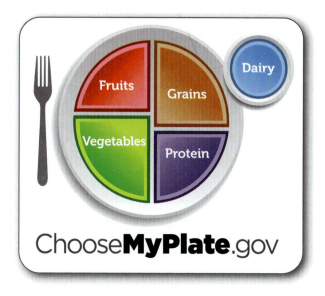

▶ **Figure 2.3 Anatomy of MyPlate**
The MyPlate icon reinforces important concepts of healthful choices, proportionality, and moderation to be used in planning a healthful diet.
Source: U.S. Department of Agriculture. 2011. ChooseMyPlate.gov.

Dietary Guidelines for Americans, 2015–2020

The *Dietary Guidelines for Americans, 2015–2020 (DGAs)* provide evidence-based guidance to Americans ages 2 and older to achieve an adequate, healthy diet. The following is a short overview of the recommendations. The complete guidelines are available at *http://health.gov/dietaryguidelines/2015/guidelines/*.

The DGAs have three primary objectives:

- Promote health
- Prevent chronic disease
- Help people reach and maintain a healthy weight

To achieve these objectives, five specific guidelines are included with accompanying key recommendations.

1. Follow a healthy eating pattern across the lifespan.

All food and beverage choices matter. Choosing a healthy eating pattern at an appropriate kilocalorie level can help individuals achieve and maintain a healthy body weight; support nutrient adequacy; and reduce the risk of chronic disease.

The *Dietary Guidelines* emphasize that healthy eating patterns are adaptable. Examples include Mediterranean-style diets, vegetarian diets, the DASH diet, and many others that we discuss later in this text.

2. Focus on variety, nutrient density, and amount.

To meet nutrient and kilocalorie needs, Americans should eat a variety of nutrient-dense foods both across and within food groups in recommended amounts.

The typical American diet does not align with the *Dietary Guidelines*. Specifically, about three-fourths (75%) of Americans eat a diet that is low in vegetables, fruits, dairy, and oils and exceeds total grain and protein recommendations. Moreover, excess weight affects two-thirds (70%) of adults and one-third (30%) of children in the United States. Thus,

Americans should focus on consuming nutrient-dense, lower-energy foods, and pay attention to portion sizes—the amount of foods and drinks they consume during meals and snacks. Individuals can determine their kilocalorie and nutrient needs based on their age, gender, and activity level, and find recommendations for portion sizes by using the ChooseMyPlate website.

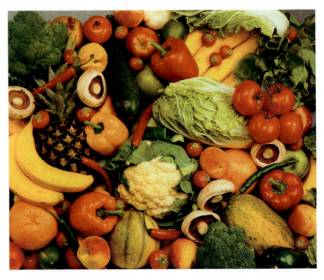

The *Dietary Guidelines* encourage consumption of a variety of fruits and vegetables.

3. Limit kilocalories from added sugars and saturated fats and reduce sodium intake.

On average, Americans consume too many kilocalories from foods high in added sugars and saturated fat, which displace healthier foods, like fruits, vegetables, and whole grains, and contribute to excessive energy intake overall. Accordingly, the *DGAs* recommend that individuals limit their intake of added sugars and saturated fat to 10 percent or less of total kilocalorie intake. To decrease added sugar intake, read labels on processed foods, especially beverages, snacks, sweets, and refined grains, as these foods contribute the majority of added sugars to the American diet. To decrease saturated fat intake, limit consumption of butter, lard, full-fat cheese, whole milk, ice cream, fatty meats, poultry skin, baked goods, and mixed dishes such as pizza, burgers, and meat dishes.

Americans should also limit their sodium intake to 2,300 mg/day. Americans of all ages consume too much sodium. Sodium is a public health concern in the United States because of its relationship with high blood pressure (hypertension) and kidney disease.

Other dietary components to limit include:

- Alcohol. Adults of legal drinking age should consume no more than one drink per day for nonpregnant women or two drinks per day for men.
- *Trans* fats. Because *trans* fats are associated with an increased risk for cardiovascular disease, Americans should keep their *trans* fat intake as low as possible by avoiding products made with partially hydrogenated oils (PHOs), such as margarines and certain processed baked goods. The FDA no longer recognizes PHOs as safe and requires that food companies remove them from their products by the summer of 2018.
- Dietary cholesterol. The DGAs do not include a recommended limit on cholesterol intake, but suggest that Americans should eat as little dietary cholesterol as possible.
- Caffeine. Moderate consumption of caffeine (400 mg/day) can be incorporated into a healthy eating pattern.

4. Shift to healthier food and beverage choices.

Replace foods and beverages that are high in kilocalories, sugar, salt, and/or saturated fats with those that are more nutrient-dense both across and within all food groups.

Examples include replacing:

- Chips and dip → Carrots and hummus
- Apple-flavored cereal bar → Apple
- White bread → Whole-wheat bread
- Sugar-sweetened beverages → Water
- Butter → oils
- Whole milk → Low-fat or skim milk

These small changes could have a big impact on health over time. Tips for changing intake habits within each food group can be found at *www.choosemy plate.gov/start-small-changes*.

5. Support healthy eating patterns for all.

In order for Americans to successfully adopt the key recommendations in the DGAs, everyone has a role to play. Collective action is needed at home, at school, at work, in the community, and at food retail outlets to ensure that all Americans have access to healthy foods that are both affordable and familiar. To help in these efforts, Americans are encouraged to create settings where healthy choices are available and affordable in the home, school/work, or community.

MyPlate Emphasizes Changes in Diet

As you can see in Figure 2.3, MyPlate shows a place setting split into five colored sections, with each representing one of five food groups: fruits, vegetables, grains, protein, and dairy. Notice that the **proportionality** of these food groups supports a plant-based diet: half of the plate is devoted to vegetables and fruits, and a quarter of the plate is devoted to grains. Lean protein foods such as fish, skinless poultry, lean meats, and legumes make up a quarter of the plate. Whereas oils are an important part of a healthy diet, they are not represented on the plate, as they are not considered a food group. The blue circle next to the plate is a visual reminder to consume fat-free and low-fat dairy foods such as milk at mealtimes.

Shifting the food proportionality on your plate can have a dramatic effect on your kilocalorie intake and thus on your weight and your risk for chronic disease. Devoting at least half of the surface of the plate to lower-kilocalorie fruits and vegetables balances higher-kilocalorie grains and protein food choices. Take the Self-Assessment to see how well proportioned your diet is.

Self-Assessment

Does Your Diet Have Proportionality?

Answer "yes" or "no" to the following questions:

1. Are grains the main food choice at all your meals?

   Yes ☐ **No** ☐

2. Do you often forget to eat vegetables?

   Yes ☐ **No** ☐

3. Do you typically eat fewer than three servings of fruit daily?

   Yes ☐ **No** ☐

4. Do you often have fewer than three cups of milk, yogurt, and/or calcium-fortified soymilk daily?

   Yes ☐ **No** ☐

5. Is the portion of meat, chicken, or fish the largest item on your dinner plate?

   Yes ☐ **No** ☐

Answer

If you answered "yes" to three or more of these questions, it is very likely that your diet lacks proportionality. You can use the information in this chapter to help improve the proportionality of your diet.

proportionality Relationship of one entity to another. Vegetables and fruits should be consumed in a higher proportion than dairy and protein foods in the diet.

Individuals who choose high-nutrient-dense and low-energy-dense foods will generally have diets that are also lower in saturated fats and added sugars. **Figure 2.4** helps you compare some nutrient-dense food choices with less healthy food choices in each food group. As you look at the figure, notice which foods are, by contrast, energy dense.

Eating a variety of foods among and within the food groups highlighted in MyPlate will increase your chances of consuming all 40 of the nutrients your body needs. **Figure 2.5** provides tips on how to choose a variety of foods from each food group.

Vegetables	Fruits	Grains	Protein	Dairy	Oils
French fries, potato chips	Fruit canned in syrup, fruit drinks, sweetened dried fruit	Buttered popcorn, cake, cookies, donuts, pastries	Fatty cuts of meat and luncheon meats, fried chicken or fish, poultry with skin	Full-fat cheeses, fried mozzarella sticks, high-fat ice cream	Butter, hydrogenated oils
Fresh, frozen and canned vegetables, dried beans and peas	Dried fruit, whole fruit, 100% fruit juice	Brown rice, bulgur, couscous, oats, pasta, popcorn, rice, whole-grain cereals, bread, crackers	Dried beans and peas, eggs, fish, lean meat, nuts, skinless poultry, seeds	Low-fat or nonfat cheese, milk or yogurt, low-fat ice cream or frozen yogurt	Vegetable oils

Foods with high amounts of added sugars and heart-unhealthy solid fats. These are less nutrient dense. →

Foods that are more nutrient dense. →

Eat **less** of these

Eat **more** of these

▲ **Figure 2.4 Nutrient-Dense Food Choices**
Choose nutrient-dense foods more often to build a balanced diet.

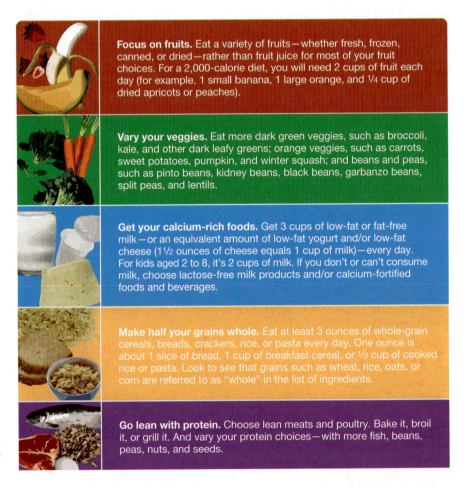

Focus on fruits. Eat a variety of fruits—whether fresh, frozen, canned, or dried—rather than fruit juice for most of your fruit choices. For a 2,000-calorie diet, you will need 2 cups of fruit each day (for example, 1 small banana, 1 large orange, and 1/4 cup of dried apricots or peaches).

Vary your veggies. Eat more dark green veggies, such as broccoli, kale, and other dark leafy greens; orange veggies, such as carrots, sweet potatoes, pumpkin, and winter squash; and beans and peas, such as pinto beans, kidney beans, black beans, garbanzo beans, split peas, and lentils.

Get your calcium-rich foods. Get 3 cups of low-fat or fat-free milk—or an equivalent amount of low-fat yogurt and/or low-fat cheese (1½ ounces of cheese equals 1 cup of milk)—every day. For kids aged 2 to 8, it's 2 cups of milk. If you don't or can't consume milk, choose lactose-free milk products and/or calcium-fortified foods and beverages.

Make half your grains whole. Eat at least 3 ounces of whole-grain cereals, breads, crackers, rice, or pasta every day. One ounce is about 1 slice of bread, 1 cup of breakfast cereal, or ½ cup of cooked rice or pasta. Look to see that grains such as wheat, rice, oats, or corn are referred to as "whole" in the list of ingredients.

Go lean with protein. Choose lean meats and poultry. Bake it, broil it, or grill it. And vary your protein choices—with more fish, beans, peas, nuts, and seeds.

▶ **Figure 2.5 Mix Up Your Choices within Each Food Group**
Source: USDA Consumer Brochure. 2005. *Finding Your Way to a Healthier You.* Based on the *Dietary Guidelines for Americans.* Accessed February 2017.

TABLE 2.4 **What Is Moderate and Vigorous Activity?**

Examples of Moderate Activities (Expend 3.5 to 7 Kilocalories per Minute):	Examples of Vigorous Activities (Expend More Than 7 Kilocalories per Minute):
• Brisk walking • Bicycling 5–9 mph • Shooting hoops • Using free weights • Yoga • Walking a dog	• Jogging or running • Bicycling more than 10 mph • Playing competitive sports like basketball, soccer, or lacrosse • Rowing on a machine vigorously • Karate, judo, or tae kwon do • Jumping rope

Source: Adapted from the Centers for Disease Control and Prevention. 2015. *Physical Activity for a Healthy Weight*. Available at www.cdc.gov. Accessed February 2017.

Lastly, physical activity is an important component of a healthy lifestyle. Being physically active (see **Table 2.4**) helps you stay fit and reduce your risk of obesity and chronic diseases such as heart disease and cancer. Advice regarding physical activity can be found at http://ChooseMyPlate.gov.

Use MyPlate to Choose Foods that Fit Your Kilocalorie Needs

You now know to eat a variety of nutrient-dense foods to be healthy and that MyPlate helps you select a diverse group of foods, but you may be wondering how much from each food group you should be eating. The ChooseMyPlate.gov interactive website will give you the exact numbers of servings to eat from each food group based on your daily kilocalorie needs. If you cannot go to the website, **Table 2.5** tells you the quantity from each food group you should consume to healthfully obtain the daily kilocalories you need.

TABLE 2.5 **How Much Should You Eat from Each Food Group?**

Kilocalorie Level	Grains (oz eq)	Vegetables (cups)	Fruits (cups)	Oils (tsp)	Dairy (cups)	Protein (oz eq)
1,400	5	1.5	1.5	4	2	4
1,600	5	2	1.5	5	3	5
1,800	6	2.5	1.5	5	3	5
2,000	6	2.5	2	6	3	5.5
2,200	7	3	2	6	3	6
2,400	8	3	2	7	3	6.5
2,600	9	3.5	2	8	3	6.5
2,800	10	3.5	2.5	8	3	7

The above are suggested amounts to consume daily from each of the basic food groups and the oils based on daily kilocalorie needs. Remember that most food choices should be fat free or low fat and contain little added sugar.

Note: Grains: Includes all foods made with wheat, rice, oats, cornmeal, or barley, such as bread, pasta, oatmeal, breakfast cereals, tortillas, and grits. In general, 1 slice of bread, 1 cup of ready-to-eat cereal, or ½ cup of cooked rice, pasta, or cereal is considered 1 ounce equivalent (oz eq) from the grains group. *At least half of all grains consumed should be whole grains such as whole-wheat bread, oats, or brown rice.*

Vegetables: Includes all fresh, frozen, canned, and dried vegetables, including legumes, as well as vegetable juices. In general, 1 cup of raw or cooked vegetables or vegetable juice, or 2 cups of raw leafy greens, is considered 1 cup from the vegetable group.

Fruits: Includes all fresh, frozen, canned, and dried fruits and fruit juices. In general, 1 cup of fruit or 100% fruit juice, or ½ cup of dried fruit, is considered 1 cup from the fruit group.

Oils: Includes vegetable oils such as canola, corn, olive, soybean, and sunflower oil, fatty fish, nuts, avocados, mayonnaise, salad dressings made with oils, and soft margarine.

Dairy: Includes all fat-free and low-fat milk and calcium-fortified soymilk, as well as yogurt and cheese. In general, 1 cup of milk or yogurt, 1½ ounces of natural cheese, or 2 ounces of processed cheese is considered 1 cup from the dairy group.

Proteins: In general, 1 ounce of lean meat, poultry, or fish, 1 egg, 1 tablespoon peanut butter, ¼ cup cooked dry beans, or ½ ounce of nuts or seeds is considered 1 ounce equivalent (oz eq) from the protein group.

Source: U.S. Department of Agriculture. 2017. Available at https://health.gov/dietaryguidelines/2015/resources/2015-2020_Dietary_Guidelines.pdf.

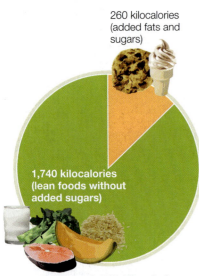

260 kilocalories (added fats and sugars)

1,740 kilocalories (lean foods without added sugars)

2,000 total daily kilocalories

▲ **Figure 2.6 How Fats and Added Sugars Fit into a Balanced Diet**
If you select mostly nutrient-dense, lean foods that contain few saturated fats and added sugars, you may have leftover kilocalories to "spend" on extra helpings or a sweet dessert.

TABLE 2.6	Choose Right	
Choosing . . .	**Over . . .**	**Will Cost You**
Whole milk (1 cup)	Fat-free milk (1 cup)	65 kilocalories
Roasted chicken thigh with skin (3 oz)	Roasted chicken breast, skinless (3 oz)	70 kilocalories
Glazed doughnut (3¾" diameter)	English muffin (one muffin)	165 kilocalories
French fries (one medium order)	Baked potato (one medium)	299 kilocalories
Regular soda (one can, 12 fl oz)	Diet soda (one can, 12 fl oz)	150 kilocalories

Note: As you can see, your daily food plan can include saturated fats and added sugars, depending on food choices.
Source: Adapted from the U.S. Department of Agriculture, MyPlate. "Empty Calories: How Do I Count the Empty Calories I Eat?" 2011. Available at www.ChooseMyPlate.gov.

For example, for a moderately active female who needs 2,000 kilocalories daily, a healthy daily diet would consist of the following:

- 6 servings from the grains group
- 2½ cups of dark green, orange, starchy, and other vegetables, including some legumes
- 2 cups of fruits
- 3 cups of fat-free or low-fat milk, calcium-fortified soymilk, and/or yogurt
- 5½ ounces of lean meat, poultry, and fish, or the equivalent in meat alternatives such as beans
- 6 teaspoons of vegetable oils

The kilocalorie levels and distribution of food groups in daily food plans are calculated using the leanest food choices with no added sugar. If all food selections are low in fat and added sugar, this menu will provide a total of about 1,740 kilocalories (**Figure 2.6**). If you pour whole milk (high in fat) over your sweetened cereal (added sugar) instead of using skim milk (fat free) to drench your shredded wheat (no added sugar), the extra fat and sugar kilocalories add up quickly to reach 2,000 kilocalories (**Table 2.6**).

Figure 2.7 shows how servings from the various food groups can create well-balanced meals and snacks throughout the day. Although this particular menu is balanced and the foods are nutrient dense, it is unlikely that every day will be this ideal. Fortunately, nutrient needs are averaged over time. If you eat insufficient servings of one food group or a specific nutrient one day, you can make up for it the next day.

Should you worry about *when* you eat? This question is debated in Examining the Evidence: Does the Time of Day You Eat Impact Your Health? on pages 56–57.

LO 2.4: THE TAKE-HOME MESSAGE MyPlate depicts the five food groups using the familiar mealtime visual of a place setting. It is part of the USDA's Web-based initiative at ChooseMyPlate.gov, providing information and tools, including personalized daily food plans, to help you build a healthy diet based on the *Dietary Guidelines for Americans*. Try to consume nutrient-dense foods—fruits, vegetables, whole grains, and lean dairy and protein foods—but limit energy-dense foods, which provide kilocalories from saturated fats and added sugars but little nutrition. Daily physical activity is encouraged to better manage your weight and health.

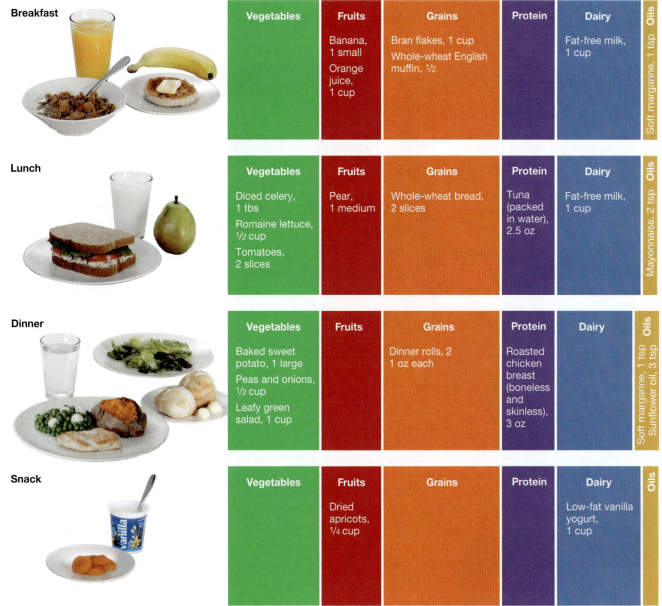

	Vegetables	Fruits	Grains	Protein	Dairy	Oils
Breakfast		Banana, 1 small; Orange juice, 1 cup	Bran flakes, 1 cup; Whole-wheat English muffin, ½		Fat-free milk, 1 cup	Soft margarine, 1 tsp
Lunch	Diced celery, 1 tbs; Romaine lettuce, ½ cup; Tomatoes, 2 slices	Pear, 1 medium	Whole-wheat bread, 2 slices	Tuna (packed in water), 2.5 oz	Fat-free milk, 1 cup	Mayonnaise, 2 tsp
Dinner	Baked sweet potato, 1 large; Peas and onions, ½ cup; Leafy green salad, 1 cup		Dinner rolls, 2 1 oz each	Roasted chicken breast (boneless and skinless), 3 oz		Soft margarine, 1 tsp; Sunflower oil, 3 tsp
Snack		Dried apricots, ¼ cup			Low-fat vanilla yogurt, 1 cup	

▲ **Figure 2.7 A Healthy Daily Food Plan**
A variety of foods from each food group creates a balanced diet.

What Is the Exchange System?

LO 2.5 Explain how the exchange system can be used as a guide to plan a balanced diet.

The **exchange lists** for meal planning were designed in 1950 to give people with diabetes a structured, balanced eating plan. The lists, which are still in use today, group foods according to their carbohydrate, protein, and fat composition and provide specific portion sizes for each food. In addition, each food in the group has a similar number of kilocalories.

There are six food groups in the exchange lists: starch, fruit, milk, vegetable, meat, and fat. You might be surprised to find some foods located in unexpected places. For example, in MyPlate, cheese is in the milk group because of its calcium content. In the exchange system, cheese is in the meat group because it has less carbohydrate than milk or yogurt but contains levels of protein and fat similar to those found in chicken or meat. Potatoes are not found in the vegetable list, but in the starch list; bacon is considered a fat exchange because it contains more fat than protein; and peanut butter is found in both the high-fat meat list and the fat list because it is high in both protein and fat.

exchange lists Diet-planning tool that groups foods together based on their carbohydrate, protein, and fat content. One food on the list can be exchanged for another food on the same list.

Does the Time of Day You Eat Impact Your Health?

We are all creatures of habit. Some of our habits, such as the time of day we eat, can either enhance or detract from our health. Do you skip a meal daily? Do you find yourself snacking late at night? Do you overload on high-fat or fried foods or drink a lot of alcohol when you go out on the weekends? These kinds of choices can affect your body weight, nutrient intake, and health.

Snacking and Skipping Breakfast

While your grandparents may have habitually had their "three square meals" (breakfast, lunch, and dinner) daily with little snacking between meals, this pattern has changed over the last several decades. In a study looking at the eating habits of over 32,000 adult women during a 40-year span, the incidence of eating three meals a day declined from 75 percent to 63 percent among the women, but the incidence of snacking increased.[1] This is a concern because snacking has been associated with the

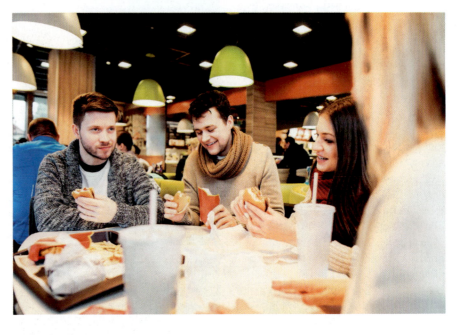

consumption of excess kilocalories and obesity.[2] Interestingly, the incidence of obesity among these women during this time period more than doubled.[3]

Skipping breakfast specifically may reduce the nutrient quality of your diet.[4] In contrast, children who eat a healthy breakfast on a regular basis are better able to meet their intake of food groups such as dairy and fruit and their daily needs for essential micronutrients such as thiamin, niacin, riboflavin, vitamins B_6 and B_{12}, calcium, iron, magnesium, potassium, and zinc.[5,6]

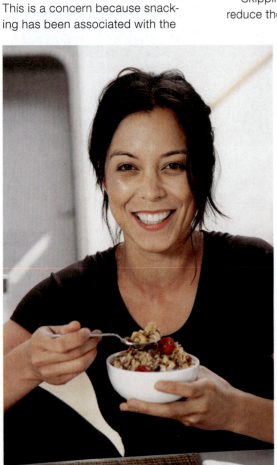

Eating More at Night and on Weekends

There may be something to the old adage to eat breakfast like a king, lunch like a prince, and dinner like a pauper when it comes to better managing your weight. Researchers studied how switching between a high-kilocalorie breakfast and a high-kilocalorie dinner, but keeping the total daily kilocalories the same, would influence body

weight.[7] In this 12-week study, 50 overweight women were randomly assigned to a 1,400-kilocalorie diet that consisted of a breakfast of 700 kilocalories, a lunch of 500 kilocalories, and a dinner of 200 kilocalories or the same kilocalories and same food choices but with the breakfast and dinner meals switched.[8]

While both groups lost significant amounts of weight, the women consuming the large breakfast lost an average of approximately 19 pounds compared to only about 8 pounds in the large dinner group. The large breakfast group also lost twice as many inches around their waists. Since the hormone ghrelin, which increases your appetite, was lower during the day in the breakfast group, these women also experienced higher levels of satiety throughout the day. In addition, large breakfast eaters also had significantly lower levels of insulin, glucose, and fat in their blood, which may help lower the risk of diabetes and heart disease.[9]

A factor in the weight-loss difference may be the body's circadian rhythms, which are hormonal, metabolic, mental, and behavioral changes that the body follows over a 24-hour cycle.[10,11] Consequently, the time of day we eat may affect the way our bodies process food. More research is needed before any strong conclusions can be drawn from these results.

Do you eat after 7:00 P.M.? Most young adults do, especially during the weekend.[12] For most students, eating schedules are influenced by hunger, pressures from work and school, convenience, and social habits. Studies suggest that the craving for late-night carbohydrate snacks is also related to your circadian rhythms.[13] Also, when eating later in the day, you are likely to eat more food, and hence consume more kilocalories, particularly from carbohydrates, fat, and alcohol.

Weekend eating patterns can also influence overall dietary intake. Haines reports that people in their study ate an average of 82 kilocalories more per day on Friday, Saturday, and Sunday compared with weekdays.[14] These increases in kilocalories were mostly due to an increase in fat (approximately 0.7 percent) and alcohol (1.4 percent); carbohydrates decreased by 1.6 percent. Over time, this increase in kilocalorie intake may lead to weight gain. Results from a similar study involving over 11,500 adults suggest that Saturday is the day with the highest kilocalorie consumption.[15] Compared to the average weekday consumption, the adults consumed 181 kilocalories more on Saturday, on average, with over 40 percent of the kilocalories coming from sugar-sweetened beverages, alcohol, sugar, and saturated fat. Not surprising, eating fast foods and dining out in restaurants was higher on Saturday than any other day of the week.[16]

Recommendations

Based on the current research on eating and time of day, it is recommended that you:

- Start your day with a nutrient-dense breakfast as part of a healthy eating pattern. Many breakfast foods—such as dry whole-grain cereals, fresh fruit, or whole-grain toast or bagels with low-fat cream cheese—can be eaten on the go. You'll have more energy and will most likely eat fewer total kilocalories by the end of the day.
- Choose breakfast foods that are more satisfying to improve your appetite control throughout the day. Enjoy foods such as whole-grain cereals and whole fruits, which are higher in fiber, protein, and water and lower in fat and sugar.
- Control kilocalorie intake on nights and weekends. Monitor your weekend eating habits to maintain a consistent balance of carbohydrates, fats, and proteins and to reduce alcohol consumption.

References

1. Kant, A., and B. Graubard. 2015. 40-Year Trends in Meal and Snack Eating Behaviors of American Adults. *Journal of the Academy of Nutrition and Dietetics* 115:50–63.
2. Piernas, C., and B. Popkin. 2010. Snacking Increased Among U.S. Adults Between 1977–2006. *Journal of Nutrition* 140:325–332.
3. Kant, 2015.
4. St-Onge, M., J. Ard, M. Baskin, S. Chiuve, H. Johnson, P. Kris-Etherton, and K. Varady. 2017. Meal Timing and Frequency: Implications for Cardiovascular Disease Prevention. A scientific Statement from the American Heart Association. DOI:10.1161.
5. USDA, Center for Nutrition Policy and Promotion. 2011. Breakfast Consumption, Body Weight, and Nutrient Intake: A Review of the Evidence. Available at https://www.cnpp.usda.gov/sites/default/files/nutrition_insights_uploads/Insight45.pdf. Accessed February 2017.
6. Dykstra, H., A. Davery, J. Fisher, H. Polonsky, S. Sherman, M. Abel, L. Dale, G. Foster, and K. Bauer. 2016. Breakfast-Skipping and Selecting Low Nutritional-Quality Foods for Breakfast Are Common Among Low-Income Urban Children, Regardless of Food Security Status. *Journal of Nutrition* 146:630–636.
7. Jakubowicz, D., M. Barnea, J. Wanstein, and O. Froy. 2013. High Caloric Intake at Breakfast vs. Dinner Differentially Influences Weight Loss of Overweight and Obese Women. *Obesity* 21:2504–2512.
8. Ibid.
9. Ibid.
10. Ibid.
11. Covassin, N., P. Singh, and V. Somers. 2016. Keeping Up With the Clock: Circadian Disruption and Obesity Risk. *Hypertension* 68:1081–1090.
12. Striegel-Moore, R. H., D. L. Franko, D. Thompson, S. Affenito, and H. C. Kraemer. 2006. "Night Eating: Prevalence and Demographic Correlates." *Obesity* 14:139–147.
13. Scheer, Frank A. J. L., Christopher J. Morris, and Steven A. Shea. 2013. "The Internal Circadian Clock Increases Hunger and Appetite in the Evening Independent of Food Intake and Other Behaviors." *Obesity* 21(3):421.
14. Haines, P. S., M. Y. Hama, D. K. Guilkey, and B. M. Popkin. 2003. "Weekend Eating in the United States Is Linked with Greater Energy, Fat, and Alcohol Intake." *Obesity Research* 11:945–949.
15. Ruopeng, A. 2016. Weekend-Weekday Differences in Diet Among U.S. Adults, 2003–2012. *Annals of Epidemiology* 26:57–65.
16. Ibid.

Using the exchange lists is a convenient method for designing a flexible meal plan that controls proportions of carbohydrate, protein, and fat intake. Because of their similar macronutrient composition, foods within each group can be exchanged or swapped with each other. **Table 2.7** presents the number of food group choices in healthy,

TABLE 2.7	Number of Exchanges per Food Group per Day by Kilocalorie Intake				
Food Group	**1,500 kcal**	**1,800 kcal**	**2,000 kcal**	**2,200 kcal**	**2,400 kcal**
Starch	8	9	10	11	12
Fruit	3	4	4	4	5
Milk, low fat	2	2	3	3	3
Nonstarchy vegetables	4	5	6	6	7
Meat and meat substitutes, lean	3	5	5	6	7
Fat	5	6	6	7	7

balanced diets of different kilocalorie levels that consist of 55 percent carbohydrate, 20 percent protein, and 25 percent fat. As you can see from the table, the higher the kilocalorie intake, the greater the number of choices from the exchange lists that are allowed. For complete exchange lists for meal planning, see Appendix C.

> **LO 2.5: THE TAKE-HOME MESSAGE** The exchange system is a convenient tool for creating meal plans based on the macronutrient content and total kilocalories of foods. The plan consists of six food groups: starch, fruit, milk, vegetables, meat, and fat. Foods within each group can be exchanged or swapped to add variety to meals and snacks.

What Information Is on the Food Label?

LO 2.6 Identify the required components of a food label and Nutrition Facts panel.

Do you pay close attention to the food labels of items you purchase at the supermarket? The information on labels can be tremendously useful when it comes to planning a healthy diet.

Food Labels Are Strictly Regulated by the FDA

To help consumers make informed food choices, the Food and Drug Administration (FDA) regulates the labeling of all packaged foods in the United States. Since the 1930s, the FDA has mandated that every packaged food (**Figure 2.8**) be labeled with:

- The name of the food
- The net weight, which is the weight of the food in the package, excluding the weight of the package or packing material
- The name and address of the manufacturer or distributor
- A list of ingredients in descending order by weight, with the heaviest item listed first

New labeling laws have been enacted to further benefit the consumer.[20] In 1990, the Nutrition Labeling and Education Act (NLEA) began mandating that labels include uniform nutrition information, serving sizes, and specific criteria for health claims. Additional requirements for food labels have since been passed to require that labels now also show:

- A Nutrition Facts panel
- Serving sizes that are uniform among similar products, which allows for easier comparison shopping
- An indication of how a serving of the food fits into an overall daily diet
- Uniform definitions for descriptive label terms such as "light" and "fat free"
- Health claims that are accurate and science based, if made about the food or one of its nutrients
- The presence of any of eight common allergens that might be present in the food, including milk, eggs, fish, shellfish, tree nuts (cashews, walnuts, almonds, etc.), peanuts, wheat, and soybeans

Whereas raw fruits and vegetables and fresh fish typically don't have a label, these foods fall under the FDA's voluntary, point-of-purchase nutrition information program. Under the guidelines of this program, the nutrition information should be displayed in

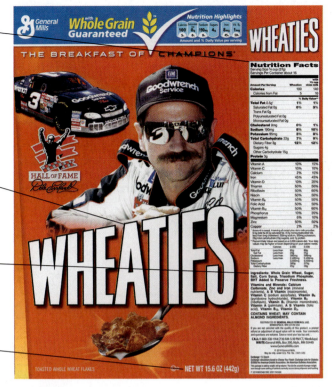

The **Nutrition Facts panel** lists standardized serving sizes and specific nutrients, and shows how a serving of the food fits into a healthy diet by stating its contribution to the percentage of the Daily Value for each nutrient.

The **name** of the product must be displayed on the front label.

The **ingredients** must be listed in descending order by weight. Whole-grain wheat is the predominant ingredient in this cereal.

The **net weight** of the food in the box is located at the bottom of the package.

▲ **Figure 2.8 Labeling Requirements Mandated by the FDA**
The nutrition facts panel—such as the one on this box of Wheaties—can help consumers make informed food choices.

close proximity to the foods.[21] The nutrition information can be displayed as a label on the food or on store shelves, signs, posters, brochures, notebooks, leaflets, or a video near the food.[22] Nutrition labeling must be provided for all meat and meat food products in the supermarket either on the label or at the point-of-purchase.[23]

Other nutrition information is sometimes available to consumers in the grocery aisle. Some supermarkets have initiated nutrition scoring systems that highlight the overall nutritional value of food products. This can also help the consumer make heathier choices.

The Nutrition Facts Panel Indicates Nutrient Values

One area of the food label in particular, the **Nutrition Facts panel**, provides a nutritional snapshot of the food inside a package. By law the panel must list amounts of specific nutrients. If an additional nutrient such as vitamin E or vitamin B_{12} has been added, or if the product makes a claim about a nutrient, then that nutrient must also be listed on the panel. The manufacturer can voluntarily list other nutrients, such as additional vitamins and minerals. The majority of packaged foods contain this nutrition information.

Very few foods are exempt from carrying a Nutrition Facts panel on the label. Such foods include plain coffee and tea; some spices, flavorings, and other foods that don't provide a significant amount of nutrients; bakery foods and other ready-to-eat foods that are prepared and sold in retail establishments; restaurant meals; and foods produced by small businesses (companies that have total sales of less than $500,000).[24]

In 2016, the FDA released a new Nutrition Facts panel. It was designed to reflect current research on the links between diet and chronic diseases and conditions, such as heart disease, stroke, type 2 diabetes, and obesity.

Because manufacturers have some time to phase in the new panel, you are likely to see a mix of the old panel and the new one on foods until this time. So let's compare the old and new Nutrition Facts panels (**Focus Figure 2.9**).

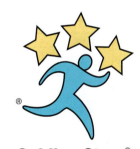

Guiding Stars®
Nutritious choices made simple™

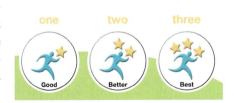

one   two   three
Good   Better   Best

The Guiding Stars in-store nutritional guidance system rates the nutrient density of foods. Foods that earn even one star are nutrient dense, but foods with three stars provide the optimal level of nutrients per kilocalories. Foods that do not meet the nutritional criteria do not display a star.

Nutrition Facts panel Area on the food label that provides a list of specific nutrients obtained in one serving of the food.

Head to **Mastering** Nutrition and watch a narrated video tour of this figure by author Joan Salge Blake.

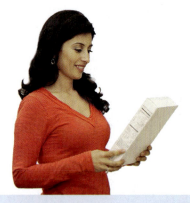

The U.S. Food and Drug Administration (FDA) has made changes to the 20-year-old nutrition labels on packaged foods. The changes to the nutrition label provide information to help compare products and make healthy food choices.

OLD LABEL

GRANOLA

Nutrition Facts
Serving Size 2/3 cup (55 g)
Servings Per Container About 8

Amount Per Serving

Calories 230   Calories from Fat 72

	% Daily Value*
Total Fat 8 g	**12**%
Saturated Fat 1 g	**5**%
Trans Fat 0 g	
Cholesterol 0 mg	**0**%
Sodium 160 mg	**7**%
Total Carbohydrate 37 g	**12**%
Dietary Fiber 4 g	**16**%
Sugars 1 g	
Protein 3 g	
Vitamin A	10%
Vitamin C	8%
Calcium	20%
Iron	45%

* Percent Daily Values are based on a 2,000 calorie diet. Your daily value may be higher or lower depending on your calorie needs.

		Calories:	2,000	2,500
Total Fat	Less than		65 g	80 g
Sat Fat	Less than		20 g	25 g
Cholesterol	Less than		300 mg	300 mg
Sodium	Less than		2,400 mg	2,400 mg
Total Carbohydrate			300 g	375 g
Dietary Fiber			25 g	30 g

SERVINGS

- Serving sizes are standardized, making comparison shopping easier.

NEW
- Serving sizes are larger and bolder.
- Serving sizes updated and more realistic.

CALORIES

- Calories per serving and the number of servings in the package are listed.

NEW
- Calories are larger to stand out more.
- "Calories from fat" is removed.

DAILY VALUES

- Daily Values are general reference values based on a 2,000 Calorie diet.
- The %DV can tell you if a food is high or low in a nutrient or dietary substance.

NEW
- Daily Values are updated.
- A shorter footnote that more clearly explains %DV is included.
- The %DV for added sugar is included.

ADDED SUGARS

NEW
- Added sugars are listed.

VITAMINS & MINERALS

- Vitamin A, vitamin C, calcium, and iron are required.
- Other vitamins and minerals are voluntary.

NEW
- Vitamin D and potassium are required, in addition to calcium and iron.
- Vitamins A and C are voluntary.
- Actual amounts of each nutrient are listed as well as the %DV.

NEW LABEL

GRANOLA

Nutrition Facts
8 servings per container
Serving size   **2/3 cup (55g)**

Amount per serving
Calories   **230**

	% Daily Value*
Total Fat 8g	**10**%
Saturated Fat 1g	**5**%
Trans Fat 0g	
Cholesterol 0mg	**0**%
Sodium 160mg	**7**%
Total Carbohydrate 37g	**13**%
Dietary Fiber 4g	**14**%
Total Sugars 12g	
Includes 10g Added Sugars	**20**%
Protein 3g	
Vitamin D 2mcg	10%
Calcium 260mg	20%
Iron 8mg	45%
Potassium 235mg	6%

* The % Daily Value (DV) tells you how much a nutrient in a serving of food contributes to a daily diet. 2,000 calories a day is used for general nutrition advice.

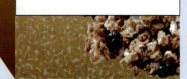

The top band of the Nutrition Facts panel indicates the **serving size**. In the new panel, this is in boldface type to help consumers see it more readily. By law, the serving size must be listed both by weight in grams and in common household measures, such as cups and ounces. Serving sizes are standardized among similar food products, making it easier to compare brands. On the new panel, the serving sizes for some foods have been updated to mirror the amounts that people *actually* eat. For example, while ½ cup of ice cream was previously the standard serving, it is now going to be ⅔ cup, an amount that people will likely scoop into a bowl.

The rest of the information on the panel is based on the listed serving size of the food. For example, if a serving were 1 cup, but you ate 2 cups, you would need to double the nutrient information on the panel. The servings-per-container information is useful for portion control.

Listed below the serving size is the kilocalories per serving. Notice that the new panel gives this information in large boldface type. Below this is a list of the nutrients that should be limited or increased in the diet. Americans typically eat too much fat, including saturated fat and *trans* fat, and too much sodium. In contrast, they tend to fall short in dietary fiber, vitamin D, and calcium, iron, and potassium. These are on the panel to remind you to choose foods rich in these substances. The old panel required manufacturers to list vitamins A and C, but these are no longer considered nutrients of concern; thus, their presence on the panel is now voluntary. A food manufacturer also may voluntarily list other nutrients, such as vitamin B_{12} or folate. Overall, the Nutrition Facts panel can be your best shopping guide to foods that are low in the nutrients you want to limit, such as saturated fat, and high in the nutrients that you need to eat in higher amounts, such as potassium.

The new panel identifies added sugars, indented as a subcategory of "Total Sugars." Recall from Chapter 1 that added sugars are not naturally occurring, but added during the manufacturing of the food. It is difficult for many Americans to meet their nutrient needs while staying within their kilocalorie limits for the day if their diets are high in added sugars. Americans are currently consuming approximately 13 percent of their daily kilocalories from added sugars. The current recommendation is to consume less than 10 percent of kilocalories from added sugars daily.

Are you wondering what determines if a food contains a "high" or "low" amount of a specific nutrient? That's where the percent Daily Values come into play.

The Percent Daily Values Help You Compare Packaged Foods

Unlike the DRIs, which are precise recommended amounts of each nutrient that you should eat, the **percent Daily Values (%DVs)** listed on the Nutrition Facts panel are general reference levels for the nutrients listed on the food label. The %DVs give an idea of how the nutrients in the foods you buy fit into your overall diet.

For example, if calcium is listed at 10 percent, a serving of that food provides 10 percent of most adults' daily requirement for calcium. Because the %DVs on the food label are based on a 2,000-kilocalorie diet, if you need more or fewer than 2,000 kilocalories daily, some of your %DV numbers may be higher or lower than those listed on the Nutrition Facts panel.

There are no %DVs listed on the label for *trans* fat, total sugars, and protein. You should consume as little *trans* fat as possible. Notice that the new panel identifies a %DV for added sugars. Although there are reference values for protein, consuming adequate amounts of protein isn't a health concern for most Americans over age 4, so listing the %DV for this nutrient isn't warranted. The %DV for protein is listed on products being marketed for children under the age of 4, such as baby food, and when a claim is made about the food, such as that it is "high in protein."[25]

serving size Recommended portion of food that is used as a standard reference on food labels.

percent Daily Values (%DVs) Reference values developed by the Food and Drug Administration and used on the Nutrition Facts panel to describe the percentage of a daily nutrient intake provided in one serving of the food.

If a serving provides 20 percent or more of the %DV, it is considered high in that nutrient. For example, a serving of the granola shown in Focus Figure 2.9 is high in calcium and iron (a healthy attribute). If a nutrient provides 5 percent or less of the %DV, it is considered low in that nutrient. A serving of this granola is low in saturated fat (another healthy attribute).

Lastly, both panels provide a footnote at the bottom of the label that explains the meaning of the %DVs. However, the old panel provided examples of %DVs for a 2,000-kilocalorie and 2,500-kilocalorie diet. These examples were eliminated from the new panel, and the explanation was revised to improve clarity.

The table inside the back cover of this book identifies the %DVs on the footnote of the Nutrition Facts panel. These are regularly updated to reflect the latest scientific evidence. For example, the %DV for fiber has increased from 25 grams to 28 grams, whereas the %DV for sodium has decreased from 2,400 milligrams to 2,300 milligrams.

Label Claims Can Reveal Potential Health Benefits

In the 1980s, the Kellogg Company ran an ad campaign for its fiber-rich All Bran cereal reminding the public of the National Cancer Institute's recommendation to eat low-fat, high-fiber foods, fresh fruits, and vegetables to maintain a healthy weight. According to the FDA, sales of high-fiber cereals increased over 35 percent within a year.[26]

For decades, manufacturers realized that putting nutrition and health claims on labels was effective in influencing consumer purchases. Supermarket shelves were soon crowded with products boasting various claims.

The FDA mandates that all claims on labels follow strict guidelines. Currently, the FDA allows the use of three types of claims on food products: (1) nutrient content claims, (2) health claims, and (3) structure/function claims. All foods displaying these claims on the label must meet specified criteria.

Nutrient Content Claims

A food product can make a claim about the amount of a nutrient it contains (or doesn't contain) by using descriptive terms such as *free* (fat-free yogurt), *high* (high-fiber crackers), *low* (low saturated fat cereal), *reduced* (reduced-sodium soup), and *extra lean* (extra lean ground beef) as long as it meets the strict criteria designated by the FDA. These terms can help identify at a glance the food items that best meet your needs. For instance, if you want to decrease or limit the amount of sodium in your diet, you could look for low-sodium claims on labels.

Look at the labels of the canned soups in **Figure 2.10**. Note that the "low-sodium" version of the chicken soup cannot contain more than 140 milligrams of sodium per serving. In contrast, the soup with the term "less sodium" on the label contains 450 milligrams of sodium per serving, which is at least 25 percent less sodium than the regular variety. The can of classic chicken soup contains almost 900 milligrams for a serving, which is likely the same or even more sodium than the average American consumes at dinner. **Table 2.8** provides some of the most common nutrient claims on food labels and the specific criteria that each claim must meet as mandated by the FDA.

Health Claims

Suppose you are sitting at your kitchen table eating a bowl of breakfast cereal. You may notice a claim on the front of the

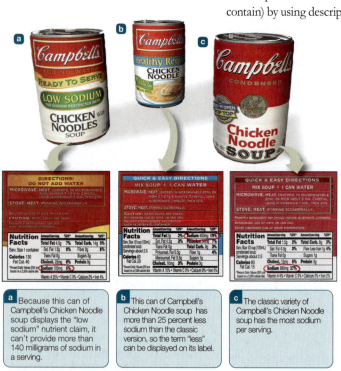

a. Because this can of Campbell's Chicken Noodle soup displays the "low sodium" nutrient claim, it can't provide more than 140 milligrams of sodium in a serving.

b. This can of Campbell's Chicken Noodle soup has more than 25 percent less sodium than the classic version, so the term "less" can be displayed on its label.

c. The classic variety of Campbell's Chicken Noodle soup has the most sodium per serving.

▲ Figure 2.10 Soup's On!
Nutrient claims on the food label must conform to strict criteria.

box that states: "The soluble fiber in oats, as part of a heart-healthy diet, can help lower your cholesterol." Do you recognize this as a health claim that links oatmeal with better heart health?

A health claim (**Figure 2.11**) must contain two important components: (1) a food or a dietary compound, such as fiber, and (2) a corresponding disease or health-related condition that is associated with the substance.[27]

In the cereal example, the soluble fiber (the dietary compound) that naturally occurs in oats has been shown to lower blood cholesterol levels (the corresponding health-related condition), which can help reduce the risk of heart disease.

There are three types of health claims: (1) authorized health claims, (2) health claims based on authoritative statements, and (3) qualified health claims. The differences between them lie in the amount of supporting research and agreement among scientists about the strength of the relationship between the food or dietary ingredient and the disease or condition. See **Table 2.9** for a definition and examples of each type of health claim.

Structure/Function Claims

The last type of label claim is the structure/function claim, which describes how a nutrient or dietary compound affects the structure or function of the human body.[28] The claims "Calcium builds strong bones" and "Fiber maintains bowel regularity" are examples of structure/function claims.[29] Structure/function claims cannot state that the nutrient or dietary compound can be used to treat a disease or a condition.

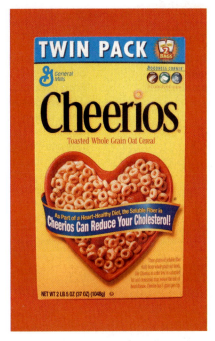

▲ **Figure 2.11 An Authorized Health Claim**
The text on this box of Cheerios is an authorized health claim stating that soluble fiber reduces the risk of heart disease.

TABLE 2.8	Nutrient Content Claims on Food Labels			
Nutrient	**Free**	**Low**	**Reduced/Less**	**Light**
Kilocalories	<5 kilocalories (kcal) per serving	<40 kcal per serving	At least 25% fewer kcal per serving	If the food contains 50% or more of its kcal from fat, then the fat must be reduced
Fat	<0.5 grams (g) per serving	<3 g per serving	At least 25% less fat per serving	Same as above
Saturated fat	<0.5 g per serving	<1 g per serving	At least 25% less saturated fat per serving	N/A
Cholesterol	<2 milligrams (mg) per serving	<20 mg per serving	At least 25% less cholesterol per serving	N/A
Sodium	<5 mg per serving	<140 mg per serving	At least 25% less sodium per serving	If the sodium is reduced by at least 50% per serving
Sugars	<0.5 g	N/A	At least 25% less sugar per serving	N/A

Other Labeling Terms

Term	**Definition**
"High," "Rich in," or "Excellent source of"	The food contains 20% or more of the DV of the nutrient in a serving. Can be used to describe protein, vitamins, minerals, fiber, or potassium.
"Good source of"	A serving of the food provides 10–19% of the DV of the nutrient. Can be used to describe protein, vitamins, minerals, fiber, or potassium.
"More," "Added," "Extra," or "Plus"	A serving of the food provides 10% of the DV. Can only be used to describe vitamins, minerals, protein, fiber, and potassium.
"Lean"	Can be used on seafood and meat that contains less than 10 g of fat, 4.5 g or less of saturated fat, and less than 95 mg of cholesterol per serving.
"Extra lean"	Can be used on seafood and meat that contains less than 5 g of fat, less than 2 g of saturated fat, and less than 95 mg of cholesterol per serving.
"Healthy"	Low in fat and saturated fat; limited in cholesterol content; sodium content can't exceed 360 mg for individual foods or 480 for meal-type foods; contains 10% of the DV of one or more of vitamins A and C, iron, calcium, protein, or fiber.

Note: N/A = not applicable.

TABLE 2.9 Health Claims on Food Labels

Type of Claim	Definition	Examples
Authorized health claims (well established)	Claims are based on a well-established relationship between the food or compound and the health benefit. Food manufacturers must submit a petition to the FDA and provide the scientific research that backs up the claim. If there is significant agreement in the supporting research and a consensus among numerous scientists and experts in the field that there is a relationship between the food or dietary ingredient and the disease or health condition, the FDA will allow an authorized health claim. Specified wording must be used.	The FDA has approved 12 authorized health claims. 1. Calcium and osteoporosis 2. Sodium and hypertension 3. Dietary fat and cancer 4. Dietary saturated fat and cholesterol and risk of coronary heart disease 5. Fiber-containing grain products, fruits, and vegetables and cancer 6. Fruits, vegetables, and grain products that contain fiber, particularly soluble fiber, and the risk of coronary heart disease 7. Fruits and vegetables and cancer 8. Folate and neural tube defects 9. Dietary sugar, alcohol, and dental caries 10. Soluble fiber from certain foods and risk of coronary heart disease 11. Soy protein and risk of coronary heart disease 12. Plant sterol/stanol esters and risk of coronary heart disease
Health claims based on authoritative statements (well established)	Claims based on statements made by a U.S. government agency, such as the Centers for Disease Control and Prevention (CDC) and the National Institutes of Health (NIH). If the FDA approves a claim submitted by the manufacturer, the wording of the claim must include "may," as in "whole grains may help reduce the risk of heart disease," to illustrate that other factors in addition to the food or dietary ingredient may play a role in the disease or condition. This type of health claim can only be used on food and cannot be used on dietary supplements.	• Whole-grain foods and risk of heart disease and certain cancers • Potassium and the risk of high blood pressure • Substitution of saturated fat in the diet with unsaturated fat and reduced risk of heart disease
Qualified health claims (less well established)	Claims based on evidence that is still emerging. However, the current evidence to support the claim is greater than the evidence suggesting that the claim isn't valid. These claims are allowed in order to expedite the communication of potential beneficial health information to the public. They must be accompanied by the statement "the evidence to support the claim is limited or not conclusive" or "some scientific evidence suggests. . . ." Many experts, including the Academy of Nutrition and Dietetics, don't support this type of health claim, as it is based on emerging evidence. Qualified health claims can be used on dietary supplements if approved by the FDA.	• Selenium and cancer • Antioxidant vitamins and cancer • Nuts and heart disease • Omega-3 fatty acids and coronary heart disease • B vitamins and vascular disease • Monounsaturated fatty acids from olive oil and coronary heart disease • Walnuts and heart disease • Psyllium husk and diabetes

Structure/function claims can be made on both foods and dietary supplements. Unlike the health claims, they don't need to be preapproved by the FDA. They do need to be truthful and not misleading, but the manufacturer is responsible for making sure that the claims are accurate.

Structure/function claims can be a source of confusion. Shoppers can easily fall into the trap of assuming that one brand of a product with a structure/function claim on its label is superior to another product without the claim. For instance, a yogurt that says "Calcium builds strong bones" on its label may be identical to another yogurt without the flashy label claim. The consumer has to understand that the yogurt with the claim is not superior to the yogurt without it.

Dietary supplements that use structure/function claims must display a disclaimer on the label stating that the FDA did not evaluate the claim and that the dietary supplement is not intended to "diagnose, treat, cure, or prevent any disease." Manufacturers of foods bearing structure/function claims do not have to display this disclaimer on the label.

Although keeping the types of health claims and the structure/function claims straight can be challenging, here's one way to remember them: Authorized health claims and health claims based on authoritative statements are the strongest, as they are based on years of accumulated research or an authoritative statement. Qualified health claims are made on potentially healthful foods or dietary ingredients but because the evidence is still emerging, the claim has to be "qualified" as such. All health claims provide information on how the food or dietary ingredient can help reduce your risk of a condition or a disease.

Structure/function claims are the weakest claims, as they are just statements or facts about the role the nutrient or dietary ingredient plays in the body. They can't claim how the food or dietary ingredient lowers the risk of developing a chronic disease such as heart disease or cancer. In general, label claims with less established scientific evidence behind them have the weakest wording.

> **LO 2.6: THE TAKE-HOME MESSAGE** The FDA regulates the labeling on all packaged foods. Every food label must contain the name of the food, its net weight, the name and address of the manufacturer or distributor, a list of ingredients, and a Nutrition Facts panel containing standardized nutrition information. The FDA allows the use of nutrient content claims, health claims, and structure/function claims on food labels. Any foods or dietary supplements displaying these label claims must meet specified criteria and the claims must be truthful.

HEALTH**CONNECTION**

Portion Distortion

LO 2.7 Compare the terms *portion* and *serving size* and summarize the health benefits of controlling your portions.

Portion distortion, or perceiving larger portions of food as appropriate sizes, may be contributing to obesity. These larger-than-recommended portion sizes, which are viewed as typical by Americans today, add kilocalories to our diets and may contribute to weight gain.

Portion versus Serving Size: What's the Difference?

The USDA defines a portion as the amount of food eaten at one sitting. In contrast, a serving size (a term that's used only on food labels) is a standard amount of food for which the nutrient composition is presented. We can illustrate the difference with a food that people often pile on their plates, such as spaghetti. A generous

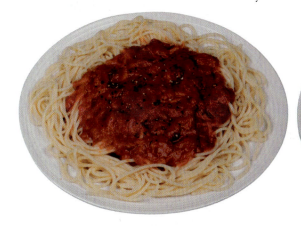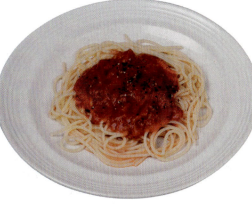

The portion of pasta (left) that Americans typically eat is larger than the serving size indicated on food labels (right).

helping of cooked spaghetti that spills over the edge of a plate is probably equal to about 3 cups. According to MyPlate, a standard serving size of pasta is ½ cup.[30] A portion of 3 cups of cooked pasta is therefore six servings, which contains more than 600 kilocalories!

How Have Portion Sizes Changed?

If your great-grandmother treated herself to a Hershey's chocolate bar when it was first introduced, at the beginning of the last century, she would have purchased a bar weighing about 0.6 ounce. Today the same milk chocolate bar is sold in 0.75-, 1.6-, 2.6-, 4.0-, 7.0-, and 8.0-ounce weights. When McDonald's first introduced French fries in 1954, the standard serving weighed 2.4 ounces. Although a small 2.4-ounce size is still on the menu, you can also choose the medium French fries weighing 5.3 ounces or the large at 6.3 ounces. Twenty years ago, a cup of coffee was 8 ounces and just 45 kilocalories with added milk and sugar. Today, consumers enjoy 16-ounce lattes on their way to work, to the tune of 350 kilocalories.[31] As you can see, portion sizes have changed across the menu.

The restaurant industry has appealed to Americans' interest in getting more food for less money with larger portion sizes at relatively low costs. Americans eat out more often than they did in the past and are often offered a wide variety of inexpensive choices sold in portion sizes that typically exceed the standards defined in MyPlate.[32] Most people are unaware of the changes in their portion sizes. And even when they are aware, they don't necessarily change their behavior. Recent studies show that posting the kilocalorie content of menu items on sign boards or on menus has little impact on consumers' behavior.[33] Though getting more food for the money may be beneficial on the wallet, the health costs may be higher than Americans realize.

In addition to restaurant and packaged foods, home-cooked meals have also bulked up over the past few decades. If you were to measure your grandmother's favorite dinner plates, they would likely be much smaller, about 9 inches in diameter, than the plates in your cupboard, which probably measure closer to 11.5 inches across. The bigger the plate, the more food you are likely to put on it. Furthermore, the larger the portion we put on that plate, the less accurate we are in our estimate of how many kilocalories we're consuming.

Health Effects of Increased Portion Size

Research has shown that an increase in the portion sizes of typical foods can lead to increased energy intake and weight gain.[34,35,36] As body weight increases, the risk of developing chronic diseases—including cardiovascular disease, diabetes, joint problems, and some cancers—also increases. Moreover, eating larger portions of foods high in added sugars and saturated fats not only increases your daily kilocalorie intake but can also decrease the amount of nutrients you consume overall. For example, eating a large portion of red meat as an entrée will increase the total fat, saturated fat, and cholesterol you consume. Instead, if the meat portion is limited and the plate is filled with large portions of vegetables, fruits, and a reasonable portion of whole grains, the result is an increase in the vitamins, minerals, phytochemicals, and dietary fiber in the meal and a decrease in the total kilocalories.

Tips for Controlling Portion Size

Unfortunately, many of us frequently underestimate the portion sizes we put on our plates or in our glasses and therefore overeat.[37] One easy way to tell if you are helping yourself to too much of a food is to use a visual that represents a standard serving size of the food, such as a cup of vegetables, three ounces of meat, or 1 tablespoon of salad dressing. Having a food scale available is not always possible. Instead, use an everyday item that you always have with you—your hand—to visualize the correct portion sizes (**Figure 2.12**). This provides an easy

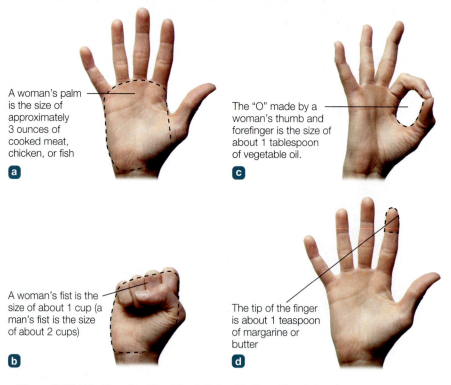

A woman's palm is the size of approximately 3 ounces of cooked meat, chicken, or fish

a

A woman's fist is the size of about 1 cup (a man's fist is the size of about 2 cups)

b

The "O" made by a woman's thumb and forefinger is the size of about 1 tablespoon of vegetable oil.

c

The tip of the finger is about 1 teaspoon of margarine or butter

d

▲ **Figure 2.12 What's a Portion Size? Eat with Your Hands!**
Your hands can help you estimate the appropriate portion size of foods.

TABLE 2.10	Controlling Portion Sizes
When You Are . . .	**Do This**
At Home	• Measure your food until you develop an "eye" for correct portion sizes, and check your measurements now and then to make sure they haven't crept up. • Use smaller plates so portions appear larger. • Plate your food at the counter before sitting down at the table. • Store leftover foods in portion-controlled containers. • Don't eat snacks directly from the box or bag; measure a portion first, then eat only that amount. • Cook smaller quantities of food so you don't pick at the leftovers. • Keep tempting foods, such as sweets and chips, out of sight.
Eating Out	• Ask for half orders when available. • Order an appetizer as your entrée. • Don't be compelled to "clean your plate"; stop eating when you're full and take the rest home.
Buying Groceries	• Divide a package of snacks into individual portion sizes and consume only one portion at any one sitting. • Be aware of the number of servings in a package; read the labels. • Buy foods that are already divided into portion sizes, such as 1 oz sliced cheese or lunch meat. • Avoid "mini" sizes of crackers, cookies, etc.; just because they're small doesn't mean you can eat the whole box!

way to approximate how much you are consuming.

Other steps that can help reduce oversized portions include buying smaller or single-portion packages of foods or dividing larger packages into individual portion sizes. In restaurants, order one meal to share with your companion, or split the food in half and take the other half home. In your cupboard, replace larger glasses and plates with smaller versions. **Table 2.10** provides further tips for controlling your portion sizes at home and elsewhere.

LO 2.7: THE TAKE-HOME MESSAGE A portion size is defined as the amount of food eaten at one sitting, whereas a serving size is the standard amount of food for nutrient comparison used on nutrient labels. Portion sizes have continued to increase over the last few decades, and increased portion sizes are thought to have contributed to America's incidence of overweight and obesity. The risk of developing chronic diseases, including cardiovascular disease, diabetes, joint problems, and even some cancers, increases as body weight increases. Measure your foods until you recognize a healthy portion size, use smaller glasses and plates, divide larger packages of food into individual portion sizes, and share meals when eating out to control portion sizes.

Visual Chapter Summary

LO 2.1 Healthy Eating Is Based on Five Key Principles

Healthy eating involves the key principles of balance, variety, and moderation. Foods should also be nutrient dense to provide adequate nutrition, but low in energy density to prevent unwanted weight gain.

LO 2.2 Dietary Reference Intakes Are Reference Values for Each Nutrient

The Dietary Reference Intakes (DRIs) are specific reference values, based on age and gender, that express the quantities of the essential nutrients needed daily. The DRIs are designed to prevent nutrient deficiencies, maintain good health, prevent chronic diseases, and avoid unhealthy excesses. The DRIs consist of the Estimated Average Requirement, Recommended Dietary Allowance, Adequate Intake, Tolerable Upper Intake Level, and the Acceptable Macronutrient Distribution Ranges. The Estimate Energy Requirement indicates how much energy an individual needs based on age, gender, and activity level.

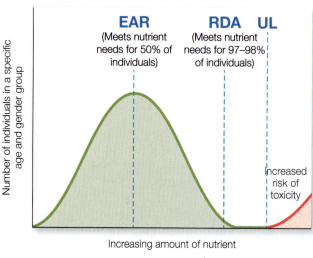

LO 2.3 *Dietary Guidelines for Americans* Are Recommendations to Lower Risk of Disease

The *Dietary Guidelines for Americans* are published every 5 years by the USDA and HHS to provide Americans with current, research-based nutrition and physical activity recommendations. The current DGAs emphasize following a healthy eating pattern such as a Mediterranean-style diet, a vegetarian diet, or another diet rich in fruits, vegetables, and whole grains. Following the DGAs can help improve the quality of the diet and lower the risk of obesity and certain chronic diseases.

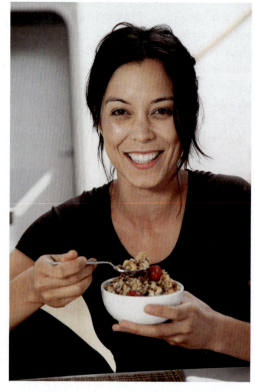

LO 2.4 MyPlate Includes an Icon for Healthy Eating and an Accompanying Website

MyPlate is an icon that serves as a reminder for healthy eating. It helps consumers plan a plant-based diet that meets the recommendations of the DGAs and the DRIs for the essential nutrients. There are five food groups: fruits, vegetables, grains, protein, and dairy. Oils are not shown on MyPlate because they are not a food group but are an important part of a healthy diet.

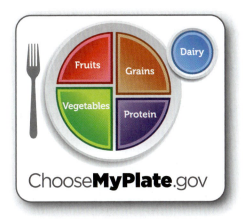

LO 2.5 The Exchange System Is Based on the Macronutrient Content of Foods

Exchange lists group foods according to their carbohydrate, protein, fat, and kilocalorie content while providing specific portion sizes. Using the exchange lists for meal planning is a convenient method for developing flexible meal plans.

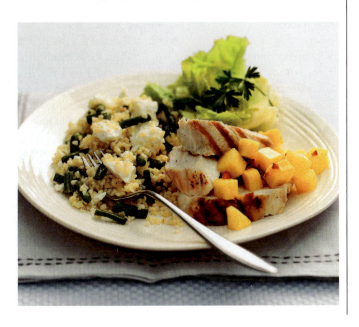

LO 2.6 The Required Components of Food Labels Provide Important Nutrition Information

The FDA regulates the information found on food labels. The Nutrition Facts panel must list the serving size of the food and the corresponding amount of kilocalories, fat, saturated fat, *trans* fat, cholesterol, sodium, sugars, added sugars, dietary fiber, protein, vitamin D, and calcium, iron, and potassium. The percent Daily Values are reference levels of intakes for the nutrients listed on the food label.

A food label can carry a nutrient content claim using descriptive terms such as *free*, *high*, and *extra lean*, as long as it meets strict FDA criteria. Health claims can also be used on food labels. These contain a food compound or a dietary ingredient and an associated disease or health-related condition. Structure/function claims describe how a food or dietary compound affects the structure or function of the body, and are not subject to FDA regulation.

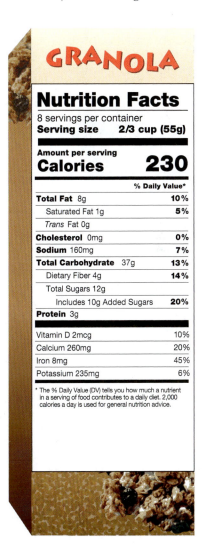

LO 2.7 Controlling Portion Size Can Reduce the Risk of Weight Gain and Chronic Disease

A portion size is the amount of food eaten at one sitting, regardless of the standard serving size printed on food labels. Larger portion sizes can lead to increased energy intake and weight gain. Over time weight gain can increase your risk for cardiovascular disease, diabetes, joint problems, and certain cancers. Learn to recognize a healthy portion size, use smaller plates and glassware, and divide large portions into individual portions to improve healthy eating and prevent weight gain.

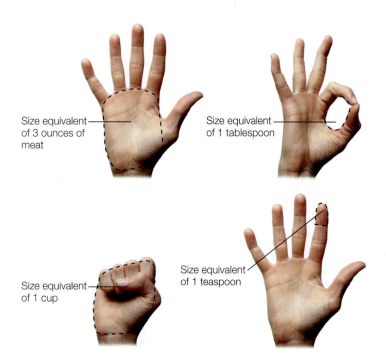

Size equivalent of 3 ounces of meat

Size equivalent of 1 tablespoon

Size equivalent of 1 cup

Size equivalent of 1 teaspoon

Terms to Know

- balance
- vary
- moderate
- nutrient density
- energy density
- portion
- satiety
- Dietary Reference Intakes (DRIs)
- nutrient requirements
- Estimated Average Requirement (EAR)
- Recommended Dietary Allowance (RDA)
- Adequate Intake (AI)
- Tolerable Upper Intake Level (UL)
- toxicity
- Acceptable Macronutrient Distribution Ranges (AMDRs)
- Estimated Energy Requirement (EER)
- *Dietary Guidelines for Americans*
- MyPlate
- proportionality
- exchange lists
- Nutrition Facts panel
- serving size
- percent Daily Values (%DVs)

Mastering Nutrition

Visit the Study Area in Mastering Nutrition to hear an MP3 chapter summary.

Check Your Understanding

LO2.1 1. Nutrient-dense foods
   a. contain an equal balance of carbohydrates, proteins, and fats.
   b. are high in nutrients and lower in kilocalories.
   c. have a nutrition label.
   d. have greater weight than volume.

LO2.1 2. Which of the following foods is the most nutrient dense?
   a. An orange ice pop
   b. An orange
   c. Orange-flavored soda
   d. Orange sherbet

LO2.2 3. The Dietary Reference Intakes (DRIs) are reference values for nutrients and are designed to
   a. only prevent nutritional deficiencies.
   b. provide a general range of nutrient needs.
   c. prevent nutritional deficiencies and toxicities and maintain good health.
   d. apply only to infants and children.

LO2.2 4. An Estimated Average Requirement (EAR) is
   a. the estimated amount of a nutrient that should be consumed daily to be healthy.
   b. the amount of a nutrient that meets the average needs of 50 percent of individuals in a specific age and gender group.
   c. the maximum safe amount of a nutrient that should be consumed daily.
   d. the amount of a nutrient that meets the needs of 99 percent of the population.

LO2.3 5. The *Dietary Guidelines for Americans* recommend that you
   a. limit the amount of saturated fat and added sugars in your diet.
   b. stop smoking and walk daily.
   c. sleep 8 hours a night and jog every other day.
   d. maintain a kilocalorie balance over time and stop smoking.

LO2.4 6. Which of the following are the food groups in MyPlate?
   a. Grains, vegetables, dairy, sweets, and protein
   b. Grains, fruits, alcohol, sweets, and proteins
   c. Grains, vegetables, fruits, dairy, and protein
   d. Grains, vegetables, oils, dairy, and proteins

LO 2.5 7. The exchange system places foods in groups based on their carbohydrate, fat, and protein content.
   a. True
   b. False

LO 2.6 8. By law, which of the following *must* be listed on the new Nutrition Facts panel?
   a. %DV for kilocalories, total sugars, and protein
   b. Saturated fat, vitamin A, and vitamin C
   c. Kilocalories, added sugars, and potassium per serving
   d. Vitamin A, vitamin E, and folate

LO 2.6 9. A yogurt that states that a serving provides 30 percent of the percent Daily Value (%DV) for calcium contains a _____ amount of calcium.
   a. high
   b. medium
   c. low
   d. negligible

LO 2.10 10. At his campus dining hall, Hamid serves himself—and eats—two heaping ladles of rice. This amount is
   a. a standard serving size.
   b. Hamid's serving size.
   c. a standard portion.
   d. Hamid's portion.

Answers

1. (b) Nutrient-dense foods are high in nutrients, such as vitamins and minerals, but low in energy (kilocalories).

2. (b) Though an orange ice pop or orange sherbet may be a refreshing treat on a hot day, the orange is by far the most nutrient-dense food among these choices. The orange-flavored soda is a sugary drink.

3. (c) The DRIs recommend the amount of nutrients needed to prevent deficiencies, maintain good health, and avoid toxicities. Values are provided for populations ranging from infants to older adults.

4. (b) The EAR is the amount of a nutrient that would meet the needs of half of the individuals in a specific age and gender group. The EAR is used to obtain the Recommended Dietary Allowance (RDA), which is the amount of a nutrient that should be consumed daily to maintain good health. The Tolerable Upper Intake Level (UL) is the maximum amount of a nutrient that can be consumed on a regular basis that is unlikely to cause harm.

5. (a) The *Dietary Guidelines for Americans* recommend that you limit the amount of saturated fat and added sugars in your diet. Walking or jogging are wonderful ways to be physically active. Though the *Dietary Guidelines* do not specifically address stopping smoking, this is a habit worth kicking. Sleeping 8 hours a night isn't mentioned in the *Dietary Guidelines* but is another beneficial lifestyle habit.

6. (c) Grains, vegetables, fruits, dairy, and protein are the five basic food groups in MyPlate. Plant and fish oils are healthful, but do not constitute a MyPlate food group. Sweets and alcohol are not food groups and should be limited in the diet.

7. (a) True. The exchange system lists the foods in groupings according to their carbohydrate, protein, and fat composition and provides specific portion sizes for each food.

8. (c) The new Nutrition Facts panel must indicate the amounts per serving of kilocalories, added sugars, and potassium. Vitamins A, C, E, and folate do not have to be listed unless they have been added to the food and/or the product makes a claim about them on the label. The panel does not indicate the %DV for kilocalories, total sugars, or protein; however, the %DV for added sugars is listed.

9. (a) Foods that provide 20 percent or more of the %DV for a nutrient are considered "high" in that nutrient. If the label states that a serving contains 5 percent or less of the %DV, it is considered "low" in that nutrient.

10. (d) A portion is the amount of food eaten at one sitting; thus, the two heaping ladles of rice is Hamid's portion. There are no standardized portions. A serving size is a standard amount of food for which the nutrient composition is presented. It is a term used on food labels.

Answers to True or False?

1. **False.** Having a balanced diet means not eating too much of any one food.

2. **False.** Because consuming too much of some essential nutrients can be harmful, the Tolerable Upper Intake Level (UL) of the DRIs was established for many nutrients.

3. **True.** The Dietary Reference Intakes are specific reference values for each nutrient according to age, gender, and life stage. They were established to prevent nutrient deficiencies and toxicities and to maintain good health and reduce the risk of developing chronic diseases.

4. **True.** These *Dietary Guidelines for Americans* are the latest recommendations for nutrition and physical activity for Americans over the age of 2.

5. **True.** The five food groups that make up the MyPlate recommendations are grains, vegetables, fruits, dairy, and protein.

6. **False.** Oils are not considered a food group but you should consume some daily for good health.

7. **True.** Exchange lists allow you to swap foods within each food group while still controlling the amount of carbohydrate, protein, fat, and kilocalories you ingest.

8. **False.** A nutrient content claim uses descriptive terms (such as low sodium or fat free) to make a claim about the amount of a nutrient a serving of the food contains (or doesn't contain). Specific terms approved by the FDA must be used.

9. **True.** The FDA requires that all packaged food items be labeled with specific information.

10. **False.** A portion of food is the amount of food you choose to eat. A standard serving size is defined by the USDA as a standard amount used on food labels.

Web Resources

■ For more tips and resources for MyPlate, visit www.ChooseMyPlate .gov.

■ For details on the latest *Dietary Guidelines for Americans*, visit Department of Health and Human Services https://health. gov/dietaryguidelines/.

■ For more on food labels, visit www .fda.gov.

References

1. Freeland-Graves, J. H., and S. Nitzke. 2013. Position of the Academy of Nutrition and Dietetics: Total Diet Approach to Healthy Eating. *Journal of the Academy of Nutrition and Dietetics.* 113(2):307–317.
2. Ibid.
3. Produce for Better Health Foundation. *Fruits and Vegetables—More Matters.* Available at www.fruitsandveggiesmorematters.org. Accessed February 2017.
4. U.S. Department of Health and Human Services and U.S. Department of Agriculture. *2015–2020 Dietary Guidelines for Americans.* 8th Edition. December 2015. Available at http://health.gov/dietaryguidelines/2015/ guidelines/. Accessed February 2017.
5. Stelmach-Mardas, Marta, Tomasz Rodacki, et al. 2016. Link Between Food Energy Density and Body Weight Changes in Obese Adults. *Nutrients* 8(4):229.
6. Ibid.
7. Eldridge, Johanna D., Carol M. Devine, et al. 2016. Environmental Influences on Small Eating Behavior Change to Promote Weight Loss among Black and Hispanic Populations. *Appetite* 96:129–137.
8. Lau, D. C., and H. Teoh. 2013. Benefits of Modest Weight Loss on the Management of Type 2 Diabetes Mellitus. *Canadian Journal of Diabetes* 37(2):128–134.
9. Williams, R. A., L. S. Roe, et al. 2013. Comparison of Three Methods to Reduce Energy Density. Effects on Energy Density Intake. *Appetite* 66:75–83.
10. Institute of Medicine. 2003. Dietary Reference Intakes: Applications in Dietary Planning. Washington, DC: The National Academies Press. Updated 2013. Available at http://fnic.nal.usda.gov. Accessed February 2017.
11. Ibid.
12. Ibid.
13. Ibid.
14. Mowry, James B., Daniel A. Spyker, et al. 2015. 2014 Annual Report of the American Association of Poison Control Centers' National Poison Data System (NPDS): 32nd Annual Report. *Clinical Toxicology* 53, Iss. 10.
15. U.S. Department of Health and Human Services and U.S. Department of Agriculture. 2015.
16. Farazo, E. 1999. *America's Eating Habits: Changes and Consequences.* Updated 2012. Available at www.ers.usda.gov. Accessed February 2017.
17. Lee, P. R. 1978. Nutrition Policy: From Neglect and Uncertainty to Debate and Action. *Journal of the American Dietetic Association* 72:581–588.

18. Report of the DGAC on the *Dietary Guidelines for Americans, 2015.* 2015. Available at https://health.gov/dietaryguidelines/2015-scientific-report/PDFs/Scientific-Report-of-the-2015-Dietary-Guidelines-Advisory-Committee.pdf. Accessed February 2017.

19. U.S. Department of Health and Human Services and U.S. Department of Agriculture. *2015–2020 Dietary Guidelines for Americans.* 8th Edition. December 2015. Available at http://health.gov/dietaryguidelines/2015/guidelines/. Accessed February 2017.

20. Food and Drug Administration. Revised 2013. *A Food Labeling Guide.* Available at www.fda.gov. Accessed February 2017.

21. Food and Drug Administration. 2016. CFR – Code of Federal Regulations Title 21. Available at www.accessdata.fda.gov/scripts/cdrh/cfdocs/cfcfr/CFRSearch.cfm?fr=101.45. Accessed February 2017.

22. Ibid.

23. USDA 2016. Nutrition Labeling Information. Available at https://www.fsis.usda.gov/wps/portal/fsis/topics/regulatory-compliance/labeling/labeling-policies/nutrition-labeling-policies/nutrition-labeling. Accessed February 2017.

24. Food and Drug Administration. 2013. *Nutrition Labeling; Questions L1 through L153. Food Labeling and Nutrition.* Available at www.fda.gov/Food/GuidanceRegulation/GuidanceDocumentsRegulatoryInformation/LabelingNutrition/ucm064904.htm#exempt. Accessed February 2017.

25. Food and Drug Administration. 2016. How to Understand and Use the Nutrition Facts Label. Available at www.fda.gov/Food/IngredientsPackagingLabeling/LabelingNutrition/ucm274593.htm. Accessed February 2017.

26. Kurtzweil, P. 1998. Staking a Claim to Good Health. *FDA Consumer.*

27. Food and Drug Administration. 2015 Guidance for Industry: A Food Labeling Guide (8. Claims). Available at http://www.fda.gov/Food/GuidanceRegulation/GuidanceDocumentsRegulatoryInformation/LabelingNutrition/ucm064908.htm. Accessed February 2017.

28. Food and Drug Administration. 2016. Structure/Function Claims. Available at www.fda.gov/Food/IngredientsPackagingLabeling/LabelingNutrition/ucm2006881.htm. Accessed February 2017.

29. Academy of Nutrition and Dietetics. 2013. Position of the Academy of Nutrition and Dietetics: Functional Foods. *Journal of the Academy of Nutrition and Dietetics* 113:1096–1103.

30. USDA Choose My Plate. 2016. Grains. Available at https://www.choosemyplate.gov/grains. Accessed February 2017.

31. Just, D. R., and B. Wansink. 2013. One Man's Tall Is Another Man's Small: How the Framing of Portion Size Influences Food Choice. *Health Economics.* DOI:10.1002/hec.2949.

32. Herman, C., J. Polivy, et al. 2016. Are Large Portions Responsible for the Obesity Epidemic? *Physiology and Behavior* 156: 177–181.

33. Downs, J. S., J. Wisdom, et al. 2013. Supplementing Menu Labeling with Calorie Recommendations to Test for Facilitation Effects. *American Journal of Public Health* 103(9):1604–1609.

34. Syrad, H., C. Llewellyn, et al. 2016. Meal Size Is a Critical Driver of Weight Gain in Early Childhood. *Scientific Reports.* DOI: 10.1038/srep28368.

35. Urban, L. E., A. H. Lichtenstein, et al. 2013. The Energy Content of Restaurant Foods without Stated Calorie Information. *Journal of the American Medical Association Internal Medicine* 173(14):1292–1299.

36. Young, L. R., and M. Nestle. 2012. Reducing Portion Sizes to Prevent Obesity. *American Journal of Preventive Medicine* 43(5): 565–568.

37. Almiron-Roig, E., I. Solis-Trapala, et al. 2013. Estimating Food Portions. Influence of Unit Number, Meal Type and Energy Density. *Appetite* 71:95–103.

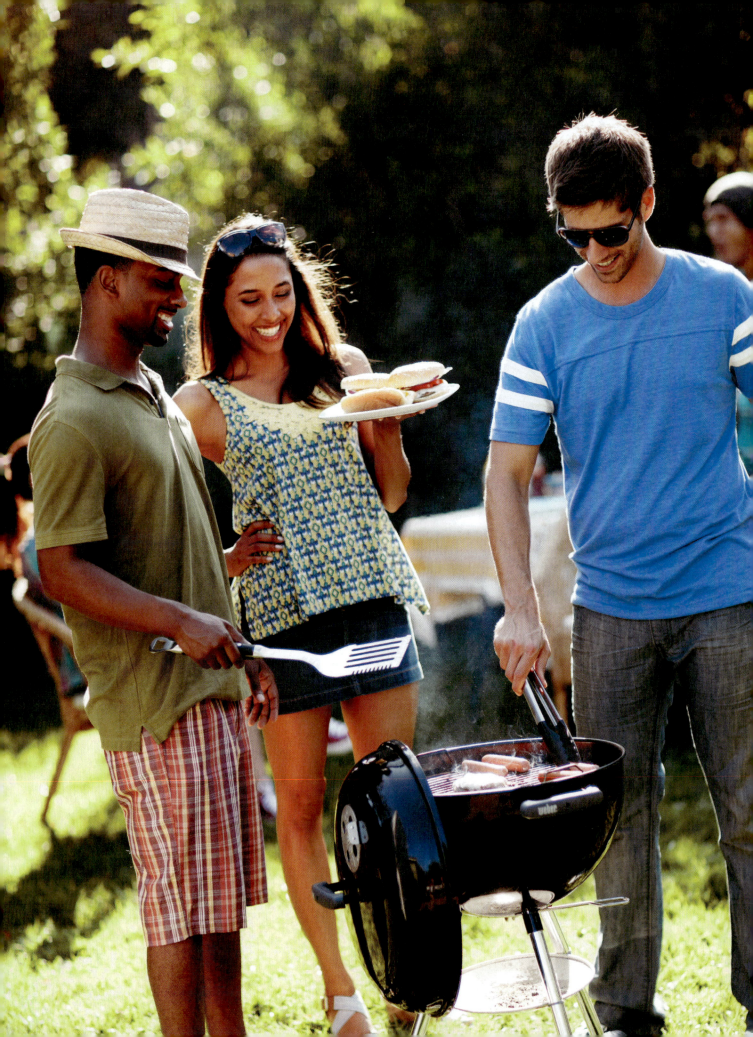

Digestion, Absorption, and Transport

Learning Outcomes

After reading this chapter, you will be able to:

3.1 Describe the processes and organs involved in digestion.

3.2 Explain how food is propelled through the gastrointestinal tract.

3.3 Identify the role of enzymes and other secretions in chemical digestion.

3.4 Describe how digested nutrients are absorbed.

3.5 Explain how hormones and the nervous system regulate digestion.

3.6 Explain how absorbed nutrients are transported throughout the body.

3.7 Discuss the most common digestive disorders.

True or False?

1. Saliva can alter the taste of food. **T**/**F**
2. Without mucus, the stomach would digest itself. **T**/**F**
3. The major function of bile is to emulsify fats. **T**/**F**
4. Acid reflux is caused by gas in the stomach. **T**/**F**
5. The primary function of the large intestine is to absorb water. **T**/**F**
6. Feces contain a high amount of bacteria. **T**/**F**
7. The lymphatic system transports all nutrients through the body once they've been absorbed. **T**/**F**
8. Hormones play an important role in digestion. **T**/**F**
9. Diarrhea is always caused by bacterial infection. **T**/**F**
10. Irritable bowel syndrome is caused by an allergy to gluten. **T**/**F**

See page 110 for the answers.

The digestion of food begins even before you take that first bite. Just the sight and smell of homemade apple pie stimulates the release of saliva in the mouth. The secretion of saliva and other digestive juices starts a cascade of events that prepares the body for **digestion**, the chemical and mechanical processes by which the body breaks food down into individual nutrient molecules ready for **absorption**. Food components that aren't absorbed are excreted as waste (feces) by **elimination**. Although these are complex processes, they go largely unnoticed. You consciously chew and swallow the pie, but you don't feel the release of chemicals or the muscular contractions that cause it to be digested or the absorption of nutrient molecules through the intestinal lining cells. In fact, you may be unaware of the entire process until about 48 hours after eating, when the body is ready to eliminate waste.

In this chapter, we explore the processes of digestion, absorption, and elimination, the organs involved, and the other biological mechanisms that regulate our bodies' processing of food and nutrients. We also discuss the causes and treatments of some common gastrointestinal conditions and disorders.

digestion Process that breaks down food into individual molecules small enough to be absorbed through the intestinal wall.

absorption Process of moving nutrients from the GI tract into the circulatory system.

elimination Excretion of undigested and unabsorbed food through the feces.

gastrointestinal (GI) tract Tubular organ system including the mouth, pharynx, esophagus, stomach, and small and large intestines, by means of which food is digested, nutrients absorbed, and wastes expelled.

lumen Channel or inside space of a vessel such as the intestine or artery.

propulsion Process that moves food along the GI tract during digestion.

sphincters Circular rings of muscle that open and close in response to nerve input.

chemical digestion Breaking down food through enzymatic reactions.

mechanical digestion Breaking down food by chewing, grinding, squeezing, and moving it through the GI tract by peristalsis and segmentation.

mastication Chewing food.

saliva Secretion from the salivary glands that softens and lubricates food and begins the chemical breakdown of starch.

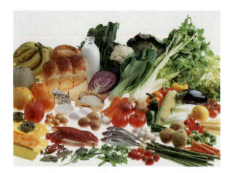

Whole foods must first be broken down into individual nutrients that can be used by the body's cells.

What Are the Processes and Organs Involved in Digestion?

LO 3.1 Describe the processes and organs involved in digestion.

Digestion, absorption, and elimination occur in the **gastrointestinal (GI) tract**, a muscular tube approximately 20–24 feet long in an adult. Stretched vertically, the tube would be about as high as a two-story building. It provides a barrier between the food within the **lumen** (the hollow interior of the tract), which is technically external, and our body cells, which are internal.

Although the prefix *gastro-* means "stomach," the GI tract actually extends from the mouth to the anus. Its six organs are the mouth, pharynx, esophagus, stomach, small intestine, and large intestine. Food moves from one organ to the next by **propulsion**. Various **sphincters** along the way allow food to pass. These muscular rings act like one-way doors, allowing the mixture of food and digestive juices to flow into the next organ but not to flow back. **Focus Figure 3.1** illustrates the organs and processes of the digestive system.

Digestion Begins in the Mouth

The body digests food *chemically,* by the actions of digestive secretions, and *mechanically,* by the actions of the teeth and the powerful muscles of the GI tract. Both **chemical digestion** and **mechanical digestion** begin in the mouth. During **mastication**, the teeth, powered by strong jaw muscles, mechanically cut and grind food into smaller pieces as the tongue mixes it with **saliva**. Saliva dissolves small food particles, which allows them to react with the taste buds so we can savor food. About 99 percent water, saliva moistens and binds food to lubricate it for comfortable swallowing and traveling down the esophagus. Saliva also contains enzymes, compounds that help accelerate the rate of chemical reactions. Enzymes are discussed in detail later in this chapter. The primary enzyme in saliva is salivary amylase, which begins to break down carbohydrates. (You can taste this enzyme working when you eat a starch-containing food such as a cracker; as the enzyme breaks down starch into sugars, the flavor becomes sweeter.)

Head to Mastering Nutrition and watch a narrated video tour of this figure by author Joan Salge Blake.

The human digestive system consists of the organs of the gastrointestinal (GI) tract and associated accessory organs. The processing of food in the GI tract involves ingestion, mechanical digestion, chemical digestion, propulsion, absorption, and elimination.

ORGANS OF THE GI TRACT

MOUTH

Ingestion Food enters the GI tract via the mouth.

Mechanical digestion Mastication tears, shreds, and mixes food with saliva, forming a bolus.

Chemical digestion Salivary amylase begins carbohydrate breakdown.

PHARYNX AND ESOPHAGUS

Propulsion Swallowing and peristalsis move the bolus from mouth to stomach.

STOMACH

Mechanical digestion This process mixes and churns the bolus with acid, enzymes, and gastric fluid into a liquid called chyme.

Chemical digestion Pepsin begins digestion of proteins.

Absorption A few fat-soluble substances are absorbed through the stomach wall.

SMALL INTESTINE

Mechanical digestion and **Propulsion** Segmentation mixes chyme with digestive juices; peristaltic waves move it along the tract.

Chemical digestion Digestive enzymes from the pancreas and brush border digest most classes of food.

Absorption Nutrients are absorbed into blood and lymph through enterocytes.

LARGE INTESTINE

Chemical digestion Some remaining food residues are digested by bacteria.

Absorption Salts, water, and some vitamins are reabsorbed.

Propulsion Compacts waste into feces.

RECTUM

Elimination Feces are temporarily stored before voluntary release through the anus.

ACCESSORY ORGANS

SALIVARY GLANDS

Produce saliva, a mixture of water, mucus, enzymes, and other chemicals

LIVER

Produces bile to digest fats.

GALLBLADDER

Stores bile before release into the small intestine through the bile duct.

PANCREAS

Produces digestive enzymes and bicarbonate ions that are released into the small intestine via the pancreatic duct.

Once food has been adequately chewed and moistened, the tongue rolls it into a **bolus** and thrusts it into the **pharynx** to be swallowed. The pharynx is the gateway to the **esophagus**, as well as to the *trachea* (or windpipe, the tube that connects to the lungs). Normally, a flap of cartilage called the **epiglottis** closes off the trachea during swallowing, so that food doesn't accidentally "go down the wrong pipe" (see **Figure 3.2**). When the epiglottis doesn't work properly, food can get lodged in the trachea and potentially cause choking.

The esophagus has only one function—to transport food and fluids from the mouth to the stomach. As food passes through the pharynx, the **upper esophageal sphincter** opens, allowing the bolus to enter the esophagus. After swallowing, rhythmic muscular contractions, with the help of gravity, move the bolus toward the stomach. The esophagus narrows at the bottom (just above the stomach) and ends at the **lower esophageal sphincter (LES)** (**Figure 3.3**). Under normal conditions, when the bolus reaches the stomach, the LES relaxes and allows food to pass into the stomach. The stomach also relaxes to comfortably receive the bolus. After food enters the stomach, the LES closes to prevent the stomach contents from regurgitating backward into the esophagus.

The Stomach Stores, Mixes, and Prepares Food for Digestion

The primary function of the **stomach** is to mix food with various gastric juices to chemically break it down into smaller and smaller pieces (**Figure 3.4**). The stomach lining includes four layers. The innermost layer contains **goblet cells** and **gastric pits** or ducts, which contain gastric glands that secrete a variety of critical digestive juices. Various other cells in the stomach lining, among them **parietal** (*puh-RAHY-i-tl*) **cells**, **chief cells**, and mucous neck cells, secrete other gastric juices and **mucus**. The gastric juices are discussed later in this chapter.

Mechanical digestion in the stomach occurs as the *longitudinal, circular,* and *diagonal* muscles that surround the organ forcefully push, churn, and mix the contents of the stomach with the gastric juices. These powerful muscles can also stretch to accommodate different volumes of food. An empty stomach can hold a little less than a cup, but the numerous folds of the stomach lining can stretch out after a large meal to hold up to 1 gallon (4 liters).[1] For several hours, food is continuously churned and mixed in the stomach.

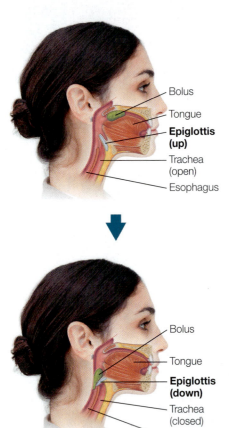

▲ **Figure 3.2 The Role of the Epiglottis**
The epiglottis prevents food from entering the trachea during swallowing.

bolus Soft mass of chewed food.

pharynx Area of the GI tract between the mouth and the esophagus; also called the *throat*.

esophagus Tube that connects the mouth to the stomach.

epiglottis Cartilage at the back of the tongue that closes off the trachea during swallowing.

upper esophageal sphincter Muscular ring located at the top of the esophagus.

lower esophageal sphincter (LES) Muscular ring located between the base of the esophagus and the stomach.

stomach J-shaped muscular organ that mixes and churns food with digestive juices and acid to form chyme.

goblet cells Cells throughout the GI tract that secrete mucus.

gastric pits Indentations or small pits in the stomach lining where the gastric glands are located; gastric glands produce gastric juices.

parietal cells Specialized cells in the stomach that secrete the gastric juices hydrochloric acid and intrinsic factor.

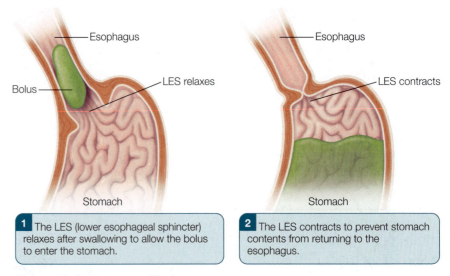

1 The LES (lower esophageal sphincter) relaxes after swallowing to allow the bolus to enter the stomach.

2 The LES contracts to prevent stomach contents from returning to the esophagus.

▲ **Figure 3.3 Sphincters at Work**
Sphincters control the passage of food by contracting or relaxing.

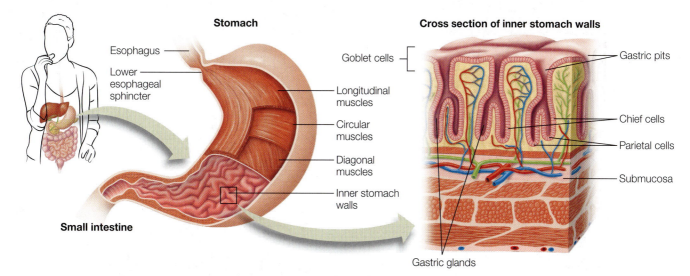

Stomach

Cross section of inner stomach walls

Esophagus

Lower esophageal sphincter

Longitudinal muscles

Circular muscles

Diagonal muscles

Inner stomach walls

Small intestine

Goblet cells

Gastric pits

Chief cells

Parietal cells

Submucosa

Gastric glands

▲ **Figure 3.4 Anatomy of the Stomach**
The cross section of the stomach illustrates the gastric cells that secrete digestive juices.

By the time the mixture reaches the lower portion of the stomach, it is a semiliquid mass called **chyme**, which contains digestive secretions plus the original food. As the chyme accumulates near the pyloric sphincter, between the stomach and the small intestine, the sphincter relaxes and the chyme gradually enters the small intestine. You eat much faster than you can digest and absorb food, so the stomach also acts as a holding tank for chyme until it can be released into the small intestine. Approximately 1–5 milliliters (1 teaspoon) of chyme is released into the small intestine every 30 seconds.[2] The pyloric sphincter prevents chyme from exiting the stomach too soon and blocks the intestinal contents from returning to the stomach.

Most Digestion Occurs in the Small Intestine

As chyme passes through the pyloric sphincter, it enters the long, coiled **small intestine**. This organ consists of three segments—the duodenum, jejunum, and ileum—and extends from the pyloric sphincter to the ileocecal valve at the beginning of the large intestine (**Figure 3.5**). The first segment, the duodenum, is approximately 10 inches long. The second, the jejunum, measures about 8 feet long, and the third, the ileum, is about 12 feet long. The "small" in "small intestine" refers to its diameter (about 1 inch), not its extended length.

As in the stomach, both mechanical and chemical digestion occur in the small intestine. Muscular contractions squeeze chyme forward while digestive secretions from the pancreas, gallbladder, and intestinal lining chemically break down the nutrients.

Numerous fingerlike projections, called **villi**, line the small intestine. They increase the surface area to maximize absorption and help mix the partially digested chyme with intestinal secretions (**Focus Figure 3.6**). Each villus contains capillaries and lymphatic vessels called *lacteals* that pick up digested nutrients during absorption. The villi extend about 1 millimeter into the lumen, creating a velvety appearance, and are arranged into hundreds of overlapping, circular folds. The circular folds cause chyme to spiral forward through the small intestine, further increasing its exposure to the villi.

chief cells Specialized cells in the stomach that secrete pepsinogen, an inactive form of the protein-digesting enzyme pepsin.

mucus Secretion produced throughout the GI tract that moistens and lubricates food and protects membranes.

chyme Semiliquid, partially digested food mass that leaves the stomach and enters the small intestine.

small intestine Long coiled chamber that is the major site of food digestion and nutrient absorption.

villi Small, fingerlike projections that line the lumen of the small intestine.

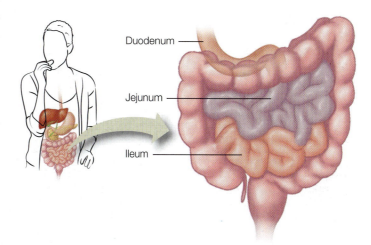

Duodenum

Jejunum

Ileum

▲ **Figure 3.5 Anatomy of the Small Intestine**
The small intestine is highly adapted for absorbing nutrients. Its length—about 20 feet—provides a huge surface area, and its wall has three structural features—circular folds, villi, and microvilli—that increase its surface area by a factor of more than 600.

Head to **Mastering** Nutrition and watch a narrated video tour of this figure by author Joan Salge Blake.

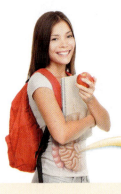

The small intestine is highly adapted for absorbing nutrients. Its length—about 20 feet—provides a huge surface area, and its wall has three structural features—circular folds, villi, and microvilli—that increase its surface area by a factor of more than 600.

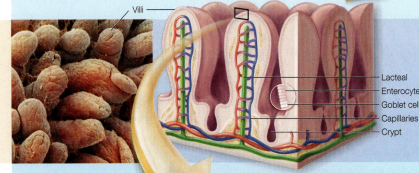

CIRCULAR FOLDS

The lining of the small intestine is heavily folded, resulting in increased surface area for the absorption of nutrients.

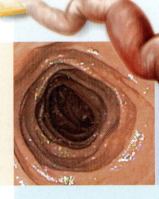

Small Intestine

VILLI

The folds are covered with villi, thousands of fingerlike projections that increase the surface area even further. Each villus contains capillaries and a lacteal for picking up nutrients absorbed through the enterocytes and transporting them throughout the body.

Villi

Lacteal
Enterocyte
Goblet cell
Capillaries
Crypt

Microvilli (brush border)

MICROVILLI

The cells on the surface of the villi, enterocytes, end in hairlike projections called microvilli that together form the brush border through which nutrients are absorbed.

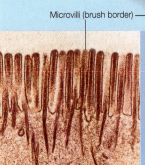

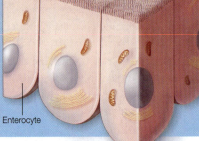

Enterocyte

Epithelial cells called **enterocytes** cover the villi. They have smaller projections called **microvilli**, referred to collectively as the *brush border,* which trap nutrients and absorb them into the enterocyte interior. There, the nutrients enter blood and lymphatic vessels that transport them throughout the body. Enterocytes also secrete several enzymes that help digest specific nutrients. We discuss these secretions in more detail later in the chapter.

Goblet cells scattered along the villi secrete lubricating mucus into the intestine. Between the villi lie glands called **crypts** that secrete intestinal juices. Within the crypts, stem cells continually divide, producing younger cells that travel up the villi to replace mature cells when they die. A constant source of nutrients is needed to replace these cells and maintain a healthy absorptive surface. Without the proper nutrients, the villi deteriorate and flatten, resulting in malabsorption.

Depending on the amount and type of food eaten, the contact time in the small intestine is between 3 and 10 hours. Usually, by the time you sit down to dinner, your breakfast is just about reaching the end of the small intestine.

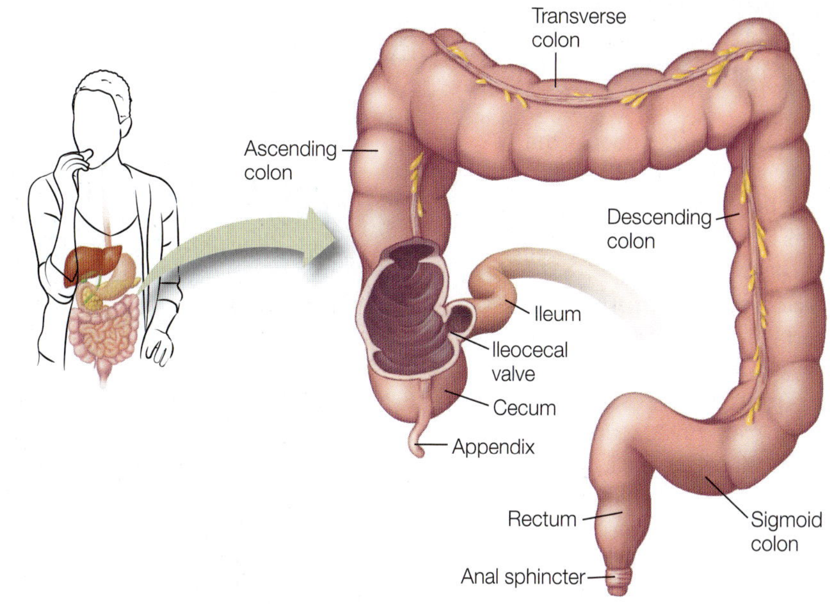

▲ **Figure 3.7 Anatomy of the Large Intestine**
By the time chyme reaches the large intestine, most of its nutrients have been absorbed. However, water and some electrolytes are absorbed in the colon. The final waste products of digestion pass out of the body through the anus.

The Large Intestine Absorbs Water and Some Nutrients

The **large intestine** is only about 5 feet long—much shorter than the small intestine—but its lumen is larger, about 2.5 inches in diameter. It has three segments: the cecum, colon, and rectum (**Figure 3.7**). The **cecum** (*SEE-kum*) marks the beginning of the large intestine. Chyme from the small intestine passes through the **ileocecal valve** into the cecum before entering the colon. The **colon** is the largest portion of the large intestine, and it is further subdivided into the ascending, transverse, descending, and sigmoid regions. These regions are relatively long and straight. Note that though the terms *colon* and *large intestine* are often used interchangeably, technically they're not the same thing.

By the time chyme enters the large intestine, the majority of the nutrients, except water and the electrolytes sodium, potassium, and chloride, have been absorbed. The cells of the large intestine absorb water and these electrolytes much more efficiently than the cells of the small intestine. The large intestine also produces mucus that protects the cells and acts as a lubricant for fecal matter.

Helpful bacteria that colonize the colon are collectively known as the **GI flora** or microflora. These GI flora produce some vitamins, including vitamin K, thiamin, riboflavin, biotin, and vitamin B_{12}. Only biotin and vitamin K can be absorbed in the colon, however. Bacteria also **ferment** some of the undigested and unabsorbed dietary carbohydrates into simpler compounds, methane gas, carbon dioxide, and hydrogen. This fermentation process is the major source of intestinal gas. Similarly, some of the colon's bacteria break down undigested fiber and produce various short-chain fatty acids. Amino acids that reach the colon are converted to hydrogen, sulfide, some fatty acids, and other chemical compounds. Given the importance of bacteria in the healthy functioning of the colon, it isn't surprising that foods containing such beneficial living microorganisms, called *probiotics,* have become popular in recent years. The Examining the Evidence feature evaluates the claims of health benefits associated with consumption of probiotic foods.

enterocytes Absorptive epithelial cells that line the lumen of the small intestine.

microvilli Tiny projections on the villi in the small intestine.

crypts Glands at the base of the villi; they contain stem cells that manufacture young cells to replace the cells of the villi when they die.

large intestine Lowest portion of the GI tract, where water and electrolytes are absorbed and waste is eliminated.

cecum Pouch at the beginning of the large intestine that receives waste from the small intestine.

ileocecal valve Sphincter that separates the small intestine from the large intestine.

colon Another name for the large intestine.

GI flora Microorganisms that live in the GI tract of humans and animals.

ferment To metabolize sugar into carbon dioxide and other gases.

Do Probiotics, Prebiotics, and Synbiotics Improve Your Health?

If you're like most people, the thought of eating food that contains living microorganisms is not appealing. But did you know that consuming certain microbes, called **probiotics,** might improve your health? Probiotics (*pro* = for, *bios* = life) are "live microorganisms, which, when administered in adequate amounts, confer a health benefit on the host."[1] They are similar to the more than 10 trillion beneficial microbes, mostly strains of bacteria, that colonize your GI tract. Medications, stress, a poor diet, and illness can disrupt the balance of friendly GI flora, and consuming them in probiotic foods can help restore their numbers. In the United States, sales of probiotic supplements and foods reached $1.14 billion in 2014, and sales are expected to nearly double by 2019.[2] Why?

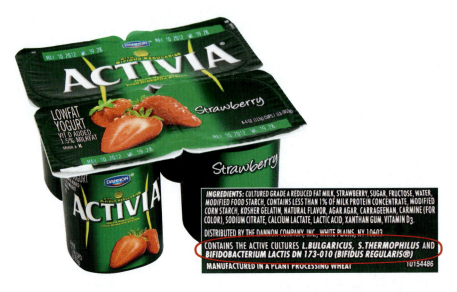

Research Supports the Health Benefits of Probiotics

Probiotics function in the same way that the native bacteria in your GI tract do. For example, they produce organic acids that inhibit the growth of disease-causing microorganisms. They also compete with these pathogens for nutrients and receptor sites, keeping the population of harmful microbes in check. Other proposed benefits of probiotics include:[3–9]

- May reduce constipation, in part by reducing transit time of chyme through the GI tract.
- May prevent or reduce the symptoms of diarrhea and the cramping and bloating associated with lactose intolerance.
- May reduce inflammation.
- May play a role in preventing food allergies.
- May shorten the duration and reduce the severity of the symptoms of the common cold, especially in academically stressed students.
- May reduce signs of colic in infants.

Prebiotics and Synbiotics Support the GI Flora

Prebiotics, which are present in thousands of plant-based foods, are nondigestible resistant starches—a form of dietary fiber—that support the growth and health of your GI flora. Because the body can't digest them, they reach the large bowel intact. There, the GI flora digest them. Eating foods rich in prebiotics thus helps build and maintain a healthy population of GI flora. The two most common prebiotics are fructo-oligosaccharides (FOS) and inulin.

Products called *synbiotics* are processed foods and supplements that contain both probiotic bacteria and prebiotic starches. For example, yogurts to which inulin has been added qualify as synbiotics. Such products both supplement your native GI flora and support their growth and activity.

Where Can You Find Probiotics, Prebiotics, and Synbiotics?

Probiotics are found primarily in fermented dairy and soy products and in dietary supplements (see the accompanying table). For example, eating Activia yogurt is one way to increase probiotics through diet. The food label should identify the strain of the bacteria used, when the product expires, the suggested serving size, and how to store the product to make sure the bacteria are still alive when you eat it. A serving should contain at least one billion CFUs (a measure of live bacteria called colony-forming units) to provide the level of probiotics found to deliver health benefits.[1] When choosing yogurt, look for brands low in saturated fat and added sugars. Plain Greek-style yogurt is a healthful and satisfying choice.

The food richest in prebiotics is bananas. Other foods containing prebiotics include garlic, onions, asparagus, leeks, squash, jicama, beets, carrots, turnips, parsnips, sweet potatoes, and artichokes. Oats, barley, and certain other whole grains also provide prebiotics.

Some yogurt producers add inulin, producing a synbiotic. You can also create your own synbiotics by eating foods rich in probiotics and prebiotics together. Consider, for example, yogurt with oatmeal and bananas, or *tempeh* (fermented soy) in a stir-fry with asparagus, garlic, and onions.

There's no downside to increasing your consumption of foods rich in probiotics, prebiotics, and synbiotics. Although there is a great deal we still don't know about their impact on our health, we do know that the dairy and plant-based foods providing them are nutrient dense and delicious.

Beneficial Bacteria

If You Have This Problem	Try This Probiotic	Found in These Foods and Dietary Supplements
Diarrhea	• *Lactobacillus reuteri* 55730 • *Saccharomyces boulardii* yeast	• BioGai tablets, drops, and lozenges • Florastor dietary supplement
Constipation, irritable bowel syndrome, and overall digestion problems	• *Bifidobacterium animalis* DN-173 010 • *Bifidobacterium infantis* 35624	• Dannon Activia yogurt • Align supplement
Poor immune system	• *Bifidobacterium lactis* Bb-12 • *Lactobacillus casei* Shirota • *Lactobacillus casei* DN-114 001	• Yo-Plus Yogurt • Yakult fermented dairy drink • Dannon's DanActive dairy drink
Vaginal infections	• *Lactobacillus rhamnosus* GR-1 combined with *Lactobacillus reuteri*	• Fem Dophilus dietary supplement

References

1. Kechagia, M. D., S. Basoulis, et al. 2013. Health Benefits of Probiotics: A Review. *ISRN Nutrition,* Article ID 481651, doi:10.5402/2013/481651. Accessed January 2017.
2. Statista: The Statistics Portal. 2016. Dollar Sales of Probiotic Supplements in the United States in 2015, By Channel (in million U.S. dollars). Available at https://www.statista.com/statistics/493536/dollar-sales-of-probiotic-supplement-in-the-us-by-channel. Accessed January 2017.
3. Ritchie, M. L., and T. N. Romanuk. 2012. A Meta-Analysis of Probiotic Efficacy for Gastrointestinal Diseases. *PLoS ONE* 7(4):e34938. doi:10.1371/journal.pone.0034938.
4. Beserra, B. T., et al. 2014. A Systematic Review and Meta-analysis of the Prebiotics and Synbiotics Effects on Glycaemia, Insulin Concentrations, and Lipid Parameters in Adult Patients with Overweight or Obesity. *Clinical Nutrition* 34(5):845–858. doi:10.1016/j.clnu.2014.10.004.
5. Spaiser, S. J., et al. 2015. Lactobacillus gasseri KS-13, Bifidobacterium bifidum G9-1, and Bifidobacterium longum MM-2 Ingestion Induces a Less Inflammatory Cytokine Profile and a Potentially Beneficial Shift in Gut Microbiota in Older Adults: A Randomized, Double-Blind, Placebo-Controlled, Crossover Study. *Journal of the American College of Nutrition* 34(6):459–469. doi:10.1080/07315724.2014.983249.
6. Savaiano, D. A., A. J. Ritter, et al. 2013. Improving Lactose Digestion and Symptoms of Lactose Intolerance with a Novel Galacto-Oligosaccharide (RP-G28): A Randomized, Double-Blind Clinical Trial. *Nutrition Journal* 12:160. doi: 10.1186/1475-2891-12-160.
7. Ritz, B. W. 2011. *Probiotics for the Prevention of Childhood Eczema.* Available at http://naturalmedicinejournal.com. Accessed January 2017.
8. Langkamp-Henken, B., et al. 2015. Bifidobacterium bifidum R0071 Results in a Greater Proportion of Healthy Days and a Lower Percentage of Academically Stressed Students Reporting a Day of Cold/Flu: A Randomised, Double-blind, Placebo-controlled Study. *British Journal of Nutrition* 113(3):426–434. doi: 10.1017/S0007114514003997.
9. Anabrees, J., F. Indrio, et al. 2013. Probiotics for Infantile Colic: A Systematic Review. *BMC Pediatrics* 13:186. doi:10.1186/1471-2431-13-186.

About 1 liter of fluid material—consisting of water, undigested or unabsorbed food particles, indigestible residue, and electrolytes—passes into the colon each day. Gradually, the material is reduced to about 200 grams of brown fecal matter (also called **stool**, or *feces*). Stool consists of the undigested food residue, as well as sloughed-off cells from the GI tract and a large quantity of bacteria. The brown color is due to unabsorbed iron mixing with a yellowish-orange substance called *bilirubin*. The greater the iron content, the darker the feces. The intestinal matter passes through the colon within 12–70 hours, depending on a person's age, health, diet, and fiber intake.

Stool is propelled through the large intestine until it reaches the final 8-inch portion called the **rectum**. The **anus** is connected to the rectum and controlled by an internal and an external sphincter. Under normal conditions, the anal sphincters are closed. When stool distends the rectum, the action stimulates stretch receptors that in turn stimulate the internal anal sphincters to relax, allowing the stool to enter the anal canal. This causes nerve impulses of the rectum to communicate with the rectum's muscles, resulting in defecation. The final stage of defecation is under voluntary control and influenced by age, diet, prescription medicines, health, and abdominal muscle tone.

probiotics Live microorganisms that, when consumed in adequate amounts, confer a health benefit on the host.

prebiotics Nondigestible starch found in plant foods that promotes the growth and health of your GI flora.

stool Waste produced in the large intestine; also called *feces*.

rectum Final 8-inch portion of the large intestine.

anus Opening of the rectum, or end of the GI tract.

The Accessory Organs Secrete Digestive Juices

The salivary glands, liver, gallbladder, and pancreas are considered accessory organs because food does not pass through them (**Figure 3.8**). These organs are still key to the digestive process, however. They contribute digestive secretions such as saliva, bile, and enzymes that help with breakdown and transport of nutrients.

The **salivary glands**, located beneath the jaw and under and behind the tongue, produce about 1 quart of saliva per day.[3] In addition to water and electrolytes, saliva contains several enzymes, including salivary amylase and lysozyme, an enzyme that destroys certain oral bacteria. It also contains mucus, which helps lubricate food, helps it stick together, and protects the inside of the mouth.

Weighing in at about 3 pounds, the **liver** is the largest organ in the body. It is located just beneath the rib cage and functions as a major player in the digestion of food and the absorption and transport of nutrients. The liver plays an essential role in carbohydrate metabolism, produces proteins, and manufactures bile salts, which contribute to the breakdown of fats. The bile produced by the liver is secreted into the gallbladder for storage. The liver also metabolizes alcohol and removes and degrades toxins and excess hormones from the circulation.

The **gallbladder** is located beneath the right side of the liver. This pear-shaped organ receives bile from the liver through the common hepatic duct, concentrates it, and secretes bile into the small intestine through the common bile duct.

The **pancreas** is a flat organ about 10–15 centimeters long that rests behind the stomach in the bend of the duodenum. The function of the pancreas is both *endocrine* (*endo* = inside) and *exocrine* (*exo* = outside). As an endocrine organ, the pancreas releases into the bloodstream hormones that help regulate blood glucose levels. As an exocrine organ, the pancreas produces and secretes digestive enzymes through the pancreatic duct into the small intestine.

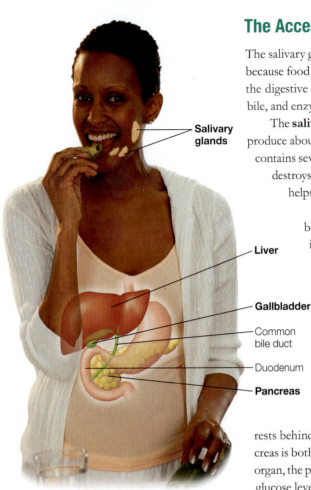

▲ Figure 3.8 The Accessory Organs
The salivary glands, liver, gallbladder, and pancreas produce digestive secretions that flow into the GI tract through various ducts.

Labels on figure: Salivary glands / Liver / Gallbladder / Common bile duct / Duodenum / Pancreas

salivary glands Cluster of glands located underneath and behind the tongue that release saliva in response to the sight, smell, and taste of food.

liver Accessory organ of digestion located in the upper abdomen and responsible for the synthesis of bile, the processing of nutrients, the metabolism of alcohol, and other functions.

gallbladder Pear-shaped organ that stores and concentrates bile produced by the liver and secretes it through the common bile duct into the small intestine.

pancreas Large gland located behind the stomach that releases digestive enzymes and bicarbonate after a meal. Also secretes the hormones insulin and glucagon, which control blood glucose.

LO 3.1: THE TAKE-HOME MESSAGE Digestion takes place in the GI tract. Chemicals break the molecular bonds in food so that nutrients can be absorbed and transported throughout the body. Saliva mixes with and moistens food in the mouth, making it easier to swallow. Once a bolus of food mixes with gastric juices in the stomach, it becomes chyme. Maximum digestion and absorption occur in the small intestine. Undigested residue enters the large intestine, where water is removed from the chyme as it is prepared for elimination. Eventually, the remnants of digestion reach the anus and exit the body in the feces. The salivary glands, liver, gallbladder, and pancreas are important accessory organs. The salivary glands produce saliva. The liver produces bile, which the gallbladder concentrates and stores. The pancreas produces digestive enzymes and hormones.

How Is Food Propelled through the GI Tract?

LO 3.2 Explain how food is propelled through the gastrointestinal tract.

Wavelike movements of the muscles throughout the GI tract propel food and liquid forward. These contractions, which depend on coordination between the muscles, nerves, and hormones in the GI tract, help mechanically digest the food by mixing and pushing

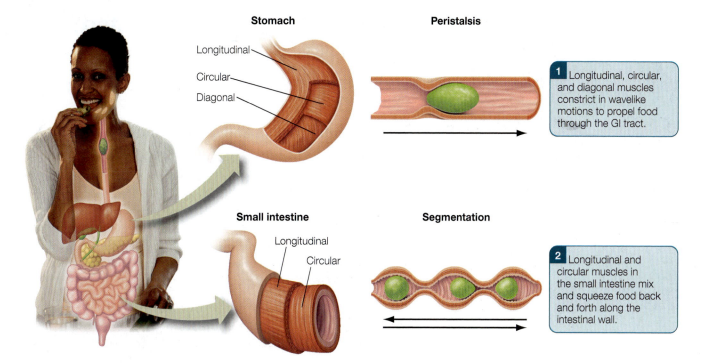

Stomach

Longitudinal
Circular
Diagonal

Peristalsis

1 Longitudinal, circular, and diagonal muscles constrict in wavelike motions to propel food through the GI tract.

Small intestine

Longitudinal
Circular

Segmentation

2 Longitudinal and circular muscles in the small intestine mix and squeeze food back and forth along the intestinal wall.

▲ **Figure 3.9 Peristalsis and Segmentation**

it at just the right pace through each organ. The two primary types of contractions are called *peristalsis* and *segmentation* (**Figure 3.9**).

Peristalsis begins in the esophagus, as contractions of circular muscles prevent food from moving backward. Repeated waves of contractions follow as the circular muscles relax and the longitudinal muscles constrict and push the food forward.

In the stomach, circular, longitudinal, and diagonal muscles move the food from the top of the stomach toward the pyloric sphincter at the base of the stomach. The waves of contractions in the stomach are slower than in other GI organs, as peristalsis mixes and churns the stomach contents with gastric juices until the food is liquefied.

As the partially digested food leaves the stomach, the second form of mechanical digestion, called **segmentation**, begins. Segmentation moves the food back and forth, helping to break it down into smaller pieces while mixing it with the chemical secretions of the intestine. Segmentation differs from peristalsis in that food is shifted (rather than squeezed) back and forth along the intestinal walls. This shifting action increases the time food is in contact with the intestinal lining, moving food through the small intestine at a rate of 1 centimeter per minute.[4]

Mass movement, also known as *mass peristalsis,* is a series of strong, slow contractions in the large intestine that move the chyme through the colon. Three or four times a day, these slow but powerful muscular contractions force the waste products toward the rectum. Meanwhile, segmentation within the colon helps dry out the feces, allowing for the maximum amount of water to be absorbed. These contractions often occur shortly after eating and are stronger when the diet contains more fiber.

LO 3.2: THE TAKE-HOME MESSAGE Food is propelled through the GI tract by strong muscular contractions. Peristalsis in the esophagus, stomach, and small intestine squeezes the food and propels it forward, while segmentation in the small and large intestines shifts food back and forth along the intestinal walls. Mass movement moves waste slowly and powerfully toward the rectum.

peristalsis Forward, rhythmic muscular contractions that move food through the GI tract.

segmentation Muscular contractions of the small intestine that move food back and forth, breaking the mixture into smaller and smaller pieces and combining it with digestive juices.

mass movement (mass peristalsis) Strong, slow peristaltic movements, occurring only three or four times a day within the colon, that force waste toward the rectum.

How Is Food Chemically Digested?

LO 3.3 Identify the role of enzymes and other secretions in chemical digestion.

While food travels through the organs of the GI tract, digestive enzymes and other chemicals break it down into nutrients. How do these chemicals work?

Enzymes Drive the Process of Digestion

Enzymes are compounds, most of which are proteins, that catalyze or speed up chemical reactions. One of the most important roles of enzymes is to accelerate **hydrolysis** (*hydro* = water, *lysis* = break) reactions, in which water breaks the bonds of digestible carbohydrates, fats, proteins, and alcohol. Hydrolysis produces single molecules small enough to be absorbed by the intestines. During hydrolysis, the hydroxyl (OH) group from water joins one of the molecules, while the hydrogen ion (H) joins the other molecule, forming two new molecules. This is illustrated in the Chemistry Boost. Enzymes aren't changed in the reaction and can thus be used over and over again.

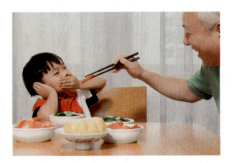

Once food enters the mouth, enzymes begin to chemically break the bonds that bind the nutrients.

Chemistry Boost

Hydrolysis

The process known as hydrolysis digests most food molecules, in which the addition of water and a specific enzyme breaks down the corresponding molecule. In the figure below, a molecule of sucrose (sugar) is digested by the enzyme sucrase when it breaks the bond with the addition of water by adding a hydroxyl group (OH) to form glucose and hydrogen (H) to form fructose.

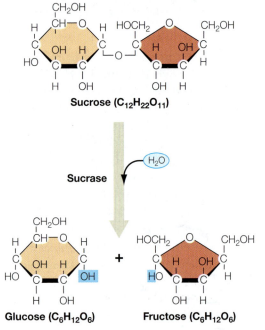

In order for enzymes to catalyze hydrolytic reactions, three conditions must be present.

1. **The compatible enzyme and nutrient must both be present.** Enzymes are compatible only with a specific compound or nutrient, referred to as a **substrate**. Each enzyme has a binding site that only fits certain substrates, much like a key fits a specific lock. When the substrate binds to the active site of the enzyme, the bond is hydrolyzed. This reaction is illustrated in **Figure 3.10**. Enzymes are often named according to the type of substrate they act upon, plus the suffix *-ase*. So, sucr*ase* hydrolyzes the sugar sucrose, and malt*ase* hydrolyzes maltose. Some enzymes, such as pepsin, were named before this new nomenclature was developed and don't follow these naming rules.

enzymes Substances, mostly proteins, that increase the rate of chemical reactions; also called *biological catalysts*.

hydrolysis Chemical reaction that breaks the bond between two molecules with water. A hydroxyl group is added to one molecule and a hydrogen ion is added to the other molecule.

substrate Substance or compound that is altered by an enzyme.

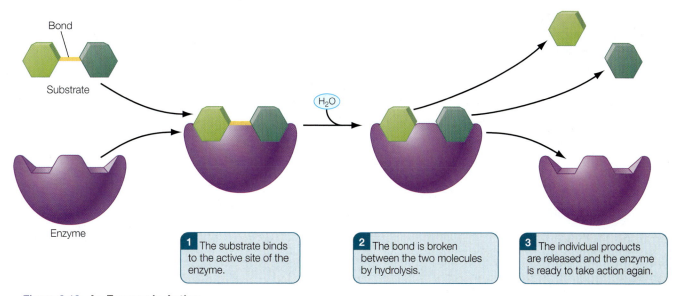

1 The substrate binds to the active site of the enzyme.

2 The bond is broken between the two molecules by hydrolysis.

3 The individual products are released and the enzyme is ready to take action again.

▲ **Figure 3.10 An Enzyme in Action**
Enzymes increase the rate of digestion without altering their shape.

2. **The pH of the environment must fall in the appropriate range.** Enzymes are most effective when the fluid environment falls within a certain **pH** range, a range of acidity or alkalinity (see the Chemistry Boost). When the pH falls outside of that range, the activity of the enzyme is decreased or even halted. For example, saliva contains bicarbonate, which neutralizes acids in foods. It has a pH of about 6.4, which is optimal for the effective action of salivary amylase. When the bolus containing the salivary enzymes reaches the stomach, where the pH is closer to 1, salivary amylase activity is stopped. However, another enzyme, pepsin, becomes activated in this acidic environment. As chyme continues to travel through the GI tract, various organs secrete digestive juices that produce the optimal range of pH for the enzymes to function.

3. **The temperature of the environment must fall within the appropriate range.** As temperature falls below optimal levels, enzyme activity slows. If the temperature becomes too high, the enzyme is inactivated. In the body, the optimal temperature for enzymatic activity is 98.6°F (35.7°C), which is considered normal body temperature. Temperature also influences enzyme activity in foods. Cooling food in a refrigerator slows enzyme activity, and cooking food completely inactivates any enzymes it contains.

Digestive enzymes are secreted all along the GI tract, but most are produced in the pancreas. The pancreas secretes digestive enzymes into the duodenum through the pancreatic duct. The brush border of the small intestine releases the last of the digestive enzymes. **Table 3.1** summarizes the digestive enzymes, the organs that secrete them, and their actions.

pH Measure of the acidity or alkalinity of a solution.

TABLE 3.1	Digestive Enzymes and Their Actions		
Organ or Gland	**Enzyme**	**Action**	**Nutrient**
Salivary glands	Salivary amylase	Begins the digestion of starch	Carbohydrates
Stomach	Pepsinogen → Pepsin	Begins the hydrolysis of polypeptides	Protein
	Gastric lipase	Begins digestion of lipids	Lipids

(continued)

TABLE 3.1 Digestive Enzymes and Their Actions *(continued)*

Organ or Gland	Enzyme	Action	Nutrient
Pancreas	Pancreatic amylase	Digests starch	Carbohydrates
	Trypsinogen → Trypsin	Catalyzes the hydrolysis of proteins in the small intestine to form smaller polypeptides	Protein
	Chymotrypsinogen → Chymotrypsin	Catalyzes the hydrolysis of proteins in the small intestine into polypeptides and amino acids	Protein
	Procarboxypeptidase → Carboxypeptidase	Hydrolyzes the carboxyl end of a peptide, releasing the last amino acid in the peptide chain	Protein
	Pancreatic lipase	Digests triglycerides	Lipids
Small Intestine	Sucrase	Digests sucrose	Carbohydrates
	Maltase	Digests maltose	Carbohydrates
	Lactase	Digests lactose	Carbohydrates
	Dipeptidase	Digests dipeptides	Protein
	Tripeptidase	Digests tripeptides	Protein
	Lipase	Digests monoglycerides	Lipids

Chemistry Boost

pH Scale

Acids and bases describe the chemical properties of a substance. Acidity level is expressed using a pH scale that measures the hydrogen ion concentration. The range of a pH scale is 0–14, with 7—the pH of pure water—considered neutral. A solution that has a pH lower than 7 is considered acidic (0 is the most acidic); one higher than 7 is basic (14 is the most basic).

The lower the number on the pH scale, the greater the concentration of hydrogen ions (H^+) in a solution. The more H^+ in a solution, the stronger the acid. For example, gastric juice, with a pH of 1, has a higher concentration of H^+ and is much more acidic than pancreatic juice, which has a pH of 8.

Bases—alkaline compounds—contain more hydroxide ions (OH^-) and have a low concentration of H^+. The more OH^- in a solution, the stronger the base. For example, sodium hydroxide, an acid, has a pH of 1, whereas bile, which is a base, has a pH of 6.8 to 8.5.

Each pH unit below 7 is 10 times more acidic than the next pH unit. For example, tomato juice, with a pH of 4, contains 10 times more H^+ than coffee, with a pH of 5, and over 100 times more H^+ than saliva, with a pH of 6.4. Each pH unit above 7 is 10 times more basic than the next pH unit.

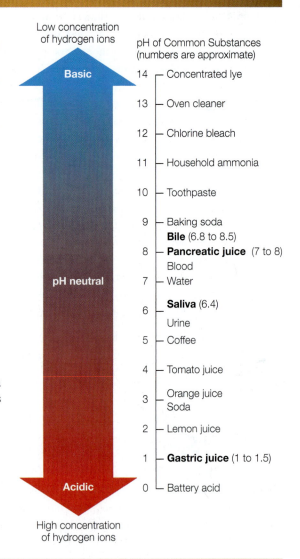

Low concentration of hydrogen ions

Basic

pH neutral

Acidic

High concentration of hydrogen ions

pH of Common Substances (numbers are approximate)

14 — Concentrated lye
13 — Oven cleaner
12 — Chlorine bleach
11 — Household ammonia
10 — Toothpaste
9 — Baking soda
  Bile (6.8 to 8.5)
8 — **Pancreatic juice** (7 to 8)
  Blood
7 — Water
6 — **Saliva** (6.4)
  Urine
5 — Coffee
4 — Tomato juice
3 — Orange juice
  Soda
2 — Lemon juice
1 — **Gastric juice** (1 to 1.5)
0 — Battery acid

Certain Secretions Are Essential for Digestion

Enzymes and other essential compounds are often contained in fluids that are secreted throughout the digestion process. These secretions include saliva, which has already been discussed, as well as gastric juices, bile, and bicarbonate ions, each of which contributes to optimal conditions for digestion to occur.

Gastric Juices

The specialized parietal and chief cells introduced earlier in the chapter produce the gastric juices secreted by the stomach. When food enters the stomach, the parietal cells produce **hydrochloric acid (HCl)** and a protein called *intrinsic factor,* which is important for the absorption of vitamin B_{12} in the ileum.

Hydrochloric acid is unique in that it can impair the activity of some proteins while activating others. It is essential for digestion because of its ability to lower the pH of gastric juice close to 1. This acidic pH denatures proteins, which means it inactivates the protein by uncoiling its strands. Once the protein is denatured, **proteases**, or protein-digesting enzymes, hydrolyze the bonds, breaking the proteins into shorter chains. Denaturing applies to all proteins, including hormones, and to bacteria found in food, which are destroyed before they can be absorbed intact.

Hydrochloric acid can also activate proteins, such as pepsinogen, a protein-digesting enzyme secreted from the chief cells lining the gastric glands. In the presence of HCl, **pepsinogen** is converted to its active form, **pepsin**, which begins the digestion of protein. HCl also enhances the absorption of certain minerals, such as calcium. In addition to pepsinogen, the chief cells also secrete *gastric lipase,* which begins to digest fats, although this enzyme is not particularly active in adults.

You might think that an acid as strong as HCl would "digest" the stomach itself, but mucus secreted by the goblet cells acts as a barrier between the HCl and the stomach lining, protecting the lining from irritation or damage. This slippery secretion is also produced in the mucous membranes lining the esophagus to lubricate food as it passes down the GI tract.

Bile

Bile, the yellowish-green substance synthesized in the liver, helps break apart dietary fats. This dilute, alkaline liquid is stored in concentrated form—up to five times its original composition—in the gallbladder. Bile, which is composed of water, bile salts, bile pigments, fat, and cholesterol, **emulsifies** fat by breaking down large fat globules into smaller globules, much like dishwashing detergent breaks up the grease in a frying pan. Emulsification increases the surface area of the fat globule, making it far more accessible to pancreatic lipase, the fat-digesting enzyme secreted by the pancreas. Pancreatic lipase is water-soluble and only works on the surface of the fat globule.

In addition to dietary fat, bile also increases the absorption of the fat-soluble vitamins A, D, E, and K. Because bile has a slightly acidic to alkaline pH (between 6.8 and 8.5), it helps neutralize excess HCl. Finally, bile salts exhibit antibacterial properties.

Unlike other digestive secretions, bile can be reused. From the large intestine, bile is recycled back to the liver through **enterohepatic** (*entero* = intestine, *hepatic* = liver) **circulation.** This recycling allows bile to be reused up to 20 times.

Bicarbonate

Bicarbonate ions alter the pH of food at various points along the GI tract. As noted earlier, the salivary glands produce enough bicarbonate to neutralize the food you eat and produce a favorable pH for salivary enzymes to hydrolyze starch. The pancreas secretes bicarbonate ions that flow into the duodenum via the pancreatic duct. The bicarbonate helps neutralize chyme as it arrives in the small intestine. The alkaline pH is critical to

hydrochloric acid (HCl) Strong acid produced in the stomach that aids in digestion.

proteases Classification of enzymes that catalyze the hydrolysis of proteins.

pepsinogen Inactive protease secreted by the chief cells in the stomach; it is converted to the active enzyme pepsin in the presence of HCl.

pepsin Active protease that begins the digestion of proteins in the stomach.

bile Secretion produced by the liver, stored in the gallbladder, and released into the duodenum to emulsify dietary fat.

emulsify To break large fat globules into smaller droplets.

enterohepatic circulation Process of recycling bile from the large intestine back to the liver to be reused during fat digestion.

bicarbonate Negatively charged alkali ion produced from bicarbonate salts; during digestion, bicarbonate ions released from the pancreas neutralize HCl in the duodenum.

TABLE 3.2	Secretions of the GI Tract and Their Actions	
Secretion	**Secretion Pathway**	**Action(s)**
Saliva	Secreted by salivary glands into mouth	Moistens food, eases swallowing; contains the enzyme salivary amylase
Hydrochloric acid (HCl)	Secreted by parietal cells into stomach	Denatures protein; activates pepsinogen → pepsin
Intrinsic factor	Secreted by parietal cells into stomach	Needed for vitamin B_{12} absorption
Mucus	Secreted throughout the GI tract, including in the stomach and intestinal glands	Lubricates and coats the internal mucosa to protect it from chemical or mechanical damage
Intestinal juice	Secreted by the crypts into small intestine	Contains enzymes that digest carbohydrate, protein, and lipid
Bile	Secreted by liver into gallbladder for storage; released from gallbladder into small intestine via common bile duct	Emulsifies large globules of lipid into smaller droplets
Bicarbonate ions	Secreted by pancreas through the pancreatic duct into the small intestine	Raise pH and neutralize stomach acid

protect the cells lining the duodenum, which are not resistant to damage by HCl, and to provide a favorable pH for the pancreatic enzymes and the brush border enzymes sucrase, maltase, and lactase.

Table 3.2 summarizes the important digestive compounds and the organs that secrete them.

LO 3.3: THE TAKE-HOME MESSAGE Foods are chemically digested by hydrolysis, which is catalyzed by enzymes. The three conditions that govern enzyme action are specific substrates (nutrients), pH, and optimal temperature. Other secretions produced in the GI tract, such as saliva, gastric juices, bile, and bicarbonate, contribute to the optimal environment for digestion to occur.

How Are Digested Nutrients Absorbed?

LO 3.4 Describe how digested nutrients are absorbed.

Although some absorption occurs in the stomach and large intestine, the small intestine absorbs most nutrients via the enterocytes lining its wall. Nutrients that are digested by the time they reach the duodenum are absorbed quickly. Nutrients that need more time to be disassembled are absorbed mainly in the jejunum. Absorption is remarkably efficient. Under normal conditions, you digest and absorb 92–97 percent of the nutrients in food. In some individuals, the tight junctions between cell membranes of the enterocytes are disrupted, inappropriately increasing the permeability of the GI tract. Read the Examining the Evidence box for more information.

There Are Four Mechanisms of Nutrient Absorption

The remarkable surface area provided by the folds and crevices in the lining of the small intestine allows for continuous, efficient absorption of most nutrients. Recall that the villi are covered with mature enterocytes—cells that absorb digested nutrients. These cells live only a few days before they are sloughed off and themselves digested.

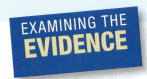
Is Increased Intestinal Permeability (aka Leaky Gut Syndrome) a Real Disorder?

Have you ever heard the term *leaky gut syndrome*? This proposed medical condition, clinically known as increased **intestinal permeability,** is characterized by a reduced ability of the GI tract to regulate the absorption of nutrients. Some researchers theorize that restoring normal functioning of the lining of the GI tract may be effective in curing many health problems. In the past, there has been little evidence to support this theory; however, new research suggests that increased intestinal permeability may exist and might contribute to a variety of conditions from simple intestinal gas and bloating, to eczema, chronic fatigue syndrome, and even cardiovascular disease and cancer. Before we explore why, let's take a closer look at how increased intestinal permeability occurs.

Physiology of Increased Intestinal Permeability

As you've learned in this chapter, the healthy lining of the GI tract is a barrier that only allows nutrients that have been properly digested to pass through the enterocyte cell membrane and enter the bloodstream. This barrier blocks the entry of allergens and microorganisms, for example, into the bloodstream.[1] As illustrated in the accompanying figure, when the tight junctions between the enterocytes become inflamed,[2] they loosen and allow large molecules to pass through into the blood. These large molecules include undigested food particles, bacteria, and even toxins. As they enter the bloodstream, the immune system releases antibodies and signaling molecules called *cytokines* that stimulate white blood cells to fight the perceived invaders. This response can trigger

inflammation throughout the body, which is a risk factor for cardiovascular disease,[3] celiac disease, Crohn's disease,[4, 5] diabetes,[6] and other disorders.[7, 8, 9]

Undigested foods, bacteria, and allergens

Disrupted junction

Healthy junction

Blood

In increased intestinal permeability, the tight junctions between the enterocytes become inflamed, loosen, and allow large molecules, including undigested food particles, bacteria, and even toxins, to pass from the lumen into the bloodstream.

Causes and Symptoms of Increased Intestinal Permeability

Little is known about the causes of increased intestinal permeability, and tests often fail to uncover the problem. The disruption of the intestinal barrier may be caused by chronic stress,[10] intestinal infections including bacterial overgrowth,[11] excessive use of alcohol,[12] poor diet,[13] or the use of certain medications.[14]

The disruption of the intestinal barrier may result in a variety of gastrointestinal symptoms, including flatulence, indigestion, constipation, bloating, and abdominal pain.[15] These symptoms aren't unique, however, and are often shared by other conditions. Symptoms beyond the GI tract have also been reported, including difficulty breathing, chronic joint and muscle pain, confusion, mood swings, poor memory, and anxiety. Moreover, asthma, recurrent infections, and chronic fatigue syndrome may be

associated with increased intestinal permeability.[16, 17]

Treatment for Intestinal Permeability

Diet is often the first approach to treating increased intestinal permeability, especially the elimination of processed foods and sugars. However, no treatment is known to restore the intestinal barrier. Moreover, it is not known whether restoration will actually resolve the patient's symptoms. Human and animal studies have not shown that intestinal barrier loss alone causes disease or that repairing the loss improves the disease state. Treatments such as nutritional supplements containing pre- and probiotics, herbal remedies, gluten-free foods, and a low-sugar diet have not been shown to be beneficial.[18] Additionally, most physicians don't know enough about the GI tract to even begin to treat increased intestinal permeability. Clearly, more research evidence is needed before an effective treatment can be found.

References

1. Brandtzaeg, P. 2011. The Gut as Communicator Between Environment and Host: Immunological Consequences. *Eur J Pharmacol* 668(Suppl 1):S16–S32.
2. Al-Sadi, R., et al. 2014. Interleukin-6 Modulation of Intestinal Epithelial Tight Junction Permeability is Mediated by JNK Pathway Activation of Claudin-2 Gene. *PLoS One* 9(3):e85345. doi: 10.1371/journal.pone.0085345
3. Schicho, R., G. Marsche, et al. 2015. Cardiovascular Complications in Inflammatory

intestinal permeability Condition in which the junctions between enterocytes allow large molecules to enter the bloodstream; also called *leaky gut syndrome.*

Bowel Disease. *Current Drug Targets* 16(3):181–188.

4. Bischof, S., et al. 2014. Intestinal Permeability: A New Target for Disease Prevention and Therapy. *BMC Gastroenterology* 14:189.

5. Sapone, A., et al. 2011. Divergence of Gut Permeability and Mucosal Immune Gene Expression in Two Gluten-associated Conditions: Celiac Disease and Gluten Sensitivity. *BMC Medicine* 9:23. doi: 10.1186/1741-7015-9-23.

6. Li, X., and M. A. Atkinson. 2015. The Role of Gut Permeability in the Pathogenesis of Type 1 Diabetes—A Solid or Leaky Concept? *Pediatric Diabetes* 16(7):485–492. doi: 10.1111/pedi.12305

7. Schulberg, J., and P. DeCruz. 2016. Characterisation and Therapeutic Manipulation of the Gut Microbiome in Inflammatory Bowel Disease. *Internal Medicine Journal* 46(3):266–273. doi: 10.1111/imj.13003.

8. Johansson, M.E., et al. 2014. Bacteria Penetrate the Normally Impenetrable Inner Colon Mucus Layer in Both Murine Colitis Models and Patients with Ulcerative Colitis. *Gut* 63(2):281–291.

9. Campbell, A. W. 2016. The Gut, Intestinal Permeability, and Autoimmunity. *Alternative Therapy in Health and Medicine* 21(1):6–7.

10. Yu, C., et al. 2016. Chronic Kidney Disease Induced Intestinal Mucosal Barrier Damage Associated with Intestinal Oxidative Stress Injury. *Gastroenterological Research and Practice.* doi: 10.1155/2016/6720575.

11. Sorobetea, D., et al. 2016. Acute Infection with the Intestinal Parasite Trichuris Muris Has Long-term Consequences on Mucosal Mast Cell Homeostasis and Epithelial Integrity. *European Journal of Immunology.* doi: 10.1002/eji.201646738.

12. Swanson, G. R., et al. 2016. Night Workers with Circadian Misalignment are Susceptible to Alcohol-induced Intestinal Hyperpermeability with Social Drinking. *American Journal of Physiology and Gatrointestinal Liver Physiology* 311(1):G192–201. doi: 10.1152/ajpgi.00087.2016.

13. Odenwald, M. A., and J. R. Turner. 2013. Intestinal Permeability Defects: Is It Time to Treat? *Clinical Gatroenterology and Hepatology* 11(9):1075–1083. doi: 10.1016/j.cgh.2013.07.001.

14. Pavlidis, P., and I. Bjarnason. 2015. Aspirin Induced Adverse Effects on the Small and Large Intestine. *Current Pharmaceutical Design* 21(35):5089–5093. Review.

15. Farré, R., and M. Vicario. 2016. Abnormal Barrier Function in Gastrointestinal Disorders. In *Handbook of Experimental Pharmacology.* doi: 10.1007/164_2016_107.

16. Claesson, M. J., Jeffery, I. B., et al. 2012. Gut Microbiota Composition Correlates with Diet and Health in the Elderly. *Nature* 488:178–184.

17. Slyepchenko, A., et al. 2017. Gut Microbiota, Bacterial Translocation, and Interactions with Diet: Pathophysiological Links Between Major Depressive Disorder and Non-Communicable Medical Comorbidities. *Psychotherapy and Psychosomantics* 86(1):31–46. doi: 10.1159/000448957.

18. NHS Choices. 2015. Leaky Gut Syndrome. Available at http://www.nhs.uk/conditions/leaky-gut-syndrome/Pages/Introduction.aspx. Accessed January 2017.

Nutrients move across cell membranes in the small intestine via one of four mechanisms: passive diffusion, facilitated diffusion, active transport, or endocytosis. **Figure 3.11** illustrates these four processes.

Passive Diffusion

passive diffusion Movement of substances across a cell membrane along their concentration gradient.

Passive diffusion is a process in which nutrients are absorbed along their concentration gradient. When the concentration of a nutrient is greater in the GI lumen than within the enterocyte, the nutrient flows passively across the cell membrane. Thus, the nutrient

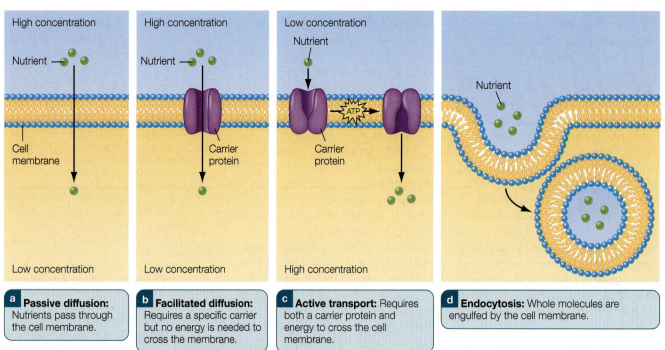

a **Passive diffusion:** Nutrients pass through the cell membrane.

b **Facilitated diffusion:** Requires a specific carrier but no energy is needed to cross the membrane.

c **Active transport:** Requires both a carrier protein and energy to cross the cell membrane.

d **Endocytosis:** Whole molecules are engulfed by the cell membrane.

▲ **Figure 3.11** **Four Methods of Nutrient Absorption in the Small Intestine**

moves from a high concentration to a low concentration. This simple process requires neither energy nor a special carrier molecule. Water, small lipids, a few minerals, and vitamin C are examples of nutrients absorbed via passive diffusion.

Facilitated Diffusion

The cell membrane of enterocytes has a lipid layer that is impermeable to most nutrients. Thus, most nutrients require an alternate method for absorption. In **facilitated diffusion**, nutrients are helped across the membrane by specific carrier proteins. This form of absorption is similar to passive diffusion in that it does not require energy, and nutrients flow from an area of higher to lower concentration. Fructose is an example of a nutrient that is absorbed with the help of a carrier protein.

Active Transport

In **active transport**, a carrier protein and energy in the form of ATP shuttle nutrients across the cell membrane from an area of lower to higher concentration. This transport mechanism allows absorption even when the concentration of nutrients outside the enterocyte is lower than the concentration inside the cell. Glucose and amino acids are examples of nutrients absorbed by active transport.

Endocytosis

Endocytosis occurs when molecules are too big to cross through a membrane using passive or active transport. This process occurs when a cell membrane folds back on itself to form a *vesicle* or pouch to surround and engulf the nutrient and bring it inside the cell using energy. Once inside the vesicle, the nutrient is dissolved in water. The membrane then disassembles and the contents are released on the other side. This type of absorption allows whole proteins, such as an immunoglobulin from breast milk, to be absorbed intact.

Fluid Absorption Occurs in the Large Intestine

By the time chyme enters the large intestine, the majority of the nutrients have been absorbed. The large intestine absorbs water and certain minerals (mainly sodium) before the remaining mass reaches the rectum for excretion. The water is absorbed via passive diffusion and sodium is absorbed via active transport.

> **LO 3.4: THE TAKE-HOME MESSAGE** The brush border of the small intestine is the major site of absorption for digested nutrients. Water and minerals not absorbed in the small intestine are absorbed in the large intestine. Nutrients are absorbed by passive diffusion, facilitated diffusion, active transport, or endocytosis.

How Do Hormones and the Nervous System Regulate Digestion?

LO 3.5 Explain how hormones and the nervous system regulate digestion.

The endocrine and nervous systems work together to control and coordinate digestion, absorption, and elimination of waste products. Endocrine glands, which are found in the stomach, small intestine, and pancreas, are specialized cells that secrete hormones into the bloodstream in response to a stimulus. For example, when the food you eat reaches your stomach, endocrine glands release gastric hormones to signal the rest of the GI tract

facilitated diffusion Movement of substances across a cell membrane with the help of a carrier protein along their concentration gradient.

active transport Movement of substances across a cell membrane against their concentration gradient with the help of a carrier protein and energy expenditure.

endocytosis Type of active transport in which the cell membrane forms an indentation, engulfs the substance to be absorbed, and releases it into the interior of the cell.

to prepare for digestion. When food is not present, these hormones are not released. Digestion, absorption, and elimination are also regulated by the **enteric nervous system**, a network of nerve fibers embedded in the layers of the GI tract. Let's take a closer look at how these two systems communicate and ultimately control the digestive process.

Hormones in the GI Tract Regulate Digestion

Hormones secreted throughout the GI tract regulate digestion by controlling the release of gastric and pancreatic secretions, peristalsis, and enzyme activity. **Enterogastrones**, for example, are hormones produced and secreted by the cells lining the stomach and small intestine. These hormones—including gastrin, secretin, cholecystokinin, and gastric inhibitory peptide (GIP)—have a powerful influence on gastrointestinal motility (the pace of digestion), stomach emptying, gallbladder contraction, intestinal absorption, and even hunger.

Certain types of food passing through the GI tract stimulate the release of hormones. For example, when a protein-containing bolus passes through the lower esophageal sphincter (LES), **gastrin** is secreted from the stomach. This hormone triggers the release of gastric secretions that contain gastric lipase and stimulates the secretion of HCl. Gastrin also increases gastric motility and emptying and increases the tone of the LES.

Cells of the duodenum release **secretin** when the acidic chyme passes through the pyloric sphincter. The release of secretin in turn stimulates the pancreas to send bicarbonate ions through the pancreatic duct to neutralize the acid. Duodenal cells also secrete **cholecystokinin (CCK)** (*koli-sis-te-KI-nin*) in response to the entry of partially digested protein and fat. This powerful hormone stimulates the pancreas to release lipase and the gallbladder to contract and release bile, while it slows down gastric motility and contributes to meal satisfaction. A third hormone released by duodenal cells is **gastric inhibitory peptide (GIP)**. Triggered by the presence of fatty acids or glucose, GIP inhibits gastric activities, allowing time for the digestive process to proceed in the duodenum before it receives more chyme. GIP also signals the pancreas to increase its secretion of insulin, which facilitates the uptake of blood glucose by body cells.

This synchronized effort by the GI tract hormones ensures the efficiency of digestion and maintains homeostasis in the body. Refer to **Table 3.3** for a summary of the individual hormones, the tissues that secrete them, and their actions.

enteric nervous system Section of the peripheral nervous system that directly controls the gastrointestinal system.

enterogastrones Group of GI tract hormones, produced in the stomach and small intestine, that controls gastric motility and secretions.

gastrin Hormone released from the stomach that stimulates the release of acid.

secretin A hormone secreted from the duodenum that stimulates the stomach to release pepsin, the liver to make bile, and the pancreas to release digestive juices.

cholecystokinin (CCK) Hormone released by the duodenum that stimulates the gallbladder to release bile.

gastric inhibitory peptide (GIP) Hormone produced by the small intestine that slows the release of chyme from the stomach.

TABLE 3.3 Hormones of the GI Tract and Their Actions

Organ	Hormone	Stimulus	Secreted from	Action(s)
Stomach	Ghrelin	Empty stomach	Gastric cells	Stimulates gastric motility; stimulates hunger
	Gastrin	Food in the stomach	Gastric cells	Stimulates parietal cells to release HCl
Small Intestine	Secretin	Acidic chyme in duodenum	Duodenum	Stimulates the pancreas to release bicarbonate ions
	Cholecystokinin (CCK)	Fats and proteins in duodenum	Duodenum	Stimulates the gallbladder to secrete bile and the pancreas to secrete bicarbonate ions and enzymes
	Gastric inhibitory peptide (GIP)	Nutrients in the small intestine	Duodenum	Stimulates secretions from the intestines and pancreas; inhibits stomach motility
	Peptide YY	Nutrients in the small intestine	Ileum	Slows stomach motility

The Enteric Nervous System Communicates Within and Beyond the GI Tract

The neurons in the enteric nervous system communicate with one another to perform certain GI functions autonomously. For example, within the walls of the GI tract, receptors of the enteric neurons sense cellular changes and trigger motor responses, which include stimulating and regulating contractions of the GI smooth muscle, motility of the GI tract, and gastrointestinal blood flow.

The enteric nervous system also works collaboratively with other branches of the nervous system, such as the central nervous system. For example, together with hormones secreted from the GI tract, enteric nerves generate signals about the fullness or emptiness of the GI tract. These signals travel to the brain, which, with the help of hormones, communicates and interprets messages of hunger or satiation and encourages you to seek food or stop eating.

The hormones ghrelin and peptide YY communicate feelings of hunger or fullness to the brain (see **Figure 3.12**). **Ghrelin**, which is referred to as the "hormone of hunger," is released from the gastric cells when the stomach is empty. It travels to the brain, where it prompts a desire to eat. **Peptide YY** is secreted by cells of the ileum and colon in response to the presence of food. It travels through the bloodstream to the brain and signals that you've eaten.

The central nervous system can also trigger enteric responses. Imagine, for example, that you walk by a bakery and smell freshly baked bread. Your brain receives this sensory data, signals the GI tract, and the enteric nerves interpret the signal and respond by stimulating the release of digestive juices.

In addition, the enteric nerves excite the muscles stimulating peristalsis, pushing the food and digestive juices through the GI tract. Once the stomach has emptied, the release of hormones and digestive juices ceases.

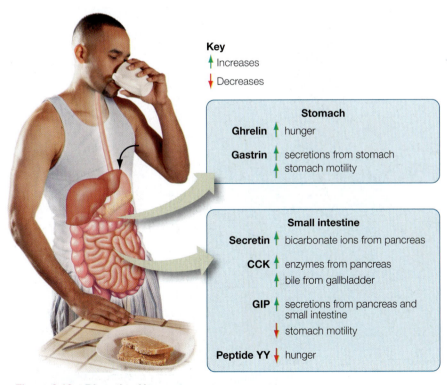

Key
↑ Increases
↓ Decreases

Stomach
Ghrelin ↑ hunger
Gastrin ↑ secretions from stomach
↑ stomach motility

Small intestine
Secretin ↑ bicarbonate ions from pancreas
CCK ↑ enzymes from pancreas
↑ bile from gallbladder
GIP ↑ secretions from pancreas and small intestine
↓ stomach motility
Peptide YY ↓ hunger

▲ Figure 3.12 **Digestive Hormones**
Digestive hormones from the stomach and small intestine control and coordinate digestive processes and hunger.

ghrelin Hormone produced in the stomach that stimulates hunger.

peptide YY Hormone produced in the small intestine that reduces hunger.

How Are Nutrients Transported throughout the Body?

LO 3.6 Explain how absorbed nutrients are transported throughout the body.

Once the nutrients have been absorbed through the lining of the small intestine, they are carried either through the cardiovascular or lymphatic system to other parts of the body (**Figure 3.13**). These two transportation systems consist of varying levels of pathways.

The Cardiovascular System Distributes Nutrients through Blood

The blood is the body's primary transport system, shuttling oxygen, nutrients, hormones, and waste products throughout the body. The heart pumps blood through this closed system of vessels through the entire body and back to the heart.

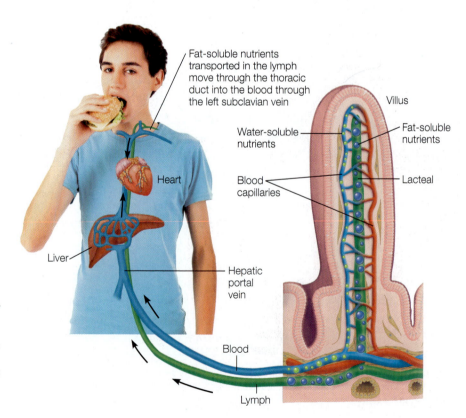

Fat-soluble nutrients transported in the lymph move through the thoracic duct into the blood through the left subclavian vein

Villus

Water-soluble nutrients

Fat-soluble nutrients

Heart

Blood capillaries

Lacteal

Liver

Hepatic portal vein

Blood

Lymph

▶ **Figure 3.13 The Cardiovascular and Lymphatic Systems**
Blood and lymph are fluids that circulate throughout the body. They both pick up nutrients absorbed by the villi of the small intestine. Water-soluble nutrients travel through the bloodstream via the hepatic portal vein to the liver for processing. Fat-soluble nutrients travel through lymphatic vessels until they are released through the thoracic duct into the bloodstream.

The heart is divided into four chambers: two upper atria and two lower ventricles. The oxygen-poor blood the heart receives from the body flows into the right atrium, through the right ventricle, and into the lungs, where it is replenished with oxygen. The oxygen-rich blood flows from the lungs to the left atrium and then into the left ventricle. As the left ventricle contracts, blood is pumped through the aorta and arteries to the capillaries, where it exchanges a variety of substances—including oxygen, water, glucose, and amino acids—with the cells. Carbon dioxide and other substances picked up by the blood are eventually returned to the heart via the veins as the blood completes its route. Carbon dioxide, a metabolic waste, is taken to the lungs and expelled.

Water-soluble nutrients, including carbohydrates, amino acids, and water-soluble vitamins, are absorbed into the enterocytes, cross into the capillaries, and travel via the **hepatic portal vein** to the liver. The portal vein branches out into capillaries, supplying all the liver cells with nutrient-rich blood. The liver further breaks down the nutrients and repackages them before releasing them into the blood. Blood leaves the liver and continues on its journey through the **hepatic vein** back to the heart. Thus, the liver plays a key role in nutrition—it is the first organ to receive water-soluble nutrients absorbed through the intestines via the hepatic portal vein.

The Lymphatic System Distributes Some Nutrients through the Lymph

The **lymphatic system** is a complex network of capillaries, small vessels, valves, nodes, and ducts that transport fat-soluble nutrients throughout the body. Lacteals in the villi collect fat-soluble vitamins, long-chain fatty acids, and some proteins too large to be transported via the blood capillaries. The vessels of the lymph system are different from those of the circulatory system. The cells of the lymph capillary overlap one another, allowing the contents of the lymph vessels to seep out under pressure and circulate between the cells. The fat-soluble nutrients are transported from the lymph capillaries through the lymphatic vessels and eventually arrive at the thoracic duct. At the junction of the thoracic duct is a valve that allows the lymph fluid to flow into the subclavian vein, where it finally enters the blood. The nutrients can then be circulated by the blood to be picked up and used by cells.

The Excretory System Eliminates Waste

After the cells have gleaned the nutrients and other useful metabolic components they need from the blood, their waste must be eliminated through the excretory system. For instance, the breakdown of proteins releases a nitrogenous waste called *urea*. The kidneys filter urea from the blood, allowing it to be excreted in urine. The nearby Table Tips provide strategies for improving your digestion.

hepatic portal vein Large vein that connects the GI tract to the liver and transports newly absorbed water-soluble nutrients.

hepatic vein Vein that carries the blood received from the hepatic portal vein away from the liver.

lymphatic system System of interconnected vessels that contains lymph fluid in which fat-soluble nutrients are carried; also includes bone marrow, lymph nodes, and other tissues and organs that produce and store defensive cells.

LO 3.6: THE TAKE-HOME MESSAGE The cardiovascular and lymphatic systems pick up absorbed nutrients in the villi of the small intestine and transport them throughout the body. Water-soluble nutrients, including carbohydrates, proteins (amino acids), and the water-soluble vitamins, are transported in the bloodstream through the hepatic portal vein to the liver; fat-soluble nutrients, including the fat-soluble vitamins and long-chain fatty acids, are transported via the lymphatic system, which eventually drains into the subclavian vein. The excretory system filters the blood and eliminates waste.

What Are Some Common Digestive Disorders?

LO 3.7 Discuss the most common digestive disorders.

When the digestive system gets "off track," the resulting symptoms can quickly catch your attention. Some of the problems are minor, like occasional heartburn or indigestion; other problems such as ulcers or colon cancer are very serious and require medical treatment.

Esophageal Problems

Several minor esophageal problems can lead to annoying symptoms such as belching, hiccups, burning sensations, or uncomfortable feelings of fullness. More serious esophageal problems include cancer, obstruction from tumors, faulty nerve impulses, severe inflammation, abnormal sphincter function, and even death.

Gastroesophageal Reflux Disease

One of the most common problems involving the esophagus is the burning sensation in the middle of the chest known as *heartburn* (also called *indigestion* or *acid reflux*). About 60 million Americans experience heartburn once a month; about 15 million report daily heartburn.[5]

Heartburn generally occurs when the lower esophageal sphincter (LES) doesn't close properly and acidic gastric juice from the stomach flows back into the esophagus and irritates its lining. Chronic heartburn is the hallmark symptom of **gastroesophageal reflux disease (GERD)**. A weak LES is often the culprit

gastroesophageal reflux disease (GERD) Chronic condition characterized by the backward flow of stomach contents into the esophagus, resulting in heartburn.

gastroenteritis Inflammation of the lining of the stomach and intestines; also known as *stomach flu*.

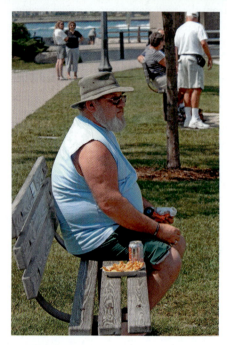

Obesity increases the risk of GERD.

in allowing this backflow. Certain foods, including chocolate, fried or fatty foods, coffee, soda, onions, and garlic, seem to be associated with this condition.[6] Lifestyle factors also play a role. For example, smoking cigarettes, drinking alcohol, wearing tight-fitting clothes, being overweight or obese, eating large evening meals, and reclining after eating tend to cause or worsen the condition.

If dietary changes and behavior modification are insufficient to relieve heartburn, over-the-counter antacids or prescription drugs may help. In rare circumstances, surgical intervention is required to treat severe, unrelenting GERD.

Esophageal Cancer

Esophageal cancer is another medical condition that has serious consequences. According to the National Cancer Institute, esophageal cancer is one of the most common cancers of the GI tract, and the seventh leading cause of cancer-related deaths worldwide. In the United States, this type of cancer is typically found among individuals older than 50 years, males, those who live in urban areas, long-term smokers, and heavy drinkers.

Treatments include surgery, radiation, and chemotherapy.[7]

Disorders of the Stomach

Stomach problems can range from the trivial, such as belching or an occasional stomachache, to life-threatening complications such as bleeding ulcers or stomach cancer. Common causes of stomachache include overeating or eating too fast. Other possible causes include eating foods that are high in fat or fiber, lactose intolerance, or swallowing air while eating.

Belching

Swallowing air usually causes belching (also called *burping*). Often, the air distends the stomach, and is then expelled up through the esophagus, pharynx, and mouth to relieve the discomfort. Swallowing large amounts of air (called *aerophagia*) is most often due to eating or drinking too fast, consuming carbonated beverages, or anxiety. However, aerophagia can occur without any act of swallowing, such as while chewing gum or smoking.

Gastroenteritis and Foodborne Illness

A stomachache can be due to a number of causes, including **gastroenteritis**, commonly known as the "stomach flu." Despite its name, stomach flu is not a form of influenza. It can be caused by a variety of bacteria and viruses, the most common of which is the norovirus. Infection causes an inflammation of the stomach or intestines. Symptoms include nausea and vomiting, diarrhea, and abdominal cramping. Sometimes the problem requires medical intervention, but usually rest, oral rehydration therapy to replace lost fluids and electrolytes, and a soft-food diet will help with the symptoms of this type of illness.

Eating food or drinking fluid that is contaminated with a pathogenic microbe usually results in foodborne illnesses. Raw meat and poultry, raw eggs, unpasteurized milk, and raw shellfish are the foods most likely to be contaminated.[8] The pathogen most commonly involved is the norovirus. The most common bacterial culprit is *Salmonella*. Symptoms such as vomiting, abdominal cramps, diarrhea, and fever occur when enough of the pathogen has been ingested to trigger the body's immune response. Most foodborne illnesses are self-limiting and may require only fluids and rest. More severe foodborne infections may require medical intervention. (You will read more about foodborne illness in Chapter 20.)

Ulcers

An **ulcer** is a sore or erosion in the lining of the lower region of the stomach or the upper part of the duodenum (**Figure 3.14**). Ulcers are named according to their location, such as gastric ulcers, duodenal ulcers, and esophageal ulcers. Whereas spicy foods and stress were once thought to cause most ulcers, researchers have since discovered that a bacterium, *Helicobacter pylori,* is often involved. The use of nonsteroidal anti-inflammatory drugs (NSAIDs), such as aspirin, ibuprofen, naproxen, and ketoprofen, may also cause or aggravate ulcers. These pain relievers inhibit the hormonelike substances that protect the stomach lining from HCl, which results in bleeding and ulceration. Nicotine increases the production of HCl, which increases the risk of developing an ulcer and slows the healing process of ulcers that have already developed. Both excess consumption of alcohol and stress can contribute to ulcer

formations, although these factors may not be directly involved.

Burning pain is the most common symptom of an ulcer, along with vomiting, fatigue, bleeding, and general weakness. Medical treatments may consist of prescription drugs and dietary changes, such as limiting alcohol and caffeine-containing beverages, and/or restricting spices and acidic foods. Surgery is necessary only when an ulcer does not respond to drug treatment. Left untreated, ulcers can result in internal bleeding and perforation of the stomach or intestinal lining, causing peritonitis, or infection of the abdominal cavity. Scar tissue can also form in the GI tract, obstructing food and causing vomiting and weight loss. People who have ulcers caused by *H. pylori* have a greater risk of developing stomach cancer.

Gallbladder Disease

The incidence of gallbladder disease is high in the United States, especially in women and older Americans. Obesity is one of the major risk factors, and this risk is even greater following rapid weight loss.[9]

A common gallbladder disorder is the presence of **gallstones** (**Figure 3.15**). Most people with gallstones have abnormally thick bile, and the bile is high in cholesterol and low in bile acids. Over time, the high-cholesterol bile forms crystals, then sludge, and finally gallstones. Some individuals with gallstones experience no pain or mild pain. Others have severe pain accompanied by fever, nausea and vomiting, cramps, and obstruction of the bile duct.

Medical treatment for gallstones may involve surgery to remove the gallbladder, prescription medicine to dissolve the stones, shock-wave therapy (a type of ultrasound treatment) to break them up, or a combination of therapies. If surgery is required to remove the gallbladder, patients typically recover quickly. After gallbladder removal surgery, the anatomy of the biliary tract adapts. The liver continues to produce the bile and secretes it directly into the duodenum.

Celiac Disease

One of the more serious malabsorption conditions to occur in the small intestine is **celiac disease**. In a healthy small intestine, millions of villi and microvilli efficiently absorb nutrients from food. In celiac disease, the lining of the small intestine flattens out, and it can no longer absorb nutrients (**Figure 3.16**). The flattening is caused by an abnormal reaction to the protein gluten, found in wheat, rye, and barley.

Celiac disease is a genetic, autoimmune disease that causes a person's own immune system to damage the small intestines when gluten is consumed. Note that celiac disease is not the same thing as gluten intolerance, which does not involve the immune system or damage the wall of the small intestine. However, individuals with gluten intolerance can experience similar symptoms such as stomachaches, diarrhea, bloating, and tiredness if gluten is consumed.

Celiac disease is most common among genetically susceptible people of European descent. The most recent estimates suggest that 1 in 133 people (less than 1 percent) have been diagnosed with celiac disease in the United States. When an individual has celiac disease, the incidence among close family members is estimated to be as high

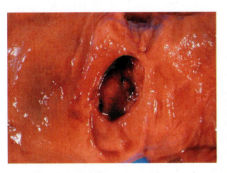

▲ **Figure 3.14 Ulcer**
An ulcer is created when the mucosal lining of the GI tract erodes.

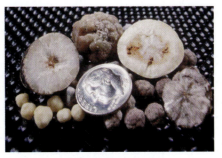

▲ **Figure 3.15 Gallstones**
The size and composition of gallstones vary.

ulcer Sore or erosion of the stomach or intestinal lining.

gallstones Stones formed from cholesterol in the gallbladder or bile duct.

celiac disease Genetic disease in which a hyperimmune response damages the villi of the small intestine when gluten is consumed.

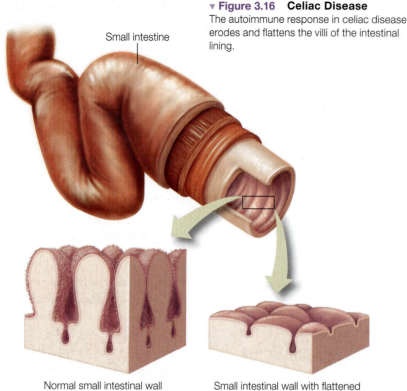

▼ **Figure 3.16** **Celiac Disease**
The autoimmune response in celiac disease erodes and flattens the villi of the intestinal lining.

Small intestine

Normal small intestinal wall with healthy villi

Small intestinal wall with flattened villi caused by celiac disease

as 4.5 percent.[10] Because of this genetic link, celiac disease is classified as a lifelong disorder.

Diagnosis of Celiac Disease

The symptoms for celiac disease vary. Classic symptoms include reoccurring abdominal bloating, cramping, diarrhea, gas, fatty and foul-smelling stools, weight loss, anemia, fatigue, bone or joint pain, and even a painful skin rash called dermatitis herpetiformis. Some people develop the symptoms of celiac disease in infancy or childhood. Others are diagnosed later in life, after being misdiagnosed with irritable bowel syndrome or various food intolerances.

In the past, diagnosing celiac disease was sometimes difficult because it resembles other similar malabsorption diseases. The contemporary method of diagnosis begins with a simple blood test measuring gluten-reactive T cells. If the test is positive, the next step is a tissue biopsy of the small intestine to confirm the diagnosis.[11]

Depending on the length of time between symptom development and diagnosis, the complications from celiac disease can be serious. Celiac patients have an increased incidence of osteoporosis from poor calcium absorption, diminished growth because of nutrient malabsorption, and even seizures due to inadequate folate absorption. Although cancers associated with celiac disease are rare, a history of celiac disease does increase the risk of developing certain types of cancer, including small intestinal adenocarcinoma, esophageal cancer, and melanoma.[12]

Treatment of Celiac Disease

The only treatment for celiac disease is a strict, lifelong gluten-free diet.[13] This should stop the symptoms from progressing, allow the intestine to heal, and prevent further damage. The symptoms often improve within a few days after beginning the gluten-free diet. If the diet is followed faithfully, the absorption area of the GI tract often returns to normal status within 3–6 months.

Avoiding all gluten-containing foods can be challenging. All breads, pasta, cereals, and other grain products made with

wheat, rye, or barley must be eliminated. Gluten-free grain products made with rice flour, bean flours, corn, quinoa, amaranth, and millet are fortunately widely available. Whole foods such as meat, milk, eggs, fruits, and vegetables are of course permissible. The Academy of Nutrition and Dietetics maintains a comprehensive list of

TABLE TIPS

Gluten Free—What Can I Eat?

Be a label reader to avoid products that contain all forms of wheat, barley, rye, triticale, or their hybrids.

Substitute whole-wheat bread with gluten-free whole grains, such as quinoa, buckwheat, amaranth, sorghum, and millet.

If you like a hot cereal for breakfast, try teff, a nutritious cereal grain from Ethiopia with a nutty, chewy texture.

Avoid packaged foods that contain modified food starch, dextrin, malt, or malt syrup, as they may be sources of gluten-containing grains.

Enjoy coffee, tea, sodas, fruit juices, and even fermented or distilled beverages, such as wine, sake, and distilled spirits on a gluten-free diet. But avoid coffee flavorings or creamers.

Look for either the GFCO or CSA Seal of Recognition marks on labels to ensure the product is gluten free.

Maintain a high fiber intake by incorporating gluten-free fresh fruits, vegetables, beans, peas, and lentils in your diet.

Consume calcium-rich milk, calcium-fortified orange juice, or calcium-fortified beverages made from soy, rice, or nuts.

Snack on gluten-free nuts, fruits, popcorn, raisins, rice cakes, and fruit smoothies.

Enjoy homemade meals to control gluten intake and eat a variety of nutrient-dense foods.

foods allowed on a gluten-free diet on its website, *www.eatright.org.*[14] The nearby Table Tips identify strategies for maintaining a gluten-free diet.

Until recently, oats had been considered a forbidden food for celiac patients. However, unprocessed oats are gluten-free. Concerns for people with celiac disease are due to the possibility that oats may be contaminated with hidden sources of gluten during processing. Purchasing oats from companies that advertise their products as gluten-free and avoiding oats sold in bulk bins can allay such concerns.

Non-Celiac Gluten Sensitivity

Many people who have tested negative for celiac disease nevertheless report a reduction in both GI and non-GI symptoms when they remove gluten from their diet. This condition, referred to as **non-celiac gluten sensitivity (NCGS)**, is currently the subject of considerable research.[15]

People without Celiac Disease or Gluten Sensitivity Should Not Avoid Gluten

Gluten-free diets have become a fad that is fueling a market of gluten-free products, with sales of more than $2 billion expected by 2020.[16] There are currently more people following a gluten-free diet than there are diagnosed with celiac disease.[17] Is this healthy?

Gluten itself isn't an essential nutrient, but the foods that contain gluten are typically rich in dietary fiber, vitamins, and minerals. Many gluten-free products are made with refined, unenriched gluten-free grains low in essential nutrients and high in kilocalories. Gluten-free foods are also typically much more expensive than similar foods made with wheat.[18] Moreover, gluten itself may provide some health benefits for individuals without celiac disease or NCGS. Recent studies have shown gluten-rich foods may improve blood lipids, control blood pressure, and boost the

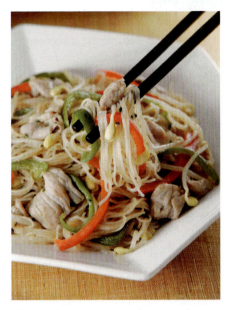

Rice noodles are a good gluten-free substitute for pasta.

immune system.[19] For this reason, there are no real benefits to eating a gluten-free diet if you are not gluten sensitive, have not been diagnosed with celiac disease, or do not have other autoimmune disorders.

Other Intestinal Disorders

Other disorders of the intestines can occur anywhere along the length of the small and large intestines.

Flatulence

Flatulence is an uncomfortable and sometimes embarrassing (but normal) condition that results from the formation of intestinal gas (*flatus*). Intestinal gas is produced for a variety of reasons, and most adults release it 10–20 times a day. Eating too fast or drinking beverages with added air such as beer or carbonated beverages can result in the intake of incidental air that makes its way through the GI tract. Beans, lentils, and other legumes can lead to gas production because they contain indigestible carbohydrates that are fermented by intestinal bacteria. The bacteria produce the gas as a by-product. Lack of exercise and smoking have also been identified as culprits in flatulence.

Flatus is a mixture of carbon dioxide, hydrogen, nitrogen, oxygen, and methane. The offending odor comes from gases that contain sulfur, chiefly hydrogen sulfide and methylmercaptan. Foods high in fiber and starches tend to produce more intestinal gas. Using products such as Beano or eating smaller meals will help reduce the amount of gas produced.

Diarrhea and Constipation

Two of the most common intestinal disorders are diarrhea and constipation. **Diarrhea** is the passage of watery, loose stools more than three times a day. Acute diarrhea lasts for up to 2 days and is usually the result of bacterial, viral, or parasitic infection. The infection results in the enterocytes becoming inflamed and secreting, rather than absorbing, fluid into the GI tract. The result is that food and fluids pass too quickly through the colon and out through the rectum.

Whereas brief episodes of diarrhea may be a sign of infection or an adverse reaction to a specific food, medication, or other compound (such as the sugar substitute sorbitol), chronic diarrhea may be a sign of celiac disease, irritable bowel syndrome (see below), or colitis, conditions that require diagnosis by a health care provider.

The loss of fluids and electrolytes in diarrhea can be mild or life-threatening. Mild diarrhea is generally treated with fluid and electrolyte replacement. Diarrhea that is severe or that lasts for an extended period can lead to dehydration, malabsorption—which in turn can lead to malnutrition—and potentially even death. The condition can be particularly dangerous for children and older adults, who are more susceptible to dehydration.

non-celiac gluten sensitivity (NCGS) Reaction to eating foods that contain gluten when celiac disease has been ruled out. Symptoms vary widely but may include abdominal pain, fatigue, headaches, rashes, or mental confusion.

flatulence Production of excessive gas in the stomach or the intestines.

diarrhea Abnormally frequent passage of watery stools.

Constipation is caused by excessively slow movements of undigested food residue through the colon, often as a result of insufficient fiber or water intake. Ignoring or putting off the need to defecate can also result in more absorption of water from fecal matter in the large intestine, leading to harder, drier stools. Stress, inactivity, cessation of smoking, and various illnesses and medications can also lead to constipation.[20,21]

Because fiber attracts water, adds bulk to stool in the colon, and stimulates peristalsis, constipation is often treated with a high-fiber, high-liquid diet. Daily exercise, establishing eating and resting routines, and using over-the-counter stool softeners are usually recommended to treat this condition without the use of laxatives or enemas.

If constipation persists, laxatives can provide some relief, but should be used sparingly. A variety of laxatives can be purchased over the counter. Bulk-forming or stool-softening laxatives trigger peristalsis by drawing water into the GI tract, which increases the bulk of the feces and stretches the circular muscles in the intestine. Stimulant laxatives, such as Ex-lax or Senokot, are the harshest form of laxative and work by irritating the lining of the GI tract to stimulate peristalsis. Because laxatives can cause dehydration, electrolyte imbalances, and laxative dependency, they should not be used routinely unless a physician supervises.

One harmful and unnecessary practice is colonic cleansing, which involves administration of an enema to flush water and feces out of the body. The practice can interfere with the absorption of fat-soluble vitamins and can be dangerous if the equipment used to administer the enema isn't sanitized or if the bowel is perforated when the rubber tube is inserted. Other problems may result from electrolyte and water imbalance and dependency.

constipation Infrequent passage of dry, hardened stools.

hemorrhoid Swelling in the veins of the rectum and anus.

irritable bowel syndrome (IBS) Intestinal disorder resulting in abdominal discomfort, pain, diarrhea, constipation, and bloating; the cause is unknown.

Hemorrhoids

A **hemorrhoid** is an inflammation and swelling of the veins in the rectum and anus. The walls of the veins dilate, become thin, and bleed. Though the exact cause of hemorrhoids is not known, several factors result in a buildup of pressure within the veins. These include constipation (straining to pass dry stools), pregnancy, and obesity. Chronic diarrhea, anal intercourse, a low-fiber diet, and aging are also risk factors. Whatever the cause, the result is that the walls of the veins dilate, become thin, and bleed. As the pressure builds, the vessels protrude. Hemorrhoids may not be noticed until they begin to bleed (following a bowel movement), itch, or become painful.

The most common treatment for hemorrhoids is the same as for constipation: increase dietary fiber and fluid intake. Other symptoms, including itching and pain, can be relieved with over-the-counter creams, ice packs to relieve swelling, and soaking in a warm bath. In severe cases of hemorrhoids, surgery may be necessary.

Irritable Bowel Syndrome

Irritable bowel syndrome (IBS) is a general term used to describe changes in colon rhythm, not an actual disease.

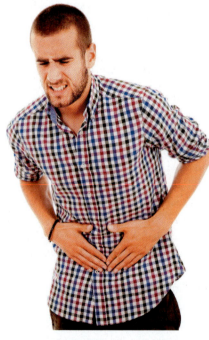

Irritable bowel syndrome can cause significant abdominal pain.

It causes a great deal of discomfort for the estimated 30 million North Americans who have it.[22] People with IBS do not have tissue damage, inflammation, or immunologic involvement of the colon. They do, however, overrespond to colon stimuli. This results in alternating patterns of diarrhea, constipation, bloating, and abdominal pain. The exact cause of IBS is unknown, but low-fiber diets, stress, consumption of foods that trigger the symptoms (such as alcohol, chocolate, and dairy products), and intestinal motility disorders are all suspected factors. Medical management includes increasing dietary fiber, managing stress, and occasional use of prescription drugs.

A diet designed to alleviate the symptoms of IBS is called the *low FODMAP diet*. The acronym FODMAP stands for *fermented, oligosaccharides, disaccharides, monosaccharides,* and *polyols*. The foods that contain these carbohydrates, which you learn more about in Chapter 4, are not completely digested and thus can trigger cramps, diarrhea, and other symptoms of IBS. They are listed in **Table 3.4**. The diet limits these carbohydrates but doesn't completely eliminate them. While the low FODMAP diet may not work for everyone with IBS, a recent study found that some participants with IBS reversed their symptoms after just 7 days on the diet.[23] See the Nutrition in Practice for more information on nutritional strategies for irritable bowel syndrome.

TABLE 3.4	FODMAP Foods
Food Components to Avoid	**Foods Containing Component**
Fructose	Fruits, honey, high-fructose corn syrup, agave
Lactose	Dairy
Fructans	Wheat, onions, garlic
Galactans	Legumes, beans, lentils, and soybeans
Polyols	Sugar alcohols, fruits with pits or seeds such as apples, avocados, cherries, figs, peaches, or plums

NUTRITION *in* PRACTICE:
Nurse Practitioner

College freshman Desiree has always had what her mother called "a nervous stomach." When she is stressed or worried about something, her bowels seem to respond first with abdominal pain followed by constipation or diarrhea. Her first semester at college has been challenging as she is trying to adjust to the rigorous demands of her pre-med curriculum and the intense schedule of science classes and labs. Her symptoms are worse right before an exam or when she eats large meals. She eats a very light breakfast because she doesn't want to feel uncomfortably full and bloated during her morning classes. Lately, Desiree has had frequent bouts of abdominal pain that are only relieved by a bowel movement, followed by several loose, watery stools. With mid-terms approaching the abdominal pain and diarrhea appear to be getting worse. She is experiencing difficulty falling asleep at night, which is causing her to become tired by midday. She decides to visit the campus health center.

After meeting with the nurse practitioner (NP) at the health center, Desiree is told that she has irritable bowel syndrome (IBS) and that stress and her diet are likely contributing to her health issue. The nurse practitioner referred Desire to the campus health center stress management program, which is designed to help students manage anxiety and stress while on campus. She also referred Desiree to the campus registered dietitian nutritionist (RDN) for an appointment. The RDN meets with Desiree to discuss her diet.

Desiree's Stats:
- Age: 18
- Height: 5 feet 4 inches
- Weight: 115 lbs
- BMI: 19.7
- Symptoms: abdominal pain; loose, watery stool with bouts of constipation

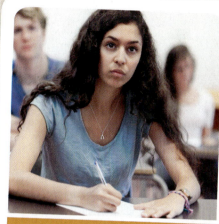

Desiree

DESIREE'S FOOD LOG

Food/Beverage	Time Consumed	Hunger Rating*	Location	Feelings/Symptoms
Large black coffee 24 oz.	7:30 a.m.	1	Walking to class	Anxious about classes and upcoming exam
Cheeseburger and fries	1 pm	5	Campus dining hall	Tired
Large diet cola	2 p.m.	1	Library	Some diarrhea
Energy drink, 12 oz.	4 p.m.	1	Walking to dorm	Tired
Fried chicken, mashed potato, and corn	6 p.m.	3	In dorm	Stressed, stomach cramps; feeling bloated

*Hunger Rating (1–5): 1 = not hungry; 5 = super-hungry.

Critical Thinking Questions
1. How do you think her eating pattern may be contributing to her IBS symptoms? What aspect of Desiree's diet and lifestyle may be contributing to her IBS symptoms?
2. Which beverages could be contributing to Desiree's bouts of diarrhea and tiredness?
3. How are Desiree's food choices contributing to her discomfort?

RDN's Observation and Plan for Desiree:
- Reinforce the NP's recommendation to visit the campus health center stress management program for guidance on dealing with stress at college. Stress is a trigger for IBS symptoms.
- Slowly reduce the caffeine (coffee, energy drinks) in her diet. Caffeine can increase jitteriness (anxiety), cause a spastic colon (diarrhea), and interfere with the ability to fall asleep (fatigue).
- Reduce the fat at her meals. Fatty foods can also trigger diarrhea in folks with IBS.
- Avoid large meals. Eat three smaller meals and two small snacks throughout the day.

Three weeks later, Desiree visits the RDN again and reports that she has reduced her caffeine intake by eliminating her daily energy drinks and is sleeping better at night. She has begun to eat a breakfast of a Greek yogurt with sliced bananas topped with a whole grain cereal. She switched to grilled chicken to reduce the fat at her lunch and is trying to eat a more balanced dinner. She listens to meditation tapes daily, as suggested in the stress management program, and is feeling less anxious. A dietary analysis of Desiree's food intake reveals she needs to add more dairy in her diet and a wider variety of vegetables and fruit. The RDN works with Desiree to make these diet changes.

Inflammatory Bowel Disease

Inflammatory bowel disease (IBD) occurs when inflammation of the GI tract impairs the ability of the colon to compact food waste and form feces. The result is diarrhea. Ulcerative colitis and Crohn's disease are forms of IBD with similar symptoms. **Ulcerative colitis** is a chronic inflammation of the large intestine that results in ulcers in the lining of the colon. The disorder usually begins between the ages of 15 and 30, occurs in both men and women, and tends to run in families, especially in Caucasians and people of Jewish descent. **Crohn's disease** is similar to ulcerative colitis except that the ulcers can occur throughout the entire GI tract, from the mouth to the anus, not just in the colon.

The cause of ulcerative colitis and Crohn's disease is not known and there is no cure. Physical examinations, laboratory tests, and a colonoscopy are often used to distinguish between the two conditions. Medical treatment includes drug therapy and, in severe cases, surgery.

Recent research findings suggest that an anti-inflammatory diet similar to the Mediterranean diet might be helpful. Foods thought to have anti-inflammatory properties include fish, olive oil, and fresh fruits and vegetables. Fish provide omega-3 fatty acids that reduce levels of inflammatory proteins in the body, including C-reactive protein, which you learn more about in Chapter 5, and interleukin-6, which plays a key role in the acute phase of the body's inflammatory response. Fresh fruits and vegetables are rich in certain vitamins and phytochemicals that also reduce inflammation; in addition, probiotics may play a role in reducing inflammation.[24,25]

Colon Cancer

Colon cancer is one of the leading forms of cancer and the second leading cause of cancer death in men and women.[26] Fortunately, colon cancer is also one of the most curable forms of cancer, if it is detected in the early stages.

Colon cancer often begins with polyps on the lining of the colon (**Figure 3.17**). They vary in size from that of a small pea to that of a mushroom or plum. The good news is that polyps are often small and benign and are routinely removed during a screening colonoscopy. This procedure has reduced the incidence of colon cancer during the past two decades.[27] If the polyps are not removed and develop into cancerous tumors, colon cancer can be difficult to cure.

Individuals diagnosed with colon cancer may require radiation therapy, chemotherapy, and surgery to remove all or part of the colon. After surgery, patients are given dietary advice regarding the foods that would be the most comfortable to eat. Survival rates vary depending on the individual's age, health, treatment response, and stage of cancer at diagnosis.[28, 29]

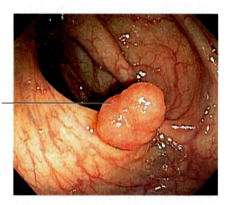

Polyp

▲ **Figure 3.17** **Colon Polyp**
Polyps on the lining of the colon can be one of the first signs of colon cancer.

LO 3.7: THE TAKE-HOME MESSAGE
Some GI disorders, such as ulcers, GERD, and irritable bowel syndrome, are not life-threatening, but can significantly reduce quality of life. Others, including celiac disease, ulcerative colitis, Crohn's disease, and colon or esophageal cancer, may cause nutrient malabsorption, malnutrition, or even death. Less serious conditions, like constipation, diarrhea, hemorrhoids, and stomach flu, are typically temporary.

inflammatory bowel disease (IBD) Chronic inflammation throughout the GI tract.

ulcerative colitis Chronic inflammation of the colon that results in ulcers forming in the lining.

Crohn's disease Form of ulcerative colitis in which ulcers form throughout the GI tract and not just in the colon.

Visual Chapter Summary

LO 3.1 Digestion Takes Place in the GI Tract, Helped by the Accessory Organs

Digestion is the process of breaking down whole food into absorbable nutrients. Digestion takes place in the GI tract, a long tube composed of the mouth, pharynx, esophagus, stomach, small intestine, and large intestine. Several sphincters control entry and exit of food and chyme through the various organs of the GI tract. Accessory organs, including the salivary glands, liver, gallbladder, and pancreas, secrete bile, hormones, and enzymes that facilitate digestion.

The small intestine is the primary organ for the absorption of digested nutrients. The large intestine absorbs water and some minerals before pushing waste through the colon and out of the body via the rectum.

Bile produced in the liver emulsifies fat, increasing its access to pancreatic lipase. The liver is the first organ to receive, process, and store absorbed water-soluble nutrients. The pancreas releases pancreatic digestive enzymes and bicarbonate into the small intestine. The gallbladder stores and concentrates bile.

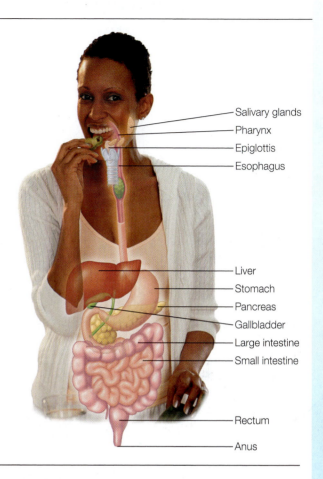

- Salivary glands
- Pharynx
- Epiglottis
- Esophagus
- Liver
- Stomach
- Pancreas
- Gallbladder
- Large intestine
- Small intestine
- Rectum
- Anus

LO 3.2 Peristalsis and Segmentation Propel Food through the Gastrointestinal Tract

Food is propelled along the GI tract by peristalsis and segmentation. Peristalsis moves food through the stomach and intestines by rhythmic contractions of longitudinal and circular muscles. Segmentation shifts the mass of food back and forth into smaller pieces while mixing it with the chemical secretions of the intestine. Segmentation in the large intestine facilitates the absorption of water from the feces and mass movements push the mass toward the rectum for excretion.

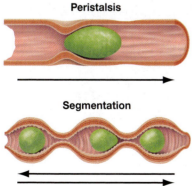

Peristalsis

Segmentation

LO 3.3 Enzymes and Other Secretions Chemically Digest Food

Chemical digestion includes mixing food with enzymes that break the bonds between molecules via hydrolysis. HCl denatures proteins and triggers the conversion of pepsinogen to pepsin, which initiates protein digestion. Bile from the gallbladder emulsifies large fat globules into smaller pieces to improve enzymatic action. Digestion is completed by the brush border enzymes maltase, sucrase, and lactase, and the proteases, breaking nutrients down into single molecules that can be absorbed into the enterocytes.

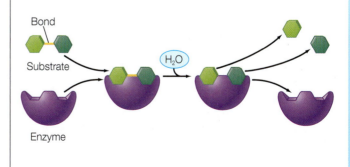

Bond

Substrate

H_2O

Enzyme

Digested Nutrients Are Absorbed Primarily through the Small Intestine

Digested nutrients pass through the brush border of the small intestinal lining via passive diffusion, facilitated diffusion, active transport, or endocytosis. The water and salts not absorbed in the small intestine are absorbed in the large intestine.

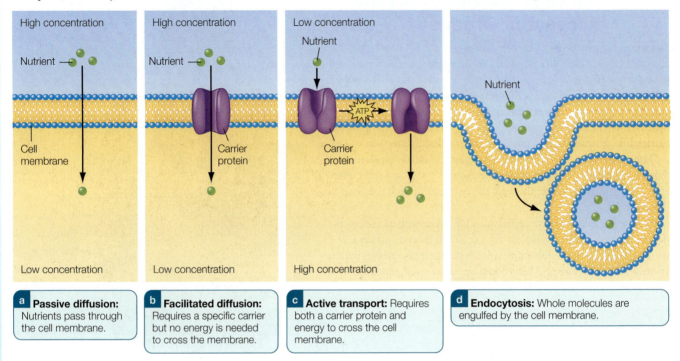

High concentration

Nutrient

Cell membrane

Low concentration

a Passive diffusion: Nutrients pass through the cell membrane.

High concentration

Nutrient

Carrier protein

Low concentration

b Facilitated diffusion: Requires a specific carrier but no energy is needed to cross the membrane.

Low concentration

Nutrient

ATP

Carrier protein

High concentration

c Active transport: Requires both a carrier protein and energy to cross the cell membrane.

Nutrient

d Endocytosis: Whole molecules are engulfed by the cell membrane.

Digestion Is Regulated by Hormones and the Nervous System

Digestive functions are regulated by hormones, including gastrin, secretin, cholecystokinin, and gastric inhibitory peptide. These hormones are chemical messengers secreted from the GI tract that direct enzymes and the release of digestive secretions during digestion. The enteric nerves embedded in the wall of the GI tract work autonomously and in collaboration with the central nervous system and other nervous system branches to achieve multiple GI functions. Nerves also interact with the GI tract to stimulate hormone release when certain foods are consumed.

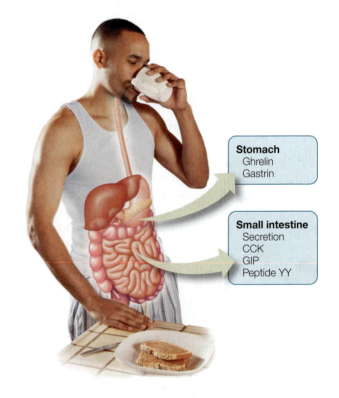

Stomach
Ghrelin
Gastrin

Small intestine
Secretion
CCK
GIP
Peptide YY

LO 3.6 Absorbed Nutrients Are Transported throughout the Body by the Cardiovascular and Lymphatic Systems

The cardiovascular system distributes water-soluble nutrients throughout the body and carries carbon dioxide and other waste products to be excreted through the lungs and the kidneys. The lymphatic system transports fat-soluble vitamins from the GI tract through the lymphatic system and into the cardiovascular system.

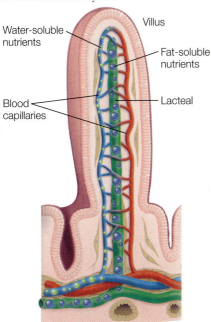

Water-soluble nutrients

Villus

Fat-soluble nutrients

Blood capillaries

Lacteal

LO 3.7 Digestive Disorders Can Result in Malabsorption and Malnutrition

Several digestive disorders can result in malabsorption and malnutrition, including celiac disease, ulcerative colitis, and Crohn's disease. Celiac disease is an autoimmune disorder that damages the villi of the small intestine following gluten ingestion. Irritable bowel syndrome is a disorder of unknown cause, the symptoms of which may improve on a low-FODMAP diet. Heartburn, constipation, diarrhea, and hemorrhoids are common, less serious digestive disorders. If left unchecked, even diarrhea can be potentially life-threatening. Common cancers of the GI tract include esophageal, stomach, and colon cancer.

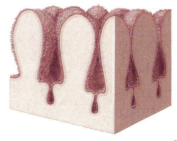

Normal small intestinal wall · Small intestinal wall with celiac disease

Terms to Know

- digestion
- absorption
- elimination
- gastrointestinal (GI) tract
- propulsion
- lumen
- sphincters
- chemical digestion
- mechanical digestion
- mastication
- saliva
- bolus
- pharynx
- esophagus
- epiglottis
- upper esophageal sphincter

- lower esophageal sphincter (LES)
- stomach
- goblet cells
- gastric pits
- parietal cells
- chief cells
- mucus
- chyme
- small intestine
- villi
- enterocytes
- microvilli
- crypts
- large intestine
- cecum
- ileocecal valve
- colon
- GI flora
- ferment

- probiotics
- prebiotics
- stool
- rectum
- anus
- intestinal permeability
- salivary glands
- liver
- gallbladder
- pancreas
- peristalsis
- segmentation
- mass movement
- enzymes
- hydrolysis
- substrate
- pH
- hydrochloric acid (HCl)
- proteases
- pepsinogen

- pepsin
- bile
- emulsify
- enterohepatic circulation
- bicarbonate
- passive diffusion
- facilitated diffusion
- active transport
- endocytosis
- enteric nervous system
- enterogastrones
- gastrin
- secretin
- cholecystokinin (CCK)
- gastric inhibitory peptide (GIP)
- ghrelin
- peptide YY
- hepatic portal vein

- hepatic vein
- lymphatic system
- gastroesophageal reflux disease (GERD)
- gastroenteritis
- ulcer
- gallstones
- celiac disease
- non-celiac gluten sensitivity (NCGS)
- flatulence
- diarrhea
- constipation
- hemorrhoid
- irritable bowel syndrome (IBS)
- inflammatory bowel disease (IBD)
- ulcerative colitis
- Crohn's disease

Check Your Understanding

LO 3.1 1. _____ is defined as breaking apart food by mechanical and enzymatic means in the stomach and the small intestine.
  a. Absorption
  b. Transport
  c. Digestion
  d. Elimination

LO 3.1 2. The protective tissue that covers the trachea during swallowing is the
  a. esophagus.
  b. tongue.
  c. pharynx.
  d. epiglottis.

LO 3.1 3. Which of the following statements about the small intestine is true?
  a. It is shorter than the large intestine.
  b. It is the primary site of both digestion and absorption.
  c. It has access to lymph vessels but not to the bloodstream.
  d. It is composed of the ileum, duodenum, and cecum, in that order.

LO 3.2 4. Food is moved through the GI tract by rhythmic muscular waves called
  a. segmentation.
  b. peristalsis.
  c. bowel movement.
  d. mastication.

LO 3.3 5. Which of the following secretions chemically breaks apart foods?
  a. Ghrelin
  b. Bicarbonate ions
  c. Cholecystokinin
  d. Enzymes

LO 3.3 6. Which of the following is a function of hydrochloric acid?
  a. Triggers the conversion of pepsinogen to pepsin
  b. Slows peristalsis
  c. Neutralizes the pH in the stomach
  d. Begins carbohydrate digestion

LO 3.4 7. Glucose and amino acids are absorbed by
  a. passive diffusion.
  b. facilitated diffusion.
  c. active transport.
  d. endocytosis.

LO 3.5 8. The hormone that is produced in the stomach and stimulates hunger is called
  a. pepsin.
  b. gastrin.
  c. cholecystokinin.
  d. ghrelin.

LO 3.6 9. Which of the following transports fat-soluble nutrients to the blood?
  a. Hepatic portal vein
  b. Lymphatic vessels
  c. Red blood cells
  d. The kidneys

LO 3.7 10. Celiac disease is caused by a reaction to gluten found in which foods?
  a. Citrus fruits
  b. Wheat, barley, and rye
  c. Legumes, nuts, and seeds
  d. Milk, cheese, and yogurt

Answers

1. (c) Digestion is defined as the process of breaking apart food by mechanical and enzymatic means. Once food is digested it can be absorbed into the blood or lymphatic system to be transported to the cells. Any waste products are eliminated through urine and feces.

2. (d) The epiglottis covers the trachea. The esophagus is a tube that carries food to the stomach. The tongue is a muscle that pushes food to the back of the mouth into the pharynx, a chamber that food passes through before being swallowed.

3. (b) The small intestine is the primary site of both digestion and absorption. With numerous villi and microvilli, it has a vast surface area to enhance absorption. It allows nutrients to pass into both blood and lymph. It consists of the duodenum, then the jejunum, and finally the ileum. It is much longer than the large intestine.

4. (b) Peristalsis is the process that moves food through the GI tract. Segmentation squeezes chyme back and forth along the intestinal walls. A bowel movement involves waves of peristalsis moving feces through the large intestine. Mastication is the process of chewing food.

5. (d) Enzymes secreted from the stomach, small intestine, and pancreas chemically break apart food. Grehlin is a hormone that stimulates gastric motility and hunger. Bicarbonate ions neutralize acid. Cholecystokinin is a hormone that slows peristalsis.

6. (a) Hydrochloric acid activates pepsinogen, which is converted to pepsin. It also breaks down connective tissue in meat and destroys some microorganisms. Cholecystokinin and gastric inhibitory hormones slow peristalsis. Bicarbonate ions neutralize pH in the duodenum. Salivary amylase begins carbohydrate breakdown in the mouth.

7. (c) Glucose and amino acids are absorbed by active transport.

8. (d) Grehlin produced by the gastric cells stimulates gastric motility and hunger. Pepsin is the active form of a protease secreted by the chief cells in the stomach. Gastrin produced in the stomach stimulates parietal cells to release HCl. Cholecystokinin (CCK) is released from the duodenum when fats and proteins enter the duodenum. CCK stimulates the gallbladder to release bile and the pancreas to secrete bicarbonate ions and digestive enzymes.

9. (b) The fat-soluble nutrients are transported through the lymphatic vessels and eventually arrive at the thoracic duct, where they enter the bloodstream at the subclavian vein. The hepatic portal vein transports water-soluble nutrients to the liver. Red blood cells transport oxygen. The kidneys filter the blood to remove and excrete waste into the urine.

10. (b) Wheat, barley, and rye contain gluten, which causes the symptoms associated with celiac disease. Fruits, legumes and other vegetables, dairy foods, meat, nuts, and seeds are free of gluten and are safe to eat on a gluten-free diet.

Answers to True or False?

1. **True.** The enzyme salivary amylase, found in saliva, begins digesting carbohydrates during chewing. As they are broken down to their simple sugars, these carbohydrates will begin to taste sweet.
2. **True.** The stomach secretes a powerful digestive acid, HCl, that is strong enough to damage the stomach lining. A thick layer of mucus protects it.
3. **True.** Bile emulsifies fat by breaking up the large globules into smaller fat droplets.
4. **False.** Acid reflux occurs when acidic stomach contents pass back through the lower esophageal sphincter into the esophagus.
5. **True.** After food has been completely broken down and its nutrients absorbed in the small intestine, the remaining mass passes into the large intestine, where water and electrolytes continue to be absorbed.
6. **True.** Fecal matter is about 50 percent bacteria, and the rest is undigested food, water, and sloughed intestinal cells.
7. **False.** Lymph transports only fat-soluble nutrients. Blood transports water-soluble nutrients.
8. **True.** Several hormones, including gastrin, secretin, cholecystokinin (CCK), and gastric inhibitory peptide, help regulate digestion.
9. **False.** Though foodborne illness can cause diarrhea, the condition can also result from an adverse reaction to stress or to certain foods, medications, or other compounds.
10. **False.** The cause of irritable bowel syndrome is not known, but low-fiber diets, stress, consumption of irritating foods, and intestinal motility disorders are all suspected factors.

Web Resources

- To learn more about the various conditions related to digestion, absorption, and elimination, visit the Center for Digestive Health and Nutrition at www.gihealth.com
- Search the National Digestive Diseases Information Clearinghouse site for more information about various digestive diseases at http://digestive.niddk.nih.gov

References

1. Marieb, E. N., and K. Hoehn. 2016. *Human Anatomy and Physiology*. 10th ed. San Francisco: Benjamin Cummings.
2. Gropper, S. S., and J. L. Smith. 2016. *Advanced Nutrition and Human Metabolism*. 7th ed. Belmont, CA: Wadsworth Cengage Learning.
3. Marieb, E. N., and K. Hoehn. 2016. *Human Anatomy and Physiology*. 10th ed. San Francisco: Benjamin Cummings.
4. Ibid.
5. Health Grades. 2013. *Prevalence and Incidence of Heartburn*. Available at www.rightdiagnosis.com. Accessed December 2016.
6. Guandalini, S., and A. Assiri. 2014. Celiac Disease: A Review. *Journal of the American Medical Association Pediatrics*. doi: 10.1001/jamapediatrics.2013.3858.
7. National Cancer Institute. 2014. *Esophageal Cancer*. Available at www.cancer.gov. Accessed December 2016.
8. Center for Disease Control and Prevention. 2016. *Foodborne Germs and Illnesses*. Available at https://www.cdc.gov/foodsafety/foodborne-germs.html. Accessed January 2017.
9. Healthline. 2017. Gallbladder Disease. Available at http://www.healthline.com/health/gallbladder-disease#Types2. Accessed January 2017.
10. Pelkowski, T. D., and A. J. Viera. 2014. Celiac Disease: Diagnosis and Management. *American Family Physician* 89(2):99–105.
11. Shenoy, S. 2016. Genetic Risks and Familial Associations of Small Bowel Carcinoma. *World Journal of Gastrointestinal Oncology* 8(6):509–519.
12. Pelkowski, T. D., and A. J. Viera, 2014.
13. Lebwohl, B., J. F. Luvigsson, and P. H. R. Green. 2015. Celiac Disease and Non-Celiac Gluten Sensitivity. *British Medical Journal*, 351:h4347.
14. Denny, S. 2015. The Gluten-Free Diet: Building the Grocery List. Available at http://www.eatright.org/resource/health/diseases-and-conditions/celiac-disease/the-gluten-free-diet-building-the-grocery-list. Accessed January 2017.
15. Lebwohl, B., J. F. Luvigsson, and P.H.R. Green. 2015.
16. Ibid.
17. Packaged Facts. 2016. Gluten-Free Foods in the U. S., 6th Edition. Available at https://www.packagedfacts.com/Gluten-Free-Foods-10378213. Accessed January 2017.
18. Jaret, P. 2017. The Truth About Gluten Free. Available at http://www.webmd.com/diet/healthy-kitchen-11/truth-about-gluten. Accessed January 2017.
19. Stein, K. 2014. Severely Restricted Diets in the Absence of Medical Necessity: The Unintended Consequences. *Journal of the Academy of Nutrition and Dietetics* 114(7):986-987.
20. Gaesser, G. A., and S. S. Angadi. 2012. Gluten Free Diet: Imprudent Dietary Advice for the General Population? *Journal of the Academy of Nutrition and Dietetics* 122(9):1330-1333.
21. Fathallah, N., D. Bouchard, et al. 2016. Diet and Lifestyle Rules in Chronic Constipation in Adults: From Fantasy to Reality . . . *La Presse Medicale* doi: 10.1016/j.lpm.2016.03.019.
22. What Is Constipation? Available at http://www.webmd.com/digestive-disorders/digestive-diseases-constipation#2. Accessed January 2017.
23. Bellini, M., et al. 2016. A Low FODMAP Diet in Irritable Bowel Syndrome Improves Symptoms Without Affecting Body Composition and Extracellular Body Water. *Gastroenterology* 150:4, S200.
24. Olendzki, B. C., et al. 2014. An Anti-inflammatory Diet as Treatment for Inflammatory Bowel Disease: A Case Series Report. *Nutrition Journal* 13:5. doi: 10.1186/1475-2891-13-5
25. Ibid.
26. U.S. Cancer Statistics Working Group. *United States Cancer Statistics: 1999–2013 Incidence and Mortality Web-based Report*. Atlanta (GA): Department of Health and Human Services, Centers for Disease Control and Prevention, and National Cancer Institute. 2016. Available at: http://www.cdc.gov/uscs. Accessed January 2017.
27. Ibid.
28. Baars, A., A. Oosting, et al. 2015. The Gut Microbiota as a Therapeutic Target in IBD and Metabolic Disease: A Role for the Bile Acid Receptors FXR and TGR5. *Microorganisms*, 3(4), 641-666. Available at http://doi.org/10.3390/microorganisms3040641
29. Joyce, S. A., and G. M. Cormac. 2016. Bile Acid Modifications at the Microbe-Host Interface: Potential for Nutraceutical and Pharmaceutical Interventions in Host Health. *Annual Review of Food Science and Technology* 7:313-333. doi: 10.1146/annurev-food-041715-033159.

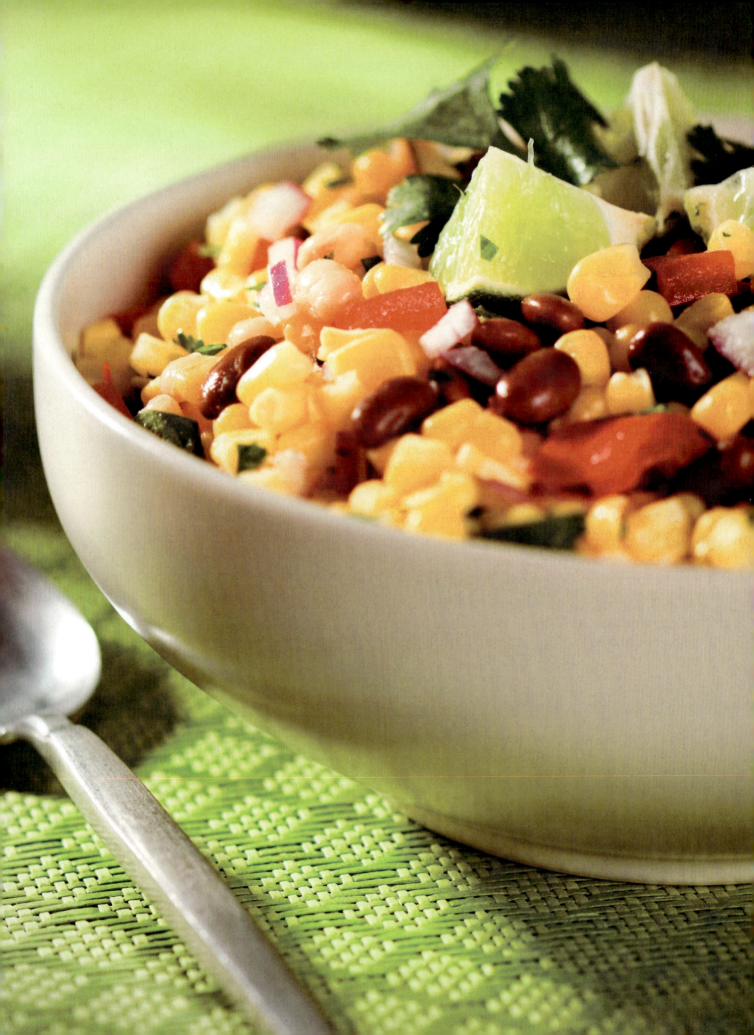

Carbohydrates

Learning Outcomes

After reading this chapter, you will be able to:

4.1 Describe and classify carbohydrates.

4.2 Explain how the body digests and absorbs carbohydrates.

4.3 List the functions of carbohydrates in the body.

4.4 Explain how the body maintains blood glucose levels.

4.5 Discuss the role of dietary fiber in promoting health.

4.6 Identify the DRIs for carbohydrate intake and the best food sources.

4.7 Compare and contrast natural sugars, added sugars, and sugar substitutes.

4.8 Describe the underlying mechanisms, symptoms, and treatment for different classifications of diabetes.

True or False?

1. Carbohydrates are the least important macronutrient. **T/F**

2. Most babies are born lactose intolerant. **T/F**

3. Carbohydrates are a main cause of obesity. **T/F**

4. Sugar causes hyperactivity in children. **T/F**

5. Whole grains are more nutrient dense than refined grains. **T/F**

6. Sugar causes tooth decay. **T/F**

7. Aspartame causes cancer in humans. **T/F**

8. Americans do not consume enough fiber. **T/F**

9. Soda and other sugar-sweetened beverages play a big role in Americans' epidemic of obesity. **T/F**

10. Obese individuals are more likely to develop type 2 diabetes. **T/F**

See page 152 for the answers.

Carbohydrates are energy-yielding macronutrients, most of which are produced in plants. Their main role in the body is to supply fuel, primarily in the form of glucose (*ose* = sugar), which cells convert to the energy molecule ATP. With such an important role in the body, it isn't surprising that foods high in carbohydrates, including rice and other grains, legumes, fruits, tubers, and nuts, make up the foundation of diets the world over.

In this chapter, you learn about different types of carbohydrates and the functions they perform in the body. We also discuss how the body digests carbohydrates and regulates blood glucose levels, and what happens when this metabolic control fails, as in the disease diabetes mellitus. We also identify the contributions that dietary fiber can make to your health and explore ways to incorporate more fiber-rich carbohydrates into your daily diet.

What Are Carbohydrates and How Are They Classified?

LO 4.1 Describe and classify carbohydrates.

Carbohydrates originate in plants. During a process called **photosynthesis** (**Figure 4.1**), plants use the **chlorophyll** in their leaves to absorb the energy in sunlight. The absorbed energy splits water molecules in the plant into their component atoms of hydrogen and

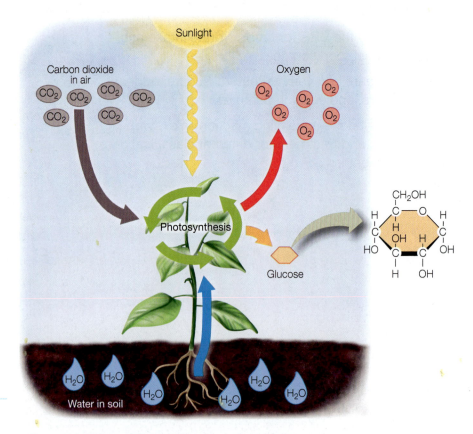

photosynthesis Process by which plants create carbohydrates using the energy from sunlight.

chlorophyll Green pigment in plants that absorbs energy from sunlight to begin the process of photosynthesis.

▲ **Figure 4.1 Photosynthesis: How Glucose Is Made**
During photosynthesis, the leaves of green plants absorb energy from sunlight. The energy splits six molecules of water (H_2O) into hydrogen and oxygen. The hydrogen joins with carbon dioxide in the plant to create glucose ($C_6H_{12}O_6$). In this process, six molecules of oxygen are released into the air.

oxygen. The hydrogen joins with the carbon dioxide that the plant has taken in from the air to form **glucose.** Thus, carbohydrates are literally hydrated carbons. The oxygen is released into the atmosphere. Plants use the glucose they produce directly for energy, store it, or combine it with minerals from the soil to make other compounds, including protein and vitamins. We then eat the plants and digest, absorb, and utilize the glucose.

The fundamental unit of all carbohydrates is a sugar (most commonly glucose). We classify carbohydrates according to how many sugar units are in the molecule. **Simple carbohydrates** consist of just one or two sugar units. **Complex carbohydrates** contain more.

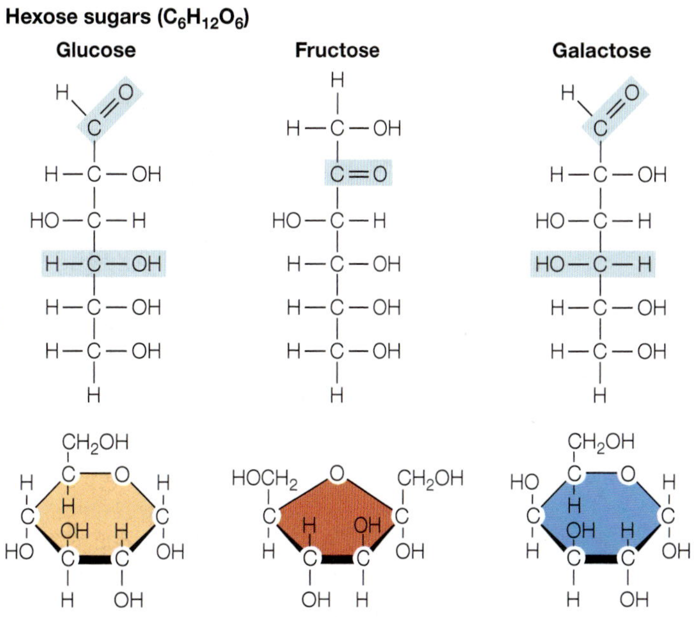

Monosaccharides Are Single Sugar Units

The first group of simple carbohydrates is the **monosaccharides** (*mono* = one, *saccharide* = sugar). They consist of a single sugar unit. There are three nutritionally important monosaccharides: glucose, fructose, and galactose. All three share the same molecular formula of six carbon atoms, 12 hydrogen atoms, and six oxygen atoms ($C_6H_{12}O_6$), referred to as a **hexose** (*hex* = six). The three monosaccharides differ in how their atoms are arranged (**Figure 4.2**). Glucose and galactose are both six-sided ring structures that, at first glance, look identical. Examine both structures carefully. On the fourth carbon, the hydroxyl group (OH) and the hydrogen (H) switch places. This slight rearrangement of atoms makes a difference in the way the body metabolizes and uses these two monosaccharides.

Glucose is the most abundant monosaccharide in foods and in the body. Brain cells and other nervous system cells in particular rely on glucose as their main source of ATP, and red blood cells can only use glucose.

Fructose contains the same number of carbon, hydrogen, and oxygen atoms as glucose and galactose but its molecular structure is arranged as a five-sided, rather than a six-sided, ring. However, fructose is still classified as a hexose because it contains six carbons (notice the location of all six carbons on the fructose molecule in Figure 4.2). The sweetest of the natural sugars, fructose is found abundantly in fruits and is also known as fruit sugar. Fructose is part of high-fructose corn syrup, a sweetener commonly used by the food industry in soft drinks and many other products.

Galactose is seldom found on its own in nature; it is most commonly bound with glucose as part of the disaccharide lactose found in milk and milk products. Several plant products, including cereals, beans and other vegetables, nuts, and seeds, contain slight amounts of galactose, but it is in the form of dietary fiber that is resistant to digestion.

Disaccharides Consist of Two Sugar Units

The second group of simple carbohydrates is the **disaccharides.** They are created when two monosaccharides are joined together. The three disaccharides, *sucrose, lactose,* and *maltose,* all have a common characteristic: At least one of their two monosaccharides is glucose. The disaccharide sucrose consists of glucose and fructose; lactose is glucose and galactose; and maltose is two glucose units linked together (**Figure 4.3**).

The two sugar units in disaccharides are joined through a chemical reaction called **condensation,** which links them with either an alpha or a beta **glycosidic bond.** (See the nearby Chemistry Boost.) The type of bond affects the digestibility of the disaccharide. Sucrose and maltose are formed with an alpha bond and are easily digested. Lactose is

Hexose sugars ($C_6H_{12}O_6$)

▲ **Figure 4.2 The Structural Differences between Glucose, Fructose, and Galactose**
The three monosaccharides are shown in their linear form (as found in foods) and in the ring structure found in the body.

glucose Primary monosaccharide and primary energy source for the body.

simple carbohydrates Carbohydrates that consist of one sugar unit (monosaccharides) or two sugar units (disaccharides).

complex carbohydrates Category of carbohydrates that contain many sugar units combined. Oligosaccharides and polysaccharides are complex carbohydrates.

monosaccharide Simple sugar that consists of a single sugar unit. The three most common monosaccharides are glucose, fructose, and galactose.

hexose Sugar that contains six carbons; glucose, galactose, and fructose are all hexoses.

fructose Sweetest of all the monosaccharides; also known as *fruit sugar* or *levulose.*

galactose Monosaccharide that links with glucose to create the disaccharide found in dairy foods.

disaccharide Simple sugar that consists of two sugar units combined. The three most common disaccharides are sucrose, lactose, and maltose.

condensation Chemical reaction in which two molecules combine to form a larger molecule, and water is released.

glycosidic bond Bond that forms when two sugar molecules are joined together during condensation.

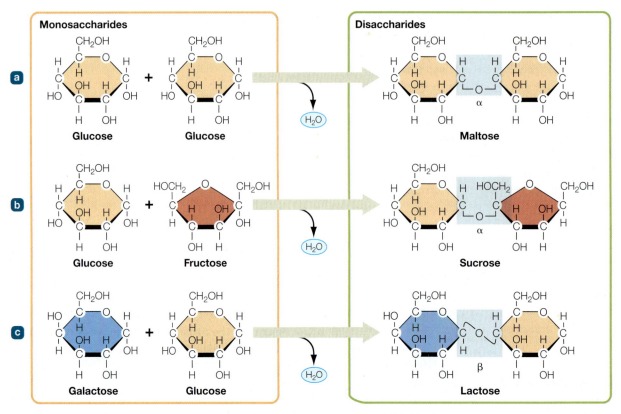

▲ **Figure 4.3 Condensation Reaction Links Monosaccharides to Form Disaccharides**
Through the process of condensation, monosaccharides join together to form disaccharides. **(a)** Two glucose units join together with an alpha bond to produce maltose. **(b)** The disaccharide sucrose is composed of a molecule of glucose linked to a molecule of fructose by an alpha bond. **(c)** The disaccharide lactose is composed of glucose and galactose. Lactose differs from sucrose and maltose in that the two monosaccharides are joined by a beta bond.

formed with a beta bond. People who are lactose intolerant lack the enzyme necessary to break the beta bond between glucose and galactose during digestion. As a result, the lactose travels through the small intestine undigested, causing a variety of uncomfortable symptoms. See the Spotlight: What Is Lactose Intolerance? for more information on this topic.

Chemistry Boost

Condensation Reaction

A condensation reaction occurs when two smaller molecules join to form a larger molecule. When two monosaccharides join together, a hydroxyl group (—OH) from one sugar gains a hydrogen and forms a molecule of water. The OH group on the second sugar loses a hydrogen and links to the other molecule where the OH group was removed.

What Is Lactose Intolerance?

lactose intolerance is a digestive disorder with symptoms of bloating, flatulence, cramps, and diarrhea. People who are lactose intolerant have a deficiency of the brush border enzyme lactase. As a result, they cannot properly digest lactose, the principal carbohydrate found in dairy products. The undigested lactose can draw water into the GI tract, causing diarrhea. Once the lactose reaches the colon, the bacteria in the colon ferment the sugar and produce various gases, and the resulting uncomfortable symptoms.[1]

As they age, many people develop **lactose maldigestion,** a reduction in the ability to digest lactose. In fact, the body reduces lactase synthesis shortly after a child is weaned. An estimated 33 percent of Americans, and 75 percent of adults around the world, have a decrease in lactase. Individuals of certain ethnic origins, such as those from northern Europe, central Africa, and the Middle East, aren't as prone to developing lactose maldigestion. They appear to have a genetic predisposition to maintaining higher levels of lactase throughout their adult life.[2]

If you have lactose maldigestion, don't despair. You don't necessarily need to eliminate dairy foods from your diet. In fact, many people continue to consume milk, yogurt, and cheese without any problems or unpleasant side effects.[3]

This is good news, as dairy products provide over 70 percent of the calcium in the diet, along with protein, potassium, and certain vitamins.[4]

However, people with lactose intolerance do need to determine their threshold for tolerating lactose-containing foods and beverages. The thresholds vary for different people, but smaller amounts of dairy foods throughout the day are usually better tolerated than a large amount at one time. Eating lactose-containing foods with a meal or snack, rather than by themselves, can also influence how much can be tolerated.[5]

People also respond differently to various types of dairy foods.[6] Whole milk tends to be tolerated better than skim milk. Cheese typically has less lactose than milk. This is especially true of hard, aged cheeses, as the amount of lactose remaining after the aging process is negligible. Yogurts that contain active cultures are better tolerated than skim or low-fat milk. Greek yogurt is thicker than regular yogurt because most of the lactose, which is in the liquid portion called *whey,* is strained out in processing. Avoid yogurts with added whey protein concentrate, which adds lactose. Or choose yogurt made with milk treated with lactase prior to processing. **Table 1** shows the amounts of lactose in some common dairy foods.

Foods that contain lactaid, including milk, yogurt, ice cream, and lactaid supplements, improve the digestion of lactose.

TABLE 1 How Much Lactose Is in Your Foods?

Food	Amount	Lactose (grams)
Milk, whole, 1%, or skim	1 cup	11
Lactaid milk	1 cup	<1
Soy milk	1 cup	0
Ice cream	$\frac{1}{2}$ cup	6
Yogurt, plain, nonfat	6 oz	14
Greek yogurt	6 oz	6
Cottage cheese	$\frac{1}{2}$ cup	2
Provolone, cheddar, or Parmesan cheese	1 oz	<1
Cream cheese	1 oz	1

Don't Forget These Hidden Sources of Lactose

Baked goods
Baking mixes for pancakes, biscuits, and cookies
Bread
Breakfast drinks
Candies
Cereals, processed
Instant potatoes
Lunch meats (other than kosher meats)
Margarine
Salad dressings
Soups

Source: Adapted from J. Joneja, *The Health Professional's Guide to Food Allergies and Intolerances* (Chicago: The Academy of Nutrition and Dietetics, 2013).

lactose intolerance When maldigestion of lactose results in symptoms such as nausea, cramps, bloating, flatulence, and diarrhea.

lactose maldigestion Inability to digest lactose due to low levels of the enzyme lactase.

In addition, lactose-reduced dairy products such as milk, cottage cheese, and ice cream are available in many supermarkets. Lactase pills or drops can also be used to break down lactose in foods before or while they are eaten. See the Table Tips for more ideas on improving your lactose tolerance.

Finally, note that lactose intolerance is not the same as having an allergy to milk. A milk allergy is a response by the immune system to one or more of the proteins in cow's milk. This condition typically affects 2.5 percent of children under the age of 3 years, and rarely occurs in adults.[7] (Food allergies are covered in Chapter 17.)

References

1. National Digestive Diseases Information Clearinghouse. 2012. *Lactose Intolerance.* Available at http://digestive.niddk.nih.gov. Accessed January 2017.
2. Ibid.
3. Nicklas, T. A., L. Jahns, et al. 2013. Barriers and Facilitators for Consumer Adherence to the *Dietary Guidelines for Americans*: The HEALTH Study. *Journal of the Academy of Nutrition and Dietetics* 113(10):1317–1331.
4. National Institutes of Health. 2013. *Calcium: Dietary Supplement Fact Sheet.* Available at http://ods.od.nih.gov. Accessed January 2017.
5. Clerfeuille, E., M. Maillot, et al. 2013. Dairy Products: How They Fit in Nutritionally Adequate Diets. *Journal of the Academy of Nutrition and Dietetics* 113(7):950–956.
6. Ibid.
7. National Institute of Allergy and Infectious Diseases. 2016. *Food Allergy: Quick Facts.* Available at www.niaid.nih.gov. Accessed January 2017.

Raffinose

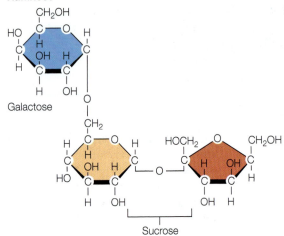

Galactose

Sucrose

▲ **Figure 4.4 The Structure of an Oligosaccharide**
The oligosaccharide raffinose consists of galactose connected to sucrose.

The white granulated sugar you add to coffee and the brown sugar you use to make cookie dough are examples of **sucrose** (brown sugar is made by adding molasses to refined sugar and is about 90 percent sucrose). Sucrose is also found naturally in sugar cane and sugar beets and is the most commonly used natural sweetener.

Lactose, or milk sugar, is present in milk and dairy products. Lactose is a particularly important carbohydrate in the diets of newborn infants because it is the first and only carbohydrate they consume in breast milk.

Maltose, or malt sugar, is the least common of the disaccharides and is formed during the digestion of starch. Manufacturers add maltose as a sweetener and to improve the shelf-life of their products. This makes processed food the main source of maltose in our diets. Maltose is also formed during the fermentation of barley used to brew beer.

In general, simple carbohydrates are sweeter than complex carbohydrates (which we discuss next). Foods such as table sugar and fruit, which are high in fructose, are perceived as especially sweet because of the structure of the fructose molecule. The five-sided ring of fructose mixes with saliva and reacts with taste buds, signaling the brain that the food is sweet.

Some of us experience a stronger taste of sweetness than others do when we eat foods high in monosaccharides and disaccharides. This may be why, across all ethnic groups, females seem to crave sweetness more than males.[1, 2] This ability to taste sweetness may be influenced by age, health problems, or genetics.[3]

Oligosaccharides Have Three to Ten Sugar Units

Oligosaccharides are short chains of 3–10 monosaccharides. They are generally classified as complex carbohydrates. Two common oligosaccharides are raffinose (**Figure 4.4**) and stachyose.

Oligosaccharides make up part of plant cell walls.[4] Humans lack the enzyme necessary to break their bonds; therefore, like dietary fiber, they pass undigested into the large intestine, where the GI flora digest and ferment them. This fermentation may result in

sucrose Disaccharide composed of glucose and fructose; also known as *table sugar*.

lactose Disaccharide composed of glucose and galactose; also known as *milk sugar*.

maltose Disaccharide composed of two glucose units joined together.

oligosaccharides Three to 10 units of monosaccharides combined.

bloating, discomfort, and flatulence. Taking a product such as Beano with a meal, which contains enzymes that digest oligosaccharides, can reduce flatulence.[5]

Oligosaccharides are found in beans and other legumes, cabbage, brussel sprouts, and broccoli. They are also present in human breast milk. Even though infants can't digest these carbohydrates, they may stimulate the immune system and support the growth of healthy GI flora.[6]

Polysaccharides Consist of Many Sugar Units

Polysaccharides consist of long chains and branches of glucose linked together. Some polysaccharides, such as starch and **glycogen,** serve as storage forms of glucose in plants and animals, whereas dietary fiber provides structure in plant cells.

Starch

Plants store glucose in chains of **starch.** These chains can be hundreds or even thousands of glucose units long. Straight chains are called **amylose,** and the branched chains are called **amylopectin** (**Figure 4.5**). Plants contain both of these polysaccharides, typically about 60 percent amylopectin and 40 percent amylose. When we eat plant foods such as corn, rice, and potatoes, we consume the stored glucose.

Some starch is resistant to digestion. In beans, for example, half of the starch is digestible and the remainder is in the form of **resistant starch.** The amylose in starch is more resistant to digestion than is the amylopectin. Linear chains of amylose are harder to break down during digestion because the molecules stack together into tight granules, which hinder the ability of enzymes to reach and break down the bonds. The branched-chain shape of amylopectin makes it impossible to compact and therefore allows for much easier digestion. Unripe bananas, baked beans, and plantains are examples of foods with

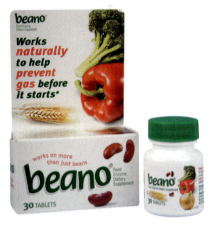

Beano helps reduce the production of gas in the large intestine.

a Two types of starch are amylose (straight chain) and amylopectin (branched).

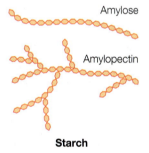

Starch

b Dietary fiber is a nondigestible food component found in the cell walls of plants. Most dietary fiber is in the form of cellulose, a straight chain of glucose units with a beta-glycosidic bond that humans lack the enzyme to digest.

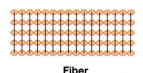

Fiber

c Glycogen, the storage form of glucose in animals, including humans, is more branched than amylopectin.

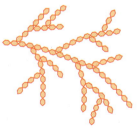

Glycogen

▲ **Figure 4.5 Comparison of Starch, Fiber, and Glycogen**

polysaccharides Many sugar units combined. Starch, glycogen, and fiber are all polysaccharides.

glycogen Storage form of glucose in animals, including humans.

starch Storage form of glucose in plants.

amylose Straight chain of polysaccharides found in starch.

amylopectin Branched chain of polysaccharides found in starch.

resistant starch Type of starch that is not digested in the GI tract but has important health benefits in the large intestine.

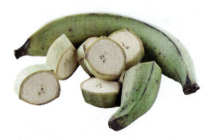

Plantains contain a fair amount of resistant starch.

high levels of resistant starch.[7] Also, once pasta or potatoes are cooked and then chilled, even if they are reheated before eating, the starch becomes resistant to the digestive enzymes in the GI tract.

Resistant starches are added to foods for health benefits.[8] Some researchers have reported that resistant starch may improve the health of the GI tract by increasing bulk, improve blood glucose regulation,[9] and stimulate the growth of the GI flora.[10]

Dietary Fiber

Most forms of **dietary fiber** are nondigestible polysaccharides and occur naturally as a structural component called **cellulose** in the cell walls of plants. Cellulose looks simple—just a straight string of glucose units (never branched like amylopectin) linked with beta-glycosidic bonds (**Figure 4.6**). When several strands stack together they give the plant cell its structure and shape, which contributes to the texture of fruits and vegetables. **Lignin,** another type of dietary fiber, is not a carbohydrate but acts as an adhesive in cell walls.

As mentioned earlier, humans lack the digestive enzyme needed to break beta-glycosidic bonds, so for the most part, dietary fiber cannot be digested and passes through the intestines intact. This means that fiber does not provide kilocalories; however, it does reduce hunger because it adds bulk. Fiber also helps maintain a healthy intestinal tract and promotes health in many other ways, discussed later in this chapter.

Dietary fiber is sometimes classified according to its affinity for water:

- **Soluble fiber** dissolves in water. Examples include pectins; beta-glucans; some gums, such as guar gum; and mucilages (e.g., psyllium). The GI flora easily ferment soluble fibers, forming carbon dioxide, methane, and some fatty acids. Soluble fibers may have numerous health benefits. They are viscous, forming gels that slow gastric emptying and may delay the absorption of some nutrients, helping to reduce blood cholesterol, improve appetite control, and normalize blood glucose levels.
- **Insoluble fiber** does not dissolve in water. Cellulose, lignin, and some hemicelluloses are examples. Insoluble fibers are not easily fermented, but like soluble fibers, they are thought to promote health. For example, they increase the bulk and weight of the stool, stimulating peristalsis, which speeds up the movement of feces through the large intestine. This increase in movement, called *transit time,* relieves constipation and keeps the GI tract healthy.

dietary fiber Food components that humans cannot digest; most are carbohydrates.

cellulose Nondigestible polysaccharide found in plant cell walls.

lignin Noncarbohydrate form of dietary fiber that binds to cellulose fibers to harden and strengthen the cell walls of plants.

soluble fiber Type of fiber that dissolves in water and is fermented by intestinal bacteria. Many soluble fibers are viscous and have thickening properties.

insoluble fiber Type of fiber that isn't dissolved in water or fermented by intestinal bacteria.

Plant cells

Cell wall

CH₂OH
C—O
C
H OH H C
HO C C OH
OH H
C
H OH

Glucose

▲ **Figure 4.6 Plants Contain Cellulose**
Found in the cell walls of plants, cellulose is a polysaccharide composed of numerous glucose units linked together.

TABLE 4.1	Forms of Dietary Fiber and Their Health Benefits	
Type	**Found in These Foods**	**Reduces the Risk of**
Insoluble Fiber		
❑ Cellulose ❑ Hemicellulose ❑ Lignins	Whole grains, whole-grain cereals, amaranth, bran, bulgur, couscous, oats, rice, quinoa, sorghum, fruits, vegetables, legumes	Constipation, diverticulosis, certain cancers, heart disease, obesity
Soluble Fiber		
❑ Pectin ❑ Beta-glucan ❑ Gums ❑ Psyllium	Citrus fruits, prunes, legumes, oats, barley, quinoa, teff, sorghum, flax seed, brussels sprouts, carrots	Constipation, heart disease, diabetes mellitus, obesity

There are exceptions to these statements: not all soluble fibers reduce serum cholesterol, and constipation may be relieved by some soluble fibers. Ultimately, whether fiber is soluble is not as important as the overall dietary fiber intake, and the good news is that most plant foods contain both soluble and insoluble fibers (**Figure 4.7**). Animal products, including meat, fish, chicken, and dairy, do not provide fiber.

Many types of dietary fiber can also be classified as **functional fiber,** which is a type of fiber that has been extracted or isolated from a plant or manufactured by the food industry, and has been shown to have health benefits.[11] For example, psyllium, used in products such as Metamucil, is isolated from psyllium seed husks. Psyllium is high in soluble fiber and has been reported to reduce total cholesterol and LDL cholesterol. Synthetic or manufactured forms of functional fiber also include some forms of resistant starch. Together, dietary fiber and functional fiber contribute to the total fiber in the diet.

Table 4.1 summarizes the various types of fiber, some of their sources, and some of their health benefits.

Glycogen

Whereas starch is the storage form of glucose in plants, glycogen is the storage form in animals, including humans. Molecules of glycogen are long, branched chains, similar to amylopectin, and are stored in muscle and in the liver. The branched structure enables the body to break glycogen down quickly and easily because there are so many sites where enzymes can attach. When blood glucose levels decrease, the liver breaks down the stored glycogen and releases the glucose into the blood. Muscle glycogen can similarly be broken down to glucose to provide energy for the muscle cells. Because glycogen breaks down quickly after an animal dies, animal products do not contain glycogen. In other words, eating meat or poultry will not provide glycogen.

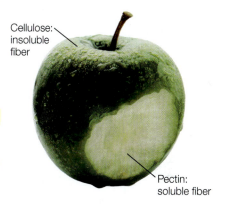

Cellulose: insoluble fiber

Pectin: soluble fiber

▲ **Figure 4.7 Most Plant Foods Contain Both Soluble and Insoluble Fibers**
The skin of an apple is high in cellulose and insoluble fiber, while the pulp is high in pectin, a soluble fiber.

LO 4.1: THE TAKE-HOME MESSAGE Carbohydrates are found primarily in plant-based foods and are used by cells for energy. Glucose is the preferred source of energy in the body. Simple carbohydrates include the monosaccharides glucose, fructose, and galactose, which combine to form the disaccharides sucrose, lactose, and maltose. Oligosaccharides contain 3–10 glucose units and are part of cellulose in cell walls. They are classified as complex carbohydrates. In contrast, the complex carbohydrates starch, fiber, and glycogen are all polysaccharides. Fiber is a nondigestible polysaccharide. Soluble fiber can be dissolved in water, is fermented by intestinal bacteria, and moves slowly through the GI tract. Insoluble fiber typically moves quickly through the GI tract, reducing constipation. Glycogen is the storage form of glucose in animals, including humans.

functional fiber Nondigestible polysaccharides that are added to foods because of a specific desired effect on human health.

How Do We Digest and Absorb Carbohydrates?

LO 4.2 Explain how the body digests and absorbs carbohydrates.

Disaccharides and starch are digested into monosaccharides that can be easily absorbed through the walls of the small intestine. Fiber generally passes through the GI tract undigested. Let's follow the carbohydrates from a sandwich through the digestive process, as illustrated in **Focus Figure 4.8**.

Digestion of Carbohydrates Begins in the Mouth

The digestion of carbohydrates begins in the mouth, where the teeth grind the sandwich and mix it with saliva, which contains the enzyme **salivary amylase** (recall that *ase* = enzyme). The amylase begins breaking down some of the amylose and amylopectin in the bread into the disaccharide maltose. The disaccharides and fiber are not altered in the mouth.

This food mixture, which now contains starch and amylase, along with the maltose, lactose, sucrose, and fiber, travels down the esophagus to the stomach. The amylase continues to break down the starch until the hydrochloric acid in the stomach deactivates this enzyme. There are no carbohydrate-digesting enzymes in the stomach; thus, little to no carbohydrate digestion takes place there.

The arrival of polysaccharides in the small intestine signals the pancreas to release an enzyme called *pancreatic amylase,* which breaks down the remaining starch units from the bread into maltose. The disaccharides maltose, lactose, and sucrose will need further dismantling by the brush border enzymes—including maltase, lactase, and sucrase—housed in the microvilli of the small intestine. These enzymes break down the disaccharides into glucose, fructose, and galactose. These monosaccharides are now readily absorbed into the bloodstream.

By the time the remnants of the sandwich reach the large intestine, all starch and simple sugars have been broken down and absorbed and only the fiber remains. The bacteria in the colon can metabolize some of the fiber, producing water, gas, and some short-chain fatty acids. The colon uses these short-chain fatty acids for energy. The majority of the fiber is eliminated from the body in the feces. Resistant starch can also be metabolized by intestinal bacteria or excreted in the feces.

Carbohydrates Are Absorbed as Monosaccharides

After carbohydrate digestion, the monosaccharides are absorbed into the enterocytes. Glucose and galactose are absorbed by active transport, which requires energy and a carrier protein (**Figure 4.9**). The carrier that helps transport glucose and galactose into the enterocyte is sodium dependent. Once glucose and galactose are absorbed into the enterocyte, they diffuse into the capillaries and are transported through the portal vein to the liver. Fructose is absorbed by facilitated diffusion, which requires no energy and is slower; thus, fructose stays in the enterocytes longer than glucose or galactose and does not raise blood glucose levels.

The fate of the monosaccharides once they've reached the liver depends on an individual's metabolic needs. The liver uses galactose and fructose for energy or converts them to glucose before releasing them into the bloodstream. Any surplus glucose that is not used immediately for energy is stored as glycogen.

The process of converting excess glucose to glycogen is called **glycogenesis** and occurs mostly in the liver and muscle cells. As you learned earlier in the chapter, the body can use this stored form of glucose when the diet lacks sufficient carbohydrate.

Once the glycogen stores are fully replenished, and presuming the diet contains sufficient kilocalories to meet energy needs, excess glucose is converted into glycerol and fatty acids. These two are combined into a triglyceride and stored in the *adipocytes* (fat cells).

salivary amylase Digestive enzyme that begins breaking down carbohydrate (starch) in the mouth; other important enzymes during carbohydrate digestion include pancreatic amylase, maltase, sucrase, and lactase.

glycogenesis Process of assembling excess glucose into glycogen in the liver and muscle cells.

FOCUS Figure 4.8 Carbohydrate Digestion and Absorption

Head to Mastering Nutrition and watch a narrated video tour of this figure by author Joan Salge Blake.

Carbohydrate digestion begins in the mouth and ends with the absorption of the monosaccharides glucose, fructose, and galactose in the small intestine.

ORGANS OF THE GI TRACT

MOUTH

Mastication mixes food with saliva. Salivary amylase breaks down amylose and amylopectin into smaller chains of carbohydrates.

Amylose → Smaller chains

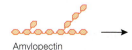

Amylopectin → Smaller chains

STOMACH

The acidity of the stomach inactivates the salivary amylase; thus, very little digestion of carbohydrates occurs in the stomach.

SMALL INTESTINE

Pancreatic amylase breaks down the amylose, amylopectin, and smaller chains of carbohydrates into maltose, a disaccharide.

Smaller amylose chains → Maltose

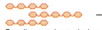

Smaller amylopectin chains → Maltose

Brush border enzymes break down all disaccharides to the monosaccharides glucose, fructose, and galactose, which are then absorbed through the enterocytes into the bloodstream.

Sucrose → Glucose Fructose

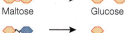

Maltose → Glucose

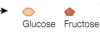

Lactose → Glucose Galactose

LARGE INTESTINE

Starches and simple sugars are broken down and absorbed in the small intestine; only fiber passes into the large intestine. Bacteria in the colon metabolize some of the fiber. The majority of fiber is eliminated in the stool.

ACCESSORY ORGANS

SALIVARY GLANDS

Produce salivary amylase.

PANCREAS

Produces pancreatic amylase that is released into the small intestine via the pancreatic duct.

LIVER

Glucose is taken up by the liver from the portal vein. Most glucose is returned to the blood to be picked up and used by body cells, or the liver can use glucose for energy, convert it to glycogen, or store it as fat.

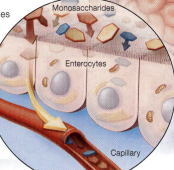

Monosaccharides

Enterocytes

Capillary

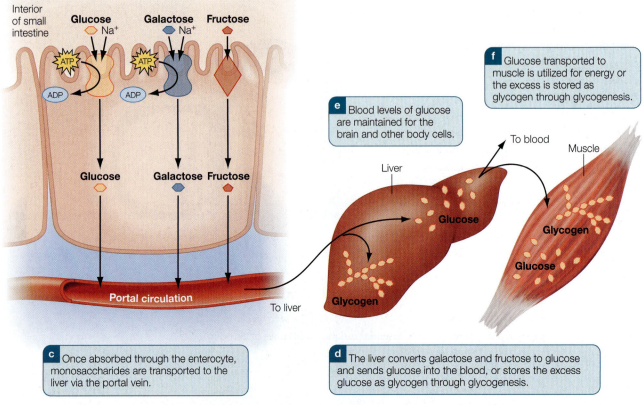

a Glucose and galactose are absorbed by active transport with sodium (Na⁺), ATP, and a carrier protein.

b Fructose is absorbed via facilitated diffusion and a carrier protein.

f Glucose transported to muscle is utilized for energy or the excess is stored as glycogen through glycogenesis.

e Blood levels of glucose are maintained for the brain and other body cells.

c Once absorbed through the enterocyte, monosaccharides are transported to the liver via the portal vein.

d The liver converts galactose and fructose to glucose and sends glucose into the blood, or stores the excess glucose as glycogen through glycogenesis.

▲ **Figure 4.9 Absorption and Storage of Monosaccharides**
Glucose and galactose are absorbed into the enterocyte via active transport, and fructose is absorbed by facilitated diffusion. Once transported to the liver, galactose and fructose are converted to glucose, which is used for energy or released into the bloodstream and transported to body cells. Excess glucose is stored in the liver and muscle cells as glycogen. The liver glycogen can be used to supply the blood with glucose when the diet is deficient in carbohydrates. Muscle glycogen provides glucose to the muscle cell.

LO 4.2: THE TAKE-HOME MESSAGE Digestion of carbohydrates begins in the mouth, where salivary amylase breaks down starch. Most carbohydrate digestion occurs in the small intestine. Pancreatic and brush border enzymes break down the carbohydrates into disaccharides and then monosaccharides so that they can be absorbed. Glucose and galactose are actively absorbed with the help of a sodium-dependent carrier and ATP. Fructose is absorbed by facilitated diffusion. All monosaccharides are converted to glucose in the liver and are used as energy, stored as glycogen in the liver and muscle cells, or converted to glycerol and fatty acids and stored as fat. Dietary fiber travels to the colon undigested and most of it is eliminated from the body.

What Functions Do Carbohydrates Perform in the Body?

LO 4.3 List the functions of carbohydrates in the body.

Carbohydrates—primarily glucose—provide about half of the energy used by the muscles and other tissues; the rest of the energy you use each day comes mostly from fats. Glucose is the only source of energy used by the red blood cells and the primary fuel source for the brain. For this reason, carbohydrates are the most desirable source of energy for the body. This section briefly describes the overall functions of carbohydrates and the variety of health benefits they provide. (A complete discussion of the metabolism of glucose appears in Chapter 8.)

Carbohydrates Provide Energy

Most of the energy we need to fuel our daily activities comes from glucose and fats. Digested carbohydrate provides 4 kilocalories of energy per gram. Stored forms of both glucose and fats come in handy between meals when you aren't eating, but the body continues to need fuel.

Under most conditions, glucose is the sole energy source for the brain, which requires a steady supply of glucose to function properly. If you haven't eaten for longer than 4 hours, blood glucose levels drop too low and the body will tap its glycogen stores by initiating **glycogenolysis** (*lysis* = loosening) to hydrolyze liver glycogen and supply glucose to the blood. Once liver glycogen stores are depleted, the body turns to other sources, such as amino acids from protein and glycerol found in stored fat, to maintain blood glucose. Note that muscle glycogen cannot be used to raise blood glucose levels because muscles lack the enzyme necessary to release glucose into the blood. Instead, muscle uses glycogen to fuel its own energy needs.

Carbohydrates Spare Protein

Glucose is the body's preferred fuel source, and as long as there is adequate glucose in the blood, protein can be spared for its many other essential functions. In times of carbohydrate deprivation, however, the body turns to noncarbohydrates, particularly amino acids (the building blocks of protein, which we discuss in Chapter 6), to generate glucose. The process of creating glucose from noncarbohydrate sources is called **gluconeogenesis** (*gluco* = sugar/sweet, *neo* = new, *genesis* = origin). Gluconeogenesis primarily occurs in the liver, but can also take place in the kidneys because these are the only organs that contain the enzymes needed for this process. The kidney is not an active site of gluconeogenesis except after long periods of fasting.

The body does not store extra protein to provide fuel during times of deprivation. Instead, the body dismantles protein from the muscles and organs to generate the needed glucose. While gluconeogenesis can provide needed glucose to the blood, the breakdown of muscle protein can have negative consequences for the body.

Carbohydrates Prevent Ketosis

After about 18 hours of fasting, liver glycogen is depleted and the body will begin to look for other sources, mostly stored fat, to meet the body's energy needs. The by-products of the incomplete breakdown of fat, called **ketone bodies,** spill into the blood. Most ketone bodies are acids and thus reduce the pH of the blood. After about 2 days of fasting, the number of ketone bodies in the blood doubles. This rise in ketones is called **ketosis.** If left unchecked, ketosis can progress to ketoacidosis, an increase in blood acidity to levels that lead to nervous system, liver, and kidney problems. This most commonly occurs in people with unmanaged diabetes, and is discussed later in this chapter. Individuals who fast or follow strict low-carbohydrate diets are often in ketosis.

> **LO 4.3: THE TAKE-HOME MESSAGE** Glucose provides a readily metabolized source of energy for muscle and other body cells. It is the only source of fuel that red blood cells can use, and is the preferred source for the brain. Adequate carbohydrate intake helps maintain normal blood glucose levels, spares protein to be used for important functions other than energy production, and prevents ketosis.

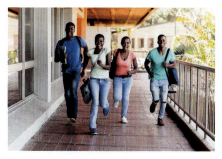

Carbohydrates provide about half the energy used by body tissues each day.

glycogenolysis Hydrolysis of glycogen to release glucose.

gluconeogenesis Creation of glucose from noncarbohydrate sources, predominantly protein.

ketone bodies By-products of the incomplete breakdown of fat.

ketosis Condition of increased ketone bodies in the blood.

How Do We Maintain Blood Glucose Levels?

LO 4.4 Explain how the body maintains blood glucose levels.

Blood glucose levels are not constant—they rise and fall according to the body's carbohydrate intake and energy needs. How does the body regulate blood glucose levels, given these changes? The answer: hormones. In fact, two hormones secreted from the pancreas, **insulin** and **glucagon,** maintain blood glucose levels between 70 and 110 milligrams per deciliter (mg/dl) (**Focus Figure 4.10**). Other hormones, including epinephrine, norepinephrine, cortisol, and growth hormone, assist in the process.

Insulin Regulates Glucose in the Blood

After eating a carbohydrate-heavy meal, the blood is flooded with glucose, which body cells cannot use until it crosses the cell membrane. The high blood glucose levels stimulate the release of insulin from the beta cells of the pancreas. Insulin travels through the bloodstream, attaching to specific receptor sites on cell membranes, where it stimulates mechanisms that result in an increase in the number of glucose transporters found on the membrane surface. These transporters then shuttle the glucose into the cell. As soon as glucose enters the cell, insulin stimulates the enzymes that will convert glucose to ATP or store it as glycogen for later use. Its role in stimulating the uptake of glucose by body cells makes insulin critical to blood glucose regulation. However, note that liver, kidney, and brain cells can use glucose without the aid of insulin.

In addition to helping glucose enter cells, insulin helps convert glucose to glycogen if the amount of glucose in the blood exceeds the body's immediate energy needs. It does this by stimulating glycogenesis in both the liver and the muscle and by inhibiting the enzymes involved in glycogenolysis and gluconeogenesis.

There is a limit to how much excess glucose the body can store as glycogen. When glycogen stores are full, excess glucose may be converted into fatty acids in a process called **lipogenesis.** The method insulin uses to promote lipogenesis is similar to the way it promotes glycogenesis: by increasing the number of glucose receptors on the surface of the fat cell. Insulin also inhibits *lipolysis* (fat breakdown) by reducing the activity of the enzyme that hydrolyzes stored fat. The result of insulin's actions is that more fat is formed and fewer fatty acids are found in the blood.

Glucagon Regulates Liver Glycogenolysis

Glucagon has the opposite effect of insulin on blood glucose levels: It stimulates release of glucose into the blood (see Focus Figure 4.10). The alpha cells of the pancreas release glucagon into the circulation when blood glucose levels are low—for example, during a period of stress or after eating a high-protein meal when blood amino acids are increased. The main target organ of glucagon is the liver, where it promotes glycogenolysis to release a burst of glucose into the blood. Under the control of glucagon, liver glycogen stores will be depleted after 10–18 hours without sufficient dietary carbohydrate intake.

Glucagon stimulates glucose production by encouraging the uptake of amino acids by the liver. The carbon skeletons of the amino acids are then used to produce glucose through gluconeogenesis.

Four Other Hormones Help Regulate Glucose Metabolism

In addition to glucagon, other hormones can increase blood glucose levels. **Epinephrine** (also known as *adrenaline*) and **norepinephrine,** both secreted from the adrenal glands, act on the liver to stimulate glycogenolysis and gluconeogenesis to raise blood glucose.

insulin Hormone secreted from the beta cells of the pancreas that stimulates the uptake of glucose from the blood into the cells.

glucagon Hormone secreted from the alpha cells of the pancreas that stimulates glycogenolysis and gluconeogenesis to increase blood levels of glucose.

lipogenesis Process that converts excess glucose into fat for storage.

epinephrine Hormone produced by the adrenal glands that signals the liver cells to release glucose; also referred to as the "fight-or-flight" hormone.

norepinephrine Hormone produced by the adrenal glands that stimulates glycogenolysis and gluconeogenesis.

FOCUS Figure 4.10 Hormones Regulate Blood Glucose

Head to **Mastering** Nutrition and watch a narrated video tour of this figure by author Joan Salge Blake.

Our bodies regulate blood glucose levels within a fairly narrow range to provide adequate glucose to the brain and other cells. Insulin and glucagon are two hormones that play a key role in regulating blood glucose levels.

HIGH BLOOD GLUCOSE

1 Insulin secretion: When blood glucose levels increase after a meal, the pancreas secretes the hormone insulin from the beta cells into the bloodstream.

2 Cellular uptake: Insulin travels to the tissues where it alters the cell membranes to allow the transport of glucose into the cells by increasing the number of glucose transporters on the cell membrane.

3 Glucose storage: Insulin also stimulates the storage of glucose in body tissues. Glucose is stored as glycogen in the liver and muscles (glycogenesis), and is stored as triglycerides in adipose tissue (lipogenesis).

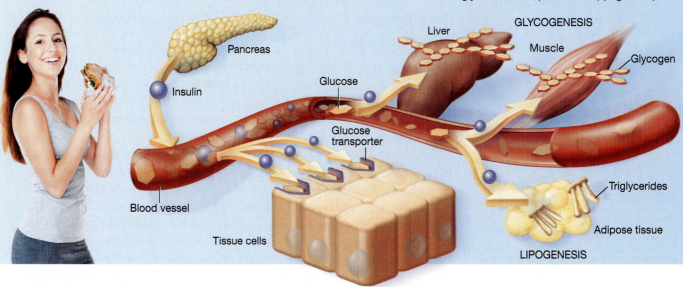

LOW BLOOD GLUCOSE

1 Glucagon secretion: When blood glucose levels are low, the pancreas secretes the hormone glucagon from the alpha cells into the bloodstream.

2 Glycogenolysis: Glucagon stimulates glycogenolysis in the liver to break down stored glycogen to glucose, which is released into the blood and transported to the cells for energy.

3 Gluconeogenesis: Glucagon also activates gluconeogenesis in the liver, stimulating the conversion of glucogenic amino acids to glucose.

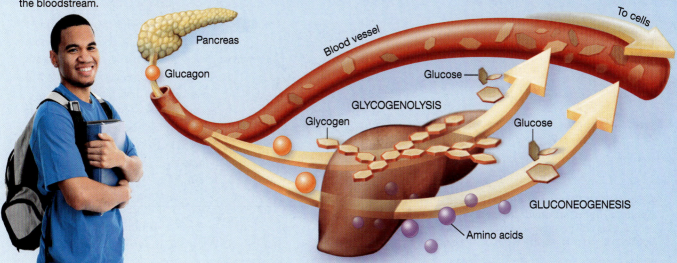

Epinephrine production can increase in the body during periods of emotional and physical stress, such as fear, excitement, and blood loss. For example, if a ferocious dog were chasing you down the street, your body would be pumping out epinephrine, thereby increasing your blood glucose to fuel your running. For this reason, epinephrine is also referred to as the "fight-or-flight" hormone.

A low blood glucose level can trigger the release of both epinephrine and norepinephrine. In fact, some of the symptoms that you may experience when your blood glucose level dips too low, such as anxiety, rapid heartbeat, pale skin, and shakiness, are caused by the release of both of these hormones.

Two other hormones—**cortisol** and **growth hormone**—also regulate glucose metabolism. Cortisol, often referred to as the "stress hormone," stimulates gluconeogenesis and reduces the uptake of glucose by the muscle cells. Both of these actions increase blood glucose levels. Growth hormone has the opposite effect of insulin: It conserves glucose by stimulating fat breakdown for energy, reducing the uptake of glucose by the muscle cells, and increasing glucose production in the liver.

Hypoglycemia Results When Blood Glucose Drops below Normal

For most healthy individuals, when the blood glucose levels drop below normal, the pancreas stops releasing insulin and begins releasing glucagon until blood glucose returns to normal. In people with **hypoglycemia,** the pancreas releases too much insulin. This causes a rapid and persistent drop in blood glucose levels to a level lower than normal (usually less than 70 mg/dl), as illustrated in **Figure 4.11**. Individuals who experience hypoglycemia may feel hungry, nervous, dizzy, light-headed, confused, weak, and shaky, and even begin to sweat. If the symptoms worsen, more severe reactions to hypoglycemia can cause seizures, coma, and even death.

Rarely, some people experience bouts of *reactive hypoglycemia* within 4 hours after a meal. The cause of reactive hypoglycemia is not known, but contributing factors may include the type of food eaten and the timing of the food as it moves through the GI tract. Some people may be overly sensitive to epinephrine, which is released when the blood glucose level begins to drop. The hormone glucagon may also play a role. Eating smaller, well-balanced meals throughout the day can help avoid reactive hypoglycemia.

Another type of hypoglycemia, called *fasting hypoglycemia,* can occur upon waking (after overnight fasting), during long stretches between meals, or after exercise. Some medications, illnesses, certain tumors, hormone imbalances, or drinking too much alcohol may cause this type of hypoglycemia.

cortisol Hormone produced by the adrenal cortex that stimulates gluconeogenesis and lipolysis.

growth hormone Hormone that regulates glucose metabolism by increasing glycogenolysis and lipolysis.

hypoglycemia Blood glucose level that drops to lower than 70 mg/dl.

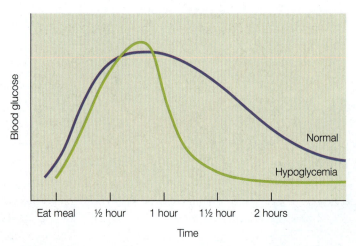

▶ **Figure 4.11 Change in Blood Glucose after Eating a High-Carbohydrate Meal**
An individual with hypoglycemia experiences a more rapid decline in blood glucose after a carbohydrate-rich meal.

Why Is Dietary Fiber So Important for Promoting Health?

LO 4.5 Discuss the role of dietary fiber in promoting health.

Even though fiber passes through the GI tract undigested, it has many powerful positive effects in the body. We discuss the most significant here.

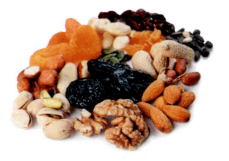

Dried fruits and nuts are excellent sources of fiber, and nuts also contribute certain types of lipids that are thought to protect the heart and blood vessels.

Dietary Fiber Helps Prevent Constipation and Diverticulosis

Over 4 million Americans report being constipated, with pregnant women, children, and adults 65 years of age and older affected more often than others.[12] Constipation is usually caused by sluggish muscle contractions in the colon that move stool along too slowly, allowing excessive water absorption along the way. This can create hard, dry stools that are more difficult and painful to expel.

A diet plentiful in insoluble fibers such as bran, whole grains, and many fruits and vegetables contributes bulk to the feces, which stretches the circular muscles in the large intestine, thus reducing the transit time in the colon and decreasing the likelihood of constipation. Some soluble fibers, such as psyllium, can also relieve constipation; psyllium's water-attracting capability allows the stool to increase in bulk and form a gel-like, soft texture, which makes it easier to pass.

Chronic constipation can lead to a disorder called **diverticulosis** (*osis* = condition), in which increased pressure in the colon causes weak spots along its wall to bulge out and form pouches called **diverticula** (see **Figure 4.12**). Infection of the diverticula, a condition known as **diverticulitis** (*itis* = inflammation), can lead to stomach pain, fever, nausea and vomiting, cramping, and chills. Approximately 50 percent of Americans ages 60–80 and the majority of individuals over 80 years of age have diverticulosis.[13] The best way to prevent both diverticulosis and diverticulitis is to eat a diet with adequate fiber.

Dietary Fiber Helps Prevent Cardiovascular Disease, Diabetes, and Cancer

A diet rich in fiber from whole grains, vegetables, and fruits is associated with a reduced risk of developing cardiovascular disease, diabetes, and cancer.

Cardiovascular Disease

A diet rich in viscous, soluble fiber has been shown to help lower elevated blood cholesterol levels, which in turn is associated with a decreased risk for heart disease and stroke (**Figure 4.13**). Bile acids contain cholesterol and are secreted by the gallbladder into the

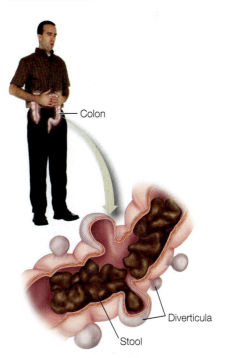

▲ **Figure 4.12 Diverticulosis**
Diverticulosis is a condition in which small pouches, or diverticula, bulge out along the colon. When stool gets trapped in these pouches, they can become inflamed, leading to diverticulitis.

diverticulosis Existence of diverticula in the lining of or colon.

diverticula Small bulges at weak spots in the colon wall.

diverticulitis Infection of the diverticula.

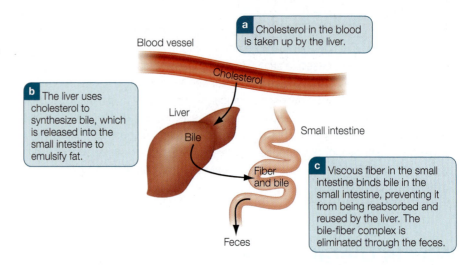

a Cholesterol in the blood is taken up by the liver.

Blood vessel

Cholesterol

b The liver uses cholesterol to synthesize bile, which is released into the small intestine to emulsify fat.

Liver

Bile

Small intestine

Fiber and bile

c Viscous fiber in the small intestine binds bile in the small intestine, preventing it from being reabsorbed and reused by the liver. The bile-fiber complex is eliminated through the feces.

Feces

intestine, where they emulsify fat. If little fiber is present in the GI tract, the bile is reabsorbed into the enterocytes. In contrast, soluble fiber in the small intestine "grabs" or sequesters the bile acids before the body can reabsorb them. They end up excreted along with the fiber in the feces. The liver then removes cholesterol from the blood to replace the bile acids that were lost. Blood cholesterol levels are lowered as a result.

Slow-moving, viscous, soluble fibers may also reduce the rate at which fat and carbohydrates are absorbed from meals. Delayed absorption can lower the surge of fat in the blood after a meal and may help improve sensitivity to the hormone insulin. Both high levels of fat in the blood and a decreased sensitivity to insulin are considered risk factors for cardiovascular disease.

Insoluble fiber also may promote cardiovascular health. Several research studies have shown that cereal grains, which contain insoluble fiber, may help to lower the risk of cardiovascular disease.

Diabetes

Research studies involving both men and women have shown that a higher consumption of fiber from cereals helped reduce the risk of developing certain types of diabetes mellitus.[14] Viscous, soluble fibers have also been shown to help individuals who already have diabetes mellitus manage the condition. As already noted, viscous fibers slow the digestion and absorption of glucose. This could help avoid a large spike in blood glucose after meals and help individuals with diabetes improve the long-term control of their blood glucose level.[15] See Health Connection: What Is Diabetes? on pages 141–147 for a complete discussion of diabetes, its prevalence, control, and prevention.

Cancer

Dietary fiber is thought to reduce the risk of certain cancers. Fiber from cereals, for example, has been shown to lower the risk of breast cancer.[16] Estrogen is associated with certain types of breast cancer, and the reduced risk may reflect fiber's ability to reduce the level of estrogen in the blood. Research suggests that fiber binds to the estrogen in bile and then eliminates the estrogen in the feces. This leads to lower blood estrogen levels. The evidence is not conclusive, but it is promising.

Research also suggests that as dietary fiber consumption increases, the incidence of colorectal cancer decreases.[17, 18] This effect may be due to the increased bulk of fiber-containing stools, which move more quickly through the colon so that potential cancer-promoting substances spend less time in contact with the colon lining. Fiber also encourages the growth in the colon of friendly bacteria and their fermentation by-products, both of which may have cancer-fighting potential. Because an increased amount of bile acids in

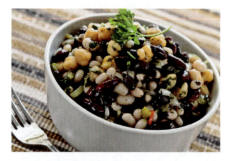

The abundant fiber found in beans and other legumes helps provide bulk to stool and may help with weight management.

the colon is thought to be associated with colon and rectal cancer, fiber's ability to bind and excrete bile acids is also viewed as a cancer deterrent.[19]

Dietary Fiber Helps Prevent Obesity

A fiber-rich diet can be a key factor in the fight against obesity. High-fiber foods, such as whole grains, fruits, and vegetables, can help you feel fuller faster (recall the concept of *satiety* from Chapter 2), helping reduce overall caloric intake. Research studies have shown that obese men and women tend to consume lower amounts of dietary fiber daily than their leaner counterparts. This lends credence to the concept that fiber plays a role in weight management.[20, 21] Some weight-loss diets restrict carbohydrates, but these plans would work better if they *increased* high-fiber carbohydrates. Results of longitudinal studies in women suggest that the intake of dietary fiber, especially whole grains, is a useful dietary tool to control body weight.[22, 23] Similar effects have been observed in men.[24, 25]

A word of caution: Initially, a high-fiber diet can have negative side effects (flatulence and bloating).[26] Consuming too much fiber may cause fluid imbalance or lead to mineral deficiencies by reducing the absorption and increasing the excretion of minerals such as iron and zinc, especially when the diet is low in these minerals or needs have temporarily increased, such as during pregnancy.[27] Gradually increase the fiber in your diet, rather than suddenly adding large amounts. Also increase your intake of fluid. These steps should help minimize these side effects. See the Table Tips for some easy ways to gradually introduce more fiber into your diet.

> **LO 4.5: THEd TAKE-HOME MESSAGE** A diet high in fiber has been found to have numerous health benefits, including reduced risk for constipation, diverticulosis, cardiovascular disease, diabetes, certain cancers, and obesity. The level of fiber in the diet should be increased gradually and accompanied by increased fluid intake.

What Are the Recommendations for Carbohydrate Intake and the Best Food Sources?

LO 4.6 Identify the DRIs for carbohydrate intake and the best food sources.

The body needs a minimum amount of carbohydrate daily to support brain and nerve function and to efficiently meet its energy needs. The RDA for carbohydrate intake for adults and children is 130 grams daily. This is based on the estimated minimum amount of glucose the brain needs to function efficiently. Though this may seem high, 130 grams is less than the amount found in the recommended daily servings for each food group in MyPlate, that is, six servings from the grain group, three servings each from the vegetable and dairy groups, and two servings from the fruit group.

In the United States, most adults consume well over the RDA. Adult males consume, on average, over 300 grams of carbohydrates daily, whereas adult females eat over 200 grams daily.

The AMDR for carbohydrates is 45–65 percent of total daily kilocalories (see Chapter 2). Adults in the United States consume at least 50 percent of their kilocalories from carbohydrate-rich foods, so they are easily within this optimal range. Practice calculating the carbohydrate content of your diet in the Calculation Corner.

Increasing Daily Fiber Intake

Choose whole-grain breakfast cereals such as shredded wheat, bran flakes, raisin bran, and oatmeal.
Enjoy a lunchtime sandwich made with a whole-wheat pita or 100 percent whole-grain bread.
Have two pieces of whole fresh fruit daily.
Layer lettuce, tomatoes, or other vegetables on sandwiches.
Include plenty of vegetables, from legumes to leafy greens to carrots, turnips, and potatoes, at lunch and dinner.

Calculation Corner

Daily Carbohydrate Intake

(a) Adam needs to eat approximately 4,000 kilocalories (kcals) daily to maintain his current weight, given his age, gender, height, weight, and activity level. Calculate how many kcals of carbohydrate Adam should eat each day to meet the AMDR.

$$4,000 \text{ (kcals)} \times 0.45 = 1,800 \text{ (kcals)}$$

$$4,000 \text{ (kcals)} \times 0.65 = 2,600 \text{ (kcals)}$$

Answer: If Adam ate between 1,800 and 2,600 kilocalories of carbohydrate each day, he would meet the AMDR for carbohydrates.

(b) How many grams of carbohydrate should Adam eat to equal 45–65 percent of his total kilocalories?

$$1,800 \text{ kcals} \div 4 \text{ kcals/gram} = 450 \text{ grams}$$

$$2,600 \text{ kcals} \div 4 \text{ kcals/gram} = 650 \text{ grams}$$

Answer: Adam should eat between 450 and 650 grams of carbohydrate each day.

(c) Would this intake of carbohydrate meet the RDA for carbohydrate?

Answer: Yes; Adam needs a minimum of 130 grams of carbohydrate.

> Go to **Mastering** Nutrition and complete a Math Video activity similar to the problem in this Calculation Corner.

TABLE 4.2 What Are Your Fiber Needs?		
	Grams of Fiber Daily*	
	Males	*Females*
Ages 14–18	38	26
Ages 19–50	38	25
Ages 51–70+	30	21
Pregnancy		28
Lactation		29

* Based on an Adequate Intake (AI) for fiber.

Source: Data from Institute of Medicine, *Dietary Reference Intakes for Energy, Carbohydrate, Fiber, Fat, Fatty Acids, Cholesterol, Protein, and Amino Acids* (Washington, DC: National Academies Press, 2005).

The AI for fiber is 25–38 grams per day for adult females and males, respectively, through age 50, or 14 grams of fiber for every 1,000 kilocalories consumed. These intake levels are based on the amount estimated to reduce the risk for cardiovascular disease (Table 4.2). Adults in the United States fall short of these recommendations and currently consume only about 12–18 grams per day. Thus, whereas most Americans consume an adequate amount of carbohydrate overall, they are getting less than the AI for dietary fiber, on average.

The American Dietetic Association and the American Heart Association do not recommend low-carbohydrate diets for weight loss.[28] Low-carbohydrate weight loss diets often restrict healthful foods, including whole grains, and promote foods low in vitamins, minerals, and dietary fiber.[29] More information on the role of carbohydrate intake in body weight is discussed in the Examining the Evidence box in Chapter 15.

Whole Plant Foods and Dairy Products Are Good Sources of Carbohydrates

The DRIs indicate the minimum amount of carbohydrate that individuals should consume daily, but it's important to note that all carbohydrates are not created equal, and some carbohydrate-rich foods are nutritionally better than others. Whole, intact foods—including grains, fruits, and legumes and other vegetables—deliver vitamins, minerals, fiber, and a host of phytochemicals. Figure 4.14 identifies excellent sources of carbohydrates.

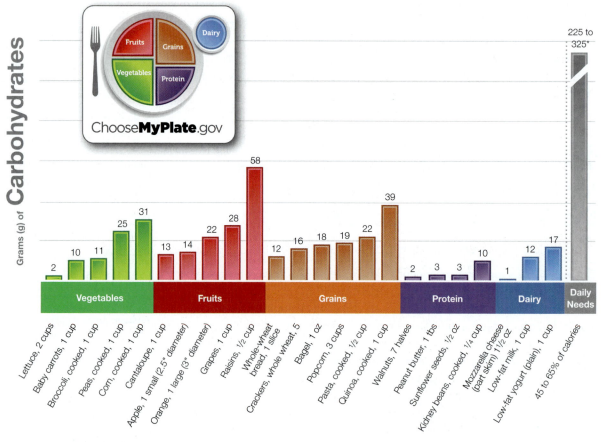

*Based on a 2,000 calorie diet

▲ Figure 4.14 Food Sources of Carbohydrates
Eating the minimum recommended servings from the grains, vegetables, fruits, and dairy groups will meet the need to consume 130 grams of carbohydrate daily.

Whole Grains

Whole grains are abundant in complex carbohydrates, including starch and dietary fiber, and they are an important staple in the diet. Moreover, a diet rich in whole grains is associated with a reduced risk of several chronic diseases.[30] In view of these potential health benefits, MyPlate recommends three servings per day of whole grains. Currently, Americans are consuming an average of 16 grams of whole grains per day, or about 60 percent of the recommended intake.[31] Choose whole-grain breads and cereals that have at least 2–3 grams of total fiber per serving, such as whole-wheat bread, bulgur, brown rice, and whole-grain pasta. Increase your dietary fiber intake with a variety of ancient whole grains including quinoa, teff, amaranth, and sorghum that all contain at least 6 grams of total fiber per serving.

What is a whole grain? Before processing, a kernel of a grain, such as wheat or oats, includes three edible parts: the **bran**, the **endosperm,** and the **germ** (**Figure 4.15**). Whole-grain foods contain all three parts of the grain.

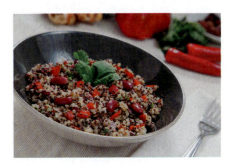

Replacing refined grains with whole grains such as quinoa provides more nutrition, including fiber, per bite.

◀ **Figure 4.15 From Wheat Kernel to Flour**
(a) The wheat grain kernel has three parts: bran, germ, and endosperm. **(b)** Whole-wheat flour is made using the entire grain kernel. It is not enriched. **(c)** Enriched wheat flour doesn't contain the bran and germ, so it is missing nutrients, phytochemicals, and fiber. Some nutrients, including folic acid, thiamin, niacin, riboflavin, and iron, are added back to the flour during an enrichment process. **(d)** Wheat flour that is not enriched lacks not only the bran and germ, but also many nutrients, phytochemicals, and fiber.

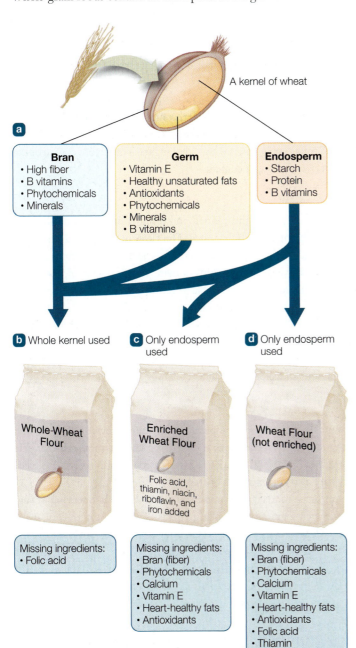

A kernel of wheat

a

Bran
• High fiber
• B vitamins
• Phytochemicals
• Minerals

Germ
• Vitamin E
• Healthy unsaturated fats
• Antioxidants
• Phytochemicals
• Minerals
• B vitamins

Endosperm
• Starch
• Protein
• B vitamins

b Whole kernel used

c Only endosperm used

d Only endosperm used

Whole-Wheat Flour

Enriched Wheat Flour

Folic acid, thiamin, niacin, riboflavin, and iron added

Wheat Flour (not enriched)

Missing ingredients:
• Folic acid

Missing ingredients:
• Bran (fiber)
• Phytochemicals
• Calcium
• Vitamin E
• Heart-healthy fats
• Antioxidants

Missing ingredients:
• Bran (fiber)
• Phytochemicals
• Calcium
• Vitamin E
• Heart-healthy fats
• Antioxidants
• Folic acid
• Thiamin
• Niacin
• Riboflavin
• Iron

whole grains Grain foods that are made with the entire edible grain kernel: the bran, the endosperm, and the germ.

bran Indigestible outer shell of the grain kernel.

endosperm Starchy inner portion of a cereal grain.

germ Vitamin-rich embryo, or seed, of a grain.

TABLE TIPS
Ways to Enjoy Whole Grains

Choose whole-grain cereal such as shredded wheat, bran flakes, raisin bran, or oatmeal in the morning.

Combine a 100% whole-wheat English muffin and low-fat cheddar cheese for a hearty breakfast cheese melt.

Enjoy your lunchtime sandwich made with a whole-wheat pita or 100 percent whole-grain bread. "Wheat" bread, even if it's brown, is not necessarily made with whole-wheat flour. Ask for whole-wheat bread specifically.

Try instant brown rice for a quick whole grain at dinner.

Snack on popcorn or 100 percent whole-wheat crackers for a high-fiber filler in the afternoon.

The grain kernel in **refined grains,** such as are found in white bread and white rice, goes through a milling process that strips out the bran and germ, leaving only the endosperm of the kernel in the end product. As a result, some, though not all, of the B vitamins, iron, phytochemicals, and dietary fiber are removed. Refining also improves the digestibility of the carbohydrate in the endosperm, resulting in a more rapid rise in blood glucose and an increased demand for insulin.[32]

To restore some of the nutrition lost from refined grains, **enriched grains** have folic acid, thiamin, niacin, riboflavin, and iron added back after the milling process. This improves their nutritional quality somewhat, but the fiber and the phytochemicals are lost.

Whole grains are potential disease-fighting allies in the diet. As little as one serving of whole grains daily may help lower the risk of dying from heart disease[33] or cancer,[34] reduce the risk of stroke,[35] improve intestinal health,[36] and improve body weight.[37] Several research studies have also shown that the fiber in whole grains may help reduce the risk of diabetes.[38] Because whole grains are rich in vitamins, minerals, fiber, and phytochemicals, it is uncertain which substances are the disease-fighting heroes or if some or all of them work in a complementary fashion to provide the protection. Try the suggestions in the Table Tips to increase your intake of tasty and nutritious whole grains.

Dairy Products

Milk and milk products, including cheese and yogurt, contain 1–17 grams of lactose per serving. Choose low-fat or fat-free dairy products whenever possible, for the sake of heart health, and avoid flavored milks and yogurts with added sugars. The lactose content is the same regardless of the fat or added sugar content.

Fruits

Whole fruits, 100 percent fruit juices, and canned and dried fruits are naturally good sources of both simple and complex carbohydrates. The flesh of fruit is rich in simple sugars, including fructose and glucose, as well as pectin, a type of fiber. Pectin makes up about 15–30 percent of the fiber in fruit. The skins of many fruits contain another fiber, cellulose; thus, eating an unpeeled fruit is preferable to eating a peeled fruit. Fruit overall contains about 2 grams of dietary fiber per serving.

When selecting fruit, fresh or frozen versions will provide more nutrients than canned fruits, which lose some vitamins and minerals during processing. If canned fruit is the only option, be sure the product is packed in fruit juice, rather than heavy syrup, to cut down on added sugar and kilocalories.

Legumes and Other Vegetables, Nuts, and Seeds

Vegetables contain abundant amounts of complex carbohydrates, including starch and fiber. In general, starchy vegetables, such as corn and potatoes, contain more carbohydrate per serving than nonstarchy vegetables like leafy greens or carrots. Legumes, such as black beans and green lentils, are also good sources of starch.

The fiber content of many foods is shown in **Figure 4.16**. Overall, a serving of vegetables contains approximately 2 grams of soluble and insoluble fiber. As with fruit, many vegetable skins are an excellent source of fiber, so consuming edible skins will increase fiber intake. Legumes are also rich in dietary fiber. Legumes provide an average of 4 grams of fiber per $1/2$ cup serving, about half of which is in the form of hemicellulose. Nuts and seeds are also good sources of fiber. Nuts provide over 1 gram of fiber in a half-ounce or small handful. A half-ounce of nuts is about 15 peanuts, 7 walnut halves, or 24 shelled pistachios.

Packaged Foods Can Be Good Sources of Carbohydrates

Packaged and processed foods, such as ready-to-eat cereals and baked crackers, can be good sources of starch and fiber, but can also contain high amounts of added sugar

refined grains Grain foods that are made with only the endosperm of the kernel. The bran and germ have been removed during milling.

enriched grains Refined grain foods that have folic acid, thiamin, niacin, riboflavin, and iron added.

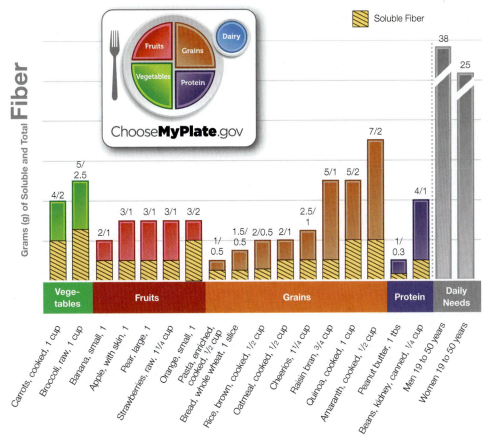

Fiber

Grams (g) of Soluble and Total

Soluble Fiber

Food	Soluble/Total
Carrots, cooked, 1 cup	4/2
Broccoli, raw, 1 cup	5/2.5
Banana, small, 1	2/1
Apple, with skin, 1	3/1
Pear, large, 1	3/1
Strawberries, raw, 1¼ cup	3/1
Orange, small, 1	3/2
Pasta, enriched, cooked, ½ cup	1/0.5
Bread, whole wheat, 1 slice	1.5/0.5
Rice, brown, cooked, ½ cup	2/0.5
Oatmeal, cooked, ½ cup	2/1
Cheerios, 1¼ cup	2.5/1
Raisin bran, ¾ cup	5/1
Quinoa, cooked, 1 cup	5/2
Amaranth, cooked, ½ cup	7/2
Peanut butter, 1 tbs	1/0.3
Beans, kidney, canned, ¼ cup	4/1
Men 19 to 50 years	38
Women 19 to 50 years	25

◀ **Figure 4.16 Food Sources of Fiber**
Adults need to consume about 25 to 38 grams of fiber daily.
Source: Hoy, M. K., and J. D. Goldman, 2014. Fiber Intake of the U.S. Population: What We Eat in America, NHANES 2009–2010. Food Surveys Research Group Dietary Data Brief No. 12. Available at https://www.ars.usda.gov/ARSUserFiles/80400530/pdf/DBrief/12_fiber_intake_0910.pdf. Accessed February 2017.

(which we discuss in depth later in this chapter), saturated fat, kilocalories, and salt, and should generally be consumed in moderation. When selecting packaged foods, choose products that contain at least 2 grams of dietary fiber per serving. If you're buying snack items, aim for baked, whole-grain crackers or low-fat pita bread rather than a box of cookies or doughnuts. The Nutrition Facts panel on all packaged foods lists the amount of total carbohydrates, including dietary fiber and added sugars, in a serving of the food (**Figure 4.17**).

Glycemic Index and Glycemic Load Can Be Used for Meal Planning

The glycemic index and glycemic load are measures of the effects of carbohydrate-containing foods on blood glucose. These measures may be helpful in dietary planning for people with diabetes.

The **glycemic index (GI)** refers to the upward rise, peak, and eventual fall of blood glucose following the consumption of a high-carbohydrate food. Some foods cause a sharp spike and rapid fall in blood glucose levels; others cause less of a spike and a more gradual decline. The GI ranks foods according to their effect on blood glucose levels compared with that of an equal amount of white bread or pure glucose (**Figure 4.18**).

A problem with using the GI is that it doesn't take into account the amount of carbohydrate consumed. For example, two slices of white bread usually weighs about 60 grams, which would be over 5 cups of puffed wheat cereal, an amount that is unlikely to be eaten in one sitting. The **glycemic load (GL)** adjusts the GI to take into account the amount of carbohydrate consumed in a typical serving of a food, and in the case of puffed wheat cereal, the normal portion size has a dramatically lower effect on blood glucose.

Nutrition Facts

8 servings per container
Serving size   2/3 cup (55g)

Amount per serving
Calories   230

	% Daily Value*
Total Fat 8g	**10%**
Saturated Fat 1g	**5%**
Trans Fat 0g	
Cholesterol 0mg	**0%**
Sodium 160mg	**7%**
Total Carbohydrate 37g	**13%**
Dietary Fiber 4g	**14%**
Total Sugars 12g	
Includes 10g Added Sugars	**20%**
Protein 3g	
Vitamin D 2mcg	10%
Calcium 260mg	20%
Iron 8mg	45%
Potassium 235mg	6%

* The % Daily Value (DV) tells you how much a nutrient in a serving of food contributes to a daily diet. 2,000 calories a day is used for general nutrition advice.

▲ **Figure 4.17 The Nutrition Facts Panel**
The new version of the Nutrition Facts panel identifies total carbohydrates, dietary fiber, and added sugars per serving of the food. How many grams of dietary fiber does a serving of this food provide? What is the %DV for fiber? Is this food a good source of dietary fiber? How many grams of added sugar does it contain?

glycemic index (GI) Rating scale of the likelihood of foods to increase the levels of blood glucose and insulin.

glycemic load (GL) Amount of carbohydrate in a food multiplied by the amount of the glycemic index of that food.

Foods	GI*
Rice, low amylose	126
Potato, baked	121
Cornflakes	119
Jelly beans	114
Green peas	107
Cheerios	106
Puffed wheat	105
Bagel, plain	103
White bread	100
Angel food cake	95
Ice cream	87
Bran muffin	85
Rice, long grain†	80
Brown rice	79
Oatmeal	79
Popcorn	79
Corn	78
Banana, overripe	74
Chocolate	70
Baked beans	69
Sponge cake	66
Pear, canned in juice	63
Custard	61
Spaghetti	59
Rice, long grain‡	58
Apple	52
Pear	47
Banana, underripe	43
Kidney beans	42
Whole milk	39
Peanuts	21

*GI = Glycemic Index

†Boiled for 25 minutes.

‡Boiled for 5 minutes.

▲ **Figure 4.18** **The Glycemic Index of Commonly Eaten Foods**
The glycemic index is a ranking of foods that indicates their potential to raise insulin and glucose levels in the blood.

The usefulness of the GI and GL for disease prevention or weight management is controversial. Research suggests that high-GI/GL foods do not raise blood glucose levels as rapidly as once believed. In fact, blood glucose levels peak at about the same level regardless of the source of the carbohydrate.[39] In general, following a diet rich in whole plant foods will result in an intake of lower GI and GL foods.

LO 4.6: THE TAKE-HOME MESSAGE The RDA for carbohydrate is 130 grams daily and the AI for fiber is 25–38 grams per day for adult females and males, respectively. Whole grains, fresh fruits, legumes and other vegetables, and low-fat dairy products are the best food sources of carbohydrates. Whole grains, fruits, legumes and other vegetables, and nuts and seeds are excellent sources of dietary fiber. Processed foods can be good sources of starches and fiber, but nutrition labels should be read carefully to avoid consuming too much added sugar, saturated fat, or energy. Foods with a low glycemic index and glycemic load may be useful for meal planning for some populations, but research is inconclusive.

How Do Natural Sugars, Added Sugars, and Sugar Substitutes Differ?

LO 4.7 Compare and contrast natural sugars, added sugars, and sugar substitutes.

Finding the taste of sweet foods pleasurable is an innate response. You don't have to fight this taste for sweetness, as a modest intake of sweet foods can easily be part of a balanced diet. However, your taste buds can't distinguish between naturally occurring sugars, like the fructose and lactose found in fruit and dairy products, and added sugars, which are added by manufacturers to foods such as soda or candy. From a nutritional standpoint, however, there is a big difference between these sugar sources.

Foods with Natural Sugars Are Generally More Nutrient Dense

Foods that contain naturally occurring sugar tend to be nutrient dense. Many fruits, for example, are among the most naturally sweet foods available. Just one bite into a ripe peach will confirm that fruit can contain more than 15 percent sugar by weight. There are many nutritional advantages of satisfying a sweet tooth with fruit, such as a whole orange, rather than with sweets that have added sugar, such as a package of candy orange slices. Let's compare these two snacks (**Figure 4.19**).

For the 65 kilocalories in six slices of a navel orange, you get more than 100 percent of the daily value for vitamin C and 3.5 grams of fiber, which is about 10 percent of the amount of fiber that adults should consume daily. These juicy slices of orange also provide fluid. In fact, *over 85 percent* of the weight of an orange is water. The hefty amounts of fiber and water make the orange a sweet snack that provides bulk. This bulk can increase satiety and reduce the likelihood of overeating.

In contrast, for the 300 kilocalories found in six candy orange slices, you'll get about 19 teaspoons of added sugar and little else: no vitamin C, no fiber, and only negligible amounts of water. Moreover, the candy is low volume, so you probably wouldn't feel satiated after consuming it and would crave more food. To consume the 300 kilocalories found in the six pieces of candy, you would have to eat almost five oranges, so it would be much easier to overeat candy orange slices than fresh oranges.

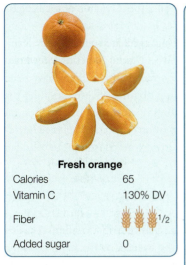

A fresh orange provides more nutrients for fewer kilocalories, and without any added sugars, compared with candy orange slices.

Fresh orange	
Calories	65
Vitamin C	130% DV
Fiber	🌾🌾🌾½
Added sugar	0

Candy orange	
Calories	300
Vitamin C	0% DV
Fiber	0
Added sugar	

🌾 = 1 gram of fiber

🥄 = 1 tsp of added sugar

Added Sugars Are Used during Food Processing

Sugars are added to foods for many reasons. In baked goods, they can hold onto water, which helps keep the product moist, and they help turn pastries a golden brown color. Sugars function as preservatives and thickeners in foods such as sauces. Fermenting sugars in dough produce the carbon dioxide that makes yeast breads rise. And of course, sugars make foods taste sweet. In the last decade, Americans' consumption of soda has decreased but that of sugar-laden sports and energy drinks tripled, from 4 to 12 percent.[40]

While sucrose and fructose are the most common added sugars in our foods, sugars can appear on the food label under a variety of names (**Figure 4.20**). To find the amount and type of added sugars in a food, read the ingredients list. If added sugars appear first or second on the list, or if the product contains many varieties of added sugars, it is likely high in sugar. Note, for example, that the ingredient label from a box of low-fat chocolate chip granola bars lists added sugars 10 different times!

As you learned in Chapter 2, the new Nutrition Facts panel used on food labels must identify added sugars in grams per serving. The panel also lists the grams of total sugars; that is, the amount of naturally occurring sugars and the added sugars, if any. For an 8-ounce carton of milk, for example, the 11 grams of sugar identified on the Nutrition Facts panel is just the

Sugar can be called a number of different names on ingredient lists and labels.

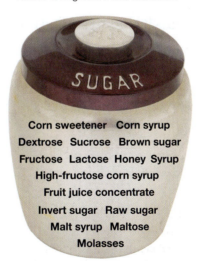

Corn sweetener   Corn syrup
Dextrose   Sucrose   Brown sugar
Fructose   Lactose   Honey   Syrup
High-fructose corn syrup
Fruit juice concentrate
Invert sugar   Raw sugar
Malt syrup   Maltose
Molasses

Ingredients: Granola (whole grain rolled oats, sugar, rice flour, whole grain rolled wheat, partially hydrogenated soybean and cottonseed oils* with TBHQ and citric acid added to preserve freshness and/or sunflower oil with natural tocopherol added to preserve freshness, whole wheat flour, molasses, sodium bicarbonate, soy lecithin, caramel color, barley malt, salt, nonfat dry milk), corn syrup, crisp rice (rice, sugar, salt, barley malt), semisweet chocolate chunks (sugar, chocolate liquor, cocoa butter, soy lecithin, vanillin [an artificial flavor]), sugar, corn syrup solids, glycerin, high fructose corn syrup, partially hydrogenated soybean and/or cottonseed oil*, sorbitol, fructose, calcium carbonate, natural and artificial flavors, salt, soy lecithin, molasses, water, BHT (a preservative), citric acid.

* Adds a dietarily insignificant amount of *trans* fat.

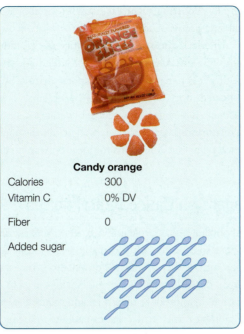

▲ **Figure 4.20** **Finding Added Sugars on the Label**
A food is likely to contain a large amount of sugar if added sugars appear first or second on the ingredients list and/or if there are many varieties of added sugars listed. The food label for these Quaker granola bars, for example, list sugar second on the ingredients list.

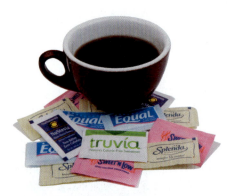

A variety of sugar substitutes, such as Truvia, Splenda, Equal, and Sweet and Low, are available to consumers.

dental caries Tooth decay.

sugar substitutes Alternatives to table sugar that sweeten foods for fewer kilocalories.

sugar alcohols Type of sweetener often used in sugar-free foods. Includes xylitol, mannitol, and sorbitol. Also known as *polyols*.

▶ **Figure 4.21 Growing Interest in Sugar-Free Foods and Beverages**
The use of sugar-free products has more than doubled since 1986.

Source: Calorie Control Council. Trends and Statistics. Copyright © 2012 by Calorie Control Council. Reprinted with permission.

naturally occurring sugar, lactose. But for chocolate milk, the 22 grams of total sugars include 11 grams of added sugars.

Americans don't eat the majority of the added sugars in their diets—they drink them. The number-one source of added sugars in the United States is sweetened soft drinks, energy drinks, and sports drinks. Sugar-sweetened beverages have been implicated in many health-related problems, including obesity.[41] See Examining the Evidence: Do Sugar-Sweetened Beverages Cause Obesity? for more information on the relationship between body weight and the consumption of sugar-sweetened beverages. Review the Table Tips for ideas on ways to cut down your consumption of added sugars.

Sugar Can Cause Dental Caries

Carbohydrates play a role in tooth decay. Sugars and starches contribute to **dental caries** because sugar is a readily available food source for the bacteria in the mouth. As the bacteria grow, they produce acids that erode the enamel of the teeth. The stickier the carbohydrate, the longer it is in contact with the teeth and the more opportunity there is for the bacteria to produce their damaging acids. Hence, hard candies that dissolve slowly in the mouth or dried fruits that can adhere to the teeth are potentially more harmful than foods that are quickly swallowed, such as whole fruits and vegetables. To avoid increased risk of dental caries, sugary snacks should be kept to a minimum, and whole fruits and raw vegetables should be chosen over candies or pastries as snacks.

Chewing sugarless gum may actually help reduce the levels of acid attacking your teeth. It encourages the production of saliva and provides a postmeal bath for your mouth.

Sugar Substitutes Add Sweetness but Not Kilocalories

Because most people perceive eating too much sugar as unhealthy, food manufacturers often use artificially created **sugar substitutes** to provide the sweet taste of sugar for fewer kilocalories. Americans' consumption of these products has increased steadily over the last two decades (**Figure 4.21**). All sugar substitutes must be approved by the FDA and deemed safe for consumption before they are allowed in food products sold in the United States.

Several sugar substitutes are presently available to consumers, including polyols (also referred to as **sugar alcohols**), stevia, saccharin, aspartame, acesulfame-K, sucralose, rebaudioside A, and neotame. Sugar alcohols are organic compounds with fewer kilocalories than table sugar, don't promote dental caries, and have less impact on blood glucose compared to other carbohydrates.

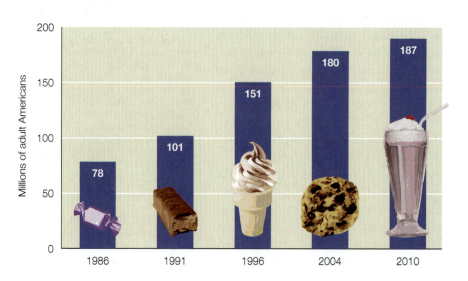

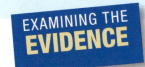

Do Sugar-Sweetened Beverages Cause Obesity?

The evidence is overwhelming: the United States is becoming an obese nation. Recent estimates suggest that 36.5 percent of adult Americans are obese.[1] Although many factors contribute to this, health professionals note that the rise in obesity rates during the past few decades coincides with an increase in consumption of sugar-sweetened beverages, at least among children, who drink more sugary beverages than they do milk.[2] This observation has prompted some municipalities to attempt to limit purchases of these drinks. For example, cities such as Berkeley, California and Boulder, Colorado have placed a tax on sugary drinks.[3] Is this effective? Are sugar-sweetened beverages the primary culprit in our obesity epidemic?

Consumption of Sugar-Sweetened Beverages in the United States

Every day, 50 percent of Americans consume some form of sugary drink equivalent to about one 12-ounce soda.[4] The top sugar-sweetened beverages reported include soda, fruit drinks, tea, coffee, energy and sports drinks, and flavored milks. Consuming one of any of these beverages adds about 180 additional kilocalories to a person's daily intake.[5] The larger the sweetened beverage, the more added sugars (see **Figure 1**). A classic (and rare) 8-ounce bottle of cola provides almost 7 teaspoons of added sugars. In today's vending machine, you are more likely to find a 12-ounce can or a 20-ounce bottle. Because people typically consume the entire can or bottle, regardless of its size, they consume more sugar.

The consumption patterns shown in **Table 1** suggest that males consume

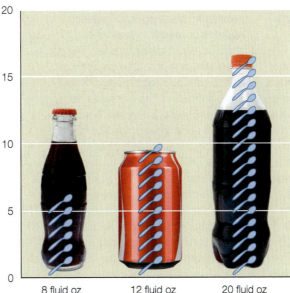

| 8 fluid oz bottle of cola | 12 fluid oz can of cola | 20 fluid oz bottle of cola |

▲ **Figure 1** The Many Sizes of Soft Drinks A single soda can provide from 6 to 17 teaspoons of added sugars, depending on the size of the container.

more of their total kilocalories per day from sugar-sweetened beverages than do females, and both genders reduce consumption of sugary beverages as they age.

The good news is that the overall consumption of sugar-sweetened soda is declining.[6] Yet while Americans are drinking fewer sodas, they have almost tripled their consumption of

sugar-sweetened sports/energy drinks,[7] and sugar-sweetened beverages are still the single largest source of added sugar in the U.S. diet. Regardless of whether Americans are drinking more soda or sports or energy drinks, do these beverages contribute to our expanded waistlines?

The Theories of Sugar-Sweetened Drink Consumption and Weight Gain

A couple of theories have been proposed to explain the possible connection between weight gain and our consumption of sugar-sweetened beverages. One theory suggests that the additional kilocalories consumed in sweetened beverages leads to excess overall kilocalorie intake and thus weight gain. The second theory is that sugar in liquid form increases our appetite, leading to an increased consumption of kilocalories from other foods. Research exploring both of these theories has yielded some interesting results.

TABLE 1	Consumption Patterns of Sugar-Sweetened Beverages			
Gender	**Age**	**Teaspoons***	**Kilocalories****	**% of Total Kcals per Day**
Males	12–19	18.4	294	11.6
	20–39	18.1	289	10.3
	40–59	12.6	202	7.7
	>60	5.9	94	4.6
Females	12–19	12.1	194	10.5
	20–39	10.8	173	9.3
	40–59	7.7	123	6.9
	>60	3.8	60	4.0

* Teaspoons of sugar consumed per day from sugar-sweetened beverages

** Total kilocalories consumed per day from sugar-sweetened beverages

Source: Adapted from P. E. Miller, et al. 2013. Sugar-Sweetened Beverage Consumption in the U.S.: Novel Assessment Methodology. *American Journal of Preventive Medicine* 45(4):416–421.

Sugar-Sweetened Drinks, Artificially Sweetened Drinks, Water, and Weight Gain

There is evidence that adding kilocalories to your daily intake by drinking sugar-sweetened beverages adds body weight. For example, normal-weight adults who drank one additional 12-ounce sugar-sweetened beverage each day gained an average of one extra pound every 4 years compared with people who did not add an extra beverage.[8] This research suggests that simply ingesting additional kilocalories through sugar-sweetened beverages is enough to contribute to weight gain. What if we replaced sugar-sweetened drinks with artificially sweetened beverages without kilocalories?

In children at least, the research is promising. Results from the Double-Blind, Randomized Intervention Study in Kids (DRINK) suggests that when the sugar in the beverage was replaced with sucralose, healthy children lost weight, mostly as body fat.[9] Other studies contradict these results and report that artificially sweetened beverages, such as diet soda, result in weight gain, not weight loss. Data from a 10-year longitudinal study reported that adults who drank two or more diet sodas a day increased their waist size by six times more than the average waist increase in those who did not drink diet sodas.[10] Another study found no effect on body weight in individuals using sweetened cocoa versus sugar-free cocoa.[11] Thus, the relationship between weight gain and sugar-sweetened beverages versus artificially sweetened beverages is still unclear.

If the increase in kilocalories from sugary beverage consumption indeed causes weight gain, perhaps the best alternative is to switch from sugary drinks to kilocalorie-free water. Again, the evidence conflicts: whereas some research suggests that adults gain less weight over time when they switch from sugar-sweetened beverages to water,[12] other research finds no effect on body weight.[13]

Sugar-Sweetened Drinks May Impact Satiation

Perhaps the answer lies in the second theory, that consuming sugar-sweetened beverages increases appetite or results in feeling less satisfied. Most beverages are sweetened with high-fructose corn syrup or sucrose, and most people who sweeten their coffee or tea do so with table sugar (sucrose). What links sucrose and high-fructose corn syrup is that both sweeteners contain fructose. Some researchers have suggested that fructose may change our appetite-control mechanisms, resulting in less satiation and a greater intake of kilocalories from other foods.[14] This theory is based on earlier studies conducted with pure crystalline fructose, which reported that fructose ingestion resulted in a decrease in the hormones insulin and leptin.[15] Both of these hormones increase satiety. Whereas glucose stimulates insulin production, thus increasing satiety, fructose alone does not stimulate insulin production.

This is significant in that the release of insulin in turn stimulates the release of leptin, a hormone that decreases appetite.[16] These two hormones also suppress the release of ghrelin, a hormone that stimulates our appetite (see Chapter 15 for more information on hormones and satiety).[17] If insulin is reduced, as would be the case with pure fructose as a sweetener, then leptin is reduced and ghrelin is not suppressed, which leads to feeling hungry and eating more kilocalories. The flaw in this theory is that we rarely consume pure fructose in our diet. This monosaccharide is consumed as part of the disaccharide sucrose or as high-fructose corn syrup, which is about 50 percent fructose and 50 percent glucose.[18]

If sugar-sweetened beverages do increase hunger, research subjects would report a decrease in satiety and an increase in kilocalorie intake compared with artificially sweetened drinks. A recent study showed that sugary beverages sweetened with either sucrose or high-fructose corn syrup versus artificially sweetened drinks

had similar satiety ratings.[19] Not only were the satiety ratings the same, but the sugar-sweetened beverage did not increase the amount of food eaten later in the day when compared with an artificially sweetened beverage. However, studies do report that sugary beverage consumption increases body weight. For example, 641 children were given either an 8-ounce sugar-sweetened beverage containing 104 kilocalories or an 8-ounce artificially sweetened beverage with zero kilocalories each day in school. After 18 months, the students who drank the sugar-sweetened beverage gained more weight and accumulated more body fat than did those who drank the artificially sweetened beverages.[20]

Not all beverages have to be sweetened with sucrose or artificial sweeteners. Using whey protein as a sweetener has shown some promise in reducing hunger and kilocalorie intake. A recent study tested this theory in normal-weight and overweight females.[21] Subjects were given beverages sweetened with glucose, whey protein, or whey protein plus glucose after an overnight fast. Their blood glucose and appetite were measured nine times for up to 2 hours following ingestion of the sweetened beverage. The kilocalorie intake was measured at a meal 3 hours after drinking the sweetened beverage. The results reported that the whey protein and whey protein plus glucose reduced the rise in blood glucose and reduced appetite and kilocalorie intake compared with glucose in both groups.

The Bottom Line: Do Sugar-Sweetened Beverages Cause Obesity?

Obesity is the result of a combination of factors, including total kilocalories consumed, genetics, physical inactivity, and aspects of our environment. Currently, there is no conclusive evidence that sugar-sweetened drinks *alone* contribute more to obesity than do other energy sources.

Although sugar-sweetened beverages may or may not be the main culprit in the dramatic rise in obesity, they clearly play a significant role in

Americans' overall increased caloric intake. A recent study reported that over a 4-year period, weight gain in adults was mostly associated with the intake of potato chips, potatoes, sugar-sweetened beverages, red meat, and processed meats, in that order.[22] Weight gain was inversely related to the ingestion of vegetables, whole grains, fruits, nuts, and yogurt. Sugar-sweetened beverages add unnecessary kilocalories and could be responsible for weight gain;[23] however, the more likely dietary factor is excessive energy intake from all foods and beverages.

References

1. Centers for Disease Control. 2016. *Adult Obesity Facts*. Available at www.cdc.gov. Accessed January 2017.
2. T. Sherman. 2013. *Examining New York City's Proposed Ban on Sugar-Sweetened Fountain Drink Sizes Greater than 16 Ounces*. Available at https://blogs.commons.georgetown.edu. Accessed January 2017.
3. *The Wall Street Journal*. 2015. Should There Be a Tax on Soda and Other Sugary Drinks? Available at http://www.wsj.com/articles/should-there-be-a-tax-on-soda-and-other-sugary-drinks-1436757039. Accessed January 2017.
4. Greenwood, D. C., et al. 2014. Association Between Sugar-sweetened and Artificially Sweetened Soft Drinks and Type 2 Diabetes: Systematic Review and Dose-response Meta-analysis of Prospective Studies. *British Journal of Nutrition* 112:725–734.
5. Han, E., and L. M. Powell. 2013. Consumption Patterns of Sugar-Sweetened Beverages in the United States. *Journal of the Academy of Nutrition and Dietetics* 113(1):43–53.
6. Miller, P. E., R. A. McKinnon, et al. 2013. Sugar-Sweetened Beverage Consumption in the U.S.: Novel Assessment Methodology. *American Journal of Preventive Medicine* 45(4):416–421.
7. Ibid.
8. Bleich, S. N., et al. 2014. Diet-beverage Consumption and Caloric Intake Among US Adults, Overall and by Body Weight. *American Journal of Public Health* 104:e72–78.
9. de Ruyter, J. C., M. R. Olthof, et al. 2012. A Trial of Sugar-Free or Sugar-Sweetened Beverages and Body Weight in Children. *New England Journal of Medicine* 367:1397–1406.
10. Fowler, S. P., K. Williams, et al. 2011. Diet Soft Drink Consumption is Associated with Increased Waist Circumference in the San Antonio Longitudinal Study of Aging. *Diabetes Pro*. Available at http://professional.diabetes.org. Accessed January 2017.
11. Fowler, S. P. 2016. Low-calorie Sweetener Use and Energy Balance: Results from Experimental Studies in Animals and Large-scale Prospective Studies in Humans. 1:164(Pt. B):517–523; doi:10.1016/j.physbeh.2016.04.047.
12. Pan, A., V. S. Malik, et al. 2013. Changes in Water and Beverage Intake and Long-Term Weight Changes: Results from Three Prospective Cohort Studies. *International Journal of Obesity* 37(10):1378–1385.
13. Muckelbauer, R., G. Sarganas, et al. 2013. Association between Water Consumption and Body Weight Outcomes: A Systematic Review. *American Journal of Clinical Nutrition* 98:282–299.
14. Page, K. A., O. Chan, et al. 2013. Effects of Fructose vs. Glucose on Regional Cerebral Blood Flow in Brain Regions Involved with Appetite and Reward Pathways. *Journal of the American Medical Association* 309(1):63–70.
15. Bray, G. A. 2013. Energy and Fructose From Beverages Sweetened with Sugar or High-fructose Corn Syrup Pose a Health Risk for Some People. *Advanced Nutrition* 4:220–225.
16. Schloegl, H., R. Percik, et al. 2011. Peptide Hormones Regulating Appetite—Focus on Neuroimaging Studies in Humans. *Diabetes Metabolism Research and Reviews* 27(2):104–112.
17. Ibid.
18. J. M. Rippe. 2013. The Metabolic and Endocrine Response and Health Implications of Consuming Sugar-Sweetened Beverages: Findings from Recent Randomized Controlled Trials. *Advanced Nutrition* 4:677–686.
19. de Ruyter, J. C. M. B. Katan, et al. 2013. The Effect of Sugar-Free versus Sugar-Sweetened Beverages on Satiety, Liking and Wanting: An 18-Month Randomized Double-Blind Trial in Children. *PLoS ONE* 8(10):e78039. doi:10.1371/journal.pone.0078039.
20. Katan, M. B., et al. 2016. Impact of Masked Replacement of Sugar-Sweetened with Sugar-free Beverages on Body Weight Increases with Initial BMI: Secondary Analysis of Data from an 18-Month Double-blind Trial in Children. *PLoS* 11(7):e0159771. Doi:10.1371/journal.pone.0159771.
21. Zafar, T. A., C. Waslien, et al. 2013. Whey Protein–Sweetened Beverages Reduce Glycemic and Appetite Responses and Food Intake in Young Females. *Nutrition Research* 33(4):303–310.
22. Fieril, D. P., P. F. Olsen, et al. 2017. Experiences in a Lifestyle Intervention in Obese Pregnant Women – A Qualitative Study. *Midwifery* 44:1–6; doi: 10.1016/j.midw.2016.10.011.
23. Hu, F. B., 2013. Resolved: There Is Sufficient Scientific Evidence that Decreasing Sugar-Sweetened Beverage Consumption Will Reduce the Prevalence of Obesity and Obesity-Related Diseases. *Obesity Review* 14(8):606–619.

Aspartame, acesulfame-K, sucralose, and neotame also don't promote dental caries and have the added advantage of not affecting blood glucose levels at all. These sugar substitutes may help people with diabetes manage their blood glucose levels. Additionally, all sugar substitutes are either reduced in kilocalories or are kilocalorie free. See **Table 4.3** for a comparison of available sweeteners.

Stevia

Stevia, one of the most popular sugar substitutes, is a natural sweetener extracted from a plant related to an aster or chrysanthemum. The sweeteners in the plant—steviol glycosides—have been used in South America and Asia to sweeten beverages such as tea. Stevia contains no carbohydrates, has zero kilocalories, and does not raise blood glucose levels.[42] Stevia registers about 250 times sweeter than table sugar, so you use much less to achieve the same sweetness.

| TABLE 4.3 | Oh So Sweet! |

Sweetener	Kilocalories/ Gram	Trade Names	Sweetening Power	The Facts
Sucrose	4.0	Table sugar	—	Sweetens food, enhances flavor, tenderizes, and contributes browning properties to baked goods
Reduced-Kilocalorie Sweeteners				
Polyols (Sugar Alcohols)				
Sorbitol	2.6	Sorbitol	50–70% as sweet as sucrose	Found in foods such as sugarless chewing gum, jams, baked goods, and candy
Mannitol	1.6	Mannitol	50–70% as sweet as sucrose	Found in foods such as chewing gum, jams, and as a bulking agent in powdered foods. May cause diarrhea.
Xylitol	2.4	Xylitol	Equally sweet as sucrose	Found in foods such as chewing gum, candies; also in pharmaceuticals and hygiene products
Hydrogenated starch hydrolysates (HSHs)	3.0	HSH	50–70% as sweet as sucrose	Found in confections and can be used as a bulking agent
Kilocalorie-Free Sweeteners				
Saccharin	0	Sweet 'N Low	200–700% sweeter than sucrose	Retains its sweetening power at high temperatures such as baking
Aspartame	4.0*	NutraSweet, Equal	Approximately 200% sweeter than sucrose	Sweetening power is reduced at high temperatures such as baking. Can be added at end stages of recipes such as cooked puddings if removed from heat source. Individuals with PKU need to monitor all dietary sources of phenylalanine, including aspartame.
Acesulfame-K	0	Sunette	200% sweeter than sucrose	Retains its sweetening power at high temperatures
Sucralose	0	Splenda	600% sweeter than sucrose	Retains its sweetening power at high temperatures
Rebaudioside A	0	Truvia, Sun Crystals, PureVia	200% sweeter than sucrose	Retains its sweetening power at high temperatures
Tagalose	1.5	Naturlose	92% as sweet as sugar	Texture and taste similar to sucrose
Neotame	0	Neotame	7,000–13,000% sweeter than sucrose	Retains its sweetening power at high temperatures

* Because so little aspartame is needed to sweeten foods, it provides negligible kilocalories.

Aspartame

In 1965, a scientist named James Schlatter was conducting research on amino acids in his quest to find a treatment for ulcers. To pick up a piece of paper in his laboratory, he licked his finger—and stumbled upon a sweet-tasting compound.[43] It was the "lick" that was soon to be "tasted" around the world. Schlatter had just discovered aspartame, a substance that has become one of the most-used sugar substitutes in the world.

Aspartame is composed of two amino acids: a modified aspartic acid and phenylalanine. Enzymes in the GI tract break down aspartame into its component parts and the amino acids are absorbed, providing 4 kilocalories per gram. Because aspartame is 200 times sweeter than sucrose, only a small amount is needed to sweeten a food.

In 1981, the FDA approved aspartame for use in tabletop sweeteners, such as Equal and NutraSweet, and to sweeten breakfast cereals, chewing gums, and carbonated beverages. The majority of the aspartame that is consumed in the United States is in soft drinks. In 1996, the FDA gave the food industry carte blanche to use aspartame in all types of foods and beverages. It is currently used as a sweetener in over 100 countries and can now be found in over 6,000 foods, pharmaceuticals, and personal care products sold in the United States.

Aspartame has undergone continual, vigorous reviews to ensure that it is safe for human consumption. Despite its intense evaluation, aspartame has been, and still is, blamed for headaches and other health problems. Major health organizations such as the Academy of Nutrition and Dietetics, the American Medical Association, and the American Diabetes Association all support aspartame's use by healthy adults, children, and pregnant women in moderation as part of a well-balanced diet.[44]

Individuals with a rare inherited disorder known as phenylketonuria (PKU) are unable to metabolize phenylalanine, one of the amino acids in aspartame, and must adhere to a special diet. Because of the seriousness of this disorder, which can lead to brain damage, the FDA mandates that all food products that contain phenylalanine carry a label declaring its content.

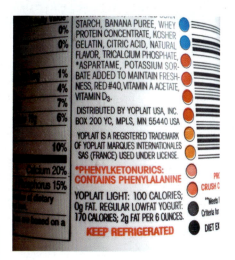

Foods, such as Yoplait, and beverages that contain aspartame must carry a label warning that phenylalanine is present.

LO 4.7: THE TAKE-HOME MESSAGE Your taste buds can't distinguish between naturally occurring and added sugars. Foods with naturally occurring sugars, such as whole fruit, tend to provide more nutrition and satiation than empty-calorie sweets such as candy. Numerous names for sugar are found on food labels, and soft drinks are the number-one contributor of added sugars to Americans' diets. Millions of Americans consume reduced-kilocalorie or kilo-calorie-free sugar substitutes. The FDA has approved several sugar substitutes for use in foods and beverages. These sugar substitutes add sweetness to your food without the added kilocalories, do not promote dental caries, and can benefit those with diabetes who need to carefully manage their blood glucose. Stevia and aspartame are two of the most popular sugar substitutes.

HEALTH CONNECTION

What Is Diabetes?

LO 4.8 Describe the underlying mechanisms, symptoms, and treatment for different classifications of diabetes.

Diabetes mellitus, or *diabetes,* is a condition related to inadequate regulation of blood glucose. An estimated 29.1 million Americans—more than 9.3 percent of the population—have diabetes.[45] Of these individuals, 8.1 million have the disease, but don't know it yet.[46] The incidence of adults being diagnosed with diabetes in the United States has more than doubled since the early 1990s and the number may be underestimated. If this trend continues, it is likely that more than one-third of Americans will develop diabetes in their lifetime, reducing their life expectancy, on average, by 10–15 years.[47]

The incidence of diabetes is rising not only among adults, but also among children. Whereas the most prevalent form of diabetes, known as type 2, used to be common only in adults, in the last two decades there has been a steady increase among those under age 20.

Over 200,000 Americans die from diabetic complications annually, and diabetes is the seventh leading cause of death in the United States. Diabetes is not only deadly, but extremely costly. Disability insurance payments, time lost from employment, and the direct medical expenses associated with diabetes cost more than $170 billion annually in the United States.[48] This is an epidemic that is spiraling out of control.

Diabetes Types and Risk Factors

There are different types of diabetes, but they all result from the inability of the body to make or properly use the hormone insulin. Insulin directs glucose into the cells to be used as immediate energy or stored for later use. Diabetes develops when the pancreas produces an inadequate amount of insulin and/or body cells develop **insulin resistance,** such that they do not respond to the insulin when it arrives. In either case, the bloodstream is flooded with glucose that can't get into the cells. When this happens, the body shifts into fasting mode. The liver begins to break down its glycogen stores (glycogenolysis) and make glucose from noncarbohydrate sources (gluconeogenesis). This floods the blood with even more glucose,

diabetes mellitus Medical condition whereby an individual either doesn't have enough insulin or is resistant to the insulin available, resulting in a rise in blood glucose levels. Diabetes mellitus is often called diabetes.

insulin resistance Inability of the cells to respond to insulin.

some of which is removed by the kidneys and enters the urine.

In addition, the body calls on its energy reserve—fat—to be used as fuel. The body needs glucose in order to thoroughly burn fat; otherwise, it makes ketone bodies. In poorly managed diabetes, acidic ketone bodies can build up in the blood to dangerous levels, causing **ketoacidosis.** Diabetic ketoacidosis can cause nausea and confusion and, if left untreated, can result in coma or death. (*Note:* Ketoacidosis occurs when insulin is lacking in the body, and is different from the condition of ketosis, which can develop in individuals who are fasting or consuming a low-carbohydrate diet; unlike diabetic ketoacidosis, ketosis is not life-threatening.)

All forms of diabetes involve a failure of blood glucose regulation. The most prevalent are type 1 and type 2 (**Focus Figure 4.22**).

Type 1 Diabetes

Type 1 diabetes is considered an autoimmune disease and is the rarer of the two main forms, affecting just 5 percent of all diabetics in the United States.[49] Approximately 1.25 million Americans—about 200,000 of them under age 20—live with type 1 diabetes. The disorder usually begins in childhood or the early adult years.[50] In people with type 1 diabetes, the immune system destroys the insulin-producing beta cells in the pancreas. An obsessive, uncontrollable thirst, excessive urination, and blurred vision are common symptoms associated with undiagnosed or untreated type 1 diabetes. Other common symptoms are hunger, weight loss, and fatigue because the glucose can't get into the cells of the body. Once they have been diagnosed, individuals with type 1 diabetes must monitor their glucose levels and inject insulin every day in order to avoid these symptoms.

The hormone insulin is a protein and is digestible by the GI tract, so it can't be taken orally. Therefore, most individuals have to inject insulin directly into their fat or muscle tissue with a syringe. Researchers are continually testing alternative, non-needle methods for those with diabetes to self-administer insulin. Insulin pens, insulin jet injectors, and insulin pumps are among the devices becoming available.

Type 2 Diabetes

Type 2 diabetes is more common than type 1, accounting for 90–95 percent of diagnoses of the disease. Being overweight increases the risk of developing type 2 diabetes.[51] People with type 2 diabetes initially produce insulin but their cells have become insulin resistant. The insulin resistance prompts the pancreas to overproduce insulin in order to compensate. After several years of increased insulin production, the pancreatic beta cells become exhausted, and the production of insulin may decrease to the point where a person with type 2 diabetes may have to take medication and/or inject insulin to manage his or her blood glucose level.

One of the major problems with type 2 diabetes is that this condition can go undiagnosed for some time. Some people may have symptoms such as fatigue, blurred vision, and increased thirst and urination; others may not have any symptoms at all. Consequently, diabetes can damage a person's vital organs without their being aware of it. Because of this, the American Diabetes Association (ADA) recommends that everyone 45 years of age and older undergo testing for diabetes every 3 years. However, people who are overweight or obese or who are genetically predisposed shouldn't wait until age 45 to be tested. Overweight children should be screened when they turn 10 years old with repeat screening every 2 years. (See the Self-Assessment to determine whether you are at risk for type 2 diabetes.)

One predictor of both type 2 diabetes and cardiovascular disease is a cluster of risk factors collectively referred to as *metabolic syndrome.* These factors include elevated blood glucose, abnormal blood lipids, high blood pressure, and abdominal obesity. The risk factors for developing metabolic syndrome, such as eating a poor diet and failing to exercise, are also risk factors for type 2 diabetes and cardiovascular disease. In fact, a diagnosis of metabolic syndrome often precedes a diagnosis of type 2 diabetes.[52]

Prediabetes

Impaired glucose tolerance, or *prediabetes,* is a condition in which an individual's blood glucose is consistently higher than normal, but not high enough to warrant a diagnosis of diabetes. In 2012, 86 million Americans age 20 and older had prediabetes. These individuals are at increased risk of developing type 2 diabetes as well as cardiovascular disease.[53] Moreover, when a person is in this prediabetic state, damage may already be occurring to body tissues.

Diagnosing Diabetes and Prediabetes

A simple blood test in a physician's office can determine whether or not a person has diabetes or prediabetes. Either of two types of tests are commonly performed.

In a fasting blood glucose test, the blood is typically drawn first thing in the morning after fasting overnight for 8–12 hours. A fasting blood glucose level of under

---

ketoacidosis Buildup of ketone bodies in the blood to dangerous levels, which can result in coma or death.

type 1 diabetes Autoimmune form of diabetes in which the pancreas does not produce insulin.

type 2 diabetes Form of diabetes characterized by insulin resistance.

impaired glucose tolerance Condition whereby a fasting blood glucose level is higher than normal, but not high enough to be classified as having diabetes mellitus. Also called *prediabetes.*

Diabetes is a chronic disease in which the body can no longer regulate glucose within normal limits, and blood glucose becomes dangerously high.

NORMAL

1 Liver releases glucose into bloodstream.

2 The cells of the pancreas release insulin into bloodstream.

3 Insulin stimulates uptake of glucose into cells.

4 As glucose is taken into interior of cells, less glucose remains in the bloodstream.

TYPE 1 DIABETES

1 Liver releases glucose into bloodstream.

2 The cells of the pancreas are damaged or destroyed. Little or no insulin is released into bloodstream.

3 In the absence of insulin, glucose is not taken up by cells.

4 High levels of glucose remain in the bloodstream.

TYPE 2 DIABETES

1 Liver releases glucose into bloodstream.

2 The cells of the pancreas release insulin into bloodstream.

3 Insulin is present, but cells fail to respond adequately. Progressively higher amounts of insulin must be produced to stimulate cells to uptake glucose.

4 High levels of glucose remain in the bloodstream.

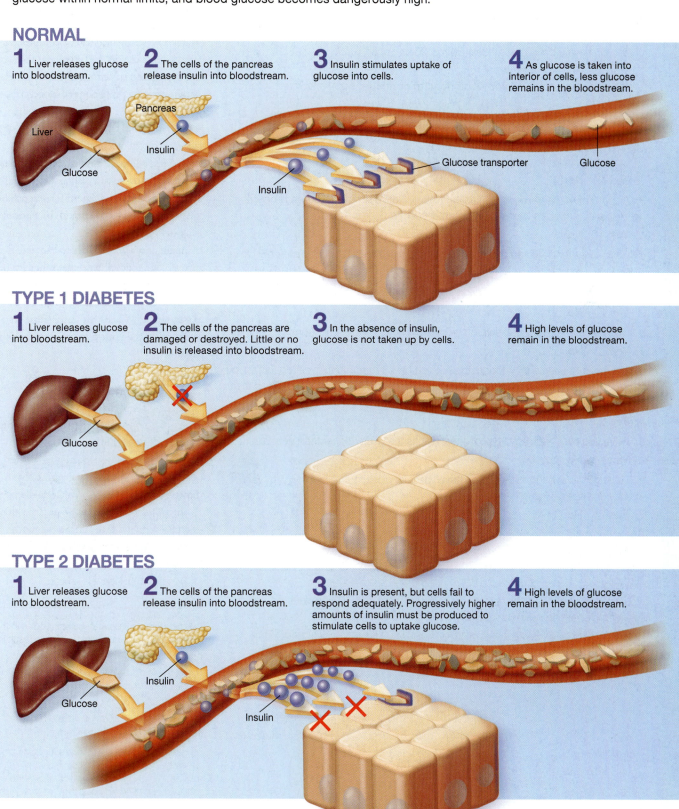

Pancreas

Liver

Glucose

Insulin

Insulin

Glucose transporter

Glucose

Glucose

Glucose

Insulin

Insulin

Self-Assessment

Are You at Risk for Type 2 Diabetes?

Take the following quiz to assess if you are at risk for developing type 2 diabetes. Whereas this list contains the presently known risk factors for type 2 diabetes, there may be others. If you have questions or doubts, check with your doctor.

Do you have a body mass index (BMI) of 25 or higher*?

Yes ☐ **No** ☐

If you answered "no," you don't need to continue. If you answered "yes," continue.

1. Does your mom, dad, brother, or sister have diabetes?

Yes ☐ **No** ☐

2. Do you typically exercise for less than 30 minutes daily?

Yes ☐ **No** ☐

3. Are you of African American, Alaskan Native, Native American, Asian American, Hispanic, or Pacific Islander American descent?

Yes ☐ **No** ☐

4. Have you ever delivered a baby that weighed more than 9 pounds at birth?

Yes ☐ **No** ☐

5. Have you ever had diabetes during pregnancy?

Yes ☐ **No** ☐

6. Do you have a blood pressure of 140/90 millimeters of mercury (mmHg) or higher?

Yes ☐ **No** ☐

7. Have you been told by your doctor that you have too much triglyceride (fat) in your blood (more than 250 mg/dl) or too little of the "good" HDL cholesterol (less than 35 mg/dl)?

Yes ☐ **No** ☐

8. Have you ever had blood glucose test results that were higher than normal?

Yes ☐ **No** ☐

9. Have you ever been told that you have vascular disease or problems with your blood vessels?

Yes ☐ **No** ☐

10. Do you have metabolic syndrome**?

Yes ☐ **No** ☐

Answers

If you are overweight and answered "yes" to any of the above 10 questions, you could benefit from speaking with your doctor.

* BMI is a measure of your weight in relationship to your height. See Chapter 14 for a chart to determine your BMI.

** Metabolic syndrome is a cluster of symptoms including elevated blood glucose and lipids, high blood pressure, and obesity. This disorder increases the risk of diabetes as well as of heart disease and stroke.

100 milligrams per deciliter (mg/dl) is considered "negative" and a fasting blood glucose of 126 mg/dl or higher is considered a "positive" test for diabetes (**Table 4.4**). A reading between 100 mg/dl and 126 mg/dl is classified as prediabetes.

An A1C test, which can be completed without an overnight fast, measures the average amount of hemoglobin (the oxygen-carrying protein in red blood cells) attached to glucose in the blood over the past 3 months. In contrast, the fasting blood sugar test typically reflects your diet only for the past 48 hours. This is why A1C tests are now being used as a diagnostic and screening tool for prediabetes. For a comparison of blood glucose and A1C tests, see Table 4.4.

Again, individuals with prediabetes have a blood glucose level that is higher than it should be but not yet high enough to be classified as diabetic. The approach to treating individuals with prediabetes is illustrated in the Nutrition in Practice on page 145.

TABLE 4.4	Interpreting Blood Glucose and A1C Levels	
If Fasting Blood Glucose and AiC Levels Are	**It Means That the Levels Are Considered**
<100 mg/dl less than 5.7%	Normal
100–125 mg/dl 5.7–6.4%	Prediabetic
126 mg/dl* 6.5% or higher	Diabetic

* There must be two "positive" tests, done on separate days, for an official diagnosis of diabetes.

Source: Data from the American Diabetes Association. 2014. Diagnosis and Classification of Diabetes Mellitus. *Diabetes Care* 37:S81–S90. doi:10.2337/dc14-S081.

NUTRITION *in* PRACTICE:
Certified Diabetes Educator

Owen has been a librarian at the campus library for over 30 years. His sedentary job of sitting the majority of the day helping students access the electronic journals and databases from the library computerized system has played a factor in his 20-pound weight gain over the past decade. His annual physical at his doctor's office uncovered that his blood glucose levels classified him as having prediabetes. According to his doctor, his blood glucose levels are higher than ideal but not high enough to be diagnosed as having diabetes. This wasn't a big surprise to Owen as diabetes "runs" in his family. His brother and father both have to take medication to control their blood glucose levels.

Due to his weight gain and family history of diabetes, Owen's doctor refers him to a certified diabetes educator (CDE) for an appointment. Owen is dreading meeting with the CDE because he and his wife are "empty nesters" so eat out in restaurants at least 3 times a week rather than cook dinner at home. The CDE meets with Owen to discuss his diet and lifestyle habits and their effect on his blood glucose levels.

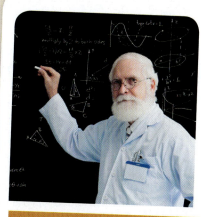

Owen

OWEN'S FOOD LOG

Food/Beverage	Time Consumed	Hunger Rating*	Location
Egg and cheese breakfast sandwich and coffee with cream	8:30 A.M.	2	Donut shop
Pizza with pepperoni, 2 slices and cola	1:00 P.M.	5	Campus pizzeria
Pretzels	4:00 P.M.	4	Vending machine on campus
Fettuccini Alfredo and Caesar salad	6:30 P.M.	4	Italian restaurant

* Hunger Rating (1–5): 1 = not hungry; 5 = super hungry.

Owen's Stats
- ❏ Age: 55
- ❏ Height: 5 feet 11 inches
- ❏ Weight: 220 pounds
- ❏ BMI: 30.7
- ❏ Fasting Blood Glucose: 124 mg/dl

Critical Thinking Questions
1. How does Owen's weight contribute to his elevated blood glucose levels?
2. What diet choices could be contributing to Owen's weight and blood glucose levels and why?
3. What role would increasing Owen's daily physical activity play in losing weight and improving his blood glucose levels?

CDE's Observation and Plan for Owen
- ❏ Discuss Owen's need to lose weight. A weight loss of as little as 5–7 percent of a person's body weight can reduce the cells' resistance to insulin. This would enable glucose to be taken up by the cells and lower his blood glucose levels.
- ❏ Consume a well-balanced, kilocalorie-reducing diet with less refined carbohydrates such as soda, chips, and pasta and fewer fatty foods such as cream and full-fat cheese to promote weight loss of approximately $\frac{1}{2}$ to 1 pound weekly. Increase intake of higher-fiber foods to promote better

glucose control. Select healthier choices when dining out.
- ❏ Increase physical activity for at least 30 minutes daily. Exercise improves the cells' sensitivity to insulin and lowers blood glucose levels.

Three weeks later, Owen visits the CDE again and is excited that he has lost 3 pounds. He brings his lunch to work so he is able to devote the majority of his lunch break walking with a fellow librarian. He and his wife also walk on the weekends. A review of his food record shows that his diet is still too low in vegetables. The CDE works with Owen to increase his vegetables at lunch and as a snack in the afternoons.

Gestational Diabetes

Gestational diabetes is a form of diabetes that may develop during pregnancy in women who have not been diagnosed as diabetic prior to the pregnancy. The cause of gestational diabetes is insulin resistance, most likely due to the influence of pregnancy-related hormones.

Blood glucose levels are screened throughout the pregnancy in women diagnosed with gestational diabetes. If blood glucose levels are controlled through a healthy diet and physical activity, there is no detrimental effect on the mother or the fetus. Uncontrolled blood glucose levels increase the risk of a larger newborn, and the birth may require cesarean section. Also, although gestational diabetes is temporary, the risk of the mother developing type 2 diabetes later in life is increased.[54]

Diabetes Can Result in Long-Term Damage

Constant exposure to high blood glucose levels can damage body tissues over time. Diabetes, especially if it is poorly managed, increases the likelihood of nerve damage, leg and foot amputations, eye diseases, blindness, tooth loss, gum problems, kidney disease, and heart disease.[54]

Nerve damage occurs in an estimated 50 percent of individuals with diabetes, and the longer the person has diabetes, the greater the risk of damage.[55] Signs and symptoms include numbness in the toes, feet, legs, and hands, as well as changes in bowel, bladder, and sexual function. Nerve damage can also affect the ability to feel a change in temperature or pain in the legs and feet. A cut or sore on the foot could go unnoticed until it becomes infected. The poor blood circulation common in persons with diabetes can also make it harder for sores or infections to heal. Over time, an infection can infiltrate the bone, causing the need for an amputation.

Diabetes can also damage the tiny blood vessels serving the retina of the eye, which can cause bleeding and cloudy vision and eventually destroy the retina and cause blindness. A high blood glucose level can cause tooth and gum problems, including the loss of teeth. Damage to the kidneys can allow protein to leak into the urine and, at the same time, cause a backup of wastes in the blood. Kidney failure could result.

Diabetes is also a risk factor for cardiovascular disease. The abnormal level of blood lipids often seen in poorly managed diabetes is likely an important factor in this increased risk. Fortunately, good nutrition plays a key role in both the prevention and management of diabetes.[56]

Control Is Key

People with diabetes can manage the disease by keeping their blood glucose level under control. Some people with type 2 may be able to do this through diet and exercise alone. Others may also need to incorporate insulin injections or other medications. People with type 1 diabetes must inject insulin to control their blood glucose level. Maintaining a healthy level of blood glucose through these means, along with monitoring blood sugar levels and routinely visiting health care professionals, can slow or, in some cases, prevent the onset of some of the complications of diabetes. For more information on dietary recommendations for controlling blood glucose, visit the American Diabetes Association link at www.diabetes.org.

The nutrition and lifestyle goals for individuals with type 1 or type 2 diabetes are the same: to minimize the complications of diabetes by adopting a healthy, well-balanced diet and participating in regular physical activity that maintains blood glucose levels in a normal or close-to-normal range.

Eat a Balanced Diet

Individuals diagnosed with diabetes should consume a combination of predominantly high-fiber carbohydrates from whole grains, fruits, and vegetables, along with low-fat milk, adequate amounts of lean protein, and unsaturated fats.[57] This diabetic diet translates into eating a moderate amount of foods that are rich in nutrients plus maintaining regular mealtimes.

The glycemic index can be a useful tool for diabetics to select carbohydrate foods; however, a less confusing approach to blood glucose control is to follow the current guidelines suggested by the American Diabetes Association (refer to Table 4.5) and using food exchange groups. As you may recall from Chapter 2, the exchange system organizes foods together by their carbohydrate, fat, and protein content. One exchange has about the same amount of each macronutrient per serving, as well as the same effect on blood glucose, as all the foods listed in the same group. For example, you could trade $1/3$ cup of pasta for one slice of whole-grain bread and ingest 15 grams of carbohydrate, 0–3 grams of protein, 0–1 gram of fat, and 80 kilocalories. See Appendix C for the lists of foods by exchange group.

Although sugar has a high glycemic index and was once thought of as a "diabetic no-no," it can be part of a diabetic's diet. Research has found that consuming sucrose doesn't cause a greater rise in a person's blood glucose level than consuming starch, so avoidance of sugar isn't necessary. However, because weight management is often a concern, especially for those with type 2 diabetes, there's little

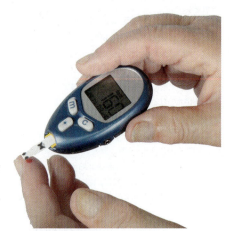

Exercise improves the control of blood glucose.

gestational diabetes Form of diabetes that may develop during pregnancy in women who were not previously diagnosed with diabetes.

room for sweets and treats in a diabetic diet (or *anyone's* diet, for that matter).

Although it's important for people with diabetes to read the Nutrition Facts panel on food labels, the serving sizes indicated may not be equivalent to those on the exchange lists. Diabetics may need to recalculate the grams of carbohydrate, protein, and fat to fit their personal meal plan.

Diabetics should not skip meals, especially if they are injecting insulin. Skipping a meal can lead to low blood glucose. The American Diabetic Association recommends diabetics eat three meals a day at regular intervals and have both a midmorning and a midafternoon snack.

Be Physically Active

Exercise is important for everyone, but especially for diabetics. Exercise on a regular basis, even brisk walking, improves insulin sensitivity. During moderate exercise, muscles take up glucose at more than 20 times the rate during inactivity, thereby lowering blood glucose levels. Any exercise that raises your heart rate for a total of 30 minutes a day will help to maintain healthy blood glucose, blood pressure, blood lipids, and body weight,[58] improve sleep, strengthen muscles and bones, including the cardiac muscle, and improve overall quality of life.

A change in exercise level may result in hypoglycemia, especially in type 1 diabetics.[59] Diabetics should check their blood glucose regularly during a workout, especially if the exercise lasts more than an hour. They should carry a small carbohydrate snack, such as fruit or fruit juice, in case blood glucose levels dip too low, and be sure to drink water before, during, and after exercise to prevent dehydration.

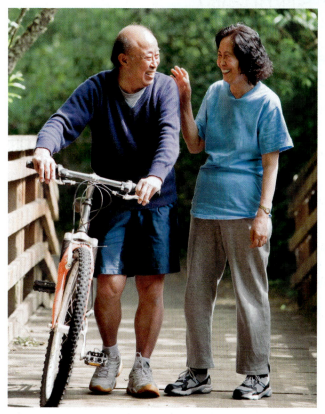

Exerercise improves the control of blood glucose.

Preventing Type 2 Diabetes

When it comes to avoiding diabetes, a healthful diet and physical activity is the best game plan. A landmark study by the Diabetes Prevention Program of over 3,000 individuals with prediabetes showed that those who made these changes in their lifestyle were 58 percent less likely to go on to develop type 2 diabetes than those who did not make these changes.[60] Losing as little as 5–7 percent of your body weight can reduce the cells' resistance to insulin. Simple steps, including exercising 150 minutes a week, eating a plant-based, heart-healthy diet, and meeting with a health professional for ongoing support and education, can also lower your risk of developing type 2 diabetes and improve your overall health.

LO 4.8: THE TAKE-HOME MESSAGE Diabetes mellitus is a complex disorder in which either the pancreas does not produce enough insulin or body cells are unable to use the insulin produced. Either factor causes the blood glucose level to rise. Type 1 diabetes is an autoimmune disorder in which the insulin-producing cells of the pancreas are destroyed. Type 2, the most common form, develops from insulin resistance, in which the body cells do not properly respond to the presence of insulin. Prediabetes can be a precursor to type 2 diabetes. Pregnancy hormones may cause gestational diabetes. In type 1 and type 2, hyperglycemia is the main characteristic. Persons with type 1 diabetes require insulin to manage their blood glucose; persons with other types of diabetes may be able to manage the condition through diet and lifestyle changes, or they may need insulin or other medications. Poorly managed diabetes increases the likelihood of nerve damage, leg and foot amputations, tooth loss, gum problems, kidney disease, and cardiovascular disease. Diabetes can also damage the retina of the eye, which can eventually lead to blindness. A moderate, well-balanced diet with regular mealtimes, exercise, and maintaining a healthy body weight are key to controlling blood glucose levels.

Visual Chapter Summary

LO 4.1 Carbohydrates Are Nutrients with Different Classifications

Carbohydrates are energy-yielding macronutrients composed of carbon, hydrogen, and oxygen that are predominant in plant-based foods.

Carbohydrates are divided into two categories: simple and complex carbohydrates. Simple carbohydrates, or sugars, include monosaccharides and disaccharides. Complex carbohydrates include oligosaccharides and polysaccharides.

The three nutritionally important monosaccharides are glucose, fructose, and galactose. Each monosaccharide is called a hexose ($C_6H_{12}O_6$). Monosaccharides linked together with a glycosidic bond form disaccharides, including sucrose, lactose, and maltose.

Oligosaccharides contain 3–10 glucose units and are part of cellulose in plant cell walls. The polysaccharide glycogen is the storage form of glucose in animals. Starch and fiber are polysaccharides found in plants. Fiber can be classified as either soluble or insoluble.

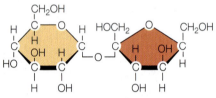

Glucose, a monosaccharide

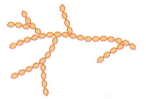

Sucrose, a disaccharide

Starch, a polysaccharide

LO 4.2 Carbohydrates Are Digested and Absorbed in the Mouth and Small Intestine

Salivary amylase begins digestion of carbohydrates in the mouth, although most carbohydrate digestion occurs in the small intestine, facilitated by pancreatic amylase. Sucrose, maltose, and lactose are broken down into monosaccharides by brush border enzymes. Glucose and galactose are absorbed into the enterocyte by active transport with the aid of sodium. Fructose is absorbed by facilitated diffusion. Once in the enterocyte, the monosaccharides are transported through the portal vein to the liver. There they can be used for energy, converted to glucose and stored as glycogen through glycogenesis, or sent into the blood for delivery to cells. Excess glucose is converted and stored as body fat. Fiber is not digestible; it travels through the colon and is eliminated.

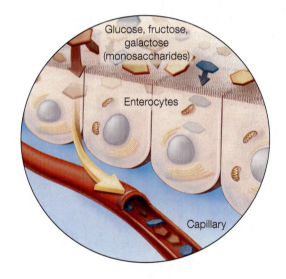

Glucose, fructose, galactose (monosaccharides)

Enterocytes

Capillary

LO 4.3 Energy Is the Key Function of Carbohydrates

The body uses carbohydrates, specifically glucose, for energy. Surplus glucose is converted to glycogen by glycogenesis and stored in the liver and muscle. Carbohydrates spare protein from being used for energy and prevent the rapid breakdown of triglycerides (lipolysis). When insufficient carbohydrates are consumed, blood glucose levels are maintained for a short time by liver glycogen through glycogenolysis, or glycerol and amino acids generate glucose through gluconeogenesis. Fasting and low-carbohydrate diets result in ketosis from the incomplete breakdown of fat used to generate energy.

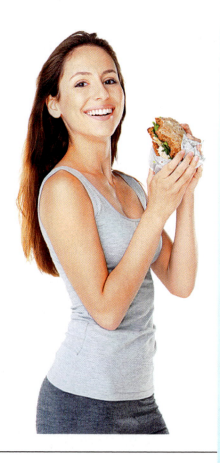

LO 4.4 Hormones Control Blood Glucose Levels

The pancreatic hormones insulin and glucagon maintain the amount of glucose in the blood at 70–110 mg/dl. Insulin directs glucose uptake by cells, which lowers the blood levels. Insulin also directs the storage of glucose as glycogen (glycogenesis) and fat (lipogenesis), both of which remove glucose from the blood and lower blood glucose levels. Glucagon stimulates the breakdown of glycogen, a process called glycogenolysis, to raise blood glucose levels. Glucagon also stimulates gluconeogenesis in the liver, which also releases glucose into the blood and raises blood glucose levels. Hypoglycemia, or low blood sugar, can occur in individuals with diabetes, especially if they are taking medication and/or insulin and are not eating properly. People without diabetes may also experience reactive hypoglycemia or fasting hypoglycemia, possibly as a result of a hormonal imbalance. The symptoms include shakiness, dizziness, light-headedness, hunger, and perspiration.

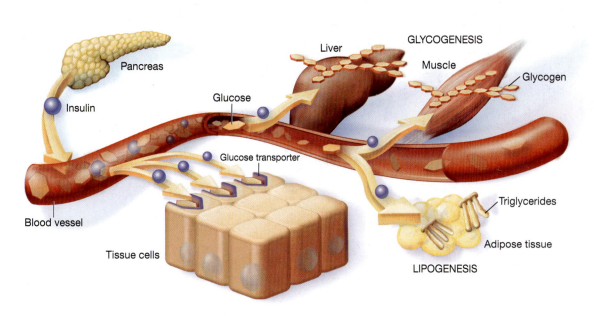

LO 4.5 Dietary Fiber Has Many Health-Promoting Benefits

Fiber may help lower the risk of developing constipation, diverticulosis, obesity, cardiovascular disease, cancer, and diabetes mellitus. Foods high in fiber can add to satiation. Viscous, soluble fibers help lower blood cholesterol levels. Insoluble fibers increase the bulk of the feces and reduce the risk of constipation and diverticulosis.

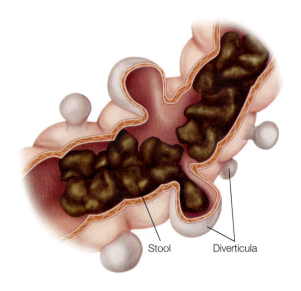

Stool   Diverticula

LO 4.6 Whole Plant Foods Are the Best Sources of Carbohydrates

The RDA for carbohydrate is 130 grams daily. The AMDR for carbohydrates is 45–65 percent of total daily kilocalories. The AI for fiber is 25 grams per day for women and 38 grams per day for men, or 14 grams per 1,000 kilocalories per day. On average, Americans consume only about 12–18 grams of dietary fiber per day.

Simple carbohydrates are found naturally in fruits, vegetables, and dairy foods or in processed foods. Soft drinks are the major source of added sugar in the American diet. Complex carbohydrates are abundant in grains, whole fruits, and vegetables. Grains and many vegetables provide starch, while fiber is found in whole grains, whole fruits, legumes and other vegetables, nuts, and seeds.

The concept of glycemic index and glycemic load can be used to plan meals. Foods with a lower glycemic index and glycemic load may not raise blood glucose levels as quickly compared with foods that have a higher glycemic index or greater glycemic load.

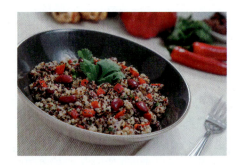

LO 4.7 There Are Differences among Natural Sugars, Added Sugars, and Sugar Substitutes

Foods with naturally occurring sugars are more nutritious than foods with a lot of added sugar. A diet too high in added sugar may increase the level of body fat.

Starch and sugary foods, especially sticky foods, can increase the risk of dental caries. Chewing sugarless gum may help reduce the risk of dental caries.

Polyols (sugar alcohols), saccharin, aspartame, acesulfame-K, stevia, sucralose, rebaudioside A, tagalose, and neotame are sugar substitutes currently deemed safe by the FDA.

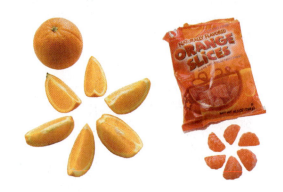

LO 4.8 Diabetes Results in Elevated Blood Glucose Levels

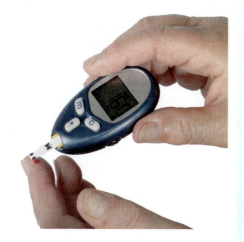

Individuals develop diabetes because they aren't producing enough insulin (type 1 diabetes) and/or they have developed insulin resistance (type 2 diabetes). Type 1 diabetes is an autoimmune disease and is not as common as type 2 diabetes. In both cases, hyperglycemia is the main characteristic. Poorly managed diabetes increases the likelihood of nerve damage, leg and foot amputations, tooth loss, gum problems, kidney disease, and cardiovascular disease. Diabetes can also damage the retina of the eye, which can cause bleeding, cloudy vision, and eventually blindness. Hypoglycemia, or low blood sugar, can occur in individuals with diabetes, especially if they are taking medication and/or insulin and are not eating properly.

Persons with type 1 diabetes must inject insulin to control blood glucose levels. Persons with type 2 diabetes may need to inject insulin or take other medications, or they may be able to control blood glucose levels through diet and lifestyle changes. A moderate, well-balanced diet with regular mealtimes, exercise, and maintaining a healthy body weight are key to controlling blood glucose levels in both type 1 and type 2 diabetics.

Terms to Know

- photosynthesis
- chlorophyll
- glucose
- simple carbohydrates
- complex carbohydrates
- monosaccharide
- hexose
- fructose
- galactose
- disaccharide
- condensation
- glycosidic bond
- sucrose
- lactose
- maltose
- lactose intolerance
- lactose maldigestion
- oligosaccharides
- polysaccharides
- glycogen
- starch

- amylose
- amylopectin
- resistant starch
- dietary fiber
- cellulose
- lignin
- soluble fiber
- insoluble fiber
- functional fiber
- salivary amylase
- glycogenesis
- glycogenolysis
- gluconeogenesis
- ketone bodies
- ketosis
- insulin
- glucagon
- lipogenesis
- epinephrine
- norepinephrine
- cortisol
- growth hormone

- hypoglycemia
- diverticulosis
- diverticula
- diverticulitis
- whole grains
- bran
- endosperm
- germ
- refined grains
- enriched grains
- glycemic index (GI)
- glycemic load (GL)
- dental caries
- sugar substitutes
- sugar alcohols
- diabetes mellitus
- insulin resistance
- ketoacidosis
- type 1 diabetes
- type 2 diabetes
- impaired glucose tolerance
- gestational diabetes

Mastering Nutrition

Visit the Study Area in Mastering Nutrition to hear an MP3 chapter summary.

Check Your Understanding

LO 4.1 1. Sucrose is a
   a. monosaccharide.
   b. disaccharide.
   c. oligosaccharide.
   d. polysaccharide.

LO 4.1 2. _____ is the storage form of glucose in animals, including humans.
   a. Glucagon
   b. Glycogen
   c. Gluconeogenesis
   d. Starch

3. Three brush border enzymes that hydrolyze carbohydrates in the small intestine are
   a. insulin, glucagon, and cortisone.
   b. salivary amylase, salivary lipase, and gastric lipase.
   c. maltase, lactase, and sucrase.
   d. fiber, starch, and glycogen.

LO 4.3 4. Carbohydrates function in the body to
   a. provide energy.
   b. prevent fat storage.
   c. regulate HCl secretion.
   d. build muscle.

LO 4.4 5. The hormones _____and _____ help to regulate and maintain blood glucose levels.
   a. peptide YY, insulin
   b. secretin, gastrin
   c. insulin, glucagon
   d. glucagon, ghrelin

LO 4.5 6. Your blood cholesterol level is too high, so you would like to eat more foods containing viscous, soluble fiber. A good choice would be
   a. whole-wheat bread.
   b. chocolate chip cookies.
   c. hard-boiled eggs.
   d. oatmeal.

LO 4.7 7. The minimum amount of carbohydrates needed daily for an adult is
   a. 75 grams.
   b. 100 grams.
   c. 120 grams.
   d. 130 grams.

LO 4.6 8. Reducing consumption of which item would have the biggest impact on decreasing the amount of added sugars that Americans consume?
   a. Fruits
   b. Candy
   c. Soft drinks
   d. Pastries

LO 4.7 9. An individual who has PKU should not consume which of the following sugar substitutes?
   a. Sucralose
   b. Acesulfame-K
   c. Aspartame
   d. Neotame

LO 4.8 10. Which of the following can help reduce your risk of type 2 diabetes?
   a. Avoiding sugar
   b. Eating a high-fiber, plant-based diet
   c. Playing computer games
   d. Eating a high-fat diet

Answers

1. (b) Sucrose contains the two monosaccharides glucose and fructose, and is therefore a disaccharide. Oligosaccharides and polysaccharides contain more than two sugar units.

2. (b) Glycogen is stored in the liver and muscles and provides a ready-to-use form of glucose for the body. Glucagon is the hormone that directs the release of glucose from the stored glycogen. Gluconeogenesis is the creation of glucose from noncarbohydrate sources. Starch is the storage form of glucose in plants.

3. (c) The enzymes maltase, lactase, and sucrase are located in the brush border of the small intestine and hydrolyze the disaccharides maltose, lactose, and sucrose, respectively. Insulin, glucagon, and cortisone are hormones, not enzymes. Salivary amylase and lipase are enzymes in saliva that begin digesting starch and lipids, and gastric lipase is a gastric enzyme that contributes to lipid digestion. Fiber, starch, and glycogen are polysaccharides, not enzymes.

4. (a) The key function of carbohydrates is to provide energy. Excess ingested carbohydrates can be converted to fatty acids, promoting fat storage, not preventing it. All macronutrients regulate hydrochloric acid (HCl) secretion. Protein is the macronutrient associated with tissue building.

5. (c) Insulin and glucagon are two hormones released from the pancreas that regulate blood glucose levels. Insulin directs the uptake of glucose by cells. When the blood glucose level drops too low, glucagon is released from the pancreas to direct the breakdown of glycogen in the liver, which provides glucose to the blood. The other hormones are produced in the GI tract. Peptide YY slows stomach motility, secretin stimulates the release of bicarbonate and water from the pancreas, gastrin stimulates the parietal cells to release hydrochloric acid, and ghrelin stimulates both gastric motility and hunger.

6. (d) Oatmeal is rich in beta-glucan, a viscous soluble fiber that can help lower cholesterol when eaten as part of a heart-healthy diet. Whole-wheat bread is high in insoluble fiber. Though nutrient dense, hard-boiled eggs do not contain fiber. Cookies, even though made with enriched flour, won't help lower cholesterol.

7. (d) The RDA for carbohydrate is 130 grams daily. This is the minimum amount needed to supply the glucose that the body, particularly the brain and red blood cells, must have to function effectively.

8. (c) Soft drinks are the number-one source of added sugars in the American diet, so reducing the intake of these sugary beverages would go a long way in reducing the amount of added sugars that Americans consume. Reducing the amount of candy and pastries would also help reduce the added sugars in the diet, but not as much as soft drinks. Fruits contain only naturally occurring sugars.

9. (c) Individuals diagnosed with PKU, or phenylketonuria, should not consume aspartame because it contains the amino acid phenylalanine.

10. (b) Eating a high-fiber, plant-based diet is the best approach, at present, to help reduce the risk of developing type 2 diabetes. If you want to prevent diabetes, getting regular exercise and not playing sedentary computer games or eating a high-fat diet are the healthiest approaches. Eating sugar doesn't cause diabetes.

Answers to True or False?

1. **False.** All macronutrients, including carbohydrate, are essential for numerous body functions.

2. **False.** In fact, infants have higher amounts of lactase, the enzyme necessary for lactose digestion, than adults. Their ability to digest lactose is critical because breast milk is high in lactose. As we age, our bodies produce less lactase, and we are more likely to become lactose intolerant.

3. **False.** Excessive intake of kilocalories, not carbohydrates specifically, is the main cause of obesity. In fact, some high-fiber carbohydrates can actually help people lose weight.

4. **False.** There is insufficient evidence to suggest that eating sugar causes hyperactivity or other behavioral problems in children.

5. **True.** Whole grains contain more nutrients (and dietary fiber) than refined grains, which have had much of the grain kernel removed during processing.

6. **True.** Simple carbohydrates, especially added sugars, encourage the growth of acid-producing bacteria in the mouth, which in turn promote dental caries.

7. **False.** There is no scientific evidence to support claims that aspartame causes cancer or other health problems in humans.

8. **True.** The average American consumes about half the amount of fiber that's recommended daily.

9. **True.** Many of the excess kilocalories in the American diet come from added sugars in sodas and other sugary beverages. Consuming more kilocalories than are necessary to meet energy needs causes weight gain.

10. **True.** Being overweight or obese can increase one's chances of developing type 2 diabetes.

Web Resources

- For more on fiber, visit the American Heart Association at www.americanheart.org
- For more on diabetes, visit the FDA's Diabetes Information site at www.fda.gov/diabetes or the American Diabetes Association website at www.diabetes.org
- For more on lactose intolerance, visit the National Institute of Diabetes and Digestive and Kidney Diseases (NIDDK) at http://digestive.niddk.nih.gov

References

1. Laeng, B., K. C. Berridge, et al. 1993. Pleasantness of a Sweet Taste During Hunger and Satiety: Effects of Gender and "Sweet Tooth." *Appetite* S21:247–254.

2. Zellner, D. A., A. Garriga-Trillo, et al. 1999. Food Liking and Craving: A Cross-Cultural Approach. *Appetite* 33:61–70.

3. Bachmanov, A. A., N. P. Bosak, et al. 2011. Genetics of Sweet Taste Preferences. *Flavour and Fragrance Journal* 26(4):286–294.

4. Jeurink, P., B. van Esch, et al. 2013. Mechanisms Underlying Immune Effects of Dietary Oligosaccharides. *American Journal of Clinical Nutrition* 98(2):572S–577S.

5. Seppo, A. E., C. Autran, et al. 2016. Human Milk Oligosaccharides and Development of Cow's Milk Allergy in Infants. *Journal of Allergy and Clinical Immunology* S0091-6749(16)31055-7. doi:http://dx.doi.org/10.1016/j.jaci.2016.08.031

6. Davis, E. C., M. Wang, et al. 2017. The Role of Early Life Nutrition in the Establishment of Gastrointestinal Microbial Composition and Function. *Gut Microbes*. doi: 10.1080/19490976.2016.1278104.

7. Landon, S., C. G. B. Colyer, et al. 2012. The Resistant Starch Report. *Food Australia Supplement*. Available at www.foodaust.com.au/wp-content/.../04/Hi_Maize-supplement_web.pdf. Accessed February 2014.

8. Birt, D. F., T. Boylston, et al. 2013. Resistant Starch: Promise for Improving Human Health. *Advanced Nutrition* 4(6):587–601.

9. Kwak, J. H., J. K. Paik, et al. 2012. Dietary Treatment with Rice Containing Resistant Starch Improves Markers of Endothelial Function with Reduction of Postprandial Blood Glucoses and Oxidative Stress in Patients with Prediabetes or Newly Diagnosed Type 2 Diabetes. *Atherosclerosis* 224(2):457–464.

10. Slizewska, K. 2013. The Citric Acid-Modified, Enzyme-Resistant Dextrin from Potato Starch as a Potential Prebiotic. *Acta Biochimica Polonica* 60(4):671–675.

11. McRorie, J. W., et al. 2017. Understanding the Physics of Functional Fibers in the Gastrointestinal Tract: An Evidence-Based Approach to Resolving Enduring Misconceptions about Insoluble and Soluble Fiber. *Journal of the Academy of Nutrition and Dietetics* 117(2):251–264.

12. National Digestive Diseases Information Clearinghouse. 2013. *Constipation*. Available at http://digestive.niddk.nih.gov/ddiseases/pubs/constipation. Accessed January 2017.

13. National Digestive Diseases Information Clearinghouse. 2013. *Diverticulosis and Diverticulitis*. Available at http://digestive.niddk.nih.gov/ddiseases/pubs/diverticulosis/index.aspx. Accessed January 2017.

14. Cho, S. S., L. Qi, et al. 2013. Consumption of Cereal Fiber, Mixtures of Whole Grains and Bran, and Whole Grains and Risk Reduction in Type 2 Diabetes, Obesity, and Cardiovascular Disease. *American Journal of Clinical Nutrition* 98(2):594–619.

15. Ibid.

16. Chen, S., et al. 2016. Dietary Fiber Intake and Risk of Breast Cancer: A Systematic review and Meta-analysis of Epidemiological Studies. *Oncotarget* 7(49):80980. doi: 10.18632/oncotarget.13140.

17. Ben, Q., Y. Sun, et al. 2013. Dietary Fiber Intake Reduces Risk for Colorectal Adenoma: A Meta-Analysis. *Gastroenterology* doi: 10.1053/j.gastro.2013.11.003.

18. Kyrø, C., A. Olsen, et al. 2014. Plasma Alkylresorcinols, Biomarkers of Whole-Grain Wheat and Rye Intake, and Incidence of Colorectal Cancer. *Journal of the National Cancer Institute* 106(1). doi: 10.1093/jnci/djt352.

19. Henderson, A. J., C. A. Ollila, et al. 2013. Chemopreventive Properties of Dietary Rice Bran: Current Status and Future Prospects. *Advanced Nutrition* 3(5):643–653.

20. Cho, S. S., et al. 2013. Consumption of Cereal Fiber.

21. Nicklas, T. A., L. Jahns, et al. 2013. Barriers and Facilitators for Consumer Adherence to the *Dietary Guidelines for Americans*: The HEALTH Study. *Journal of the Academy of Nutrition and Dietetics* 113(10):1317–1331.

22. Ramage, S., A. Farmer, et al. 2014. Healthy Strategies for Successful Weight Loss and Weight Management: A Systematic Review. *Applied Physiology, Nutrition, and Metabolism* 39:1–20.

23. Giacco, R., J. Lappi, et al. 2013. Effects of Rye and Whole Wheat versus Refined Cereal Foods on Metabolic Risk Factors: A Randomized Controlled Two-Centre Intervention Study. *Clinical Nutrition* 32(6):941–949.

24. Jung, Chan-Hee, and Kyung Mook Choi. "Impact of High-Carbohydrate Diet on Metabolic Parameters in Patients with Type 2 Diabetes." *Nutrients* 9.4 (2017): 322.

25. Turner-McGrievy, G. M., et al. 2015. Comparative Effectiveness of Plant-based Diets for Weight Loss: A Randomized Controlled Trial of Five Different Diets. *Nutrition* 31(2):350–358. doi: 10.1016/j.nut.2014.09.002.

26. Ramage, S., A. Farmer, et al. 2014. Healthy Strategies for Successful Weight Loss and Weight Management: A Systematic Review. *Applied Physiology, Nutrition, and Metabolism* 39:1–20.

27. Donazar-Ezcurra, M., C. López-Del Burgo, et al. 2017. Primary Prevention of Gestational Diabetes Mellitus Through Nutritional Factors: A Systematic Review. *Bio Med Central Pregnancy and Childbirth* 17(1):30. doi: 10.1186/s12884-016-1205-4.

28. American Heart Association. 2014. Long Term Benefits of Popular Diets Are Less Than Evident. Available at http://news.heart.org/long-term-benefits-popular-diets-less-evident. Accessed February 2017.

29. Paz-Tal, O., et al. 2015. Effect of Changes in Food Groups Intake on Magnesium, Zinc, Copper, and Selenium Serum Levels During 2 years of Dietary Intervention. *Journal of the American College of Nutrition* 34(1):1–14. doi: 10.1080/07315724.2013.875432.

30. Giacco, R., J. Lappi, et al. 2013. Effects of Rye and Whole Wheat Versus Refined Cereal Foods on Metabolic Risk Factors: A Randomized Controlled Two-Centre Intervention Study. *Clinical Nutrition* 32(6):941-949.

31. McGill, C., D. Liska, et al. 2014. Trends in Fiber and Whole Grain Intake in the U.S. NHANES 2001-2010: What's Changing? *FASEB Journal* 28:810. Available at http://www.fasebj.org/content/28/1_Supplement/810.5.short. Accessed February 2017.

32. Golozar, A., et al. 2017. White Rice Intake and Incidence of Type-2 Diabetes: Analysis of Two Prospective Cohort Studies from Iran. *MC Public Health* 17(1):133. doi: 10.1186/s12889-016-3999-4.

33. Lillioja, S., et al. 2013. Whole Grains, Type 2 Diabetes, Coronary Heart Disease, and Hypertension: Links to the Aleurone Preferred over Indigestible Fiber. *Biofactors* 39(3): 242–258. doi: 10.1002/biof.1077.

34. Aune, D., et al. 2016. Whole Grain Consumption and Risk of Cardiovascular Disease, Cancer, and All Cause and Cause Specific Mortality: Systematic Review and Dose-response Meta-analysis of Prospective Studies. *BMJ* 353: i2716. doi: 10.1136/bmj.i2716.

35. Foroughi, M., et al. 2013. Stroke and Nutrition.

36. Cho, S. S., et al. 2013. Consumption of Cereal Fiber.

37. Wycherley, T.P., et al. 2016. Long-term Effects of Weight Loss with a Very-low Carbohydate, Low Saturated Fat Diet on Flow Mediated Dilatation in Patients with Type 2 Diabetes: A Randomized Controlled Trial. *Atherosclerosis* 252:28-31. doi: 10.1016/j.atherosclerosis.2016.07.908.

38. Yamini, S., and P. R. Trumbo, 2016. Qualified Health Claim for Whole-Grain Intake and Risk of Type 2 Diabetes: An Evidence-based Review by the US Food and Drug Administration. *Nutrition Reviews* 74(10):601-11. doi: 10.1093/nutrit/nuw027.

39. Sluijs, I., J. W. J. Beulens, et al. 2013. Dietary Glycemic Index, Glycemic Load, and Digestible Carbohydrate Intake Are Not Associated with Risk of Type 2 Diabetes in Eight European Countries. *Journal of Nutrition* 143:93–99.

40. Han, E., and L. M. Powell. 2013. Consumption Patterns of Sugar-Sweetened Beverages in the United States. *Journal of the Academy of Nutrition and Dietetics* 113(1):43–53.

41. Hu, F. B. 2013. Resolved: There is Sufficient Scientific Evidence that Decreasing Sugar-Sweetened Beverage Consumption Will Reduce the Prevalence of Obesity and Obesity-Related Diseases. *Obesity Review* 14(8):606–619.

42. Tey, S. L., N. B. Salleh, et al. 2017. Effects of Aspartame, Monk Fruit, Stevia, and Sucrose-sweetened Beverages on Postprandial Glucose, Insulin and Energy Intake. *International Journal of Obesity* doi: 10.1038/ijo.2016.225.

43. Ajinomoto USA, Inc. 2017. *The History of Aspartame*. Available at www.aspartame.net. Accessed January 2017.

44. Popkin, B.M. and C. Hawkes. 2016. Sweetening of the Global Diet, Particularly Beverages: Patterns, Trends, and Policy Responses. *Lancet Diabetes Endocrinology* 4(2):174-86. doi: 10.1016/S2213-8587(15)00419-2.

45. American Diabetes Association. 2017. Statistics About Diabetes. Available at http://www.diabetes.org/diabetes-basics/statistics. Accessed January 2017.

46. Ibid.

47. Busco, M. 2017. Diabetes Contribution to Deaths Underestimated; Third Leading Cause. Available at http://www.medscape.com/viewarticle/875135?src=soc_lk_share. Accessed February 2017.

48. Kochanek, K. D., S. L. Murphy, et al. Final Data for 2014. National Vital Statistics Reports. Available from http://www.cdc.gov/nchs/data/nvsr/nvsr65/nvsr65_04.pdf. Accessed January 2017.

49. American Diabetes Association. 2017. Type 1 Diabetes. Available at http://www.diabetes.org/diabetes-basics/type-1. Accessed January 2017.

50. Centers for Disease Control and Prevention. 2015. Annual Number (in Thousands) of New Cases of Diagnosed Diabetes Among Adults Aged 18-79 Years, United States, 1980-2014. Available at https://www.cdc.gov/diabetes/statistics/incidence/fig1.htm. Accessed January 2017.

51. American Diabetes Association. 2017. Type 2. Available at http://www.diabetes.org/diabetes-basics/type-2. Accessed January 2017.

52. Ibid.

53. van Wissen, K., et al. 2017. Cardiovascular Disease and Prediabetes As Complex Illness: People's Perspectives. *Nursing Inquiry* doi: 10.1111/nin.12177.

54. National Institute of Diabetes and Digestive and Kidney Disease. 2016. *Diabetes* Available at https://www.niddk.nih.gov/health-information/diabetes. Accessed January 2017.

55. Ibid.

56. National Diabetes Information Clearinghouse. 2013. *Diabetes Prevention Program* Available at http://diabetes.niddk.nih.gov/dm/pubs/preventionprogram. Accessed January 2017.

57. American Diabetes Association. 2017. Diabetes Meal Plans and a Healthy Diet. Available at http://www.diabetes.org/food-and-fitness/food/planning-meals/diabetes-meal-plans-and-a-healthy-diet.html. Accessed January 2017.

58. Metcalf, K. M., A. Singhvi, et al. 2014. Effects of Moderate- to Vigorous-Intensity Physical Activity on Overnight and Next-Day Hypoglycemia in Active Adolescents with Type 1 Diabetes. *Diabetes Care* doi:10.2337/dc13-1973.

59. Ibid.

60. American Diabetes Association. 2017. Diabetes Meal Plans and a Healthy Diet.

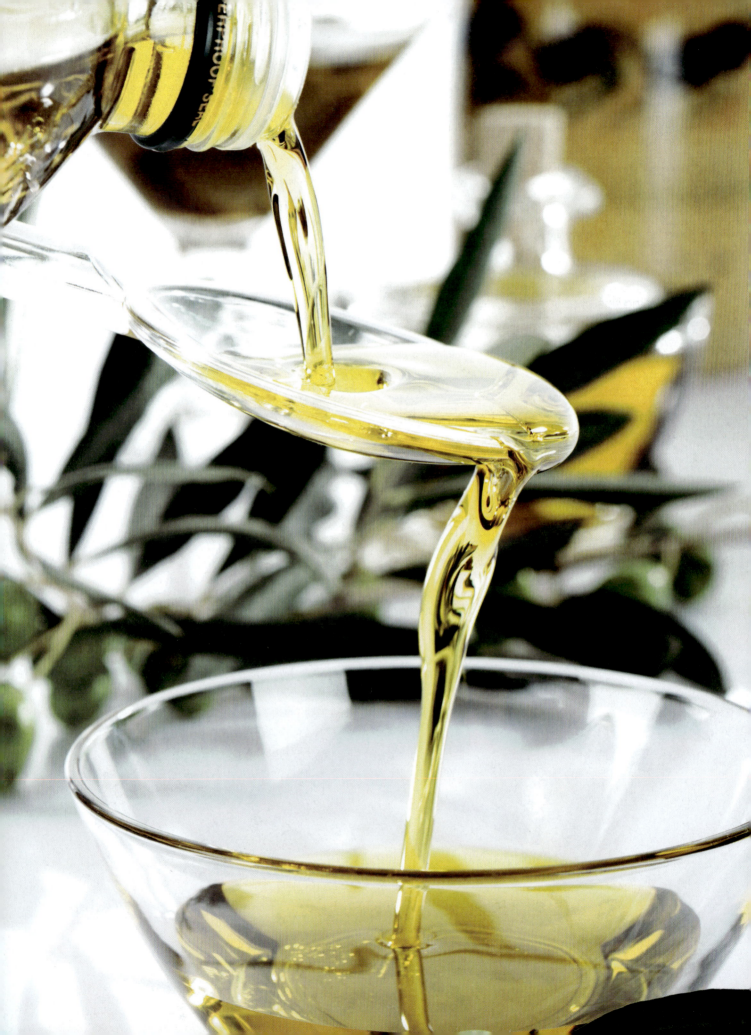

Lipids

5

Learning Outcomes

After reading this chapter, you will be able to:

5.1 Define the term *lipid* and classify lipids according to their structure.

5.2 Explain how lipids are digested, absorbed, and transported in the body.

5.3 Describe the functions of lipids in the body.

5.4 Identify the dietary recommendations for total fat, saturated fat, *trans* fat, the essential fatty acids, and cholesterol.

5.5 Identify the best, worst, and alternative food sources of dietary fats.

5.6 Describe the development of atherosclerosis and coronary heart disease, and explain how lifestyle factors can affect the risk.

True or False?

1. Cholesterol should be consumed daily to meet the body's needs. **T**/**F**

2. A healthy diet is very low in fat. **T**/**F**

3. Only commercially made fried foods and snack items contain *trans* fats. **T**/**F**

4. A diet high in saturated fat is a risk factor for elevated blood cholesterol. **T**/**F**

5. Fat-free cookies tend to have half the kilocalories of full-fat varieties. **T**/**F**

6. A high level of HDL cholesterol in the blood is considered heart healthy. **T**/**F**

7. Butter is a healthier choice than margarine. **T**/**F**

8. Nuts are high in cholesterol. **T**/**F**

9. Taking fish oil supplements is the best way to consume adequate omega-3 fatty acids. **T**/**F**

10. The LDL cholesterol present in foods is harmful to the heart. **T**/**F**

See page 204 for the answers.

When you go shopping, what is on your grocery list? If you're like many Americans, you probably have the best intentions of filling your grocery cart with low-fat, nonfat, or cholesterol-free items to eat a more healthful diet. Even just saying the words *fat* or *cholesterol* brings up negative images of foods that we should avoid. The truth is, a moderate amount of dietary fat is essential to the body.

In this chapter, we discuss the structure and functions of the different types of lipids, how they are handled in the body, and the amounts of each that should be consumed in a healthy diet. We also explore the role of dietary fat in the development of coronary heart disease.

What Are Lipids and How Do They Differ in Structure?

lipid Category of carbon, hydrogen, and oxygen compounds that are insoluble in water.

hydrophobic "Water fearing." In nutrition, the term refers to compounds that are not soluble in water.

fatty acid Most basic unit of triglycerides and phospholipids; fatty acids consist of carbon chains ranging from 2 to 80 carbons in length.

LO 5.1 Define the term *lipid* and classify lipids according to their structure.

When you think of the word **lipid,** you may think it is a synonym for *fat*. But that's only partly correct. *Lipo* means "fatty," but lipids are a broader category of compounds than fats alone. Lipids all contain carbon, oxygen, and hydrogen, and they are all **hydrophobic** (*hydro* = water, *phobic* = fearing). In other words, they do not dissolve in water. If you drop lipids like butter or olive oil into a glass of water, they rise to the top and sit on the water's surface. This repelling of water allows lipids to play a unique role in foods and in the body.

Whereas the popular press often portrays lipids as bad or unhealthy, the reality is that lipids serve several basic functions for maintaining health. For example, lipids store and provide energy and are essential components of many body compounds. The functions of lipids are described later in this chapter.

We begin the discussion of lipids by introducing the chemical structure of fatty acids, the basic building blocks of most lipids. We then classify lipids into three main types: triglycerides are the most common lipid in foods and in the body; phospholipids are critical to the structure of the cell membrane and to lipid transport; and sterols are ring-shaped lipids that do not contain fatty acids.

Most Lipids Are Composed of Fatty Acids

Triglycerides and phospholipids are built from a basic unit called a **fatty acid.** All fatty acids (**Figure 5.1**) are organic compounds that consist of chains of carbon and hydrogen atoms. The basic structure of every individual fatty acid has an acid group (specifically a carboxylic acid group, abbreviated as COOH) at one end, called the *alpha* end, and a methyl group (CH₃) on the other end, called the *omega* end. The carboxylic acid consists of a carbon atom attached with a double bond to an oxygen atom and single bonded to a hydroxyl group (OH).

The ratio of carbon and hydrogen to oxygen in the chain of a fatty acid accounts for the higher number of kilocalories in fat (9 kilocalories per gram) than in carbohydrates and proteins (4 kilocalories per gram). In short, a fatty acid requires 50 percent more oxygen per carbon atom to release energy. Thus, the fatty acid takes longer to oxidize and has more energy or kilocalories than either carbohydrates or proteins. We cover this in more detail in Chapter 8.

There are hundreds of naturally occurring fatty acids. They vary in structure by the length of the carbon chain, degree of saturation, location of double bonds, if any, and shape.

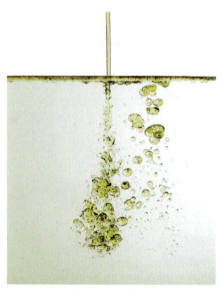

Because of their chemical properties, fats and oils don't dissolve in water.

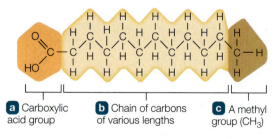

a Carboxylic acid group

b Chain of carbons of various lengths

c A methyl group (CH₃)

▲ **Figure 5.1 Chemical Structure of a Fatty Acid** The basic chemical structure of a fatty acid is composed of three different parts.

Length of Fatty Acids

The carbon chains of most naturally occurring dietary fatty acids contain 4–24 carbons (usually in even numbers), with the most common fatty acids containing 12–24 carbons. If the fatty acid is fewer than eight carbons long, it is a **short-chain fatty acid.** An example is acetic acid, which contains two carbons (**Figure 5.2a**). Fatty acids with 8–12 carbons are

short-chain fatty acid Fatty acid with a chain of less than eight carbons.

a Acetic acid (C2:0)

b Palmitic acid, a saturated fatty acid (C16:0)

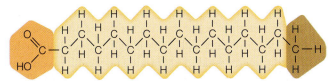

c Oleic acid, a monounsaturated fatty acid (C18:1)

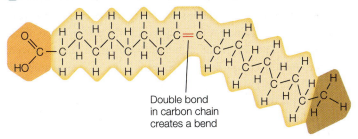

Double bond in carbon chain creates a bend

d Linoleic acid, a polyunsaturated fatty acid (C18:2)

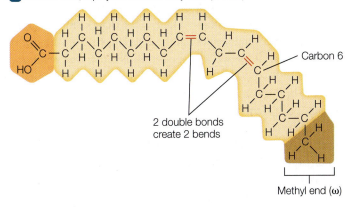

Carbon 6

2 double bonds create 2 bends

Methyl end (ω)

e Alpha-linolenic acid, a polyunsaturated, omega-3 fatty acid (C18:3)

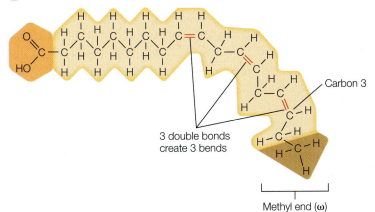

Carbon 3

3 double bonds create 3 bends

Methyl end (ω)

◄ **Figure 5.2 Fatty Acids Vary by Length, Degree of Saturation, and Shape**
Fatty acids differ by the number of carbons in the chain, whether or not the chain contains any double bonds (the saturation of the fatty acid), and the shape of the carbon chains on either side of the double bonds.

called **medium-chain fatty acids,** and those with 12 or more carbons are called **long-chain fatty acids** (Figure 5.2b–e). Long-chain fatty acids are the most common type of fatty acid found in foods.

Chain length is important because it affects the way we digest, absorb, and metabolize fatty acids. Long-chain fatty acids take longer to digest and absorb than do short- or medium-chain fatty acids. Shorter-chain fatty acids are more water-soluble than fatty acids with more carbons. The length of the chain also changes the way the body transports the fatty acids. We cover the details of fat digestion later in the chapter.

Saturation of Fatty Acids

The degree of saturation of a fatty acid refers to the presence or absence of a carbon-carbon double bond. Every carbon within the molecule has four bonds. The bonds between each carbon in the fatty acid chain can be either single or double, and the remaining bonds are to hydrogen atoms. The presence of a carbon-carbon double bond implies that the carbons are not *saturated* with hydrogens or have less than the number of hydrogens that are capable of bonding with each carbon. A fatty acid in which each of the carbons in the carbon chain are bound with two hydrogens is called a **saturated fatty acid.** In contrast, a carbon chain with carbons that are not bound to two hydrogens so that there are one or more double bonds is called an **unsaturated fatty acid.**

Palmitic acid (Figure 5.2b), which is present in palm oil and used in some processed foods, is an example of a saturated fatty acid because all the carbons in its central chain are bound with hydrogens with no double bonds to each other. In contrast, two of the 18 carbons in oleic acid (Figure 5.2c) are paired with each other rather than hydrogen, forming one double bond. This lone double bond makes oleic acid a **monounsaturated fatty acid (MUFA)** (*mono* = one).

A **polyunsaturated fatty acid (PUFA)** (*poly* = many) contains two or more double bonds and is less saturated with hydrogen. Linoleic acid, shown in Figure 5.2d, is an example of a polyunsaturated fatty acid.

The length of the fatty acid chain and the presence of double bonds between the carbons also determine the melting point of a fat, or the temperature at which it changes from a solid to a liquid (**Figure 5.3**). Double bonds cause a kink in the chain of the fatty acid, which prevents fatty acids from packing together tightly. Bends in the chain are due to double bonds and reduce the interaction between the molecules. This produces a fatty acid with a lower melting point. The lower melting points of shorter-chain and unsaturated fatty acids mean they tend to be liquid at room temperature. Fats that are liquid at room temperature are called **oils.** The monounsaturated fatty acid oleic acid is found in olive oil, and the polyunsaturated fatty acids, linoleic acid and alpha-linolenic acid (Figure 5.2e), are found in soybean oil. In general, straight, long-chain saturated fatty acids have higher melting points than do unsaturated fatty acids. This is because the saturated fatty acids can stack closer together and bond with one another. Examples are butter, lard, coconut oil, and palm oil, all of which are solid at room temperature.

Stability of Fatty Acids

When exposed to oxygen, or *oxidized,* foods containing fatty acids may develop a bitter, pungent smell or taste, a condition called **rancidity.** The double bonds of an unsaturated fatty acid are the most reactive sites on the fatty acid chain. Notice in **Figure 5.4** that during the first step of this oxidation reaction, a H^+ is extracted from the unstable fatty acid and forms a **free radical,** an atom or molecule that has at least one unpaired electron. This unpaired electron makes the free radical both unstable and destabilizing; that is, a free radical is highly likely to capture an electron from the nearest stable atom or molecule. When it does, the atom or molecule that loses an electron becomes a free radical itself and goes on to destabilize other atoms and molecules. Once this chain reaction has begun, it can cascade, and a food can quickly become rancid.

medium-chain fatty acids Fatty acids with a chain of 8–12 carbons.

long-chain fatty acids Fatty acids with a chain of more than 12 carbons.

saturated fatty acid Fatty acid in which all of the carbons are bound with hydrogen.

unsaturated fatty acid Fatty acid in which there are one or more double bonds between carbons.

monounsaturated fatty acid (MUFA) Fatty acid that has one double bond.

polyunsaturated fatty acid (PUFA) Fatty acid with two or more double bonds.

oils Lipids that are liquid at room temperature.

rancidity Spoiling of lipids through oxidation.

free radicals Atoms or molecules that have an unpaired electron and are thus chemically unstable and destabilizing.

a Saturated fatty acids

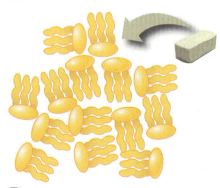

b Unsaturated fatty acids

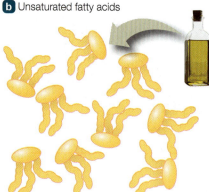

▲ **Figure 5.3 Saturated and Unsaturated Fatty Acids Help Shape Foods**
The straight chains of saturated fatty acids pack tightly together and are solid at room temperature. The double bonds in unsaturated fatty acids cause kinks in their shape and prevent them from packing tightly together, so they tend to be liquid at room temperature.

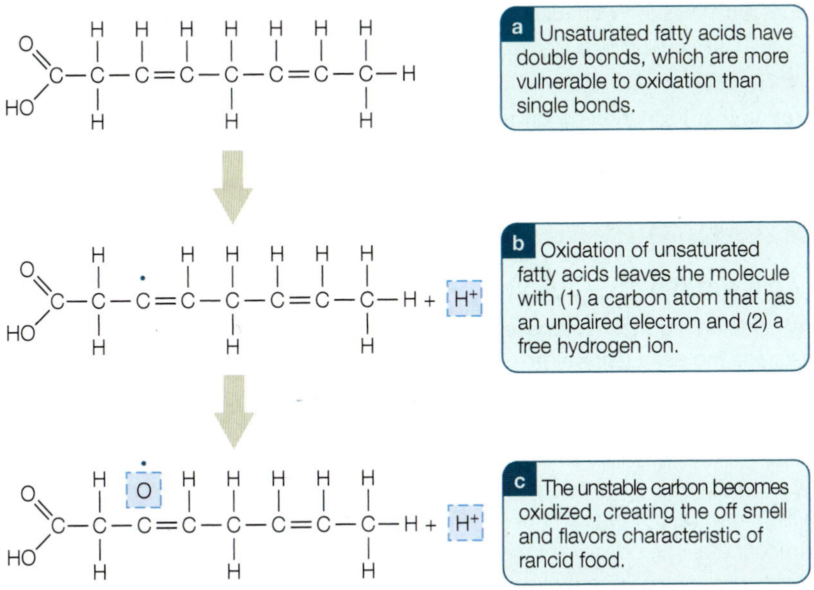

a Unsaturated fatty acids have double bonds, which are more vulnerable to oxidation than single bonds.

b Oxidation of unsaturated fatty acids leaves the molecule with (1) a carbon atom that has an unpaired electron and (2) a free hydrogen ion.

c The unstable carbon becomes oxidized, creating the off smell and flavors characteristic of rancid food.

◄ **Figure 5.4 Rancidity Reaction of a Fatty Acid**
When fatty acids become oxidized, the chemical structure is altered, creating the off smell and flavors characteristic of rancid food.

Because double bonds are less stable than single bonds, foods that contain unsaturated fatty acids become rancid faster than foods that contain saturated fatty acids. Similarly, polyunsaturated fatty acids are more susceptible to rancidity than monounsaturated acids because they have more double bonds (see Figure 5.4). Flax oil, which is rich in polyunsaturated fatty acids, is more susceptible to oxidation than corn oil, which contains more saturated and monounsaturated fatty acids. Saturated fatty acids have no double bonds and are thus much less susceptible to oxidation.

Food manufacturers have tested various ways to reduce rancidity, including adding antioxidants to hinder the oxidation process. Antioxidants bond with the free radicals (more on antioxidants in Chapter 9), thereby preventing oxygen from attacking the double bonds. Vitamins such as C and E are natural antioxidants, but lack the shelf-life of synthetic antioxidants such as butylated hydroxyanisole (BHA) and butylated hydroxytoluene (BHT).

Limiting a food's exposure to oxygen, heat, and light can also reduce rancidity. Storing oils and fats in airtight containers in a cool, dry, and dark location will lessen the formation of free radicals, which contribute to the rancidity of foods.

Another method used to stabilize unsaturated fatty acids is a process called **hydrogenation.** Hydrogenation involves heating oil and exposing it to hydrogen gas, which adds hydrogen to the carbons in the double bonds, making the fatty acids more saturated. Food manufacturers hydrogenate oils for several reasons. The process gives crackers and snack foods a longer shelf-life, improves the texture of pastries, makes fried foods crisper, and provides a "mouthfeel" like butter at a lower cost. We discuss the use of hydrogenation in more detail later in the chapter.

Location of the Double Bond

The location of the double bond in the fatty acid chain also affects the properties of a fatty acid (see Figure 5.2d and 5.2e). A polyunsaturated fatty acid in which the first double bond is located between the third and fourth carbon from the methyl (or *omega*) end is referred to as an **omega-3 fatty acid.** When the first double bond is between carbons six and seven from the omega end, the fatty acid is called an **omega-6 fatty acid.**

Linoleic acid, shown in Figure 5.2d, is an omega-6 fatty acid. It has 18 carbons with two double bonds, the first of which is located on carbon 6 from the omega end. **Alpha-linolenic acid,** shown in Figure 5.2e, is an omega-3 fatty acid. It also has

hydrogenation Adding hydrogen to an unsaturated fatty acid to make it more saturated and solid at room temperature.

omega-3 fatty acid Family of polyunsaturated fatty acids with the first double bond located at the third carbon from the omega end.

omega-6 fatty acid Family of polyunsaturated fatty acids with the first double bond located at the sixth carbon from the omega end.

linoleic acid Polyunsaturated essential fatty acid; part of the omega-6 fatty acid family.

alpha-linolenic acid Polyunsaturated essential fatty acid; part of the omega-3 fatty acid family.

18 carbons, but it has three double bonds, with the first double bond on carbon 3 from the omega end. These two fatty acids are called **essential fatty acids** because the body cannot synthesize them; that is, they must be obtained from foods. See the nearby Chemistry Boost for more information on the notation of fatty acids.

Chemistry Boost

Fatty Acid Notations

Fatty acids are frequently represented by two different methods of notation. Chemists use the delta (Δ) system (see figure below). In this form, the first number indicates the number of carbons in the chain. The second number, after the colon, notes how many double bonds are in the molecule. The two superscript numbers indicate the location of the two double bonds from the carboxyl end of the fatty acid.

The second method, called the omega (ω) system, is similar to the delta system. This system uses either the symbol ω or the letter *n* after the number of double bonds. This symbol notes the position of the first double bond from the omega (methyl) end of the fatty acid. In polyunsaturated fatty acids, three carbons usually separate double bonds. Using this notation makes it easy to locate the rest of the double bonds in a fatty acid molecule. With linoleic acid, the first double bond is located on carbon 6, followed by the second double bond on carbon 9.

Delta system describing linoleic acid:

$$18:2 \ \Delta^{9,12}$$

Omega system describing linoleic acid:

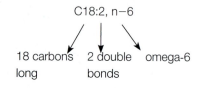

C18:2, n−6

18 carbons long · 2 double bonds · omega-6

Shape of Fatty Acids

Unsaturated fatty acids form two different shapes based on the position of the hydrogen atoms around the double bond. A fatty acid with the hydrogen atoms on the same side of the double bond, as illustrated at the top of **Figure 5.5**, has a *cis* configuration. A fatty acid with the hydrogen atoms on opposite sides of the double bond, as illustrated at the bottom of Figure 5.5, has a *trans* configuration. In nature, most fatty acids are in the *cis* configuration. There are a few *trans* fatty acids found naturally in milk and meat, but most are the result of hydrogenation during food processing. This is important because, as discussed later in the chapter, consumption of foods with commercially produced *trans* fatty acids is linked to an increased risk for cardiovascular disease.

Triglycerides Are the Most Common Lipid

The most common lipid in both foods and the body is the **triglyceride,** commonly called *fat*. It makes up about 95 percent of the lipids found in food. A triglyceride molecule consists of three fatty acids connected to a **glycerol** (*glyc* = sweet, *ol* = alcohol) backbone made of three alcohol (OH) groups. Through a condensation reaction, a hydrogen from the glycerol bonds with the hydroxyl group (OH) of the fatty acid and attaches the fatty acid to the glycerol (**Figure 5.6**). A molecule of water is released in the process for each fatty acid. A variety of fatty acids can bond with the same glycerol backbone, so a triglyceride usually contains a mixture of fatty acids. For example, canola oil is not just composed of polyunsaturated fatty acids; small amounts of saturated and monounsaturated fats are also present.

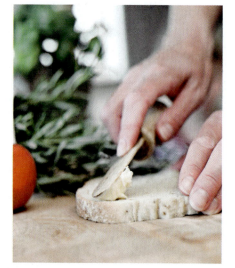

Many margarines are made by hydrogenating vegetable oils to make them spreadable.

essential fatty acids Two polyunsaturated fatty acids that the body cannot make and that therefore must be eaten in foods: linoleic acid and alpha-linolenic acid.

cis Configuration of a fatty acid in which the carbon atoms on each side of the double bond are on the same side.

trans Configuration of a fatty acid in which the carbon atoms are on opposite sides of the double bond.

triglycerides Type of lipid commonly found in foods and the body; also known as *fat*. Triglycerides consist of three fatty acids attached to a glycerol backbone.

glycerol Three-carbon backbone of a triglyceride.

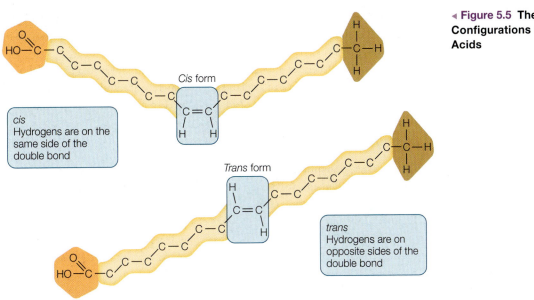

◂ **Figure 5.5** The *Cis* and *Trans* Configurations of Unsaturated Fatty Acids

Cis form

cis
Hydrogens are on the same side of the double bond

Trans form

trans
Hydrogens are on opposite sides of the double bond

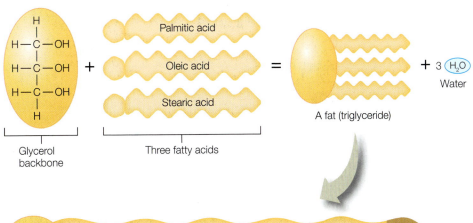

◂ **Figure 5.6** Structure of a Triglyceride
A triglyceride is formed when three fatty acids attach to a glycerol backbone with a condensation reaction.

Palmitic acid

Oleic acid

Stearic acid

Glycerol backbone

Three fatty acids

A fat (triglyceride)

$+ \ 3 \ H_2O$
Water

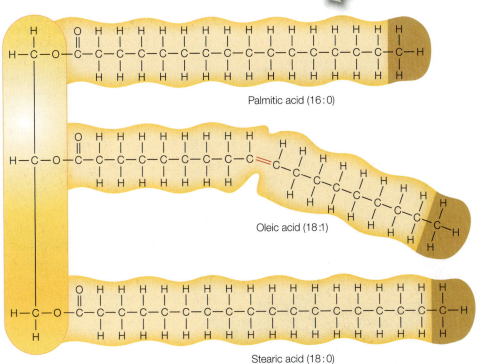

Palmitic acid (16:0)

Oleic acid (18:1)

Stearic acid (18:0)

Triglycerides perform a variety of functions in food. They make pie crusts flaky and meat tender. Triglycerides can also preserve freshness, which makes them important in food processing.

In the body, triglycerides are carried through the blood and stored in the adipose tissue to provide a major source of available energy. High concentrations of triglycerides in the blood are a risk factor for heart disease. We cover this topic later in the chapter.

Phospholipids Differ from Triglycerides

Like triglycerides, **phospholipids** contain a glycerol backbone, but instead of three fatty acids, the glycerol is linked to two fatty acids, a phosphate group, and different nitrogen-containing compounds such as **choline** (**Figure 5.7**). The glycerol backbone and phosphate group form a polar head, which attracts charged particles such as water. The fatty acid–containing tail is nonpolar and therefore soluble with other nonpolar molecules, such as fats. In other words, one end of the phospholipid is hydrophilic (*philic* = loving) and the other end is hydrophobic.

As discussed later in this chapter, phospholipids are essential structural components of the cell membrane. One of the body's major functional phospholipids is **lecithin,** also called *phosphatidylcholine*. Lecithin contains a choline group attached to the phosphate on the third carbon of the glycerol backbone. The fatty acids and the phosphate and choline give the phospholipid both fat-soluble and water-soluble properties, which allow it to shuttle other lipids across the cell membrane.

phospholipids Category of lipids that consists of two fatty acids and a phosphate group attached to a glycerol backbone. Lecithin is an example of a phospholipid found in food and in the body.

choline Member of the B vitamin family that is a component of the phospholipid lecithin.

lecithin Phospholipid made in the body that is integral in the structure of cell membranes; also known as *phosphatidylcholine.*

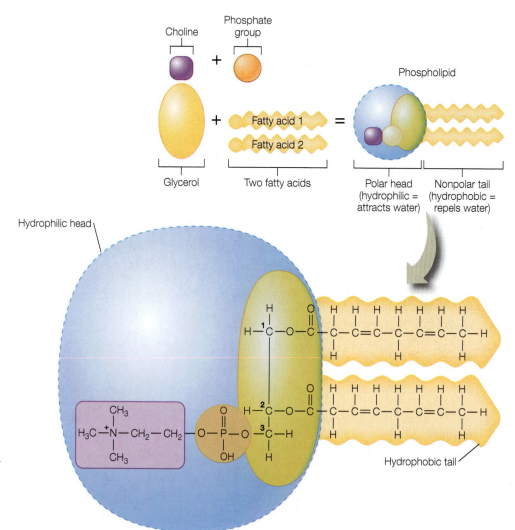

▶ **Figure 5.7 Structure of a Phospholipid**
Phospholipids, such as the lecithin shown here, are similar in structure to triglycerides but they have only two fatty acids. A phosphate group connected to the glycerol backbone replaces the third fatty acid. The tail is nonpolar and repels water whereas the polar head attracts water.

Because of its unique water- and fat-loving attributes, lecithin is used in many foods as an **emulsifier,** which helps keep incompatible substances, such as water and oil, mixed together. An emulsifier is sometimes added to commercially made salad dressings to prevent the fat from separating and rising to the top of the dressing (**Figure 5.8**). The emulsifier's nonpolar, fat-attracting tail surrounds the droplets of fat, which orients the polar, water-attracting head toward the watery solution of the dressing. This keeps the fat droplet suspended and allows the water and the oil to stay blended together.

Sterols Are More Complex than Triglycerides

Sterols are a much more complex molecule than phospholipids or triglycerides. They do not contain glycerol or fatty acids, but rather are composed mainly of four connecting rings of carbon and hydrogen (**Figure 5.9**). Unlike the other lipids, sterols do not provide energy.

The best-known sterol, **cholesterol,** is composed of four carbon rings with a tail of carbons and hydrogens on one end and a hydroxyl group on the other end. It is found in the body as well as in foods from animals, including meat, eggs, and dairy. The majority of sterols found in plants are **phytosterols** and **phytostanols,** which are similar in structure to cholesterol. Phytosterols have a double bond in the sterol ring. An example is sitosterol (see Figure 5.9). Phytostanols lack the double bond in the sterol ring. Phytosterols may provide health benefits, as they inhibit the intestinal absorption of cholesterol.[1]

> **LO 5.1: THE TAKE-HOME MESSAGE** Lipids are hydrophobic compounds composed of carbon, hydrogen, and oxygen. The three types of lipids are triglycerides, phospholipids, and sterols. Fatty acids, which consist of a carbon-and-hydrogen chain, a carboxylic acid group, and a methyl group, are the basic structural units of triglycerides and phospholipids. Fatty acids differ in chain length, degree of saturation, and shape. Triglycerides consist of three fatty acids attached to a glycerol backbone by condensation reactions. Triglycerides are found in blood and are stored in the adipose tissue. They are a major source of energy to the body. Phospholipids are made of two fatty acids and a phosphate and sometimes a nitrogen-containing group attached to a glycerol backbone. Sterols are made up of four connected rings of carbon and hydrogen. Cholesterol is present in animals and foods derived from animals, whereas phytosterols and phytostanols are present in foods derived from plants.

How Are Lipids Digested, Absorbed, and Transported in the Body?

LO 5.2 Explain how lipids are digested, absorbed, and transported in the body.

The lipids found in food are primarily in the form of fat (triglycerides) and, to a lesser extent, phospholipids and sterols. During the digestion of fat, the fatty acids are removed from the glycerol backbone by hydrolysis to form a combination of free fatty acids, glycerol, and monoglycerides (**Focus Figure 5.10**). This action is accomplished by a group of

◄ **Figure 5.8 Keeping a Salad Dressing Blended**
Emulsifiers are often added to salad dressing to keep the oil part of the dressing blended in the watery solution. When a salad dressing does separate, it is usually because it doesn't contain an emulsifier.

Water

Fat droplet

Emulsifier
(lecithin, a
phospholipid)

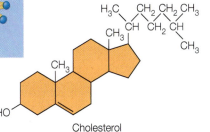

Cholesterol

Sitosterol

▲ **Figure 5.9 Structure of a Sterol**
Sterols have a carbon ring configuration with hydrogens and an oxygen attached. Cholesterol is the best-known sterol found in animal products. Sitosterol is a common sterol found in plants.

emulsifier Compound that keeps two incompatible substances, such as oil and water, mixed together.

sterols Category of lipids that contains four connecting rings of carbon and hydrogen. Cholesterol is the most common sterol.

cholesterol Common sterol found only in animal products and made in the liver from saturated fatty acids.

phytosterols Naturally occurring sterols found in plants.

phytostanols Type of plant sterol similar in structure to cholesterol.

Head to **Mastering** Nutrition and watch a narrated video tour of this figure by author Joan Salge Blake.

Most lipid digestion occurs in the small intestine with the aid of bile and lipase enzymes. The absorbed lipids are transported via chylomicrons into the lymphatic system.

ORGANS OF THE GI TRACT

MOUTH
Mastication begins the mechanical digestion of food. Solid fat melts with the warmth of the body. Lingual lipase in the saliva begins the chemical digestion of triglycerides.

STOMACH
Peristalsis mixes and churns the fat-containing food with gastric juices. Gastric lipase hydrolyzes some triglycerides, creating diglycerides and free fatty acids. In infants, lingual lipase also continues hydrolyzing triglycerides in the stomach.

SMALL INTESTINE
Bile secreted from the gallbladder through the common bile duct into the duodenum emulsifies fat into smaller globules.

Pancreatic lipase hydrolyzes triglycerides into monoglycerides, glycerol, and free fatty acids.

Phospholipases hydrolyze phospholipids.

The products of lipid hydrolysis are packaged into micelles for transport to enterocytes of the intestinal wall.

As they are absorbed into enterocytes, micelles separate into their component parts. Short-chain fatty acids enter the bloodstream directly. Long-chain fatty acids, cholesterol, phospholipids, and other remnants are repackaged into chylomicrons for transport into the lymphatic system.

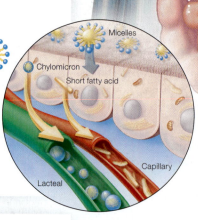

Micelles
Chylomicron
Short fatty acid
Capillary
Lacteal

LARGE INTESTINE
Any lipids not digested and absorbed in the small intestine bind to fiber and move into the large intestine to be eliminated in the feces.

ACCESSORY ORGANS

SALIVARY GLANDS
Produce saliva.

LIVER
Produces bile, which is stored in the gallbladder.

GALLBLADDER
Upon stimulation by CCK, releases bile into the duodenum through the common bile duct.

PANCREAS
Produces pancreatic lipase and phospholipases, which are secreted into the small intestine via the pancreatic duct.

enzymes called **lipases** (*ase* = enzyme), which act on a specific site along the glycerol backbone. The digested fat is absorbed through the small intestine and transported by lipoproteins.

Triglyceride Digestion Begins in the Mouth and Stomach

Lipid digestion begins in the mouth as the warmth of the body begins to melt the triglycerides. As chewing continues and food mixes with saliva, lingual lipase (secreted from the glands located at the base of the tongue) begins to hydrolyze the medium-chain fatty acids. Lingual lipase, which plays only a minor role in adults, is structurally different from the other lipases found in the body, and can hydrolyze fatty acids from any of the three carbons of the glycerol molecule. Lingual lipase travels with the bolus through the esophagus and into the stomach where it can function in the acidic environment of the stomach before being deactivated.

The presence of the bolus as it enters the stomach stimulates the release of the hormone gastrin from the gastric pits lining the stomach. Gastrin in turn stimulates the release of gastric juices, rich in gastric lipase, from the chief cells. Fat mixes with the gastric lipase, and the enzyme hydrolyzes one fatty acid from the triglyceride, which produces a free fatty acid and a **diglyceride.**

Most Triglycerides Are Digested and Prepared for Absorption in the Small Intestine

The majority of triglyceride digestion occurs in the small intestine. When the triglyceride in chyme enters the duodenum, the hormone cholecystokinin (CCK) is secreted, which, in turn, stimulates the gallbladder to release bile through the bile duct into the duodenum. Just as oil can't disperse in water without the help of an emulsifier, the fat globules in chyme tend to cluster together rather than disperse in the watery digestive juices. Bile, a greenish liquid made in the liver and stored in the gallbladder, begins to break up these fat globules. Hydrophobic portions of bile combine with the fat, while hydrophilic portions attract the water in the digestive juices (**Figure 5.11**). This action breaks up the fat globules into smaller droplets and prevents the droplets from merging again. Reducing the size of the fat globules provides more surface area to expose the bonds to the enzyme pancreatic lipase, which hydrolyzes the fat into free fatty acids and **monoglycerides.** These bond with cholesterol and biliary phospholipids to form smaller lipid complexes called **micelles,** which diffuse into the enterocyte.

Bile also emulsifies phospholipids during digestion. A group of enzymes called *phospholipases* then hydrolyze the phospholipids, dismantling them and producing two free fatty acids and the phospholipid remnant, which become part of micelles.

Bile emulsifies sterols as well. Unlike triglycerides and phospholipids, however, sterols are not digested. Instead, they remain intact and become part of the center of micelles.

Any lipids that are not digested and prepared for absorption in the small intestine bind to fiber and move into the large intestine, where they are eliminated in the feces. The large intestine does not have the enzymes necessary to digest lipids.

Chylomicrons Facilitate Lipid Absorption into the Lymph

Micelles transport digested fats, phospholipids, and sterols from the lumen of the GI tract into the enterocyte. Once inside, the various lipids are absorbed differently according to their structure.

Glycerol and short- to medium-chain fatty acids pass into the bloodstream directly through the mucosa of the small intestine because they are more water-soluble. They then enter the portal vein and go directly to the liver.

lipases Group of lipid-digesting enzymes.

diglyceride Remnant of fat digestion that consists of a glycerol with two attached fatty acids; also the form of fat used as an emulsifier in food production.

monoglyceride Remnant of fat digestion that consists of a glycerol with only one fatty acid attached to one of the three carbons.

micelle Transport carrier in the small intestine that enables fatty acids and other compounds to be absorbed.

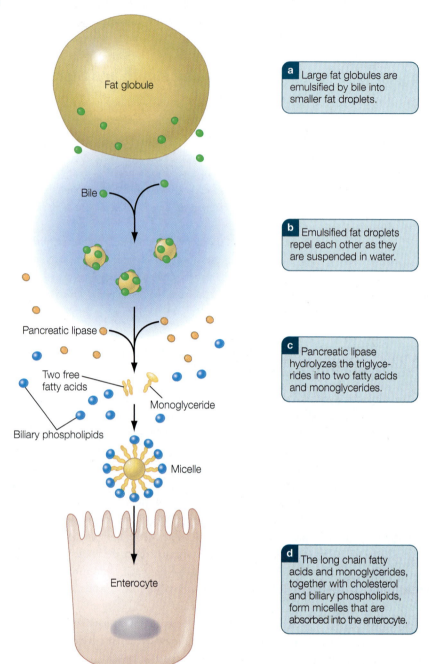

▶ **Figure 5.11 Role of Bile in Emulsifying Fat**

Fat globule

Bile

a Large fat globules are emulsified by bile into smaller fat droplets.

b Emulsified fat droplets repel each other as they are suspended in water.

Pancreatic lipase

c Pancreatic lipase hydrolyzes the triglycerides into two fatty acids and monoglycerides.

Two free fatty acids

Monoglyceride

Biliary phospholipids

Micelle

Enterocyte

d The long chain fatty acids and monoglycerides, together with cholesterol and biliary phospholipids, form micelles that are absorbed into the enterocyte.

lipoprotein Capsule-shaped transport carrier that enables fat and cholesterol to travel through the lymph and blood.

chylomicron Type of lipoprotein that carries digested fat and other lipids through the lymph system into the blood.

lipoprotein lipase (LPL) Enzyme that hydrolyzes triglycerides in lipoproteins into three fatty acids and glycerol.

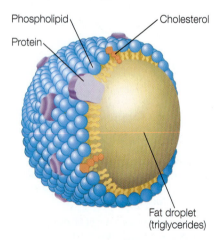

Phospholipid

Cholesterol

Protein

Fat droplet (triglycerides)

▲ **Figure 5.12 Structure of a Chylomicron**
A chylomicron contains a core of triglycerides and dietary lipids, surrounded by a coat of protein, phospholipids, and cholesterol.

In contrast, long-chain fatty acids and monoglycerides must be reassembled before they can pass into the bloodstream. Inside the enterocyte, free long-chain fatty acids reattach to monoglycerides to form new triglycerides. Together with phospholipids and cholesterol, these triglycerides are combined with carrier proteins to form a type of protein-containing transport compound (or **lipoprotein**) called a **chylomicron** (**Figure 5.12**).

Chylomicrons are too large to be absorbed directly into the bloodstream. Instead, they are absorbed via the lacteals into the lymph (**Figure 5.13**), which transports them through the lymphatic system until they enter the bloodstream through the thoracic duct located near the heart. As the chylomicrons travel through the blood en route to the liver, they interact with the enzyme **lipoprotein lipase (LPL),** located in the walls of the capillaries. This enzyme hydrolyzes the triglycerides in the chylomicrons, separating the fatty acids from the glycerol backbone so they can be stored in the cells.

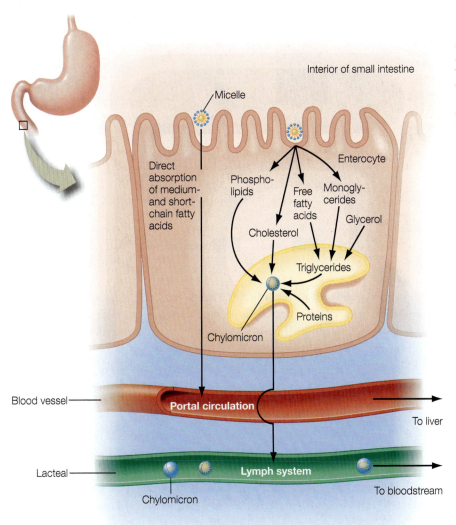

◀ Figure 5.13 **Absorption of Dietary Lipids**
Short- and medium-chain fatty acids are absorbed from the enterocytes directly into the bloodstream. Longer-chain fatty acids, cholesterol, phospholipids, and other remnants are reassembled into chylomicrons and enter lymph before being routed into the bloodstream.

Fatty acids are used by muscles (including the heart) as energy or stored as an energy reserve in the fat cells. After the fat is removed from the chylomicrons, the remnants of these lipoproteins travel to the liver to be dismantled.

Lipoproteins Transport Lipids

Chylomicrons are one form of lipoprotein, and they are made in the enterocytes to transport dietary lipids. The liver synthesizes three other lipoproteins important to the transport of fat in the body:

- **Very low-density lipoproteins (VLDLs)** are formed from chylomicron remnants and lipids already present in the liver
- **Low-density lipoproteins (LDLs)** are formed from VLDLs
- **High-density lipoproteins (HDLs)** are formed from cholesterol gathered from the tissues and arterial walls

Like chylomicrons, these lipoproteins consist of a lipid center surrounded by a shell of phospholipids and proteins. The density of each lipoprotein is determined by the amount of lipid and protein it contains (**Figure 5.14**). The more protein there is in a lipoprotein, the higher its density. Moreover, density influences how each lipoprotein functions.

Chylomicrons and VLDLs are both composed mostly of triglycerides, but VLDLs have more protein than chylomicrons, which makes them denser. The role of the VLDLs is to transport triglycerides and cholesterol from the liver to the cells, where they interact

very low-density lipoproteins (VLDLs) Lipoproteins that deliver fat made in the liver to the tissues. VLDL remnants are converted into LDLs.

low-density lipoproteins (LDLs) Lipoproteins that deposit cholesterol in the walls of the arteries. Because this can lead to heart disease, LDL is referred to as the "bad" cholesterol.

high-density lipoproteins (HDLs) Lipoproteins that remove cholesterol from the tissues and deliver it to the liver to be used as part of bile and/or to be excreted from the body. Because of this, HDL is known as the "good" cholesterol.

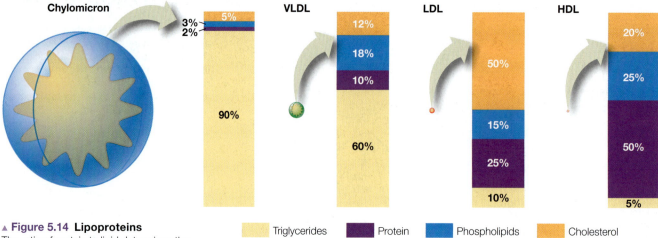

▲ Figure 5.14 Lipoproteins
The ratio of protein to lipid determines the density of the lipoprotein (as well as its name). Chylomicrons are the largest of the lipoproteins and contain the least amount of protein.

Chylomicron — 5%, 3%, 2%, 90%

VLDL — 12%, 18%, 10%, 60%

LDL — 50%, 15%, 25%, 10%

HDL — 20%, 25%, 50%, 5%

Triglycerides   Protein   Phospholipids   Cholesterol

with lipoprotein lipase (**Focus Figure 5.15**). The enzyme lipoprotein lipase (LPL) resides on the surface of the cells and hydrolyzes the fatty acids and glycerol from the core of the lipoprotein. As fat is deposited in cells and tissues, the ratio of protein to lipid increases. What began as a VLDL becomes an LDL.

LDLs continue to transport triglycerides to the cells. The LDLs are often referred to as the "bad" cholesterol carriers because they deposit cholesterol in the walls of the arteries, which can lead to heart disease. To help remember this, think of the first "**L**" in **L**DL as being "**L**ousy."

HDLs are small and contain equal amounts of protein and lipid, which makes them the densest of the lipoproteins. The primary role of HDLs is to pick up cholesterol from the body cells and return it to the liver. The liver uses the cholesterol to make bile and other functional compounds. In fact, approximately 25 percent of the cholesterol in blood is carried by HDLs back to the liver. Because of this function, HDLs are often referred to as the "good" cholesterol. An easy way to remember this is to think of the "**H**" in **H**DL as referring to "**H**ealthy." HDLs begin as high-density molecules, but as they pick up cholesterol from the cells, the percentage of lipid to protein changes and the density decreases. Thus, lipoproteins are constantly changing as they transport lipids throughout the body.

The level of LDL cholesterol relative to HDL cholesterol in the blood can be useful in determining the health of arteries. Essentially, a high concentration of HDL cholesterol is healthful because the HDL carriers in the blood are working to remove cholesterol from arterial-lining cells and contribute to its excretion from the body. A high concentration of LDL cholesterol indicates that more lipids are being delivered to cells and more cholesterol is being deposited in arterial-lining cells, which may contribute to blocked arteries, as discussed later in this chapter.

LO 5.2: THE TAKE-HOME MESSAGE Lipid digestion begins in the mouth and stomach with the help of lingual lipase and gastric lipase. Most triglycerides are digested in the small intestine with the help of bile and pancreatic lipase. Micelles transport digested lipids from the lumen of the GI tract into the enterocytes. Short- and medium-chain fatty acids are absorbed directly into the bloodstream. Longer-chain fatty acids and other remnants of fat digestion are packaged into chylomicrons, which transport them through the lymphatic system until they enter the bloodstream. Lipoproteins transport triglycerides, cholesterol, and other lipids through the lymph and bloodstream. LDLs deposit cholesterol in artery walls, whereas HDLs remove cholesterol from arteries and deliver it to the liver, which uses it in the synthesis of bile and other compounds.

Head to Mastering Nutrition and watch a narrated video tour of this figure by author Joan Salge Blake.

Dietary and endogenous lipids are transported in the body via several different lipoprotein compounds, such as chylomicrons, VLDLs, LDLs, and HDLs.

CHYLOMICRONS

Chylomicrons are formed in the enterocytes to transport lipids from a meal. Lipoprotein lipase, which is located on the surface of non-liver cells (mostly muscle and adipose cells), catalyzes the uptake of fatty acids into the cells through hydrolysis. The remaining chylomicron remnant is dismantled in the liver.

VLDLs

The liver produces VLDLs (very-low-density lipoproteins), which transport triglycerides to the cells. Lipoprotein lipase catalyzes the uptake of fatty acids into the cells, primarily those in muscle and adipose tissue, transforming VLDLs to LDLs (low-density lipoproteins).

LDLs

Low-density lipoproteins interact with receptor sites on body cells and release cholesterol into those cells. LDLs not taken up by cells degrade over time, releasing cholesterol that may then adhere to blood vessel walls.

HDLs

HDLs (high-density lipoproteins) produced by the liver circulate in the blood, picking up cholesterol from cells. The cholesterol is returned to the liver to be recycled or excreted, removing it from the bloodstream.

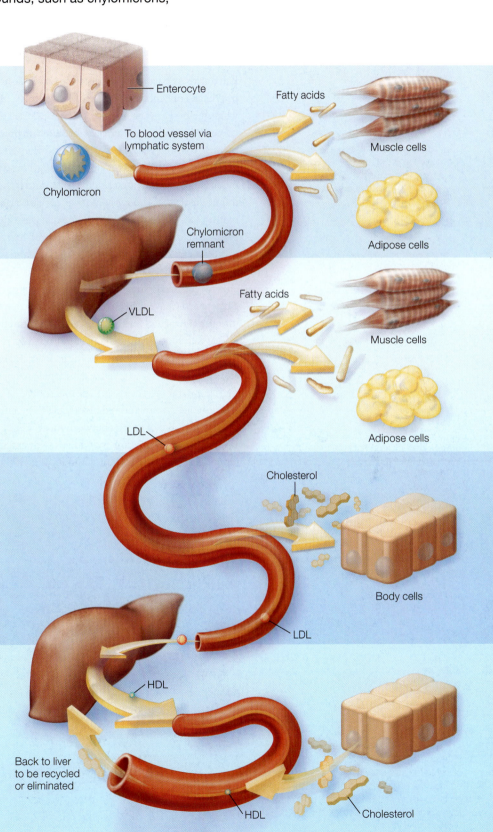

Enterocyte

Fatty acids

To blood vessel via lymphatic system

Muscle cells

Chylomicron

Chylomicron remnant

Adipose cells

Fatty acids

VLDL

Muscle cells

LDL

Adipose cells

Cholesterol

LDL

Body cells

HDL

Back to liver to be recycled or eliminated

HDL

Cholesterol

What Are the Functions of Lipids in the Body?

LO 5.3 Describe the functions of lipids in the body.

Once lipids are delivered to the cells by lipoproteins, they serve several critical roles in the body.

Fatty Acids Are Used for Energy

Fatty acids as part of the triglyceride molecule are a powerful source of fuel because they provide a concentrated source of kilocalories, are easily stored, and are readily available when the body needs energy. At 9 kilocalories per gram, dietary fat provides more than twice the energy of either carbohydrates or protein. In fact, dietary fat is a good source of energy throughout the day. The body has an *unlimited* ability to store excess energy as triglycerides in **adipocytes** (**Figure 5.16**). These fat cells have the capacity to enlarge to as much as 1,000 times their original size. And if they fill to capacity, the body manufactures more adipocytes. Though some triglyceride is also stored in the muscle, and a small amount of fatty acids are found in blood, the majority of fat is stored in adipose tissue. Adipocytes store more than 60 times the energy stored in liver and muscle glycogen combined.

Fatty acids are deposited into adipose (and some muscle) cells from the chylomicrons and VLDLs that carry it through the blood. As mentioned earlier, the lipoprotein lipase enzyme located on the outside of adipocytes and muscle cells reacts with the lipoprotein carriers and cleaves the fatty acids from the triglyceride. This allows the fatty acid to move into the adipocytes and muscle cells to be stored for later use.

When blood glucose concentrations begin to decline, the hormone glucagon promotes the release of glucose from the liver and fatty acids from the triglyceride molecule stored in adipocytes to provide additional energy for the body. The heart, liver, and resting muscles prefer fatty acids as their fuel source, which spares glucose to be used by the central nervous system and red blood cells. The fatty acids stored in the adipocytes provide a backup source of energy between meals.

In a famine situation, individuals with extensive triglyceride stores and adequate fluids could survive for months without eating if they consumed at least some carbohydrate.

adipocytes Cells in adipose tissue that store fat; also known as *fat cells.*

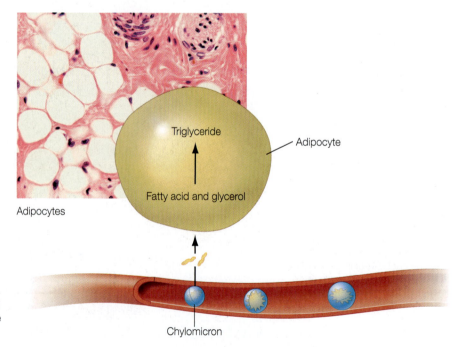

▶ **Figure 5.16 Adipocytes**
Excess triglycerides are stored in the adipocytes for later use. When the body needs energy, the enzyme lipoprotein lipase, located on the outside of the adipocyte, breaks off the fatty acids from the chylomicron or VLDL.

Adipocytes

Triglyceride

Adipocyte

Fatty acid and glycerol

Chylomicron

Stores of triglycerides alone cannot sustain life because glucose cannot be made from fatty acids or ketone bodies. Glycerol is the only part of the stored triglycerides that can be used for gluconeogenesis. Proteins provide glucogenic amino acids that can also be used for gluconeogenesis; however, the body has no mechanism for protein storage.

Dietary Fat Aids the Absorption of Lipid Compounds

Several essential nutrients, including the fat-soluble vitamins A, D, E, and K, as well as cholesterol, phospholipids, other lipid compounds, and a large group of phytochemicals called *carotenoids*, require dietary fat in order to be absorbed. Twenty grams of dietary fat is needed daily to stimulate the formation of the chylomicrons that transport the fat-soluble vitamins. Consuming less than this amount may impede fat-soluble vitamin absorption.

Triglycerides Stored in Adipose Tissue Insulate the Body and Protect Vital Organs

The stored triglycerides located in the subcutaneous tissue, just under the skin, help to insulate the body and maintain body temperature, especially in cold environments. However, excess body fat may actually hinder temperature regulation in hot weather, as the excess layer of stored fat prevents heat from flowing to the skin for release.

Stored triglycerides also act as a protective cushion against trauma for the bones and vital organs, including the brain, liver, kidneys, and spinal cord. Stored triglycerides in the abdomen act like a fatty apron protecting the abdominal organs from injury. However, too much stored fat eliminates the protective benefits because of the accompanying increased risk of heart disease, hypertension, and diabetes.

Essential Fatty Acids Manufacture Eicosanoids and Maintain Cell Membranes

The essential fatty acids discussed earlier in the chapter, linoleic acid and alpha-linolenic acid, are needed as precursors to form **eicosanoids,** hormonelike substances such as prostaglandins, thromboxanes, and leukotrienes (**Figure 5.17**). These compounds regulate the immune system, blood clotting, inflammation, and blood pressure.

eicosanoids Hormonelike substances in the body. Prostaglandins, thromboxanes, and leukotrienes are all eicosanoids.

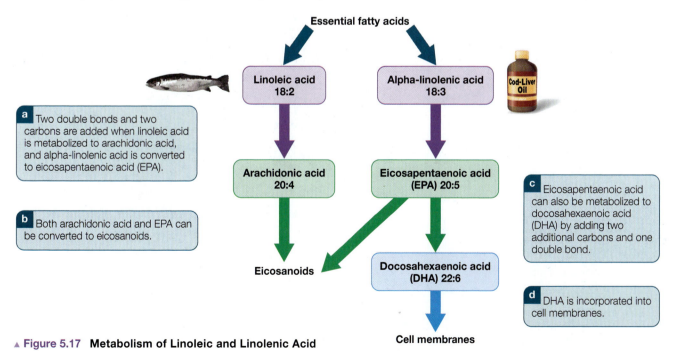

a Two double bonds and two carbons are added when linoleic acid is metabolized to arachidonic acid, and alpha-linolenic acid is converted to eicosapentaenoic acid (EPA).

b Both arachidonic acid and EPA can be converted to eicosanoids.

c Eicosapentaenoic acid can also be metabolized to docosahexaenoic acid (DHA) by adding two additional carbons and one double bond.

d DHA is incorporated into cell membranes.

Essential fatty acids

Linoleic acid 18:2 → Arachidonic acid 20:4 → Eicosanoids

Alpha-linolenic acid 18:3 → Eicosapentaenoic acid (EPA) 20:5 → Eicosanoids, Docosahexaenoic acid (DHA) 22:6 → Cell membranes

▲ Figure 5.17 **Metabolism of Linoleic and Linolenic Acid**

Specifically, linoleic acid can be elongated and desaturated to **arachidonic acid,** a 20-carbon, four-double-bond polyunsaturated fatty acid that is a precursor to eicosanoids. Alpha-linolenic acid is desaturated into the omega-3 fatty acid **eicosapentaenoic acid (EPA),** which is also an eicosanoid precursor. Moreover, EPA can be elongated to a second omega-3 fatty acid, **docosahexaenoic acid (DHA),** which is essential for the healthy development and function of the brain. EPA and DHA can also be obtained by eating cold-water fish such as salmon, herring, tuna, and halibut.

Alpha-linolenic acid is also needed for the structure of healthy cell membranes, particularly in nerve tissues, including the retina. A lack of this essential fatty acid in the diet can result in depression, impaired vision, and scaly skin.

Cholesterol Is Used to Make Hormones, Bile, and Vitamin D

Cholesterol is also a precursor for some very important compounds. A key role of cholesterol is to serve as the starting material in the synthesis of steroid hormones, including the sex hormones estrogen and testosterone, and the adrenal corticoids such as cortisol and aldosterone. The liver uses cholesterol to manufacture bile. In addition, a type of cholesterol in the skin is converted to a precursor of vitamin D using energy from the ultraviolet rays of the sun.

Phospholipids and Cholesterol Make Up Cell Membranes

Phospholipids make up the phospholipid bilayer in cell membranes. Their hydrophilic polar heads are attracted to the watery fluids both outside and inside of the cells, and their hydrophobic tails line up with each other in the center, creating a phospholipid barrier that surrounds the cell (**Figure 5.18**). This structure of the cell membrane allows

arachidonic acid Omega-6 fatty acid formed from linoleic acid; used to synthesize the eicosanoids, including leukotrienes, prostaglandins, and thromboxanes.

eicosapentaenoic acid (EPA) and docosahexaenoic acid (DHA) EPA (C20:5n–3) and DHA (C22:6n–3) are omega-3 fatty acids that are synthesized in the body and found in cold-water fish. These compounds may be beneficial in reducing heart disease.

▼ Figure 5.18 **The Role of Phospholipids and Cholesterol in Cell Membranes**
The two-layer cell membrane surrounding the cell is composed of a polar head and nonpolar tail. Cholesterol keeps the phospholipids separate.

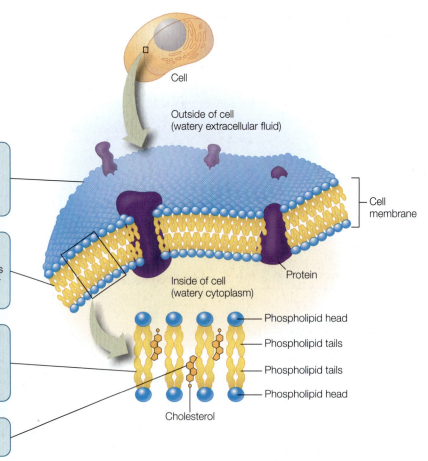

Cell

Outside of cell (watery extracellular fluid)

1 Because the phosphate-containing head is polar, it attracts charged particles, such as water, located both outside and inside your cells.

2 Its fatty acid-containing tail is nonpolar, so it mingles and lines up with other nonpolar molecules such as the fatty acid-containing ends of other phospholipids.

3 This creates a two-layer membrane that surrounds the cell and acts as a barrier, allowing certain substances to enter the cell but keeping others from leaving.

4 Cholesterol adds stability and fluidity to the cell.

Cell membrane

Inside of cell (watery cytoplasm)

Protein

Phospholipid head

Phospholipid tails

Phospholipid tails

Phospholipid head

Cholesterol

certain substances, such as water, to enter the cell but keeps others, like protein, from leaking out.

Cholesterol is also a structural component in cell membranes, where it improves cell fluidity and firmness. In cell membranes, cholesterol is interwoven with phospholipids, helping to keep them separate from each other so that their fatty acid tails don't crystallize. In this way, cholesterol improves cell fluidity and integrity. Moreover, the unique shape of cholesterol makes the cell membrane less soluble to very small molecules that otherwise could cross it too easily.

LO 5.3: THE TAKE-HOME MESSAGE Fatty acids are an energy-dense source of fuel for the body. Stored triglycerides cushion and protect bones, organs, and nerves and help maintain body temperature. Dietary fat provides essential fatty acids and is needed for the absorption of fat-soluble vitamins and carotenoids. Essential fatty acids are precursors to arachidonic acid and EPA, which are used to synthesize a variety of eicosanoids, substances that regulate several body functions. Cholesterol is used to make sex hormones, bile, and vitamin D. Phospholipids and cholesterol are part of cell membranes.

What Are the Recommendations for Daily Intake of Triglycerides and Cholesterol?

LO 5.4 Identify the dietary recommendations for total fat, saturated fat, *trans* fat, the essential fatty acids, and cholesterol.

Americans' fat consumption has gone up and down over the last century. In the 1930s, Americans were consuming about 34 percent of their kilocalories from fat; this number climbed to 42 percent in the mid-1960s, but has now fallen to about 33 percent of total kilocalories.[2] Although this consumption level is in line with current recommendations, we can't break out the hot fudge sundaes just yet. Measuring fat consumption as a percentage of total kilocalories, without considering the type or total amount of fat, can be misleading. You will soon read that the amount of heart-unhealthy saturated fat that we are eating could use some adjusting.

Dietary Fat Intake Is Based on a Percentage of Total Kilocalories

The current AMDR (Acceptable Macronutrient Distribution Range) for fat is 20–35 percent of daily kilocalories. For help converting the AMDR for fat to grams of fat, see the Calculation Corner. Consuming a diet that provides less than 20 percent of kilocalories from fat and that is high in carbohydrates may increase LDL cholesterol and triglyceride concentrations in the blood and lower HDL cholesterol—blood lipid levels that increase the risk for heart disease.

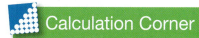 Calculation Corner

Calculating the AMDR for Fat
Approximately how many grams of total fat does an individual with a 2,000-kilocalorie energy requirement need to consume to meet the recommendations?

The AMDR recommends that 20–35 percent of daily kilocalories (kcal) come from fat, so the range for an individual who needs 2,000 kilocalories per day would be:

$$2{,}000 \text{ kcal} \times 0.20 \ (20\%) = 400 \text{ kcal}; \ 9 \text{ kcal/g} = 44 \text{ g}$$
$$2{,}000 \text{ kcal} \times 0.35 \ (35\%) = 700 \text{ kcal}; \ 9 \text{ kcal/g} = 78 \text{ g}$$

Answer: This person's range of fat intake should be 44–78 grams daily.

To find the maximum grams of saturated and trans fats that this person should consume daily, calculate 10 percent of total kcal:

$$2{,}000 \text{ kcal} \times 0.10 \ (10\%) = 200 \text{ kcal}; \ 9 \text{ kcal/g} = 22 \text{ g}$$

Answer: The total amount of saturated fat and trans fat should be no more than 22 grams daily.

> Go to Mastering Nutrition and complete a Math Video activity similar to the problem in this Calculation Corner.

Overconsumption of dietary fat won't increase your body weight unless it's coupled with overconsumption of kilocalories. However, because dietary fat is more concentrated in kilocalories than either carbohydrates or protein, a diet high in fat is likely to result in eating too many kilocalories, and could make for a weight-management problem. Numerous research studies have shown that reducing dietary fat can also reduce dietary kilocalories, which can result in weight loss.[3] Consequently, controlling fat intake may help control body weight.

For heart health, the recommendation is to consume no more than 10 percent of total kilocalories from saturated fats (and ideally less than 7 percent) and to limit *trans* fats to less than 1 percent.[4] (*Trans* fats are discussed in detail shortly.) Individuals are encouraged to use more monounsaturated and polyunsaturated fats to replace saturated fats. For example, if you consume 30 percent of your total kilocalories as fat, about 6 percent should be derived from saturated fats, 1 percent or less from *trans* fat, about 10 percent from polyunsaturated fats, and 13 percent from monounsaturated fats. This is because monounsaturated fats are the best at lowering LDL cholesterol and either maintaining or slightly increasing HDL cholesterol.

When it comes to keeping track of fat intake, counting grams of fat in foods is a good strategy. Use the Self-Assessment to estimate how much total fat you currently consume daily.

Self-Assessment

How Much Fat Is in Your Diet?

Are you consuming too much fat, saturated fat, *trans* fat, or all three? Use a diet analysis program, the food tables in the appendix, or food labels to track your fat consumption for a day and fill out the food log below. How does your intake compare with the grams you calculated you need according to the AMDR?

Food Log				
Meal	**Food/Drink**	**Total Fat (g)**	**Saturated Fat (g)**	***Trans* Fat (g)**
Breakfast				
Snack				
Lunch				
Snack				
Dinner				
Snack				
Total				

Essential Fatty Acids Have Specific Recommendations

The two essential fatty acids are linoleic acid and alpha-linolenic acid. The Adequate Intake (AI) for linoleic acid is 17 grams per day for adult men and 12 grams per day for adult women.[5] The AI for alpha-linolenic acid for men and women is 1.6 and 1.1 grams, respectively. There is no AI for EPA and DHA specifically, but Americans currently consume only about 0.1–0.2 grams of EPA and DHA in their daily diet.

The AMDR for linoleic acid is set at 5–10 percent of total kilocalories, while alpha-linolenic acid should make up 0.6–1.2 percent of total kilocalories. These recommended amounts are based on the estimated daily kilocalorie needs according to gender and age.

Based on randomized trials, the American Heart Association recommends that people diagnosed with heart disease consume about 1 gram of essential fatty acids each day. For those who have been diagnosed with **hypertriglyceridemia** (elevated blood triglycerides), 2–4 grams per day of EPA and DHA supplements may lower blood triglycerides.[6]

Dietary Cholesterol and Phospholipids Are Not Essential

Many people are confused about the merits of cholesterol. While high blood cholesterol is unhealthy, cholesterol is used in the synthesis of bile, hormones, and vitamin D and is part of the cell membrane. But do we need to eat cholesterol to accomplish these tasks?

The answer is no. Dietary cholesterol is not necessary because the liver synthesizes all that the body needs. The liver manufactures about 900 milligrams of cholesterol per day. This is three times greater than the 300 milligrams the average American consumes daily. However, if cholesterol is consumed, the body adjusts the amount it synthesizes. Normally, the total amount of cholesterol remains constant because the rate of cholesterol synthesis in the liver is under feedback control. When the dietary intake is high, liver synthesis is low; when intake is low, synthesis increases.

Previous editions of the *Dietary Guidelines for Americans (DGAs)* included a precise limit on dietary cholesterol intake to reduce the risk of developing cardiovascular disease. Healthy individuals over the age of 2 were advised to limit their dietary cholesterol to less than 300 milligrams (mg) daily, on average. The new *2015–2020 DGAs* did not bring forward this recommendation because available evidence shows no appreciable relationship between consumption of dietary cholesterol and serum cholesterol concentrations.[7] However, the current DGAs still suggest that Americans should eat as little dietary cholesterol as possible. Adult males in the United States currently consume about 358 milligrams daily, whereas adult females take in about 237 milligrams, on average. **Table 5.1** lists a variety of foods and their cholesterol content.

A diet low in saturated and *trans* fats but rich in unsaturated fats may reduce the risk of developing cardiovascular disease. One such diet is the Mediterranean diet. For more on this diet, see the Spotlight, "The Mediterranean Diet: What Do People Living in the Mediterranean Do Differently?" on page 179.

Even though lecithin, the most common phospholipid in our diet, plays an important role in the body, it does not need to be consumed in foods or in supplements. The liver is able to synthesize all phospholipids, including lecithin. In fact, dietary lecithin is digested in the GI tract, which means it does not reach the cell membranes intact.

Lecithin supplements, which are commonly marketed as a miracle solution for weight loss, fat metabolism, cardiovascular health, exercise performance, and arthritis relief, have not been scientifically proven to be effective in weight loss or improving health. In addition, the fatty acids present in lecithin supplements (which, like all lipids, contain 9 kilocalories per gram) can add unwanted kilocalories.

hypertriglyceridemia Presence of high concentrations of triglycerides in the blood. Defined as triglyceride concentrations between 400 and 1,000 milligrams per deciliter.

TABLE 5.1	How Much Cholesterol Is in Foods?
	Cholesterol (mg)
Liver, 3 oz	324
Breakfast biscuit with egg and sausage, 1	290
Egg, 1 large	186
Shrimp, canned, 3 oz	147
Fast-food hamburger, large, double patty	122
Ice cream, soft serve, vanilla, $\frac{1}{2}$ cup	78
Beef, ground, cooked, 3 oz	77
Salmon, cooked, 3 oz	74
Chicken or turkey, breast, cooked, 3 oz	72
Lobster, cooked, 3 oz	61
Turkey, light meat, cooked, 3 oz	59
Egg noodles, 1 cup	53
Butter, 1 tbs	31
Cheddar cheese, 1 oz	30
Frankfurter, beef, 1	24
Milk, whole, 1 cup	24
Cheddar cheese, low fat, 1 oz	6
Milk, skim, 1 cup	4

Source: Data from USDA. 2015. *National Nutrient Database for Standard Reference, Release 28.* Available at www.ars.usda.gov. Accessed January 2017.

LO 5.4: THE TAKE-HOME MESSAGE Dietary lipids, particularly the essential fatty acids, are key for a healthy diet, but intake of saturated fats, *trans* fats, and cholesterol should be limited. Dietary fat intake should range from 20 to 35 percent of total kilocalories. To meet essential fatty acid needs, 5–10 percent of total daily kilocalories should come from linoleic acid and 0.6–1.2 percent of total daily kilocalories should come from alpha-linolenic acid. Dietary intake of saturated fat should be limited to no more than 10 percent of total fat consumption, and less than 1 percent of fat consumption should be from *trans* fats. Dietary cholesterol and phospholipids are both made in the body and are not essential nutrients.

The Mediterranean Diet: What Do People Living in the Mediterranean Do Differently?

The Mediterranean diet doesn't refer to the diet of a specific country but to the dietary patterns found in several areas of the Mediterranean region, specifically Crete (a Greek island), other areas of Greece, and southern Italy, circa 1960. Researchers were first drawn to these areas in the early 1990s because the adults living there had very low rates of chronic diseases, such as heart disease and cancer, and a very long life expectancy. For example, the natives of Greece had a rate of heart disease that was 90 percent lower than that of Americans at that time.[1]

The people in Crete, in particular, were less educated and affluent than Americans, and less likely to obtain good medical care, so their greater health and life expectancy could not be explained by education level, financial status, or a superior health care system. Early research did find, however, that compared with the diets of affluent Americans, the Cretans' diet was dramatically lower in foods from animal sources, such as meat, eggs, and dairy products, and higher in monounsaturated fats (mostly from olive oil and

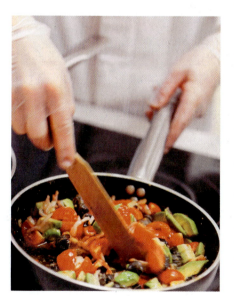

olives) and inexpensive grains, fruits, and vegetables.[2]

The latest research continues to support the health benefits of a Mediterranean-style diet. Numerous recent studies have found that adopting a Mediterranean-style diet reduces cardiovascular risk factors such as high blood pressure, high LDL cholesterol, and low HDL cholesterol.[3] People who follow the Mediterranean diet are more likely to live longer,[4] have lower blood glucose, less abdominal fat,[5] and reduce blood markers of certain inflammatory chemicals linked to cardiovascular disease.[6]

Figure 1 illustrates the dietary patterns and lifestyle habits characteristic of the Mediterranean diet.[7] Let's look more closely at this Mediterranean diet pyramid, the dietary and lifestyle changes that augment it, and some potential changes that you could make in your diet and lifestyle to reap similar benefits.[8]

Mediterranean Lifestyle

First, notice that the Mediterranean diet pyramid portrays the relative importance and frequency of each group of foods as it contributes to the whole diet. It identifies recommendations for every main meal, as well as daily and weekly choices, but does not dictate rigid amounts or precise foods from each food group.

Next, notice that physical activity is depicted at the base of this pyramid, reflecting the traditional Mediterranean habits of walking, hiking, bicycling, and engaging in physical labor such as farming, fishing, and gardening. Mediterranean citizens also traditionally enjoyed other lifestyle habits associated with mental and physical health. They had a supportive community of family and friends, long relaxing family meals, and afternoon *siestas* (naps). Exercising daily, resting, and relaxing with family and friends is good health advice for all, no matter what food plan you follow.

Daily Plant Foods, Olive Oil, Fish, and Dairy

Plant-based foods such as whole grains, fruits, legumes and other vegetables, and nuts are the focus of the Mediterranean diet. In fact, more than 60 percent of the recommended kilocalories are supplied by these high-fiber, nutrient-dense plant foods. In traditional Mediterranean-style eating, a combination of plant foods, such as legumes, green vegetables, and a small amount of pasta, is the focus of the meal. Fruit is typically served as dessert. Spices, herbs, garlic, and onions add flavor to foods while reducing the need for salt.

Olives and olive oil supply more than 75 percent of the fat in the Mediterranean diet. As previously discussed, vegetable oils are low in saturated fat, and olive oil in particular is high in monounsaturated fat. At least two servings of fish and seafood should be enjoyed weekly.

Nonfat milk and yogurt and low- or reduced-fat cheeses can be enjoyed on a daily basis when eating a Mediterranean-style diet. A small amount of grated Parmesan cheese sprinkled over vegetables and a grain can provide a distinct Mediterranean flavor.

Occasional Poultry, Eggs, and Meat

Foods from animal sources are limited. The Mediterranean diet relegates red meat consumption to less than two servings weekly. No more than two to four servings of eggs should be eaten weekly and poultry should be limited to about two servings per week.

Sweets, Water, and Wine

Historically, fruit was the standard daily dessert and sweets were prevalent only during the holidays. Consequently, the Mediterranean diet includes fewer than

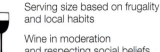

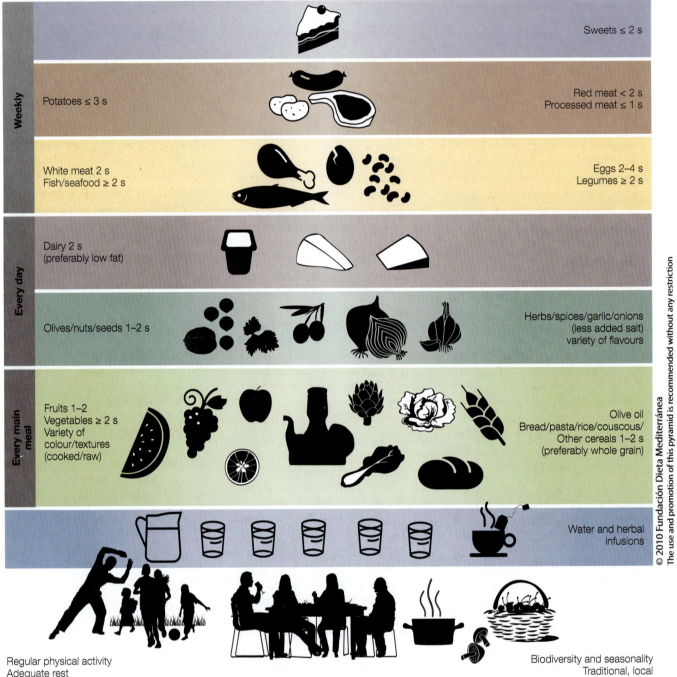

▲ **Figure 1 The Healthy Mediterranean Diet Pyramid**
A plant-based diet with minimal amounts of high-saturated-fat, high-sugar foods, coupled with daily physical activity, reflects the healthy habits of the Mediterranean lifestyle.

Source: Fundacion Dieta Mediterranea. 2010. *Mediterranean Diet Pyramid Today: Science and Cultural Updates.* Available at http://dietamediterranea.com/en. Accessed March 2017.

two servings a week of honey- or sugar-based sweets.

Water is recommended daily. Though many Mediterranean people drink wine daily, alcohol consumption is optional. The choice should be based on personal preferences, family and medical history, and social situations.

How Does the Mediterranean Diet Pyramid Compare with MyPlate?

The Mediterranean diet is a perfect example of a food plan that is easy to follow. Like MyPlate, it is not based on specific foods but is flexible, allowing for the social, economic, and environmental factors that influence food choices. This symbiotic approach to eating and lifestyle combines the old food ways of the Mediterranean with contemporary concerns for nutrition, health benefits, locally grown foods, and culture into a sustainable, healthy cuisine.[9]

There are many other similarities between the Mediterranean diet pyramid and MyPlate. Both emphasize the importance of regular physical activity, and both encourage a plant-based diet rich in whole grains, fruits, and vegetables, and daily consumption of dairy products. Mediterranean-style eating encourages the use of olive oil, a fat source that is rich in heart-healthy, unsaturated fat, and fish and seafood. Vegetable oils are also encouraged on MyPlate, but more modestly. Whereas poultry, eggs, and meat are recommended more modestly in the Mediterranean diet pyramid than in MyPlate, both advise minimizing intake of sweets. Both tools can be used as a foundation for a healthy diet.

References

1. Helsing, E. 1995. Traditional Diets and Disease Patterns of the Mediterranean, circa 1960. *American Journal of Clinical Nutrition* 61:1329S–1337S.
2. Ibid.
3. Di Daniele, N., et al. 2016. Impact of Mediterranean Diet on Metabolic Syndrome, Cancer, and Longevity. *Oncotarget* doi: 10.18632/oncotarget.13553.
4. Ibid.
5. Ibid.
6. Bihuniak, J. D., et al. 2016. Adherence to a Mediterranean-Style Diet and Its Influence on Cardiovascular Risk Facts in Postmenopausal Women. *Journal of the Academy of Nutrition and Dietetics* 116(11):1767–775. doi: 10.1016/j.jand.2016.06.377.
7. Bach-Faig, A., E. M. Berry, D. Lairon, J. Reguant, A. Trichopoulou, S. Dernini, F. X. Medina, et al. 2011. Mediterranean Diet Pyramid Today. Science and Cultural Updates. *Public Health Nutrition* 14(12A): 2274–2284.
8. Guasch-Ferré, M., M. Bulló, M. A. Martínez-González, E. Ros, D. Corella, R. Estruch, M. Fitó, et al. 2013. Frequency of Nut Consumption and Mortality Risk in the PREDIMED Nutrition Intervention Trial. *BMC Medicine* 11:164 doi: 10.1186/1741-7015-11-164.
9. Martínez-González, M.A. 2016. Benefits of the Mediterranean Diet Beyond the Mediterranean Sea and Beyond Food Patterns. *BMC Medicine* 14(1):157.

What Are the Best, Worst, and Alternative Food Sources for Fat?

LO 5.5 Identify the best, worst, and alternative food sources of dietary fats.

Eating foods that contain unsaturated fats (which also contain essential fatty acids) is better for health than eating foods high in saturated fat, cholesterol, and/or *trans* fat. So, which foods contain the healthier fats?

The Best Food Sources Are Low in Saturated Fat

Unsaturated fats are abundant in vegetable oils, such as soybean, corn, and canola oils, as well as in soybeans, walnuts, flaxseeds, and wheat germ. These foods are also all good sources of linoleic acid. Walnuts, flaxseeds, and canola oil also contain alpha-linolenic acid. **Figure 5.19** lists examples of foods that are excellent sources of unsaturated fats and essential fatty acids.

Fish are generally good sources of omega-3 fatty acids, and all fish contain EPA and DHA, with fatty fish being especially rich sources (**Figure 5.20**). Eating fish at least twice a week has been shown to improve heart health.[8]

Individuals are sometimes hesitant to consume fish because of concerns about mercury, a toxic heavy metal. Although all fish and shellfish contain a trace of mercury, only a few fish are high in mercury. These include shark, ahi tuna, mackerel, and swordfish. In general, mercury contamination from fish consumption is considered a health risk only for pregnant women and young children.

Foods high in saturated fat should be limited in the diet. Most saturated fat comes from animal foods, such as fatty cuts of meat, whole-milk dairy products (including

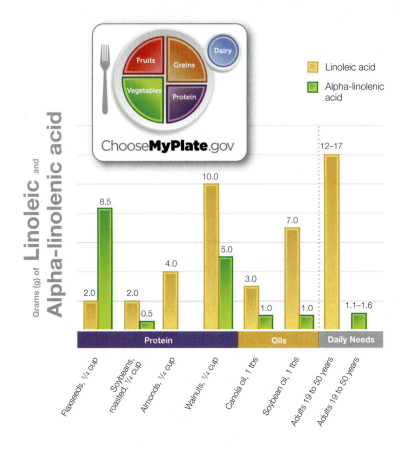

▶ **Figure 5.19** Food Sources of the Essential Fatty Acids

Many oils and nuts are good sources of the two essential fatty acids.

Source: Data from *USDA What's In The Food You Eat?* 2016. Available at https://www.ars.usda.gov. Accessed March 2017.

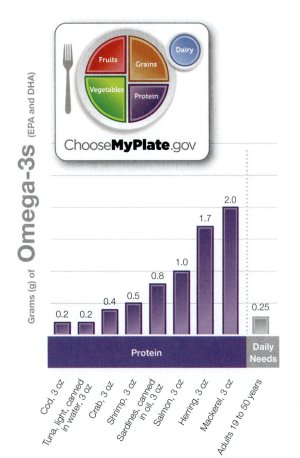

◀ **Figure 5.20** Food Sources of Omega-3 Fatty Acids

Several types of fish, particularly fatty fish, are high in the heart-healthy omega-3 fatty acids.

Source: Data from *USDA What's In The Food You Eat?* 2016. Available at https://www.ars.usda.gov. Accessed March 2017.

cheese, butter, and ice cream), and the skin on poultry. Certain tropical oils, such as coconut, palm, and palm kernel oils, are also very high in saturated fat. These oils are sometimes found in candies, commercially made baked goods, and gourmet ice cream. Reading the ingredient label on food packages is the best way to check for these oils. Currently, many consumers are choosing coconut oil for cooking and baking, and some are even adding it to coffee, oatmeal, or smoothies! Read more on the science behind this fad in Examining the Evidence: Is Coconut Oil the Next Superfood? on page 183.

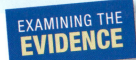
Is Coconut Oil the Next Superfood?

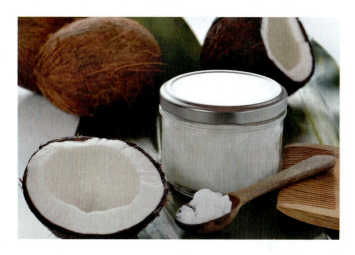

You've probably noticed coconut oil on the ingredients list of milk, spreads, and yogurt, or even seen jars filled with this solid milky-white fat on the grocery shelves. Once thought of as a fat to avoid, coconut oil is making a comeback and is being touted as a healthy alternative to other oils.

Coconut oil used in some brands of microwave popcorn, coffee creamer, and candy is made from dried coconut that is treated to yield the refined oil used in these foods. In contrast, today's "virgin" coconut oil found on grocery store shelves is extracted from the fresh meat of the coconut. When this is heated, the fat rises to the top and is skimmed off, much as cream is separated from milk. Whether the process begins with dried or fresh coconut, the composition of the coconut oil is the same.[1]

The Composition of Coconut Oil

The key difference between coconut oil and other, more commonly used vegetable oils is its saturation (see **Figure 1**). About 91 percent of the fatty acids in coconut oil are saturated. Because its fatty acids are mostly saturated, coconut oil is solid at room temperature and isn't as susceptible to rancidity.[2] In fact, coconut oil is actually classified as a solid fat, not an oil. Olive oil,

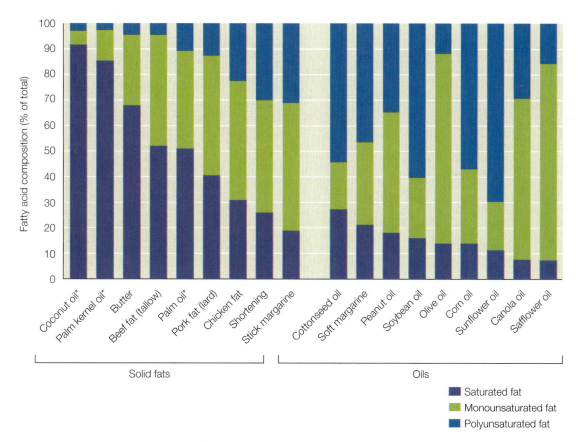

▲ **Figure 1 Composition of Various Oils**
Oils used for cooking and in food preparation vary in their saturation.

in comparison, is 15 percent saturated and liquid at room temperature.

In addition, coconut oil differs from common vegetable oils in its chain length. About 72 percent of the fatty acids in coconut oil are medium-chain fatty acids 8–12 carbons long. The majority of these medium-chain fatty acids (45 percent) are lauric acid, which is 12 carbons long. In contrast, most of the fatty acids in other oils are long-chain fatty acids between 12 and 18 carbons long. Soybean oil, for example, is 100 percent long-chain fatty acids. The chain length is what gives coconut oil its advantage over other oils in food processing. Its high concentration of lauric acid makes coconut oil highly resistant to oxidation at high heats, which makes it a good choice for frying (see **Table 1**).

Possible Health Benefits of Coconut Oil

Coconut oil does not contain any polyunsaturated essential fatty acids, but it is rich in vitamin E and a variety of phytochemicals.[3] Does coconut oil's composition provide unique health benefits beyond those nutrients?

In spite of its high concentration of saturated fatty acids, there is evidence that coconut oil may provide some health benefits, including reducing the risk of heart disease,[4,5] improving weight loss,[6] improving Alzheimer's,[7] or protecting against infections.[8]

The original research supporting this idea came from studies indicating an absence of heart disease in individuals who live in the Polynesian islands, where most of the fat consumed is from coconuts.[9] Recently, there have been more studies to support the use of coconut oil for health benefits.

One such study reported the results of comparing LDL and HDL cholesterol blood concentrations in young adults fed 20 percent of their total kilocalories from either coconut oil or olive oil for 5 weeks.[10] A high LDL cholesterol level combined with a low HDL cholesterol level seems to increase risk of heart disease. Both LDL cholesterol and HDL cholesterol were higher with coconut oil than olive oil. Olive oil appeared to have a neutral effect on both LDL cholesterol and HDL cholesterol. In other research comparing people who used coconut oil versus sunflower oil, the amount of plaque buildup in the arteries was the same.[11] In another study, coconut oil consumption increased HDL cholesterol and lowered the LDL:HDL ratio, while soybean oil increased both the total blood cholesterol and LDL cholesterol and decreased HDL cholesterol.[12]

This study also indicated that coconut oil may have an effect on weight loss: Using coconut oil versus soybean oil did result in a significantly reduced waist circumference in overweight women.[13] Does this mean that coconut oil may melt the pounds away? If so, how? The answer may lie in the way the body absorbs medium-chain fatty acids compared with long-chain fatty acids. Long-chain fatty acids are absorbed as part of chylomicrons, which deposit fatty acids in the adipose tissue en route to the liver. However, medium-chain fatty acids are absorbed directly into the bloodstream and not transported through the lymphatic system. Medium-chain fatty acids are used directly by the liver for energy and are not stored in the adipose tissue. A 6-week pilot study reported that obese males significantly reduced their waist circumference after consuming coconut oil for 4 weeks.[14] One theory was that these subjects felt more satisfied after eating coconut oil and because they were less hungry, they consumed fewer kilocalories.[15] A similar study was reported in overweight men who consumed medium-chain triglycerides prior to eating lunch. The researchers were surprised by the results in that the participants' food intake, blood glucose, and serum triglcyerides were lower, while the levels of leptin and other satiety hormones were higher following the ingestion of medium-chain triglycerides.[16] Consuming medium-chain triglycerides as part of a weight loss diet may promote weight loss.[17]

Dementia is an umbrella term used to describe impaired mental abilities. Alzheimer's disease is the most common and most severe form of dementia. Inflammation is emerging as a trigger for Alzheimer's disease. The initial inflammatory response is prompted by the immune system to defend tissues against viruses, cancerous cells, and harmful amyloid protein deposits that damage the neurons. However, chronic inflammation damages the ability of healthy brain cells to utilize glucose. The brain switches to ketone bodies for fuel.[18] The medium-chain fatty acids in coconut oil are metabolized to ketone bodies and may provide the fuel for the brain that was normally provided by glucose. In addition, ketones may reduce the amyloid levels that disrupt the brain, thus protecting the neurons from amyloid damage.[19] Research continues to study the question of whether or not consuming coconut oil can prevent or slow the progression of Alzheimer's disease.

TABLE 1	Saturated Fatty Acid Composition of Common Vegetable Oils					
Oil	**Caprylic C8:0**	**Capric C10:0**	**Lauric C12:0**	**Myristic C14:0**	**Palmitic C16:0**	**Linoleic C18:0**
Coconut oil	1.0	0.8	6.1	2.3	1.1	0.4
Olive oil	0	0	0	0	11.2	1.9
Soybean oil	0	0	0	0	10.4	4.4
Canola oil	0	0	0	0	4.4	6.8
Corn oil	0	0	0	0	10.6	1.8
Flaxseed oil	0	0	0	0.1	5.1	3.4

Source: Adapted from the Position Statement of the Academy of Nutrition and Dietetics: Dietary Fatty Acids for Healthy Adults. 2014. *Journal of the Academy of Nutrition and Dietetics* 114:136–153.

The Bottom Line

Limited research evidence suggests that medium-chain triglycerides found in coconut oil may lower blood LDL cholesterol concentration, a significant factor in heart disease risk. Some research also suggests that coconut oil may be beneficial for weight loss and possibly for age-related dementia. At this point, the body of research on coconut oil and health is still inconclusive, however, and health professionals are divided over whether to recommend replacing heart-healthy polyunsaturated vegetable oils with coconut oil.

References

1. Tropical Traditions. 2013. *What Is Virgin Coconut Oil?* Available from www.tropicaltraditions.com. Accessed February 2014.
2. Lekshmi, S. D., et al. 2016. In Silico and Wet Lab Studies Reveal the Cholesterol Lowering Efficacy of Lauric Acid, a Medium-Chain Fat of Coconut Oil. *Plant Foods Human Nutrition* 71(4):410–415.
3. Marina, A. M., Y. B. Man, S. A. Nazimah, and I. Amin. 2009. Antioxidant Capacity and Phenolic Acids of Virgin Coconut Oil. *International Journal of Food Science and Nutrition* 60(Suppl 2):114–123.
4. Newgent, Jackie. 2013. *Coconut Oil: What Is It All About?* Available at www.eatright.org. Accessed January 2017.
5. Eyres, L., Eyres, M. F., Chisholm, A., and Brown, R. C. 2016. Coconut Oil Consumption and Cardiovascular Risk Factors in Humans. *Nutrition Reviews* 74(4):267–280. 10.1093/nutrit/nuw002S.
6. Lemarié, F., Beauchamp, E., Legrand, P., and Rioux, V. 2016. Revisiting the Metabolism and Physiological Functions of Caprylic Acid (C8:0) with Special Focus on Ghrelin Octanoylation. *Biochimie* 120:40–48. doi: 10.1016/j.biochi.2015.08.002.
7. Fernando, W. M., et al. 2015. The Role of Dietary Coconut for the Prevention and Treatment of Alzheimer's Disease: Potential Mechanisms of Action. *British Journal of Nutrition* 114(1):1–14. doi: 10.1017/S0007114515001452.
8. Vysakh, A., M. Ratheesh, T. P. Rajmohanan, C. Pramod, S. Premlal, K. B. Girish, and P. Sibi. 2014. Polyphenolics Isolated from Virgin Coconut Oil Inhibits Adjuvant Induced Arthritis in Rats through Antioxidant and Anti-inflammatory Action. *International Immunopharmacology* 20(1):124–130.
9. Prior, I. A., Davidson, F., Salmond, E. E., and Czochanska, Z. 1981. Cholesterol, Coconuts, and Diet on Polynesian Atolls: A Natural Experiment: The Pukapuka and Tokelau Island Studies. *American Journal of Clinical Nutrition* 34(8):1552–1561.
10. Voon, P. T., T. K. Ng, V. K. Lee, and K. Nesaretnam. 2011. Diets High in Palmitic Acid (16J), Lauric and Myristic Acids (12:0 + 14:0) or Oleic Acid (18:1) Do Not Alter Postprandial or Fasting Plasma Homocysteine and Inflammatory Markers in Healthy Malaysian Adults. *American Journal of Clinical Nutrition* 94(6):1451–1457.
11. Palazhy, S., P. Kamath, P. C. Rajesh, K. Vaidyanathan, S. K. Nair, and D. M. Vasudevan. 2012. Composition of Plasma and Atheromatous Plaque among Coronary Artery Disease Subjects Consuming Coconut Oil or Sunflower Oil as the Cooking Medium. *Journal of the American College of Nutrition* 31(6): 392–396.
12. Assunção, M. L., H. S. Ferreira, A. F. dos Santos, C. R. Cabral, Jr., and T. M. Florêncio. 2009. Effects of Dietary Coconut Oil on the Biochemical and Anthropometric Profiles of Women Presenting Abdominal Obesity. *Lipids* 44(7):593–601.
13. Ibid.
14. Liau, K. M., Y. Y. Lee, C. K. Chen, and A. H. Rasool. 2011. An Open-Label Pilot Study to Assess the Efficacy and Safety of Virgin Coconut Oil in Reducing Visceral Adiposity. *ISRN Pharmacology* 2011:949686. doi: 10.5402/2011/949686.
15. Poppitt, S. D., C. M. Strik, A. K. MacGibbon, B. H. McArdle, S. C. Budgett, and A. T. McGill. 2010. Fatty Acid Chain Length, Postprandial Satiety and Food Intake in Lean Men. *Physiological Behavior* 101(1):161–167.
16. St-Onge, M.P., et al. 2014. Impact of Medium and Long Chain Triglycerides Consumption on Appetite and Food Intake in Overweight Men. *European Journal of Clinical Nutrition* 68(10):1134–1140. doi: 10.1038/ejcn.2014.145.
17. Mumme, K. 2015. Effects of Medium-Chain Triglcyerides on Weight Loss and Body Composition: A Meta-Analysis of Randomized Controlled Trials. *Journal of the Academy of Nutrition and Dietetics* 115:249–263.
18. Fernando, W. M., et al. The Role of Dietary Coconut for the Prevention and Treatment of Alzheimer's Disease: Potential Mechanisms of Action. *British Journal of Nutrition* 114(1): 1–14. doi: 10.1017/S0007114515001452.
19. Yin, J. X., et al. 2016. Ketones Block Amyloid Entry and Improve Cognition in an Alzheimer's Model. *Neurobiological Aging* 39:25–37. doi: 10.1016/j.neurobiolaging.2015.11.018.

While it's important to limit saturated fat in the diet, it's impossible to eliminate it entirely. All fats and oils contain a variety of fatty acids, some of which are saturated. Avoiding all foods and oils containing saturated fats could lead to the unnecessary exclusion of healthy foods, such as soybean and canola oils, lean meats, fish, poultry, and low-fat dairy foods. The result may be an inadequate intake of important nutrients such as essential fatty acids, fat-soluble vitamins, protein, and calcium. A better strategy is to consume lower-fat versions of a variety of foods. **Figure 5.21** compares similar foods high and low in saturated fat.

In the supermarket, read the Nutrition Facts panel to help you choose foods that are low in saturated fat. For reasons discussed next, you should also scan the ingredient list to make sure the product has little or no partially hydrogenated oil.

Reduce Foods That Contain *Trans* Fat

Recall that, in a *trans* fatty acid, the hydrogen atoms are on opposite sides of the double carbon bond. This configuration occurs naturally in meat and dairy products, which account for about 15–20 percent of the ***trans* fats** in the American diet. Ground beef, for example, contains approximately one gram of *trans* fats per 100 grams (3.5 ounces) of beef, while butter fat has double that amount.[9] Even some plant products contain small

trans fats An unsaturated fatty acid formed as the result of hydrogenation. This type of fatty acid causes a reconfiguring of some of its double bonds. A small amount of *trans* fats occur naturally in foods from animal sources.

Grams (g) of saturated fat

Breakfast

Food	Saturated fat (g)
Cream (2 oz) in coffee	7.0
Low-fat milk (2 oz) in coffee	0.5
Whole milk, 1 cup	5.0
Skim milk, 1 cup	< 0.5
Bagel with 2 oz cream cheese	13.0
English muffin with 1 tbs light margarine	2.0

Lunch

Food	Saturated fat (g)
Cheeseburger on hamburger roll	13.5
Veggie burger on hamburger roll	1.5
Pepperoni pizza, 2 slices	4.5
Mushroom and pepper pizza, 2 slices	1.5
Steak and cheese sub	10.0
Roast beef sandwich on roll	2.0

Dinner

Food	Saturated fat (g)
Beef hot dog on roll	6.5
Turkey hot dog on roll	3.0
Mashed potatoes with butter and milk, 1 cup	6.0
Baked potato (small) with 1 tbs light margarine	2.0
Prime rib, 3 oz	13.0
Grilled salmon, 3 oz	2.0

Snacks

Food	Saturated fat (g)
Nachos with cheese, 2 oz chips and 3 oz cheese	21.0
Vegetables with salsa, 1 cup vegetables and 1/2 cup salsa	0
Gourmet vanilla ice cream, 1 cup	21.0
Gourmet lemon sorbet, 1 cup	0

Scale: 0, 5, 10, 15, 20, 25

■ Choices high in saturated fat
■ Choices low in saturated fat

▲ **Figure 5.21 Where's the Saturated Fat in Foods?**
Choosing less-saturated-fat versions of foods can dramatically lower the amount of saturated fat consumed in the diet.

amounts of *trans* fats. Pomegranates are low in fat but almost 70 percent of the fat they do contain is a *trans* fatty acid called punicic acid.[10] (Pomegranates are still considered a healthy fruit.) However, the great majority of the *trans* fatty acids we consume are derived from processed foods.

Hydrogenation of Oils Creates *Trans* Fats

At one time, saturated fats from animal sources, like lard, and highly saturated tropical plant oils, like coconut and palm oils, were staples in home cooking and commercial food preparation. These saturated fats worked well in commercial products because they

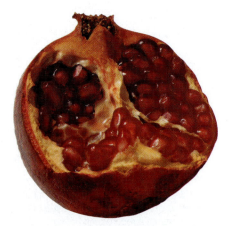

Pomegranates, while low in total fat, contain the *trans* fatty acid punicic acid.

provided a rich, flaky texture to baked goods and were more resistant to rancidity than the unsaturated fats found in oils. Later, food manufacturers developed the technique of hydrogenation of oils, which was inexpensive and performed a similar function.

Hydrogenation came into widespread commercial use when saturated fat fell out of favor in the 1980s. Research had confirmed that saturated fat played a role in increasing the risk of heart disease, so food manufacturers reformulated many of their products to contain less saturated fat. The easiest solution was to replace the saturated fat with partially hydrogenated oils (PHOs). During the hydrogenation process, hydrogen is added to some of the unstable *cis* fatty acids in a vegetable oil such as corn oil, converting some of them to *trans* fatty acids and making the oil partially hydrogenated. This process increases the level of *trans* fat found in the processed food. Commercially prepared baked goods, margarines, fried potatoes, chips and other snacks, shortenings, and salad dressings are often major sources of PHOs. They are also frequently used for frying at fast-food restaurants. Why is this a concern?

Consumption of *Trans* Fats Increases the Risk of Cardiovascular Disease

In 2015, the U.S. Food and Drug Administration (FDA) ruled that partially hydrogenated oils are no longer generally recognized as safe for consumption. The ruling followed years of research linking PHOs, and the *trans* fats they create, to an increased risk for cardiovascular disease. Research shows that *trans* fats raise blood concentrations of LDL cholesterol and triglycerides, lower HDL cholesterol concentrations, and increase inflammation of the arterial wall.[11] For these reasons, *trans* fats are thought to pose a greater risk for heart health than saturated fats. Food manufacturers have until July 26, 2018, to remove PHOs from their products.

In the meantime, you can determine whether or not a processed food contains PHOs by checking the Nutrition Facts panel. Since 2006, the FDA has mandated that most foods, and even some dietary supplements such as energy bars list the grams of *trans* fats per serving.[12] Food labels are allowed to state that the product is free of *trans* fat if it contains 0.5 grams or less of *trans* fat per serving. If the ingredients list includes partially hydrogenated oils, then the food contains *trans* fat.

Despite the fact that the health effects of *trans* fats are now well known, they currently provide an estimated 2.5 percent of the daily kilocalories in the diets of American adults. Of this amount, about 25 percent are derived from cakes, cookies, pies, and snacks such as chips.[13] Whether naturally occurring *trans* fats have the same heart-unhealthy effects as do those that are created through hydrogenation has yet to be determined. The bottom line is that *trans* fats should be kept as low as possible in the diet. Reducing the amount of food sources of solid fats in your diet will help reduce the consumption of both saturated fats and *trans* fats.

Increase Plant Sterols and Stanols

Most of the dietary cholesterol we consume comes from animal products, such as meat, chicken, fish, shellfish, eggs, and dairy products. Some plants also produce cholesterol as part of the cell walls and oils in their leaves.[14] However, the quantity of cholesterol in plants is so small when it is expressed as a percent of the total lipid content (about 5 milligrams per 100 grams in plants, versus as much as 500 milligrams per 100 grams in foods from animal sources) that plant oils are considered cholesterol free. Thus the main lipid in plant fats and oils is a triglyceride.

Phytosterols and phytostanols lower LDL cholesterol concentrations by competing with cholesterol for absorption in the intestinal tract. These lipids occur naturally in soybean oil, many fruits, legumes and other vegetables, sesame seeds, nuts, cereals, and other plant foods.[15] In addition, food manufacturers fortify foods such as margarine with plant sterols and stanols to help lower blood cholesterol.

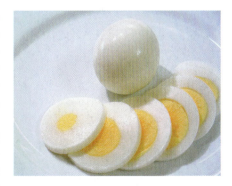

Eggs are an excellent source of protein, but egg yolks are high in dietary cholesterol.

Fat Substitutes Lower Fat in Foods

If you enjoy the taste and texture of creamy foods but don't want the extra fat, you're not alone. A research survey found that over 160 million Americans (79 percent of the adult population) choose lower-fat foods and beverages. Respondents cited their health as the major reason they were actively shopping for these foods.[16] To meet this demand, food manufacturers introduced more than 1,000 reduced-fat or low-fat products, from margarine to potato chips, each year during the 1990s.[17] Today, with few exceptions, almost any high-fat food on the grocery store shelves will be sitting next to its lower-fat counterpart. The keys to these products' lower fat content are **fat substitutes.**

Fat substitutes are designed to provide all the creamy properties of fat but with fewer kilocalories and total fat grams. Because fat has more than double the kilocalories per gram of carbohydrates or protein, fat substitutes have the potential to reduce kilocalories from fat by more than 50 percent without sacrificing taste and texture.

Carbohydrate-, Protein-, or Fat-Based Fat Substitutes

No single fat substitute works in all foods and with all cooking preparations, so several types of fat substitutes have been developed. Depending on their primary ingredient, fat substitutes fall into three categories (**Table 5.2**):

- **Carbohydrate-based substitutes** The majority of fat substitutes are carbohydrate based and use plant polysaccharides such as fiber, starches, gums, and cellulose to help retain moisture and provide a fatlike texture.[18] For example, low-fat muffins might have fiber added to them to help retain the moisture that is lost when fat is reduced. Carbohydrate-based substitutes have been used for years and work well under heat preparations other than frying.

- **Protein-based substitutes** Protein-based fat substitutes are created from the protein in eggs and milk. The protein is heated and broken down into microscopic balls that tumble over each other during chewing, providing a creamy

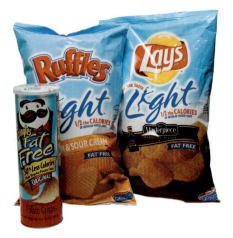

Foods made with fat substitutes, such as Ruffles, Lay's, and Pringles potato chips, aren't kilocalorie free.

fat substitutes Substances that replace added fat in foods; provide the creamy properties of fat for fewer kilocalories and total fat grams.

carbohydrate-based fat substitutes Substances that use polysaccharides to retain moisture and provide a fatlike texture.

protein-based fat substitutes Substances created from the protein in eggs and milk.

TABLE 5.2	The Lighter Side of Fat: Fat Substitutes		
Name (Trade Names)	**Kilocalories per Gram**	**Properties**	**Used for**
Carbohydrate Based			
Fibers from grains (Betatrim)	1–4	Gelling, thickener	Baked goods, meats, spreads
Fibers, cellulose (Cellulose gel)	0	Water retention, texture, mouthfeel	Sauces, dairy products, frozen desserts, salad dressings
Gums	0	Thickener, texture, mouthfeel, water retention	Salad dressings, processed meats
Polydextrose (Litesse)	1	Water retention, adds bulk	Baked goods, dairy products, salad dressings, cookies, and gum
Modified food starch (Sta-Slim)	1–4	Thickener, gelling, texture	Processed meats, salad dressings, frostings, fillings, frozen desserts
Protein Based			
Microparticulated protein (Simplesse)	1–4	Mouthfeel	Dairy products, salad dressings, spreads
Fat Based			
Mono- or diglycerides (Dur-Lo)	9*	Mouthfeel, moisture retention	Baked goods
Short-chain fatty acids (Salatrim)	5	Mouthfeel	Confections, baked goods
Olestra (Olean)	0	Mouthfeel	Savory snacks

Source: Data from R. D. Mattes. 1998. Fat Replacers. *Journal of the American Dietetic Association* 98:463–468; J. Wylie-Rosett. 2002. Fat Substitutes and Health: An Advisory from the Nutrition Committee of the American Heart Association. *Circulation* 105:2800–2804.

*Less of this fat substitute is needed to create the same effect as fat, so the kilocalories are reduced in foods using this product.

feel in the mouth that's similar to fat. Protein-based substitutes break down under high temperatures and lose their creamy properties, which makes them unsuitable for frying and baking.[19]

- **Fat-based substitutes** Fat-based substitutes are fats that have been modified to either provide the physical attributes of fat for fewer kilocalories or to interfere with the absorption of fat.[20] Mono- and diglycerides are used as emulsifiers in products such as baked goods and icings to provide moistness and mouthfeel. These emulsifiers are used with water to replace part of the fat in bakery goods and ice creams. Though fat-based substitutes have the same number of kilocalories per gram as fat, a smaller quantity is needed to create the same effect, so the total number of kilocalories is reduced.

One fat substitute, olestra (also known as Olean), approved in 1996 by the FDA, is a mixture of sucrose and long-chain fatty acids. Unlike fat, which contains three fatty acids connected to a glycerol backbone, olestra contains six to eight fatty acids connected to sucrose. The enzymes that normally break apart fatty acids from their glycerol backbones during digestion cannot hydrolyze the fatty acids in olestra. Instead, olestra moves through the GI tract unabsorbed. Thus, this fat substitute has zero kilocalories. Because olestra travels through the GI tract untouched, there was concern that it may cause stomach cramps and loose bowels. Though there have been anecdotal reports of individuals experiencing diarrhea and cramps after eating olestra-containing foods, controlled research studies don't support these side effects.[21] Olestra is very heat stable, so it can be used in baked and fried foods.

Reduced-Fat Products

Despite their intended purpose, the use of fat substitutes doesn't seem to curb Americans' kilocalorie intake or help with weight management. One explanation for this may be that individuals feel a false sense of entitlement when eating low-fat and fat-free foods, and thus overeat. Research indicates that people who snack on olestra-containing products may be reducing their overall fat intake, but not their intake of total kilocalories.[22] As with sugar substitutes, consumers should recognize that using reduced-fat or fat-free products does not mean they can eat unlimited amounts of those foods. The foods still contain kilocalories, and overconsuming kilocalories leads to weight gain.

LO 5.5: THE TAKE-HOME MESSAGE Lean meat and poultry, fish, low-fat or non-fat dairy products, and limited amounts of nuts and cheese are the best food sources to obtain the essential fatty acids and limit saturated and *trans* fats. Commercially prepared baked goods and snack items are high in kilocalories, saturated fat, and *trans* fats, and should be consumed rarely. Vegetable oils should be used in place of butter. *Trans* fats are found in commercially prepared foods made with partially hydrogenated oils (PHOs). Any *trans* fats in a food must be listed on the Nutrition Facts panel. The FDA has banned all PHOs from processed foods by July 2018. Cholesterol is found mostly in animal-based foods, whereas plant-based foods contain mostly phytosterols. Fat substitutes can be carbohydrate based, protein based, or fat based. Reduced-fat or fat-free foods still contain kilocalories and should be eaten in limited amounts.

fat-based substitutes Substances that resemble triglycerides and are either chemically synthesized or derived from conventional fats and oils by enzymatic modification.

What Is Heart Disease and What Factors Increase Risk?

LO 5.6 Describe the development of atherosclerosis and coronary heart disease, and explain how lifestyle factors can affect the risk.

Cardiovascular disease (CVD) is a term that encompasses several disorders affecting the heart and blood vessels, including problems with heart valves, heartbeat irregularities, infections, and the blood vessels serving the brain, the abdominal organs, or the extremities. The most common type of cardiovascular disease, and the type we focus on in this chapter, is *coronary heart disease,* which affects the blood vessels that serve the heart muscle and can lead to a heart attack or a sudden cardiac arrest. Stroke and peripheral vascular disease are also forms of cardiovascular disease.

Coronary heart disease (or simply *heart disease*) has been the number-one killer of adults in the United States since 1918. While the death rate from heart disease dropped by 31 percent between 2000 and 2010, one in three Americans still dies of heart disease every 40 seconds.[23]

Heart Disease Begins with Atherosclerosis

Coronary heart disease develops when the coronary arteries, the large blood vessels that lead to the heart, accumulate substances such as fat and cholesterol along their walls. As the artery narrows, blood flow is impeded and less oxygen and nutrients are delivered to the heart. If the heart doesn't receive enough oxygen, chest pains can result. Narrowed arteries increase the likelihood that a blood clot can get caught and block the vessel, leading to a **heart attack.** If the artery supplies blood to the brain, a **stroke** can occur. Clinically known as *cerebrovascular accidents,* strokes are the

fifth leading cause of death in the United States.[24]

The exact cause of the narrowed arteries, known as **atherosclerosis** (*athero* = porridge, *sclera* = hardening, *sis* = condition), is unknown, but researchers believe it begins with an injury to the lining of the arteries. Just as with a cut finger or sprained ankle, the injury results in inflammation. Inflamed arterial walls may develop weak areas that can rupture easily, increasing the risk of blood clots and a heart attack. High blood concentrations of cholesterol and fat, high blood pressure, and smoking likely contribute to this damage.

Over time, LDLs and other lipid substances infiltrate the injured artery wall. Reacting with free radicals and metal ions such as iron, the LDLs that accumulate become oxidized; moreover, they attract *macrophages* (white blood cells), which become enlarged with cholesterol-laden LDLs, transforming into foam cells. The foam cells stick to the walls of the artery and build up, along with *platelets* (fragments of cells in the blood) and other substances, into **plaque.** The plaque narrows the passageway of the artery (see **Focus Figure 5.22**).

Some Risk Factors Are Not Controllable

The known risk factors for heart disease are listed in **Table 5.3**. Some of these risk factors are beyond your control. These include age, gender, family history, and type 1 diabetes.

Total blood cholesterol, along with the risk of a heart attack, tends to rise with age until it stabilizes around age 65. Gender also plays a role. Until menopause (usually around age 50), women tend to have a lower blood cholesterol level than men and a reduced risk of heart disease. After menopause, the blood cholesterol level in women tends to catch up and even surpass that of men of the same age.[25]

Genetics can also be a risk factor for heart disease, as high LDL cholesterol concentrations are partly determined by genes

and can run in families.[26] An individual whose father or brother had early signs of heart disease before age 55, or whose mother or sister had them before age 65, is at a greater risk. This may be due to a genetic defect in the LDL receptor that regulates the amount of LDL cholesterol in the blood. Family members who have this defective gene have elevated LDL concentrations in the blood, which may produce premature atherosclerosis.[27]

Some individuals have normal concentrations of LDL cholesterol in their blood, yet still develop heart disease, which points to other factors that must be affecting their heart health. These other potential risk factors, referred to as *emerging risk factors,* include high blood concentrations of **C-reactive protein (CRP),** which the body produces in response to inflammation.[28] Because inflammation is a factor in atherosclerosis, a high CRP concentration suggests an increased risk of heart disease. Another blood marker associated with atherosclerosis is a high blood concentration of the amino acid *homocysteine,* a condition often seen with deficiencies of the B vitamins folate, vitamin B_{12}, and/or vitamin B_6.[29] High concentrations of this amino acid may injure the arteries, decrease their flexibility, and increase the likelihood of blood clots. The presence in the blood of *Chlamydia pneumoniae,* a bacterium that can cause pneumonia and respiratory infections, may also damage or inflame the vessel walls.[30] Lastly, another lipoprotein, **Lp(a) protein,** is being investigated for its

---

cardiovascular disease (CVD) General term for diseases of the heart and blood vessels.

heart attack Permanent damage to the heart muscle that results from a sudden lack of oxygen-rich blood; also called a *myocardial infarction (MI).*

stroke Interruption or cessation of circulation to a region of the brain that deprives the area of oxygen and nutrients and can result in paralysis and possibly death.

atherosclerosis Narrowing of the coronary arteries due to buildup of debris along the artery walls.

plaque Hardened buildup of cholesterol-laden foam cells, platelets, cellular waste products, and calcium in the arteries that results in atherosclerosis.

Head to **Mastering** Nutrition and watch a narrated video tour of this figure by author Joan Salge Blake.

Plaque accumulation within coronary arteries narrows their interior and impedes the flow of oxygen-rich blood to the heart.

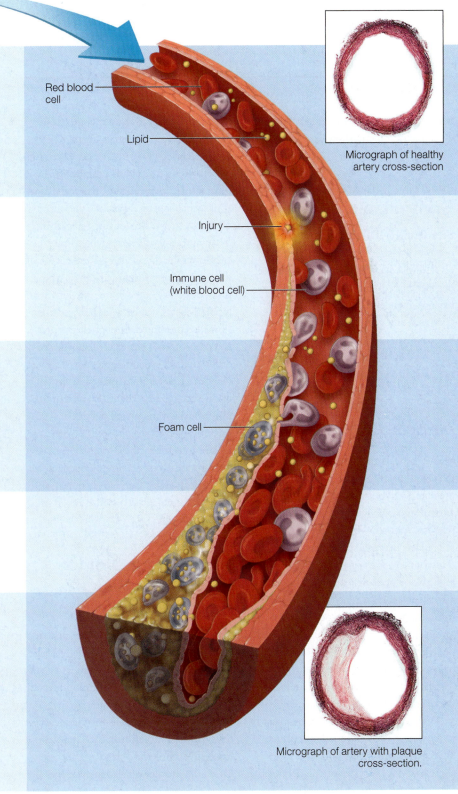

Red blood cell

Lipid

Injury

Immune cell (white blood cell)

Foam cell

Micrograph of healthy artery cross-section

Micrograph of artery with plaque cross-section.

HEALTHY ARTERY

Blood flows unobstructed through a normal, healthy artery.

ARTERIAL INJURY

The artery's lining is injured, attracting immune cells, and prompting inflammation.

LIPIDS ACCUMULATE IN WALL

Lipids, particularly cholesterol-containing LDLs, seep beneath the wall lining. The LDLs become oxidized. Immune cells, attracted to the site, engulf the oxidized LDLs and are transformed into foam cells.

FATTY STREAK

The foam cells accumulate to form a fatty streak, which releases more toxic and inflammatory chemicals.

PLAQUE FORMATION

The foam cells, along with platelets, calcium, protein fibers, and other substances, form thick deposits of plaque, stiffening and narrowing the artery. Blood flow through the artery is reduced or obstructed.

TABLE 5.3	Risk Factors for Heart Disease	
Uncontrollable Risk Factors	**Controllable Risk Factors**	**Emerging Risk Factors**
• Age • Gender • Family history of heart disease • Type 1 diabetes mellitus	• Type 2 diabetes mellitus • High blood pressure • Smoking • Physical activity • Excess body weight • Low HDL blood cholesterol • High LDL blood cholesterol	• Blood concentrations of C-reactive protein • High amount of homocysteine • Presence of *Chlamydia pneumoniae* in the blood • Lp(a) protein • Metabolic syndrome

role in causing excessive blood clotting and exacerbating inflammation.[31]

Some Risk Factors Are Controllable

Because high HDL cholesterol can help protect against heart disease, having an HDL level of less than 40 milligrams per deciliter (mg/dl) increases risk. In contrast, having a high level of HDL cholesterol, 60 mg/dl or higher, is considered a negative risk factor; in other words, there is so much of this good cholesterol helping to protect against heart disease that it counteracts another risk factor on the list. While genetics plays a large role in determining blood cholesterol concentrations, diet is also a factor.

Blood pressure (the force of blood against the walls of the arteries) can affect the risk of heart disease. Chronic high blood pressure, or **hypertension,** can damage the arteries and begin the progression of atherosclerosis. A **normal blood pressure** is considered less than 120 millimeters mercury (Hg) for the *systolic pressure* (the top number in the blood pressure reading) and less than 80 millimeters Hg for the *diastolic pressure* (the bottom number). A blood pressure reading of 120/80 to 139/89 is considered prehypertension, and a reading of 140/90 or higher is considered hypertension.

Chronic high blood pressure thickens the arteries and causes them to become stiff and less flexible, which may initiate injury to the arterial walls and accelerate plaque buildup. Chronic high blood pressure also causes the heart to work harder than

normal and can lead to an enlarged heart. (The Health Connection in Chapter 19 provides a detailed discussion of hypertension.)

Diabetes is a significant risk factor for heart disease; an estimated 75 percent of adults with diabetes die from either heart disease or stroke. It's not surprising, then, that controlling diabetes can help dramatically lower the risk of heart disease. Though the less common form of diabetes, type 1, is not preventable, the more prevalent form, type 2 diabetes, can be managed, and possibly even prevented, through diet, exercise, and other lifestyle changes. Metabolic syndrome, introduced in Chapter 4, is a cluster of risk factors for both cardiovascular disease and type 2 diabetes. Recall that these factors include abdominal obesity.[32]

Smoking damages the walls of the arteries and accelerates atherosclerosis. Female smokers are two to six times more likely to have a heart attack than female nonsmokers.[33] Male smokers also increase their risk for heart disease.

Modify Your Diet to Lower Your Risk of Heart Disease

The primary risk factor for heart disease is abnormal blood lipids, especially a high LDL cholesterol level.[34] Starting at age 20, individuals should have their blood tested at least once every 5 years to obtain a **blood lipid profile.** This profile includes tests for total cholesterol, HDL cholesterol, LDL cholesterol, and triglycerides. Often the profile will also include the

cholesterol-to-HDL ratio or a risk score calculated from lipid measurements, age, gender, and other risk factors.[24] **Table 5.4** indicates the optimal blood concentrations for total cholesterol, LDL cholesterol, and HDL cholesterol. The best way to impact blood concentrations of these lipids is through diet, exercise, and other lifestyle factors as described in the Nutrition in Practice on page 197.

Consume Less Saturated and *Trans* Fat

The ideal dietary pattern to reduce your risk of heart disease is one that lowers LDL cholesterol and raises HDL cholesterol simultaneously. In general, blood concentrations of LDL cholesterol increase on a high-saturated-fat and high-*trans*-fat diet, not a high-cholesterol diet.[35] Per kilocalorie, *trans* fats appear to increase the risk of heart disease more than any other food component, one reason that the FDA has banned the use of partially hydrogenated oils in foods sold in the United States after July 2018.[36] Controlled studies have shown that a diet containing *trans* fats raises LDL cholesterol concentrations, lowers HDL cholesterol concentrations, and increases the ratio of total cholesterol to HDL cholesterol. These fats also increase blood triglyceride concentrations and inflammation along the arterial wall.[37]

C-reactive protein (CRP) Protein found in the blood that is released from the cells during inflammation; used as a marker for the presence of atherosclerosis.

Lp(a) protein Lipoprotein containing LDL cholesterol found in the blood; has been correlated to increased risk of heart disease.

hypertension High blood pressure; defined as a systolic blood pressure higher than 140 mm Hg and/or a diastolic blood pressure greater than 90 mm Hg.

normal blood pressure Systolic blood pressure less than 120 mm Hg (the top number) and a diastolic blood pressure less than 80 mm Hg (the bottom number); referred to as 120/80.

blood lipid profile Measurement of blood lipids used to assess cardiovascular risk.

TABLE 5.4 | What Blood Cholesterol Concentrations* Indicate

Total Cholesterol (mg/dl)	Interpretation
< 200	Desirable
200–239	Borderline high
≥ 240	High

LDL Cholesterol (mg/dl)	Interpretation
< 100	Optimal
100–129	Near or above optimal
130–159	Borderline high
160–189	High
≥ 190	Very high

HDL Cholesterol (mg/dl)	Interpretation
> 60	Desirable
40–60	Adequate
< 40	Low

*All lipoprotein concentrations are measured in milligrams of cholesterol per deciliter of blood (mg/dl).

Source: Data from National Cholesterol Education Program. 2001. Detection, Evaluation, and Treatment of High Blood Cholesterol in Adults (Adult Treatment Panel III). National Institutes of Health Publication No. 01-3290.

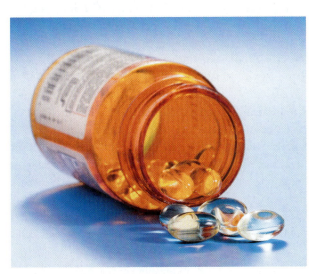

Although fish oil supplements contain omega-3 fatty acids, excessive omega-3 intake can be unhealthy; thus, fish oil supplements should be used only in consultation with a physician.

The best grocery list for lowering blood cholesterol concentrations includes foods that are low in saturated fats, *trans* fats, and cholesterol. Specifically, lean meats, fruits and vegetables, whole grains, fish, shellfish, and fat-free and low-fat dairy products are healthy choices. Snacks and bakery items that contain *trans* fats plus saturated fats increase the risk of heart disease and therefore should be strictly limited or avoided entirely.

Although limiting total saturated fat intake is important, the type of saturated fatty acid may have a greater influence on heart health. Saturated fatty acids such as myristic acid, found in butterfat, may decrease LDL cholesterol when substituted for other saturated fatty acids such as palmitic acid, which raises LDL cholesterol.[38] The same is true for stearic acid, which is good news for chocolate lovers.[39] Though the cocoa butter in chocolate is high in saturated fatty acids, the predominant fat is stearic acid, which neither raises nor lowers LDL cholesterol. Keep in mind that chocolate is still high in kilocalories and shouldn't be consumed in excessive amounts. Reducing saturated fat intake overall, regardless of the type of fatty acid in the molecule, will reduce LDL cholesterol and the risk of heart disease.

Eat More Fish and Plant-Based Foods

The American Heart Association (AHA) encourages Americans to increase their fish and plant-based food consumption as part of a heart-healthy diet. This dietary pattern increases omega-3 fatty acids, reduces saturated fat and LDL cholesterol, and boosts dietary fiber and heart-healthy phytochemicals.

Fish and Other Seafood

In general, seafood contains an abundance of healthy fats. It is true that some shellfish, such as shrimp, are high in cholesterol, but they are very low in saturated fat and contain some heart-healthy omega-3 fatty acids. Lobster has less than one-third the

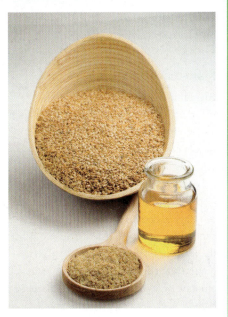

Flaxseeds and flaxseed oil are low in saturated fat.

amount of cholesterol of shrimp and is very low in total fat.

The AHA recommends consuming at least two servings of fish (especially fatty fish) per week to obtain omega-3 fatty acids. These recommendations should be met with baked, poached, or broiled fish. Fried fish that is commercially prepared tends to have few omega-3 fatty acids and is often fried in unhealthy fat. The Table Tips provide a few quick ways to add fish to your diet.

Though consuming some omega-3 fatty acids is good, more may not be better. Because EPA and DHA interfere with blood clotting, consuming more than 3 grams, which typically only happens by taking supplements, could raise both blood glucose and LDL cholesterol concentrations, increase the risk of excessive bleeding, and cause other related problems such as hemorrhagic stroke (*hemo* = blood, *rhagic* = ruptured flow) in which a cerebral artery ruptures, releasing blood into the brain.[40] Because of these potential adverse effects, omega-3 fatty acid supplements (fish oil supplements) should only be consumed with the advice and guidance of a doctor. Eating one gram of EPA and DHA daily from fish may provide some protection against heart disease without any known adverse effects.[41]

Plant-Based Foods

In addition to fish, the AHA recommends consuming plant-based foods such as walnuts, flaxseeds, and soybean and canola oils, which are all high in alpha-linolenic acid.

Eating more plant-based foods high in viscous, soluble fiber may be one of the easiest ways to decrease LDL cholesterol concentrations and lower risk of stroke.[42] While the DRI for fiber ranges from 20 to 38 grams daily, consuming about half of this amount, or 10–25 grams, can help decrease high LDL cholesterol concentrations.

Increasing another plant-based food—soy—may lessen your risk of heart disease by lowering blood pressure.[43] The benefits of soy consumption are discussed in more detail in Chapter 6.

Plant foods are not only cholesterol free but they also contain phytosterols, which are plant sterols similar to cholesterol that are found in the plant's cell membranes. Plant sterols can help lower LDL cholesterol concentrations by competing with cholesterol for absorption in the intestinal tract. With less cholesterol being absorbed, there will be

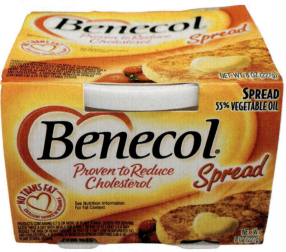

Benecol, a margarine made with plant sterols, may reduce LDL cholesterol concentrations in the blood.

less in the blood. Plant sterols occur naturally in soybean oil, many fruits, legumes, other types of vegetables, sesame seeds, nuts, cereals, and several other plant-based foods. Consuming 2 grams of plant sterols per day lowers LDL cholesterol concentrations by 10 percent and may cut heart disease risk up to 15 percent.[44] Products such as margarines, yogurt, cream cheese spreads, cereals, fruit juices, and soft-gel tablets that contain plant sterols are now available.

Increase Your Intake of Antioxidant Nutrients and Phytochemicals

A diet rich in plants contains antioxidant nutrients such as vitamins E and C, as well as antioxidant phytochemicals. You might think that a substance that begins with the prefix -anti couldn't be good for you. However, antioxidants protect cells from oxidative damage by neutralizing free radicals, which not only cause rancidity of fats in foods but can also damage body cells. They also stimulate your immune system to repair tissue damage and reduce the risk of heart disease.[45] (For more information on antioxidants, see Chapter 9.)

Nuts are one type of food that is rich in antioxidants and fiber and can have a positive effect on LDL cholesterol concentrations. In one study, a diet with 20 percent

of kilocalories from walnuts lowered LDL cholesterol by a little over 15 percent in healthy men.[46] In women, those who ate one ounce of nuts at least five times a week had a 35 percent reduction in the risk of heart disease compared with women who rarely ate nuts.[47] The only downside to nuts is that they are high in kilocalories. A mere ounce of nuts can contribute a hefty 160–200 kilocalories to your diet. However, there is evidence that the potential kilocalorie content of nuts is not as high as the actual kilocalories the body obtains. It's thought that chewing and other forms of mechanical and chemical digestion don't fully release the energy found within the cell walls of nuts.[48] The Table Tips provide ideas on how to enjoy a modest amount of nuts in your diet.

Other antioxidant phytochemicals may also boost heart health. Garlic contains organosulfur compounds that have been found in some studies to reduce high blood cholesterol concentrations by inhibiting cholesterol synthesis in the body, decreasing the clustering of platelets, interfering with blood clotting, and helping to lower blood pressure. Black and green tea are high in **flavonoids,** antioxidant phytochemicals that are believed to prevent LDL cholesterol from becoming oxidized in the body. Drinking tea is associated with a lower incidence of dying from heart disease.[49] Green tea is particularly high in catechins, antioxidants that may also reduce total and LDL cholesterol.[50]

When it comes to reducing the risk of heart disease, the whole diet may be greater than the sum of its parts. Consume a diet low in saturated fat and cholesterol and high in soluble fiber, soy protein, plant sterols, and nuts to lower total cholesterol and LDL cholesterol. The Table Tips summarize several eating tips for a heart-healthy diet.

TABLE TIPS
Easy Ways to Add Fish to the Diet

Flake canned salmon over a lunch or dinner salad.

Add tuna to cooked pasta and vegetables and toss with a light salad dressing for a quick pasta salad meal.

Order baked, broiled, or grilled fish when dining out.

Try a shrimp cocktail for added omega-3 fatty acids.

---

flavonoids Phytochemicals found in fruits, vegetables, tea, nuts, and seeds that have antioxidant properties and neutralize free radicals.

Nuts about Nuts?

Toss some nuts into a mealtime salad. Use less oil or salad dressing and more nonfat vinegar to adjust for the added kilocalories.

Swap nuts for meat, like chicken or beef, in meals such as stir-fries. A third of a cup of nuts is equal in protein to an ounce of red meat or chicken.

Add a tablespoon of nuts to morning cereal, and use skim rather than reduced-fat milk to offset some of the extra kilocalories.

Add a tablespoon of chopped nuts to an afternoon yogurt.

Add a handful of peanuts to air-popped popcorn for a snack.

Moderate Alcohol Consumption Has Protective Effects

Some researchers have shown that drinking alcohol in moderate amounts (no more than one drink for females, two drinks for males daily) can reduce the risk of heart disease.[51] The heart-protective action of alcohol may occur through three different mechanisms. First, alcohol can increase the level of the heart-protective HDL cholesterol. In fact, approximately 50 percent of alcohol's heart-protective effect is probably due to this positive effect on HDL cholesterol. Second, alcohol may decrease blood clotting by affecting the coagulation of platelets or by helping the blood to break up clots.[52] Third, the antioxidants in wine as well as in dark beer may stabilize free radicals and thereby contribute to the heart-protective effects of alcohol.[53]

The health benefits of alcohol have only been demonstrated in middle-aged individuals. In addition, the problems associated with overconsumption far outweigh the health benefits of moderation. In fact, individuals who consume three or more drinks per day *increase* their risk of dying prematurely.[54] (Alcohol is the subject of Chapter 7.)

Exercise, Manage Your Weight, and Quit Smoking

Regular exercise is one way to help lower LDL cholesterol, raise HDL cholesterol, reduce hypertension and insulin resistance, and lose weight.[55] A review of over 50 studies involving more than 4,500 people found that exercise training for more than 12 weeks increased HDL cholesterol concentrations by about 4.5 percent. Currently, the AHA recommends that healthy individuals engage in 30 minutes or more of moderate exercise on most days, if not every day. This amount of physical activity is considered sufficient to help reduce the risk of heart disease, but exercising longer than 30 minutes or at higher intensity could offer greater protection, especially when it comes to maintaining a healthy body weight.[56] Sedentary individuals should "move" and sedentary, overweight individuals should "move and lose" to lower their risk of heart disease. **Table 5.5** summarizes the diet and lifestyle changes that can help lower LDL cholesterol concentrations and risk for heart disease.

In addition to regular exercise and losing excess weight, quit smoking. Smoking damages the walls of the arteries and accelerates atherosclerosis. In fact, individuals who smoke are three times more likely to have a heart attack than nonsmokers.[57]

Eating for a Healthy Heart

Choose only lean meats (round, sirloin, and tenderloin cuts) and skinless poultry, and keep portions to about 6 ounces. Eat fish at least twice a week.

Use two egg whites in place of a whole egg when baking.

Use reduced-fat or nonfat dairy products, such as low-fat or skim milk, reduced-fat cheese, and low-fat or nonfat ice cream. Sprinkle cheese on top of food rather than mixing it in, so as to use less. Be sure to keep ice cream servings small.

Substitute cooked beans for half the meat in chili, soups, and casseroles.

Use canola, olive, soybean, or corn oil, and *trans* fat–free margarine instead of butter or shortening.

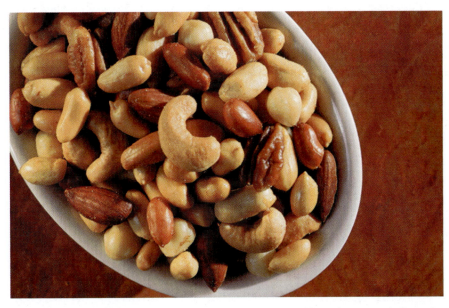
Though high in kilocalories, nuts are an excellent source of antioxidants, have zero cholesterol, and are low in saturated fat.

TABLE 5.5	To Decrease Excess LDL Cholesterol
Dietary Changes	**Lifestyle Changes**
• Consume less saturated fat • Strickly limit *trans* fats • Consume less dietary cholesterol • Consume more foods rich in soluble fiber • Consume a plant-based diet	• Lose excess body weight • Exercise more

LO 5.6: THE TAKE-HOME MESSAGE Heart disease is primarily caused by athero-sclerosis, a narrowing of the arteries due to a buildup of plaque. Uncontrollable risk factors for heart disease include age, gender, and genetics; controllable risk factors include high LDL blood cholesterol, low HDL blood cholesterol, high blood pressure, excess body weight, inactivity, type 2 diabetes, and smoking. Limiting saturated fat, cholesterol, and *trans* fat and increasing fish consumption, as well as consuming antioxidant-rich fruits, vegetables, whole grains, and nuts, are dietary choices associated with a reduction in the risk of heart disease. Drinking a moderate amount of alcohol may help reduce the risk of heart disease in middle-aged and older adults. Regular exercise and maintaining a healthy body weight can also help lower LDL cholesterol concentrations and raise HDL cholesterol concentrations. If you currently smoke, quit, because smoking damages the walls of the arteries.

NUTRITION *in* PRACTICE:
Physical Therapist and MD

During spring break, Brendan, a 20-year-old junior in finance, visited his doctor because of a re-occurring pain in his foot whenever he worked out at the gym as well as his annual physical. The doctor referred Brendan to a physical therapist (PT) for his foot pain, which he diagnosed as plantar fasciitis. Because Brendan's family has a history of heart disease, the doctor also order a blood test to assess his blood cholesterol levels. Within a few days of his physical, the nurse at his doctor's office called with the laboratory results. Similar to his parents, Brendan's blood cholesterol levels were not in a healthy range. The nurse suggested that he meet with a local registered dietitian nutritionist (RDN) to see if he could change his diet to lower his levels. Because he has an unlimited meal plan at college, his mom suggested that he set up an appointment with the campus RDN for nutrition counseling and advice about what to eat at the dining hall.

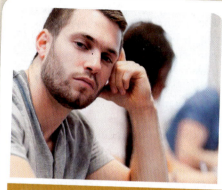

Brendan

BRENDAN'S FOOD LOG

Food/Beverage	Time Consumed	Hunger Rating*	Location
Egg, sausages, hash browns with a glass of whole milk	9:30 A.M.	5	Campus dining hall
Hot dogs and fries Whole milk	1:30 P.M.	3	Campus dining hall
Cookies	3:00 P.M.	4	Watching in dorm room
Steak, rice, corn	6:30 P.M.	4	Campus dining hall
Ice cream	11:00 P.M.	4	His dorm room

*Hunger Rating (1–5): 1 = not hungry; 5 = super hungry.

Brendan's Stats:
- Age: 20
- Height: 6 feet 1 inch
- Weight: 220 pounds
- BMI: 29
- Total Cholesterol: 240 mg/dl
- LDL Cholesterol: 185 mg/dl
- HDL Cholesterol: 37 mg/dl. Suggest putting a real number rather than under 40

Critical Thinking Questions
1. How could Brendan's food choices potentially contribute to his high blood cholesterol level?
2. What foods could be added to Brendan's diet to help lower his cholesterol?
3. What lifestyle changes could Brendan make to possibly increase his HDL cholesterol?
4. What is your assessment of Brendan's weight?

RDN's Observation and Plan for Brendan:
- Discuss the need to reduce saturated fat to less than 10 percent of total kilocalories and dietary cholesterol to less than 300 milligrams (mg) per day to help lower his blood cholesterol. Order an egg white omelet with vegetables, and switch from whole to low fat milk. Order a turkey sandwich at lunch and grilled poultry or fish more often at dinner. Try to consume at least two fish meals weekly. Opt for reduced calorie ice milk or frozen yogurt rather than ice cream for an occasional treat.
- Increase the soluble fiber at his meals to further lower his cholesterol. Consider eating oatmeal for breakfast twice a week and add a salad bar salad of fresh vegetables with beans at lunch with his sandwich. Keep fruit in dorm room for an evening snack.
- Increase physical activity to at least 2.5 hours weekly under the guidance of a PT. Exercise may help increase the HDL cholesterol.

Three weeks later, Brendan visits the RDN again. He has made the switch from whole milk to low fat milk and trying to eat oatmeal for breakfast on most days. A review of his food record shows that his saturated fat is a little over 10 percent of his total calorie intake but his dietary cholesterol is less than 300 mg. He is having difficulty eating two fish meals weekly so the RDN suggests that Brendan consume tuna fish sandwiches made with tuna packed in water and reduced fat mayonnaise at lunch at least twice a week. Use low fat mayo or salad dressing to prepare and purchase tuna in water vs. tuna in oil for calorie control.

PT's Observation and Plan for Brendan:
- Explained that plantar fasciitis is a chronic inflammation of the plantar fascia, which is the thick band of tissue that connects the heel bone to the toes. This inflammation is causing pain and tightness in the bottom of the foot.
- Recommends that he wear shoes, such as sneakers, that support the arch of the foot.
- Provided stretching program that he should in the morning and at night.

Brendan returns to the PT in two weeks and is experiencing some improvement. The PT adjusts his stretching program.

Visual Chapter Summary

LO 5.1 Lipids Are Hydrophobic Compounds That Vary in Structure

Lipids refer to a category of carbon, oxygen, and hydrogen compounds that don't dissolve in water. There are three types: triglycerides, phospholipids, and sterols. Triglycerides and phospholipids are built from fatty acids, which consist of a chain of carbon and hydrogen atoms with an acid group (COOH) at the alpha end and a methyl group (CH₃) at the omega end.

Short-chain fatty acids contain fewer than six carbons; medium-chain fatty acids have 6–10 carbons; and long-chain fatty acids have 12 or more carbons. A saturated fatty acid has all of its carbons bound with hydrogen. An unsaturated fatty acid that has one double bond is called a monounsaturated fatty acid. A polyunsaturated fatty acid contains two or more double bonds. If the first double bond is located between the third and fourth carbon from the omega end it is called an omega-3 fatty acid. The first double bond for an omega-6 fatty acid is between carbons 6 and 7 from the omega end.

Unsaturated fatty acids have either a *cis* (hydrogen atoms are on the same side of the double bond) or a *trans* configuration (one hydrogen atom is on the opposite side of the double bond). Phospholipids are made of two fatty acids and a phosphate-containing group attached to a glycerol backbone. Sterols do not contain glycerol or fatty acids but are composed of four connecting rings of carbon and hydrogen.

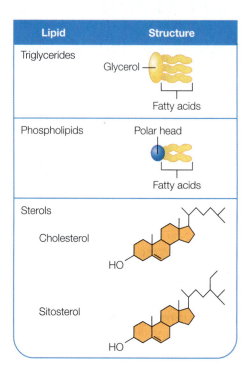

Lipid	Structure
Triglycerides	Glycerol — / Fatty acids
Phospholipids	Polar head / Fatty acids
Sterols	
Cholesterol	HO
Sitosterol	HO

LO 5.2 Most Lipid Digestion Occurs in the Small Intestine

Most fat digestion occurs in the small intestine. Fat globules are emulsified by bile before pancreatic lipase hydrolyzes the fatty acids, producing two free fatty acids and a monoglyceride. Sterols are absorbed intact. Phospholipids are hydrolyzed by phospholipases.

Glycerol and short- and medium-chain fatty acids enter the portal vein and go directly to the liver. Free long-chain fatty acids are absorbed into enterocytes within micelles. They are then disassembled and recombined with other dietary lipids into chylomicrons, which are released into the lymph fluid.

Chylomicrons transport dietary fat to the cells. Very low-density lipoproteins (VLDLs) and low-density lipoproteins (LDLs) carry lipids from the liver to the cells. High-density lipoproteins (HDLs) pick up cholesterol from the body cells and return it to the liver.

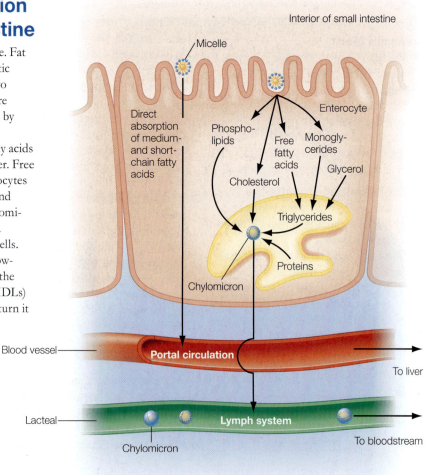

LO 5.3 Lipids Play Many Key Roles in the Body

Lipids provide essential fatty acids, enhance the absorption of the fat-soluble vitamins, provide a layer of insulation, and cushion the major organs. Essential fatty acids are needed for healthy cell membranes and to produce eicosanoids that regulate certain body functions. Fat is also an important source of energy, providing 9 kilocalories per gram.

Phospholipids and cholesterol make up the cell membranes. Cholesterol is also a precursor for vitamin D, bile, and sex hormones such as estrogen and testosterone.

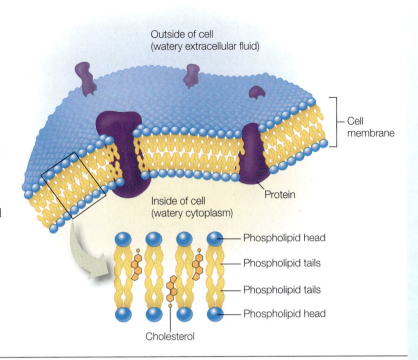

Outside of cell (watery extracellular fluid)

Cell membrane

Inside of cell (watery cytoplasm)

Protein

Phospholipid head

Phospholipid tails

Phospholipid tails

Phospholipid head

Cholesterol

LO 5.4 Moderate Consumption of Dietary Fat Is Essential for Health

The AMDR for fat is 20–35 percent of daily kilocalories. No more than 10 percent of energy should come from saturated fat and less than 1 percent from *trans* fats. A minimum of 5–10 percent of the total kilocalories should come from linoleic acid and 0.6–1.2 percent from alpha-linolenic acid.

Men ages 19–50 need 17 grams and women need 12 grams of linoleic acid daily. Men ages 14–70 need 1.6 grams and women need 1.1 grams of alpha-linolenic acid daily.

Cholesterol and phospholipids are both made in the body and are not considered essential nutrients.

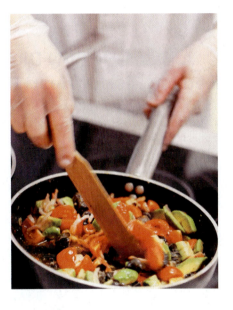

LO 5.5 The Best Food Sources of Fat Contain Unsaturated Fats and Essential Fatty Acids

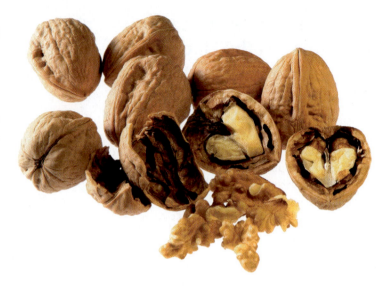

Unsaturated fats are abundant in vegetable oils, soybeans, walnuts, flaxseeds, and wheat germ, and these are also all good sources of linoleic acid. Walnuts, flaxseeds, and canola oil are good sources of alpha-linolenic acid.

Most saturated fat comes from animal foods such as fatty cuts of meat, whole-milk dairy products, butter, ice cream, and the skin of poultry. Certain vegetable oils, such as coconut, palm, and palm kernel oils, are very high in saturated fat. *Trans* fats are mostly found in processed foods and must be listed on the food label. The FDA has banned foods containing partially hydrogenated oils—the source of most *trans* fats in the diet—from commercially prepared foods. Dietary cholesterol is found only in foods from animal sources such as egg yolks, meats, and whole-fat dairy. Fat substitutes can be carbohydrate based, protein based, or fat based. Reduced-fat or fat-free foods still contain kilocalories and should be eaten in limited amounts.

LO 5.6 A Heart-Healthy Diet and Lifestyle Changes Can Reduce Risk of Heart Disease

Atherosclerosis, the narrowing of arteries due to plaque buildup, is a primary cause of cardiovascular disease, including coronary heart disease. Consuming too much saturated and *trans* fat can increase blood cholesterol concentrations, a factor in atherosclerosis. The goal is to lower the LDL level to less than 100 milligrams per deciliter (mg/dl) and raise the HDL level to greater than 40 mg/dl.

To lower LDL cholesterol, eat a balanced plant-based diet. Limit commercially prepared baked goods, snack items, and fried foods to decrease *trans* fat intake. Consume plenty of foods providing soluble fiber, such as oats and legumes. Drinking a moderate amount of alcohol may help reduce the risk of heart disease in middle-aged and older adults.

Regular exercise and maintaining a healthy weight can also help lower LDL cholesterol concentrations and raise HDL cholesterol concentrations. If you currently smoke, quit.

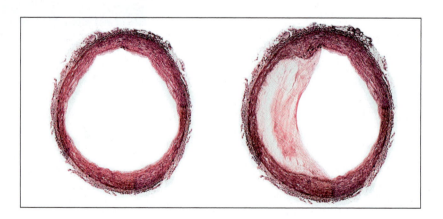

Terms to Know

- lipid
- hydrophobic
- fatty acid
- short-chain fatty acid
- medium-chain fatty acid
- long-chain fatty acid
- saturated fatty acid
- unsaturated fatty acid
- monounsaturated fatty acid
- polyunsaturated fatty acid
- oils
- rancidity
- free radical
- hydrogenation
- omega-3 fatty acid
- omega-6 fatty acid
- linoleic acid
- alpha-linolenic acid
- essential fatty acids
- *cis*
- *trans*
- triglycerides
- glycerol
- phospholipids
- choline
- lecithin
- emulsifier
- sterols
- cholesterol
- phytosterols
- phytostanols
- lipases
- diglyceride
- monoglyceride
- micelle
- lipoprotein
- chylomicron
- lipoprotein lipase (LPL)
- very low-density lipoproteins (VLDLs)
- low-density lipoproteins (LDLs)
- high-density lipoproteins (HDLs)
- adipocytes
- eicosanoids
- arachidonic acid
- eicosapentaenoic acid (EPA) and docosahexaenoic acid (DHA)
- hypertriglyceridemia
- *trans* fats
- fat substitutes
- carbohydrate-based substitutes
- protein-based substitutes
- fat-based substitutes
- cardiovascular disease (CVD)
- heart attack
- stroke
- atherosclerosis
- plaque
- C-reactive protein (CRP)
- Lp(a) protein
- hypertension
- normal blood pressure
- blood lipid profile
- flavonoids

Mastering Nutrition

Visit the Study Area in Mastering Nutrition to hear an MP3 chapter summary.

Check Your Understanding

LO 5.1 1. Fatty acids vary in structure based on all of the following *except*
   a. shape.
   b. degree of saturation.
   c. length of carbon chain.
   d. presence or absence of hydrogen.

LO 5.2 2. Which statement best describes the characteristics of foods high in unsaturated fatty acids?
   a. They are solid at room temperature.
   b. They are more stable than saturated fatty acids and resist oxidation.
   c. They tend to be liquid at room temperature.
   d. They are higher in kilocalorie content than a saturated fatty acid.

LO 5.2 3. The type of lipoprotein that carries absorbed dietary fat and other lipids through the lymph system is called
   a. a micelle.
   b. a VLDL.
   c. an LDL.
   d. a chylomicron.

LO 5.3 4. Arachidonic acid and eicosapentaenoic acid (EPA) are
   a. used to manufacture hormonelike substances called eicosanoids.
   b. stored as part of the subcutaneous tissue needed to insulate the body.
   c. the main fatty acids used to manufacture bile in the liver.
   d. used by the body to manufacture the essential fatty acids linoleic acid and alpha-linolenic acid.

LO 5.4 5. The AMDR for dietary fat intake is
   a. less than 10 percent of daily kilocalories.
   b. 20–35 percent of daily kilocalories.
   c. 40–45 percent of daily kilocalories.
   d. as low as possible.

LO 5.5 6. At least two fish meals should be consumed weekly to obtain the heart-healthy omega-3 fatty acids. Examples of heart-healthy fish meals include
   a. a tuna fish sandwich and a Burger King fish sandwich.
   b. boiled or grilled shrimp and grilled salmon.
   c. fish and chips and flounder.
   d. fried fish sticks and steamed lobster.

LO 5.5 7. Which of the following foods does not contain dietary cholesterol?
   a. Steak
   b. Chicken
   c. Low-fat milk
   d. Peanut butter

LO 5.5 8. Which of the following foods are good sources of the essential fatty acids linoleic acid and alpha-linolenic acid?
   a. Ground flaxseeds
   b. Cheese
   c. Butter
   d. Oranges

LO 5.6 9. The major dietary component that raises blood LDL cholesterol is
   a. viscous soluble fiber.
   b. C-reactive protein.
   c. saturated fat.
   d. plant sterols.

LO 5.6 10. To raise the level of HDL cholesterol,
- a. increase the viscous, soluble fiber in the diet.
- b. increase exercise.
- c. maintain a healthy body weight.
- d. do all of the above.

Answers

1. (d) All lipids contain carbon, hydrogen, and oxygen. Lipids vary in shape, saturation, and length of their carbon chains.

2. (c) Foods high in unsaturated fats are typically liquid at room temperature. Plant oils are an example. Foods high in saturated fats are solid at room temperature. Butter is an example. Because unsaturated fatty acids contain double bonds, they are more unstable and tend to oxidize easier than saturated fatty acids. All fatty acids have the same number of kilocalories per serving.

3. (d) Chylomicrons are capsule-shaped carriers that enable insoluble fat as well as cholesterol and phospholipids to travel through the watery lymph system to the bloodstream. Micelles enable dietary fats to cross from the lumen of the GI tract into the enterocytes. VLDLs and LDLs are lipoproteins that transport fat and other lipids through the bloodstream.

4. (a) Arachidonic acid and eicosapentaenoic acid (EPA) are used to manufacture eicosanoids such as prostaglandins, thromboxanes, and leukotrienes. They are not stored in subcutaneous tissue or used to synthesize cholesterol. These two compounds are made from the essential fatty acids linoleic acid and alpha-linolenic acid.

5. (b) The AMDR for daily fat intake is 20–35 percent of total daily kilocalories. Saturated fat intake should be less than 10 percent of daily kilocalories. *Trans* fat intake should be as low as possible.

6. (b) While tuna fish is a wonderful way to enjoy fish at lunch, the commercially prepared fried fish sandwich, fish and chips, and fish sticks have little of the heart-healthy omega-3 fatty acids. Boiled shrimp and grilled salmon are much healthier ways to enjoy fish.

7. (d) Because plant sources are not a significant source of dietary cholesterol, peanut butter, which is made from peanuts, is free of dietary cholesterol.

8. (a) Ground flaxseeds are a good source of essential fatty acids.

9. (c) Saturated fat is the key culprit behind elevated LDL cholesterol in the blood. Viscous, soluble fiber, such as psyllium, as well as plant sterols can help lower LDL cholesterol. C-reactive protein is not a dietary component, but a protein produced in the body during inflammation.

10. (b) Increasing exercise can help increase the HDL cholesterol level. Increasing soluble fiber intake and maintaining a healthy body weight can help lower the LDL cholesterol level but do not affect the level of HDL cholesterol.

Answers to True or False?

1. **False.** While the body *does* need cholesterol for important functions, it can be synthesized in the liver in sufficient amounts. Thus, consuming dietary cholesterol is not necessary.

2. **False.** Whereas too much dietary fat may cause weight gain, eating too little isn't healthy, either. A diet low in fat but high in added sugars may increase the level of triglycerides in the blood.

3. **False.** Though the majority of *trans* fats are made from hydrogenated oils that are found in commercially prepared, processed foods, *trans* fats also occur naturally in foods such as meat and dairy products.

4. **True.** A diet high in saturated fat can raise blood cholesterol.

5. **False.** Fat-free foods often have added carbohydrates, which add back kilocalories. The savings in fat kilocalories is usually not much of a savings in total kilocalories.

6. **True.** High concentrations of HDL cholesterol can help reduce the risk of heart disease.

7. **False.** Although a limited number of stick margarines still contain heart-unhealthy *trans* fats, and these may legally be sold through July 2018, most margarines are now formulated to be heart-healthy. In contrast, butter is high in cholesterol-raising saturated fats, and so is ultimately less healthy.

8. **False.** Because nuts are plant foods, they do not contain cholesterol but are rich sources of essential fatty acids and plant sterols.

9. **False.** Consuming too much fish oil can be unhealthy. The best source of omega-3 fatty acids is fresh fish.

10. **False.** LDL cholesterol is a lipoprotein carrier found in the blood and is not found in foods.

Web Resources

To learn more about lipids and health, visit

- National Cholesterol Education Program at www.nhlbi.nih.gov
- EPA Fish Advisories at www.epa.gov
- American Heart Association at www.americanheart.org
- EFA Education at http://efaeducation.nih.gov
- National Heart, Lung, and Blood Institute at www.nhlbi.nih.gov
- Centers for Disease Control and Prevention, Physical Activity, Energize Your Life! at www.cdc.gov
- Heart Healthy Women at www.hearthealthywomen.org
- WebMD Heart Health Center at www.webmd.com
- Lipid Corner for the Lipid Research Division of ASBMB at www.asbmb.org
- MEDLINE Plus Health Information at www.nlm.nih.gov/medlineplus
- Seafood Watch at www.seafoodwatch.org

References

1. Gylling, H., and P. Simonen. 2015. Phytosterols, Phytostanols, and Lipoprotein Metabolism. *Nutrients* 7(9):7965–7977. doi: 10.3390/nu7095374.

2. Centers for Disease Control and Prevention: National Center for Health Statistics. 2016. *Diet/Nutrition.* Available at https://www.cdc.gov/nchs/fastats/diet.htm. Accessed February 2017.

3. Ibid.

4. Institute of Medicine. 2006. *Dietary Reference Intakes: The Essential Guide to Nutrient Requirements.* Washington, DC: National Academies Press.

5. Ibid.

6. Ulven, S. M., and K. B. Holven. 2015. Comparison of Bioavailability of Krill Oil Versus Fish Oil and Health Effect. *Vascular Health and Risk Management* 11:511–524. doi: 10.2147/VHRM.S85165.

7. USDA Center for Nutrition Policy and Promotion. 2015-2020 Dietary Guidelines for Americans. Available at https://www.cnpp.usda.gov/2015-2020-dietary-guidelines-americans. Accessed February 2017.

8. Yang, Z. H., B. Emma-Okon, and A.T. Ramely, 2016. Dietary Marine-Derived Long Chain Monounsaturated Fatty Acids and

Cardiovascular Disease Risk: A Mini Review. *Lipids in Health and Disease* 15(1):201.

9. Da Silva, M. S., P. Julien, L. Pérusse, M. C. Vohl, and I. Rudkowska, 2015. Natural Rumen-Derived *Trans* Fatty Acids Are Associated with Metabolic Markers of Cardiac Health. *Lipids* 50(9):873–882. doi: 10.1007/s11745-015-4055-3.

10. Asghari, G., et al. 2012. Effect of Pomegranate Seed Oil on Serum TNF-α Level. *International Journal of Food Sciences and Nutrition* 63(3):368–371. doi: 10.3109/09637486.2011.631521.

11. Brouwer, I. A., A. J. Wanders, and M. B. Katan. 2013. *Trans* Fatty Acids and Cardiovascular Health: Research Completed? *European Journal of Clinical Nutrition* 67:541–547.

12. Food and Drug Administration. 2017. Trans *Fat Added to Nutrition Labels.* Available at www.fda.gov. Accessed February 2017.

13. Kris-Etherton, P. M., M. Lefere, and B. D. Flickinger. 2012. *Trans*-Fatty Acid Intakes and Food Sources in the U.S. Population: NHANES 1999–2002. *Lipids* 47(10):931–940.

14. Jaceldo-Siegl, K., et al. 2017. Variations in Dietary Intake and Plasma Concentration of Plant Sterols Across Plant-based Diets Among North American Adults. *Molecular Nutrition and Food Research* doi: 10.1002/mnfr.201600828.

15. Gylling, H., et al. 2013. The Effects of Plant Stanol Ester Consumption on Arterial Stiffness and Endothelial Function in Adults: A Randomised Controlled Clinical Trial. *BMC Cardiovascular Disorders* 13:50. doi: 10.1186/1471-2261-13-50.

16. Calorie Control Council. 2017. *Fat Replacers.* Available at www.caloriecontrol.org. Accessed February 2017.

17. Ibid.

18. Wylie-Rosett, J. 2002. Fat Substitutes and Health: An Advisory from the Nutrition Committee of the American Heart Association. *Circulation* 105:2800–2804.

19. Calorie Control Council. 2014. *Fat Replacers.*

20. Ibid.

21. Patterson, R. E., A. R. Kristal, J. C. Peters, M. L. Neuhouser, C. L. Rock, L. J. Cheskin, D. Neumark-Sztainer, and M. D. Thornquist. 2000. Changes in Diet, Weight, and Serum Lipid Levels Associated with Olestra Consumption. *Archives of Internal Medicine* 160:2600–2604.

22. Kris-Etherton, P. M., et al. 2012. *Trans* Fatty Acid Intakes and Food Sources.

23. American Heart Association. 2014. *Heart Disease and Stroke Statistics—2014 Update.* Available at www.myamericanheart.org. Accessed February 2017.

24. National Vital Statistics Report. 2016. Deaths, Leading Causes for 2014. Available at https://www.cdc.gov. Accessed February 2017.

25. Goldstein, J. L., and M. S. Brown. 1987. Regulation of Low-Density Lipoprotein Receptors: Implications for Pathogenesis and Therapy of Hypercholesterolemia and Atherosclerosis. *Circulation* 76:504–507.

26. Pendyal, A., and S. Fazio. 2015. The Severe Hypercholesterolemia Phenotype: Genes

and Beyond, In De Groot, L. J., Chrousos, G., Dungan, K., et al., editors. South Dartmouth (MA): MDText.com, Inc. Available from https://www.ncbi.nlm.nih.gov/books/NBK343488. Accessed February 2017.

27. Ibid.

28. Tanveer, S., et al. 2016. Clinical and Angiographic Correlation of High-sensitivity C-reactive Protein with Acute ST Elevation Myocardial Infarction. *Experimental and Therapeutic Medicine* 12(6):4089–4098. doi:10.3892/etm.2016.3882.

29. Ganguly, P., and S. F. Alam. 2015. Role of Homocysteine in the Development of Cardiovascular Disease. *Nutrition Journal.* doi:10.1186/1475-2891-14-6.

30. Joshi, R., B. Khandelwal, D. Joshi, and O.P. Gupta. 2013. *Chlamydophila pneumoniae* Infection and Cardiovascular Disease. *North American Journal of Medicine* (5)3:169–181.

31. Tsimikas, S, and J. L. Hall. 2012. Lipoprotein(a) as a Potential Causal Genetic Risk Factor of Cardiovascular Disease: A Rationale for Increased Efforts to Understand Its Pathophysiology and Develop Targeted Therapies. *Journal of the American College of Cardiology* 60(8):716–721.

32. American Heart Association. 2016. *About Metabolic Syndrome.* Available at www.heart.org. Accessed February 2017.

33. Psaltopoulou, T., et al. 2017. Socioeconomic Status and Risk Factors for Cardiovascular Disease: Impact of Dietary Mediators. *Hellenic Journal of Cardiology.* doi: 10.1016/j.hjc.2017.01.022.

34. American Heart Association. 2013. *Why Cholesterol Matters.* Available at www.heart.org. Accessed February 2017.

35. Ibid.

36. Neddleton, J. A., I. A. Brower, J. M Geleijnse, and Hornstra G. 2017. Saturated Fat Consumption and Risk of Coronary Heart Diseae and Ischemic Stroke: A Science Update. *Annuals of Nutrition Metabolism* 70(1):26–33. doi: 10.1159/000455681.

37. American Heart Association. 2014. *Trans Fats.* Available at www.heart.org. Accessed February 2014.

38. Brouwer, I. A., A. J. Wanders, and M. B. Katan. 2013. *Trans* Fatty Acids and Cardiovascular Health: Research Completed? *European Journal of Clinical Nutrition* 67:541–547.

39. Zong, G., et al. 2016. Intake of Individual Saturated Fatty Acids and Risk of Coronary Heart Disease in US Men and Women: Two Prospective Longitudinal Cohort Studies. *BMJ* 355:i5796. doi: 10.1136/bmj.i5796.

40. Ibid.

41. Mozaffarian, D. R., N. Lemaitre, I. B. King, X. Song, H. Huang, F. M. Sacks, E. B. Rimm, et al. 2013. Plasma Phospholipid Long-Chain ω-3 Fatty Acids and Total and Cause-Specific Mortality in Older Adults: A Cohort Study. *Annals of Internal Medicine* 158(7):515–525.

42. American Heart Association. 2016. *Fish and Omega-3 Fatty Acids.* Available at www.heart.org. Accessed February 2017.

43. American Heart Association. 2013. *Eating More Fiber May Lower Risk of First-Time Stroke.* Available at http://newsroom.heart.org. Accessed February 2017.

44. Melendez, G. C., et al. 2015. Beneficial Effects of Soy Supplementation on Postmenopausal Atherosclerosis Are Dependent on Pretreatment Stage of Plaque Progression. *Menopause.* 22(3):289-96. doi: 10.1097/GME.0000000000000307.

45. Gylling, H., J. Plat, S. Turley, et al. 2014. Plant Sterols and Plant Stanols in the Management of Dyslipidaemia and Prevention of Cardiovascular Disease. *Atherosclerosis* 232(2):346–360.

46. Shaghaghi, A. M., S. S. Abumweis, and P. J. Jones. 2013. Cholesterol-Lowering Efficacy of Plant Sterols/Stanols Provided in Capsule and Tablet Formats: Results of a Systematic Review and Meta-analysis. *Journal of the Academy of Nutrition and Dietetics* 113(11):1494–1503.

47. Wu, L., K. Piotrowski, T. Rau, et al. 2013. Walnut-Enriched Diet Reduces Fasting Non-HDL Cholesterol and Apolipoprotein B in Healthy Caucasian Subjects: A Randomized Controlled Cross-Over Clinical Trial. *Metabolism* doi: 10.1016/j.metabol.2013.11.005.

48. Eilat-Adar, S., T. Sinai, C. Yosefy, and Y. Kenkin. 2013. Nutritional Recommendations for Cardiovascular Disease Prevention. *Nutrients* 5(9):3646–3683.

49. Grundy, M.M., et al. 2015. Effect of Mastication on Lipid Bioaccessibility of Almonds in a Randomized Human Study and Its Implications. *American Journal of Clinical Nutrition* 101(1):25–33. doi: 10.3945/ajcn.114.088328.

50. Miller, P. E., et al. 2017. Associations of Coffee, Tea, and Caffeine Intake with Coronary Artery Calcification and Cardiovascular Events. *American Journal of Medicine* 130(2):188–197.e5. doi: 10.1016/j.amjmed.2016.08.038.

51. Appelhans, B. M., et al. 2016. Beverage Intake and Metabolic Syndrome Risk Over 14 Years: The Study of Women's Health Across the Nation. *Journal of the Academy of Nutrition and Dietetics* pii: S2212-2672(16)31293-X. doi: 10.1016/j.jand.2016.10.011.

52. Ibid.

53. Ibid.

54. Zaridze, D., S. Lewington, D. Phil, A. Boroda, G. Scelo, et al. 2014. Alcohol and Mortality in Russia: Prospective Observational Study of 151,000 Adults. *The Lancet.* doi: 10.1016/S0140-6736(13)62247-3.

55. Brekke, H. K., F. Bertz, K. M. Rasmussen, et al. 2014. Diet and Exercise Interventions Among Overweight and Obese Lactating Women: Randomized Trial of Effects on Cardiovascular Risk Factors. *PLoS One* 9(2):e88250. doi: 10.1371/journal.pone.0088250.

56. Ibid.

57. American Heart Association. 2015. *Why Quit Smoking?* Available at www.heart.org. Accessed February 2017.

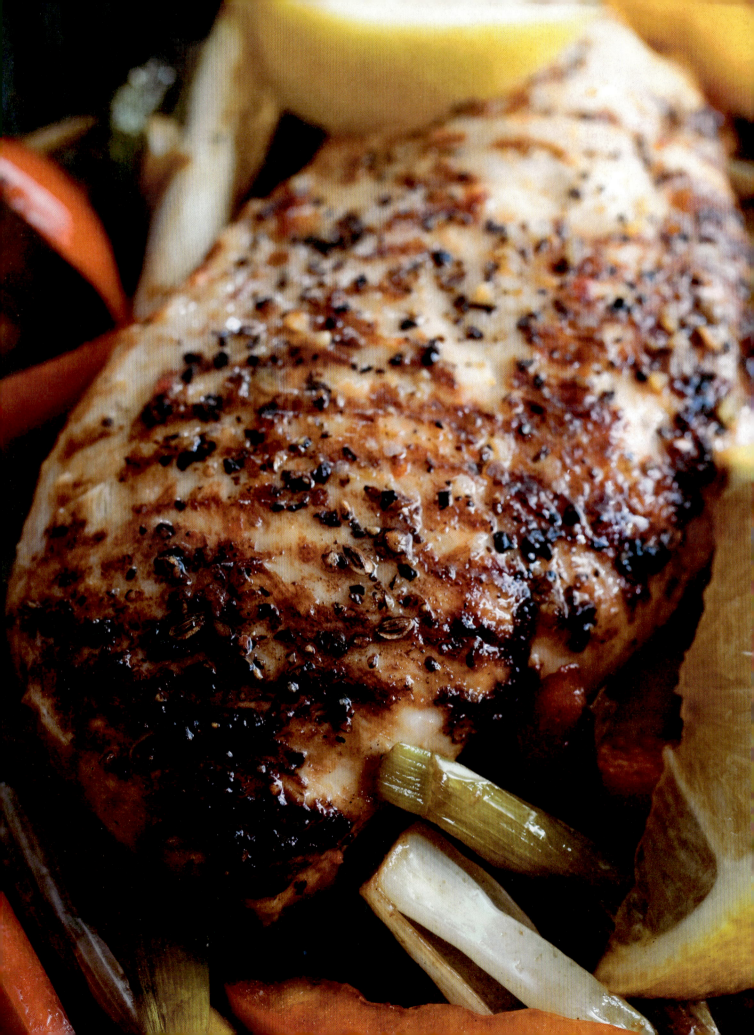

Proteins

Learning Outcomes

After reading this chapter, you will be able to:

6.1 Describe protein, its basic structure and shape, and the classification of amino acids.

6.2 Identify the key steps in digesting proteins and absorbing amino acids.

6.3 Explain the metabolism of amino acids and the role of the amino acid pool.

6.4 Describe the functions of protein in the body.

6.5 Calculate the daily amount of protein recommended based on the Dietary Reference Intakes.

6.6 Describe the best food sources of protein and the methods available to determine protein quality.

6.7 Explain the health consequences of consuming too much or too little protein.

6.8 Describe the benefits and risks of a vegetarian diet.

True or False?

1. Proteins are chemically different from carbohydrates or lipids because they contain nitrogen. **T/F**

2. Proteins are made up of 20 essential amino acids. **T/F**

3. The first step in the chemical digestion of protein occurs in the mouth with the enzyme pepsin. **T/F**

4. Hydrochloric acid denatures protein in the stomach. **T/F**

5. The body can use protein as a source of glucose. **T/F**

6. The primary function of protein is to provide energy to the cells. **T/F**

7. Growing children are in a state of negative nitrogen balance. **T/F**

8. Animal products are a good source of incomplete protein. **T/F**

9. Eating too much protein is associated with high blood cholesterol levels. **T/F**

10. Consuming a diet inadequate in protein may lead to a disease called kwashiorkor. **T/F**

See page 244 for the answers.

Proteins are the predominant structural and functional materials in every cell of the body. In fact, protein alone makes up 50 percent of your body's dry weight. Proteins carry out most of the work of body cells. Your protein-rich muscles enable you to swim, jog, walk, and hold your head up so you can read this chapter. Without adequate protein, your body couldn't replace the skin cells that slough off when you shower or produce sufficient antibodies to fight off infections. Your hair and fingernails wouldn't grow and you wouldn't be able to digest food. Many enzymes and some hormones, which control essential metabolic processes, are made of proteins. They direct how fast the body burns kilocalories, how quickly the heart beats, and possibly your attraction to another person.[1] In short, proteins are involved in all of the body's functions, and without them, you wouldn't survive.[2]

In this chapter we discuss the structure and roles of proteins and how they are digested, absorbed, and synthesized. We also cover the health risks associated with consuming too much or too little protein and the pros and cons of different eating patterns, including vegetarian diets.

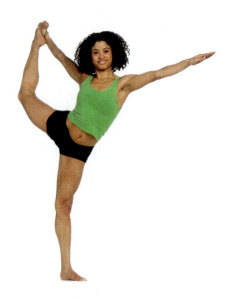

Protein-rich muscles enable you to perform daily activities.

What Are Proteins?

LO 6.1 Describe protein, its basic structure and shape, and the classification of amino acids.

Chemically, the structure of **proteins** is similar to that of carbohydrates and lipids in that all three nutrients contain atoms of carbon (C), hydrogen (H), and oxygen (O). Protein is unique, however, because 16 percent of each protein molecule is nitrogen (N). In fact, protein is the only food component that provides the nitrogen the body needs for important processes, such as the synthesis of neurotransmitters. Some proteins also contain the mineral sulfur (S), which is not found in either carbohydrates or lipids.

The Building Blocks of Proteins Are Amino Acids

In Chapters 4 and 5, you learned that dietary carbohydrates are chains of glucose units and that most dietary lipids contain fatty acid chains (**Figure 6.1**). Proteins are also made up of chains, but the units (or building blocks) of these chains are **amino acids.**

proteins Large molecules, made up of chains of amino acids, found in all living cells.

amino acids Fundamental units of proteins; composed of carbon, hydrogen, oxygen, and nitrogen.

▶ **Figure 6.1 Macronutrient Structure** Carbohydrates, some lipids, and proteins are similar in their chainlike structures. The main difference is that proteins contain nitrogen and carbohydrates and lipids do not. Carbohydrates are composed of glucose chains; triglycerides and phospholipids contain fatty acids; and proteins are made of chains of amino acids.

Macronutrients	Composed of	Example
Carbohydrates	Monosaccharides	Polysaccharide — Glucose units
Lipids	Fatty acids	Triglyceride — Fatty acids
Proteins	Amino acids	Peptide — Amino acids

All proteins in the body consist of a unique combination of up to 20 different amino acids and are classified according to the number of amino acids in the chain. Proteins typically contain between 100 and 10,000 amino acids in a sequence. For instance, the protein that forms the hemoglobin in red blood cells consists of 574 amino acids. In contrast, collagen, a protein found in connective tissue, contains approximately 1,000 amino acids.

Amino acids are like numeric digits: Their specific sequence determines a specific function of the protein. Consider that telephone numbers, Social Security numbers, and bank PIN numbers are all made up of the same digits (0–9) arranged in different sequences of varying lengths. Each of these numbers has a specific purpose. Similarly, amino acids can be linked together to make unique sequences of varying lengths, giving each protein a specific function.

As illustrated in **Figure 6.2**, each amino acid contains a central carbon (C) surrounded by a carboxylic acid group (COOH), which is why it is called an amino "acid"; an **amine group** (NH₂) that contains the nitrogen; a hydrogen atom; and a distinctive **side chain** also referred to as the "R" group. All amino acids contain the same five parts, and the side chain makes each amino acid unique.

Side chains can be as simple as a single hydrogen atom, as in the amino acid glycine, or they can be as complex as the ring structure in phenylalanine (see **Figure 6.2b**). Though each side chain is distinct, some have similar properties. For example, some side chains cause their amino acids to be basic, such as those found in arginine and histidine, whereas others, such as the side chain in aspartic acid, cause their amino acid to be acidic. The side chains of two amino acids, methionine and cysteine, contain sulfur. Some side chains are branched, as in the case of leucine, isoleucine, and valine.

Side chains influence the function of each amino acid, whether the body can make the amino acid, and the metabolic pathway the amino acid follows after absorption. Side chains also influence the shape of the protein because of the way they bond with the side chains of other amino acids. Certain side chains are attracted to certain others; some are neutral; and some repel each other, causing the protein to be either linear or globular in shape. Because the shape of the protein determines its function in the body, anything that alters the attractions between the side chains will alter the protein's shape and thus its function.

Any amino acid chain that contains fewer than 50 amino acids is called a **peptide**. If a chain consists of two joined amino acids it is called a **dipeptide**; three joined amino acids form a **tripeptide**; more than 10 amino acids joined together is called a **polypeptide**. A polypeptide chain that contains 50 or more amino acids is called a *protein*.

Peptide Bonds

Peptide bonds link amino acids into unique chains. They form when the carbon from the acid group (COOH) of one amino acid bonds with the nitrogen atom from the amine group (NH₂) of another amino acid by a condensation reaction (**Figure 6.3**), releasing a molecule of water. In contrast, peptide bonds are broken by hydrolysis, which is particularly important during digestion. In this process, a molecule of water is used to split the bond, adding the hydroxyl (OH) group to one amino acid and hydrogen to the other.

Essential, Nonessential, and Conditional Amino Acids

Nine of the 20 amino acids that the body uses to make protein are classified as **essential amino acids.** It is *essential* that the diet provide them because these amino acids either cannot be made by the body or cannot be made in sufficient quantities to sustain the body's needs.

The remaining 11 amino acids are considered **nonessential amino acids** because the body can make them. It is not essential to consume them. **Table 6.1** lists the 20 known, nutritionally important amino acids by their classification.

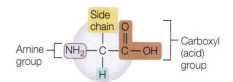

a **Amino acid structure.** All amino acids contain a central carbon surrounded by a side chain, carboxylic acid (COOH), a hydrogen, and an amine group (NH₂).

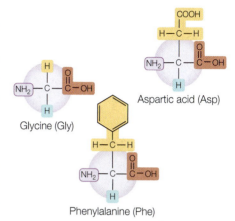

Aspartic acid (Asp)

Glycine (Gly)

Phenylalanine (Phe)

b **Different amino acids with their unique side chains.** A unique side chain (shown in yellow) distinguishes the various amino acids.

▲ **Figure 6.2 The Anatomy of an Amino Acid**

amine group Nitrogen-containing compound (NH₂) connected to the central carbon of an amino acid.

side chain Part of an amino acid that provides its unique qualities; also referred to as the R group.

peptide Chain of amino acids.

dipeptide Chain of two amino acids joined together by a peptide bond.

tripeptide Chain of three amino acids joined together by peptide bonds.

polypeptide Chain consisting of 10 or more amino acids joined together by peptide bonds.

peptide bonds Bonds that connect amino acids; created when the acid group of one amino acid is joined with the amine group of another through condensation.

essential amino acids Nine amino acids that the body cannot synthesize; they must be obtained through dietary sources.

nonessential amino acids Eleven amino acids the body can synthesize and that therefore do not need to be consumed in the diet.

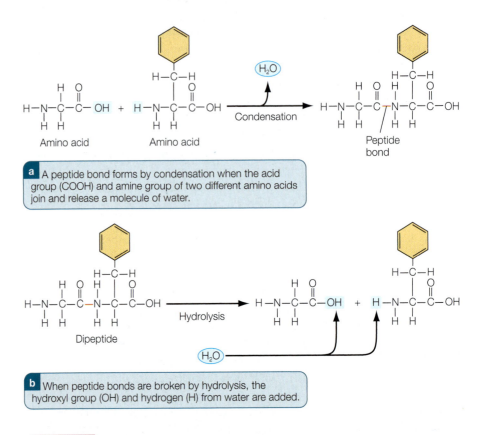

a A peptide bond forms by condensation when the acid group (COOH) and amine group of two different amino acids join and release a molecule of water.

b When peptide bonds are broken by hydrolysis, the hydroxyl group (OH) and hydrogen (H) from water are added.

TABLE 6.1	The Mighty Twenty	

Essential Amino Acids	Nonessential Amino Acids (Conditionally Essential[b] Amino Acids in Italics)
Histidine (His)[a]	Alanine (Ala)
Isoleucine (Ile)	*Arginine (Arg)*
Leucine (Leu)	Asparagine (Asn)
Lysine (Lys)	Aspartic acid (Asp)
Methionine (Met)	*Cysteine (Cys)*
Phenylalanine (Phe)	Glutamic acid (Glu)
Threonine (Thr)	*Glutamine (Gln)*
Tryptophan (Trp)	*Glycine (Gly)*
Valine (Val)	*Proline (Pro)*
	Serine (Ser)
	Tyrosine (Tyr)

[a]Histidine was once thought to be essential only for infants. It is now known that small amounts are also needed for adults.

[b]These amino acids can be "conditionally essential" if there are either inadequate precursors or inadequate enzymes available to create these in the body.

Some nonessential amino acids may become **conditionally essential amino acids** if the body cannot make them because of illness or because the body lacks the necessary precursors or enzymes. In such situations, the amino acid involved is considered essential and must be consumed. An example of this is when premature infants are not able to make enough of the enzymes needed to synthesize arginine; they need to get this amino acid in their diet.

The Organization and Shape of Proteins Affect Their Function

Every protein has four different levels of structure: primary, secondary, tertiary, and quaternary; each level must be correct in order for the protein to function (**Figure 6.4**).

conditionally essential amino acids Nonessential amino acids that become essential (and must be consumed in the diet) when the body cannot make them.

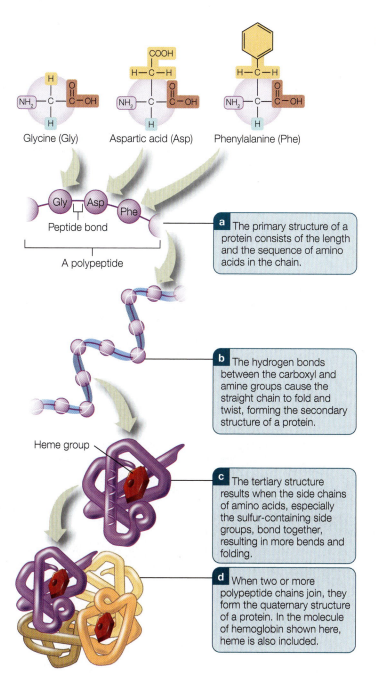

COOH

H—C—H

H—C—H

NH₂—C—C—OH

Glycine (Gly)   Aspartic acid (Asp)   Phenylalanine (Phe)

Gly   Asp   Phe

Peptide bond

A polypeptide

a The primary structure of a protein consists of the length and the sequence of amino acids in the chain.

b The hydrogen bonds between the carboxyl and amine groups cause the straight chain to fold and twist, forming the secondary structure of a protein.

Heme group

c The tertiary structure results when the side chains of amino acids, especially the sulfur-containing side groups, bond together, resulting in more bends and folding.

d When two or more polypeptide chains join, they form the quaternary structure of a protein. In the molecule of hemoglobin shown here, heme is also included.

The **primary structure** is the order in which the amino acids are assembled and the total length—up to thousands of amino acids—of the chain. The amino acids are held together by peptide bonds in a sequence that is unique to that protein. The gene that codes for that protein determines the sequence. A change in just one amino acid in the sequence results in a dramatic change in the eventual shape of the protein and, therefore, its function, in the same way that a telephone number with digits out of order or missing will no longer work.

Once the sequence is formed, the amino acids either attract and form bonds with one another or repel each other. The formation of hydrogen bonds between the carboxyl and amine groups of amino acids in the chain creates the **secondary structure.** The hydrogen bonding causes the straight chain to fold, twist, and coil.

Side chains—especially sulfur-containing side chains—can be attracted to (*hydrophilic*) or repelled by (*hydrophobic*) water in the cells. This property affects how they interact

primary structure First stage of protein synthesis after transcription when the amino acids have been linked together with peptide bonds to form a simple linear chain.

secondary structure Shape of a protein in which hydrogen bonding between carboxyl and amine groups has caused the straight chain to fold and twist.

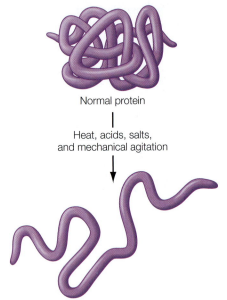

Normal protein

|

Heat, acids, salts,
and mechanical agitation

↓

Denatured protein

▲ **Figure 6.5 Denaturing a Protein**
A protein can be denatured, or unfolded, by exposure to heat, acids, or salts or by mechanical agitation. Any change in a protein's shape will alter its function.

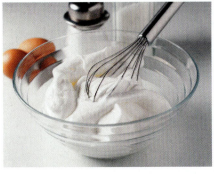

Whipping egg whites denatures the protein.

with their environment. Hydrophobic side chains cluster together on the inside of the protein, combining to form a globular shape called the **tertiary structure.** Hydrophilic side chains assemble on the outside of the protein and interact with the watery portion of blood and other body fluids.

Finally, the **quaternary structure** of a protein forms when two or more polypeptide chains bond together with a hydrogen bond, or when there is a reaction between the sulfur-containing side chains of the amino acids methionine and cysteine. A good example of a quaternary structure of a protein is hemoglobin (**Figure 6.4d**). Notice that the iron-containing heme groups shown in red in the illustration assist in binding oxygen and are not part of the normal quaternary structure of proteins.

Denaturation of Proteins Changes Their Shape

Heat, acids, bases, salts, or mechanical agitation can unfold, or **denature,** proteins (**Figure 6.5**). Denaturation doesn't alter the primary structure of the protein (the amino acids stay in the same sequence), but does change the shape.

You can see denaturation in action when you cook an egg. When you apply heat to a raw egg, such as by frying it, the heat denatures the protein in both the yolk and the egg white. Heat disrupts the bonds between the amino acid side chains, causing the protein in the egg to uncoil. New bonds then form between the side chains, changing the shape and structure of the protein and the appearance and texture of the egg.

Similarly, mechanical agitation, such as beating egg whites when you prepare a meringue, can denature protein. Beating an egg white uncoils the protein, allowing the hydrophilic side chains to react with the water in the egg white, while the hydrophobic portions of the side chains form new bonds, trapping the air from the beating. The stiffer the peaks of egg white, the more denatured the protein. Whether you cook an egg, or whip egg whites, the change in the protein's shape and structure is permanent because new bonds between the amino acids have been formed.

Salts and acids can also denature proteins. For example, when you marinate a chicken breast or a steak before cooking, you might use salt (such as in soy sauce) or acid (such as wine or vinegar), which denatures its protein. The end result is juicier, more tender meat. During digestion, acidic stomach juices help denature and untangle proteins to reveal the peptide bonds. This allows digestive enzymes to break the bonds apart.

tertiary structure Protein structure that occurs when the side chains of the amino acids, most often containing sulfur, form bonds resulting in loops, bends, and folds in the molecule.

quaternary structure Rod-like or globular structure of a protein formed when two or more polypeptide chains cluster together.

denature To alter a protein's secondary, tertiary, or quaternary structure, thereby disabling its function; the amino acids of the primary structure remain linked together by peptide bonds.

LO 6.1: THE TAKE-HOME MESSAGE Proteins are chains of amino acids linked together with peptide bonds. Amino acids, which contain carbon, hydrogen, oxygen, nitrogen, and, in some cases, sulfur, are composed of a central carbon with a carboxyl group, a hydrogen, a nitrogen-containing amine group, and a unique side chain. There are 20 different side chains and therefore 20 unique amino acids. Eleven are classified as nonessential and nine are classified as essential. Under certain circumstances, some nonessential amino acids become conditionally essential. Interactions between the side chains cause the protein to fold into a precise three-dimensional shape that determines its function. Heat, mechanical agitation, acids, bases, and salts can denature a protein and alter its shape and function.

What Are the Key Steps in Digesting and Absorbing Protein?

LO 6.2 Identify the key steps in digesting proteins and absorbing amino acids.

When you eat a peanut butter sandwich, what happens to the protein in the peanut butter and the whole-wheat bread after it has been chewed and swallowed? How do proteins in food become body proteins?

Protein Digestion Begins in the Stomach

The peanut butter sandwich is prepared for digestion in the mouth, where teeth tear and shred the food, breaking the sandwich into smaller pieces while mixing it with saliva (**Focus Figure 6.6**). This mechanical digestion helps make the food easy to swallow and is the only digestion of protein that takes place in the mouth. No chemical or enzymatic digestion of proteins occurs in the mouth.

After you eat a meal, the hormone gastrin directs the release of hydrochloric acid (HCl) from the parietal cells in the stomach wall. At the same time, gastrin directs the release of pepsinogen, an inactive protein enzyme, from the chief cells. Once the bolus enters the stomach, HCl begins to denature the protein strands. HCl also converts the pepsinogen to the active enzyme pepsin, which begins breaking the polypeptides into shorter chains via hydrolysis. As part of chyme, they are then propelled into the small intestine. **Table 6.2** provides a complete list of enzymes that participate in protein digestion.

Protein Digestion Continues in the Small Intestine

When the protein-rich chyme reaches the small intestine, the intestinal cells release the hormone cholecystokinin into the blood. This hormone stimulates the pancreas to secrete proteases such as trypsin, chymotrypsin, and carboxypeptidase, through the pancreatic duct into the small intestine (see Table 6.2). Trypsin and chymotrypsin continue to break apart the peptide bonds in the center of the polypeptide chain, resulting in smaller and smaller peptide chains. The enzyme carboxypeptidase breaks apart the first peptide bond closest to the carboxylic end of the chain. What started out in the peanut butter as a very large protein molecule has now been reduced to tripeptides and dipeptides. Dipeptidases and tripeptidases help break these small peptide chains into single amino acids.

Amino Acids Are Absorbed in the Small Intestine

The single amino acids are absorbed into and pool inside the enterocytes, where they can be used for energy or to synthesize new compounds. Most enter the bloodstream and are transported via the portal vein to the liver. After reaching the liver, amino acids can be used to synthesize new proteins or can be converted to adenosine triphosphate (ATP), glucose, or fat. When other cells need them, the liver releases amino acids into the bloodstream and they are transported throughout the body.

Almost all dietary proteins are digested, absorbed, and transported via the portal vein as single amino acids. However, newborns have a limited ability to absorb whole proteins—for example, the antibodies in breast milk—intact.

Head to **Mastering** Nutrition and watch a narrated video tour of this figure by author Joan Salge Blake.

Protein digestion begins in the stomach with the aid of hydrochloric acid (HCl) and the enzyme pepsin. Proteases continue the digestion in the small intestine, releasing single amino acids to be absorbed into the portal vein for delivery to the liver.

ORGANS OF THE GI TRACT

ACCESSORY ORGANS

MOUTH

Mechanical digestion of protein begins with chewing, tearing, and mixing food with salivary juices to form a bolus.

STOMACH

Hydrochloric acid denatures protein and activates pepsinogen to form pepsin.

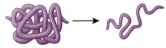

Pepsin breaks the polypeptide chain into smaller polypeptides.

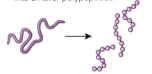

SMALL INTESTINE

Proteases continue to cleave peptide bonds, resulting in dipeptides, tripeptides, and single amino acids.

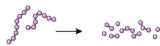

Tripeptidases and dipeptidases on the surface of the enterocytes finish the digestion to yield single amino acids, which can then be absorbed into the bloodstream and travel through the portal vein to the liver.

PANCREAS

Produces proteases that are released into the small intestine via the pancreatic duct.

LIVER

Uses some amino acids to make new proteins or converts them to glucose. Most amino acids pass through the liver and return to the blood to be picked up and used by body cells.

Amino acids

Enterocytes

Capillary

TABLE 6.2 Enzymes Involved in Protein Digestion

Digestive Enzyme	Where Released	Purpose
Pepsinogen	From chief cells in the stomach (activated to pepsin by HCl)	Breaks apart polypeptides into shorter polypeptide chains
Trypsin	From pancreas into small intestine	Breaks apart peptide bonds
Chymotrypsin	From pancreas into small intestine	Breaks apart peptide bonds
Carboxypeptidase	From pancreas into small intestine	Breaks free one amino acid at a time from the carboxyl end of a peptide chain
Aminopeptidase	Brush border of the small intestine	Breaks free the end amino acids from tri- and dipeptides into single amino acids
Tripeptidase	Brush border of the small intestine	Breaks tripeptides into single amino acids
Dipeptidase	Brush border of the small intestine	Breaks dipeptides into single amino acids

LO 6.2: THE TAKE-HOME MESSAGE Chemical digestion of protein begins in the stomach. Gastrin stimulates the release of HCl from the parietal cells and the inactive enzyme pepsinogen from the chief cells. HCl denatures the protein and converts pepsinogen to pepsin, which breaks polypeptides into shorter chains. Cholecystokinin from the duodenum stimulates release of trypsinogen, carboxypeptidase, and chymotrypsinogen from the pancreas. These proteases hydrolyze the shorter chains into tripeptides and dipeptides. Dipeptidases and tripeptidases hydrolyze the tripeptides and dipeptides into single amino acids that are absorbed through the enterocytes via the portal vein to the liver. Absorbed amino acids are used to synthesize new proteins or are converted to nonessential amino acids, ATP, glucose, or fat.

How Are Amino Acids Metabolized?

LO 6.3 Explain the metabolism of amino acids and the role of the amino acid pool.

How the liver metabolizes newly absorbed amino acids depends on the needs of the body. For example, amino acids might be used to replace old proteins or synthesize new ones or, if necessary, they may be used as an energy source. If an individual is not eating sufficient carbohydrates, amino acids can be converted to glucose through gluconeogenesis, as discussed in Chapter 4. However, most amino acids travel back out to the blood to be picked up and used by cells.

Amino Acid Pools Allow Protein Synthesis on Demand

Proteins don't last indefinitely. The daily wear and tear on the body causes the breakdown of hundreds of grams of proteins each day. For example, the protein-rich cells in the skin are constantly sloughed off, and proteins help create a new layer of outer skin every 25 to 45 days.[3] Because red blood cells have a short lifespan—only about 120 days—new red blood cells must be continually regenerated. The cells that line the inner surfaces of the organs, such as the lungs and intestines, are recycled and replaced every 3 to 5 days, thanks to protein synthesis.

In addition to regular maintenance, extra protein is sometimes needed for emergency repairs. Protein is essential in healing, and a person with extensive wounds, such as severe burns, may have dietary protein needs that are more than triple his or her normal needs.

Newly absorbed amino acids collect in limited amounts in **amino acid pools** found in the blood and inside cells. When cellular proteins are degraded or broken down into

amino acid pools Limited supplies of amino acids that accumulate in the blood and cells; amino acids are pulled from the pools and used to build new proteins.

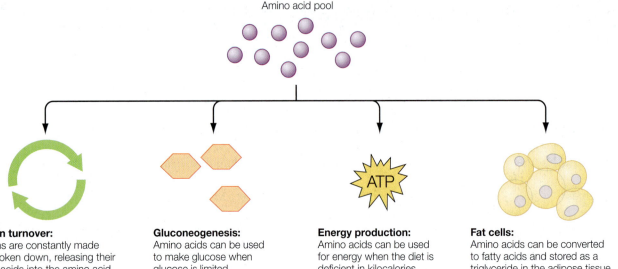

Amino acid pool

Protein turnover:
Proteins are constantly made and broken down, releasing their amino acids into the amino acid pool or using the amino acids for protein synthesis and other important compounds such as niacin and serotonin.

Gluconeogenesis:
Amino acids can be used to make glucose when glucose is limited.

Energy production:
Amino acids can be used for energy when the diet is deficient in kilocalories.

Fat cells:
Amino acids can be converted to fatty acids and stored as a triglyceride in the adipose tissue when kilocalorie intake is sufficient.

▲ **Figure 6.7** **Metabolic Fate of Amino Acids**
Once in the amino acid pool, most amino acids are used for protein synthesis. Under certain conditions, amino acids can be used for gluconeogenesis or energy production, or converted to fatty acids and stored in fat cells.

their component parts, the resulting amino acids also enter the amino acid pools. The body can then use the amino acids in the pool to create proteins on demand. This process of degrading and synthesizing protein is called **protein turnover** (**Figure 6.7**). More than 200 grams of protein are turned over daily. The proteins in the intestines and liver—two tissue types with rapid degradation and resynthesis rates—account for as much as 50 percent of this turnover. Some of the amino acids in the pools are also used to synthesize nonproteins, including thyroid hormones, which contain iodine, and melanin, a complex pigment that gives color to dark skin and hair.

Protein Synthesis Is Regulated by Genes

When the cell is ready to synthesize new or repair old proteins, it uses the instructions for assembly coded in the **genes** that you inherited from your parents. Unless you have an identical twin, your specific *genotype* or genetic makeup is unique to you.

Genes are segments of deoxyribonucleic acid (DNA), which is stored in the nucleus of most body cells. DNA is a two-stranded compound. Each strand is made of combinations of four bases (nucleotides): adenine (A), thymine (T), guanine (G), and cytosine (C). Bases on opposite strands of DNA pair specifically: an A always pairs with a T and a C always pairs with a G. Within a gene, each group of *three* nucleotide bases codes for a *single* amino acid. For example, A-T-G codes for the amino acid methionine. In this way, the order of the As, Ts, Cs, and Gs that make up a gene code for the precise protein to be synthesized.

The body is made up of over 100,000 different proteins. When the body requires a protein, the cells receive a signal to begin the process of protein synthesis. This signal is communicated to a cell receptor by hormones, cell-to-cell contact, or neurotransmitters. Cells can "turn on" and "turn off " protein synthesis as needed.

Because the DNA cannot leave the nucleus of the cell and protein is synthesized outside the nucleus in the cytoplasm, a gene's code must be copied and delivered to the cytoplasm. There, cellular organelles called **ribosomes** translate the message and assemble the exact sequence of amino acids described in the code. Let's walk through the process of protein synthesis (**Focus Figure 6.8**).

protein turnover Continual process of degrading and synthesizing protein.

genes A segment of DNA that codes for a protein; genes are inherited from our parents and determine a variety of characteristics.

ribosomes Organelles found in the cytoplasm that read the mRNA and build the protein in the proper sequence during elongation.

FOCUS Figure 6.8 Protein Synthesis

Head to Mastering Nutrition and watch a narrated video tour of this figure by author Joan Salge Blake.

Protein synthesis is the process by which the DNA code within a cell's nucleus is transcribed and translated to produce specific proteins.

1 In the nucleus, DNA unwinds to allow a copy of the code, called messenger RNA (mRNA) to be made. This process is called **transcription**.

2 The mRNA leaves the nucleus and travels to the cytoplasm.

3 Once the mRNA reaches the cytoplasm, it binds to a ribosome.

4 **Translation** is initiated as the ribosome moves along the mRNA, reading the code. Transfer RNA (tRNA) brings specific amino acids to the ribosome based on the code.

5 The process of **elongation** occurs as translation continues. The ribosome builds a chain of amino acids (the protein) in the proper sequence, based on the code in the mRNA.

6 Translation and elongation are terminated when all the appropriate amino acids are added and the protein is complete. The protein is released from the ribosome.

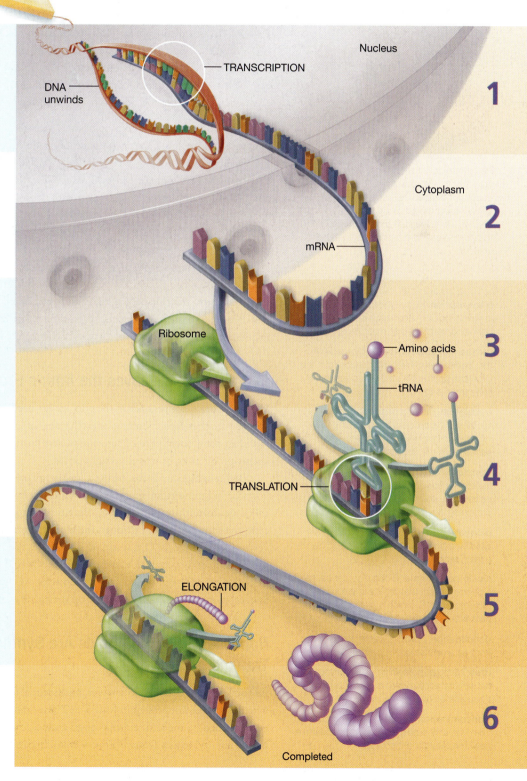

Cell

Nucleus

Nucleus

DNA unwinds

TRANSCRIPTION

1

Cytoplasm

mRNA

2

Ribosome

Amino acids

tRNA

3

TRANSLATION

4

ELONGATION

5

Completed

6

How Are Amino Acids Metabolized? **215**

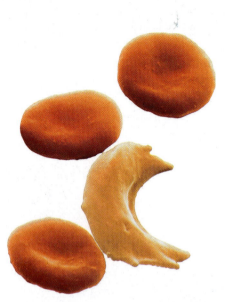

Red blood cells with normal hemoglobin are smooth and round, like the three red doughnut-shaped cells. A person with sickle cell anemia has red blood cells that are stiff and form a sickle (half-moon) shape, like the orange cell, when blood oxygen levels are low.

transcription First stage in protein synthesis, in which the DNA sequence is copied from the gene and transferred to messenger RNA.

messenger RNA (mRNA) Type of RNA that copies the genetic information from the DNA and carries it from the nucleus to the ribosomes in the cell.

translation Second phase of protein synthesis; the process of converting the information in mRNA to an amino acid sequence in the ribosomes.

transfer RNA (tRNA) Type of RNA that transfers a specific amino acid to a growing polypeptide chain in the ribosomes during protein synthesis.

elongation Phase of protein synthesis in which the polypeptide chain grows longer by adding amino acids.

sickle cell anemia Blood disorder caused by a genetic defect that results in the synthesis of hemoglobin S, which makes the red blood cells likely to distort into a sickle shape.

deamination Removal of the amine group from an amino acid.

urea Nitrogen-containing waste product of protein metabolism that is mainly excreted through the urine via the kidneys.

transamination Transfer of an amino group from one amino acid to a keto acid to form a new nonessential amino acid.

1. **Transcription.** The first step in making a new polypeptide chain is to transcribe (or copy) the DNA into ribonucleic acid (RNA). This is somewhat similar to transcribing Chinese characters into English words. The information transcribed is the nucleotide sequence, which as noted earlier determines the amino acids in the protein chain. The bonds between the two strands of DNA break, the strands unwind, and the nucleotide code is transcribed into an RNA molecule called **messenger RNA (mRNA).**

2. **Translation.** Once the code has been transcribed from DNA to mRNA, the new mRNA detaches from the DNA, leaves the nucleus, enters the cytoplasm, and attaches to a ribosome. The ribosome moves along the mRNA, reading the nucleotide instructions recorded in the mRNA. The ribosome then sends a second type of RNA, called **transfer RNA (tRNA),** to collect the corresponding amino acid from the cytoplasm and transport it to the ribosome. Note that 20 unique tRNAs exist, each of which can bind to one and only one of the 20 different amino acids. This gathering and building step is called **elongation** and continues until the full sequence of amino acids has been completed and a new protein is released.

When the sequence of amino acids is incorrect, abnormalities occur and medical conditions can result. One such condition is **sickle cell anemia.** The most common inherited blood disorder in the United States, sickle cell anemia is caused by an abnormal variant of the gene that codes for the assembly of the protein hemoglobin. The displacement of just *one* amino acid, glutamine, with another amino acid, valine, in polypeptide chains of hemoglobin makes the chains likely to stick to one another and form crescent-shaped blood cells. Whereas red blood cells with normal hemoglobin are smooth and round, those with this mutation are stiff and form a sickle shape under certain conditions, such as after vigorous exercise, when oxygen levels in the blood are low. These abnormal sickle cells are recognized and destroyed by the immune system, causing anemia; moreover, because of their shape, they can build up in blood vessels, causing painful blockages and damage to tissues and organs. Approximately one in 12 African Americans and one in 100 Hispanic Americans are carriers of the mutated gene that causes the disease.[4]

Deamination Removes the Amine Group from Amino Acids

What happens if amino acids in the pool are not used for protein synthesis? As the amino acid pool reaches capacity, amino acids that are not used to build proteins are broken down into their component parts. These component parts are used for other purposes, such as energy production, or stored as triglycerides.

Before amino acids can be used for energy production or converted to other compounds, the amine group must be removed and converted to ammonia (NH_3) in a process called **deamination** (**Figure 6.9a**). Because ammonia in high amounts can be toxic to cells, the ammonia is sent through the bloodstream to the liver, where it is quickly converted to **urea,** CH_4N_2O, a waste product that is released into the blood, filtered out by the kidneys, and eventually excreted in urine. Once the nitrogen has been removed, the carbon-containing remnants of the amino acids are eventually converted to glucose, used as energy, or stored as fat, depending on the needs of the body.

Nonessential Amino Acids Are Synthesized through Transamination

As you learned earlier in this chapter, nonessential amino acids can be made in the body when needed or not present in your diet. These amino acids can be made from the nitrogen provided by the amine group of an amino acid or by ammonia, and another compound referred to as a *keto acid* (**Figure 6.9b**). In this process, called **transamination,** the

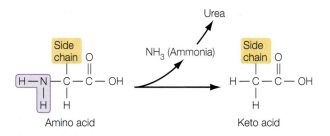

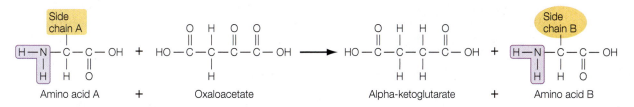

a Deamination: In the liver, the amine group is removed, producing ammonia and a keto acid. The ammonia is used to form urea, which is excreted in the urine.

b Transamination: An amine group from an essential amino acid is transferred to a keto acid, producing a nonessential amino acid and a new keto acid.

liver transfers the amine group to the keto acid, creating a nonessential amino acid and a different keto acid. This reaction requires vitamin B_6 and will be discussed in greater detail in Chapter 8.

Excess Protein Is Converted to Body Fat

If you add too much water to a swimming pool, the excess overflows. The same is true of an amino acid pool. When the diet contains sufficient carbohydrates, and protein intake exceeds requirements, the amino acid pool becomes saturated. The "overflow" amino acids are deaminated, and the remaining carbon remnants are converted to fatty acids and stored as triglycerides in adipose tissue.

LO 6.3: THE TAKE-HOME MESSAGE During digestion, proteins are broken down into amino acids with the help of gastric juices, enzymes in the stomach and small intestine, and enzymes from the pancreas and small intestinal lining. A limited supply of amino acids exists in the amino acid pools, which act as a reservoir for protein synthesis. Surplus amino acids are deaminated, with the carbon-containing remnants used for glucose or energy or stored as fat, depending on the body's needs. The nitrogen in the amine groups is eventually converted to the waste product urea and excreted in urine. Nonessential amino acids are synthesized through transamination.

What Are the Functions of Protein in the Body?

LO 6.4 Describe the functions of protein in the body.

Proteins play many important roles in the body, from providing structural and mechanical support and maintaining body tissues to functioning as enzymes and hormones and helping maintain acid–base, and fluid balance. They also transport nutrients, assist the immune system, and, when necessary, are a source of energy. Let's examine each of these vital functions in more depth.

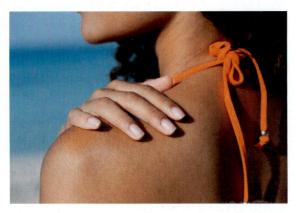

Proteins play an important role in keeping skin healthy and nails strong.

Proteins Provide Structural Support and Enable Movement

Proteins provide much of the structural and mechanical support that keeps the body upright, moving, and flexible. Collagen, the most abundant protein in the body, is found in all connective tissues, including bones, tendons, and ligaments, which support and connect joints and other body parts. This fibrous protein is also responsible for the skin's elasticity and forms the scar tissue necessary to repair injuries.

The proteins actin and myosin enable movement by contracting muscle fibers. They are also involved in nonmuscle movement, such as when cells divide during mitosis or when chemicals are transported along actin filaments in the cell cytoplasm.

Proteins Act as Catalysts

Recall that enzymes are biological catalysts that speed up reactions. Most enzymes are proteins, although to be activated, some may also need a coenzyme, such as a vitamin. Without enzymes, reactions would occur so slowly that you couldn't survive.

Each of the thousands of enzymes in the body catalyzes a specific reaction. Some enzymes, such as digestive enzymes, are **catabolic** enzymes: They break compounds apart. The enzyme lactase is needed to break down the milk sugar lactose (see Chapter 4). Other enzymes are **anabolic,** and build substances. For example, the anabolic enzyme glycogen synthetase converts excess glucose units one by one into a chain of glycogen that is then stored. Enzymes aren't changed, damaged, or used up in the process of speeding up a particular reaction (see **Figure 3.10** on page 87). Thus, an enzyme is available to catalyze additional reactions.

Proteins Act as Chemical Messengers

Recall that hormones are chemical messengers with regulatory functions. There are over 70 trillion cells in the body, and all of these cells interact with at least one of over 50 known hormones.[5] Although some hormones are made from cholesterol, many are proteins or peptides (amino acid based). Familiar examples include insulin and glucagon, which regulate blood glucose levels, and leptin and ghrelin, which regulate appetite. Antidiuretic hormone (ADH) contributes to blood pressure regulation, whereas growth hormone (GH) supports childhood development and many other body functions.

Proteins Help Regulate Fluid Balance

The body is made up predominantly of water, which is distributed both outside (extracellular) and inside (intracellular) the cells. Fluid can generally flow easily in and out of cells. However, proteins are too large to move across the cell membranes and thus stay either within the cells or outside in the extracellular fluid. Normally, blood pressure forces nutrient- and oxygen-rich fluids out of *capillaries* (the smallest blood vessels of the body) and into the spaces between the cells (called *interstitial spaces*). But proteins, including an important blood protein called **albumin,** remain in the blood. As fluid is forced out of the blood with each heartbeat, the concentration of albumin increases, drawing the fluid from the interstitial spaces back into the blood by osmosis. (*Osmosis* is described in detail in Chapter 11.) Hence, albumin and other blood proteins play an important role in keeping body fluids dispersed evenly inside and outside of cells, helping to maintain a state of fluid

catabolic Energy-releasing process that breaks larger molecules into smaller parts.

anabolic Energy-requiring process in which smaller molecules are combined to form larger molecules.

albumin Protein produced in the liver and found in the blood that helps maintain fluid balance.

balance. (*Note:* Sodium and other minerals, discussed in Chapter 12, also play a major role in fluid balance.)

When fewer proteins are available to draw the fluid from between the cells back into the bloodstream, as during severe malnutrition, a fluid imbalance results. The interstitial spaces between the cells become bloated and the body tissue swells, a condition known as **edema** (**Figure 6.10**).

Proteins Help Regulate Acid–Base Balance

Proteins can alter the pH of the body fluids. Normally, the blood has a pH of about 7.4. Even a small change in the pH of the blood in either direction can be harmful or even fatal. A blood pH below 7.35, a condition called **acidosis,** can result in a coma. A blood pH above 7.45, known as **alkalosis,** can cause convulsions.

Proteins act as **buffers** and minimize the changes in acid–base levels by picking up hydrogen ions in the blood or donating hydrogen ions to the blood. Should the blood become too basic (contain too few hydrogen ions), the carboxyl groups of amino acids lower the pH of the blood by donating hydrogen ions; if blood becomes too acidic (too many hydrogen ions), the amine groups bind the excess hydrogen ions and restore the pH to an optimal level. This dual buffering role helps maintain the acid–base balance in the cells and the blood.

Proteins Transport Substances throughout the Body

Transport proteins shuttle oxygen, waste products, lipids, some vitamins, sodium and potassium, and other substances through the blood and across cell membranes. For example, hemoglobin is a transport protein that carries oxygen to cells from the lungs; hemoglobin also picks up carbon dioxide for delivery to the lungs to be exhaled. Lipoproteins are another example; they transport fat-soluble nutrients through the bloodstream (see Chapter 5).

Some nutrients, such as vitamin A, are fat soluble and need assistance to move through the water-based blood. Vitamin A attaches to the blood protein albumin for transport to the liver and other cells. Essential minerals—for example, iron and zinc—have specialized transport proteins whose sole function is to escort them across the enterocytes.

Channel proteins in cell membranes form passageways that allow ions such as sodium and potassium to pass in and out of cells (**Figure 6.11**). In contrast, carrier proteins change their shape to allow the entry of substances such as glucose into cells. Without channel and carrier proteins, cells would be unable to maintain an optimal concentration of such nutrients or remove waste from the cell. If your diet is deficient in essential amino acids,

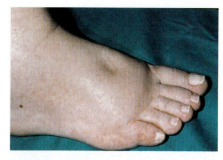

▲ **Figure 6.10 Edema**
Inadequate protein in the blood can cause edema.

edema Accumulation of excess water in the spaces surrounding the cells, which causes swelling of the body tissue.

acidosis Condition in which the blood pH is too low, generally due to excessive hydrogen ions.

alkalosis Condition in which the blood pH is too low due to a low concentration of hydrogen ions.

buffers Substances that help maintain the proper pH in a solution by accepting or donating hydrogen ions.

transport proteins Proteins that carry other substances, mainly nutrients, through the blood to various organs and tissues. Proteins can also act as channels through which some substances enter your cells.

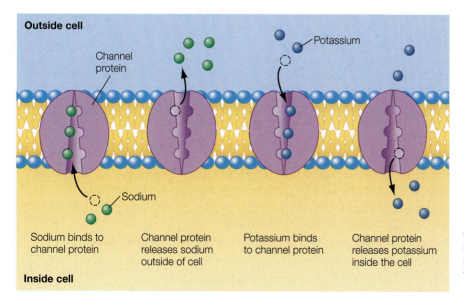

Outside cell

Potassium

Channel
protein

Sodium

Sodium binds to
channel protein

Channel protein
releases sodium
outside of cell

Potassium binds
to channel protein

Channel protein
releases potassium
inside the cell

Inside cell

◀ **Figure 6.11 Proteins as Ion Channels**
Channel proteins form tunnels through which ions such as sodium and potassium can move from one side of the cell membrane to the other.

fewer such proteins are produced, causing an unhealthy balance of nutrients inside and outside of the cell membrane.

Proteins Contribute to a Healthy Immune System

The immune system protects the body from pathogens. Once pathogens, including bacteria and viruses, enter the cells, they can multiply rapidly, eventually causing illness. An army of specialized protein "soldiers," called **antibodies,** quickly recognize and assist in the destruction of pathogens before they have a chance to multiply.

Once the body knows how to create antibodies against a specific foreign substance, such as a particular virus, it stores that information, giving the body **immunity** to that pathogen. The next time the invader enters the body, the body can respond very quickly (producing up to 2,000 precise antibodies per second!) to fight it.

Sometimes, the body incorrectly perceives a nonthreatening substance, typically a protein, as harmful and attacks it. A substance of this type is called an **allergen.** Proteins in certain foods, such as peanuts, wheat, and eggs, commonly act as allergens. Food allergies are discussed in detail in Chapter 17.

Proteins Can Provide Energy

Because proteins provide 4 kilocalories per gram, they can be used as an energy source. After amino acids are deaminated, the remaining carbon remnants can enter the energy cycle to produce ATP. (We cover this process in depth in Chapter 8.)

When an individual eats too few kilocalories or carbohydrates, the stores of glycogen in the liver and muscle become depleted and blood glucose levels drop. To raise blood glucose levels, the body turns to specific amino acids called **glucogenic amino acids.** These amino acids are converted to glucose through gluconeogenesis. (Remember that the red blood cells and brain need glucose to function properly.)

However, the last thing you want to do is use this valuable nutrient, which plays so many important roles in the body, as a regular source of fuel because carbohydrates and fats are far better suited to providing energy. When the diet contains adequate amounts of kilocalories from carbohydrates and fat, proteins are spared and used for their more important roles. For optimal health, individuals need to eat enough protein daily to meet the body's needs and enough carbohydrates and fats to prevent protein from being used as energy.

Table 6.3 summarizes the many structural and functional roles proteins play in the body.

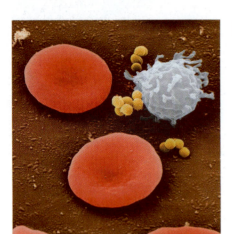

Certain white blood cells of the immune system (see upper right) produce antibodies, proteins that defend against harmful agents such as the Staphylococcus bacteria shown (in yellow) in this photo. (The red cells are red blood cells.)

TABLE 6.3   The Many Roles of Proteins

Role of Protein	How It Works
Structural and mechanical support and maintenance	Proteins are the body's building materials, providing strength and flexibility to tissues, tendons, ligaments, muscles, organs, bones, nails, hair, and skin. Proteins are also needed for the ongoing maintenance of the body.
Enzymes and hormones	Proteins are needed to make most enzymes that speed up reactions in the body and many hormones that direct specific activities, such as regulating blood glucose levels.
Fluid balance	Proteins play a major role in ensuring that body fluids are evenly dispersed in the blood and inside and outside cells.
Acid–base balance	Proteins act as buffers to help keep the pH of body fluids within a tight range. A drop in pH will cause body fluids to become too acidic, whereas a rise in pH can make them too basic.
Transport	Proteins shuttle substances such as oxygen, waste products, and nutrients (such as sodium and potassium) through the blood and into and out of cells.
Antibodies and the immune response	Proteins create specialized antibodies that attack pathogens that may cause illness.
Energy	Because proteins provide 4 kilocalories per gram, they can be used as fuel or energy.
Satiety	Protein increases satiety, which can help control appetite and weight.

Protein Improves Satiety and Appetite Control

In addition to its structural and functional roles, protein also improves satiety after a meal more than either carbohydrate or fat.[6] Eating a meal that contains a good source of protein will leave you more satisfied than will a high-carbohydrate meal with the same number of kilocalories. The satiety following a high-protein meal may be due to dietary protein suppressing the release of ghrelin.[7] Recall that ghrelin, which is produced in the stomach, stimulates the hypothalamus to sense hunger. Including protein in each meal helps to control appetite, which in turn can help maintain a healthy weight.

> **LO 6.4: THE TAKE-HOME MESSAGE** Proteins play many important roles in the body: (1) synthesizing, repairing, and maintaining structural tissues; (2) helping facilitate muscular contraction; (3) catalyzing reactions as enzymes; (4) acting as hormones; (5) maintaining fluid balance; (6) maintaining acid–base balance; (7) transporting nutrients throughout the body; (8) providing antibodies for a strong immune system; (9) providing energy when kilocalorie intake doesn't meet daily energy needs; and (10) promoting satiety and appetite control.

How Much Protein Do You Need Daily?

LO 6.5 Calculate the daily amount of protein recommended based on the Dietary Reference Intakes.

Healthy, nonpregnant adults should consume enough dietary protein to replace the amount they use each day. However, pregnant women, people recovering from surgery or an injury, and growing children need more protein to supply the necessary amino acids and nitrogen to build new tissue. **Nitrogen balance** studies are often used to determine how much protein individuals need to replace or build new tissue.

Healthy Adults Should Be in Nitrogen Balance

A person's protein requirement can be estimated by using what we know about the structure of an amino acid. We know that 16 percent of every dietary protein molecule is nitrogen. And we know that the body retains this nitrogen during protein synthesis. It follows that we can assess a person's protein status by checking their nitrogen balance—measuring the amount of nitrogen they consume and subtracting the amount of nitrogen they excrete, mostly as urea. The goal is to achieve nitrogen balance. See the Calculation Corner for an example of the calculation done to assess nitrogen balance.

 ## Calculation Corner

Nitrogen Balance

(a) Using the fact that protein is 16 percent nitrogen, a common factor of 6.25 is used to calculate how much nitrogen is in a given amount of food (100/16 = 6.25).

We analyzed the food and beverages from a meal and found that it contained 73 grams (g) of protein. Divide this by 6.25 to determine the nitrogen content of the meal:

$$\text{Nitrogen} = \frac{73 \text{ g protein}}{6.25 \text{ g nitrogen}} = 11.6 \text{ g nitrogen}$$

antibodies Proteins that identify and participate in the destruction of pathogens as part of the body's immune response.

immunity State of having built up memory immune cells that target a particular pathogen so that any subsequent encounter with that pathogen prompts rapid production of specific antibodies.

allergen Substance, such as wheat protein, that causes an allergic reaction.

glucogenic amino acids Amino acids that can be used to form glucose through gluconeogenesis.

nitrogen balance Difference between nitrogen intake and nitrogen excretion.

(b) Now calculate the amount of nitrogen lost from the body. First, nitrogen is lost in the urine as urea nitrogen, and in other nitrogen sources that are not part of the urea molecule. Because it's difficult to account for the nonurea sources directly, a factor of 0.2 grams × urinary urea nitrogen (UUN) is used to determine these losses. In this example, let's assume we analyzed the urine and found 8 grams of UUN. The total nitrogen lost in the urine would be calculated as follows:

8 g UUN + (0.2 × 8 g UUN) = 9.6 g nitrogen lost

(c) Next, we must account for nitrogen lost through other means, including hair, skin, and feces—approximately 2 grams per day. Add this to the equation.

8 g UUN + (0.2 × 8 g UUN) + 2 g = 11.6 g nitrogen lost

(d) Now let's put it all together with the equation:

Nitrogen balance = nitrogen in − nitrogen out
Nitrogen balance = (73 g protein/6.25) − (8 g UUN + [0.2 × 8 g UUN] + 2 g)
= 0 g of nitrogen

The calculation for nitrogen balance can be useful to dietitians as well as researchers to determine protein requirements.

Go to **Mastering** Nutrition and complete a Math Video activity similar to the problem in this Calculation Corner.

Once we know the amount of nitrogen consumed, we can compare that to the amount of nitrogen excreted to determine if an individual is in nitrogen balance (**Figure 6.12**). If the nitrogen intake from dietary protein is equivalent to the amount of nitrogen excreted as urea in the urine, then a person is in nitrogen balance. Healthy, nonpregnant adults are typically in nitrogen balance.

A body that retains more nitrogen than it excretes is in positive nitrogen balance. Rapidly growing babies, children, and adolescents are all in positive nitrogen balance. They excrete less nitrogen than they take in because their bodies incorporate nitrogen

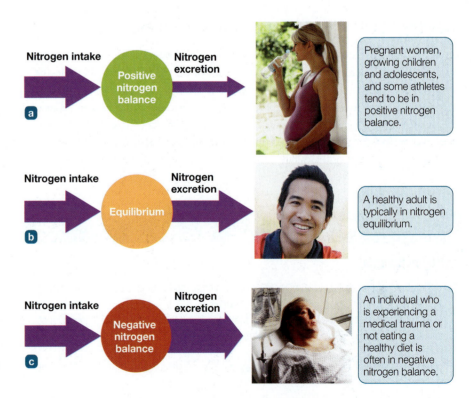

Nitrogen intake → Positive nitrogen balance → Nitrogen excretion
a
Pregnant women, growing children and adolescents, and some athletes tend to be in positive nitrogen balance.

Nitrogen intake → Equilibrium → Nitrogen excretion
b
A healthy adult is typically in nitrogen equilibrium.

Nitrogen intake → Negative nitrogen balance → Nitrogen excretion
c
An individual who is experiencing a medical trauma or not eating a healthy diet is often in negative nitrogen balance.

▶Figure 6.12 **Nitrogen Balance and Imbalance**

into new tissues as they grow, build muscles, and expand their supply of red blood cells. When a woman is pregnant, she, too, is in positive nitrogen balance because her body is building a robust baby.

An individual is in negative nitrogen balance when nitrogen losses are greater than nitrogen intake. This occurs immediately following surgery, when fighting an infection, or when experiencing severe emotional trauma. These situations all increase the body's need for both kilocalories and protein. If the kilocalories and protein in the diet are inadequate to cover these increased demands, then proteins from tissues are broken down to meet the body's needs.

You Can Determine Your Own Protein Needs

There are two ways to determine whether or not your protein intake falls within recommended levels. The RDA measures grams of protein per kilogram of body weight, and the AMDR measures protein intake as a percentage of total kilocalories.

The RDA for Protein

The RDA for protein has been established to provide adequate amounts of essential amino acids and nitrogen. This ensures the body will have the materials necessary to make the nonessential amino acids and body proteins necessary to meet daily needs. The RDAs for the essential amino acids are illustrated in **Figure 6.13**. As you can see, the RDA per day for each of the nine essential amino acids is based on grams per kilogram of body weight. This is also true for the RDA for protein. Adults older than 19 years of age should consume 0.8 grams of protein for each kilogram of body weight. For individuals under the age of 19, the RDA is somewhat higher (see the tables in the front cover of this textbook).

In the United States, men age 20 and older consume, on average, more than 100 grams of protein daily, and women on average consume more than 70 grams. In general, Americans are meeting, and even exceeding, their dietary protein needs. Follow the steps in the Calculation Corner to calculate your RDA for protein.

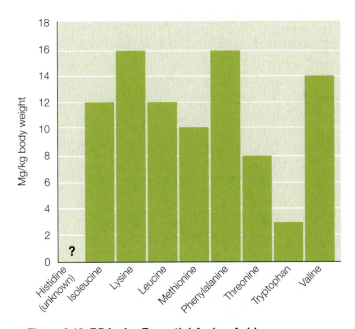

▲ **Figure 6.13 RDAs for Essential Amino Acids**
Recommended Dietary Allowances for the nine essential amino acids based on body weight.
Source: Data from Institute of Medicine. 2005. *Dietary Reference Intakes for Energy, Carbohydrate, Fiber, Fat, Fatty Acids, Cholesterol, Protein, and Amino Acids* (Washington, DC: National Academies Press).

Protein Requirements

(a) To calculate protein requirements, the first step is to convert body weight in pounds to kilograms. The conversion factor is 2.2. For example, an adult who weighs 176 pounds (lb) would weigh 80 kilograms (kg):

176 lb ÷ 2.2 = 80 kg

(b) Next, multiply weight in kilograms × 0.8 grams of protein. In this example, a healthy adult who weighs 80 kg should consume 64 grams (g) of protein per day.

80 kg × 0.8 g = 64 g protein

(c) How much protein should a healthy adult who weighs 130 pounds consume each day?

Source: Data from Institute of Medicine, National Academy of Science. 2002. *Dietary Reference Intakes for Energy, Carbohydrate, Fiber, Fat, Fatty Acids, Cholesterol, Protein, and Amino Acids* (Washington, DC: National Academies Press).

Go to **Mastering** Nutrition and complete a Math Video activity similar to the problem in this Calculation Corner.

The AMDR for Protein

Total protein intake is also measured as a percentage of total kilocalories. The latest AMDR for protein, based on data from numerous nitrogen balance studies, is 10–35 percent of total daily kilocalories. Currently, even though many adults in the United States are consuming more grams of protein than they need, they consume about 15 percent of their daily kilocalories from protein, which falls within the AMDR. This is because Americans are overconsuming kilocalories from carbohydrates and fats, which lowers the percentage of the total kilocalories coming from protein.

An overweight individual's protein needs are not much greater than those of a normal-weight person of similar height because the RDA for dietary protein is based on a person's need to maintain protein-dependent tissues, like lean muscle and organs, and to perform protein-dependent body functions. Because people who are overweight carry more of their weight as fat, they do not need to consume significantly more protein than normal-weight people.

The American College of Sports Medicine, the Academy of Nutrition and Dietetics, and other experts have advocated an increase of 50–100 percent more protein for competitive athletes participating in endurance exercise (marathon runners) or resistance exercise (weight lifters).[8, 9] However, athletes typically maintain a higher intake of food and thus already consume higher amounts of both kilocalories and protein.

LO 6.5: THE TAKE-HOME MESSAGE When protein intake equals the amount of nitrogen excreted, a healthy body is in nitrogen balance. Nitrogen balance studies suggest adults should consume 0.8 gram of protein for each kilogram of body weight, and 10–35 percent of their daily energy intake as protein. In the United States, men typically consume more than 100 grams of protein daily and women more than 70 grams—in both cases, far more than is needed—but their AMDR is about 15 percent, which is within the recommended range. Athletes have higher protein needs than nonathletes, but their higher food intake means that they typically meet or exceed these higher needs.

What Are the Best Food Sources of Protein?

LO 6.6 Describe the best food sources of protein and the methods available to determine protein quality.

The protein content of foods varies greatly. Although fruits are an excellent dietary choice, most contain one gram or less of protein per serving. Other foods, especially animal products, can contribute substantial amounts of protein to the diet.

Not All Protein Is Created Equal

A high-quality protein is digestible, contains all the essential amino acids, and provides a sufficient quantity of amino acids to be used to synthesize the nonessential amino acids and support the body's requirements for growth and maintenance. If a single essential amino acid is in low supply in the diet and thus in the amino acid pool, the body's ability to synthesize proteins will be limited. Thus, while it is important to eat enough protein, the quality of protein also matters.

Which protein is best? Several methods have been used to yield chemical scores to answer this question. These methods include the amino acid score, the protein digestibility corrected amino acid score, and the biological value.

Amino Acid Score

The **amino acid score** is used to determine if a protein is complete. To calculate an amino acid score, the amount of an essential amino acid per gram of food protein (mg/g) being tested is divided by the standard amount for that same amino acid in a gram of the reference protein. Egg white protein is typically used as the reference because it is known to have a balance of all of the essential amino acids needed to support growth. Amino acid scores range from 0 to 1, with 1 representing an optimal score. The Calculation Corner provides an example of how to calculate this score for peanut butter using the information shown in **Table 6.4**.

amino acid score Composition of essential amino acids in a protein compared with a standard, usually egg protein.

TABLE 6.4	Amino Acid Scores for Peanut Butter		
Essential Amino Acid	**Peanut Butter (mg/g)**	**Egg Protein (mg/g)**	**Amino Acid Score**
Histidine	30	22	1.36
Isoleucine	40	54	0.74
Leucine	77	86	0.90
Lysine	39	70	0.56
Methionine plus cysteine	24	57	0.42
Phenylalanine plus tyrosine	108	93	1.16
Threonine	30	47	0.64
Tryptophan	12	17	0.71
Valine	46	66	0.71

Source: Data from Institute of Medicine. 2002. *Dietary Reference Intakes for Energy, Carbohydrate, Fiber, Fat, Fatty Acids, Cholesterol, Protein, and Amino Acids* (Washington, DC: National Academies Press).

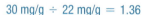
Amino Acid Score

The formula used to calculate the amino acid score for any food is:

$$\text{Amino acid score} = \frac{\text{essential amino acid for protein (mg/g)}}{\text{essential amino acid for standard (mg/g)}}$$

We can use peanut butter to illustrate this calculation. Table 6.4 shows the essential amino acid content for peanut butter in column two. The third column shows the essential amino acid content for egg protein, which is most often used as the standard for this calculation. As you read across the table to column four, you can see the amino acid score. This means that peanut butter contains 136 percent of the histidine that egg protein does. This is how you calculate the amino acid score. Begin with histidine and divide the amount of histidine in peanut butter by the amount found in egg protein:

$$30 \text{ mg/g} \div 22 \text{ mg/g} = 1.36$$

Continue the calculation for each of the amino acids. Each of the nine essential amino acid scores is calculated individually and presented in column four in Table 6.4. Now add together all the amino acid scores found in peanut butter and compare with egg protein using the total mg/g for each as follows:

$$406 \text{ mg/g peanut butter} \div 674 \text{ mg/g egg protein} = 0.60 \text{ or } 60\%$$

This amino acid score means that overall, peanut butter contains 60 percent of the essential amino acids that egg protein does.

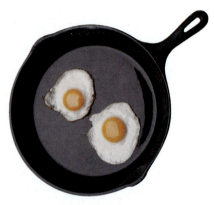

Egg protein is the highest quality protein in the diet.

The essential amino acid that has the lowest score is called the **limiting amino acid.** In the case of peanut butter, the limiting amino acid is methionine, with a score of 0.42. This score means that peanut butter contains 42 percent of the methionine found in egg protein.

The amino acid score is one method for comparing food proteins and their essential amino acid composition. Though it is a useful method of comparison, it doesn't take into consideration how protein is digested.

Protein Digestibility Corrected Amino Acid Score (PDCAAS)

The **protein digestibility corrected amino acid score (PDCAAS)** combines the chemical score with the digestibility of a food protein to give a more accurate indication of quality. This is important because only amino acids that are digested and absorbed can contribute to the amino acid pool and be used to build and maintain body proteins. An example of the PDCAAS calculation for peanut butter is presented in the Calculation Corner.

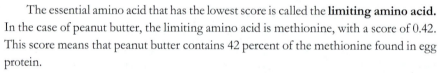
Calculation Corner

PDCAAS

The digestibility of a food has a major impact on the protein quality. This calculation, called the Protein Digestibility Corrected Amino Acid Score (PDCAAS), compares the amino acid content of a food with the amino acid requirement for humans and then corrects for digestibility. This is how the calculation works:

(1) First you need to know the amino acid score of the food. For this calculation you use the lowest amino acid score. From Table 6.4 you see that the lowest amino acid score for peanut butter is methionine plus cysteine, or 0.42.

limiting amino acid Essential amino acid that is in the shortest supply, relative to the body's needs, in an incomplete protein

protein digestibility corrected amino acid score (PDCAAS) Score measured as a percentage that takes into account both digestibility and amino acid score and provides a good indication of the quality of a protein.

(2) Next, to determine the PDCAAS for peanut butter, multiply the score for its lowest limiting amino acid (0.42) by the protein digestibility of peanut butter (95%):

$$\text{PDCAAS for peanut butter} = 0.42 \times 0.95 = 0.40$$

In other words, because the protein in peanut butter is not completely digested, the amino acid score for methionine plus cysteine has been corrected from 0.42 to 0.40.

These calculations are used by the Food and Drug Administration to determine the %DV represented on food labels. For example, one serving (2 tbsp) of peanut butter contains 8 grams (g) of protein. To calculate the %DV, this number is multiplied by the PDCAAS:

$$8 \text{ g} \times 0.40 = 3.2$$

Next, divide this by 50 grams, which is the recommended intake of protein for adults used on the label:

$$3.2 \div 50 \text{ g} = 0.064 \text{ or } 6.4\%$$

In this example, a serving of peanut butter would represent 6.4 percent of the %DV for protein.

In general, animal proteins are more digestible than plant proteins. Some plant proteins, especially when consumed raw, are protected by the plant's cell walls and cannot be broken down by the enzymes in the intestinal tract, whereas 90–99 percent of the proteins from animal sources (cheese and other dairy foods, meat, poultry, and eggs) are digestible. Plant proteins, such as in oatmeal (86 percent digestible) and soybeans (78 percent digestible), are generally only 70–90 percent digestible.[10]

Milk protein, which is easily digested and provides all essential amino acids, has a PDCAAS of 1.00. In comparison, kidney beans garner a PDCAAS of 0.68, and wheat has a score of only 0.40. However, when wheat is combined with another protein source, such as peanut butter, the protein quality of the meal is improved.

The PDCAAS is used by the Food and Drug Administration to calculate the % Daily Value of protein used on food labels. Manufacturers use 50 grams of protein as the standard to calculate the %DV for a serving of a food for adults and children 4 or more years of age. Recall from Chapter 2 that the %DV for protein is only required on the Nutrition Facts panel if the manufacturer has made a nutrient claim for the protein in the food.

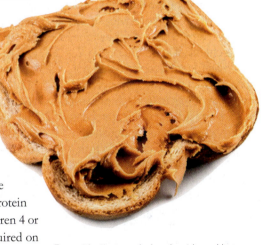

Peanut butter on whole-wheat bread is a protein-rich snack.

Complementary and Complete Proteins

Protein from animal products is considered a high-quality, **complete protein** that provides all nine of the essential amino acids, along with some of the 11 nonessential amino acids. Plant proteins are considered to be **incomplete protein** because plants are deficient in one or more essential amino acids. Some exceptions to this generalization are gelatin, quinoa, and soy. Gelatin, an animal protein, is not a complete protein because it is missing the amino acid tryptophan. Quinoa and soy, plant proteins, have amino acid profiles that resemble those of animal proteins, and are considered complete proteins. Examining the Evidence: Does Soy Reduce the Risk of Disease? discusses a variety of soy products to incorporate into a vegetarian diet to improve the quality of your meals.

complete protein Protein that provides all the essential amino acids, along with some nonessential amino acids. Soy protein and protein from animal sources are complete proteins.

incomplete protein Protein that is low in one or more of the essential amino acids. Proteins from plant sources tend to be incomplete.

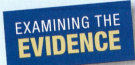
Does Soy Reduce the Risk of Heart Disease and Cancer?

Soy consumption in the United States, in foods ranging from soy milk to soy burgers, has been increasing in recent decades at a rate of 5 percent annually.[1] According to a survey conducted by the United Soybean Board, 81 percent of U.S. consumers perceive soy foods as being healthy.[2] The popularity of soy foods has increased 14 percent among many age groups and ethnic groups, including baby boomers; Asian populations in the United States looking for traditional soy-based foods; and young adults with an increasing interest in vegetarian diets.[3]

Soy is a complete, high-quality protein source that is low in saturated fat and that contains **isoflavones,** which are naturally occurring phytoestrogens (*phyto* = plant). These plant estrogens have a chemical structure similar to human estrogen, a reproductive hormone present in lower levels in males and higher levels in females. However, they are considered weak estrogens, as they have less than a thousandth the potential activity of human estrogen. Though isoflavones can also be found in other plant foods, such as grains, vegetables, and other types of legumes, soybeans contain the largest amount found in food.

Epidemiological studies have suggested that eating soy protein as part of a heart-healthy diet may reduce the risk of heart disease by lowering cholesterol levels. Research suggests that soy protein can lower LDL cholesterol and raise HDL cholesterol levels.[4] Soy protein may also help lower blood pressure, a risk factor for heart disease.[5]

Observational studies suggest that isoflavones may help relieve

isoflavones Naturally occurring phytoestrogens, or weak plant estrogens, that function in a similar fashion to the hormone estrogen in the human body.

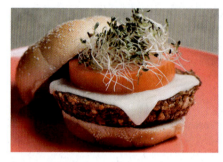

Soy meat analogs, such as hot dogs, sausages, burgers, and cold cuts, are made using soy.

menopausal symptoms, although a well-designed, double-blind study reported no benefit.[6] At the same time, because isoflavones act as weak estrogens in the body, some concern exists that they may have a harmful impact on certain estrogen-sensitive cancers (tumors that use estrogen for growth), including an estrogen-sensitive form of breast cancer. Recently, however, several new reports have found no link between breast cancer prognosis and soy isoflavones.[7] In fact, some studies have suggested that isoflavones may actually *reduce* the risk of breast cancer, possibly by competing with the hormone estrogen for its binding site on tumor cells.[8]

Timing may be an important part of the preventative role that soy plays in breast cancer. A study of Chinese women revealed that those who ate the most soy during their adolescent years had a reduced risk of breast cancer in adulthood.[9] Early exposure to soy foods may be protective by stimulating the growth of cells in the breast, enhancing the rate at which the glands mature, and altering the tissues in beneficial ways.

Research supports the safety of soy isoflavones when consumed in soy foods and beverages such as soymilk.[10] According to the American Cancer Society, soy foods and beverages are healthy and safe, and women with

breast cancer may consume them in moderate amounts. They should, however, avoid soy-containing pills, powders, and supplements with high levels of isoflavones.[11]

Soy can be an inexpensive, heart-healthy protein source that may also help lower your LDL cholesterol and blood pressure, raise HDL cholesterol, and reduce your risk of certain cancers.

References

1. United Soybean Board. 2014. Bite. *The Data is Delicious.* Available at www.soyconnection.com/sites/default/files/Consumer%20Attitudes_Med_062714.pdf. Accessed February 2017.
2. United Soybean Board. 2016. *Consumer Attitudes About Nutrition, Health, and Soy Foods.* Available at www.soyconnection.com. Accessed February 2017.
3. United Soybean Board. 2016.
4. Wofford, M. R., C. M. Rebholz, et al. 2012. Effect of Soy and Milk Protein Supplementation on Serum Lipid Levels: A Randomized Controlled Trial. *European Journal of Clinical Nutrition* 66:419–425.
5. He, J., M. Wofford, K. Reynolds, et al. 2011. Effect of Dietary Protein Supplementation on Blood Pressure: A Randomized Controlled Trial. *Circulation* 124:589–595.
6. Levis, S., N. Strickman-Stein, et al. 2011. Soy Isoflavones in the Prevention of Menopausal Bone Loss and Menopausal Symptoms: A Randomized Double-Blind Trial. *Archives of Internal Medicine* 171(15):1363–1369.
7. Messina, M. 2016. Soy and Health Update: Evaluation of the Clinical and Epidemiologic Literature. *Nutrients* 8(12):754. doi:10.3390/nu8120754.
8. Fritz, H., D. Seely, et al. 2013. Soy, Red Clover, and Isoflavones and Breast Cancer: A Systematic Review. *PLoS One* 8(11):e81968. doi: 10.1371/journal.pone.0081968.
9. Maskarinec, G., D. Ju, et al. 2017. Soy Food Intake and Biomarkers of Breast Cancer Risk: Possible Difference in Asian Women? *Nutrition and Cancer* 69(1):146–153. doi: 10.1080/01635581.2017.1250924.
10. American Cancer Society. 2015. How Your Diet May Affect Your Risk of Breast Cancer. Available at www.cancer.org. Accessed March 2017.
11. Ibid.

Does this mean that most plant proteins are of less value in the diet? Absolutely not. When incomplete proteins are eaten with modest amounts of animal proteins or soy, or combined with other plant proteins that are rich in the incomplete protein's limiting amino acids, the incomplete protein is *complemented*. In other words, the amino acid profile of the meal is complete. For example, when rice, which is low in lysine but high in methionine, is combined with beans, which provide lysine, they complement each other and provide all nine essential amino acids. In addition, adding a small amount of cheese or meat to a plant protein, such as in macaroni and cheese or a shrimp stir-fry, provides the amino acid that is limited in the plant food.

Complementary proteins do not need to be consumed at the same meal to improve the quality of the protein source. As long as the foods are consumed in the same day, all the essential amino acids will be available to meet your biological needs. Vegetarian diets can contain a sufficient quality as well as quantity of protein in carefully planned meals. Read more on this topic in the Health Connection later in this chapter.

Chickpeas are short of the limiting amino acid methionine. The addition of sesame seed paste, which has an abundance of methionine, completes the protein. Add garlic and lemon as seasonings for a *completely* delicious hummus.

Many Healthy Foods Provide Significant Protein

The best sources of protein are low-fat dairy foods, lean meats, fish, poultry, and meat alternatives such as dried beans, peanut butter, nuts, quinoa, and soy (**Figure 6.14**). A 3-ounce serving of lean meat, poultry, or fish (about the size of a deck of cards) provides 21–25 grams of protein, or about 7 grams per ounce. Grains and vegetables are less robust protein sources, providing about 3–4 grams per serving, but as part of a varied, balanced diet, they can contribute significantly to daily needs.

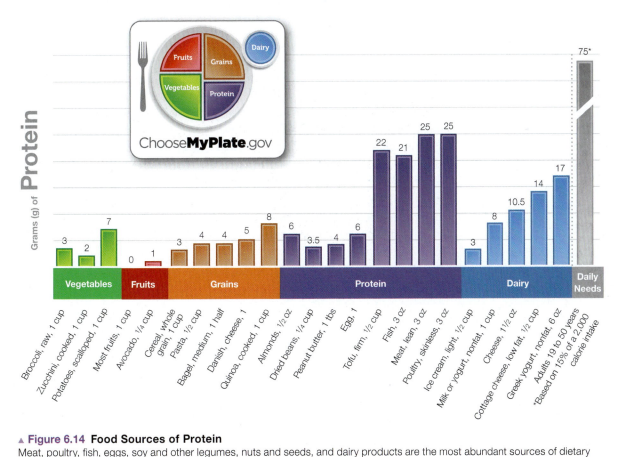

▲ **Figure 6.14 Food Sources of Protein**
Meat, poultry, fish, eggs, soy and other legumes, nuts and seeds, and dairy products are the most abundant sources of dietary protein. Grains and vegetables provide less protein per serving, but as part of a varied, balanced diet can contribute to daily needs.

Source: Data from *USDA National Nutrient Database for Standard Reference Release 28*. Revised 2016. Available at www.nal.usda.gov/fnic. Accessed March 2017.

Eating a wide variety of foods is the best approach to meeting protein needs. A diet that consists of the recommended servings from the five food groups based on 1,600 kilocalories (which is far less than most adults consume daily) will supply an adequate amount of protein for adult women and most adult men. In fact, many people have met their daily protein needs before they even sit down to dinner.

Most People Don't Need Protein Supplements

Some of the most popular supplements in the United States are protein and amino acids, often marketed especially to athletes (see Spotlight: Protein Supplements). Physically active people may take protein supplements as an ergogenic aid to increase muscle size and strength and endurance performance. However, the DRIs for protein are based on healthy food choices and you do not need additional protein in the form of supplements. (We discuss protein and sport performance in greater detail in Chapter 16.)

LO 6.6: THE TAKE-HOME MESSAGE Protein quality is determined by the digestibility of protein and the amino acid profile, which includes the types and amounts of amino acids it contains. Protein from animal foods is more digestible than plant proteins. Complete protein, found in animal foods, quinoa, and soy, provides a complete set of essential amino acids and some nonessential amino acids. Incomplete plant proteins can be complemented with protein from other plant sources or animal food sources to improve their protein quality. Low-fat dairy, eggs, lean meat, fish, poultry, and meat alternatives such as dried beans, peanut butter, nuts, and soy are healthy foods rich in protein.

Protein Supplements

The sale of protein supplements has skyrocketed over the last decade, fueling an industry that now generates almost $2 billion annually.[1] These products are marketed with promises to give you an energy boost, help shed those unwanted pounds, build muscle, fight aging, and cure a host of health problems. Their manufacturers use phrases such as "scientifically proven," but dietary supplements do not undergo rigorous testing for quality, efficacy, or safety. So how do you know if these supplements contain what they say they contain, do what they say they do, and are safe? Is more protein always better?

Protein Shakes and Powder

Most protein shakes and powders use whey, soy, or rice protein as a key ingredient. The amount of protein their label claims they contain ranges from 10 to 40 grams per serving, along with added vitamins and minerals. Muscle Milk® lists 25 grams of protein per serving and suggests 3 servings per day for a total of 75 grams of protein, almost 100 percent of the total RDA for protein for a male weighing 176 pounds.

Do these products actually contain what is listed on the label? Recently, a consumer research lab found that a popular brand of protein powder provided 16 fewer grams of protein per scoop than stated on the label. Instead, it contained an extra 16 grams of carbohydrates, including 3 grams of sugar, not accounted for on the label.[2] Other labs have found arsenic, cadmium, lead, and mercury in 15 tested samples.[3] Chronic ingestion of these toxic metals can cause severe health consequences, including organ damage, anemia, and osteoporosis.

Protein intake enhances muscle synthesis,[4] but athletes consume enough protein for muscle growth and repair in an average mixed diet. The same whey protein used in protein supplements is abundant in milk and dairy products, including Greek yogurt.[5] Any protein not used for protein synthesis is either burned for energy or stored as fat.

The key to increasing muscle mass is a well-designed strength-training program combined with additional kilocalories from all three macronutrients. These kilocalories allow dietary protein to be used for muscle synthesis instead of energy. Another important key is timing. Research suggests that ingestion of protein with carbohydrate before and immediately after a workout improves muscle synthesis.[6] A glass of low-fat chocolate milk, rather than a protein supplement, before and after a workout will provide both key amino acids and carbohydrate.

Protein shakes and powders are also marketed as meal replacers. Dieters might lose weight using a high-protein meal replacer, but the same results can be obtained with a kilocalorie-controlled meal of whole foods, without the health risks and the added expense.

There are instances where protein shakes and supplements may be advised. Older adults, who may have limited appetites and be less likely to consume adequate nutrients in foods, may benefit from drinking a protein shake every day. However, these products should be used to *supplement* meals, not replace them.

Amino Acid Supplements

Amino acid supplements, including those containing individual amino acids such as tryptophan and lysine, are marketed as remedies for a range of health issues, including chronic pain, depression, insomnia, and certain infections. Typically, these supplements contain single amino acids in amounts

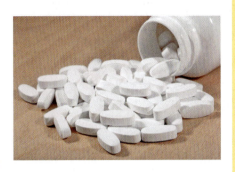

or combinations not found naturally in foods. High amounts of single amino acids can compete with other amino acids for absorption, possibly causing a deficiency of other amino acids. Furthermore, over-consuming specific amino acids can lead to side effects such as nausea, lightheadedness, vomiting, and drowsiness.

Protein Bars and Energy Bars

Protein bars and energy bars are commonly marketed as a portable snack or a quick meal, but if convenience is the main attraction, consider a peanut butter sandwich. It can be made in a snap, and since it doesn't have to be refrigerated, it can travel anywhere. From a price standpoint, a peanut butter sandwich is a bargain compared with protein bars and energy bars, which can cost 5–10 times as much. Whereas the kilocalories and protein content of the sandwich and most bars are similar, the sandwich is lower in saturated fat and has no added sugars. In contrast, some bars contain up to 7 teaspoons (about 28 grams) of added sugar. Many bars are also low in fiber. Thus, the peanut butter sandwich is the healthier choice.

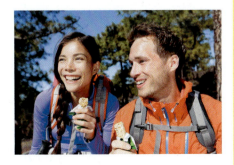

References

1. Euromonitor International. 2014. The Rise of Protein in the Global Health and Wellness and Supplement Arenas: Examining the Global Protein Surge. Available at http://globalfoodforums. com/wp-content/uploads/2014/04/Chris-Schmidt-Euromonitor-2014-Protein-Trends-Technologies.pdf. Accessed February 2017.
2. ConsumerLab.com. 2015. 31% of Protein Powders and Drinks Flunk Test of Quality. Available at www.consumerlab. com/reviews/Protein_Powders_Shakes_ Drinks_Sports_%20Meal_Diet/Nutrition-Drinks/. Accessed February 2017.
3. Consumer Reports Magazine. 2010. Alert! You Don't Need the Extra Protein or the Heavy Metals Our Tests Found. *Consumer Reports* 75:24.
4. R. J. Maughan and S. M. Shirreffs. 2012. "Nutrition for Sports Performance: Issues and Opportunities." *Proceedings of the Nutrition Society* 71:112–119.
5. Oosthuyse, T., M. Carstens, and A. M. Millen. 2015. Whey or Casein Hydrolysate with Carbohydrate for Metabolism and Performance in Cycling. *International Journal of Sports Medicine* 36(8):636–646. doi: 10.1055/s-0034-1398647.
6. Naclerio, F., et al. 2016. Effects of Protein-carbohydrate Supplementation on Immunity and Resistance Training Outcomes: A Double-blind, Randomized, Controlled Clinical Trial. *European Journal of Applied Physiology*. doi: 10.1007/s00421-016-3520-x.

What Happens If You Eat Too Much or Too Little Protein?

LO 6.7 Explain the health consequences of consuming too much or too little protein.

Most people in industrialized nations consume more than enough protein, while people from less developed countries may struggle to meet even the minimum requirements. Let's look at what happens to the human body when it gets too much or too little protein.

Eating Too Much Protein May Contribute to Chronic Disease

Eating too great a percentage of the diet as protein could cause the displacement of other nutrient-dense foods such as whole grains, fruits, and vegetables, all of which also provide disease-fighting phytochemicals and dietary fiber. Moreover, a diet with excessive protein has long been thought to increase the risk of heart disease, kidney stones, osteoporosis, and some types of cancer. However, recent research provides some reassurance that eating too much protein (0.9–2.0 g/kg per day) may not be as bad as once thought. [11]

Heart Disease

Recent research reports that the type of protein is more important in reducing the risk of heart disease than the quantity.[12] A diet low in red meat that contains nuts, low-fat dairy, poultry, or fish lessens the risk for heart disease compared with a diet high in red meat and high-fat dairy. A high-red-meat diet may mean overloading on heart-unhealthy saturated fat (see **Figure 6.15**). Even lean meats and skinless poultry, which contain less saturated fat than some other cuts of meat, are not free of saturated fat. A diet high in saturated fat can raise LDL cholesterol levels in the blood, whereas lowering the saturated fat may lower the risk of heart disease. While the overall effect of high protein intake on heart disease is still not clear, it is clear that eating a variety of plant proteins low in saturated fat is the best heart-healthy approach.

Kidney Stones

A high-protein diet may increase the risk of kidney stones. Eating a diet high in animal protein and low in carbohydrate lowers the pH of the urine, which raises the risk of developing kidney stones, especially in people who are more susceptible to the condition.[13] This change in pH may be due to higher levels of oxalates in the urine from oxalic acid;

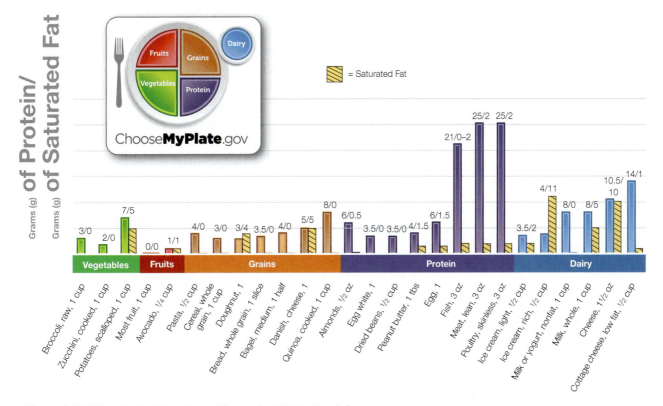

Grams (g) of Protein/ Grams (g) of Saturated Fat

= Saturated Fat

| Vegetables | | | Fruits | | Grains | | | | | | | | Protein | | | | | | | | | Dairy | | | | | |

Broccoli, raw, 1 cup: 3/0
Zucchini, cooked, 1 cup: 2/0
Potatoes, scalloped, 1 cup: 7/5
Most fruit, 1 cup: 0/0
Avocado, 1/4 cup: 1/1
Pasta, 1/2 cup: 4/0
Cereal, whole grain, 1 cup: 3/0
Doughnut, 1: 3/4
Bread, whole grain, 1 slice: 3.5/0
Bagel, medium, 1 half: 4/0
Danish, cheese, 1: 5/5
Quinoa, cooked, 1 cup: 8/0
Almonds, 1/2 oz: 6/0.5
Egg white, 1: 3.5/0
Dried beans, 1/2 cup: 3.5/0
Peanut butter, 1 tbs: 4/1.5
Egg, 1: 6/1.5
Fish, 3 oz: 21/0–2
Meat, lean, 3 oz: 25/2
Poultry, skinless, 3 oz: 25/2
Ice cream, light, 1/2 cup: 3.5/2
Ice cream, rich, 1/2 cup: 4/11
Milk or yogurt, nonfat, 1 cup: 8/0
Milk, whole, 1 cup: 8/5
Cheese, 1½ oz: 10.5/10
Cottage cheese, low fat, 1/2 cup: 14/1

▲ **Figure 6.15 Where's the Protein and Saturated Fat in Foods?**
Though many foods, in particular dairy foods and meats, can provide a hefty amount of protein, they can also provide a large amount of saturated fat. Choose nonfat and low-fat dairy foods, lean cuts of meat, and skinless poultry to avoid overloading on saturated fat.
Source: USDA National Nutrient Database for Standard Reference (www.nal.usda.gov). 2016. Accessed March 2017.

oxalic acid combines with other compounds, including calcium, to form kidney stones. The impact of protein on the change in pH may be the type of protein, not the amount of protein, consumed. A diet that contains plenty of fluid, a lower protein intake (not greater than 0.8 g/kg), a proper calcium intake, and a balance of fruits and vegetables may be beneficial, especially for people who already have kidney disease.

Osteoporosis

Though still controversial, past studies have shown that bones lose calcium when a person's diet is too high in protein. The loss seems to occur because calcium is removed from bone to neutralize the acid generated when specific amino acids are broken down. In fact, in a study of individuals on a low-carbohydrate, high-protein diet, researchers observed a 50 percent loss of calcium in the subjects' urine.[14] The calcium loss was not observed when these individuals were on a lower-protein diet, so the researchers concluded that it was due to the buffering effect.

More recent research suggests a more positive effect of high protein intake on bone health as long as dietary calcium is sufficient.[15, 16] Foods such as low-fat milk, yogurt, and cheese can add both protein and calcium to the diet.[17] Unfortunately, many American adults are falling short of their recommended calcium intake, and if their diets are also high in protein, the combination may not be healthy for their bones.

Eating too little protein can also lead to loss of bone mass. A study of more than 900 elderly men and women showed that higher protein consumption was associated with denser bone.[18] Similar results were also reported in younger adults. When it comes to our bones, too much protein coupled with low calcium intake, or too little protein intake, can both be unhealthy.[19]

Cancer

The relationship between high-protein diets and cancer is also less than clear. Although large amounts of meat, especially red and processed meats, may increase the risk for colon cancer, research doesn't support a connection between high amounts of total protein and increased colon cancer risk.[20] Processed meats have also been associated with an increased risk for bladder cancer.[21]

The *Dietary Guidelines for Americans* recommend avoiding processed meats that have been preserved by smoking, curing, salting, or adding chemical preservatives. If you are in the habit of eating bacon, sausage, ham, deli meats, and other processed meats, try replacing them with other high-protein foods, including peanut butter, low-fat dairy foods, eggs, soy-based meat alternatives, or low-fat yogurt with berries and nuts.

Eating Too Little Protein Can Lead to Protein-Energy Malnutrition

Whereas many individuals have the luxury of worrying about consuming too much protein, others are desperately trying to meet their daily needs. Every day, 795 million people, or one in nine (many of them children), around the world don't have access to enough food.[22] These children's diets are inadequate in either protein or energy or both, a condition known as **protein-energy malnutrition (PEM).** When kilocalories and protein are inadequate, dietary protein is used for energy rather than for its other roles in the body. Moreover, other important nutrients, such as vitamins and minerals, also tend to be in short supply, which further compounds PEM.

Many factors can lead to PEM, including poverty, poor food quality, insufficient food intake, unsanitary living conditions (causing diarrhea and infection), ignorance regarding the proper feeding of children, and the cessation of breastfeeding in the first few months of age.[23] Because infants and children are growing, they have higher nutritional needs for their size than adults. They are also dependent on others to provide them with food. For these reasons, PEM is more frequently seen in infants and children than in adults.

Because protein is needed for so many body functions, it isn't surprising that chronic protein deficiency can lead to numerous health problems. Without adequate dietary protein, cells lining the gastrointestinal tract aren't sufficiently replaced as they're sloughed off. The inability to regenerate these cells inhibits digestive function. Absorption of the little amount of food that may be available is reduced, and bacteria that normally stay in the intestines can contaminate the blood, causing septicemia. Malnourished individuals frequently have a compromised immune system, which can make fighting infection, such as a respiratory infection or diarrhea, impossible. Malnourished children have a much greater risk of death after exposure to measles or after bouts of diarrhea.[24, 25]

Though deficiencies of kilocalories and protein often occur simultaneously, sometimes one may be more prevalent than the other. A severe deficiency of protein is called **kwashiorkor,** whereas a severe deficiency of kilocalories is called **marasmus.** A condition that is caused by a chronic deficiency of both kilocalories and protein is called marasmic kwashiorkor.

Kwashiorkor

Kwashiorkor was first observed in the 1930s in tribes in Ghana (a republic of West Africa) when firstborn toddlers became malnourished following the birth of a sibling. Typically, when the newborn began receiving the mother's nutritionally balanced breast milk, the firstborn child was relegated to an inadequate and unbalanced diet high in

protein-energy malnutrition (PEM) Lack of sufficient dietary protein and/or kilocalories.

kwashiorkor State of PEM in which there is a severe deficiency of dietary protein.

marasmus State of PEM in which there is a severe deficiency of kilocalories, which perpetuates wasting; also called *starvation.*

carbohydrate-rich grains but severely deficient in protein. This breast milk displacement set the stage for a serious decline in the child's health.

A classic symptom of severe kwashiorkor is edema in the legs, feet, and stomach (**Figure 6.16**). Because protein plays an important role in maintaining fluid balance in the blood and around the cells, a protein deficiency can cause fluid to accumulate in the spaces surrounding the cells, causing swelling. In addition, as muscle proteins are broken down to generate the amino acids needed to synthesize other body proteins, muscle tone and strength diminish. Those with kwashiorkor may also have skin that is dry and peeling. Rashes or lesions can also develop. Their hair is often brittle and can be easily pulled out. Children with kwashiorkor often appear pale, sad, and apathetic, and cry easily. They are prone to infections, rapid heartbeat, excess fluid in the lungs, pneumonia, septicemia, and fluid and electrolyte imbalances—all of which can be deadly.

Marasmus

The bloating seen in kwashiorkor is the opposite of the frail, emaciated appearance of marasmus (**Figure 6.17**). Because they are not consuming enough kilocalories, marasmic individuals are literally starving. They are often not even at 60 percent of their desirable body weight. Marasmic children's bodies use all available kilocalories to stay alive; thus, growth is interrupted. Such children are weakened and appear apathetic. Many can't stand without support. They look old beyond their years, as the loss of fat in their face—one of the last places that the body loses fat during starvation—diminishes their childlike appearance. Their hair is thin and dry and lacks the sheen found in healthy children. Their body temperature and blood pressure are both low, and they are prone to dehydration, infections, and unnecessary blood clotting.

Individuals with marasmic kwashiorkor have the worst of both conditions. They often have edema in their legs and arms, yet have a "skin and bones" appearance in other parts of the body. When these individuals are provided with medical and nutritional treatment, such as adequate protein, the edema subsides and their clinical symptoms more closely resemble that of a person with marasmus.

Appropriate medical care and treatment can dramatically reduce the 22–40 percent mortality rate seen among children with severe PEM worldwide.[26] The treatment for PEM should be carefully and slowly implemented using a three-step approach. The first step addresses the life-threatening factors, such as severe dehydration and fluid imbalances, using electrolyte solutions. The second step is to restore the individual's depleted tissues by gradually providing nutritionally dense kilocalories and high-quality protein. The third step involves transitioning the person to solid foods and introducing physical activity.

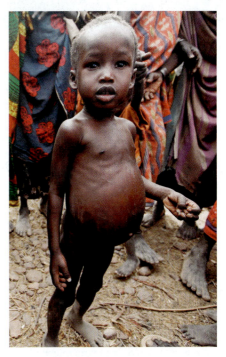

▲ **Figure 6.16 Kwashiorkor**
The edema in this child's belly is a classic sign of kwashiorkor.

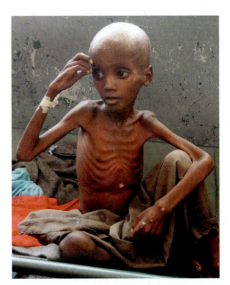

▲ **Figure 6.17 Marasmus**
The emaciated appearance of this child is a sign of marasmus.

LO 6.7: THE TAKE-HOME MESSAGE Too many protein-rich foods can displace whole grains, fruits, and vegetables, which have been shown to help reduce many chronic diseases. A high-protein diet may increase the risk of heart disease, kidney problems, and calcium loss from bone. Consuming too much protein from animal sources can increase the amount of saturated fat in the diet. A low-protein diet has also been shown to lead to loss of bone mass. PEM is caused by an inadequate amount of protein, kilocalories, or both in the diet. A severe deficiency of protein results in kwashiorkor; a severe deficiency of kilocalories causes marasmus.

What Is a Vegetarian Diet?

LO 6.8 Describe the benefits and risks of a vegetarian diet.

Whereas many people choose to become a **vegetarian** for ethical, religious, or environmental reasons, others follow a vegetarian diet for health reasons.[27] An estimated 3.3 percent of Americans consider themselves vegetarians.[28] There are several types of vegetarians and associated ranges of acceptable foods. See **Table 6.5** for a description of different vegetarian diets and the foods associated with each.

Because vegetarians avoid meat, poultry, and fish, which are high in complete protein, they need to be sure to get adequate protein from other food sources. Vegetarians can meet their daily protein needs by consuming a varied plant-based diet that contains meat alternatives such as soy, dried beans and other legumes, and nuts. Vegetarians who consume some animal products, such as milk, eggs, and/or fish, can use these foods to help meet their protein needs.

In the United States, the vegetarian food market continues to grow as manufacturers accommodate increased consumer demand with an array of new vegetarian products each year.[29] Many sit-down restaurants offer vegetarian entrées on their menus, and even some fast-food restaurants now offer veggie burgers. University food services are increasingly making vegetarian options available to meet growing student demand.

Balanced Vegetarian Diets Confer Health Benefits

A plant-based vegetarian diet can be rich in high-fiber whole grains, legumes and other vegetables, fruits, and nuts; naturally

vegetarian Person who avoids eating animal foods. Some vegetarians only avoid meat, fish, and poultry, while others (vegans) avoid all animal products, including eggs and dairy.

TABLE 6.5	The Many Types of Vegetarians	
Type	**Eats**	**Avoids**
Lacto-vegetarian	Grains, vegetables, fruits, legumes, seeds, nuts, dairy foods	Meat, fish, poultry, and eggs
Lacto-ovo-vegetarian	Grains, vegetables, fruits, legumes, seeds, nuts, dairy foods, eggs	Meat, fish, and poultry
Ovo-vegetarian	Grains, vegetables, fruits, legumes, seeds, nuts, eggs	Meat, fish, poultry, dairy foods
Vegan	Grains, vegetables, fruits, legumes, seeds, nuts	Any animal foods (meat, fish, poultry, dairy foods, eggs)
Pescetarian	Grains, vegetables, fruits, legumes, seeds, nuts, dairy foods, eggs, and fish	Meat and poultry
Semivegetarian	A vegetarian diet that occasionally includes meat, fish, and poultry	Meat, fish, and poultry on occasion

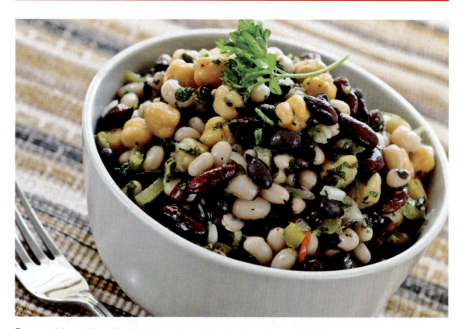

Beans add protein, antioxidants, and a variety of minerals to a healthful plant-based diet.

lower in saturated fat; and cholesterol free. These qualities are fundamental for reducing the risk of heart disease, high blood pressure, diabetes, cancer, stroke, and obesity, assuming the diet is not limited or unbalanced in nutrients.

Vegetarian food staples such as soy, nuts, and soluble fiber–rich foods including beans and oats have all been shown to reduce blood cholesterol levels. Research collected from numerous studies has shown that deaths from heart disease are about 29 percent lower among vegetarians than among nonvegetarians.[30]

Vegetarians also tend to have lower blood pressure than those who consume meat. The incidence of high blood pressure has been shown to be over two times higher in nonvegetarians.[31] High blood pressure is a risk factor not only for heart disease but also for stroke.

A plant-based diet can help reduce the risk of type 2 diabetes, and vegetarians as a population group tend to have a lower incidence of diabetes. Among people who already have diabetes, the predominance of foods rich in fiber and low in saturated fat and cholesterol in a vegetarian diet can help manage the disease.[32]

Vegetarians also have lower cancer rates compared with the general population. The latest World Cancer Research Fund Report advocates a plant-based diet that is high in nutrients and dietary fiber yet low in energy-dense foods (highly processed foods with added sugars and saturated fat, as well as sugary beverages) to reduce the risk for cancer.[33]

Also, a plant-based diet that contains mostly fiber-rich whole grains and low-kilo-calorie, nutrient-dense vegetables and fruits tends to be one that "fills you up before it fills you out," which means that you are likely to eat fewer overall kilocalories. Consequently, eating the plant-based foods of a vegetarian diet can be a healthy and satisfying strategy for fighting the battle against obesity. **Figure 6.18** can help vegetarians easily incorporate these foods into their diet.

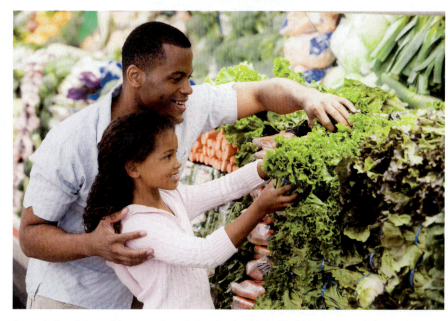

A vegetarian diet combines a variety of plant foods with fortified foods or supplements rich in vitamin B_{12}.

A Healthy Vegetarian Diet Requires Planning

The biggest risk of a vegetarian diet is underconsuming certain nutrients, such as protein, or certain vitamins and minerals. Vegetarian foods contain protein, but the amount per serving is lower than that found in animal sources. For example, 100 grams, or a serving, of kidney beans contains 7 grams of protein, whereas 100 grams of cooked chicken breast, or the size of a medium boneless chicken breast, contains 17 grams. Most plant foods also do not contain complete protein. A vegetarian's protein needs can be met by consuming a *variety* of plant foods. A combination of protein-rich soy foods, legumes, nuts, or seeds should be eaten daily.

The form of iron in plants is not as easily absorbed as the form of iron in meat, fish, and poultry. Also, phytate in grains and rice, and polyphenols in tea and coffee, can inhibit iron absorption. The iron needs of vegetarians are about 1.5 times higher than those of nonvegetarians. Consuming iron-fortified cereals, enriched grains, pasta, wheat germ, and nuts and seeds can improve iron intake in vegetarians. Consuming animal protein enhances the absorption of zinc. Following a vegetarian diet means that you lose out on this benefit and are more likely to develop a zinc deficiency. Phytates found in grains and rice also bind zinc, making it less bio-available. A vegan's zinc needs may be as much as 50 percent higher than a nonveg-etarian's. A diet rich in soybeans, fortified soy burgers, legumes, nuts, and seeds will increase the zinc content of the diet.

Calcium is abundant in low-fat dairy foods such as nonfat or low-fat milk, yogurt, and cheese. If you follow a lacto-vegetarian diet, these foods would meet your calcium needs; however, if you follow a vegan diet, you may have more difficulty meeting your calcium needs. Calcium-forti-fied soymilk and orange juice as well as tofu can provide about the same amount of cal-cium per serving as is found in dairy foods. Adding calcium-rich vegetables including bok choy, broccoli, kale, collard greens, and okra will enhance calcium intake.

Vitamin A and vitamin D may be low in a vegetarian diet. Preformed vitamin A is found only in animal foods. However, veg-etarians can meet their needs by consum-ing the vitamin A precursor beta-carotene found in vegetables such as carrots and spinach. Some vegetarians will need to consume vitamin D–fortified milk, yogurt, or soymilk to maintain adequate levels of

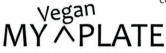

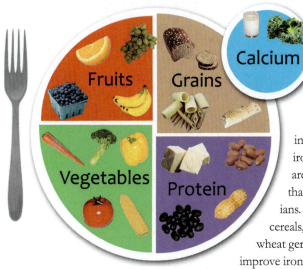

▲ **Figure 6.18 My Vegan Plate**
Source: The Vegetarian Resource Group, www.vrg.org.

vitamin D. Egg yolk and ready-to-eat cereals, in addition to a vitamin supplement, will add sufficient vitamin D to the diet.

Vitamin B_{12} is also a concern in vegetarian diets because it is only found in animal-based foods.[34] If the vegetarian diet contains eggs and dairy products, the diet may contain some vitamin B_{12}. If the diet plan is strictly vegan, fortified foods or supplements should be included. Plant foods that are fermented or sprouted may contain a little vitamin B_{12} but the amount is not consistent or dependable. Foods fortified with vitamin B_{12} such as cereals, fortified soy products, nutritional yeast, and yeast extracts should be incorporated into the menu. Vitamin B_{12} supplements can also be used or vitamin B_{12} intramuscular injections from a physician will prevent vitamin B_{12} deficiencies.

If your vegetarian diet doesn't include fish, you may not be consuming enough of the essential omega-3 fatty acid alpha-linolenic acid, which is a precursor to eicosanoids. Moreover, fatty fish such as salmon and sardines are direct sources of both EPA and DHA. Walnuts, flaxseed and flaxseed oil, and soybean and canola oil are other good vegetarian food sources to increase the omega-3 content of the diet.

To avoid nutrient deficiencies, vegetarians must consume adequate amounts of a wide variety of foods. Monitor those nutrients found in abundance in animal-based foods, including protein, iron, zinc, calcium, vitamin D, vitamin B_{12}, vitamin A, and omega-3 fatty acids. A vitamin and mineral supplement may be necessary. The tips in **Table 6.6** can help vegetarians increase these nutrients in their diet. Analyze the dietary habits of Megan, a college sophomore who has recently become a vegan, in the Nutrition in Practice on page 239.

TABLE 6.6 Suggested Servings for a Healthy Vegetarian Diet

Food Group	Number of Servings	Serving Size	Calcium-Rich Foods (8 servings daily)
Grains	6	Bread, 1 slice	Whole-wheat bread, 1 slice
		Cooked grain or cereal, $\frac{1}{2}$ cup	Calcium-fortified cereal, 1 oz
		Ready-to-eat cereal, 1 oz	
Legumes, nuts, and other protein-rich foods	5	Cooked beans, peas, or lentils, $\frac{1}{2}$ cup Tofu or tempeh, $\frac{1}{2}$ cup Nut or seed butter, 2 tbsp Nuts, $\frac{1}{4}$ cup Meat analog, 1 oz Egg, 1	Cow's milk or yogurt, $\frac{1}{2}$ cup Calcium-fortified soy milk, $\frac{1}{2}$ cup Cheese, $\frac{3}{4}$ oz
Vegetables	4	Cooked vegetables, $\frac{1}{2}$ cup	Bok choy, collards, broccoli, Chinese cabbage, kale, mustard greens, or okra; 1 cup cooked or 2 cups raw
		Raw vegetables, 1 cup	Calcium-fortified tomato juice, $\frac{1}{2}$ cup
		Vegetable juice, $\frac{1}{2}$ cup	
Fruits	2	Medium fruit, 1 Cut-up or cooked fruit, $\frac{1}{2}$ cup Fruit juice, $\frac{1}{2}$ cup Dried fruit, $\frac{1}{4}$ cup	Calcium-fortified fruit juice, $\frac{1}{2}$ cup Figs, 5
Fats	2	Oil, 1 tsp Soft margarine, 1 tsp Mayonnaise, 1 tsp	

LO 6.8: THE TAKE-HOME MESSAGE Some vegetarians abstain from all animal foods, whereas others may eat eggs and dairy products or even fish or poultry in limited amounts. A balanced vegetarian diet may reduce the risk of heart disease, high blood pressure, diabetes, cancer, stroke, and obesity. All vegetarians must take care in planning a varied diet that meets their nutrient needs, especially for protein, iron, zinc, calcium, vitamin A, vitamin D, vitamin B_{12}, and omega-3 fatty acids.

NUTRITION *in* PRACTICE:

Registered Nurse and MD

Megan, a college sophomore, has a micro-fridge in her dorm room so she eats breakfast in her room daily. Her lunch and dinner are eaten in the campus dining hall. Even though she eats breakfast and lunch before her classes, she is often fatigued by midafternoon. Megan has lost 5 pounds over the last 2 months, and her worried parents convinced her to make an appointment at the college student health center. During the initial screening, the health center registered nurse (RN) uncovered that Megan had recently become a vegan. Megan was following a vegan diet that she found on the Internet, which restricted her food choices to only grains, vegetables, and fruit. The nurse communicated this finding to the doctor, and after his physical examination of Megan, a blood test was ordered to rule out any underlying health issue. The test results were negative.

Based on the results of the laboratory test and the findings from the RN's initial screening, the doctor referred Megan to the campus registered dietitian nutritionist (RDN) to receive guidance about her diet. The nurse called Megan with the contact information for the RDN.

Megan's Stats
- ❏ Age: 19
- ❏ Height: 5 feet 3 inches
- ❏ Weight: 110 pounds
- ❏ BMI: 19.3

Critical Thinking Questions

1. Why do you think Megan is hungry and tired during the day?
2. Based on her food log, which nutrients are likely to be low in Megan's diet?
3. Based on her food log, which other food group is Megan falling short of daily?

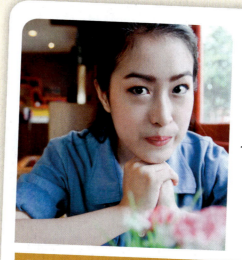

Megan

MEGAN'S FOOD LOG

Food/Beverage	Time Consumed	Hunger Rating*	Location
English muffin with jam and a banana	8:00 A.M.	5	In dorm room
Salad bar salad: lettuce, tomato, carrots, peppers, and cucumbers with Italian dressing. Diet soda.	12:30 P.M.	5	Campus dining hall
Popcorn	3:00 P.M.	5	Studying in dorm room
Veggie stir-fry over rice. Diet soda.	6:30 P.M.	5	In dining hall

* Hunger Rating (1–5): 1 = not hungry; 5 = super hungry.

RDN's Observation and Plan for Megan

- ❏ Discuss the need to add vegan protein sources at each meal to meet her daily protein needs. Add peanut butter on her morning English muffin. Top her salad bar lunch with the chickpeas that are available in the dining hall. Add tofu to her veggie stir-fry, which is always available at the salad bar.
- ❏ Discuss the need to consume three servings of a vegan equivalent of dairy foods in order to meet her calcium, vitamin D, and vitamin B$_{12}$ needs.

Drink a fortified soy beverage at each meal.

A month later, Megan returns for a follow-up visit with the RDN. By incorporating all of the RDN's suggestions, she was feeling less fatigued and hungry. She had also gained 1.5 pounds. A review of her food record shows that she is meeting her daily protein needs and her diet is more balanced. However, she is still a little hungry late in the afternoon. The RDN recommends that Megan add some soy cheese with her afternoon popcorn snack to curb her hunger.

Visual Chapter Summary

LO 6.1 Proteins Are Made of Amino Acids Linked with a Peptide Bond

Proteins are made up of 20 amino acids, 11 nonessential and nine essential. Nonessential amino acids can be made in the body, but the essential amino acids must be consumed in the diet. A third category, conditionally essential, contains those amino acids that under certain conditions must be supplied by food.

Amino acids are composed of carbon, hydrogen, oxygen, nitrogen, and, in some cases, sulfur. Every amino acid contains a central carbon, an acid group (COOH), an amine group (NH₂), a single hydrogen, and a unique side chain that gives each amino acid its distinctive qualities.

Amino acids are joined together by peptide bonds through condensation. Two amino acids joined together form a dipeptide, three form a tripeptide, and a polypeptide consists of many amino acids joined together. The unique sequence of amino acids in the chain is the primary structure of a protein. Hydrogen bonding between the carboxyl and amine groups of the amino acids causes the chain to twist and coil, forming the secondary structure. The hydrophobic side chains cluster together on the inside and combine to the globular tertiary structure. The quaternary structure forms when two or more polypeptide chains bond. Heat, acids, bases, salts, or mechanical agitation denature proteins. The primary structure doesn't change but the shape of the protein does, and it no longer functions.

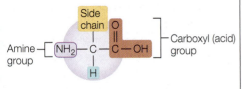

LO 6.2 Protein Digestion Occurs in the Stomach and Small Intestine

The chemical digestion of protein begins in the stomach. Gastrin stimulates the release of HCl from the parietal cells and the inactive enzyme pepsinogen from the chief cells. HCl denatures the protein and converts pepsinogen to pepsin, which breaks polypeptides into shorter chains. Cholecystokinin from the duodenum stimulates trypsinogen, carboxypeptidase, and chymotrypsinogen from the pancreas. These proteases hydrolyze the shorter chains into tripeptides and dipeptides. Dipeptidases and tripeptidases hydrolyze the tripeptides and dipeptides into single amino acids that are absorbed through the enterocytes via the portal vein to the liver. Absorbed amino acids are used to synthesize new proteins, or are converted to energy (ATP), glucose, or fat and stored in the adipose tissue.

LO 6.3 The Metabolism of Protein Is Based on the Body's Needs

During protein synthesis, the cell derives amino acids from the amino acid pools throughout the body. Proteins are assembled by ribosomes in the cell cytoplasm, using instructions encoded in genes in the DNA in the cell nucleus and transported to the cytoplasm by messenger RNA. Excess amino acids can be deaminated and then converted into ATP, glucose, or fatty acids. Transamination is used to synthesize nonessential amino acids.

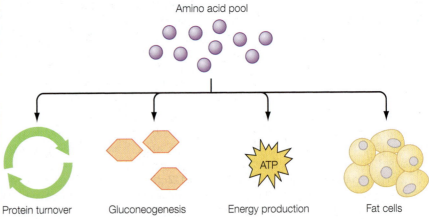

LO 6.4 Protein Plays Key Roles in the Body

Proteins provide structural and mechanical support and help maintain body tissues. Most enzymes and many hormones are proteins, as are antibodies and certain other chemicals involved in the immune response. Proteins help maintain fluid and acid–base balance, transport substances throughout the body, and act as channels in cell membranes. Proteins also provide energy, improve satiety, and help control appetite.

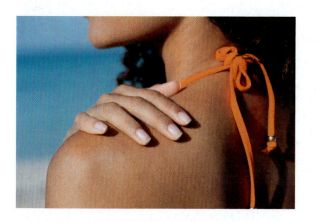

LO 6.5 Protein Needs Are Based on the Dietary Reference Intakes and Determined by Nitrogen Balance Studies

For a healthy adult, the amount of dietary protein consumed every day should equal the amount of protein used. Nitrogen balance studies suggest an RDA for adults of 0.8 grams of protein per kilogram of body weight daily. Men typically consume more than 100 grams of protein daily, and women more than 70 grams—in both cases, far more than is needed. The AMDR for protein intake is between 10 and 35 percent of total daily kilocalories.

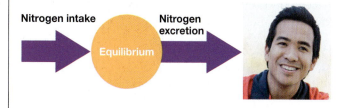

LO 6.6 Protein Foods Are Evaluated by Their Digestibility, Amino Acid Score, and Essential Amino Acid Content

Protein quality is determined by the body's ability to digest the protein and the essential or nonessential amino acids that the protein contains, called the amino acid score. A protein's digestibility and its amino acid score are combined to yield a protein digestibility corrected amino acid score (PDCAAS). The essential amino acid with the lowest score is called the limiting amino acid. Proteins with a higher PDCAAS are of higher quality. A complete protein, found in animal foods, quinoa, and soy, provides a complete set of the essential amino acids. Plant proteins are typically incomplete, as they are missing or low in one or more of the essential amino acids. Combining complementary protein sources can yield a high-protein meal. Healthy food sources of proteins include eggs, lean meats, low-fat or fat-free dairy products, quinoa, soy, other legumes, nuts, and seeds. Grains and vegetables also supply protein to the diet. Most people consume more than enough protein each day and thus protein supplements are not necessary.

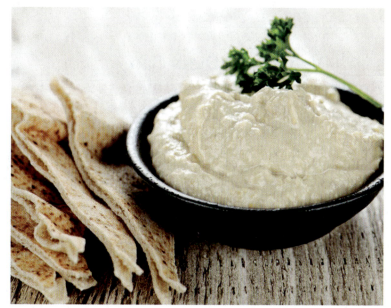

LO 6.7 Too Much or Too Little Protein Is Linked to Health Problems

A diet too high in protein is linked to health problems such as cardiovascular disease, kidney stones, osteoporosis, and some types of cancer. An excess of protein-rich foods can displace whole grains, fruits, and vegetables in the diet. Eating too little protein can also compromise bone health.

Diets that are inadequate in protein, kilocalories, or both lead to protein-energy malnutrition (PEM), two forms of which are marasmus and kwashiorkor. Marasmus is a severe wasting disease caused by insufficient intake of kilocalories. Kwashiorkor occurs when a person consumes sufficient kilocalories but not sufficient protein. PEM significantly increases vulnerability to infectious disease. It is treated with careful refeeding.

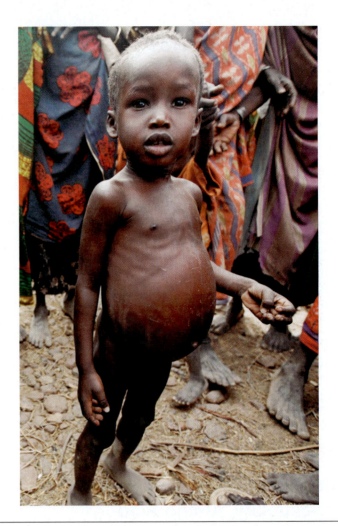

LO 6.8 Vegetarian Diets Can Reduce the Risk of Certain Diseases

Healthy vegetarian diets can reduce the risk of heart disease, high blood pressure, diabetes, cancer, stroke, and obesity. All vegetarians must take care to eat a varied diet that meets all of their nutrient needs, especially for protein, iron, zinc, calcium, vitamin D, vitamin B$_{12}$, vitamin A, and omega-3 fatty acids.

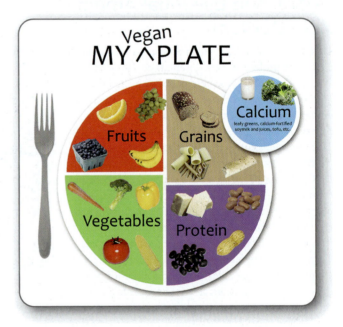

Terms to Know

- proteins
- amino acids
- amine group
- side chain
- peptide
- dipeptide
- tripeptide
- polypeptide
- peptide bonds
- essential amino acid
- nonessential amino acid
- conditionally essential amino acid
- primary structure
- secondary structure
- tertiary structure
- quaternary structure
- denature

- amino acid pools
- protein turnover
- genes
- ribosomes
- transcription
- messenger RNA (mRNA)
- translation
- transfer RNA (tRNA)
- elongation
- sickle cell anemia
- deamination
- urea
- transamination
- catabolic
- anabolic
- albumin
- edema
- acidosis
- alkalosis

- buffers
- transport proteins
- antibodies
- immunity
- allergen
- glucogenic amino acids
- amino acid score
- limiting amino acid
- nitrogen balance
- protein digestibility corrected amino acid score (PDCAAS)
- complete protein
- incomplete protein
- isoflavones
- protein-energy malnutrition (PEM)
- kwashiorkor
- marasmus
- vegetarian

Mastering Nutrition
Visit the Study Area in Mastering Nutrition to hear an MP3 chapter summary.

Check Your Understanding

LO 6.1 1. Proteins differ from carbohydrates and lipids because
  a. they contain carbon–carbon bonds.
  b. they contain nitrogen.
  c. they contain carbon, hydrogen, and oxygen.
  d. only proteins vary in chain length.

LO 6.1 2. Which of the following nonessential amino acids can also be considered a conditionally essential amino acid?
  a. Alanine
  b. Serine
  c. Glutamic acid
  d. Proline

LO 6.2 3. The enzyme that begins the chemical digestion of protein in the stomach is
  a. carboxypeptidase.
  b. pepsin.
  c. alcohol dehydrogenase.
  d. ghrelin.

LO 6.3 4. Gluconeogenesis is stimulated when
  a. the diet is high in carbohydrate.
  b. the diet is high in fat.
  c. the diet is low in protein.
  d. the diet is low in carbohydrate.

LO 6.3 5. Before excess amino acids can be used for energy or stored as fat, they must be
  a. deaminated.
  b. digested.
  c. denatured.
  d. deactivated.

LO 6.4 6. Proteins play important roles in the body, but do not
  a. regulate fluid balance.
  b. enable movement.
  c. act as chemical messengers.
  d. constitute part of bile used to emulsify fat.

LO 6.5 7. Connie is a healthy 22-year-old student who weighs 155 pounds. What is her Recommended Dietary Allowance (RDA) for protein?
  a. 56 grams per day
  b. 70 grams per day
  c. 86 grams per day
  d. 140 grams per day

LO 6.6 8. Protein is found abundantly in
  a. fruits and nuts.
  b. milk, eggs, meat, and beans.
  c. vegetables and whole grains.
  d. oils and sugars.

LO 6.7 9. Kwashiorkor is a type of PEM that develops when
  a. there is a severe deficiency of protein in the diet but adequate kilocalories.
  b. intake of both protein and kilocalories is inadequate.
  c. there is an inadequate amount of animal protein in the diet but sufficient plant protein.
  d. there are adequate amounts of both protein and kilocalories in the diet.

LO 6.8 10. Which of the following is a characteristic of a lacto-vegetarian diet?
  a. Calcium is likely to be deficient in this diet.
  b. This diet is likely to be low in fiber.
  c. The risk of developing heart disease is reduced on this diet.
  d. This diet includes eggs and dairy.

Answers

1. (b) Proteins differ from carbohydrates because they contain nitrogen found in the amine group. All three macronutrients contain carbon, hydrogen, and oxygen. The chains of glucose units or fatty acids vary in length as do chains of amino acids.

2. (d) Proline can be a conditionally essential amino acid under certain conditions.

3. (b) Pepsin is the active form of the enzyme that begins protein digestion. Carboxypeptidase and alcohol dehydrogenase are other digestive enzymes. Ghrelin is a hormone that stimulates appetite.

4. (d) If an individual does not eat an adequate amount of carbohydrate, the body can break down proteins to create glucose.

5. (a) Before amino acids can be converted to glucose or fatty acids, or enter the energy cycle, the amine group must first be removed through deamination. Denaturing is the process of unfolding or changing the shape of proteins.

6. (d) The body needs adequate amounts of protein to maintain fluid balance, to provide structural and mechanical support for movement, and as hormones, which act as chemical messengers. Protein is not part of bile used to emulsify fat.

7. (a) Adults need 0.80 gram protein per kilogram of body weight daily. To calculate Connie's daily protein needs, convert her body weight to kilograms and multiply by 0.8 gram per kg of body weight. She needs 56 grams per day.

8. (b) Animal foods and some plant-based proteins, such as beans and nuts, are protein rich. There is some protein in vegetables, but little in fruits. Oils and sugars do not contain protein.

9. (a) Kwashiorkor occurs when protein is deficient in the diet even though kilocalories may be adequate. Marasmus occurs when kilocalories are inadequate in a person's diet. Protein from animal sources is not necessary because people can meet their protein needs from a combination of plant proteins.

10. (c) Consuming a lacto-vegetarian diet reduces the risk for heart disease. Because a lacto-vegetarian diet includes dairy products, it is likely to provide sufficient calcium. Because it is a vegetarian diet, it is likely to provide sufficient dietary fiber. Eggs are excluded on a lacto-vegetarian diet.

Answers to True or False?

1. **True.** Proteins are the only macronutrients that contain nitrogen.

2. **False.** Of the 20 amino acids that make up protein, nine are considered essential and 11 are nonessential.

3. **False.** Chemical digestion of protein begins in the stomach with the enzyme pepsin, which is secreted by the chief cells lining the stomach.

4. **True.** When proteins arrive in the stomach, hydrochloric acid uncoils them, revealing the peptide bonds that connect the amino acids.

5. **True.** Amino acids can be converted to glucose through gluconeogenesis.

6. **False.** The primary function of protein is to build new tissues and repair proteins that have been degraded or sloughed off in the body.

7. **False.** Growing children are in a state of positive nitrogen balance, which means that more nitrogen is being retained by the body than excreted in the urine.

8. **False.** Animal proteins are considered complete proteins because they contain all nine essential amino acids.

9. **False.** Protein itself doesn't raise blood cholesterol levels. It depends on the type of protein food you consume.

10. **True.** A diet that is inadequate in protein results in kwashiorkor, characterized by edema and body wasting.

Web Resources

- For information on specific genetic disorders, including those that affect protein use in the body, visit the National Human Genome Research Institute at www.nhgri.nih.gov

- For more information on protein bars and supplements, visit the Center for Science in the Public Interest at www.cspinet.org

- For more information on vegetarian diets, visit the Vegetarian Resource Group at www.vrg.org

References

1. Marieb, E. N., and K. Hoehn. 2016. *Human Anatomy and Physiology.* 10th ed. San Francisco: Benjamin Cummings.
2. Ibid.
3. Marieb. 2016. *Human Anatomy and Physiology.*
4. National Human Genome Research Institute. 2014. *Learning About Sickle-Cell Disease.* Available at www.genome.gov. Accessed February 2017.

5. Berg, J. M., J. L. Tymoczko, and L. Stryer. 2013. *Biochemistry.* 7th ed. New York: W. H. Freeman and Company.

6. Kranz, S., et al. 2017. High-Protein and High-Dietary-Fiber Breakfasts Result in Equal Feelings of Fullness and Better Diet Quality in Low-Income Preschoolers Compared with Their Usual Breakfast. *Journal of Nutrition* pii: jn234153. doi: 10.3945/jn.116.234153.

7. Missimer, A., et al. 2017. Consuming Two Eggs per Day, as Compared to an Oatmeal Breakfast, Increases Plasma Ghrelin While Maintaining the LDL/HDL Ratio. *Nutrients* 9(2). pii: E89. doi: 10.3390/nu9020089.

8. Breen, L., and S. M. Phillips. 2012. Nutrient Interaction for Optimal Protein Anabolism in Resistance Exercise. *Current Opininion in Clinical Nutrrition and Metabolic Care* 15:226–232.

9. Beelen, M., A. Zorenc, B. Pennings, J. M. Senden, H. Kuipers, and L. J. van Loon. (2011b). Impact of Protein Coingestion on Muscle Protein Synthesis during Continuous Endurance Type Exercise. *American Journal of Physiology* 300:E945–E954.

10. Stipanek, M., and M. A. Caudill. 2013. *Biochemical, Physiological, and Molecular Aspects of Human Nutrition.* 3rd ed. St. Louis, MO: Elsevier Sanders.

11. Aldrich, N. D., C. Perry, W. Thomas, S. K. Raatz, and M. Reicks. 2013. Perceived Importance of Dietary Protein to Prevent Weight Gain: A National Survey among Midlife Women. *Journal of Nutrition Education and Behavior* 45(3):213–221.

12. Haring, B., et al. 2014. Dietary Protein Intake and Coronary Heart Disease in a Large Community Based Cohort: Results from the Atherosclerosis Risk in Communities (ARIC) Study. *PLoS One* 9(10):e109552. doi: 10.1371/journal.pone.0109552.

13. National Kidney and Urologic Diseases Information Clearinghouse (NKUDIC). 2013. *Diet for Kidney Stone Prevention.* Available at http://kidney.niddk.nih.gov. Accessed February 2017.

14. Allen, L. H., E. A. Oddoye, and S. Margen. 1979. Protein-Induced Calciuria: A Longer-Term Study. *American Journal of Clinical Nutrition* 32:741–749.

15. Mangano, K. M., S. Sahni, D. P. Kiel, K. L. Tucker, A. B. Dufour, and M. T. Hannan. 2017. Dietary Protein Is Associated with Musculoskeletal Health Independently of Dietary Pattern: The Framingham Third Generation Study. *American Journal of Clinical Nutrition* pii: ajcn136762. doi: 10.3945/ajcn.116.136762.

16. Ibid.

17. Jesudason, D., C. Nordin, J. Keogh, and P. Clifton. 2013. Comparison of Two Weight-Loss Diets of Different Protein Content on Bone Health: A Randomized Trial. *American Journal of Clinical Nutrition* 98(5):1343–1352.

18. Mangano, K. M., 2017. Dietary Protein Is Associated with Musculoskeletal Health Independently of Dietary Pattern: The Framingham Third Generation Study. *American Journal of Clinical Nutrition* pii: ajcn136762. doi: 10.3945/ajcn.116.136762.

19. Cao, J. J., S. M. Pasiakos, L. M. Margolis, E. R. Sauter, L. D. Whigham, J. P. McClung, A. J. Young, and G. F. Combs, Jr. 2014. Calcium Homeostasis and Bone Metabolic Responses to High-Protein Diets during Energy Deficit in Healthy Young Adults: A Randomized Controlled Trial. *American Journal of Clinical Nutrition* 99(2):400–407.

20. Egeberg, R., A. Olsen, J. Christensen, J. Halkjaer, M. U. Jakobsen, K. Overvad, and A. Tjønneland. 2014. Associations between Red Meat and Risks for Colon and Rectal Cancer Depend on the Type of Red Meat Consumed. *Journal of Nutrition* 143(4):464–472.

21. Crippa, A., S. C. Larsson, A. Discacciati, A. Wolk, and N. Orsini. 2016. Red and Processed Meat Consumption and Risk of Bladder Cancer: A Dose-response Meta-analysis of Epidemiological Studies. *European Journal of Nutrition.* doi: 10.1007/s00394-016-1356-0.

22. Food and Agriculture Organization of the United Nations. 2013. *The State of Food Insecurity in the World, 2015.* Available at www.fao.org. Accessed February 2017.

23. World Health Organization. 2012. *WHO Global Database on Child Growth and Malnutrition Introduction.* Available at www.who.int. Accessed February 2017.

24. Denno, D. M. 2013. Child Health Part 2: Interventions to Combat the Major Childhood Killers. *Global Health Education Consortium.* Available at www.cugh.org. Accessed February 2017.

25. GBD 2015 Risk Factors Collaborators. 2016. Global, Regional, and National Comparative Risk Assessment of 79 Behavioural, Environmental and Occupational, and Metabolic Risks or Clusters of Risks, 1990-2015: A Systematic Analysis for the Global Burden of Disease Study 2015. *Lancet* 388(10053):1659–1724. doi: 10.1016/S0140-6736(16)31679-8.

26. Agozie, C. U., N. S. Ibeziako, C. I. Ndiokwelu, C. M. Uzoka, and C. A. Nwafor. 2012. Under-Five Protein Energy Malnutrition Admitted at the University of Nigeria Teaching Hospital, Enugu: A 10-Year Retrospective Review. *Nutrition Journal* 11:43–50.

27. Nordin, S., M. Boyle, and T. Kemmer. 2013. Position of the Academy of Nutrition and Dietetics: Nutrition Security in Developing Nations: Sustainable Food, Water, and Health. *Journal of the Academy of Nutrition and Dietetics* 113:581–595.

28. Vegetarian Resource Group. 2016. How Many Adults in the U.S. Are Vegetarian and Vegan? Available at www.vrg.org/nutshell/Polls/2016_adults_veg.htm. Accessed February 2017.

29. Ginsberg, C. 2017. *The Market for Vegetarian Foods.* Available at www.vrg.org. Accessed February 2017.

30. Dinu, M., R. Abbate, G. F. Gensini, A. Casini, and F. Sofi. 2016. Vegetarian, Vegan Diets and Multiple Health Outcomes: A Systematic Review with Meta-analysis of Observational Studies. *Critical Reviews in Food Science and Nutrition.* doi.org/10.1080/10408398.2016.1138447.

31. Yokoyama, Y., K. Nishimura, N. D. Barnard, et al. 2013. Vegetarian Diets and Blood Pressure: A Meta-Analysis. *Journal of the American Medical Association Internal Medicine.* doi:10.1001/jamainternmed.2013.14547.

32. Tonstad, S., K. Stewart, K. Oda, M. Batech, R. P. Herring, and G. E. Fraser. 2013. Vegetarian Diets and Incidence of Diabetes in the Adventist Health Study-2. *Nutrition, Metabolism, and Cardiovascular Diseases* 23(4):292–299.

33. Collins, K., and S. Palmer. 2013. *Eating Patterns to Lower Cancer Risk: More Than One Route to a Plant-Based Diet.* Available at www.aicr.org. Accessed February 2017.

34. Pawlak, R., S. J. Parrott, S. Raj, D. Cullum-Dugan, and D. Lucus. 2013. How Prevalent Is Vitamin B_{12} Deficiency among Vegetarians? *Nutrition Reviews* 71(2):110–117.

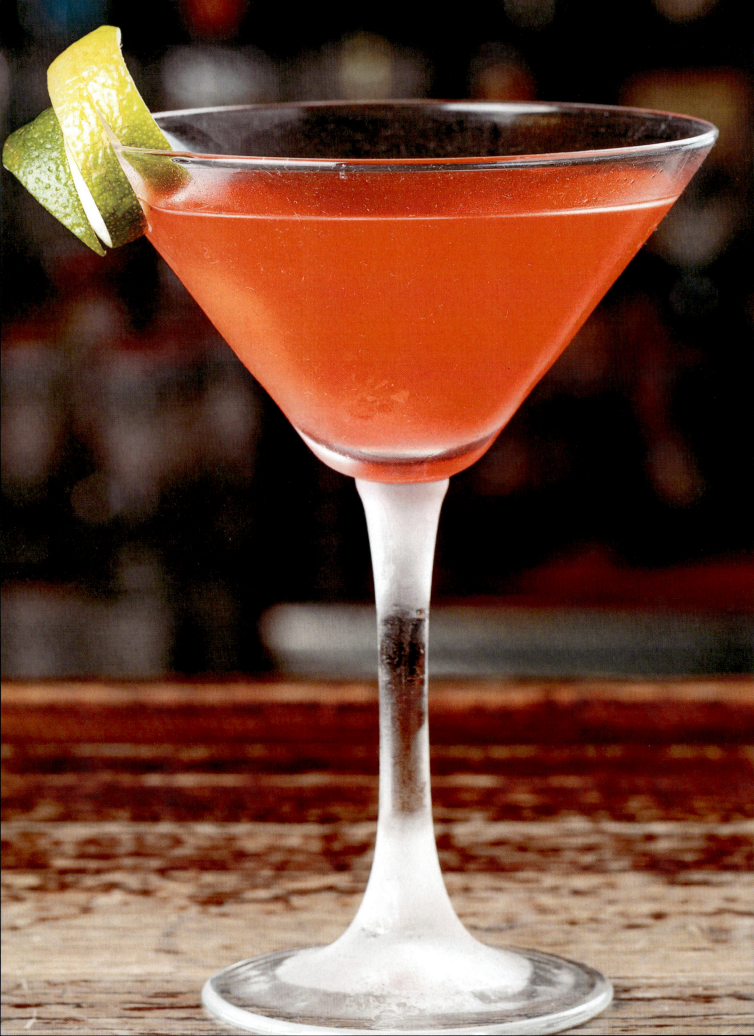

Alcohol

Learning Outcomes

After reading this chapter, you will be able to:

7.1 Describe the sources of alcohol and how alcohol is made.

7.2 Explain why people drink alcohol, and define a standard drink.

7.3 Explain how alcohol is absorbed and metabolized and how it circulates throughout the body.

7.4 Describe the short-term effects of alcohol consumption on the body.

7.5 Describe the effects of chronic excessive alcohol consumption on the body.

7.6 Summarize alcohol use disorder.

True or False?

1. Alcohol is an essential nutrient. **T**/**F**
2. A shot of whiskey contains more alcohol than a can of beer. **T**/**F**
3. Red wine contains phytochemicals that are beneficial for the heart. **T**/**F**
4. Women feel the effects of alcohol sooner than men. **T**/**F**
5. The body can metabolize three alcoholic beverages per hour. **T**/**F**
6. The best way to cure a hangover is to drink a Bloody Mary. **T**/**F**
7. Alcohol provides 7 kilocalories per gram. **T**/**F**
8. Drinking too much alcohol can lead to malnutrition. **T**/**F**
9. Moderate drinking means consuming six or more drinks once a week. **T**/**F**
10. Alcohol use disorders can be cured through counseling. **T**/**F**

See page 276 for the answers.

A lcohol is not classified as an essential nutrient because your body doesn't need alcohol to survive. But alcohol does contain kilocalories. In fact, alcohol contributes more energy per gram than either carbohydrates or protein. For example, a 12-ounce beer contains almost as much energy as a Hershey's chocolate bar and more than two large hard-boiled eggs. For this reason, we cover alcohol following the chapters on the three energy-yielding macronutrients.

Alcohol is legally sold in the United States to adults age 21 and older, but teenagers often feel under social pressure to consume it. Some medical reports say that in moderation, alcohol can provide health benefits, at least in older adults; however, drinking too much alcohol can be fatal.

Understanding alcohol warrants a more detailed look. In this chapter, we discuss how the body handles alcohol, its positive and negative health effects, and how to tell when someone has an alcohol use disorder. We begin with the basic definition of alcohol.

What Is Alcohol and How Is It Made?

LO 7.1 Describe the sources of alcohol and how alcohol is made.

An **alcohol** is an organic compound in which one or more hydroxyl (OH) groups are attached to the carbon atoms in place of hydrogen atoms (**Figure 7.1**). Alcohol compounds tend to be soluble in water because the OH is polar and attracts water.

Alcohol Has Many Forms

What is the first image that comes to mind when you hear the word *alcohol*? Do you envision a bottle of beer, a glass of wine, or a stiff martini? These beverages all contain a form of alcohol called *ethyl alcohol,* or **ethanol** (C_2H_5OH). (See Figure 7.1a.)

In Chapter 5, we covered another type of alcohol, *glycerol,* which is found in food and the body as part of the triglyceride molecule. (See Figure 7.1b.) The difference between glycerol and ethanol is that glycerol has three hydroxyl groups (one attached to each of the three carbons that make up the glycerol backbone), while ethanol contains only one hydroxyl group.

Another alcohol compound, methanol (CH_3OH), is used in antifreeze, fuel, and other industrial compounds. (See Figure 7.1c.) Methanol and isopropanol (C_3H_7OH), used in rubbing alcohol, are both poisonous when ingested. Ethanol is considered safe for consumption, but it is not harmless; consuming excessive amounts of ethanol can be toxic, even lethal.

alcohol Class of organic compounds that contain one or more hydroxyl groups attached to carbons. Examples include ethanol, glycerol, and methanol. Ethanol is often referred to as "alcohol."

ethanol Type of alcohol, specifically ethyl alcohol (C_2H_5OH), found in alcoholic beverages such as wine, beer, and liquor.

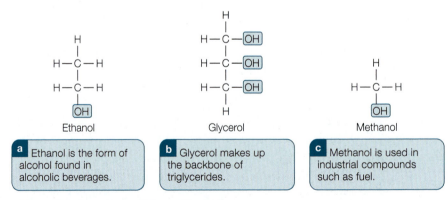

Ethanol

a Ethanol is the form of alcohol found in alcoholic beverages.

Glycerol

b Glycerol makes up the backbone of triglycerides.

Methanol

c Methanol is used in industrial compounds such as fuel.

▲ **Figure 7.1** **Structure of Three Alcohols**

Although ethanol is the scientific name for the alcohol found in consumable beverages, we use the more common term *alcohol* throughout this chapter.

Alcohol Begins with Sugar

Ethanol is made when yeasts **ferment** the natural sugars in grains (glucose and maltose) and fruits (fructose and glucose). Yeasts are single-celled organisms that metabolize glucose into ethanol and carbon dioxide (see the Chemistry Boost). Yeast is used in the production of all alcoholic beverages at some point in the fermentation process.

Chemistry Boost

Fermentation

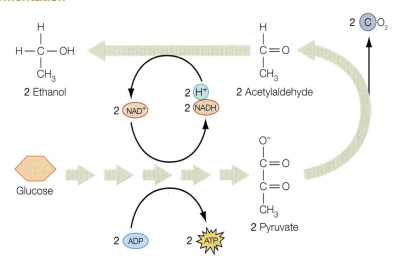

The process of fermentation involves converting glucose ($C_6H_{12}O_6$) into alcohol (CH_3CH_2OH) and carbon dioxide gas (CO_2). The basic reaction of fermentation happens within the yeast as shown below.

$$C_6H_{12}O_6 \rightarrow 2\ (CH_3CH_2OH) + 2\ (CO_2) + 2\ ATP$$
Glucose $\rightarrow$ Ethyl alcohol + Carbon dioxide gas + Energy

Fermentation begins with glucose, the main energy source for yeast. The enzymes in the yeast convert the glucose first to pyruvate, which generates energy in the form of ATP. Once pyruvate is formed, the enzymes in the yeast convert it to acetaldehyde and carbon dioxide. In the final step of ethyl alcohol production, acetaldehyde is converted into ethanol. The hydrogen needed to convert the acetaldehyde to ethanol is provided by the coenzyme form of the B vitamin niacin NADH + H$^+$.

The most common form of yeast used to make alcohol, brewer's yeast, can tolerate up to about 5 percent alcohol. Beyond this level of alcohol, the yeast dies. Wine yeast is still active in 12 percent alcohol and some cultured strains of yeast can tolerate up to 21 percent alcohol. Depending on the type of yeast that is used, the fermentation reaction stops once the alcohol content reaches 11–14 percent because the level of alcohol becomes toxic to the yeast and the yeast itself dies. The carbon dioxide formed during fermentation bubbles through the liquid and evaporates, leaving an alcohol-containing beverage.

Fermenting the glucose and fructose in grapes and other fruits makes wine. The characteristics of wines—whether the wine is spicy, zesty, acidic, or sweet—vary depending on the types of grapes or fruit that are used, where they are grown, and the climate.

ferment (fermentation) Process by which yeast converts sugars in grains or fruits into ethanol and carbon dioxide.

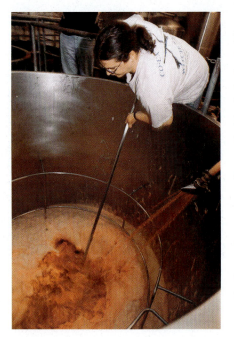

Beer is made when yeast converts the glucose in grain to ethyl alcohol and carbon dioxide gas.

Malted cereal grains, such as barley, are used to make beer. In malting, the barley partially germinates, releasing enzymes that hydrolyze the starch in the endosperm into smaller sugar molecules, or maltose. The brewer stops germination before the plant uses all the sugars. The brewing process hydrolyzes maltose further into glucose, which then undergoes fermentation. The carbon dioxide is captured and used to carbonate the brew. The basic ingredients added to beer include *hops,* the dried flowers of a plant similar to hemp, which add flavor and antibacterial properties; sugar; water; and different types of yeast. Variations in these ingredients account for the varying types of beer.

Like beer and wine, liquors begin with the fermentation of sugars from an initial food item. Vodka begins with potatoes or grains, rum begins with molasses or sugarcane juice, and tequila begins with the blue agave plant. After fermentation, the alcoholic liquids undergo **distillation**: the liquid is heated, causing the ethanol to vaporize. The vapor is collected, cooled, and condensed into a concentrated beverage called *liquor* (or, more accurately, distilled spirits). The alcohol content of these beverages is indicated by its **proof**, a number that reflects twice the alcohol content in the beverage. For example, 80 proof vodka contains 40 percent alcohol. **Table 7.1** identifies the average alcohol content for various alcoholic beverages including beer, wine, and spirits.

TABLE 7.1	Alcohol Content of Various Beverages	
Beverage	**Amount, fluid oz.**	**Alcohol Content, g**
Beer		
Light beer	12	10
Regular beer	12	12
Wine (white, red, and rose)	5	14
Spirits (tequila, vodka, whiskey, rum) 80 proof	1.5	14

LO 7.1: THE TAKE-HOME MESSAGE Ethanol is the type of alcohol consumed in alcoholic beverages. It is an organic chemical produced by the fermentation of sugars by yeast. Wine is made from fruits; beer from malted cereals; and distilled spirits from potatoes, grains, molasses, or other ingredients that, following fermentation, yield liquids that undergo distillation. Alcohol provides kilocalories but very little nutritional value. It is not a nutrient because your body doesn't need it to survive.

Why Do People Drink Alcohol and What Is Considered a Standard Drink?

LO 7.2 Explain why people drink alcohol, and define a standard drink.

Alcohol is a drug that alters your conscious mind. Within minutes of sipping an alcoholic beverage, a person feels more relaxed. After a few more sips, a mild, pleasant euphoria sets in and inhibitions begin to loosen. By the end of the first or second drink, a person often feels more outgoing, happy, and social. This initial effect is just one reason people drink alcohol.[1]

People Drink to Relax, Celebrate, and Socialize

People around the world drink alcohol in many different forms and for many different reasons. The Japanese drink *sake* (rice wine) during tea and Shinto ceremonies, while Irish pub patrons consume dark beer to celebrate their favorite sport. Russians enjoy vodka and the French appreciate wine to relax and for pleasure. Wine is part of many religious traditions, including the Catholic Mass and the Jewish Sabbath, and in some cultures, it's the beverage of choice during the main meal of the day. For parts of human history, wine and beer were safer to drink than water, which was often contaminated with disease-causing microbes.

In the United States, more than half of adults consume at least one alcoholic beverage per month.[2] Americans drink alcohol for many of the same reasons people in other

distillation Evaporation and then collection of a liquid by condensation. Liquors are made using distillation.

proof Measure of the amount of ethanol contained in alcoholic beverages.

parts of the world do: to relax, celebrate, and socialize. Although many college students are under age 21, they may drink alcohol to meet new friends, relax their social inhibitions, and have more fun.[3]

Having a drink with another person also symbolizes social bonding.[4] **Social drinking** is defined as drinking patterns that are considered acceptable by society. Social drinking is not necessarily light drinking, as people can and do consume too much alcohol in social situations. Later in this chapter we discuss binge drinking, which often occurs in social settings.

Advertisements Encourage Alcohol Consumption

Alcohol advertising is everywhere. One need only drive down a major highway or turn on the television to see billboards and commercials for beer, wine, or liquor. In some popular magazines like *Rolling Stone* and *Sports Illustrated,* alcohol ads can outnumber non–alcohol ads by almost three to one.[5] Some studies have shown that advertisements for alcoholic beverages increase drinking among adolescents.[6] Many ads tend to emphasize sexual and social stereotypes. When targeted to underage drinkers, this type of message has been shown to increase adolescents' desire to emulate those portrayed in the advertisements.[7] **Figure 7.2** shows a typical alcohol advertisement that may appear in a magazine. These ads should be viewed with caution, as the messages in them are often misleading and in some cases blatantly false.

Moderate Drinking Is Measured in Terms of a Standard Drink

Moderate drinking is considered the amount of alcohol that puts the individual and others at the lowest risk of alcohol-related problems. Moderation is defined in the latest *Dietary Guidelines for Americans* as up to one drink per day for women and up to two drinks a day for men. In order to be a moderate drinker, an individual must limit both the size of drinks and the frequency of drinking.

A standard drink, whether it's in a 12-ounce bottle of beer, a shot of liquor, or a 5-ounce glass of wine, contains about ½ ounce of alcohol (**Figure 7.3**). Sometimes, the drinks poured at a bar or restaurant appear to be a standard size, but are actually larger, allowing the customer to consume multiple standard drinks in one glass or mug (**Figure 7.4**). Mixed drinks also often contain more than one standard drink. A rum and coke, for example, could provide the equivalent of over 2½ standard alcoholic drinks.

Another very important point about drinking in moderation is that abstaining from alcohol on weekdays and then drinking 10 beers on Saturday night does not count as moderate drinking. There isn't any "banking" allowed when it comes to alcohol; drinking excessive quantities in a short amount of time is called *binge drinking* (which we discuss in more detail later in the chapter).

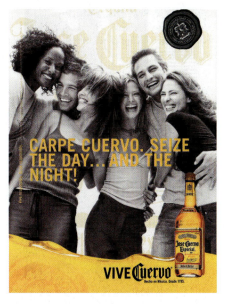

▲ Figure 7.2 **Alcohol Advertisements Target Young Adults**
Alcohol advertisements, including advertisements such as this one for Cuervo tequila, often portray people who drink as happy, successful, attractive, and popular.

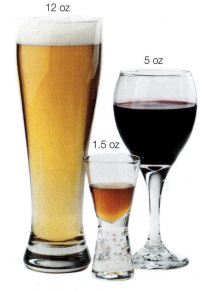

▲ Figure 7.3 **What Is a Standard Drink?**
One standard drink of beer, liquor, or wine contains about ½ ounce of alcohol.

LO 7.2: THE TAKE-HOME MESSAGE People drink alcohol to relax, celebrate, socialize, and to feel more "adult." The *Dietary Guidelines for Americans* emphasize moderation for those who choose to drink alcohol, defined as up to one drink a day for women and two drinks a day for men. One standard drink contains ½ ounce of alcohol, the amount in a typical 12-ounce bottle of beer, a shot of liquor, or a 5-ounce glass of wine. Drinking excessive amounts of alcohol in a short time is binge drinking.

social drinking Moderate drinking of alcoholic beverages in social settings within safe limits.

moderate drinking According to the *Dietary Guidelines for Americans,* up to one drink per day for women and up to two drinks a day for men.

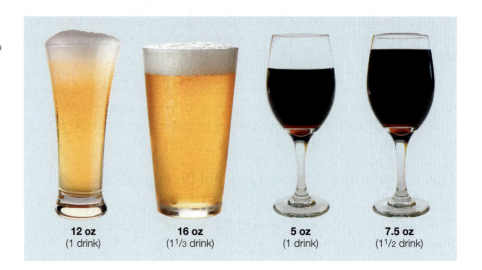

12 oz	16 oz	5 oz	7.5 oz
(1 drink)	(1¹/₃ drink)	(1 drink)	(1¹/₂ drink)

How Is Alcohol Absorbed, Circulated, and Metabolized in the Body?

LO 7.3 Explain how alcohol is absorbed and metabolized and how it circulates throughout the body.

Alcohol is a toxin, and the body treats it differently from any other substance, working quickly to metabolize and eliminate it.

Alcohol Is Absorbed in the Stomach and Small Intestine

Alcohol doesn't require digestion, so it can be absorbed by simple diffusion through the gastric mucosa into the bloodstream. About 20 percent of alcohol is absorbed through the stomach, while the majority is absorbed through the duodenum of the small intestine. As soon as alcohol enters the blood, it travels through the body and is distributed throughout the watery tissues (**Figure 7.5**). This means that it quickly reaches the brain.

Many factors, including gender, age, ethnicity, and the amount of alcohol consumed, affect how quickly alcohol is absorbed; however, a key factor influencing alcohol absorption is the amount and type of food in the stomach.[8] If a swallow of beer chases a cheeseburger and fries, the alcohol takes longer to leave the stomach and enter the small intestine than if the beer were consumed on an empty stomach. This is partly due to the fact that food in the stomach keeps some of the alcohol away from the stomach wall, thereby reducing the amount that diffuses through the gastric lining. Fat- and carbohydrate-containing foods have additional effects. Fat slows down peristalsis, which slows the departure of food from the stomach, and carbohydrates slow the absorption of alcohol through the stomach lining.[9]

Keep in mind, however, that while a full stomach delays the arrival of alcohol in the small intestine, the alcohol will still eventually arrive there. If a person drinks several glasses of beer with dinner, the alcohol will be absorbed once the stomach starts emptying.

Alcohol Is Metabolized in the Stomach and the Liver

The stomach gets the first pass at metabolizing alcohol before it is absorbed into the bloodstream. The rate at which alcohol is metabolized in the stomach is affected by how quickly the stomach empties into the duodenum. The longer alcohol lingers in the

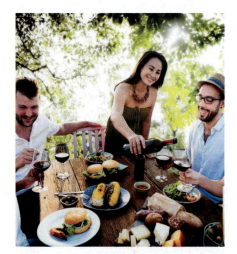

Eating food while drinking alcohol affects the rate at which the alcohol is absorbed.

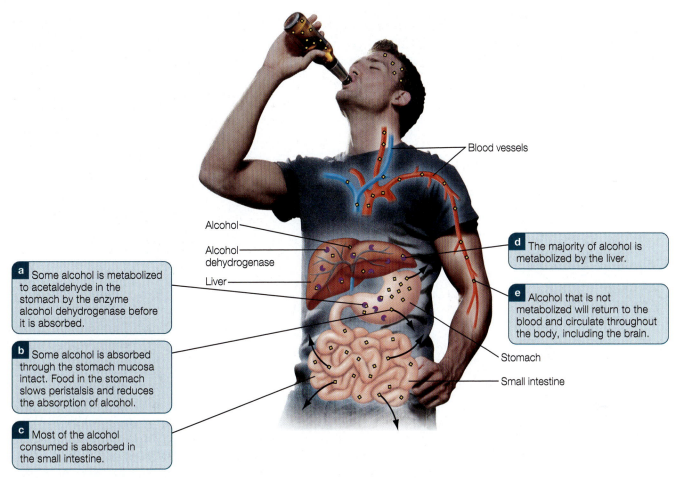

Blood vessels

Alcohol

Alcohol dehydrogenase

Liver

d The majority of alcohol is metabolized by the liver.

e Alcohol that is not metabolized will return to the blood and circulate throughout the body, including the brain.

Stomach

Small intestine

a Some alcohol is metabolized to acetaldehyde in the stomach by the enzyme alcohol dehydrogenase before it is absorbed.

b Some alcohol is absorbed through the stomach mucosa intact. Food in the stomach slows peristalsis and reduces the absorption of alcohol.

c Most of the alcohol consumed is absorbed in the small intestine.

▲ **Figure 7.5 The Absorption, Circulation, and Metabolism of Alcohol**

stomach, the more time the enzyme **alcohol dehydrogenase (ADH)**, which is secreted by the gastric cells, has to metabolize it,[10] and the less alcohol directly enters the blood and eventually reaches the brain.

The liver, however, is the main site for alcohol metabolism. The liver can metabolize a limited amount of alcohol every hour, and the amount depends on body mass and liver size.

There are two pathways that metabolize alcohol in the liver. The ADH pathway metabolizes the majority of alcohol, using the same enzyme secreted by the gastric cells when alcohol is metabolized in the stomach. The second alcohol metabolism pathway is the microsomal ethanol oxidizing system (MEOS), which uses niacin in the form of NADPH.

The Alcohol Dehydrogenase Pathway

The initial pathway to oxidize alcohol is an anaerobic, two-step enzyme process in the cytoplasm, or fluid portion of the cell. The enzyme ADH with the help of NAD^+ converts ethanol to **acetaldehyde** by removing two hydrogen atoms (**Figure 7.6**). During the second step, the enzyme **acetaldehyde dehydrogenase (ALDH)** removes more hydrogen atoms from acetaldehyde to form acetate. Once the acetate is produced, it can continue through the metabolic pathways to produce energy or be converted to a fatty acid and stored as body fat in the adipocytes. (See Chapter 8 for more details on the metabolic pathways for alcohol.)

alcohol dehydrogenase (ADH) One of the alcohol-metabolizing enzymes, found in the stomach and the liver, that converts ethanol to acetaldehyde.

acetaldehyde One of the first compounds produced in the metabolism of ethanol. Eventually, acetaldehyde is converted to carbon dioxide and water and excreted.

acetaldehyde dehydrogenase (ALDH) Alcohol-metabolizing enzyme found in the liver that converts acetaldehyde to acetate.

The liver rapidly breaks down ethanol to acetyl CoA through either the alcohol dehydrogenase (ADH) pathway or the microsomal enzyme oxidizing system (MEOS).

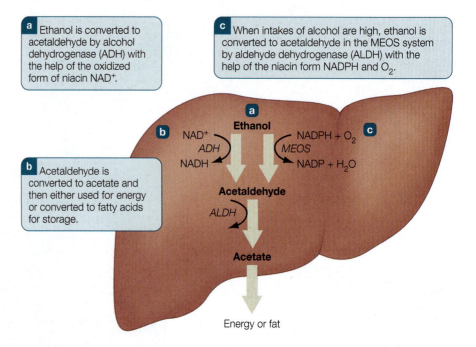

a Ethanol is converted to acetaldehyde by alcohol dehydrogenase (ADH) with the help of the oxidized form of niacin NAD$^+$.

c When intakes of alcohol are high, ethanol is converted to acetaldehyde in the MEOS system by aldehyde dehydrogenase (ALDH) with the help of the niacin form NADPH and O$_2$.

b Acetaldehyde is converted to acetate and then either used for energy or converted to fatty acids for storage.

A Breathalyzer is used to measure a person's blood alcohol concentration.

microsomal ethanol oxidizing system (MEOS) Second major enzyme system in the liver that metabolizes alcohol.

alcohol tolerance State in which the body has adjusted to long-term alcohol use by becoming less sensitive to the alcohol. More alcohol needs to be consumed in order to get the same euphoric effect.

microsomes Small vesicles in the cytoplasm of liver cells where oxidative metabolism of alcohol takes place.

blood alcohol concentration (BAC) Amount of alcohol in the blood. BAC is measured in grams of alcohol per deciliter of blood, usually expressed as a percentage.

The Microsomal Ethanol Oxidizing System (MEOS)

When an individual consumes too much alcohol, the ADH enzymes become overwhelmed and can't keep up with the need to oxidize ethanol into acetaldehyde. Under these circumstances, a second major enzyme system in the liver that usually metabolizes drugs—the **microsomal ethanol oxidizing system (MEOS)**—takes over. Chronic alcohol abuse increases the liver's production of the enzymes making up the system, which in turn increases the liver's ability to metabolize alcohol, so that a larger dose of alcohol is needed to achieve the same effects. The more alcohol you drink, the more active the MEOS becomes, a state that contributes to **alcohol tolerance**. Moreover, using the MEOS to metabolize alcohol reduces the body's ability to metabolize drugs. Alcohol takes precedence over drugs, so consuming drugs and alcohol together can allow the drugs to build up to lethal levels while the MEOS is metabolizing the alcohol.

Another difference between the MEOS and the ADH pathway is that the MEOS takes place in the **microsomes** of the cell rather than in the cytoplasm. The reactions in these small vesicles use oxygen (aerobic) and produce water as a by-product; use a different form of the B vitamin niacin, NADPH, rather than NAD$^+$; and consume energy rather than produce it to convert ethanol to acetaldehyde.

Alcohol Circulates in the Blood

If the liver cannot metabolize alcohol as fast as it is consumed, some of the alcohol remains in the blood and is continually circulated in the fluid portions of the body. Though the liver eventually metabolizes 95 percent of the alcohol that is consumed, the other 5 percent is excreted intact either through the lungs, the skin in perspiration, and/or the kidneys through the urine. The amount of alcohol expelled through the lungs correlates with the amount of alcohol in the blood. For this reason, a Breathalyzer test can be used by police officers if they suspect that a person has consumed too much alcohol.

The **blood alcohol concentration (BAC)** is the amount of alcohol in the blood measured in grams of alcohol per deciliter, usually expressed as a percentage (**Table 7.2**). Because alcohol infiltrates the brain, as the BAC increases so does the level of mental impairment and intoxication. For a closer look at the equation behind the BAC, see the Calculation Corner.

TABLE 7.2 Blood Alcohol Concentration Tables

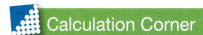

For Women
Body Weight in Pounds

Drinks Per Hour	100	120	140	160	180	200
1	0.05	0.04	0.03	0.03	0.03	0.02
2	0.09	0.08	0.07	0.06	0.05	0.05
3	0.14	0.11	0.10	0.09	0.08	0.07
4	0.18	0.15	0.13	0.11	0.10	0.09
5	0.23	0.19	0.16	0.14	0.13	0.11
6	0.27	0.23	0.19	0.17	0.15	0.14
7	0.32	0.27	0.23	0.20	0.18	0.16
8	0.36	0.30	0.26	0.23	0.20	0.18
9	0.41	0.34	0.29	0.26	0.23	0.20
10	0.45	0.38	0.32	0.28	0.25	0.23

For Men
Body Weight in Pounds

Drinks Per Hour	100	120	140	160	180	200
1	0.04	0.03	0.03	0.02	0.02	0.02
2	0.08	0.06	0.05	0.05	0.04	0.04
3	0.11	0.09	0.08	0.07	0.06	0.06
4	0.15	0.12	0.11	0.09	0.08	0.08
5	0.19	0.16	0.13	0.12	0.11	0.09
6	0.23	0.19	0.16	0.14	0.13	0.11
7	0.26	0.22	0.19	0.16	0.15	0.13
8	0.30	0.25	0.21	0.19	0.17	0.15
9	0.34	0.28	0.24	0.21	0.19	0.17
10	0.38	0.31	0.27	0.23	0.21	0.19

Notes: Shaded area indicates the condition of being mentally and physically impaired; the definition of legal intoxication. Blood alcohol concentrations are expressed as percent, meaning grams of alcohol per 10 milliliters (per deciliter) of blood.

Source: Tables are adapted from those of the Pennsylvania Liquor Control Board, Harrisburg, PA.

Gender, Genetics, and Ethnicity Affect Alcohol Metabolism

When women consume the same amount of alcohol as men, they have a higher alcohol concentration in the blood, even when the difference in body size is taken into account. This is because women have about 20–30 percent less ADH secreted from their gastric mucosa than men, so more ethanol enters the blood through a female's gastric lining. In essence, every alcoholic beverage that a man consumes is equivalent to about 1⅓ alcoholic beverages for a woman.

In addition to a reduced first-pass metabolism of alcohol in the stomach, women have less muscle mass, and thus less body water, than men (recall that fat tissue has less water than muscle). Because alcohol mixes in water, muscular individuals are able to distribute more of the alcohol throughout their bodies than those who have more fat tissue and, consequently, less body water. So even if a woman is the same height and weight as a man, the female, drinking the same amount of alcohol, will have a higher concentration of alcohol in her blood than the male.

Because of these two factors—less gastric ADH and less body water in which to distribute the ingested alcohol—women feel alcohol's narcotic effects sooner than men. Women take note: Females can't keep up, drink for drink, with their male friends.

Estimate Blood Alcohol Concentration

The current BAC estimation calculators are based on the original equation developed by Widmark 80 years ago.[1] The estimation of BAC takes into account the amount of alcohol in a drink, the individual's metabolism rate of alcohol, the amount of body water (recall that males have more body water than females), and the time since the alcohol was consumed and metabolized. In the equation below, use 7.5 for the gender constant for males and 9.0 for the gender constant for females. Body weight is in pounds (lbs), and 0.017 g/dl per hour is the average rate of alcohol metabolism.[2]

$$BAC = [(\text{\# of standard drinks} \div 2) \times (\text{gender constant} \div \text{body weight})] - (0.017 \times \text{hours})$$

Example #1: Calculate Mark's BAC if he weighs 175 lbs and drank three regular 12-ounce beers in 2 hours.

Mark's estimate of BAC:

$$= [(3 \div 2) \times (7.5 \div 175)] - (0.017 \times 2)$$
$$= [(1.5 \times 0.04)] - (0.03)$$
$$= 0.06 - 0.03$$
$$= 0.03$$

Does Mark's BAC indicate he would be legally impaired?

Example 2: Calculate Ruby's percent BAC if she weighs 120 lbs and drank three regular 12-ounce beers in 2 hours.

Ruby's estimate of BAC:

$$= [(3 \div 2) \times (9.0 \div 120)] - (0.017 \times 2)$$
$$= [(1.5 \times 0.075)] - (0.034)$$
$$= 0.11 - 0.034$$
$$= 0.08$$

Does Ruby's estimate of BAC indicate she would be legally impaired?

References

1. Widmark, E. M. P. 1932. *Principles and Applications of Medicolegal Alcohol Determination,* translated into English by R. C. Baselt, Department of Pathology, University of California, Davis, 1981, p. 163.
2. Hustad, J. T. P., and K. B. Carey. 2005. Using Calculations to Estimate Blood Alcohol Concentrations for Naturally Occurring Drinking Episodes: A Validity Study. *Journal of Studies on Alcohol* 66:130–138.

Go to Mastering Nutrition and complete a Math Video activity similar to the problem in this Calculation Corner.

Genetics and ethnicity may also influence alcohol metabolism. There are several genes that code for ADH activity. These genes have variations that affect how quickly ADH metabolizes alcohol. People whose genes have certain variations may be at greater risk of feeling the effects of alcohol than those whose genes have other variations.[11] Some ethnic groups, including Hispanics, Asian Americans, and American Indians/Alaska Natives, also have lower ADH activity levels and feel the effects of alcohol much sooner than Caucasians.[12]

LO 7.3: THE TAKE-HOME MESSAGE Alcohol is absorbed in the stomach and small intestine. Some alcohol is metabolized in the stomach by the enzyme alcohol dehydrogenase before it can be absorbed through the gastric mucosa. Alcohol is mainly metabolized in the liver by two enzyme systems. The initial pathway is controlled by alcohol dehydrogenase. This anaerobic pathway converts ethanol to acetate. The MEOS system kicks into play when too much alcohol is consumed and overwhelms alcohol dehydrogenase. Both enzyme pathways use the B vitamin niacin. Alcohol circulates in the blood until the liver metabolizes it. The blood alcohol concentration is the amount of alcohol in the blood expressed as a percentage. A person's gender, genetics, ethnicity, and the amount of food and alcohol consumed affect the rate of absorption and metabolism in the body.

What Are the Short-Term Effects of Alcohol Consumption on the Body?

LO 7.4 Describe the short-term effects of alcohol consumption on the body.

Alcohol can have many harmful effects on the body and the brain, caused mostly by the products of metabolism: acetaldehyde and acids. The more alcohol consumed, the more acetaldehyde is formed. These effects can be acute and short term, occurring while an individual is intoxicated, or they can occur within 72 hours following intoxication.

Drinking in moderation allows the body time to eliminate alcohol and to repair the damage it causes. Even at low doses, alcohol can impair judgment and coordination, but moderate drinkers typically do not experience serious physiological consequences of their drinking. In contrast, drinking in excess can have quick, dangerous consequences and put personal safety at risk.

Alcohol Affects the Brain

Alcohol is considered a *drug* because of its effects on the central nervous system and other body systems. Although many people think alcohol is a stimulant because it has the effect of lowering inhibitions, it is actually a central nervous system *depressant,* which means it slows communication between neurons. The brain is very sensitive to alcohol, which can easily cross the blood–brain barrier. The depressant effect of alcohol on the brain is also what slows down a person's reaction time to stimuli (such as an oncoming car on the road) after drinking.

Brain Areas Affected

The more alcohol consumed, the more areas of the brain are affected. Look at **Figure 7.7** to see how increasing alcohol levels impact specific areas of the brain.

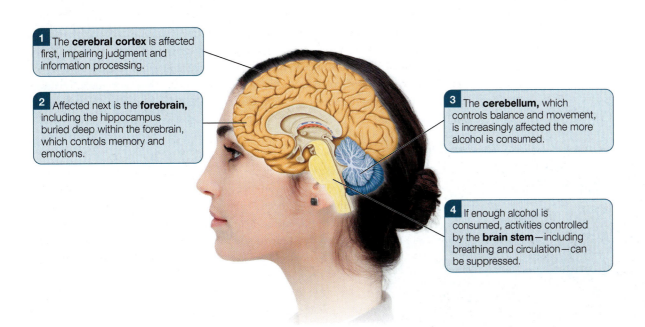

1 The **cerebral cortex** is affected first, impairing judgment and information processing.

2 Affected next is the **forebrain,** including the hippocampus buried deep within the forebrain, which controls memory and emotions.

3 The **cerebellum,** which controls balance and movement, is increasingly affected the more alcohol is consumed.

4 If enough alcohol is consumed, activities controlled by the **brain stem**—including breathing and circulation—can be suppressed.

▲ Figure 7.7 **The Brain and Alcohol**
As more alcohol is consumed, additional areas of the brain are affected. The cerebral cortex is affected first, followed by the forebrain, cerebellum, and brainstem. The greater the alcohol intake, the greater the physical and behavioral changes in the body.

The area of the brain affected by alcohol first is the cerebral cortex, where you process information received from your senses, including sight, smell, and hearing. When alcohol reaches this part of the brain, individuals become more talkative and less inhibited and have more confidence. However, the ability to think clearly or make good judgments is reduced. The higher the BAC, the more noticeable the effects.

Affected next is the hippocampus, which is buried deep inside the forebrain and is responsible for memory. Alcohol impairs formation and storage of long-term memories. Even a small amount of alcohol can make you forget what you were doing (or learning) while drinking. Excessive alcohol intake may even result in a **blackout**, the loss of all memory of an event. The hippocampus also controls emotions. As alcohol intake is increased, feelings such as sadness and anger become exaggerated.

The cerebellum controls your balance and movements such as walking and talking. The more alcohol consumed, the more difficult it is to control body movements and speech. The result is an inability to stand, walk in a straight line, or speak clearly.

With continued alcohol intake, the activities of the brainstem, which controls breathing and circulation, can be suppressed, impairing breathing and heart rate and ultimately causing death. A particular area at the top of the brainstem, called the *reticular activating system (RAS),* controls whether an individual is awake or asleep. Excessive quantities of alcohol can shut down the RAS, causing loss of consciousness. This reaction to excessive alcohol intake is beneficial in that it prevents further drinking.

Alcohol Poisoning

Drinking to excess without stopping, even when you feel the effects of alcohol, can result in **alcohol poisoning** even before you pass out. Alcohol in the stomach and intestines is still being absorbed into the bloodstream, raising BAC even after you've stopped drinking. Alcohol poisoning results when the BAC is so high that basic physiological functions, including breathing, heart rate, and the gag reflex, which prevents choking, are depressed. Alcohol irritates the stomach and can cause vomiting. Because the gag reflex is depressed, an unconscious person can choke on the vomit, leading to asphyxiation, which can result

blackout Amnesia for events that occurred while a person was intoxicated.

alcohol poisoning State in which the BAC rises to the point that a person's central nervous system is affected and his or her breathing and heart rate are interrupted.

in death. Even if an individual survives alcohol poisoning, he or she can still experience brain damage. A person who has passed out after drinking should never be left to "sleep it off," because BAC can continue to rise from nearly toxic to fatally toxic levels while the person is unconscious. Cool, pale, or bluish skin, abnormally slow or irregular breaths, and inability to rouse the person are signs that he or she needs immediate medical care. Call 9-1-1.[13]

Injuries

Because even moderate alcohol consumption reduces brain function, the risk of unintentional injuries is much greater when an individual has been drinking. Each year nearly 600,000 students between the ages of 18 and 24 are unintentionally injured because of drinking. One of the most significant risks is driving while intoxicated. Every day in the United States, 27 people die each day in automobile accidents that involved an alcohol-impaired driver.[14] Driving in the United States with a BAC of 0.08 or higher is illegal (some states have set their legal limit even lower), but the level of alcohol in the blood doesn't need to get that high to impair driving. Even the lowest level of BAC, the level that occurs after one alcoholic beverage, impairs alertness, judgment, and coordination (see Table 7.2).

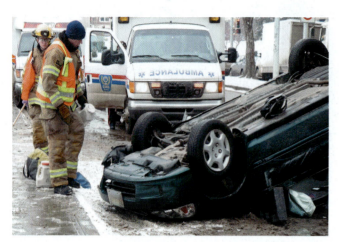

Drinking and driving can be deadly.

Intentional injuries also increase with alcohol consumption. Each year, close to 696,000 college students are assaulted by another student who is intoxicated.[15] Sexual assault, unsafe sex, suicide attempts, and property damage are also much more common when students are under the influence of alcohol. More than 1,800 students die each year as a result of drinking alcohol.[16]

Sleep Disruption

Having a drink within an hour before bed may help an individual fall asleep more quickly, but it disrupts the sleep cycle, causes middle-of-night wakefulness, and makes returning to sleep a challenge.[17] Even a moderate amount of alcohol consumed at dinner or even late in the afternoon during happy hour can disrupt that evening's sleep.

After a poor night's sleep, it's a bad idea to drink alcohol the next day. Studies have shown that a night of sleep disruption followed by even small amounts of alcohol the next day reduces reaction time and alertness in individuals performing a simulated driving test.[18] Fatigue exacerbates alcohol's sedating effect.[19]

Alcohol Causes Hangovers

A **hangover** is the body's way of saying, "Don't do that to me again." After a bout of heavy drinking, individuals can experience hangover symptoms ranging from a pounding headache, fatigue, nausea, and increased thirst to a rapid heartbeat, tremors, sweating, dizziness, depression, anxiety, and irritability. A hangover begins within hours of the last drink, as the BAC begins to drop. The symptoms appear in full force once all the alcohol is cleared from the blood and can linger for up to an additional 24 hours.[20] In other words, a few hours of excessive alcohol consumption on a Saturday night can ruin not only an entire Sunday, but even part of Monday.

Alcohol causes the symptoms of a hangover in several ways. Acetaldehyde, the intermediate by-product of alcohol metabolism, is mildly toxic. In large enough amounts, acetaldehyde causes nausea, headache, fatigue, and irritability, all the symptoms of a hangover. But this is not the only cause of hangovers. Alcohol is also a diuretic, so it can cause dehydration, and thus electrolyte imbalances. It inhibits the release of antidiuretic hormone

hangover Collective term for the unpleasant symptoms, such as a headache and dizziness, that occur after drinking an excessive amount of alcohol; many of the symptoms are caused by high levels of acetaldehyde in the blood.

from the pituitary gland, which in turn causes the kidneys to excrete water, as well as electrolytes, into the urine. Vomiting and sweating during or after excessive drinking contributes further to dehydration and electrolyte loss. Dehydration also increases thirst and can cause feelings of lightheadedness, dizziness, and weakness. Increased acid production in the stomach and secretions from the pancreas and intestines can cause stomach pain and nausea and vomiting.

Lastly, alcoholic beverages often contain compounds called **congeners** that are produced during the fermentation process. Congeners contribute to the taste and appearance of the drink, but are also thought to contribute to hangover symptoms. The greatest amounts of congeners are found in red wine and darker liquors such as tequila, brandy, or bourbon. Bourbon has more than 40 times the quantity of congeners in vodka. Combining alcoholic beverages that contain different levels of congeners can cause severe hangover symptoms. Drinking beer, which is carbonated, along with liquor that contains congeners speeds up the absorption of the alcohol, which gives the body less time to eliminate the congeners.

Forget the idea of consuming an alcoholic beverage to "cure" a hangover. Drinking more alcohol, even if it is mixed with tomato or orange juice, during a hangover only prolongs the recovery time. Nor do caffeine, hot showers, and long walks improve the symptoms. The only cure for a hangover is time.

Whereas aspirin and other nonsteroidal anti-inflammatory medications, such as ibuprofen, can ease a headache, these medications can also contribute to stomachache and nausea. Taking acetaminophen (Tylenol) during and after alcohol consumption, when the alcohol is being metabolized, has been shown to intensify the pain reliever's toxicity to the liver and may cause severe liver damage.[21] The FDA recently changed regulations on acetaminophen, limiting the amount in combination prescription drugs to 325 milligrams, to reduce the risk of liver damage, especially when drinking alcohol.[22] The best strategy for dealing with a hangover is to avoid it by limiting the amount of alcohol you consume.

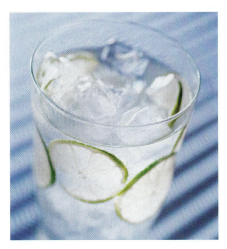

Staying hydrated by drinking water between alcoholic beverages can help you avoid the effects of a hangover.

LO 7.4: THE TAKE-HOME MESSAGE Alcohol is a central nervous system depressant, impairing brain function and behavior. Excessive drinking can cause alcohol poisoning, which can be fatal. Someone who has passed out after drinking and cannot be roused requires immediate medical attention. Alcohol can also result in unintentional injuries, disrupt your sleep, and cause hangovers. Congeners are thought to contribute to hangover symptoms. The only cure for a hangover is time.

What Are the Effects of Chronic Excessive Alcohol Consumption on the Body?

LO 7.5 Describe the effects of chronic excessive alcohol consumption on the body.

Research suggests that chronic excessive consumption of alcohol may result in malnutrition, affect metabolism and hormones, and increase the risk of developing depression, cardiovascular disease, and some cancers. **Figure 7.8** summarizes both the short-term effects of excessive alcohol intake just discussed, and the many harmful effects of chronic excessive drinking.

congeners Fermentation by-products in alcoholic beverages that may contribute to hangover symptoms.

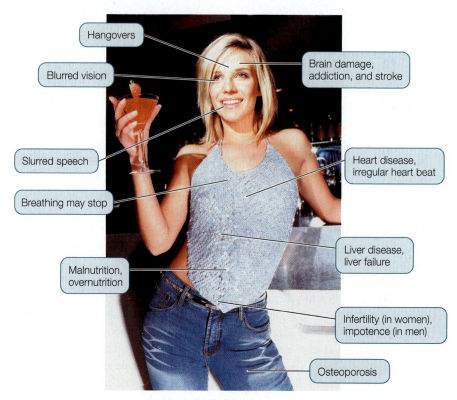

Hangovers

Blurred vision

Brain damage, addiction, and stroke

Slurred speech

Heart disease, irregular heart beat

Breathing may stop

Liver disease, liver failure

Malnutrition, overnutrition

Infertility (in women), impotence (in men)

Osteoporosis

▲ **Figure 7.8 Effects of Alcohol on the Body**
Consuming more than a moderate amount of alcohol leads to both short-term and long-term adverse health effects.

Alcohol Can Interfere with Digestion, Absorption, and Nutrition

Even if an individual consumes a healthy meal while drinking, excessive alcohol can interfere with the digestion and absorption of the nutrients consumed. Individuals who drink heavily tend to eat poorly, and a major concern is that alcohol's effects on the digestion of food and use of nutrients may shift a mildly malnourished person toward severe malnutrition.

Impaired Digestion, Absorption, and Nutrient Metabolism

Alcohol can inhibit chemical digestion by decreasing secretion of digestive enzymes from the pancreas, thereby inhibiting the breakdown of nutrients such as dietary triglycerides.[23] This in turn impairs the absorption and transport of fat-soluble vitamins. Alcohol also impairs nutrient absorption by damaging the cells lining the stomach and intestines, thereby reducing transport of some nutrients into the blood. Nutritional deficiencies themselves may lead to further absorption problems. For example, folate deficiency alters the cells lining the small intestine, which in turn impairs absorption of water and other essential nutrients such as glucose, sodium, and vitamin B_{12}.[24] Heavy drinkers also have increased incidences of **gastritis** (*gastr* = stomach, *itis* = inflammation) and stomach ulcers,[25] which can impair digestion. Chronic consumption of alcohol can also cause pancreatitis, a painful inflammation of the pancreas that reduces its ability to function.[26]

Malnutrition and Wernicke-Korsakoff Syndrome

Individuals who consume more than 30 percent of their daily kilocalories from alcohol over the long term often have some form of **primary malnutrition**. Fueling their energy needs with alcohol, they cut nutritious foods from their diet and can fall short of meeting

gastritis Inflammation of the lining in the stomach.

primary malnutrition State of being malnourished due to poor diet, consuming either too much or too little of a nutrient or energy.

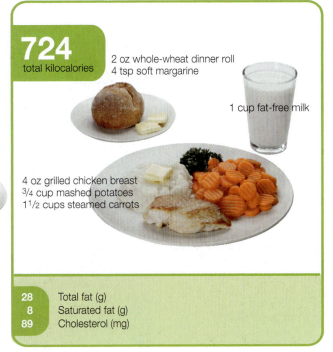

Dinner 1

5 12-oz beers

1,719 total kilocalories

8 BBQ chicken wings

1 large serving nachos with cheese

1 handful Goldfish crackers

	Total fat (g)	51
	Saturated fat (g)	16
	Cholesterol (mg)	154

Dinner 2

724 total kilocalories

2 oz whole-wheat dinner roll
4 tsp soft margarine

1 cup fat-free milk

4 oz grilled chicken breast
3/4 cup mashed potatoes
1 1/2 cups steamed carrots

28	Total fat (g)	
8	Saturated fat (g)	
89	Cholesterol (mg)	

▲ Figure 7.9 **Too Much Alcohol Costs Good Nutrition**
A dinner of several alcoholic beverages and bar foods not only adds kilocalories, fat, and saturated fat to the diet, but displaces healthier foods that would provide better nutrition.

their specific nutrient needs (**Figure 7.9**). Their diets tend to be low in protein, fiber, vitamins A, C, D, riboflavin, and thiamin, and the minerals calcium and iron.[27]

Excessive alcohol consumption can also interfere with nutrient metabolism even after the nutrients have been absorbed, resulting in **secondary malnutrition**. Alcohol can alter transport, storage, and excretion of a variety of nutrients, including protein, zinc, and magnesium, and the B vitamins thiamin, folate, and B_{12}, as well as the fat-soluble vitamins A, D, E, and K. Decreased liver stores of vitamins such as vitamin A and increased excretion of nutrients such as fat in the feces indicate impaired use of nutrients by long-term heavy drinkers.

Chronic alcohol abuse is the number-one cause of **Wernicke-Korsakoff syndrome**, a condition that includes mental confusion and uncontrolled muscle movement.[28] This syndrome is due to a thiamin deficiency that affects brain function, including memory loss. Thiamin helps the brain convert glucose to energy. When the levels of thiamin in the body fall too low, the brain can't generate enough energy to function. Alcoholics are at risk for thiamin deficiency because their diet is often poor in thiamin content and because chronic alcoholism reduces the absorption of thiamin and may reduce the activation of thiamin. While the actual mechanism by which Wernicke-Korsakoff syndrome manifests is unclear, the severe lack of thiamin may destroy brain cells and cause bleeding in the brain and scar tissue buildup.[29]

Weight Gain

At 7 kilocalories per gram, alcohol provides almost as much energy as fat (9 kilocalories per gram) and more than either carbohydrates or protein (4 kilocalories per gram). On top of that, mixed drinks almost always contain more kilocalories than just those from the alcohol (**Table 7.3**). For example, in a rum and coke, the added cola almost triples the calories of the rum alone. In many mixed drinks, depending on the mixers and other ingredients, the kilocalorie count can rival that of a meal. The popular Mudslide, for

secondary malnutrition State of being malnourished due to interference with nutrient absorption or metabolism.

Wernicke-Korsakoff syndrome Severe brain disorder associated with chronic excessive alcohol consumption; symptoms include vision changes, loss of muscle coordination, and loss of memory; the cause is a thiamin deficiency.

TABLE 7.3 Kilocalories in Selected Alcoholic Drinks

Beer

Serving size: 12 oz

Alcohol serving: 1

Kilocalories per drink: 150

Light beer

Serving size: 12 oz

Alcohol serving: 1

Kilocalories per drink: 110

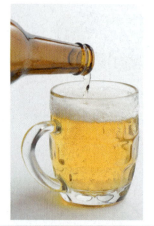

Mudslide

Serving size: 12 oz

Alcohol servings: 4

Kilocalories per drink: 820

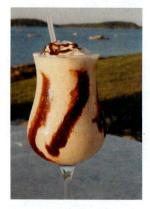

Distilled spirits (whiskey, vodka, gin, rum)

Serving size: 1.5 oz

Alcohol serving: 1

Kilocalories per drink: 100

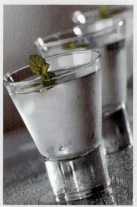

Bloody Mary

Serving size: 5.5 oz

Alcohol serving: 1

Kilocalories per drink: 97

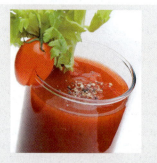

Red or white wine

Serving size: 5 oz

Alcohol serving: 1

Kilocalories per drink: 100–105

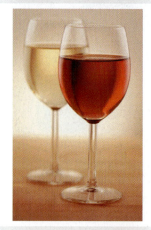

Margarita

Serving size: 6.3 oz

Alcohol servings: 3

Kilocalories per drink: 327

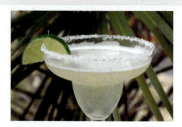

Cosmopolitan

Serving size: 2.5 oz

Alcohol servings: 1.7

Kilocalories per drink: 131

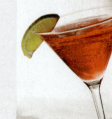

Rum and Coke

Serving size: 12 oz

Alcohol servings: 2.7

Kilocalories per drink: 361

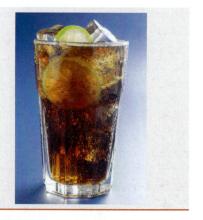

Note: Alcohol servings are per beverage.

Source: Data from U.S. Department of Agriculture. 2015. *Dietary Guidelines for Americans, 2015–2020.* Available at www.health.gov. Accessed February 2017.

example, made with vodka, Irish cream, coffee liqueur, ice cream, and cream, provides more than 800 kilocalories.

Consistently consuming kilocalories above daily energy needs will cause weight gain. However, epidemiological data from the National Health and Nutrition Examination Survey (NHANES) suggests that alcohol consumption does not contribute to obesity. In fact, in a 10-year follow-up study, people who consumed alcohol did not gain weight but rather had more stable weight than those who didn't drink alcohol.[30] Even consuming as much as two drinks or more a day did not appear to increase the risk of weight gain. However, a 2014 study of male college students reported weight gain associated with a higher intake of kilocalories from both alcohol and food.[31] At this point, there is no clear relationship between drinking alcohol and an expanding waistline. Other factors, not just alcohol, may also be responsible for the weight gain.[32]

Interaction with Hormones

When individuals who overindulge in alcohol don't eat enough while they are drinking, their body's glucose stores can become depleted and their blood glucose levels can fall. Typically, the hormones insulin and glucagon would automatically be released to control blood glucose, but chronic alcohol consumption reduces insulin sensitivity and can result in hyperglycemia. Acute alcohol consumption, such as when binge drinking, has the opposite effect. In this case, insulin secretion is overstimulated and can cause hypoglycemia. Because the brain needs glucose to function properly, a low blood glucose level can contribute to the feelings of fatigue, weakness, mood changes, irritability, and anxiety often experienced during a hangover.[33]

Alcohol can interfere with other hormones in addition to those that regulate blood glucose levels. Alcohol negatively affects parathyroid hormone and other bone-strengthening hormones, increasing the risk of osteoporosis.[34] Alcohol can also increase estrogen levels in women, which may increase the risk of breast cancer.[35] Drinking alcohol can affect reproductive hormones and is associated with both male[36] and female sexual dysfunction and infertility.[37]

Alcohol Can Cause Liver Disease

The liver bears the brunt of the impact of overconsumption of alcohol, so it's not surprising that individuals who drink in excess over a long period of time are likely to develop **alcoholic liver disease**, a condition that kills more than 12,000 people each year.[38] The disease develops in three stages, although some stages can occur simultaneously.

The first stage is **fatty liver** (**Figure 7.10**), which can result from just a weekend or a few days of excessive drinking. Because alcohol metabolism takes top priority in the liver, the metabolism of other nutrients, including fats, slows.[39] The metabolic reactions of alcohol cause a buildup of the coenzymes NADH and NADP, which disrupts the breakdown of fatty acids for energy. Fatty acids that are not metabolized accumulate in the liver cells, resulting in fatty liver. The liver tries to reduce this accumulation of fatty acids by transporting them away from the liver into the blood. The result is *hyperlipidemia*—an excess of lipids in the blood, which contributes to atherosclerosis (see Chapter 5).

As fat accumulates in the liver, the liver's ability to perform vital functions is impaired. For example, the liver can't make bile for fat digestion, produce proteins needed for blood clotting, or remove dangerous toxins from the blood. In addition, the hydrogen ions created during the conversion of ethanol to acetaldehyde and acetaldehyde to acetate lowers the pH, making the liver more acidic. The good news is that at this stage a fatty liver can reverse itself *if* the alcohol consumption is stopped.

If the drinking doesn't stop, the second stage of liver disease, **alcoholic hepatitis**, can develop. In alcoholic hepatitis, the various by-products of alcohol metabolism, such as acetaldehyde and free radicals, irritate the liver. Acetaldehyde inhibits liver function,

alcoholic liver disease Degenerative liver condition that occurs in three stages: (1) fatty liver, (2) alcoholic hepatitis, and (3) cirrhosis.

fatty liver Stage 1 of alcoholic liver disease, in which fat begins to build up in the liver cells.

alcoholic hepatitis Stage 2 of alcoholic liver disease, in which the liver becomes inflamed.

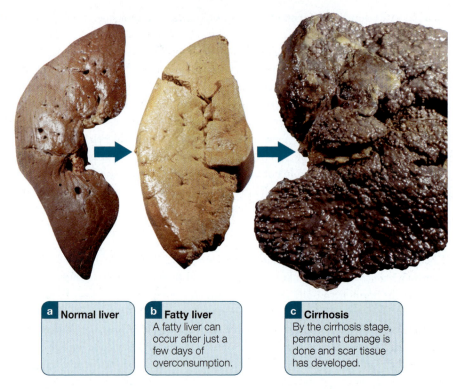

► **Figure 7.10** The Progression of Alcoholic Liver Disease

a Normal liver

b Fatty liver
A fatty liver can occur after just a few days of overconsumption.

c Cirrhosis
By the cirrhosis stage, permanent damage is done and scar tissue has developed.

while free radicals damage cells by reacting with their proteins, lipids, and DNA. Nausea and vomiting, fever, jaundice, and loss of appetite are signs of alcoholic hepatitis. Chronic, excessive amounts of alcohol may also impair the immune system, which can contribute to liver damage and increase the susceptibility to infectious diseases.

Heavy drinking can also cause the increased passage of destructive **endotoxins**, found in the cell walls of bacteria that live in your intestines, into the blood. When these bacteria die, the release of these endotoxins triggers a series of reactions that further damages liver cells. Studies have reported that alcoholics have elevated levels of endotoxins in their blood, which may lead to further liver damage and eventually alcoholic hepatitis.[40]

Alcoholic hepatitis can last for years before progressing to the most serious stage of liver disease. If someone is diagnosed with alcoholic hepatitis, alcohol use must cease to reverse this condition or, in more advanced cases, prevent it from progressing to cirrhosis.

As many as 70 percent of individuals with alcoholic hepatitis develop **cirrhosis**, the final stage of alcoholic liver disease.[41] Cirrhosis occurs with continued bouts of heavy drinking, as chronic inflammation destroys more liver cells and causes more scarring. The scar tissue prevents the liver from performing its many critical metabolic roles, including detoxifying alcohol, medications, and metabolic wastes. As these substances build up, the person can experience mental confusion, nausea, tremors or shakiness, and even coma.

By the time scar tissue develops, the liver is permanently damaged. The survival rate for those with cirrhosis is grim: more than 50 percent of individuals with the condition die within 4 years.[42]

Alcohol and Depression

Alcohol use, especially excessive alcohol consumption, may result in depression. This theory has been reported mainly from observational studies in which the more alcohol a population consumes, the greater their incidence of depression. For example, one study reported that 43 percent of patients who were classified as alcoholics were clinically depressed. But when these patients were abstinent, only 6 percent remained depressed after 4 weeks.[43]

endotoxins Damaging products released from the cell wall of dead bacteria, such as those in the GI tract. They can travel in the blood to the liver and initiate liver damage.

cirrhosis Stage 3 of alcoholic liver disease, in which liver cells die and are replaced by scar tissue.

Whether alcohol consumption causes depression or whether people drink because they're depressed is still unclear. One study suggests that the relationship between alcohol ingestion and depression is explained by other factors, such as genetics, rather than the alcohol itself.[44] That is, a certain genetic makeup may increase an individual's risk of developing depression with greater alcohol consumption. The researchers also proposed that a glass of wine or beer once in a while could actually reduce the risk of developing depression.[45]

Alcohol and Cardiovascular Disease

Alcohol has both favorable and adverse effects on the risks associated with cardiovascular disease (CVD). Higher intakes of alcohol (more than three drinks per day) can increase the risk of developing or dying from CVD.[46] Studies have reported that alcohol may stimulate the synthesis of cholesterol in the liver, which increases blood lipids.[47]

Drinking more than two drinks a day is considered an important determinant of hypertension. The Nurses' Health Study reported that adult women between 30 and 55 years of age who drank more than 20 grams of alcohol per day (about two drinks) had an increase in hypertension.[48] In fact, heavy drinkers who cut back to moderate drinking can lower their systolic blood pressure by 2–4 mm Hg, and lower their diastolic blood pressure 1–2 mm Hg.[49]

Excessive amounts of alcohol can trigger a **cardiac arrhythmia**, which likely plays a role in the sudden deaths of some heavy drinkers.[50] In addition, alcohol can cause **cardiac myopathy**, a condition in which the heart enlarges and becomes weak, thin, and unable to pump blood effectively throughout the body. Excessive drinking plus a poor diet can result in heart failure over time.

Moderate alcohol intake (up to two drinks a day for males and one for females) may have the opposite effect and lower CVD risk by increasing HDL cholesterol, decreasing LDL cholesterol and lipoprotein(a), and/or reducing clot formations.[51] For more information on the possible health benefits of moderate alcohol intake, see the Examining the Evidence feature on page 266.

cardiac arrhythmia Disturbance in the beating and rhythm of the heart; can be caused by excessive alcohol consumption.

cardiac myopathy Condition in which the heart becomes thin and weak and is unable to pump blood throughout the body; also called *disease of the heart muscle*.

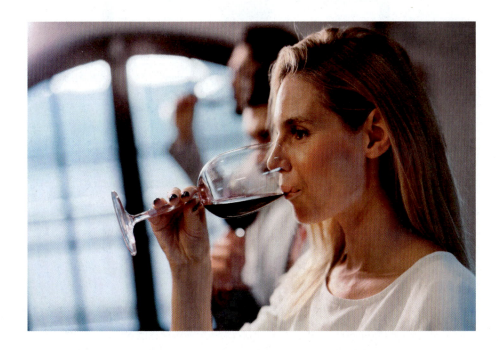

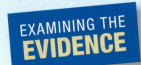

Does Moderate Alcohol Consumption Provide Health Benefits?

Although a consistent body of research supports the health benefits of moderate alcohol consumption, some caution is in order. Most of this research is epidemiological in nature.[1] In addition, alcohol consumption in excess of moderate levels is known to be harmful. With these cautions in mind, let's look at some recent controlled trials that shed new light on the physiological benefits of moderate alcohol intake.

Wine and Beer Provide Phytochemicals

Red wine contains resveratrol, the same beneficial polyphenol phytochemical found in grapes and purple grape juice. Large amounts of resveratrol and other polyphenols are found in the skins of the grape and the bark, leaves, and twigs of the grapevine. When red wine is produced, the grape skins and other parts of the plant are included in the fermentation process. This is in contrast to white wine, which is fermented without the skins. Liquors are distilled, a process that removes the polyphenols. Resveratrol and the other polyphenols in red wine are powerful antioxidants that neutralize free radicals and are associated with reduced risk for heart disease and cancer. White wine is not entirely without benefit, however. It contains a number of polyphenols that are also thought to have antioxidant properties.

Though its nutrient content is still negligible, beer contains more protein and B vitamins (B_6 and folate) than wine and a similar concentration of antioxidant phytochemicals.[2] The precise types differ, however, because beer is made from barley and hops whereas wine is made mostly from grapes. Beer also contains more kilocalories and carbohydrates than wine.

Moderate Alcohol Consumption May Reduce Cardiovascular Risk in Older Adults

Since the 1990s, researchers have explored a health phenomenon known as the "French Paradox." The French,

even though they eat as much saturated fat as Americans, have much lower rates of cardiovascular disease.[3] The paradox may be partially explained, however, by the fact that the French consume fewer *trans* fats than Americans do and have a less stressful lifestyle and better-developed social networks—all factors known to confer a reduced risk for cardiovascular disease.[4] They also drink more red wine.

Scientists report that drinking moderate amounts of alcohol, especially red wine, may reduce the incidence of cardiovascular disease (**Figure 1**). The lowest risk is associated with daily consumption of only one to two drinks, or 12.5–25 grams of alcohol, as compared to zero or more than two drinks per day.[5] These statistics may reflect the effect of a moderate intake of red wine on blood pressure. The greatest blood pressure reduction is seen with one 5-ounce glass of red wine per day for females and two glasses per day

for men.[6] At higher intakes, blood pressure increases in a J-shaped curve; that is, the larger the dose, the higher the blood pressure. Moderate intakes of red wine may also lower LDL cholesterol and raise HDL cholesterol, reduce the stickiness of platelets and thus the formation of blood clots, and reduce inflammation.[7] Like the reduction in blood pressure, these benefits are also J-shaped, with higher intakes actually increasing risk.

Age may play a factor in the cardiovascular benefits of alcohol. Some research suggests that moderate alcohol consumption is beneficial among women age 55 and older and men age 45 and older, but another study suggests that women as young as 45 may also benefit.[8] For people younger than 45, no beneficial effects have been found.[9] In fact, drinking heavily in college may lead to cardiovascular disease later in life.[10]

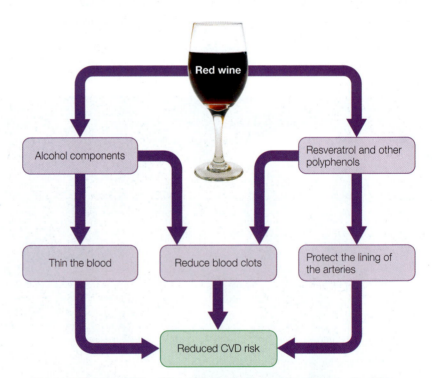

▲ **Figure 1** **How Red Wine May Affect the Risk of Cardiovascular Disease**
Red wine contains phenolic compounds that appear to be beneficial by reducing LDL oxidation; the alcohol itself affects the risk of CVD by thinning the blood.
Source: Adapted from Wollin, S. D., and P. J. H. Jones. 2001. Alcohol, Red Wine and Cardiovascular Disease." *Journal of Nutrition* 131:1401–1404.

Moderate Alcohol Consumption May Reduce the Risk of Diabetes and Metabolic Syndrome

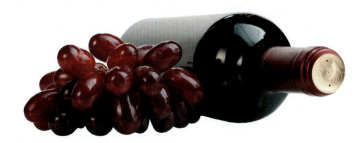

In studies involving individuals with type 2 diabetes, moderate alcohol intake may increase insulin sensitivity.[11] However, diabetics should be sure to drink alcohol with a meal to reduce the risk of hypoglycemia. For those who have been diagnosed with type 1 diabetes, alcohol ingestion of greater than three drinks per day may reduce blood glucose levels to dangerously low levels, causing hypoglycemia.[12]

Alcohol consumption and its effects on metabolic syndrome are related to the amount of alcohol consumed. An analysis of more than 28,000 participants reported that light alcohol intake of less than 10 grams of alcohol per day, or the amount in about 4.5 ounces of wine, was significantly related to a lower risk for metabolic syndrome.[13] Heavy drinking (greater than 35 grams of alcohol per day) increased the risk.

Moderate Alcohol Consumption Is Associated with Longevity

Moderate drinkers appear to live longer. In fact, the lowest death rate from any cause has been reported in those who drink one to two drinks per day.[14] A meta-analysis that reviewed 34 studies involving more than a million older adults from countries around the world reported that one to two drinks per day for women and two to four drinks per day for men increased life expectancy by 2 years when compared with the mortality risk for those who don't drink at all.[15] The other side of the spectrum tells a different story: Chronic alcohol abuse is a leading risk factor for premature death.[16]

The type of alcoholic beverage that increases longevity is still unclear. Although not all health professionals agree, the results in the meta-analysis suggest that living longer is more closely related to consumption of wine than consumption of liquor.[17] When red wine, white wine, beer, and liquor were compared, red wine and dark-colored beer were found to be more protective.[18] Liquor was linked to greater incidence of both cirrhosis and heart disease.[19] Researchers suggest this is because liquor is distilled, and thus does not contain the polyphenols linked to a reduced cardiovascular disease risk.[20]

The bottom line is, if you consume alcohol, limit your intake to one drink per day if you are a female and two if you are a male. In addition, choose red wine and dark beer more often.

References

1. Gow, P. 2016. Open a Nice Bottle of Wine: Randomized Controlled Trials Show Promising Results for the Health Benefits of Moderate Alcohol. *Journal of Studies on Alcohol and Drugs* 77(5):837.
2. Hansel, B., R. Roussel, et al. 2013. Relationships between Consumption of Alcoholic Beverages and Healthy Foods: The French Supermarket Cohort of 196,000 Subjects. *European Journal of Preventive Cardiology* doi: 10.1177/2047487313506829.
3. Vendrame, S. 2013. The French Paradox: Was It Really the Wine? *American Society for Nutrition.* Available at www.nutrition.org.
4. Ibid.
5. Gepner, Y., R. Golan, et al. 2015. Effect of Initiating Moderate Alcohol Intake on Cardiometabolic Risk in Adults with Type 2 Diabetes: A 2-Year Randomized, Controlled Trial. *Annals of Internal Medicine* 163:569–579. doi:10.7326/M14-1650.
6. Zachariah, J. P. 2017. Alcohol Consumption Patterns and Vascular Properties: The Value of Repeatedly Measured Longitudinal Data. *Journal of the American Heart Association* 6(2), pii:e005594. doi: 10.1161/JAHA.117.005594.
7. Barden, A. E., K. D. Croft, et al. 2013. Acute Effects of Red Wine on Cytochrome P450 Eicosanoids and Blood Pressure in Men. *Journal of Hypertension* 31(11):2195–2202.
8. King, D. E., A. G. Mainous, et al. 2013. Impact of Healthy Lifestyle on Mortality in People with Normal Blood Pressure, LDL-cholesterol, and C-reactive Protein. *European Journal of Preventive Cardiology* 20(1):73–79. doi: 10.1177/1741826711425776.
9. Ibid.
10. Vogel, R. A. 2013. Binge Drinking and Vascular Function: A Sober Look at the Data. *Journal of the American College of Cardiology* 62(3):208–209.
11. Schrieks, I. C., A. L. Heil, et al. 2015. The Effect of Alcohol Consumption on Insulin Sensitivity and Glycemic Status: A Systematic Review and Meta-analysis of Intervention Studies. *Diabetes Care* 38(4):723–732. doi: 10.2337/dc14-1556.
12. Desjardins, K., A. S. Brazeau, et al. 2013. Are Bedtime Nutritional Strategies Effective in Preventing Nocturnal Hypoglycemia in Patients with Type 1 Diabetes? *Diabetes Obesity Metabolism* doi:10.1111/dom.12232.
13. Sun, K., M. Ren, et al. 2013. Alcohol Consumption and Risk of Metabolic Syndrome: A Meta-Analysis of Prospective Studies. *Clinical Nutrition.* doi:10.1016/ j.clnu.2013.10.003.
14. Giacosa, A., R. Barale, et al. 2016. Mediterranean Way of Drinking and Longevity. *Critical Reviews in Food Science and Nutrition* 56(4):635–640. doi: 10.1080/10408398.2012.747484.
15. Ibid.
16. O'Keefe, J. H., S. K. Bhatti, et al. 2014. Alcohol and Cardiovascular Health: The Dose Makes the Poison . . . or the Remedy. *Mayo Clinic Proceedings* 89(3):382–393.
17. Chiva-Blanch, G., S. Arranz, et al. 2013. Effects of Wine, Alcohol and Polyphenols on Cardiovascular Disease Risk Factors: Evidences from Human Studies. *Alcohol and Alcoholism* 48(3):270–277. doi: 10.1093/alcalc/ agt007.L.
18. Ibid.
19. Askgaard, G., M. Grønbæk, et al. 2015. Alcohol Drinking Pattern and Risk of Alcoholic Liver Cirrhosis: A Prospective Cohort Study. *Journal of Hepatology* 62(5):1061–1067. doi: 10.1016/j.jhep.2014.12.005.
20. Adjemian, M. K., R. J. Volpe, et al. 2015. Relationships Between Diet, Alcohol Preference, and Heart Disease and Type 2 Diabetes Among Americans. *PLoS One* 10(5):e0124351. doi: 10.1371/journal. pone.0124351.

Alcohol Contributes to Cancer Risk

Chronic excessive alcohol consumption increases the risk of developing cancers, including cancers of the mouth, esophagus, liver, colon or rectum, and breast. Cancer of the mouth, for example, is six times greater in people who drink alcohol. Chronic consumption of alcohol is strongly associated with esophageal cancer: Alcohol promotes inflammation, which reduces the effectiveness of the lower esophageal sphincter in contracting and preventing gastroesophageal reflux. Individuals who smoke while drinking alcohol further increase their risk of developing esophageal cancer, as well as mouth and throat cancer, as the alcohol exacerbates the cancer-causing effects of cigarettes.[52] Alcohol is the primary cause of liver cancer, which is often preceded by cirrhosis of the liver.[53] A meta-analysis suggests that there is a link between drinking more than one alcoholic beverage a day and colorectal cancer.[54] Breast cancer studies have also shown a relationship to alcohol intake.[55] The more alcohol consumed, the greater the risk.

How alcohol contributes to cancer is not well understood, but it probably relates to the toxic effects of acetaldehyde.[56] Research is currently studying whether or not folate supplements may reduce cancer risk in those who consume alcohol.

Alcohol Can Put a Pregnancy at Risk

When a pregnant woman drinks, she is never drinking alone—her fetus becomes her drinking partner. Alcohol easily crosses the placenta and enters the bloodstream of the fetus through the umbilical cord. Because the underdeveloped fetal organs don't efficiently metabolize the alcohol, the fetal BAC rises higher and remains higher longer than the mother's, potentially damaging its central nervous system, particularly the brain. Because no safe level of drinking is known, zero alcohol ingestion during pregnancy is the only safe approach to ensure zero risk for the fetus.

Ultimately, children exposed to alcohol *in utero* may be born with **fetal alcohol syndrome (FAS)**, a cluster of physical, mental, and behavioral signs and symptoms, including the facial abnormalities shown in **Figure 7.11**. They may not develop physically at the pace of other children their age, and they are at increased risk for deficits in attention span, memory, and coordination, as well as for low IQ and learning disabilities.[57] Thus, it's not surprising that children with FAS often have problems in school, in interacting socially with others, and in activities of daily living.

fetal alcohol syndrome (FAS) Most severe of the fetal alcohol spectrum disorders (FASDs); children with FAS display physical, mental, and behavioral abnormalities.

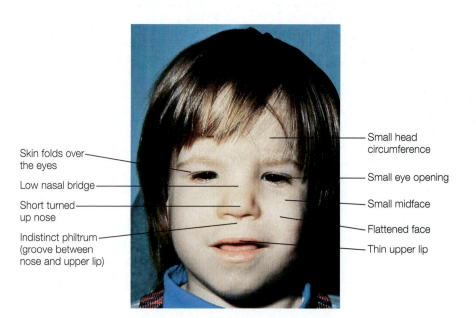

Skin folds over the eyes

Low nasal bridge

Short turned up nose

Indistinct philtrum (groove between nose and upper lip)

Small head circumference

Small eye opening

Small midface

Flattened face

Thin upper lip

▶ **Figure 7.11 Fetal Alcohol Syndrome** Children born with fetal alcohol syndrome often have facial abnormalities.

FAS affects an estimated 2–7 of every 1,000 U.S. children born each year, making FAS the most common and preventable cause of mental retardation and birth defects in the United States.[58] Moreover, another 20–50 of every 1,000 children born each year are thought to have experienced some degree of *in utero* exposure to alcohol and manifest some of the physical, mental, and behavioral abnormalities characteristic of FAS.[59] Recently a new term, **fetal alcohol spectrum disorders (FASDs)**, which includes FAS, has been adopted by major health organizations to describe the wide range of conditions that can occur in children exposed to alcohol *in utero*.[60] No matter the degree of abnormalities, FASDs are permanent. The only proven, safe amount of alcohol a pregnant woman can consume is *none*. Women should avoid alcohol if they think they are, or could become, pregnant.

fetal alcohol spectrum disorders (FASDs) Range of conditions that can occur in children who are exposed to alcohol in utero.

LO 7.5: THE TAKE-HOME MESSAGE Long-term consequences of chronic excessive alcohol consumption can include damage to the digestive organs, heart, and liver; malnutrition and weight gain; hormone imbalances; increased risk of cancer and heart disease, depression, and irreversible damage to a developing fetus during pregnancy. Individuals with alcoholic liver disease can experience a fatty liver and deterioration of the liver that develops into alcohol-related hepatitis and cirrhosis.

HEALTHCONNECTION

What Is Alcohol Use Disorder (AUD)?

LO 7.6 Summarize alcohol use disorder.

Whereas most people drink alcohol responsibly, some abuse it. Problem drinking that has become severe is medically known as **alcohol use disorder (AUD)**. The illness is characterized by impaired control over alcohol intake. Individuals with AUD continue to drink excessively even though they know the negative consequences of their drinking; moreover, they neglect their job, academic, family, or other responsibilities because of their drinking. Individuals with AUD are also at serious risk of

alcohol use disorder (AUD) Pattern of alcohol intake characterized by lack of control over drinking; preoccupation with drinking; continuation of drinking despite negative consequences; tolerance; or withdrawal symptoms when drinking is discontinued.

Self-Assessment

Red Flags for AUD

Complete the following CAGE self-assessment to see if you may be at increased risk for AUD.

1. Have you ever felt you needed to **C**ut down on your drinking?
   Yes ☐ **No** ☐

2. Have people **A**nnoyed you by criticizing your drinking?
   Yes ☐ **No** ☐

3. Have you ever felt **G**uilty about drinking?
   Yes ☐ **No** ☐

4. Have you ever felt you needed a drink first thing in the morning (**E**ye-opener) to steady your nerves or to get rid of a hangover?
   Yes ☐ **No** ☐

Answers

The NIAAA says: If you answered "yes" to two or more questions, you are strongly advised to consult an alcohol assessment and treatment specialist.

Source: J.A. Ewing, "Detecting Alcoholism: The CAGE Questionnaire," JAMA. 1984 Oct 12;252(14):1905–7. Accessed February 2017.

suffering one or more of the alcohol-related health problems just discussed. Among U.S. adults age 18 and older, approximately 11.2 million men and 5.7 million women have been diagnosed with AUD.[61]

Alcohol Use Disorder Includes Alcohol Abuse and Alcoholism

AUD has two forms: alcohol abuse and alcohol dependence, also known as *alcoholism*. Alcohol abuse includes drinking too much or too often; drinking under the age of 21; any alcohol consumption by women of childbearing age who may become pregnant or who are pregnant or lactating; and alcohol consumption by anyone engaging in activities that require attention, skill, or coordination, such as driving or operating machinery. On college campuses, binge drinking and underage drinking are common forms of alcohol abuse. Are you at risk for AUD? Take the nearby Self-Assessment and find out.

Binge Drinking

Binge drinking is a pattern of drinking that brings BAC levels to 0.08 g/dl or higher. This occurs when a male consumes five or more drinks and when a woman consumes four or more drinks in about 2 hours.[62] The incidence of binge drinking is highest in individuals 18–24 years of age. These drinkers report binge drinking more than four times per month and consuming nearly eight alcoholic drinks each time they binge.[63]

The consequences of binge drinking can be severe. College students who binge-drink are more likely to miss classes, have hangovers, and experience potentially fatal unintentional injuries such as falling, motor vehicle accidents, and drowning (see

binge drinking Pattern of consuming five or more alcoholic drinks by men or four or more drinks by women in about 2 hours that raises BAC to 0.08 g/dl or more.

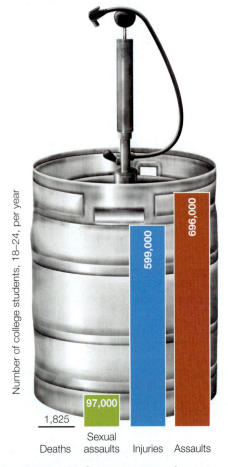

▲ **Figure 7.12 Consequences of College Binge Drinking**
Alcohol use by college students results in numerous assaults, injuries, and deaths each year.
Source: National Institute on Alcohol Abuse and Alcoholism. 2015. College Drinking. Available at https://pubs.niaaa.nih.gov/publications/CollegeFactSheet/CollegeFactSheet.pdf. Accessed February 2017.

Figure 7.12).[64] Research also indicates that binge drinkers engage in more unplanned sexual activity and fail to use safe-sex strategies more frequently than non–binge drinkers.[65] Sexual aggression and assaults on campus increase when drinking enters the picture. Alcohol is involved in over 70 percent of the reported rapes of women on college campuses,[66] victims are often too drunk to consent to or refuse the actions of the other person.

Binge drinking is associated with many health problems, such as hypertension, heart attack, sexually transmitted infection,

suicide, homicide, and child abuse. Binge drinking can also cause blackouts, as discussed earlier in the chapter. A research study of over 2,300 students ages 14–20, found that in the past 3 months, 8 percent of students reported having one or more blackouts per month. Many reported risky health behaviors during the blackout period.[67] Binge drinking can also lead to alcohol poisoning, which, as noted earlier, can lead to brain damage or death.

While binge drinking, some students consume energy drinks to counteract the sedative effects of the alcohol. This is dangerous. College-age drinkers who mix alcohol with energy drinks are three times more likely to leave the bar drunk and four times more likely to drive drunk.[68] Moreover, without the sedating effect of alcohol, the drinker can drink more total alcohol before passing out, and is thus more likely to reach a toxic or potentially lethal BAC.

For strategies to moderate your alcohol intake, see the nearby Table Tips.

Underage Drinking

One of the risk factors for AUD is underage drinking, a form of alcohol abuse common on college campuses. By the age of 15, about 33 percent of American teens have had at least one drink.[69] By the time they graduate from high school, that figure has risen to over 60 percent. Underage drinking not only increases the risk of violence, injuries, and other health risks as discussed earlier, but alcohol consumption at this age can also interfere with brain development and lead to permanent cognitive and memory damage in teenagers.

There is another danger in consuming alcohol at a young age. The earlier a person starts drinking, the higher the chances that alcohol will become a problem later in life. A person who starts drinking at age 15 is six times more likely to suffer from alcoholism than an individual who doesn't start drinking until age 21.[70]

TABLE TIPS
Moderate Your Drinking

Never drink on an empty stomach. The alcohol will be absorbed too quickly, which will impair judgment and lower willpower to decline the next drink.

Keep track of how many beverages you drink using one of the free apps available for smartphones.

Make your first drink at a party a glass of water. This helps you pace yourself and reduces the chance that you will guzzle your first alcoholic drink because you are thirsty. Drink another glass of water before you have a second alcoholic drink.

Drink fun nonalcoholic drinks. Try a Virgin Mary (a Bloody Mary without the vodka), a tame frozen margarita (use the mix and don't add the tequila), or a Tom Collins without the gin.

Don't drink a lot of junk; drink a little of the good stuff. Rather than consume excessive amounts of cheap beer or jug wine, have a single microbrewed beer or one glass of fine wine.

Become the standing Designated Driver among your friends and make your passengers reimburse you for the cost of the gasoline.

Alcoholism

Over time, any form of alcohol abuse can lead to **alcoholism**, a disease characterized by a level of alcohol intake that causes physical, mental, social, and sometimes legal problems. A person who suffers from alcoholism exhibits four classic symptoms of the disease. He or she:

1. Craves alcohol
2. Has developed a higher tolerance for it; that is, the person can drink more without experiencing the same effects as someone who does not have the disease
3. Can't control or limit his or her intake once drinking starts

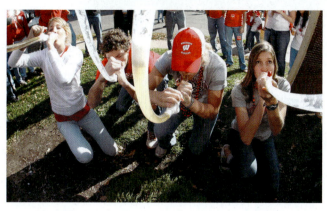

Cultural norms that encourage drinking, for example in drinking games, are among many factors that increase the risk for alcoholism.

4. Suffers withdrawal symptoms such as nausea and tremors if drinking is discontinued

A family history of alcoholism puts a person at a higher than average risk for alcoholism. Research has shown that several genes, not just one, may influence the risk for alcoholism.[71] However, genetics are not destiny. Home life, the drinking habits of family and friends, social pressures, cultural norms related to drinking, and access to alcohol all influence whether a person develops the disease.

Alcohol Use Disorder Can Be Treated But Not Cured

There is no cure for alcohol use disorder. However, AUD can be treated using a combination of approaches.

Support groups such as Alcoholics Anonymous (AA; *www.aa.org*) or Secular Organizations for Sobriety (SOS; *www.sossobriety.org*) can be invaluable to an alcoholic on the road to recovery. In addition, most U.S. colleges and universities support students in recovery from alcohol addiction. For more information, check the Association of Recovery in Higher Education website at http://collegiaterecovery.org/programs/.

Medication can be helpful in reducing withdrawal symptoms such as nausea, insomnia, and anxiety. Three medications

are FDA approved for treating alcoholism: Naltrexone works by blocking the "high" people experience when they drink alcohol; Acamprosate reduces alcohol cravings and withdrawal symptoms by restoring balance to levels of neurotransmitters in the brain, which become imbalanced by chronic alcohol abuse; and Disulfiram prevents the breakdown of alcohol by the liver, thereby causing a person to vomit after drinking alcohol.

Because people with alcoholism can't limit their consumption once they start drinking, merely reducing alcohol consumption is rarely possible. To maintain recovery, most alcoholics must entirely eliminate alcohol from their lives.

Certain personality characteristics have been found to be more common among those who relapse during treatment. These include lower levels of persistence, dependence, and cooperativeness than seen among those who don't relapse.[72] People who relapse despite treatment may need to seek specialized counseling as well as medical support. See **Table 7.4** to review the progressive effects, including the changes in personality that may occur when drinking alcohol.

alcoholism Chronic disease influenced by genetic, psychosocial, and environmental factors and characterized by a level of alcohol intake that causes physical, mental, social, and sometimes legal problems.

TABLE 7.4	Progressive Effects of Alcohol		
Blood Alcohol Concentration	**Changes in Feelings and Personality**	**Brain Regions Affected**	**Impaired Functions (continuum)**
0.01–0.05	Relaxation, sense of well-being, loss of inhibition	Cerebral cortex	Alertness; judgment
0.06–0.10	Pleasure, numbing of feelings, nausea, sleepiness, emotional arousal	Cerebral cortex and forebrain	Coordination (especially fine-motor skills); visual tracking
0.11–0.20	Mood swings, anger, sadness, mania	Cerebral cortex, forebrain, and cerebellum	Reasoning and depth perception; appropriate social behavior
0.21–0.30	Aggression, reduced sensations, depression, stupor	Cerebral cortex, forebrain, cerebellum, and brainstem	Speech; balance; temperature regulation
0.31–0.40	Unconsciousness, coma, death possible	Entire brain	Bladder control; breathing
0.41 and greater	Death		Heart rate

Source: National Institute on Alcohol Abuse and Alcoholism. 2013. *Understanding Alcohol: Investigations into Biology and Behavior.* Available at http://science.education.nih.gov. Accessed February 2017.

LO 7.6: THE TAKE-HOME MESSAGE Problem drinking that has become severe is medically known as alcohol use disorder (AUD). Its two forms are alcohol abuse and alcoholism. Binge drinking and underage drinking are forms of alcohol abuse common on college campuses. All forms of alcohol abuse can lead to alcoholism, a disease characterized by cravings, tolerance, lack of control, and withdrawal symptoms. Alcoholism is a disease that can't be cured, but it can be treated with medical help and psychological support. People with alcoholism typically need to abstain from drinking alcohol entirely.

Visual Chapter Summary

LO 7.1 Alcohol Is Produced by Fermentation of Sugars

Ethanol is the type of alcohol in alcoholic beverages. In the production of beer, wine, and distilled spirits, alcohol is produced by the fermentation of sugars in grains, fruits, potatoes, and other starter substances. In distilled spirits, distillation concentrates the alcohol produced by fermentation. Alcohol is not a nutrient, but it does provide 7 kilocalories per gram.

```
        H
        |
  H — C — H
        |
  H — C — H
        |
       OH
     Ethanol
```

LO 7.2 People Drink Alcohol to Relax, Celebrate, and Socialize

Alcohol produces an initial euphoric, pleasurable state of mind. Adults drink alcohol to relax, celebrate, and socialize. A standard drink (½ ounce of alcohol) is equal to 12 ounces of beer, 5 ounces of wine, or 1.5 ounces of liquor. For adults who choose to drink, moderate alcohol consumption is up to one drink daily for women and up to two drinks daily for men.

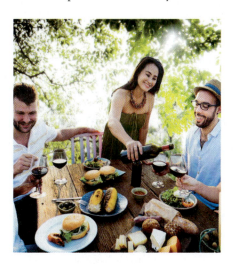

LO 7.3 Alcohol Is Absorbed in the Stomach and Small Intestine, Metabolized in the Stomach and Liver, and Circulated by the Blood

Some alcohol is absorbed into the bloodstream directly from the stomach, but most alcohol is absorbed in the small intestine. Alcohol mixes with water and is distributed in the watery tissues of the body. Some of the alcohol remains in the blood and is circulated until it is metabolized by the liver. The amount of alcohol in a person's blood is called blood alcohol concentration (BAC). A person's gender, age, ethnicity, the amount of food in the stomach, and the quantity of alcohol consumed affect the rate of absorption and metabolism in the body. Some alcohol in the blood is lost in the breath and urine.

Some alcohol is metabolized in the stomach before it is absorbed. However, most of the alcohol is metabolized in the liver by the enzymes alcohol dehydrogenase (ADH) and acetaldehyde dehydrogenase (ALDH). The microsomal ethanol oxidizing system (MEOS) is a secondary pathway that takes over when the ADH pathway is overwhelmed. MEOS is also the primary pathway for drugs and pharmaceuticals, but alcohol takes precedence over these substances.

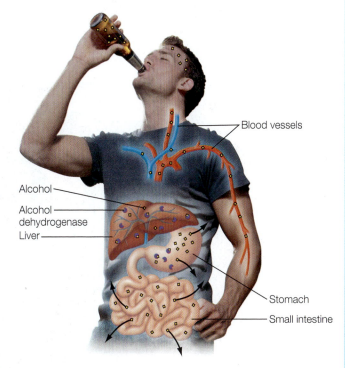

LO 7.4 Alcohol Has Immediate Effects on the Body

Alcohol is a central nervous system depressant. The brain's cerebral cortex, forebrain, cerebellum, and brainstem are sensitive to the effects of alcohol, and, depending on the amount consumed, alcohol can cause numerous mental, behavioral, and physical changes in the body. Alertness, judgment, and coordination are initially affected. Higher BACs can cause impaired vision, speech, reasoning, balance, and memory. Alcohol poisoning (usually at a BAC of 0.30 or higher) can result in impaired breathing and heart rate and can ultimately lead to death. Alcohol consumption is a risk factor for unintentional and intentional injuries, disrupted sleep, and hangovers.

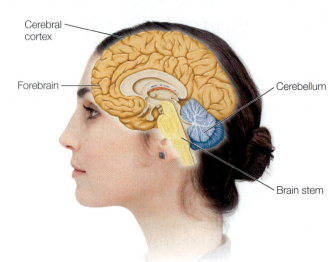

LO 7.5 Excessive Alcohol Consumption Can Have Severe Health Consequences

Excess alcohol can interfere with digestion, absorption, and hormone function. Alcohol can contribute to excess kilocalorie intake and displace healthy foods from the diet. Chronically consuming excessive amounts of alcohol can harm the digestive organs, heart, and liver, can promote heart disease and cancer, and may increase the risk of depression in genetically predisposed individuals. Alcohol can put a fetus at risk for fetal alcohol spectrum disorders.

The liver is damaged from excess alcohol consumption. The three stages of alcoholic liver disease are fatty liver, alcoholic hepatitis, and cirrhosis.

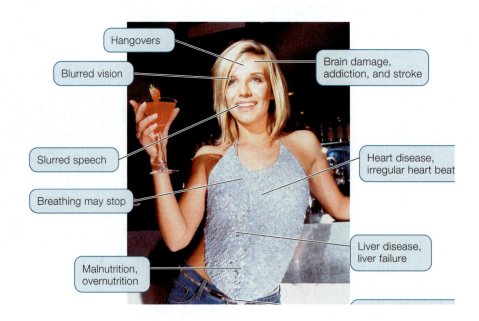

LO 7.6 Alcohol Use Disorder Can Negatively Affect One's Life and Health

Alcohol use disorder is a medical term for problem drinking that has become severe. Its two forms are alcohol abuse and alcohol dependence, more commonly known as alcoholism. Binge drinking and underage drinking are common forms of alcohol abuse on college campuses. Alcoholism is characterized by cravings, tolerance, loss of control, and withdrawal symptoms. Individuals with AUD should seek support. Though alcoholism can't be cured, it can be treated with counseling, medications, and participation in support groups.

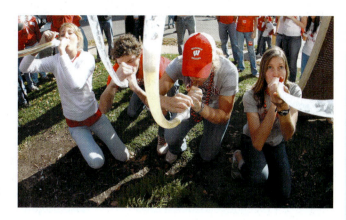

Terms to Know

- alcohol
- ethanol
- fermentation
- distillation
- proof
- social drinking
- moderate drinking
- alcohol dehydrogenase (ADH)
- acetaldehyde
- acetaldehyde dehydrogenase (ALDH)
- microsomal ethanol oxidizing system (MEOS)

- alcohol tolerance
- microsomes
- blood alcohol concentration (BAC)
- blackout
- alcohol poisoning
- hangover
- congeners
- gastritis
- primary malnutrition
- secondary malnutrition
- Wernicke-Korsakoff syndrome
- alcoholic liver disease
- fatty liver

- alcoholic hepatitis
- endotoxins
- cirrhosis
- cardiac arrhythmia
- cardiac myopathy
- fetal alcohol syndrome (FAS)
- fetal alcohol spectrum disorders (FASDs)
- alcohol use disorder
- binge drinking
- alcoholism

Mastering Nutrition
Visit the Study Area in Mastering Nutrition to hear an MP3 chapter summary.

Check Your Understanding

LO 7.1 1. Alcohol, also known as ethanol, is made by the process known as
   a. distillation.
   b. fermentation.
   c. malting.
   d. germination.

LO 7.2 2. Which of the following is *not* considered a standard drink?
   a. A 12-ounce can of beer
   b. A 7-ounce glass of wine
   c. A shot (1.5 ounces) of liquor
   d. A mixed drink made with a shot (1.5 ounces) of liquor

LO 7.3 3. Once ingested, the majority of alcohol is
   a. absorbed through the mucosa lining the mouth.
   b. absorbed slowly on an empty stomach.
   c. absorbed mainly through the small intestine into the blood.
   d. absorbed directly into the liver through the lymph system.

LO 7.3 4. Which of the following factors affect(s) your rate of alcohol absorption and metabolism?
   a. The individuals you are drinking with
   b. The place where you are drinking
   c. The time of day you drink
   d. Whether you're male or female

LO 7.3 5. The enzyme that begins metabolizing alcohol in the liver and the stomach is
   a. sucrase.
   b. insulin.
   c. alcohol dehydrogenase (ADH).
   d. ethanol.

LO 7.3 6. MEOS is
   a. the enzyme system found in the liver that metabolizes alcohol and drugs.
   b. an intermediate compound formed during the metabolism of alcohol.
   c. the chemical that causes the symptoms related to a hangover.
   d. a form of liver disease.

LO 7.4 7. Which of the following statements about alcohol consumption is true?
   a. All areas of the brain are affected equally even when only a small amount of alcohol is consumed.
   b. Drinking an excessive amount of alcohol can shut down the reticular activating system (RAS) in the brain that controls consciousness.
   c. The more alcohol you consume, the less the forebrain is able to control your walking and talking.
   d. Alcohol stimulates the central nervous system.

LO 7.5 8. The first stage of alcoholic liver disease is
   a. malnutrition.
   b. a fatty liver.
   c. cirrhosis.
   d. alcoholic hepatitis.

LO 7.5 9. Drinking four to five alcoholic beverages on one occasion in a span of 2 hours would qualify as
   a. alcoholism.
   b. moderate drinking.
   c. chronic excessive alcohol intake.
   d. binge drinking.

LO 7.6 10. The two forms of AUD are
   a. heavy drinking and drinking while driving.
   b. alcohol abuse and alcoholism.
   c. binge drinking and underage drinking.
   d. drinking too much and drinking too often.

Answers

1. (b) Alcohol found in alcoholic beverages is made by fermentation of natural sugars by yeast. After fermentation, distilled spirits go through a distillation process, which concentrates the beverage. Beer is made by germinating cereal grains to convert starch into sugar, referred to as malting. The sugar is then fermented by yeast to make beer.

2. (b) Five ounces of wine is considered a standard drink, so a 7-ounce glass of wine is the equivalent of almost 1.5 drinks. A 12-ounce beer and a single 1.5-ounce shot, whether or not it is in a mixed drink, are also standard drinks.

3. (c) Most alcohol is absorbed through the small intestine into the blood, where it is taken up by the liver and metabolized. Some alcohol is also absorbed through the stomach on an empty stomach, but absorption is reduced after eating. Alcohol is water-soluble and therefore is not absorbed through the lymph system. Alcohol is not absorbed through the mouth.

4. (a) Your biological sex—male or female—will affect your rate of absorption and metabolism of alcohol. Females have less alcohol dehydrogenase in the stomach, which means they metabolize less alcohol in the stomach and more alcohol will be absorbed into the blood. They also have less body water, so the concentration of alcohol in their systems is higher. The time of day and the place where you drink do not have any effect on the absorption and metabolism of alcohol. Your drinking partners also won't alter the absorption or metabolism of alcohol; of course, they could influence the *amount* of alcohol you drink.

5. (c) ADH is the enzyme in the stomach and the liver that begins metabolizing alcohol. Sucrase is an enzyme that breaks down the sugar sucrose. Insulin is a hormone, not an enzyme; it regulates blood glucose levels. Ethanol is the chemical name for the form of alcohol found in alcoholic beverages.

6. (a) The term *MEOS* (microsomal ethanol oxidizing system) refers to a set of enzymes found in the liver that oxidize ethanol when the consumption is greater than the ADH enzymes can handle. This system also oxidizes drugs. The MEOS does not refer to an intermediate compound or a compound that causes the symptoms of a hangover.

7. (b) Excessive alcohol can shut down the reticular activating system in the brain, causing unconsciousness. The more alcohol you consume, the more areas of the brain are affected. Alcohol affects the cerebellum, which controls walking, while the forebrain controls behavior. Alcohol is a depressant, not a stimulant.

8. (b) The first stage of alcoholic liver disease is a fatty liver. Alcoholic hepatitis is the second stage, followed by cirrhosis. Some people who have alcoholic liver disease are also malnourished.

9. (d) Consuming that much alcohol in 2 hours would qualify as binge drinking. Moderate drinking is no more than one drink per day for females and two for males. Binge drinking over time can lead to alcoholism. Drinking to excess on a single occasion does not qualify as chronic excessive intake.

10. (b) The two forms of AUD are alcohol abuse and alcoholism. Binge drinking, underage drinking, drinking while driving, drinking too much, and drinking too often are forms of alcohol abuse, as is heavy drinking, which is drinking too much and too often.

Answers to True or False?

1. **False.** Although alcohol provides kilocalories, the body does not need it to function and it is therefore not an essential nutrient.

2. **False.** A straight shot of liquor may look and taste more potent than a can of beer, but they contain the same amount of alcohol.

3. **True.** Red wine does contain heart-healthy phytochemical compounds.

4. **True.** Women have less body water and less of the enzyme that metabolizes alcohol in the stomach; they therefore respond more quickly to the narcotic effects of alcohol than do men.

5. **False.** In general, the body can only metabolize about one drink per 1½ hours.

6. **False.** Drinking more alcohol isn't going to take away the ill effects of a hangover. The only cure for a hangover is time.

7. **True.** However, not all alcoholic beverages contain equal amounts of kilocalories. In fact, some mixed drinks can contain almost as many kilocalories as a meal.

8. **True.** Overconsumption of alcohol can lead to displacement of more nutritious foods and diminish the body's ability to absorb or use some essential nutrients.

9. **False.** Moderate drinking is defined as up to one drink per day for women and up to two drinks per day for men. Drinking several alcoholic beverages in one sitting is binge drinking, not moderate drinking.

10. **False.** Although counseling is an important component of recovery from alcohol use disorders, there is no cure.

Web Resources

- For research-based information about alcohol abuse and binge drinking among college students, visit www.collegedrinkingprevention.gov
- For more information about alcohol and your health, visit the National Institute on Alcohol Abuse and Alcoholism (NIAAA) at www.niaaa.nih.gov
- For more information about alcohol consumption and its consequences, visit the National Center for Chronic Disease Prevention and Health Promotion, Alcohol and Public Health, at www.cdc.gov/alcohol/index.htm
- For an overview of the risks and benefits of alcohol, visit the Harvard School of Public Health, The Nutrition Source, *Alcohol: Balancing Risks and Benefits* at www.hsph.harvard.edu

References

1. Holmes, A., P. J. Fitzgerald, et al. 2012. Chronic Alcohol Remodels Prefrontal Neurons and Disrupts NMDAR-Mediated Fear Extinction Encoding. *Nature Neuroscience.* doi: 10.1038/nn.3204.
2. Centers for Disease Control and Prevention. 2016. *Fact Sheets: Alcohol Use and Your Health.* Available at www.cdc.gov. Accessed February 2017.
3. Boynton Health Service. 2015. *2015 College Student Health Survey Report.* Available at www.bhs.umn.edu. Accessed February 2017.
4. Fairbairn, C. E., M. A. Sayette, et al. 2015. Alcohol and Emotional Contagion: An Examination of the Spreading of Smiles in Male and Female Drinking Groups. *Clinical Psychological Science* 3(5):686–671.
5. Centers for Disease Control. 2013. *Youth Exposure to Alcohol Advertising on Television—25 Markets, United States 2010.* Available at www.cdc.gov. Accessed March 2017.
6. Ross, C. S., J. Ostroff, et al. 2014. Evidence of Underage Targeting of Alcohol Advertising on Television in the United States: Lessons from the Lockyer v. Reynolds Decisions. *Journal of Public Health Policy* 35(1):105–118.
7. Grenard, J. L., C. W. Dent, et al. 2013. Exposure to Alcohol Advertisements and Teenage Alcohol-Related Problems. *Pediatrics* 131(2):e369–e379.
8. National Institute on Alcohol Abuse and Alcoholism. 2007. *Alcohol Metabolism: An Update.* Available at http://pubs.niaaa.nih.gov. Accessed February 2017.
9. Finnigan, F., R. Hammersley, et al. 1998. Effects of Meal Composition on Blood Alcohol Level, Psychomotor Performance and Subjective State after Ingestion of Alcohol. *Appetite* 31:361–375.
10. Oneta, C., U. Simanowski, et al. 1998. First-Pass Metabolism of Ethanol Is Strikingly Influenced by the Speed of Gastric Emptying. *Gut* 43:612–619.
11. Enoch, M. A. 2013. Genetic Influences on Response to Alcohol and Response to Pharmacotherapies for Alcoholism. *Pharmacological Biochemical Behavior* doi:10.1016/j.pbb.2013.11.001.
12. Vaeth, P. A., M. Wang-Schweig, et al. 2017. Drinking, Alcohol Use Disorder, and Treatment Access and Utilization Among U.S. Racial/Ethnic Groups. *Alcoholism, Clinical, and Experimental Research* 41(1):6–19. doi:10.1111/acer.13285.
13. National Institute on Alcohol Abuse and Alcoholism. 2017. *Drinking Levels Defined.* Available at https://www.niaaa.nih.gov. Accessed March 2017.
14. National Highway Traffic Safety Administration. 2016. *Traffic Safety Facts 2014: Alcohol-Impaired Driving.* Washington DC: National Highway Traffic Safety Administration. Available at http://www.nrd.nhtsa.dot.gov/Pubs/812231.pdf. Accessed February 2017.
15. College Drinking—Changing the Culture. 2013. *Snapshot of High-Risk College Drinking Consequences.* Available at www.collegedrinking prevention.gov. Accessed February 2017.
16. Ibid.
17. Ebrahim, I. O., C. M. Shapiro, et al. 2013. Alcohol and Sleep I: Effects on Normal Sleep. *Alcoholism: Clinical and Experimental Research* 37(4):539–540.
18. Fell, J. C., D. A. Fisher, et al. 2017. Evaluation of a Responsible Beverage Service and Enforcement Program: Effects on Bar Patron Intoxication and Potential Impaired Driving by Young Adults. *Traffic Injury Prevention* doi: 10.1080/15389588.2017.1285401.
19. Ibid.
20. Mayo Clinic. 2014. *Hangovers.* Available at http://www.mayoclinic.org. Accessed March 2017.
21. WebMD. 2015. *Acetaminophen and Alcohol a Bad Mix, Study Suggests.* Available at http://www.webmd.com/mental-health/addiction/news/20131104/tylenol-and-alcohol-a-bad-mix-study-suggests#2. Accessed February 2017.
22. U.S. Food and Drug Administration. 2016. *FDA Reminds Health Care Professionals to Stop Dispensing Prescription Combination Drug Products with More than 325 mg of Acetaminophen.* Available at https://www.fda.gov/Drugs/DrugSafety/ucm394916.htm. Accessed February 2017.
23. Nikkola, J. 2013. Abstinence After First Acute Alcohol-Associated Pancreatitis Protects Against Recurrent Pancreatitis and Minimizes the Risk of Pancreatic Dysfunction. *Alcohol and Alcoholism* 49(4): 483–486.
24. Lieber, C. S. 2000. Alcohol: Its Metabolism and Interaction with Nutrients. *Annual Review of Nutrition* 20:394–430.
25. Ibid.
26. Nokkola, J. 2013. Abstinence After First Acute Alcohol-Associated Pancreatitis.
27. Campagnolo, N., et al. 2017. Fluid, Energy, and Nutrient Recovery via Ad Libitum Intake of Different Fluids and Food. *Physiology and Behavior* 171:228-235. Available at http://dx.doi.org/10.1016/j.physbeh.2017.01.009.
28. Logan, C., H. Asadi, et al. 2016. Neuroimaging of Chronic Alcohol Misuse. *Journal of Medical Imaging and Radiation Oncology* doi: 10.1111/1754-9485.12572.
29. Hagnäs, M. P., J. Jokelainen, et al. 2017. Alcohol Consumption and Binge Drinking in Young Men as Predictors of Body Composition Changes During Military Service. *Alcohol and Alcoholism* doi: 10.1093/alcalc/agx002.
30. Ibid.
31. Andréasson, S., T. Chikritzhs, et al. 2014. Evidence About Health Effects of "Moderate" Alcohol Consumption: Reasons for Skepticism and Public Health Implications. *Swedish Society of Medicine.* Available at http://iogt.se/wp-content/uploads/Alkoholrapp-2014_ENG-s%c3%a4rtryck.pdf. Accessed February 2017.
32. Ibid.
33. National Institute on Alcohol Abuse and Alcoholism. 2017. *Sex Hormone-sensitive Gene Complex Linked to Premenstrual Mood Disorder.* Available at https://www.niaaa.nih.gov. Accessed February 2017.
34. Schuster, R., A. Koopmann, et al. 2017. Association of Plasma Calcium Concentrations with Alcohol Craving: New Data on Potential Pathways. *European Neuropsychopharmocology* 27(1):42-47. doi: 10.1016/j.euroneuro.2016.11.007.

35. van Erkelens, A., L. Derks, et al. 2016. Lifestyle Risk Factors for Breast Cancer in BRCA1/2-Mutation Carriers Around Childbearing Age. *Journal of Genetic Counseling* doi:10.1007/s10897-016-0049-4.

36. Čulić, V., Ž. Bušić, and M. Bušić. 2016. Circulating Sex Hormones, Alcohol Consumption and Echocardiographic Parameters of Cardiac Function in Men with Heart Failure. *International Journal of Cardiology* 224:245–251. doi: 10.1016/j.ijcard.2016.09.050.

37. Kaya, Y., Beji N. Kizilkaya, et al. 2016. The Effect of Health-Promoting Lifestyle Education on the Treatment of Unexplained Female Infertility. *European Journal of Obstetrics, Gynecology, and Reproductive Biology* 207:109–114. doi: 10.1016/j.ejogrb.2016.10.050.

38. National Institute on Alcohol Abuse and Alcoholism. 2014. *Hepatitis C and Alcohol Exacerbate Livery Injury by Suppression of FOX03.* Available at http://pubs.niaaa.nih.gov. Accessed February 2017.

39. Ibid.

40. Kawaratani, H., T. Tsujimoto, et al. 2013. The Effect of Inflammatory Cytokines in Alcoholic Liver Disease. *Mediators of Inflammation.* doi: 10.1155/2013/495156.

41. American Liver Foundation. 2016. *Cirrhosis.* Available at http://www.liverfoundation.org/abouttheliver/info/cirrhosis. Accessed February 2017.

42. National Institute on Alcohol Abuse and Alcoholism. 2014. *Alcohol's Effects on the Body.* Available at https://www.niaaa.nih.gov. Accessed February 2017.

43. Paulus, D. J., A. Vujanovic, et al. 2017. Main and Interactive Effects of Depression and Posttraumatic Stress in Relation to Alcohol Dependence Among Urban Male Firefighters. *Psychiatry Research* 251:69-75. doi: 10.1016/j.psychres.2017.02.011

44. Almeida, O. P., G. J. Hankey, et al. 2013. The Triangular Association of ADH1B Genetic Polymorphism, Alcohol Consumption and the Risk of Depression in Older Men. *Molecular Psychiatry* doi:10.1038/mp.2013.117.

45. Ibid.

46. Matsumoto, C., M. D. Miedema, et al. 2014. An Expanding Knowledge of the Mechanisms and Effects of Alcohol Consumption on Cardiovascular Disease. *Journal of Cardiopulmonary Rehabilitation and Prevention* doi: 10.1097/HCR.0000000000000042.

47. Bulle, S., V. D. Reddy, et al. 2017. Association Between Alcohol-Induced Erthyrocyte Membrane Alterations and Hemolysis in Chronic Alcoholics. *Journal of Clinical Biochemistry and Nutrition* 60(1):63-69. doi: 10.3164/jcbn.16-16.

48. Appelhans, B. M., A. Baylin, et al. 2016. Beverage Intake and Metabolic Syndrome Risk Over 14 Years: The Study of Women's Health Across the Nation. *Journal of Academy of Nutrition and Dietetics* pii: S2212-2672(16)31293-X. doi: 10.1016/j.jand.2016.10.011.

49. Huang, C., et al. 2014. Association Between Alcohol Consumption and Risk of Cardiovascular Disease and All-cause Mortality in Patients with Hypertension: A Meta-analysis of Prospective Cohort Studies. Mayo Clinic Proceedings 80(9) 1201–1210.

50. Rosenqvist, M. 1998. Alcohol and Cardiac Arrhythmias. *Alcoholism: Clinical and Experimental Research* 22:318s–322s.

51. Barden, A. E., K. D. Croft, et al. 2013. Acute Effects of Red Wine on Cytochrome P450 Eicosanoids and Blood Pressure in Men. *Journal of Hypertension* 31(11):2195–2202.

52. American Cancer Society. 2014. *Alcohol Use and Cancer*. Available at www.cancer.org. Accessed March 2017.

53. Turati, F., C. Galeone, et al. 2014. Alcohol and Liver Cancer: A Systematic Review and Meta-Analysis of Prospective Studies. *Annals of Oncology* doi:10.1093/annonc/mdu020.

54. Yang, B., S. M. Gapstur, et al. 2017. Alcohol Intake and Mortality Among Survivors of Colorectal Cancer: The Cancer Prevention Study II Nutrition Cohort. *Cancer* doi: 10.1002/cncr.30556.

55. Scoccianti, C., B. Lauby-Secretan, et al. 2014. Female Breast Cancer and Alcohol Consumption: A Review of the Literature. *American Journal of Preventative Medicine* 46(3 Supplement 1):S16–S25.

56. Ibid.

57. Jones, K., and D. Smith. 1973. Recognition of the Fetal Alcohol Syndrome in Early Infancy. *The Lancet* 2:999–1001.

58. National Institute on Alcohol Abuse and Alcoholism. 2017. *Alcohol Facts and Statistics*. Available at https://www.niaaa.nih.gov. Accessed February 2017.

59. Ibid.

60. Ibid.

61. National Institute on Alcohol Abuse and Alcoholism. 2017. *Alcohol Use Disorder*. Available at https://www.niaaa.nih.gov. Accessed February 2017.

62. National Institute on Alcohol Abuse and Alcoholism. 2017. *Drinking Levels Defined*. Available at http://niaaa.nih.gov. Accessed March 2017.

63. Centers for Disease Control and Prevention. 2015. *Binge Drinking*. Available at www.cdc.gov. Accessed March 2017.

64. World Health Organization. 2017. *Alcohol and Injuries*. Available at www.who.int. Accessed March 2017.

65. Glatter, R. 2014. *Update on Binge Drinking and Risky Sex among College Students*. Available at https://www.forbes.com/. Accessed March 2017.

66. Parkhill, M. R., J. Norris, et al. 2016. The Effects of Sexual Victimization History, Acute Alcohol Intoxication, and Level of Consensual Sex on Responses to Sexual Assault in a Hypothetical Scenario. *Violence and Victims* 31(5):938-956.

67. Voloshyna, D. M., E. E. Bonar, et al. 2016. Blackouts Among Male and Female Youth Seeking Emergency Department Care. *American Journal of Drug and Alcohol Abuse* 29:1-11. doi: 10.1080/00952990.2016.1265975.

68. Reuters. 2013. *Energy Drinks and Alcohol A Dangerous Combo For College Kids: Study*. Available at http://www.nydailynews.com/life-style/health/energy-drinks-alcohol-dangerous-combo-college-kids-study-article-1.1546930. Accessed February 2017.

69. Centers for Disease Control and Prevention. 2016. *Fact Sheets: Underage Drinking*. Available at https://www.cdc.gov. Accessed March 2017.

70. Ibid.

71. Rietschel, M., and J. Treutlein, 2013. The Genetics of Alcohol Dependence. *Annals of the New York Academy of Sciences* 1282():39-70.

72. Foulds, J. A., G. M. Newton-Howes, et al. 2017. Dimensional Personality Traits and Alcohol Treatment Outcome: A Systematic Review and Meta-Analysis. *Addiction* doi: 10.1111/add.13810.

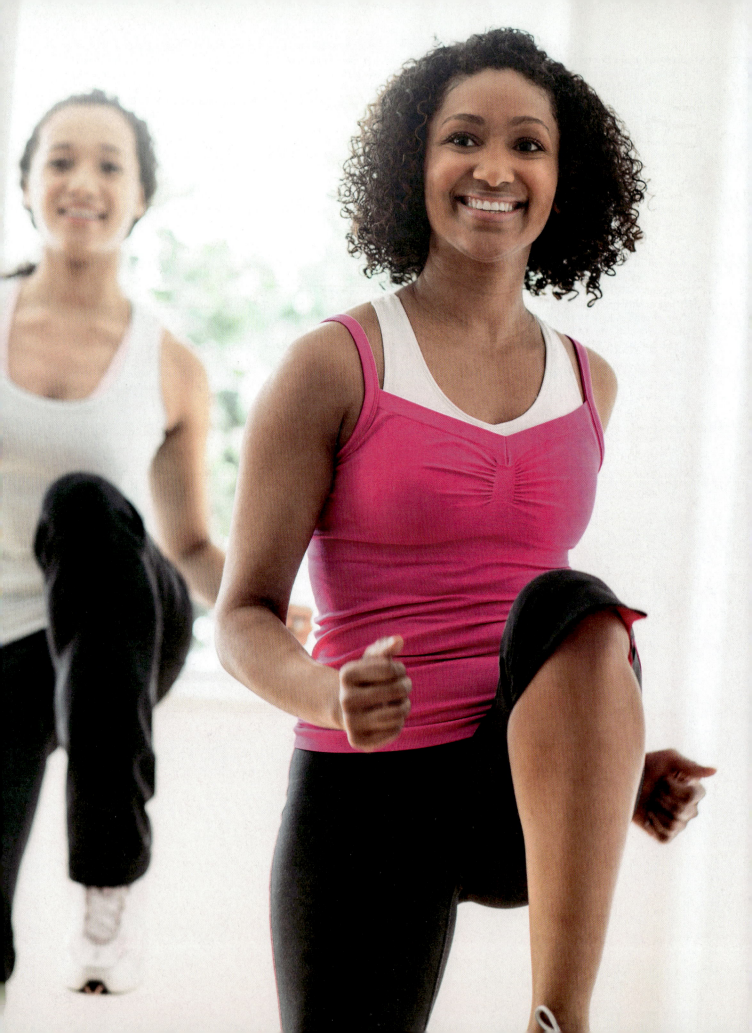

Energy Metabolism

Learning Outcomes

After reading this chapter, you will be able to:

8.1 Define *metabolism* and provide examples of anabolic and catabolic reactions and the hormones that regulate these reactions.

8.2 Explain the role of adenosine triphosphate (ATP) as an energy source for cells.

8.3 Compare and contrast the major metabolic pathways that carbohydrates, fatty acids, glycerol, and amino acids follow to produce ATP.

8.4 Explain how metabolism changes during the absorptive, postabsorptive, and starvation stages of food intake.

8.5 Describe the metabolism of alcohol.

8.6 Describe the causes, diagnosis, symptoms, and dietary treatments of the most common genetic disorders of metabolism.

True or False?

1. Metabolism takes place within cells. **T**/**F**

2. The body prefers to use carbohydrates for fuel because, as compared to fats or proteins, their metabolism requires less energy. **T**/**F**

3. Fructose is preferable to glucose as an energy source. **T**/**F**

4. Lactate buildup during exercise causes a burning sensation in the legs. **T**/**F**

5. Excess dietary protein is stored in the muscle and therefore increases muscle size. **T**/**F**

6. Fat is the main fuel used during high-intensity exercise. **T**/**F**

7. Alcohol is converted to blood glucose during metabolism. **T**/**F**

8. B vitamins provide energy. **T**/**F**

9. Kilocalories consumed after 7:00 P.M. are automatically stored as fat and contribute to weight gain. **T**/**F**

10. Children with inborn errors of metabolism outgrow such disorders when they reach puberty. **T**/**F**

See page 314 for the answers.

nergy is defined as the capacity to perform work. In the body, it includes mechanical energy to move muscles, heat to warm you, electrical energy to conduct nerve impulses, and chemical energy in your stores of glycogen and fat.

Every second of every day, your cells produce a steady supply of energy from the foods you eat. Hundreds of complex chemical reactions transform the energy-yielding macronutrients to a form of energy the cells can use. Understanding these intricate reactions is an important aspect of the study of nutrition. This goal may at first seem a little daunting, but the process is not unlike assembling a jigsaw puzzle. Once the first pieces are in place, the larger picture begins to take shape and the later pieces are easier to understand.

In this chapter we discuss the chemical reactions within the pathways of energy metabolism and how the individual nutrients—the pieces—flow into this larger metabolic puzzle. We also discuss how the body adapts to the day-to-day changes in dietary intake and what happens when metabolic processes fail to work properly.

What Is Metabolism?

LO 8.1 Define *metabolism* and provide examples of anabolic and catabolic reactions and the hormones that regulate these reactions.

How does a kilocalorie from food transform into the energy required to throw a baseball, open a door, or think through a math equation? The answer can be summed up in one word: **metabolism**.

Metabolism Is a Series of Chemical Reactions

Metabolism is the sum of all the chemical reactions that take place within the 10 trillion cells in the body. These chemical reactions follow **metabolic pathways** in which the product of one reaction is the starting substance for the next reaction. This chapter focuses on the metabolic pathways involved with the production of **adenosine triphosphate (ATP)**, the energy currency for body cells. **Figure 8.1** illustrates the main stages in which food is transformed into metabolic by-products and ATP.

Metabolic pathways can be as simple as only two to three chemical reactions or they can be much more complex, requiring multiple reactions to complete. These reactions may be **aerobic**, meaning they require oxygen to proceed, or **anaerobic**, meaning they can proceed when oxygen is not available to the cell. In addition, chemical reactions involved in metabolism are either anabolic or catabolic (**Figure 8.2**).

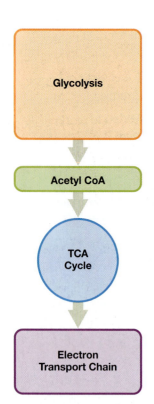

▲ Figure 8.1 **The Stages of Metabolism**
The chemical reactions of energy metabolism include glycolysis, the intermediate reaction of pyruvate to acetyl CoA, the TCA cycle, and the electron transport chain.

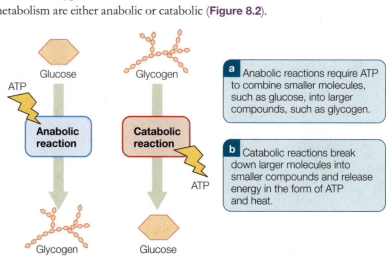

a Anabolic reactions require ATP to combine smaller molecules, such as glucose, into larger compounds, such as glycogen.

b Catabolic reactions break down larger molecules into smaller compounds and release energy in the form of ATP and heat.

▲ Figure 8.2 **Anabolic and Catabolic Reactions**
Metabolic processes involve both anabolic and catabolic reactions.

Anabolic Reactions

Anabolic reactions generally use or absorb energy to combine simpler molecules into larger, more complex ones. For example, single amino acids join to form proteins, excess glucose molecules combine to form glycogen, and excess fatty acids attach to glycerol molecules to make triglycerides. These reactions involve the formation of new bonds, which requires energy.

Catabolic Reactions

Catabolic reactions are the opposite of anabolic processes: They generally release energy as they break down large molecules into simple structures. The breakdown products of catabolism can be used for energy, recycled, or excreted. For example, glycogen molecules are hydrolyzed to yield molecules of glucose, and triglycerides are disassembled to yield fatty acids and glycerol. The smaller glucose, fatty acid, and glycerol molecules are then broken down through the stages of energy metabolism to produce ATP. Note in both a catabolic and an anabolic reaction, some energy is released as heat.

Metabolism Takes Place within Cells

The chemical reactions involved in energy production and storage take place within the body's cells. Even though different cells perform different metabolic functions, their fundamental structure is similar (**Figure 8.3**). All cells have an outer envelope, called the *cell membrane,* which holds in the cell's contents, and several specialized internal structures, called *organelles.* The organelles shown in Figure 8.3 include two you encountered in Chapter 6: the nucleus, the location of the cell's DNA, and ribosomes, which are sites of protein assembly in the cytoplasm, the fluid portion of cells. Also shown is the smooth endoplasmic reticulum, which produces lipids used by other organelles.

One particular organelle, the **mitochondrion** (plural: mitochondria), is referred to as the powerhouse of the cell. The mitochondria generate most of the cell's energy through aerobic metabolism. Almost all body cells contain mitochondria. The exception is the red blood cells, which produce energy anaerobically in the cytoplasm.

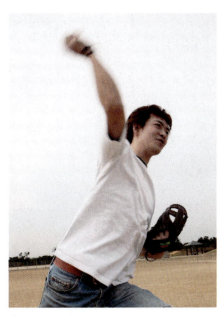

Metabolism allows the body to convert energy from foods into energy needed for physical activity.

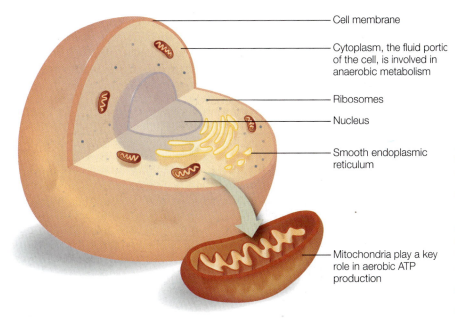

- Cell membrane
- Cytoplasm, the fluid portic of the cell, is involved in anaerobic metabolism
- Ribosomes
- Nucleus
- Smooth endoplasmic reticulum
- Mitochondria play a key role in aerobic ATP production

▲ Figure 8.3 **Metabolism Takes Place within Cells**
The mitochondrion is a metabolically active organelle located in the cytoplasm. Other common cell structures include the nucleus, the location of DNA; the ribosomes, which help manufacture proteins; and the smooth endoplasmic reticulum, which produces lipids used by the organelles.

metabolism Sum of all chemical reactions in the body.

metabolic pathway Sequence of reactions that convert compounds from one form to another.

adenosine triphosphate (ATP) High-energy molecule composed of adenine, ribose, and three phosphate molecules; used by cells to fuel all biological processes.

aerobic Reaction that requires oxygen.

anaerobic Reaction that does not require oxygen.

mitochondrion Cellular organelle that releases energy from carbohydrates, proteins, and fats to make ATP; *pl.* mitochondria.

The Liver Plays a Central Role in Metabolism

The most metabolically active organ in the body is the liver. In previous chapters you learned that the proteins, carbohydrates, and fats in foods are digested and absorbed as amino acids, monosaccharides, glycerol, and fatty acids, respectively. Once these nutrients have been absorbed, the liver is the first organ to metabolize them or send them through the blood to other tissues. The liver also uses these nutrients to synthesize new compounds—for instance, converting essential amino acids into nonessential amino acids. The liver also stores some of these nutrients—glycogen, for example—to use in the future.

Enzymes and Hormones Regulate Metabolism

Enzymes and their assistant coenzymes enable the chemical reactions of metabolism to occur at fast enough rates to maintain normal body function. Nearly every metabolic reaction requires a specific enzyme to catalyze the reaction and, in some cases, a coenzyme, or helper, that is often a vitamin, assists the enzyme.

Two B vitamins, niacin and riboflavin, are key players in energy metabolism, assisting enzymes by accepting or donating electrons and hydrogen ions produced during oxidation-reduction reactions (see the Chemistry Boost):

- Niacin is found in the cells in an oxidized form, **nicotinamide adenine dinucleotide (NAD^+)**, and a reduced form, called NADH. NAD^+ accepts one hydrogen ion and two electrons during metabolism to become $NADH + H^+$.
- The oxidized coenzyme form of riboflavin, **flavin adenine dinucleotide (FAD)**, is reduced during metabolism to $FADH_2$. This reduced form gains two hydrogen ions and two electrons.

Without these two essential B vitamins in the diet, the coenzyme forms NAD^+ and FAD would not be made in the body and metabolism would come to a halt. We cover the functions of all the B vitamins in Chapter 10.

nicotinamide adenine dinucleotide (NAD^+) Coenzyme that is a hydrogen carrier as NADH in oxidation-reduction reactions.

flavin adenine dinucleotide (FAD) Electron carrier similar to NAD that picks up a hydrogen ion from the TCA cycle and carries it to the electron transport chain.

Chemistry Boost

Oxidation-Reduction Reactions

We obtain energy during metabolism by oxidation-reduction reactions (also called *redox reactions*), which involve the transfer of electrons. Oxidation reactions involve the loss of an electron, while reduction reactions gain an electron. These reactions happen in sets: When an oxidation reaction occurs and one molecule loses an electron, another molecule is reduced and gains an electron.

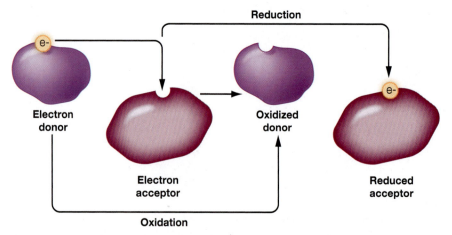

Redox reactions involve the transfer of electrons. During glycolysis, for example, glucose is oxidized to pyruvate and the coenzyme form of the B vitamin niacin (NAD^+) is reduced to $NADH + H^+$.

TABLE 8.1	The Major Hormones That Control Metabolism					
Hormone	Produced by	Type of Reaction	Control of Protein Metabolism	Control of Carbohydrate Metabolism	Control of Fat Metabolism
Insulin	Pancreas	Anabolic	Stimulates protein synthesis	Stimulates glycogen synthesis	No effect
Glucagon	Pancreas	Catabolic	Stimulates protein degradation	Stimulates glycogenolysis	Stimulates lipolysis
Epinephrine	Adrenal glands	Catabolic	No effect	Stimulates glycogenolysis	Stimulates lipolysis
Cortisol	Adrenal glands	Catabolic	Stimulates protein degradation	Stimulates gluconeogenesis	No effect

Hormones can also regulate anabolic and catabolic reactions. When the endocrine system detects a change in the concentration of nutrients, such as when blood glucose levels rise, hormones are released that influence whether enzymes that regulate metabolism are activated or deactivated. For instance, the hormone insulin lowers blood glucose levels by enabling the movement of glucose into the cells. Furthermore, within the cells, insulin controls the metabolic fate of glucose. Three other hormones, namely glucagon, epinephrine, and cortisol, can also influence metabolism and result in an increase in blood glucose by stimulating glycogenolysis. **Table 8.1** outlines the major hormones controlling anabolic and catabolic reactions.

LO 8.1: THE TAKE-HOME MESSAGE Metabolism is the sum of all metabolic processes that occur in cells. Most of these reactions take place within the mitochondria. Anabolic reactions require energy to build new substances whereas catabolic reactions break molecules apart, yielding energy. Enzymes catalyze the reactions involved in metabolism along with the aid of coenzymes, especially forms of niacin and riboflavin, as well as hormones, including insulin, glucagon, epinephrine, and cortisol.

How Does ATP Fuel Metabolism?

LO 8.2 Explain the role of adenosine triphosphate (ATP) as an energy source for cells.

All body actions require energy, whether you're running a marathon or lying in bed. Furthermore, the more strenuous the action, the more energy the body requires. For example, your body burns more energy to lift a 50-pound bag of dog food than to lift a 5-pound bag of flour. You know by now that the source of fuel for all this energy is food.

However, before your body can use the energy in the cereal, fruit, and toast you ate for breakfast, it must first disassemble the macronutrients, break them into smaller compounds, and transfer their energy into the high-energy molecule adenosine triphosphate (ATP).

Adenosine Triphosphate Is the Cell's Energy Source

ATP is the only source of energy that cells can use directly for work. The process of disassembling food to create ATP actually requires some ATP to convert the food into energy and more ATP. (In other words, you have to "spend" ATP to make ATP.) The cells then use that ATP to fuel other metabolic processes.

ATP has three components: adenine, a nitrogen-containing compound that you may recall from Chapter 6 is one of the four bases of DNA; ribose, a five-carbon sugar; and three phosphate groups (which contain phosphorus and oxygen). The energy in ATP is stored in the bonds that connect the phosphate groups to each other.

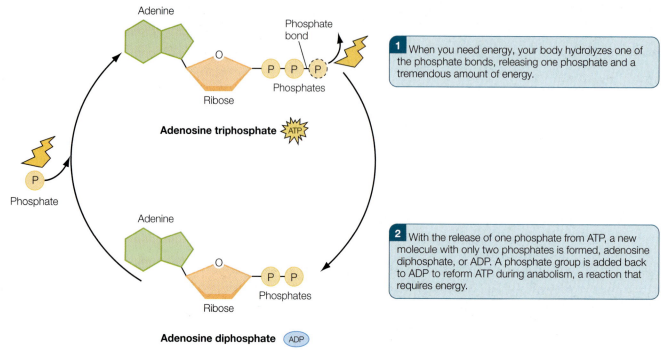

Adenosine triphosphate (ATP)

① When you need energy, your body hydrolyzes one of the phosphate bonds, releasing one phosphate and a tremendous amount of energy.

② With the release of one phosphate from ATP, a new molecule with only two phosphates is formed, adenosine diphosphate, or ADP. A phosphate group is added back to ADP to reform ATP during anabolism, a reaction that requires energy.

Adenosine diphosphate (ADP)

▲ **Figure 8.4 ATP to ADP**
The high-energy molecule adenosine triphosphate (ATP) releases energy to be used by the cells when the phosphate bond is broken, producing adenosine diphosphate (ADP).

As **Figure 8.4** illustrates, when you need energy, one of the bonds connecting the phosphate groups is hydrolyzed. This releases one phosphate *plus* a tremendous amount of energy. The new molecule that is formed is called **adenosine diphosphate (ADP)**.

At any given moment, cells only have 3–5 seconds' worth of ATP available for immediate use. Therefore, the body must continually produce ATP to provide a constant supply of energy.

ATP Can Be Regenerated from ADP and Creatine Phosphate

Regenerating ATP from ADP requires a source of phosphate. As illustrated in Figure 8.4, the phosphate produced from the initial breakdown of ATP is one source. Another source of phosphate is **creatine phosphate (PCr)**, also called *phosphocreatine*. PCr is a high-energy compound formed in muscle cells when *creatine* (a nitrogenous organic acid found in foods and produced in the body) combines with phosphate. This phosphate can be released from creatine phosphate and added to ADP to form ATP. In addition, when the phosphate bond is broken, energy is released, which provides the fuel needed to restore ATP. These two sources of phosphate, ATP and PCr, can provide enough ATP to sustain a sprint for about 10 seconds. (See Chapter 16's Chemistry Boost on page 586 for further discussion of creatine phosphate.)

As the available ATP dwindles and creatine phosphate in the muscle cell is exhausted, the body relies on anaerobic and aerobic metabolism to produce the needed ATP. Anaerobic metabolism produces more ATP per minute than aerobic metabolism, but it is very limited in its use (it only provides about 1–1.5 minutes of maximal activity). Activities that primarily involve anaerobic metabolism are high-intensity, short-duration activities such as sprinting or heavy weightlifting. When the demand for ATP is greater than the rate at which metabolism can produce it, the activity slows down or stops completely. This is one reason why individuals who lift weights have to rest between sets; it gives the body time to form more ATP to be used for the next set of lifts. Aerobic metabolism produces less ATP per minute than anaerobic metabolism, but it can continue indefinitely.

adenosine diphosphate (ADP) Nucleotide composed of adenine, ribose, and two phosphate molecules; formed when one phosphate molecule is removed from ATP.

creatine phosphate (PCr) Compound that provides a reserve of phosphate to regenerate ADP to ATP.

Low-intensity, long-duration activities, such as walking or slow jogging, primarily involve aerobic metabolism.

The transformations that convert energy stored in carbohydrates, proteins, and fats into ATP are tightly integrated and somewhat complex. To learn this material, we break down these integrated processes by stages.

LO 8.2: THE TAKE-HOME MESSAGE ATP is the energy source cells use to fuel metabolic reactions. Cells only have 3–5 seconds' worth of ATP; thus, ATP must be regenerated from ADP and phosphate (which can be donated by creatine phosphate) or produced during anaerobic metabolism, which can fuel the body for no more than 1.5 minutes, or aerobic metabolism, which can continue indefinitely.

How Do the Macronutrients Provide ATP?

LO 8.3 Compare and contrast the major metabolic pathways that carbohydrates, fatty acids, glycerol, and amino acids follow to produce ATP.

All three macronutrients—carbohydrates, proteins, and fats—fuel the production of ATP by entering the metabolic pathway at some point in the stages of metabolism. Their metabolic fate is determined by the chemical reactions within each metabolic pathway (**Figure 8.5**). The major energy nutrient, glucose, fuels metabolism from the first stage through the final stage, much like electricity flowing through wires. Fatty acids and amino acids contribute to metabolism as they are transformed into different substrates along the pathway.

Carbohydrates are unique in that they are oxidized anaerobically in stages 1 and 2 of metabolism (see Figure 8.5) and also aerobically in stage 3. Fatty acids from triglycerides are only oxidized aerobically (see Figure 8.5, stage 2), a process that is slower than anaerobic metabolism. The fatty acids are split from the glycerol backbone before they are metabolized and converted to acetyl CoA, whereas glycerol enters metabolism through glycolysis.

When amino acids from proteins are needed for energy, the structure of their side group determines where they enter the metabolic pathway. As you know, the glucogenic amino acids can be transformed into glucose through gluconeogenesis when carbohydrate intake is low. They can also be converted to substrates and enter glycolysis (see Figure 8.5, stage 1). **Ketogenic** amino acids (*keto* = ketone, *genic* = forming) can be converted to acetyl CoA (stage 2), and a few amino acids can be converted to intermediate substrates in the TCA cycle (stage 3).

Regardless of the stage in which energy nutrients enter metabolism, they eventually all converge at acetyl CoA. Let's take a closer look at each stage.

Glycolysis Transforms Glucose to Pyruvate

The first step in forming ATP from glucose is **glycolysis** (*glyco* = glucose, *lysis* = break apart), the universal pathway for glucose oxidation. Glucose metabolism is an essential energy source for all cells and particularly the brain and red blood cells. As you follow the metabolic pathway illustrated in **Figure 8.6**, track the carbons through the process from beginning to end.

Notice that glucose is depicted here as a row of six carbons, rather than a six-sided ring structure as shown in Chapter 4. This representation makes it easier to see the movement of carbon during metabolism.

ketogenic Describing molecules that can be transformed into ketone bodies.

glycolysis Breakdown of glucose; for each molecule of glucose, two molecules of pyruvate and two ATP molecules are produced.

After the energy-containing nutrients have been absorbed through the small intestine, they can enter a metabolic pathway and be converted to energy or be stored as fat for later use.

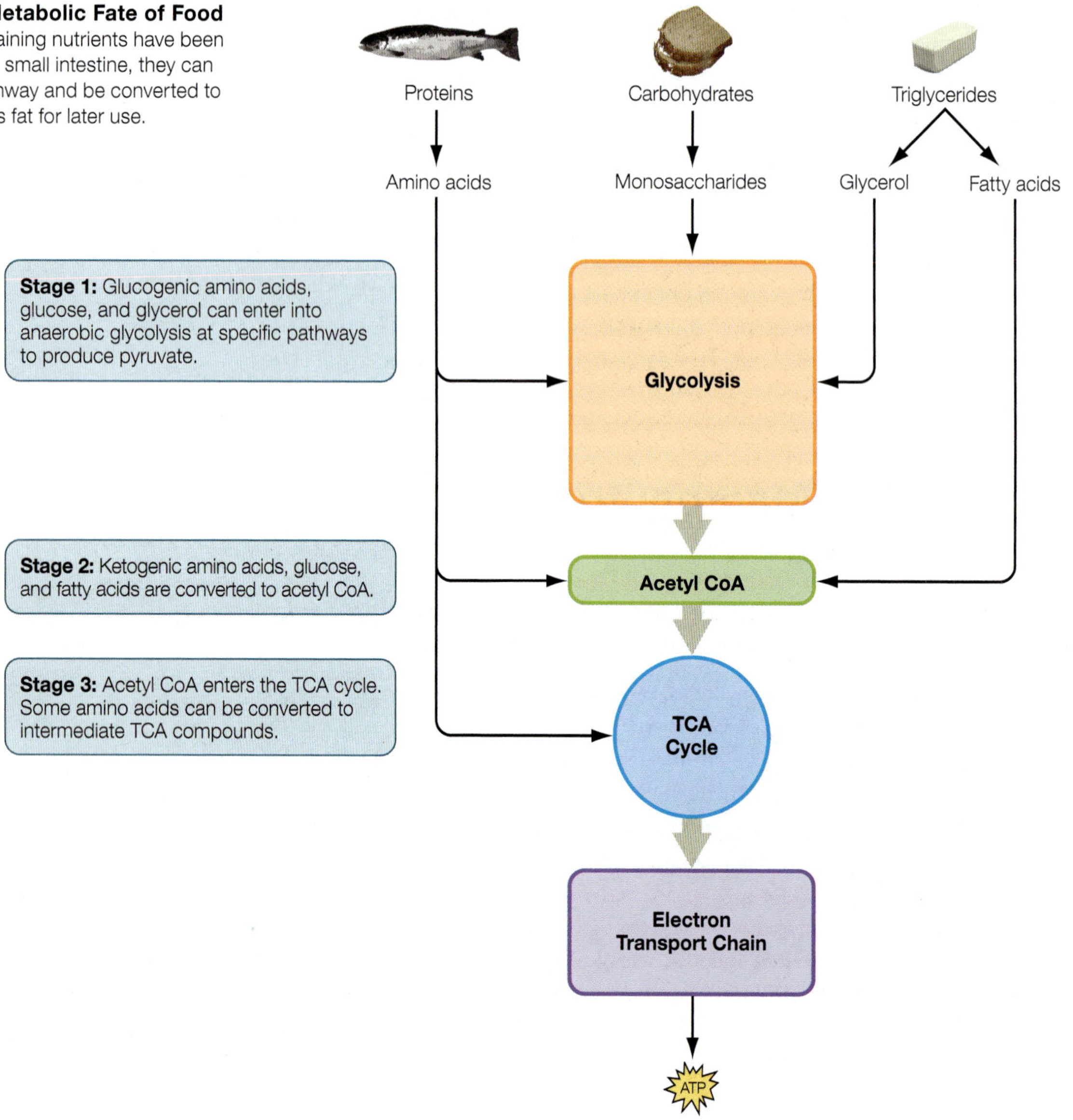

Proteins   Carbohydrates   Triglycerides

Amino acids   Monosaccharides   Glycerol   Fatty acids

Stage 1: Glucogenic amino acids, glucose, and glycerol can enter into anaerobic glycolysis at specific pathways to produce pyruvate.

Glycolysis

Stage 2: Ketogenic amino acids, glucose, and fatty acids are converted to acetyl CoA.

Acetyl CoA

Stage 3: Acetyl CoA enters the TCA cycle. Some amino acids can be converted to intermediate TCA compounds.

TCA Cycle

Electron Transport Chain

ATP

Glucose to Pyruvate

Glycolysis is a 10-step anaerobic catabolic pathway that takes place in the cytoplasm of the cells. It begins with one six-carbon glucose molecule and ends with two three-carbon molecules of **pyruvate** and a net of two molecules of ATP.

The initial step of glycolysis absorbs or uses ATP. In this reaction, a phosphate is transferred from ATP to the sixth carbon of glucose as the glucose enters the cell, forming glucose 6-phosphate and ADP. Once glucose 6-phosphate is formed, it continues through nine more reactions until the anaerobic stage of glycolysis is complete and pyruvate is created (see Figure 8.6).

In addition to ATP, glycolysis also generates hydrogen ions (H^+). As you can see in Figure 8.6, step 6, the coenzyme NAD^+ picks up a hydrogen ion, thereby reducing NAD^+ to NADH. The NADH eventually carries the hydrogen ion to the final stage of energy production, the electron transport chain.

Notice that the coenzyme form of riboflavin, FAD, plays no role in glycolysis. FAD is reduced to $FADH_2$ in the TCA cycle. Like NADH, $FADH_2$ carries its hydrogen ion to the electron transport chain. There, the hydrogen ions are used to produce ATP from ADP.

pyruvate Three-carbon molecule formed from the oxidation of glucose during glycolysis.

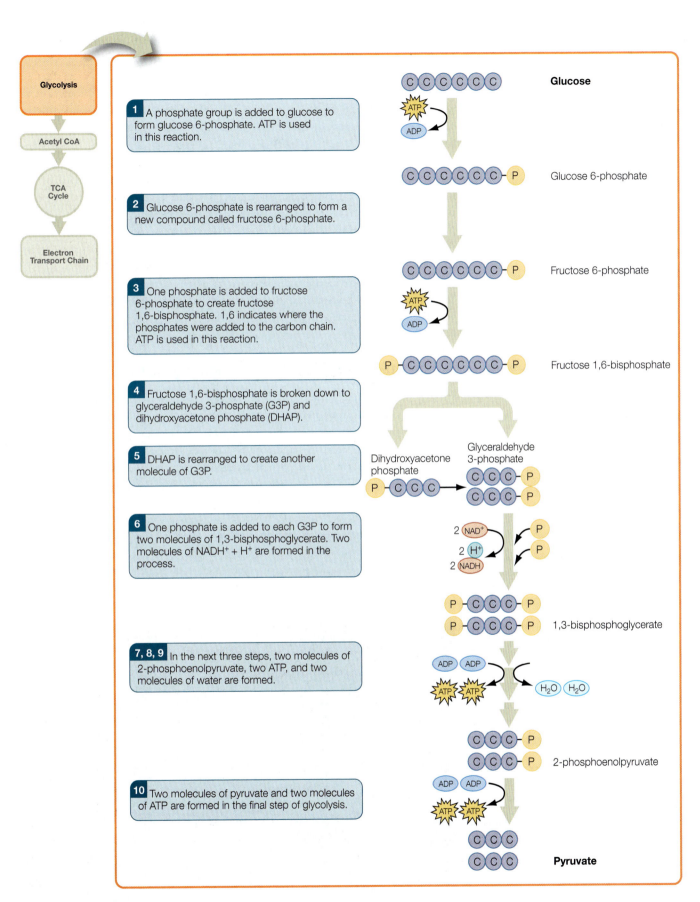

Glycolysis

Glycolysis

Acetyl CoA

TCA Cycle

Electron Transport Chain

1 A phosphate group is added to glucose to form glucose 6-phosphate. ATP is used in this reaction.

2 Glucose 6-phosphate is rearranged to form a new compound called fructose 6-phosphate.

3 One phosphate is added to fructose 6-phosphate to create fructose 1,6-bisphosphate. 1,6 indicates where the phosphates were added to the carbon chain. ATP is used in this reaction.

4 Fructose 1,6-bisphosphate is broken down to glyceraldehyde 3-phosphate (G3P) and dihydroxyacetone phosphate (DHAP).

5 DHAP is rearranged to create another molecule of G3P.

6 One phosphate is added to each G3P to form two molecules of 1,3-bisphosphoglycerate. Two molecules of NADH$^+$ + H$^+$ are formed in the process.

7, 8, 9 In the next three steps, two molecules of 2-phosphoenolpyruvate, two ATP, and two molecules of water are formed.

10 Two molecules of pyruvate and two molecules of ATP are formed in the final step of glycolysis.

Glucose

Glucose 6-phosphate

Fructose 6-phosphate

Fructose 1,6-bisphosphate

Dihydroxyacetone phosphate

Glyceraldehyde 3-phosphate

1,3-bisphosphoglycerate

2-phosphoenolpyruvate

Pyruvate

▲ **Figure 8.6 Glycolysis**
Glycolysis is a 10-step process that takes place in the cytoplasm of the cell; it converts glucose to pyruvate.

Metabolism of Fructose and Galactose

In addition to glucose, other monosaccharides, including fructose and galactose, can be used to produce ATP, but they are converted to substrates in glycolysis at different points. In muscle, fructose is first phosphorylated before it enters glycolysis as fructose 6-phosphate (see step 3 in Figure 8.6). In the liver, however, fructose passes through a more complex conversion before it becomes a substrate in glycolysis. It is first phosphorylated to form fructose 1-phosphate, which is then split into glyceraldehyde and dihydroxyacetone phosphate (DHAP), and then enters glycolysis as glyceraldehyde 3-phosphate (see steps 4 and 5 in Figure 8.6).

Galactose is also metabolized in the liver and must be converted to glucose before it can enter glycolysis. The first step is to add a phosphate to galactose to produce galactose 1-phosphate. After four more metabolic steps, galactose enters glycolysis as glucose 6-phosphate (see step 1 in Figure 8.6).

A specific enzyme directs each step of converting each monosaccharide into an intermediate substrate in glycolysis. Although rare, deficiencies in any of these enzymes due to genetic mutations have a debilitating effect on metabolism. For example, a deficiency in the enzyme that converts galactose into glucose results in a condition known as *galactosemia*, which can lead to mental retardation and liver damage unless dietary intake of galactose is controlled. We discuss genetic errors of metabolism in more detail at the end of this chapter.

Amino Acids and Glycerol Can Yield Pyruvate

Pyruvate sits at the junction between several significant pathways in energy metabolism. It is the end product for anaerobic glycolysis and the beginning molecule for gluconeogenesis. It can be converted to acetyl CoA and enter the TCA cycle or provide the basis for long-chain fatty acids to be stored in the adipose tissue as a triglyceride. In other words, pyruvate serves as an intermediate substrate that helps balance the energy needs of the cells.

Pyruvate to Lactate

In certain circumstances, pyruvate is converted to **lactate**. Most people associate the term *lactate* with muscle; however, the conversion of pyruvate to lactate happens in any human cell. For this discussion we use the muscle cell as an example.

When mitochondria lack sufficient oxygen, such as during intense exercise, pyruvate is reduced to lactate, preventing the buildup of hydrogen ions in the cell (**Figure 8.7**).

lactate Three-carbon compound generated from pyruvate when mitochondria lack sufficient oxygen.

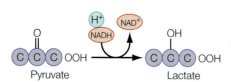

▲ **Figure 8.7 The Conversion of Pyruvate to Lactate**
Pyruvate is reduced to lactate during anaerobic metabolism and NADH is oxidized to NAD$^+$ that can be used in glycolysis.

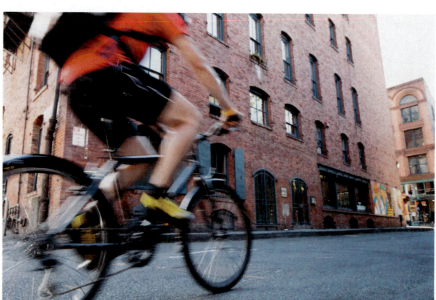

Strenuous exercise can cause a buildup of hydrogen ions in the muscle.

When lactate is not produced fast enough to keep up with the production of hydrogen ions, their buildup reduces the pH in the muscle cell, making the cell more acidic. Contrary to popular belief, it is this buildup of hydrogen ions, not lactate, that produces the uncomfortable "burning" sensation in the muscles after exercise.

Lactate diffuses out of the cell into the blood, which transports it to the liver. Once in the liver cells, enzymes convert the lactate back to pyruvate, which is then transformed by gluconeogenesis into glucose through the **Cori cycle** (**Figure 8.8**) and released back into the blood as glucose. The glucose is picked up by the muscle to begin glycolysis over again. This gluconeogenic mechanism occurs mainly in the liver and to a lesser extent in the kidneys. The muscles do not contain the necessary gluconeogenic enzymes to catalyze the conversion of lactate to glucose.

Glucogenic Amino Acids to Pyruvate

Eighteen out of 20 amino acids are considered glucogenic because they can be transformed into pyruvate and other TCA cycle intermediates that enter gluconeogenesis. Six of these amino acids—alanine, serine, glycine, threonine, tryptophan, and cysteine—enter the metabolic pathway at pyruvate. The pyruvate formed can be converted to glucose, through gluconeogenesis, and enter glycolysis to produce ATP through the later stages of metabolism (**Figure 8.9a**). Or the pyruvate can be transported into the mitochondria and

Cori cycle Metabolic pathway in the liver that regenerates glucose from lactate released from the muscle.

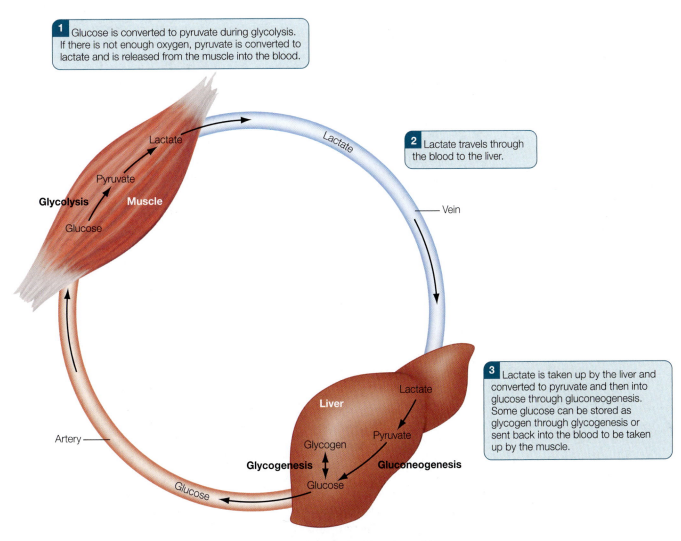

1 Glucose is converted to pyruvate during glycolysis. If there is not enough oxygen, pyruvate is converted to lactate and is released from the muscle into the blood.

2 Lactate travels through the blood to the liver.

3 Lactate is taken up by the liver and converted to pyruvate and then into glucose through gluconeogenesis. Some glucose can be stored as glycogen through glycogenesis or sent back into the blood to be taken up by the muscle.

▲ **Figure 8.8 The Cori Cycle Is a Metabolic Pathway between the Muscle and Liver**
The Cori cycle in the liver regenerates glucose from lactate released from the muscle.

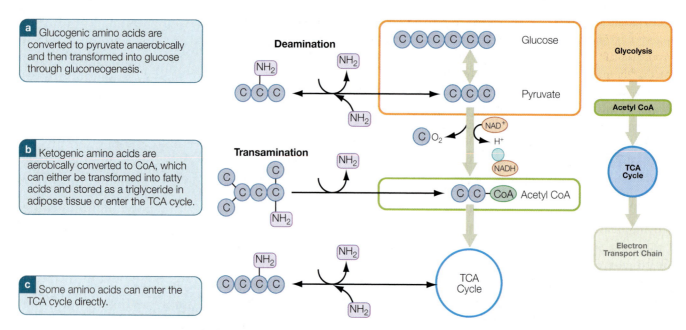

a Glucogenic amino acids are converted to pyruvate anaerobically and then transformed into glucose through gluconeogenesis.

b Ketogenic amino acids are aerobically converted to CoA, which can either be transformed into fatty acids and stored as a triglyceride in adipose tissue or enter the TCA cycle.

c Some amino acids can enter the TCA cycle directly.

▲ **Figure 8.9** **Glucogenic and Ketogenic Amino Acid Metabolism**

TABLE 8.2	Glucogenic and Ketogenic Amino Acids	
Glucogenic Amino Acids	**Ketogenic Amino Acids**	**Amino Acids That Are Both Glucogenic and Ketogenic**
Alanine	Leucine	Isoleucine
Arginine	Lysine	Phenylalanine
Asparagine		Tryptophan
Aspartate		Tyrosine
Cysteine		
Glutamate		
Glutamine		
Glycine		
Proline		
Serine		
Histidine		
Methionine		
Threonine		
Valine		

Source: Adapted from Berg, J. M., J. L. Tymoczko, et al. 2015. *Biochemistry.* 8th ed. (New York: W. H. Freeman).

transformed into acetyl CoA. The other 12 glucogenic amino acids enter the metabolic pathway at points along the TCA cycle (Figure 8.9c). Glucogenic amino acids, which come not only from food but also from the breakdown of proteins in muscle, are a major source of blood glucose when the diet is lacking in carbohydrate. **Table 8.2** classifies the amino acids.

Glycerol to Pyruvate

Triglycerides are a concentrated source of kilocalories and yield about six times more energy than either carbohydrates or proteins. Both the glycerol and fatty acids can be used for fuel, but only the glycerol is glucogenic and thus able to contribute to blood glucose levels. Glycerol produces very little energy, however, compared with fatty acids.

Glycerol can enter the main pathway at two distinct points. First, glycerol can be taken up by the liver cells and converted to glucose via gluconeogenesis. The first step in this pathway uses ATP to phosphorylate the three-carbon glycerol into DHAP (dihydroxyacetone phosphate), one of the intermediate substrates in glycolysis. Once glycerol is converted to DHAP it can be changed into glucose in one direction or it can follow a different series of chemical reactions to produce pyruvate, depending on the body's need for glucose.

Pyruvate Is Transformed into Acetyl CoA

At the end of glycolysis, what began as one six-carbon molecule of glucose has produced two three-carbon molecules of pyruvate, a net of two ATP, two coenzyme molecules in the form of NADH, two hydrogen ions (which enter the electron transport chain), and two molecules of water. Now let's continue down the metabolic pathway with the newly formed pyruvate as it is transformed into **acetyl CoA**.

Acetyl CoA is often called the "gateway" molecule for aerobic metabolism because all energy-producing nutrients—glucose, amino acids, fatty acids, glycerol, even alcohol—are usually transformed to acetyl CoA before entering the TCA cycle. Until this point along the metabolic pathway, energy is produced anaerobically. When cells contain an ample supply of oxygen, pyruvate now continues down the aerobic energy pathway to create acetyl CoA.

In the presence of oxygen, the two molecules of pyruvate formed during glycolysis cross the outer mitochondrial membrane and enter the mitochondria, where they each lose a carbon. Next, coenzyme A, an organic compound synthesized from the B vitamin pantothenic acid, attaches to the remaining two carbons from each pyruvate molecule to form acetyl CoA (**Figure 8.10**). Thus a three-carbon pyruvate molecule is changed into a two-carbon acetyl CoA. The third carbon combines with oxygen to form carbon dioxide and is expelled through the lungs as waste.

Once acetyl CoA is formed it can continue down the pathway to enter the TCA cycle if ATP is scarce. If there is sufficient ATP to meet the body's needs, the acetyl CoA is transported out of the mitochondria and into the cytoplasm to be converted into a fatty acid, which can be stored as fat through lipogenesis. Thus, energy needs determine whether acetyl CoA enters the TCA cycle (stage 3).

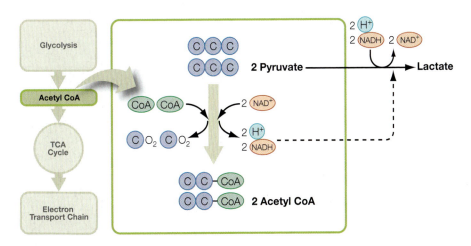

▲ Figure 8.10 **The Fate of Pyruvate**
At the end of glycolysis, two molecules of pyruvate are formed for every molecule of glucose. These three-carbon molecules can be converted to acetyl CoA and enter the TCA cycle or be transformed into lactate, which diffuses out of the cell into the blood.

acetyl CoA Two-carbon compound formed when pantothenic acid combines with acetate.

Fatty Acids Can Be Converted to Acetyl CoA

Before they can be used for energy, fatty acids are hydrolyzed from triglycerides by lipolysis (*lipo* = fat, *lysis* = break apart). **Figure 8.11** illustrates this process. An enzyme called **hormone-sensitive lipase** in the adipose tissue catalyzes the reaction. The activity of this enzyme is stimulated by the hormone glucagon when blood glucose levels are low (as when the diet is low in carbohydrate or kilocalories) or by the adrenal hormones epinephrine or cortisol when an individual is under stress. The free fatty acids are released into the blood and taken up by various tissues, including the muscle and the liver.

Just as you put on a coat to prepare to step outside on a cold day, fatty acids are "prepared" or activated before they cross into the mitochondria. In this step, which uses ATP, coenzyme A joins the carboxylic end of the fatty acid chain. The resulting long-chain fatty acetyl CoA can then cross the mitochondrial membrane with the help of a carrier molecule.

The fatty acid is disassembled inside the mitochondrion by a series of chemical reactions called **beta-oxidation**. During beta-oxidation the fatty acid is taken apart two carbon fragments at a time, beginning at the carboxyl end of the molecule. The two-carbon fragments are joined with a molecule of CoA and converted to acetyl CoA. This process continues, forming a new acetyl CoA and a shorter fatty acid chain, until all of the carbons have been oxidized.

As each pair of carbons is cleaved from the fatty acid chain, hydrogen ions and electrons are released and picked up by two coenzymes, NAD^+ and FAD, forming

hormone-sensitive lipase Enzyme that catalyzes lipolysis of triglycerides.

beta-oxidation Series of metabolic reactions in which fatty acids are oxidized to acetyl CoA; also called *fatty acid oxidation*.

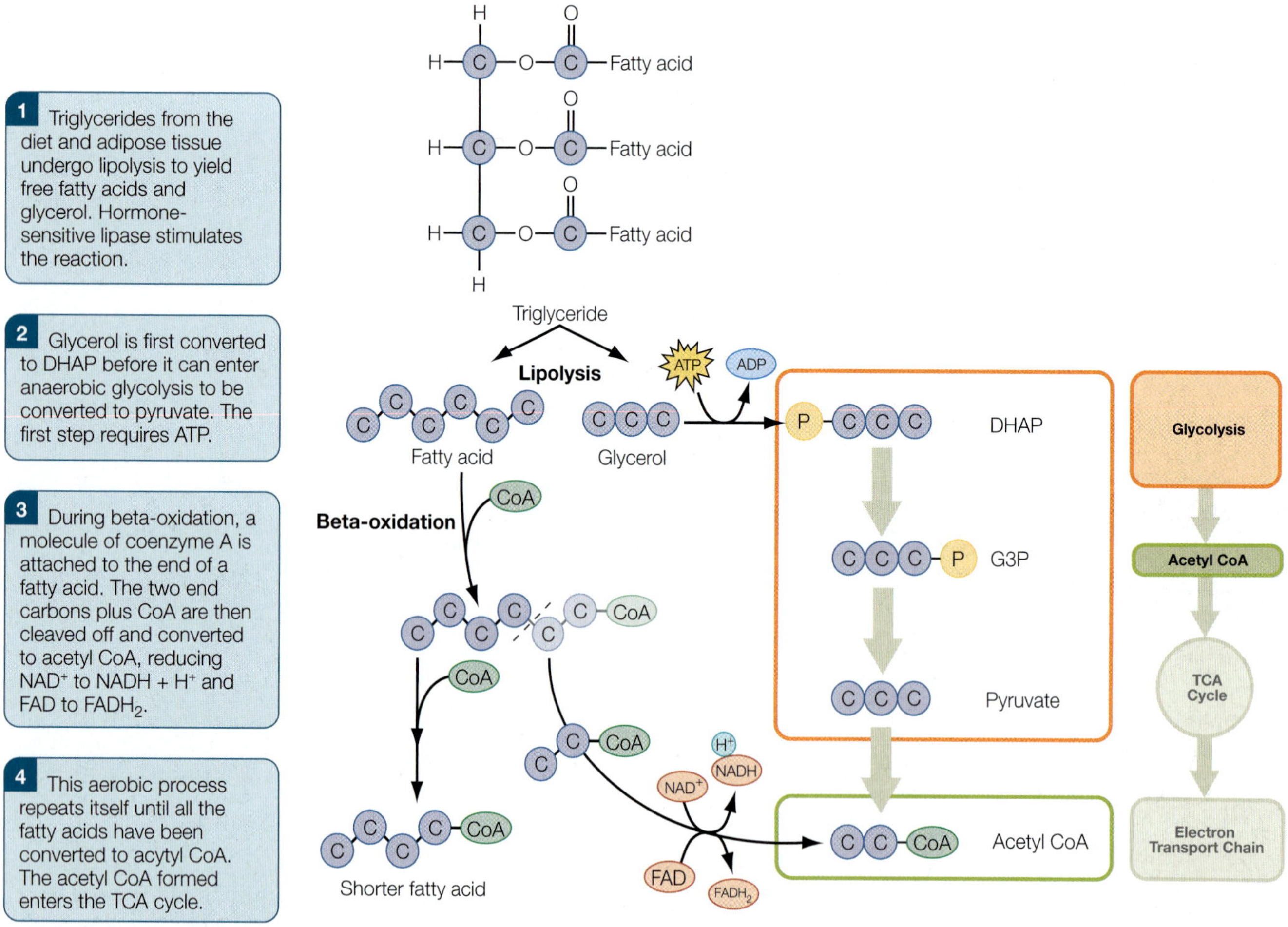

1 Triglycerides from the diet and adipose tissue undergo lipolysis to yield free fatty acids and glycerol. Hormone-sensitive lipase stimulates the reaction.

2 Glycerol is first converted to DHAP before it can enter anaerobic glycolysis to be converted to pyruvate. The first step requires ATP.

3 During beta-oxidation, a molecule of coenzyme A is attached to the end of a fatty acid. The two end carbons plus CoA are then cleaved off and converted to acetyl CoA, reducing NAD^+ to $NADH + H^+$ and FAD to $FADH_2$.

4 This aerobic process repeats itself until all the fatty acids have been converted to acytyl CoA. The acetyl CoA formed enters the TCA cycle.

▲ Figure 8.11 **Fatty Acids Are Oxidized for Energy**
Stored triglycerides can be used for energy after the fatty acids are first hydrolyzed from the glycerol backbone.

$NADH + H^+$ and $FADH_2$. As mentioned earlier, these coenzymes eventually unload the electrons they carry in the electron transport chain.

Fatty acids are considered ketogenic, not glucogenic; that is, they can be used to produce ketone bodies, which are used as backup fuel for the brain and nerve functions when glucose is limited. (We discuss ketogenesis later in the chapter.) There is no metabolic pathway to convert fatty acids to glucose.

Amino Acids Can Be Converted to Acetyl CoA

Recall that 18 of the 20 amino acids are considered glucogenic. The other two amino acids, leucine and lysine, are considered strictly ketogenic (see Figure 8.9b and Table 8.2), while four of the glucogenic amino acids—isoleucine, tryptophan, phenylalanine, and tyrosine—can also be ketogenic.[1]

The conversion begins when leucine and lysine undergo transamination (review Chapter 6 on the transamination reaction). The TCA acid **alpha-ketoglutarate** accepts the amino group that is transferred. After several more steps, leucine and lysine are ultimately converted to acetyl CoA, which can be converted into a fatty acid or acetoacetate and then into ketone bodies, depending on cellular needs.

Isoleucine and tryptophan are converted to acetyl CoA using the same pathway as leucine. Phenylalanine and tyrosine are transformed into acetoacetyl CoA first before they are converted to acetyl CoA.

Remember that acetyl CoA cannot be used to make glucose, so once these amino acids are transformed, they are committed to continue through the energy pathway, to be converted to fatty acids and stored as a triglyceride in the adipocyte, or to undergo ketogenesis.

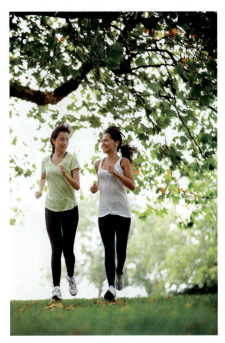

Walking or low-intensity exercise uses mostly fatty acids and glucose to produce ATP through aerobic metabolism.

The Tricarboxylic Acid (TCA) Cycle Releases High-Energy Electrons

The **tricarboxylic acid (TCA) cycle**, also known as the *citric acid cycle* or the *Kreb's cycle,* is the third stage of energy metabolism. It results in the oxidation of acetyl CoA (**Figure 8.12**) and occurs in the mitochondria. Up to this point, the macronutrients have followed different pathways and entered the energy pathway at different points; now, they have all arrived at acetyl CoA. Recall that fuel molecules are carbon-containing compounds that can be oxidized or lose electrons. During each turn of the TCA cycle, hydrogen ions, which carry high-energy electrons, are released and gathered up by NAD^+, forming $NADH + H^+$, and FAD, forming $FADH_2$. These electron carriers release the electrons in the electron transport chain. Hydrogen ions released in the TCA cycle drive the production of ATP in the electron transport chain.

One molecule of acetyl CoA enters the cycle at a time. The first step is to remove the CoA and combine the two remaining carbons with a four-carbon molecule called **oxaloacetate**. Together, oxaloacetate and acetyl CoA form a new six-carbon compound called citrate. The cycle continues with seven more reactions, ending with oxaloacetate as the last molecule formed at the end of every turn of the TCA cycle. This brings us back to the beginning of the cycle. You'll notice as you track the carbons in Figure 8.12 that for every acetyl CoA that enters the TCA cycle, two carbons are lost as CO_2.

In addition to the two carbons lost as CO_2, three $NADH + H^+$ and one $FADH_2$ are produced during each turn of the TCA cycle. For example, notice that in the third step of the cycle, the coenzyme carrier NAD^+ grabs a hydrogen ion. In the succeeding steps of the cycle, three more coenzymes are reduced, NADH in step 4 and step 8 and $FADH_2$ in step 6. In total, for each turn of the TCA cycle, four coenzymes are reduced, along with the formation of carbon dioxide.

Also notice in step 5, a molecule called *guanosine triphosphate (GTP)* is generated. This energy molecule is readily converted to ATP.

alpha-ketoglutarate Compound that participates in the formation of nonessential amino acids during transamination.

tricarboxylic acid (TCA) cycle Cycle of aerobic chemical reactions in the mitochondria that oxidize glucose, amino acids, and fatty acids, producing hydrogen ions to be used in the electron transport chain, some ATP, and by-products carbon dioxide and water.

oxaloacetate Starting molecule for the TCA cycle.

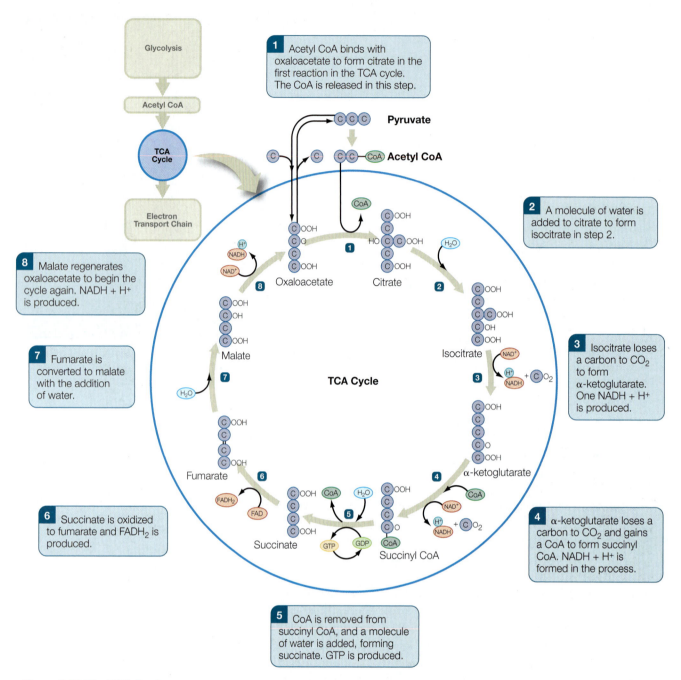

▲ Figure 8.12 The TCA Cycle
(**1**) The TCA cycle begins with oxaloacetate combining with acetyl CoA to form citrate. (**2–8**) The cycle continues through seven more steps, changing the molecules and releasing hydrogen atoms. Pyruvate can provide some oxaloacetate as a starting molecule for the cycle.

Text from the figure:

1. Acetyl CoA binds with oxaloacetate to form citrate in the first reaction in the TCA cycle. The CoA is released in this step.

2. A molecule of water is added to citrate to form isocitrate in step 2.

3. Isocitrate loses a carbon to CO_2 to form α-ketoglutarate. One NADH + H⁺ is produced.

4. α-ketoglutarate loses a carbon to CO_2 and gains a CoA to form succinyl CoA. NADH + H⁺ is formed in the process.

5. CoA is removed from succinyl CoA, and a molecule of water is added, forming succinate. GTP is produced.

6. Succinate is oxidized to fumarate and $FADH_2$ is produced.

7. Fumarate is converted to malate with the addition of water.

8. Malate regenerates oxaloacetate to begin the cycle again. NADH + H⁺ is produced.

The Electron Transport Chain and Oxidative Phosphorylation Produce the Majority of ATP

electron transport chain Final stage of energy metabolism in which NADH and $FADH_2$ transport high-energy electrons to the protein complexes in the electron transport chain, resulting in the formation of ATP and water.

The **electron transport chain** is composed of a series of protein complexes located in the inner mitochondrial membrane that function as electron carriers (**Figure 8.13**). The high-energy electrons delivered to the electron transport chain by NADH + H⁺ and $FADH_2$ are passed from one protein complex to the next. As the electrons are passed along the chain, hydrogen ions are pumped out of the mitochondrial matrix into the intermembrane space. The hydrogen ions accumulate, creating a high concentration gradient that forces

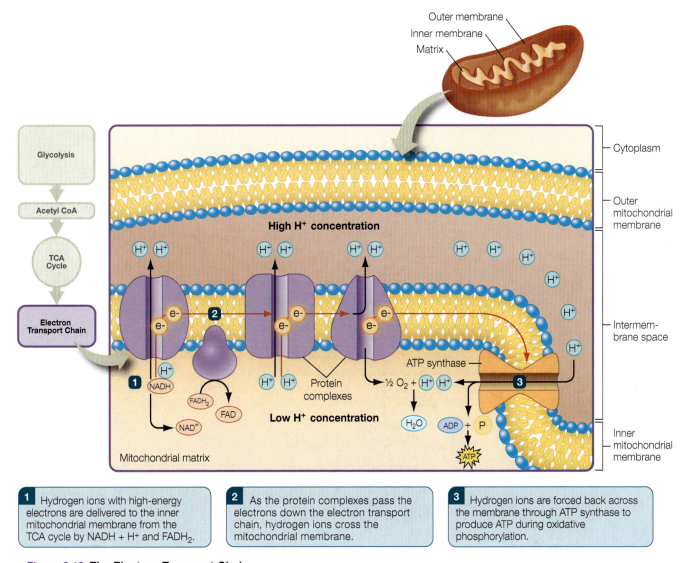

Outer membrane
Inner membrane
Matrix

Glycolysis

Acetyl CoA

TCA Cycle

Electron Transport Chain

Cytoplasm

Outer mitochondrial membrane

High H⁺ concentration

Intermembrane space

ATP synthase

Protein complexes

Low H⁺ concentration

½ O_2 + H⁺ H⁺

H_2O

ADP + P

ATP

Mitochondrial matrix

Inner mitochondrial membrane

1 Hydrogen ions with high-energy electrons are delivered to the inner mitochondrial membrane from the TCA cycle by NADH + H⁺ and FADH₂.

2 As the protein complexes pass the electrons down the electron transport chain, hydrogen ions cross the mitochondrial membrane.

3 Hydrogen ions are forced back across the membrane through ATP synthase to produce ATP during oxidative phosphorylation.

▲ **Figure 8.13 The Electron Transport Chain**

them back across the mitochondrial membrane into the matrix. There, the enzyme ATP synthase uses the energy generated by the concentration gradient to add a phosphate to ADP, forming ATP through a process called **oxidative phosphorylation**. At the same time, oxygen, electrons, and hydrogen ions combine to form water. The ATP produced flows into the cytoplasm to be used by the body.

The protein complexes that transfer the electrons through the electron transport chain are classified as **flavoproteins**, which contain the B vitamin riboflavin, and **cytochromes**, which contain the minerals iron and copper. If you are iron deficient, the cytochromes are less able to pass the electrons along the chain to complete the production of ATP. This is one of the reasons someone with inadequate iron intake feels tired or fatigued. This illustrates the point that though vitamins and minerals do not provide energy, they are essential for energy production in the body.

Figure 8.14 provides a detailed review of all four stages of energy metabolism. Look at the figure closely and check your understanding; can you describe what's happening in each stage? **Table 8.3** summarizes the role of individual nutrients in producing ATP, glycogen, nonessential amino acids, and fat.

oxidative phosphorylation Metabolic pathway in the mitochondria in which ATP is formed using energy from the oxidation-reduction reactions in the electron transport chain.

flavoproteins Protein complexes that move electrons down the electron transport chain; contain the B vitamin riboflavin.

cytochromes Protein complexes that move electrons down the electron transport chain; contain the minerals iron and copper.

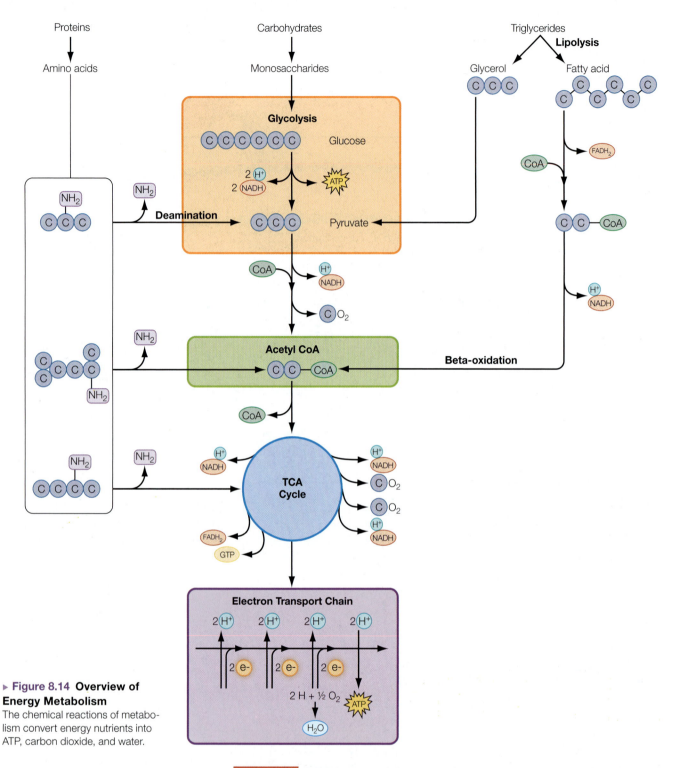

▶ Figure 8.14 **Overview of Energy Metabolism**
The chemical reactions of metabolism convert energy nutrients into ATP, carbon dioxide, and water.

TABLE 8.3	Role of Individual Nutrients and Alcohol in Energy Metabolism			
Nutrient	Produces ATP?	Can Produce Glucose?	Can Be Used in Transamination (To Produce Amino Acids)?	Excess Can Be Stored as Fat?
Glucose	Yes	Yes	Yes	Yes
Amino acid	Yes	Yes	Yes	Yes
Fatty acid	Yes	No	No	Yes
Glycerol	Yes	Yes	Yes	Yes
Alcohol	Yes	No	No	Yes

The metabolism of the macronutrients and tissues involved in various metabolic pathways is summarized in **Table 8.4**. Carbohydrates provide energy to cells through glycolysis, a 10-step anaerobic pathway that yields two molecules of pyruvate, a net of two ATP, two coenzymes, two hydrogen ions, and two molecules of water. Pyruvate is either converted to lactate during anaerobic metabolism or converted to acetyl CoA during aerobic metabolism. Glycerol can produce energy by entering glycolysis or can be used to form glucose through gluconeogenesis. Fatty acids are ketogenic and cannot be used to form glucose. Fatty acids are broken down into two-carbon fragments and converted into acetyl CoA through beta-oxidation. Glucogenic amino acids can be used to produce glucose and ketogenic amino acids can be converted to acetyl CoA and then to fatty acids. All of the energy nutrients come together in the gateway molecule acetyl CoA. Once acetyl CoA is formed, it combines with oxaloacetate to form citrate in the first step of the TCA cycle. One turn of the TCA cycle produces two coenzymes, one molecule of CO_2, and a small amount of energy in the form of guanosine triphosphate (GTP), which is readily converted to ATP. The electrons generated are carried by coenzymes to the electron transport chain, where they are passed along the chain by protein complexes. During this process, the hydrogen ions are used to form ATP during oxidative phosphorylation and join with oxygen to make water.

TABLE 8.4	Summary of Metabolic Processes in the Cells			
Metabolic Pathway	**Nutrient(s) Involved in the Pathway**	**Description of the Pathway**	**Major Tissues Involved**	**Type of Pathway**
Glycolysis	Carbohydrates	Metabolism of glucose to produce pyruvate and two ATP	All cells	Catabolic and anabolic
Glycogenesis	Carbohydrates	Producing glycogen from excess glucose	Muscle and liver	Anabolic
Glycogenolysis	Carbohydrates	Breakdown of glycogen to glucose	Muscle and liver	Catabolic
Gluconeogenesis	Noncarbohydrates, including glucogenic amino acids, glycerol, pyruvate, and lactate	Producing glucose from noncarbohydrate sources	Liver and kidneys	Anabolic
Beta-oxidation	Fatty acids	Fatty acid oxidation to acetyl CoA	Liver and muscle	Catabolic
Lipolysis	Fatty acids	Breakdown of triglycerides to yield fatty acids and glycerol	Adipose tissue and liver	Catabolic
Lipogenesis	Fatty acids	Synthesis of fatty acids and triglycerides	Adipose tissue and liver	Anabolic
Ketogenesis	Fatty acids and ketogenic amino acids	The conversion of fatty acids and ketogenic amino acids to acetyl CoA and to ketone bodies	Liver	Catabolic
Transamination	Amino acids	Formation of nonessential amino acids produced by transferring an amine group from one amino acid to an alpha-keto acid	Liver	Catabolic and anabolic
TCA cycle	All nutrients	Oxidation of acetyl CoA releases hydrogen ions with high-energy electrons; carbon dioxide; and GTP	All cells (except RBCs)	Catabolic and anabolic
Electron transport chain and oxidative phosphorylation	All nutrients	ATP is generated from the energy released in glycolysis and the TCA cycle and delivered by NADH + H^+ and $FADH_2$. Process is aerobic. Oxygen accepts 2 H^+ and forms water.	All cells (except RBCs)	Catabolic and anabolic

Important Advice for Maintaining Energy Levels

Eat a nutritious breakfast! It's the most important meal and improves energy levels throughout the day.

Don't skip meals; instead, be sure to eat at least three meals and one to two small snacks throughout the day.

Be sure each meal includes a combination of protein, carbohydrates, and some fat.

Enjoy carbohydrate-rich foods such as whole-grain crackers, baby carrots, or fresh grapes as snacks when you need a pick-me-up between meals.

Drink plenty of fluid, especially water, so you're sure to stay hydrated.

absorptive state Period after you eat when the stomach and small intestine are full and anabolic reactions exceed catabolic reactions.

postabsorptive state Period when you haven't eaten for more than 4 hours and the stomach and intestines are empty. Energy needs are met by the breakdown of stores.

How Does Metabolism Change during the Absorptive and Postabsorptive States?

LO 8.4 Explain how metabolism changes during the absorptive, postabsorptive, and starvation stages of food intake.

Once food has been digested, the amino acids, monoglycerides, and triglycerides are absorbed and available to be used by the body. We refer to this as the **absorptive state**, or that period within 4 hours following a meal in which anabolic processes exceed catabolic processes. During the absorptive state, the body uses glucose as the primary source of energy (see the Table Tips, Important Advice for Maintaining Energy Levels). Later, when you need energy during sleep, between meals, or when you're too busy to eat, your body uses the glucose stored as glycogen, and the fatty acids and glycerol stored in triglycerides, for fuel. This is referred to as the **postabsorptive state**, or the period of time usually more than 4 hours after eating, such as during the late afternoon or overnight. Hormones regulate both the absorptive and postabsorptive states.

During the Absorptive State, Metabolism Favors Energy Storage

Metabolism adjusts to either provide energy for immediate use or store it for later, depending on your energy needs and intake. In the normal process of eating, if you consume more kilocalories than you require for your immediate energy needs, your metabolism favors anabolic reactions for the sake of storing the excess kilocalories for later use. For instance, if you eat excess protein, the excess is converted to fatty acids and stored as a triglyceride. If you overconsume carbohydrates, the anabolic reactions include converting the excess carbohydrates to glycogen. Once the glycogen stores are full, carbohydrates are converted to fatty acids.

Take a close look at **Focus Figure 8.15**, which illustrates the catabolic and anabolic pathways of the absorptive state.

Carbohydrates Are Stored as Glycogen

Although glucose is essential to red blood cells and *neural* (nervous system) cells, neither of these cell types can convert glucose to its storage form, glycogen, nor can they convert excess glucose to fat. Only liver and muscle cells can convert excess glucose to glycogen for storage.

Remember that dietary glucose arrives first at the liver from the portal vein. If glucose levels are high, the liver converts glucose to glycogen through glycogenesis or releases the glucose for circulation to other tissues. Enzymes in muscle cells can also convert excess glucose to glycogen. The body has a limited ability to store glycogen, however, and only about 1 percent of body weight is in the form of glycogen.

Liver glycogen plays an important role in maintaining glucose homeostasis. When intake of dietary carbohydrate is low, blood glucose levels drop. The glycogen stored in the liver can be broken down into glucose through glycogenolysis and released into the blood. However, about 12–18 hours after eating, liver glycogen levels are nearly depleted.

Even though muscle cells have a high storage capacity for glycogen, they lack the enzyme that can release glucose into the blood. In essence, glucose is "trapped" in the muscle to be used for energy or stored as glycogen; it is not used to maintain blood glucose levels.

The absorptive (fed) state is generally an anabolic state: After digestion, absorption, and transport in the body, the end products of digestion can be synthesized into important biological compounds, used for energy, or converted to storage forms of energy.

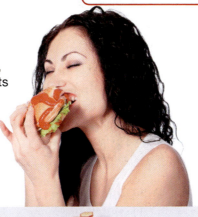

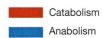

🟥 Catabolism

🟦 Anabolism

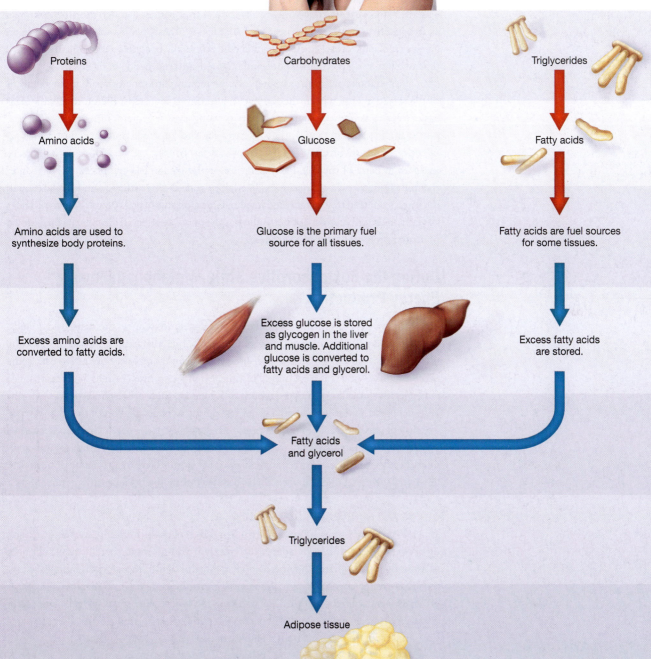

Proteins

Amino acids

Amino acids are used to synthesize body proteins.

Excess amino acids are converted to fatty acids.

Carbohydrates

Glucose

Glucose is the primary fuel source for all tissues.

Excess glucose is stored as glycogen in the liver and muscle. Additional glucose is converted to fatty acids and glycerol.

Triglycerides

Fatty acids

Fatty acids are fuel sources for some tissues.

Excess fatty acids are stored.

Fatty acids and glycerol

Triglycerides

Adipose tissue

Excess Carbohydrates and Amino Acids Are Stored as Triglycerides

Carbohydrates are first stored as glycogen. After those stores are full and energy needs are met, excess carbohydrates form triglycerides. Once glucose has been oxidized to acetyl CoA, it enters lipogenesis, forming fatty acids that are stored in the adipocytes. This conversion is very costly—almost 25 percent of the kilocalories glucose provides must be used to generate enough ATP to convert the glucose to fatty acids—and inefficient.

The same is true for excess amino acids. Protein is first used for the numerous functions it provides to the body before excess is converted to fatty acids. In this process, amino acids are first deaminated, then the remaining carbons are converted to acetyl CoA and formed into fatty acids. Both ketogenic and glucogenic amino acids can be catabolized and converted to fatty acids through pyruvate and acetyl CoA pathways, but the process is highly inefficient.

Fatty Acids Are Stored as Triglycerides

The body stores excess kilocalories in any form as triglycerides through the process known as lipogenesis, or fatty acid synthesis. Fatty acid synthesis begins with the two-carbon gateway molecule acetyl CoA. This molecule eventually becomes a long-chain fatty acid that attaches to a glycerol backbone and is stored as a triglyceride in fat cells.

The metabolic pathway to store dietary fat requires little energy (only about 5 percent of the stored energy within the fatty acid) and only a few steps; therefore dietary fat is easier to store as body fat than are dietary carbohydrate or protein. Lipogenesis is a separate anabolic pathway that synthesizes fatty acids to be stored and is not just a reversal of the reactions involved in the breakdown of fat. In fact, the two processes take place in different parts of the cell. Fatty acids are synthesized in the cytoplasm rather than in the mitochondria, where fats are oxidized. Lipogenesis also differs from fat oxidation in the way it's affected by glucagon and insulin. Glucagon stimulates lipolysis, which provides the fatty acids for beta-oxidation. Insulin has the opposite effect: It inhibits the breakdown of fat and promotes fatty acid synthesis.

During the Postabsorptive State, Metabolism Favors Energy Production

Many Americans consume more than enough kilocalories to meet their energy demands, a fact which is reflected in the current obesity crisis. But what happens when the opposite is true? That is, you're too busy to consume enough food or you choose not to eat? Some people choose not to eat for a period of time, often for spiritual or religious reasons. For example, Muslims fast during the month of Ramadan, there are seven fasting days in the Jewish religion, and some Christians may fast during Lent. Regardless of the reason, when you do not consume enough kilocalories to meet your energy needs, your body enters a postabsorptive state—usually more than 4 hours after eating. The stomach and small intestine are empty and the need for energy is met from stored energy. **Focus Figure 8.16** illustrates the metabolic pathways that are active during the postabsorptive state.

Stores Are Depleted during Fasting

Whereas glycogen stores supply energy during short periods of fasting, such as overnight or between meals, the body adapts differently if you go more than 18 hours without consuming carbohydrates. Again, the body maintains blood glucose levels initially by tapping into liver glycogen through glycogenolysis. At the same time, an increase in lipolysis provides fatty acids for energy, thus reducing the use of glucose by the cell. Once liver glycogen has been depleted, gluconeogenesis is initiated, using amino acids, glycerol, pyruvate, and lactate to meet the body's glucose needs.

Head to Mastering Nutrition and watch a narrated video tour of this figure by author Joan Salge Blake.

The postabsorptive (fasting) state is generally a catabolic state: After a period of fasting, when the body's glycogen stores are reduced, the body increases its use of stored fatty acids.

🟥	Catabolism
🟦	Anabolism
🟪	Nutrient Transport

SHORT-TERM FASTING

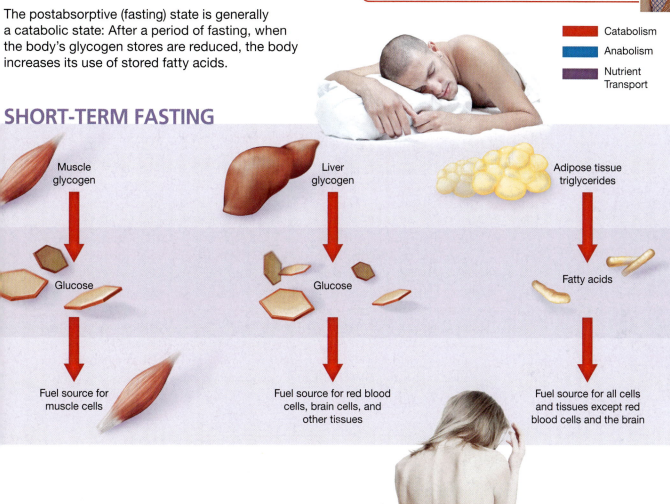

Muscle glycogen → Glucose → Fuel source for muscle cells

Liver glycogen → Glucose → Fuel source for red blood cells, brain cells, and other tissues

Adipose tissue triglycerides → Fatty acids → Fuel source for all cells and tissues except red blood cells and the brain

LONG-TERM FASTING

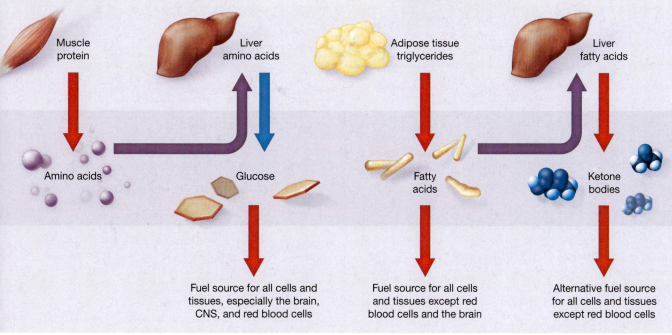

Muscle protein → Amino acids → Liver amino acids → Glucose → Fuel source for all cells and tissues, especially the brain, CNS, and red blood cells

Adipose tissue triglycerides → Fatty acids → Fuel source for all cells and tissues except red blood cells and the brain

Liver fatty acids → Ketone bodies → Alternative fuel source for all cells and tissues except red blood cells

Fat reserves are broken down faster as fasting continues. The brain must switch to an alternative source of energy—ketone bodies—derived from the fatty acids. A severe, prolonged fast, or starvation, depletes fat reserves and begins to break down muscle tissue to provide energy.

Ketogenesis Generates Energy during Prolonged Fasting

As you've learned in this chapter, acetyl CoA is generated from glucose (glycolysis) or fatty acid breakdown (lipolysis), both of which produce oxaloacetate that enters the TCA cycle. When deprived of carbohydrates, less oxaloacetate is available. The body depends less and less on glucose, and the TCA cycle slows. This allows acetyl CoA to accumulate because it is not metabolized in the TCA cycle. Some of the acetyl CoA produced by fatty acid oxidation in the liver is converted to ketone bodies, namely acetone, acetoacetate, and β-hydroxybutyrate.

Ketogenesis (the formation of ketone bodies, illustrated in **Figure 8.17**) occurs when there is an excess buildup of acetyl CoA. Ketogenesis reaches peak levels after an individual has fasted or consumed a limited-carbohydrate diet for 3 days. By the fourth day of a fast, the ketone bodies are providing almost half of the fuel used by the mitochondria.[2] The presence of ketone bodies is referred to as *ketosis* (described in Chapter 4). As you continue to fast, your brain switches from glucose to ketone bodies for fuel, thereby preserving blood glucose. Eventually, about 30 percent of the brain's energy comes from ketone bodies, with the rest provided by blood glucose.

Ketogenesis is a normal metabolic response to fasting, and ketosis is not life-threatening. The kidneys reabsorb ketone bodies to be used by other tissues for energy or excrete excess ketone bodies in the urine, thereby maintaining a balanced pH. Ketogenesis can be used therapeutically: A ketogenic diet is sometimes prescribed to control seizures in patients who have epilepsy and don't respond to medications. A ketogenic diet is difficult

ketogenesis Formation of ketone bodies from excess acetyl CoA.

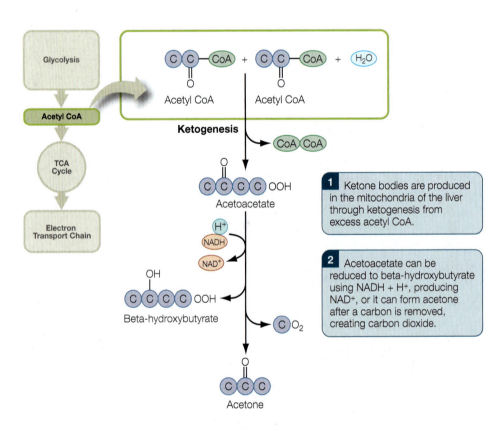

▶ **Figure 8.17 The Formation of Ketone Bodies**

to follow and must be strictly monitored by a registered dietitian nutritionist. It is much stricter than the Atkins diet, another form of a ketogenic diet, requiring careful control of kilocalorie intake, fluids, and proteins.[3]

When very high concentrations of ketone bodies—which are acidic—accumulate in the blood, they lower the body's pH to dangerous levels. This condition, called **ketoacidosis**, most commonly occurs in individuals with untreated type 1 diabetes because, without insulin, glucose is not available to the cells. The body responds with hyperventilation, rapid and shallow breathing that increases excretion of CO_2, which in turn increases the blood pH. If the level of ketone bodies continues to rise, diabetic ketoacidosis can lead to deep and labored breathing, impaired heart activity, coma, and even death.

LO 8.4: THE TAKE-HOME MESSAGE The differences in metabolism between the absorptive, or feeding, state and the postabsorptive, or fasting, state are listed in **Table 8.5**. During the absorptive state, anabolic reactions are favored. Carbohydrates are first used for ATP synthesis with excess stored as glycogen or triglycerides in the adipose tissue. Excess amino acids and dietary fat are also converted to triglycerides and stored. During the postabsorptive state, metabolism shifts to favor catabolic reactions. Fat is broken down to fatty acids to be used for ATP synthesis, while liver glycogen, glycerol, and glucogenic amino acids are used to maintain blood glucose levels. As fasting continues, glycogen stores are depleted, and muscle is broken down to provide amino acids for energy and gluconeogenesis. A lack of sufficient glucose in the blood can lead to excess breakdown of fat and the synthesis of ketone bodies, which can be used by the brain and muscles for energy, but are acidic. If ketogenesis is prolonged, ketoacidosis—an excessive level of ketones in the blood—can develop, leading to coma and even death.

TABLE 8.5	Metabolism during Feeding and Fasting		
	Feeding: Metabolism Following a Meal in the Absorptive State	**Fasting: Metabolism Several Hours after a Meal in the Postabsorptive State**	**If Fasting Continues after Liver and Muscle Glycogen Stores Are Depleted**
Proteins	Amino acids are used for protein synthesis or stored as a triglyceride in the adipose tissue		Amino acids are used for gluconeogenesis or catabolized for energy
Carbohydrates	Glucose is used for energy or stored as glycogen in the liver or muscle	Liver and muscle glycogen is broken down to provide glucose for energy	
Triglycerides	Fatty acids and glycerol are stored as a triglyceride in the adipose tissue	Triglycerides in adipose tissue are broken down to glycerol and fatty acids to be used for energy metabolism	Fatty acids are used to produce ketone bodies and oxidized for energy

ketoacidosis Form of metabolic acidosis, or pH imbalance due to excess acid, that occurs when excess ketone bodies are present in the blood; most often seen in individuals with untreated type I diabetes.

How Does the Body Metabolize Alcohol?

LO 8.5 Describe the metabolism of alcohol.

Recall from Chapter 7 that alcohol can be a significant source of energy. In fact, it provides almost twice the amount of energy (7 kilocalories per gram) of an equal amount of carbohydrate or protein (4 kilocalories per gram). Moreover, alcohol doesn't have to be digested before the body absorbs it. Although some of the alcohol an individual consumes is metabolized in the stomach, most is absorbed directly through the stomach mucosa and through the enterocytes. This means that alcohol makes its way into the blood quickly and, through the blood, is transported to the liver, where it is metabolized.

The body can easily metabolize about half an ounce of alcohol, the amount in a standard drink, in an hour and a half. When more than half an ounce is consumed in this period of time, the excess alcohol circulates throughout the body until the liver enzymes can break it down.

Alcohol Is Metabolized via Three Pathways

Alcohol is metabolized through three distinct pathways. The primary pathway involves the oxidation of ethanol by the enzyme alcohol dehydrogenase (ADH) (described in Chapter 7), which is found in both the stomach and the liver. As soon as the capillaries deliver the alcohol to the liver cells, it is converted to acetaldehyde (**Figure 8.18**). In this reaction, ADH removes hydrogen ions from alcohol, which are picked up by the coenzyme NAD^+. More hydrogens are removed as acetaldehyde is quickly changed to acetate by a similar enzyme called *acetaldehyde dehydrogenase (ALDH)*. The final step converts acetate to acetyl CoA. The acetyl CoA can then either be used to produce energy in the TCA cycle if needed or be transformed into fatty acids and stored as a triglyceride in the adipocytes.

The alternative alcohol metabolism pathway is the microsomal ethanol oxidizing system (MEOS). This system is not as significant as ADH for small amounts of alcohol,

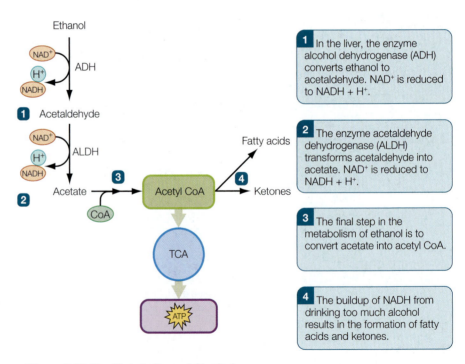

1 In the liver, the enzyme alcohol dehydrogenase (ADH) converts ethanol to acetaldehyde. NAD^+ is reduced to $NADH + H^+$.

2 The enzyme acetaldehyde dehydrogenase (ALDH) transforms acetaldehyde into acetate. NAD^+ is reduced to $NADH + H^+$.

3 The final step in the metabolism of ethanol is to convert acetate into acetyl CoA.

4 The buildup of NADH from drinking too much alcohol results in the formation of fatty acids and ketones.

▲ **Figure 8.18 The Metabolism of Alcohol**
The liver is the main organ involved in the metabolism of alcohol.

but becomes more important with the chronic consumption of alcohol. As explained in Chapter 7, this system also metabolizes many prescription and over-the-counter medications. If you drink alcohol while taking certain medications, the liver metabolizes the alcohol first, which causes the effects of the drugs to be felt over a longer period of time. This is the reason drugs and alcohol should never be taken together.

Not all alcohol is metabolized in the liver or stomach. A third metabolic pathway for alcohol takes place in the brain, where alcohol is oxidized to acetaldehyde by the enzyme catalase. This pathway may be responsible for some of the psychological effects people experience, such as reduced inhibitions, when they consume alcohol.

Excess Alcohol Is Stored as Fat

Fat metabolism shifts after you drink alcohol in two key ways. First, fewer fatty acids are used for energy. At the same time, the excess kilocalories in alcohol are metabolized and stored as fatty acids in the adipose tissue and liver. In chronic alcoholics, excess fatty deposits in the liver can eventually result in cirrhosis (see the discussion of this dangerous condition in Chapter 7). Note that fat can begin to accumulate in the liver after a single bout of binge drinking.

LO 8.5: THE TAKE-HOME MESSAGE Alcohol is primarily absorbed and metabolized in the liver by two enzyme systems. The most efficient enzyme system is alcohol dehydrogenase (ADH) and acetaldehyde dehydrogenase (ALDH), which convert the ethanol to acetaldehyde in the initial stages of metabolism and ultimately to acetyl CoA. The MEOS system, which is used with chronic consumption of alcohol, also metabolizes drugs. A third system is found in the brain and metabolizes alcohol to acetaldehyde. Alcohol is not stored, but the excess kilocalories from alcohol not used for ATP production are converted to fatty acids and stored as a triglyceride.

HEALTHCONNECTION

What Are Genetic Disorders of Metabolism?

LO 8.6 Describe the causes, diagnosis, symptoms, and dietary treatments of the most common genetic disorders of metabolism.

Genes code for all of the enzymes needed to control metabolism. However, some people inherit a genetic defect in one or more of these genes. Thus, the enzyme is not properly synthesized. The lack of a functional enzyme prevents one metabolic substrate from being converted to another. The result is a buildup of abnormal by-products that can be toxic. These genetic disorders of metabolism are fairly rare and cannot be cured, although they can be controlled through careful dietary treatment.

Each genetic disorder presented here is named for either the enzyme that is dysfunctional or a symptom that is caused by the disorder. Some of these disorders, such as phenylketonuria, are monogenic,

phenylketonuria (PKU) Genetic disorder characterized by the inability to metabolize the essential amino acid phenylalanine.

hyperphenylalanemia Elevated levels of blood phenylalanine due to a lack of the enzyme phenylalanine hydroxylase.

or caused by a mutation in just one gene. Others, such as maple syrup urine disease, involve more than one gene. Some of the most common genetic disorders involving protein and carbohydrate metabolism are presented in **Table 8.6**.

Phenylketonuria

A simple newborn screening test can detect **phenylketonuria (PKU)**, a rare monogenic disorder that causes serious health problems if untreated. Classic PKU is the most severe form of the genetic disorder. If it is left untreated, it can result in behavior problems and brain damage before the child's first birthday. The milder form of PKU has a lower risk of brain damage.

Individuals with PKU lack the enzyme *phenylalanine hydroxylase* that converts the essential amino acid phenylalanine to the nonessential amino acid tyrosine, which is used for the production of certain neurotransmitters, thyroid hormones, and other important biological compounds (see Table 8.6). This conversion reaction

removes phenylalanine from the blood. In people with PKU, any phenylalanine consumed in the diet accumulates in the blood, a condition called **hyperphenylalanemia**. At the same time, production of compounds requiring tyrosine is impaired.

All babies born in the United States and Canada are screened for PKU with a simple blood test shortly after birth. If the initial test is positive for PKU, further blood and urine tests are completed to confirm the diagnosis. The treatment for PKU is a controlled-phenylalanine diet designed to limit blood levels of phenylalanine and provide sufficient tyrosine, energy, and protein to grow and develop normally. Because breast milk contains phenylalanine, infants are fed a special phenylalanine-free formula. Children and adults must follow a lifelong diet

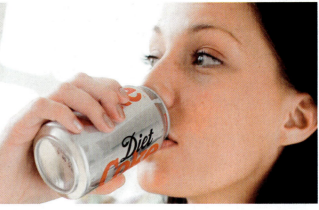

Many diet sodas, such as Diet Coke, contain phenylalanine, a major ingredient in the artificial sweetener aspartame, also called Equal or NutraSweet.

TABLE 8.6	Five Genetic Disorders in Metabolism			
Disorder	**Incidence**	**Enzyme That Is Lacking**	**Examples of Acceptable Foods**	**Examples of Foods to Avoid**
Phenylketonuria	1:15,000	Phenylalanine hydroxylase	Fruits, vegetables, breads, cereals, special formulas	Meat, chicken, fish, eggs, dairy, nuts, legumes
Maple syrup urine disease	1:185,000	Branched-chain alpha-keto acid dehydrogenase	Foods low in branched-chain amino acids, fruits, vegetables, breads, cereals, specialized formulas	Meats, eggs, dairy, nuts, legumes
Homocystinuria	1:300,000	Cystathionine beta-synthase	Fruits, vegetables, special formulas	Meats, eggs, dairy
Galactosemia	1:60,000	Galactose 1-phosphate uridyltransferase	Fruits, vegetables, breads, cereals, eggs, meats	Milk, cheese, milk chocolate, organ meats, legumes, hydrolyzed protein made from milk, casein, fermented soy products
Glycogen Storage Disease	1:50,000	Glucose 6-phosphatase	Corn starch and continuous overnight feeds	Milk, cheese, fruits

that strictly limits high-protein foods and entirely eliminates any products containing aspartame (the sugar substitute found in NutraSweet), which contains phenylalanine.

Maple Syrup Urine Disease

Another protein-related disorder is **maple syrup urine disease (MSUD)**. The disorder results from mutations of four different genes that provide the instructions for making proteins from the branched-chain amino acids leucine, isoleucine, and valine. The mutated genes eliminate or reduce the ability to metabolize these three amino acids. The result is a buildup of the amino acids and their by-products in the blood. Excessive blood levels of these three amino acids are toxic to several organs, including the brain. Not all states require screening for MSUD, and babies with MSUD appear normal at birth. Within a few weeks, however, they begin to show signs of the disease, such as a maple syrup smell to their urine (hence the name). If left untreated, the condition can result in seizures, coma, and even death.[4] The prescribed diet includes a specially

designed infant formula and avoidance of foods such as beef, chicken, fish, eggs, nuts, and legumes, which are high in the three affected amino acids.[5] Unfortunately, such a restrictive diet often means the child subsists solely on specially designed formulas or medically created foods.

Homocystinuria

Homocystinuria is an inherited monogenic disorder that occurs when the enzyme cystathionine beta-synthase, which converts homocysteine to cystathionine, is lacking or not working properly.

A diet rich in the essential amino acid methionine promotes the buildup of homocysteine because methionine is converted to homocysteine during metabolism. The prescribed treatment is therefore a diet low in methionine, along with a supplement of B vitamins, including folate, vitamin B_6, and vitamin B_{12}, which are important in homocysteine metabolism and are often low in individuals with homocystinuria. The low-methionine diet must be followed for life. If left untreated, the disorder can result in dislocation of the lens in the eye, nearsightedness, and blood clots in the veins

and arteries.[6] In adults, the high rate of blood clots and atherosclerosis, especially in the carotid artery, could cause premature cardiovascular disease.[7]

Galactosemia

The genetic disorder **galactosemia** results in the inability to convert galactose to glucose. Any of several genetic mutations may prompt the disorder, which therefore has several variants; however, the fundamental result is improper synthesis of the enzyme galactose 1-phosphate uridyltransferase (GALT), which normally facilitates the conversion of galactose to glucose (**Figure 8.19**). The result is a buildup of galactose in the

maple syrup urine disease (MSUD) Genetic disorder characterized by the inability to metabolize branched-chain amino acids; symptoms include a maple syrup smell in the urine.

homocystinuria Genetic disorder characterized by the inability to metabolize the essential amino acid methionine.

galactosemia Genetic disorder characterized by high levels of galactose in the blood; due to the inability to convert galactose to glucose.

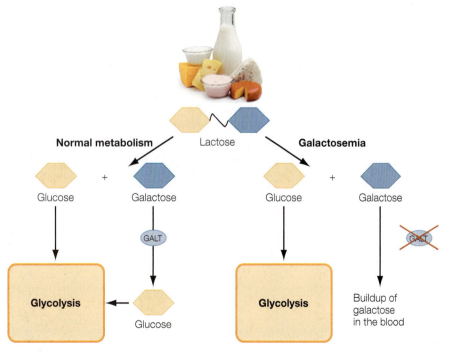

▲ Figure 8.19 **Metabolic Disruption of Galactose Metabolism in Galactosemia**
The lack of the enzyme galactose-1-phosphate uridyltransferase (GALT) blocks the conversion of galactose to glucose. Galactose builds up in the blood and can cause serious complications.

blood, which can damage several different organs if left untreated, including the liver, brain, kidneys, and eyes.[8]

Not all states screen newborns for galactosemia. Affected newborns develop diarrhea and vomiting within a few days of drinking milk or formula containing lactose. They will show signs of irritability, failure to grow, lethargy, and poor sucking response to feeding. Untreated babies may develop mental retardation or die from liver disease.[9]

The treatment focuses mainly on restricting dietary lactose and galactose, which means avoiding milk and all dairy products and products that contain milk chocolate, whey protein or whey solids, casein, and dry milk solids, all of which may contain galactose.

glycogen storage disease Genetic disorder characterized by a lack of glucose 6-phosphatase, which impairs the body's ability to break down glycogen.

Glycogen Storage Disease

Glycogen storage disease is a genetic disorder that disrupts glycogenolysis in the liver. The gene mutation causes a deficiency of the enzyme glucose 6-phosphatase, the enzyme that converts liver glycogen to glucose. If glycogen is trapped in the liver, the body is unable to maintain normal blood glucose levels between meals. Babies with glycogen storage disease can have hypoglycemia, which can lead to seizures. They can also develop high levels of lactic acid in the blood, high levels of uric acid in the urine, and excessive blood lipids, or hyperlipidemia.[10]

To treat glycogen storage disease, foods that contain sucrose, lactose, galactose, and fructose are restricted because these carbohydrates are often stored as glycogen in the liver. Individuals diagnosed with glycogen storage disease must follow the dietary recommendations for life.

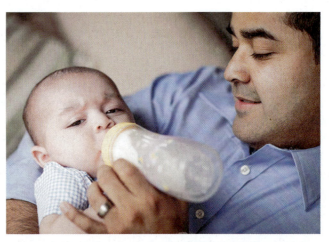

Infants with genetic disorders of metabolism such as galactosemia and glycogen storage disease require special formulas and medically designed foods to meet their nutritional needs.

LO 8.6: THE TAKE-HOME MESSAGE Genetic disorders of metabolism result from an inherited genetic defect in one or more genes that code for enzymes that control metabolic processes. Metabolism is disrupted when the enzyme is improperly synthesized or lacking, allowing metabolic intermediaries to accumulate to toxic levels in the blood. Infants with these disorders generally require feeding with special formulas designed to control the amount of the nutrient affected. Once the infant begins to take solid food, a special diet typically must be followed for life.

Visual Chapter Summary

LO 8.1 Metabolism Is the Sum of All Chemical Reactions in the Body

Metabolism is the term given to all chemical reactions in the cells. The mitochondria are the organelles within the cells that generate most of the cell's ATP. Metabolism balances anabolic reactions that create large molecules, such as glycogen, from smaller parts, such as glucose, with catabolic reactions that break apart large molecules, such as triglycerides to glycerol and fatty acids, to produce ATP. Aerobic metabolism requires oxygen, whereas anaerobic metabolism does not. These reactions are turned on and off by enzymes and coenzymes and are stimulated by hormones.

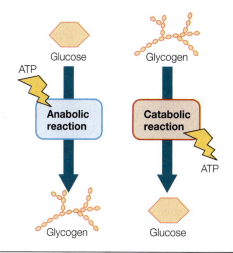

LO 8.2 ATP Is the Energy Source That Fuels Metabolism

Adenosine triphosphate, or ATP, is the energy source used by body cells. ATP is not stored and must be regenerated. Energy is released when one of ATP's phosphate bonds is broken, producing adenosine diphosphate, or ADP. This energy is used to fuel anabolic reactions. ATP is regenerated from ADP plus a phosphate molecule, which can be donated from creatine phosphate.

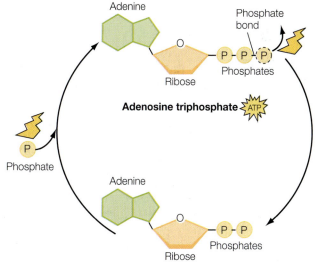

LO 8.3 Carbohydrates, Triglycerides, and Amino Acids Follow Metabolic Pathways

Glucose, the main monosaccharide in metabolism, is oxidized in the cytoplasm through glycolysis to form pyruvate. If there is sufficient oxygen in the cell, pyruvate continues down the pathway to acetyl CoA and enters the TCA cycle.

Triglycerides are hydrolyzed to glycerol and fatty acids. Glycerol enters the metabolic pathway through glycolysis, while fatty acids undergo beta-oxidation to form acetyl CoA.

Deaminated amino acids can be oxidized in the TCA cycle. Glucogenic amino acids can be transformed into pyruvate and participate in gluconeogenesis. Ketogenic amino acids are converted to acetyl CoA and are either oxidized in the TCA cycle or converted into fatty acids and stored as triglycerides.

The TCA cycle, which occurs in the mitochondria, begins with acetyl CoA. Its products include hydrogen atoms with their high-energy electrons, which are transferred to the electron transport chain and ultimately to ATP synthase, through which the majority of ATP is generated via oxidative phosphorylation.

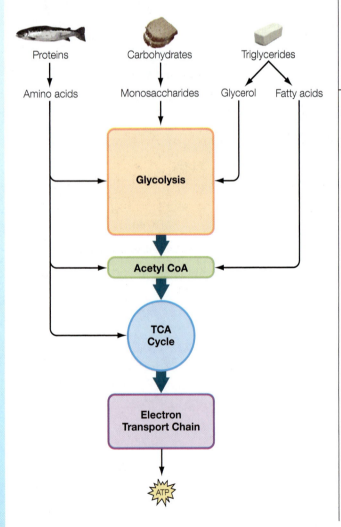

LO 8.4 Metabolism Switches between Anabolic Processes and Catabolic Processes during the Absorptive State, Postabsorptive State, and Starvation

During the absorptive state, excess kilocalories stimulate fat synthesis and are stored as triglycerides. Excess carbohydrates can also be stored as glycogen.

Fasting during the postabsorptive state shifts the metabolism to catabolic reactions to maintain energy balance. The body uses stored glycogen and fatty acids from stored triglycerides in the early stages of fasting. As fasting continues, the body increases the breakdown of fats for energy and conversion to ketone bodies, which can be used by the brain and muscle. Blood glucose levels are maintained using amino acids, pyruvate, lactate, and glycerol as precursors in gluconeogenesis.

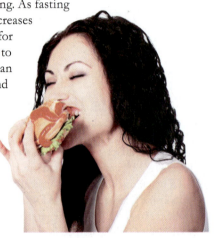

LO 8.5 The Liver Metabolizes Alcohol

Alcohol is metabolized in the liver to acetyl CoA by the enzyme system ADH. The acetyl CoA enters the TCA cycle to produce ATP. When an excess of alcohol builds up, the acetyl CoA is converted to fatty acids and can be stored as a triglyceride in the liver or sent out into the blood. The consumption of excess alcohol can result in the buildup of stored fat in the liver, eventually leading to a condition called cirrhosis.

LO 8.6 Genetic Disorders Can Disrupt Metabolism

In genetic disorders of metabolism, a genetic defect impairs the assembly of an enzyme involved in either protein or carbohydrate metabolism. Lack of a functional enzyme allows the buildup of certain metabolites to toxic levels in the body. Examples are phenylketonuria, maple syrup urine disease, and galactosemia. Serious health consequences, including brain damage, can occur if an affected newborn is not fed with a special infant formula or a child or adult fails to follow strict dietary treatment.

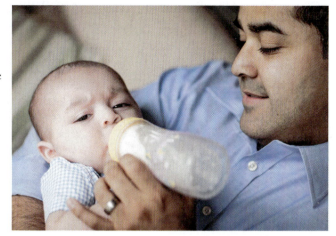

Terms to Know

- metabolism
- metabolic pathway
- adenosine triphosphate (ATP)
- aerobic
- anaerobic
- mitochondrion
- nicotinamide adenine dinucleotide (NAD$^+$)
- flavin adenine dinucleotide (FAD)
- adenosine diphosphate (ADP)
- creatine phosphate (PCr)

- ketogenic
- glycolysis
- pyruvate
- lactate
- Cori cycle
- acetyl CoA
- hormone-sensitive lipase
- beta-oxidation
- alpha-ketoglutarate
- tricarboxylic acid (TCA) cycle
- oxaloacetate
- electron transport chain
- oxidative phosphorylation

- flavoproteins
- cytochromes
- absorptive state
- postabsorptive state
- ketogenesis
- ketoacidosis
- phenylketonuria (PKU)
- hyperphenylalanemia
- maple syrup urine disease (MSUD)
- homocystinuria
- galactosemia
- glycogen storage disease

Mastering Nutrition
Visit the Study Area in Mastering Nutrition to hear an MP3 chapter summary.

Check Your Understanding

LO8.1 1. Metabolism is defined as
   a. the breakdown of large compounds into smaller particles.
   b. the synthesis of new compounds.
   c. the sum of all chemical reactions in the body.
   d. the storage of fat in the adipocytes.

LO8.1 2. Your metabolism is regulated by
   a. hormones and enzymes.
   b. hydroxylase activity.
   c. the amount of creatine phosphate in your cells.
   d. ketone bodies.

LO8.2 3. The energy molecule that fuels metabolism is
   a. adenosine diphosphate.
   b. adenosine triphosphate.
   c. creatine phosphate.
   d. acetyl CoA.

LO8.3 4. Glycolysis is a metabolic pathway that breaks down glucose. This is an example of a(n)
   a. redox reaction.
   b. anabolic reaction.
   c. catabolic reaction.
   d. glucogenic reaction.

LO8.3 5. The compounds that can be used for gluconeogenesis include
   a. fatty acids.
   b. lactate.
   c. ketogenic amino acids.
   d. acetaldehyde.

LO8.3 6. Fatty acids cannot be used for gluconeogenesis because
   a. they lack sufficient carbons to form glucose.
   b. they enter the TCA cycle through citrate.
   c. they are converted to oxaloacetate, which can't reform pyruvate.
   d. they are converted to acetyl CoA, which can't reform pyruvate.

LO8.4 7. During periods of prolonged starvation, the body uses glucose as a fuel source for the brain in a pathway called gluconeogenesis.
   a. True
   b. False

LO8.5 8. Which pathway metabolizes drugs and oxidizes ethanol when alcohol intake is high?
  a. Acetaldehyde dehydrogenase oxidizing system
  b. Catalase oxidizing system
  c. Microsomal ethanol oxidizing system
  d. Alcohol dehydrogenase oxidizing system

LO8.5 9. What is the first compound produced by the oxidation of ethanol by alcohol dehydrogenase?
  a. Acetaldehyde
  b. Oxaloacetate
  c. Lactate
  d. Pyruvate

LO8.6 10. Homocystinuria is a genetic disorder caused by
  a. a buildup of galactose.
  b. a lack of the enzyme cystathionine beta-synthase.
  c. the inability to break down glycogen.
  d. a deficiency in the amino acid methionine.

Answers

1. (c) Metabolism is defined as the sum of all chemical reactions in the body. This includes anabolic reactions that build larger compounds from smaller molecules, catabolic reactions that break molecules apart, or lipogenesis—storing fat in the adipocyte.

2. (a) Metabolism is regulated by hormones, which are released in response to changes in blood glucose levels and other internal conditions, and by the activity of enzymes and their related coenzymes. Phenylalanine hydroxylase is a particular enzyme active in phenylalanine metabolism. The amount of creatine phosphate in your cells is strictly limited. Ketone bodies are fuels produced from fatty acids.

3. (b) Adenosine triphosphate (ATP) is a high-energy molecule that, when hydrolyzed to adenosine disphosphate (ADP), provides energy to cells. ATP can be reformed by adding an inorganic phosphate to ADP donated from the initial reaction or from creatine phosphate (PCr).

4. (c) Catabolic reactions are those that break larger molecules into smaller molecules. Anabolic reactions are the opposite and build larger molecules from smaller molecules. Redox reactions, or oxidation-reduction reactions, involve the transfer of electrons, and glucogenic reactions produce glucose.

5. (b) Lactate can be transformed into glucose through gluconeogenesis. Fatty acids, ketogenic amino acids, and acetaldehyde are not gluconeogenic substrates.

6. (d) Fatty acids contain sufficient carbons but they are converted to acetyl CoA, which is not able to form the pyruvate needed for gluconeogenesis.

7. (b) During prolonged starvation, the brain uses ketone bodies produced from the breakdown of stored fatty acids for fuel.

8. (c) When alcohol intake is high, the oxidation of ethanol is accomplished by the microsomal ethanol oxidizing system (MEOS).

9. (a) The compound produced from the oxidation of ethanol by alcohol dehydrogenase is called acetaldehyde.

10. (b) Homocystinuria is caused by the lack or impaired function of the enzyme cystathionine beta-synthase that converts homocysteine to cystathionine. Homocysteine and certain amino acids, such as methionine, build up in the blood. Controlling methionine intake is essential to reducing the buildup of homocysteine. A buildup of galactose is called galactosemia and glycogen storage disease results in the inability to break down stored glycogen.

Answers to True or False?

1. **True.** All chemical reactions involved in metabolism take place within the mitochondria or the cytoplasm of cells.

2. **True.** The metabolism of carbohydrates is more efficient than the metabolism of either fatty acids or amino acids.

3. **False.** Most fructose is converted to glucose before entering the metabolic pathway.

4. **False.** A burning sensation in muscles during strenuous exercise is caused by a reduction in pH, which reflects a buildup of hydrogen ions, not a buildup of lactate.

5. **False.** Once protein and energy needs have been met, excess amino acids are converted to fatty acids and stored as triglycerides in adipocytes. Thus excess intake of dietary protein will not result in larger muscles.

6. **False.** Fatty acids are oxidized when cells contain sufficient oxygen. Under the anaerobic conditions of high-intensity exercise, a larger percentage of glucose, rather than fatty acids, is used for energy production.

7. **False.** During alcohol metabolism in the liver, ethanol is converted to acetate, which is metabolized for energy or is transformed into fatty acids. Ethanol cannot be used to produce glucose.

8. **False.** Vitamins and minerals in foods do not provide energy. However, certain B vitamins are essential for energy production because they act as coenzymes, facilitating the activity of enzymes during metabolism.

9. **False.** Regardless of what time of day you eat, an excess of total kilocalories favors anabolic metabolism, which means you store the excess kilocalories as body fat or glycogen. If you consume fewer kilocalories than you need each day, catabolic reactions are favored, resulting in a breakdown of triglycerides.

10. **False.** Inborn errors of metabolism are the result of a genetic mutation

that causes a specific metabolic enzyme to be either missing or produced in inadequate amounts. The gene is not repaired during puberty, and the disorders cannot be outgrown.

Web Resources

- For general information on genetic disorders, visit the National Human Genome Research Institute at www.nhgri.nih.gov
- For more information on phenyl-ketonuria, visit the National PKU Alliance at www.npkua.org

- For more information on galactose-mia, visit the Galactosemia Foundation at http://galactosemia.org
- For more information about metabolism from a peer-reviewed online journal, visit *Nutrition and Metabolism* at www.nutritionandmetabolism.com

References

1. Gropper, S. S., and J. L. Smith. 2018. *Advanced Nutrition and Human Metabolism.* 7th ed. (Belmont, CA: Wadsworth/Cengage Learning).
2. Ibid.
3. Sampaio, L. P. 2016. Ketogenic Diet for Epilepsy Treatment. *Aquivos de Neuropsiquiatria* 74(10):842–848. doi: 10.1590/0004-282X20160116.
4. Genetics Home Reference. 2017. *Maple Syrup Urine Disease.* Available at http://ghr.nlm.nih.gov. Accessed February 2017.
5. Ibid.
6. National Institutes of Health. 2017. *Homocystinuria.* Available at www.nlm.nih.gov. Accessed February 2017.
7. Ibid.
8. American Liver Foundation. 2015. *Galactosemia.* Available at www.liverfoundation.org. Accessed February 2017.
9. Ibid.
10. Genetics Home Reference. 2017. *Glycogen Storage Disease Type 1.* Available at http://ghr.nlm.nih.gov. Accessed February 2017.

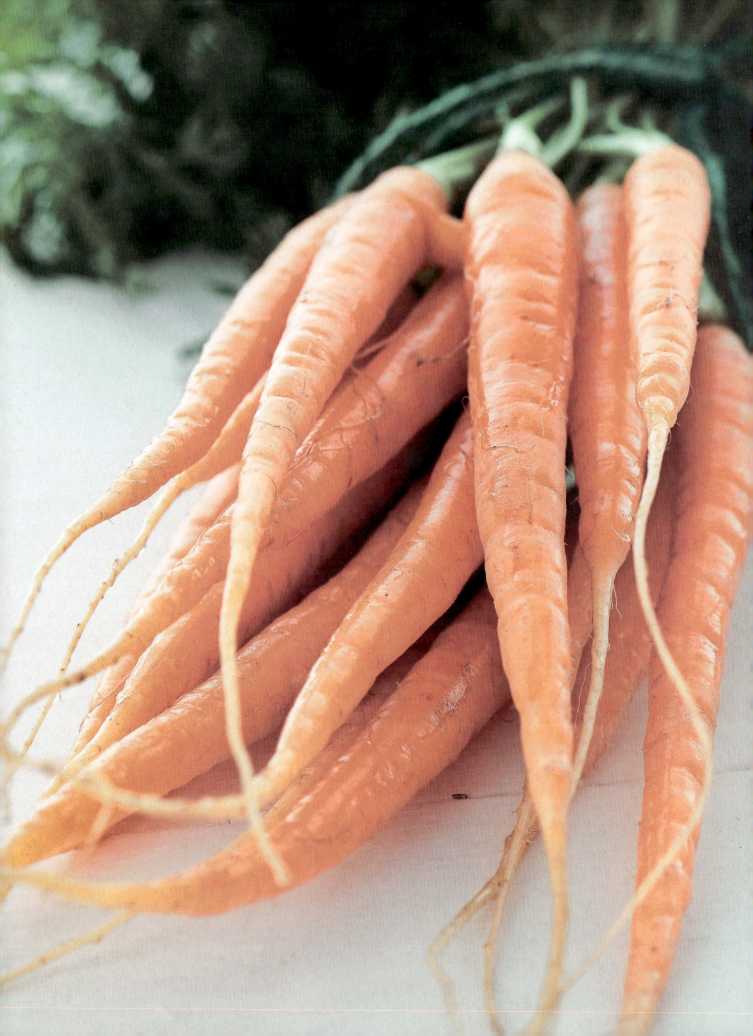

Fat-Soluble Vitamins

Learning Outcomes

After reading this chapter, you will be able to:

9.1 Explain the characteristics of vitamins and classify vitamins according to their solubility.

9.2 Compare and contrast the absorption and storage of fat-soluble and water-soluble vitamins.

9.3 Define the term *antioxidant* and explain which vitamins perform this function.

9.4 Describe the best sources of vitamins and the factors that affect the vitamin content of foods.

9.5 Describe the functions, recommended intakes, food sources, and deficiency and toxicity effects of vitamin A.

9.6 Describe the functions, recommended intakes, food sources, and deficiency and toxicity effects of vitamin D.

9.7 Describe the functions, recommended intakes, food sources, and deficiency and toxicity effects of vitamin E.

9.8 Describe the functions, recommended intakes, food sources, and deficiency and toxicity effects of vitamin K.

9.9 Explain the role of dietary supplements in maintaining a healthy diet.

True or False?

1. Vitamins provide the body with energy. **T/F**

2. Fat-soluble vitamins are found in fatty foods. **T/F**

3. Taking vitamin supplements is never harmful. **T/F**

4. Most people can meet their vitamin needs through food, so supplements are unnecessary. **T/F**

5. Steaming is the best cooking method to retain the vitamins in vegetables. **T/F**

6. Carrots, winter squash, and broccoli are good sources of vitamin A. **T/F**

7. The body makes vitamin D with the help of sunlight. **T/F**

8. Vitamin K is an anticoagulant. **T/F**

9. Vitamin E helps keep bones strong. **T/F**

10. Antioxidants are a magic pill that will prevent aging. **T/F**

See page 357 for the answers.

Vitamins remained undiscovered until the early part of the twentieth century, when scientists sought cures for diseases such as beriberi, scurvy, and rickets. These may sound like the names of rock bands, but they are actually devastating diseases caused by deficiencies of thiamin (for beriberi), vitamin C (for scurvy), and vitamin D (for rickets). In the early decades of the twentieth century, scientists discovered the vitamins that cured these and other diseases. By the 1940s, the U.S. government had mandated the addition of several vitamins to grain products and milk to improve the nation's health.

In the latter part of the twentieth century, improved diets meant that vitamin deficiencies were less of an issue for most Americans. Scientists shifted their focus from using vitamins to cure disease to using them to prevent disease. Today, researchers seek to find out how vitamins affect and prevent everything from birth defects to heart disease and cancer.

In this chapter, we begin with an overview of vitamins, followed by a discussion of differences between the fat-soluble and water-soluble vitamins. We then cover the four fat-soluble vitamins in detail, including their functions, recommended intakes, food sources, and the effects of deficiency and toxicity. (We cover water-soluble vitamins in Chapter 10.)

What Are Vitamins?

LO 9.1 Explain the characteristics of vitamins and classify vitamins according to their solubility.

Vitamins are tasteless organic compounds the body requires in small amounts for normal metabolic functions. Vitamins act as coenzymes to help regulate metabolism and assist the body to convert the energy in fat, carbohydrates, and protein into ATP. They do not provide energy themselves, but a deficiency of any vitamin can cause a lack of energy and other serious health problems. Vitamins also preserve tissues, promote growth and reproduction, act as antioxidants, and perform many other functions.

Vitamins Were Discovered about 100 Years Ago

During the eighteenth century alone, an estimated 2 million sailors died of scurvy, a deficiency disease caused by a lack of vitamin C. The mottled skin, spongy gums, and bleeding that are characteristic of the disease frequently occurred among men on long sea voyages, during which supplies of fresh foods would be depleted before the end of the trip. Eventually, the acid in citrus fruit was recognized as a curative factor, and British sailors came to be known as "limeys" because of the British Navy's policy of issuing lime juice to sailors to prevent scurvy. What they didn't recognize was that the citrus fruit provides vitamin C, which is the vitamin needed to ward off scurvy.

In the early part of the twentieth century, scientists searching for substances to cure diseases such as beriberi and rickets[1] eventually identified thiamin as the curative vitamin for beriberi and vitamin D as the cure for rickets. As they associated additional vitamins with other diseases and conditions, scientists realized their value in promoting public health.

The term *vitamin* is derived from two words, *vital* and *amine,* because some of the first vitamins identified contain an amine group. As each new vitamin was discovered, it was given a temporary name until its structure was isolated. Researchers started at the beginning of the alphabet with vitamins A, B, C, D, E, and K. The letters F, G, and H were dropped once those substances were determined to be unnecessary to support life. This nomenclature changed after vitamin B was found to have more than one chemical compound, and chemists began adding a subscript number to each newly isolated

vitamins Thirteen essential, organic micronutrients that are needed by the body for normal functions.

structure. Together, these vitamins became known as the B complex, with individual vitamins labeled B_1, B_2, and so forth. While vitamins B_6 and B_{12} still retain their numeric names, most of the B vitamins are now better known by their scientific names, such as thiamin (for B_1) and riboflavin (for B_2).

There Are Criteria for Classifying Vitamins

Whereas all carbohydrates are made up of saccharides and all proteins of amino acids, vitamins do not share a fundamental chemical structure. They also do not share similar functions. How, then, are vitamins classified?

An organic, non-energy-providing compound is classified as a vitamin when it cannot be synthesized in sufficient amounts in the body, yet is essential to human health. For instance, vitamin K and two of the B vitamins (niacin and biotin) can be made in the body, but not in amounts sufficient to meet the body's metabolic needs, so they must also be consumed in the diet. The second requirement for a compound to be called a vitamin is that a chronic deficiency of the compound is likely to cause physical symptoms, from fatigue or confusion to scaly skin or blindness. The symptoms are likely to disappear once the vitamin has been sufficiently restored to the diet and absorbed into the body, provided the deficiency has not caused permanent damage.

Based on these criteria, 13 compounds are classified as vitamins. The vitamins are further organized into two groups according to their solubility. There are four fat-soluble (hydrophobic) vitamins—A, D, E, and K—and nine water-soluble (hydrophilic) vitamins—including the B vitamin complex and vitamin C (**Figure 9.1**). The distinction in solubility is important because it influences how the body digests, absorbs, transports, stores, and excretes these essential nutrients. Choline, a water-soluble compound some researchers recognize as a new vitamin, is discussed briefly in Chapter 10.

All Vitamins Are Organic, but Differ in Structure and Function

All vitamins are organic because they contain carbon. Vitamins also contain hydrogen and oxygen and, in some cases, nitrogen, cobalt, or sulfur. Again, the chemical structure of each vitamin is unique. There are no bonds for the body to hydrolyze during digestion, and vitamins are absorbed into the enterocytes intact.

Vitamins perform numerous essential functions in the body. Some, including thiamin, riboflavin, and niacin, participate in releasing energy from the macronutrients. Vitamin D helps regulate bone metabolism, while vitamins E and C donate or accept electrons as antioxidants. Several vitamins play more than one role in metabolism. **Table 9.1** illustrates the variety of functions vitamins play in maintaining health.

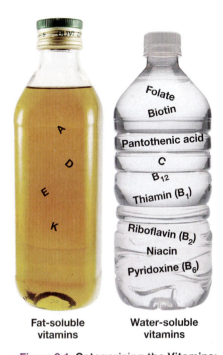

▲ **Figure 9.1 Categorizing the Vitamins: Fat Soluble and Water Soluble**
A vitamin is either fat soluble or water soluble, depending on how it is absorbed and handled in the body. Fat-soluble vitamins need dietary fat to be properly absorbed, whereas water-soluble vitamins are absorbed with water.

TABLE 9.1	The Many Roles of Vitamins in Maintaining Health
Metabolic Function	**Vitamins That Play a Role**
Antioxidants	Vitamin C, vitamin E
Blood clotting and red blood cell synthesis	Folate, vitamin B_6, vitamin B_{12}, vitamin K
Bone health	Vitamin A, vitamin C, vitamin D, vitamin K
Energy production	Biotin, niacin (B_3), pantothenic acid, riboflavin (B_2), thiamin (B_1), vitamin B_6, vitamin B_{12}
Growth and reproduction	Vitamin A, vitamin D
Immune function	Vitamin A, vitamin C, vitamin D
Protein metabolism and synthesis	Folate, vitamin B_6, vitamin B_{12}, vitamin C

Provitamins are substances found in foods that are not in a form directly usable by the body, but that can be converted into an active form once they are absorbed. The best-known example of this is beta-carotene, which is split into two molecules of vitamin A in the enterocytes or in the liver cells. Vitamins found in foods that are already in the active form, called **preformed vitamins**, do not undergo conversion.

Overconsumption of Some Vitamins Can Be Toxic

Vitamin **toxicity**, or **hypervitaminosis**, results when a person ingests more of a vitamin than the body needs, to the point at which tissues become saturated. The excess vitamin can damage cells, sometimes permanently. Vitamin toxicity does not occur in people who eat a normal balanced diet. It can result when individuals consume **megadose** levels of vitamin supplements, usually in the false belief that "more is better." Many individuals, for example, overload on vitamin C tablets to ward off a cold, despite the lack of evidence that vitamin C prevents the common cold, and they may suffer unpleasant side effects, including diarrhea. In general, however, vitamin C and most other water-soluble vitamins do not cause toxicity because the excess is excreted in the urine. Vitamin B_6 is sometimes linked to toxicity, and the fat-soluble vitamins A, D, and E, which are stored in the body's tissues, can be toxic in megadoses.

To prevent excessive intake, the Dietary Reference Intakes include a tolerable upper intake level for most vitamins. Even though sufficient evidence to establish a Tolerable Upper Intake Level (UL) is lacking for some vitamins, there still may be risks in taking them in megadose amounts.

> **LO 9.1: THE TAKE-HOME MESSAGE** Vitamins are essential organic compounds that the body cannot synthesize in adequate amounts to maintain health. All vitamins are either fat soluble (A, D, E, and K) or water soluble (the B vitamins and vitamin C). Provitamins such as beta-carotene are converted to their active form before they can be directly used in the body. Most water-soluble vitamins are not toxic because excesses are excreted in the urine. Vitamins A, D, and E are stored in the body's tissues and can be toxic if taken in megadose amounts.

How Do Vitamins Differ in Their Absorption and Storage?

LO 9.2 Compare and contrast the absorption and storage of fat-soluble and water-soluble vitamins.

All vitamins are absorbed in the small intestine, but they differ in their level of absorption and their storage. Let's take a closer look at these differences.

Vitamins Differ in Bioavailability

Not all of the vitamins consumed in foods are completely absorbed. The **bioavailability** of individual vitamins varies according to several factors, including the amount of the vitamin in the food; whether the food is cooked, raw, or refined; how efficiently the food is digested and absorbed; the individual's nutritional status and general health; and whether or not the vitamin is natural or synthetic. In general, if the body needs more of a certain vitamin, a greater percentage is absorbed. For example, a young child or pregnant woman absorbs a higher percentage of vitamins than does a nonpregnant adult consuming the same food.

provitamin Vitamin precursor that is converted to a vitamin in the body.

preformed vitamins Vitamins found in food.

toxicity Accumulation of a substance to a harmful level.

hypervitaminosis Condition resulting from the presence of excessive amounts of vitamins in the body; also referred to as *vitamin toxicity*.

megadose Amount of a vitamin or mineral that's at least 10 times the amount recommended in the DRI.

bioavailability Degree to which a nutrient is absorbed from foods and used in the body.

In general, fat-soluble vitamins are less bioavailable than water-soluble vitamins because fat-soluble vitamins require bile and the formation of micelles in order to be absorbed. Vitamins in plant foods are typically less bioavailable than those in animal foods because plant fiber can trap vitamins.

Fat-Soluble Vitamins Are Stored after They Are Absorbed

Fat-soluble vitamins are often attached to food components, usually protein, in foods. To be absorbed, the vitamin must be released from the protein with the help of pepsin and hydrochloric acid (refer to Chapter 3). The freed fat-soluble vitamins are then ready to be absorbed, primarily in the duodenum (**Figure 9.2**). They are packaged with fatty acids and bile in micelles that transport them close to the intestinal mucosa. Once there, the fat-soluble vitamins travel through the enterocytes and are repackaged with fat and other lipids into chylomicrons. The vitamins then travel through the lymph system before they enter the bloodstream.

Note that absorption of fat-soluble vitamins can be compromised in the absence of adequate fatty acids. This is why having some fat in the diet is absolutely necessary to avoid fat-soluble vitamin deficiencies. The absorption of fat-soluble vitamins can also be compromised in certain malabsorption diseases such as celiac disease[2] and cystic fibrosis.[3] Diseases that impair the synthesis of bile can also reduce the absorption of the fat-soluble vitamins, especially vitamins D and K.[4]

Fat-soluble vitamins are stored in the body and used as needed when dietary intake falls short of the body's needs. The liver is the main storage depot for vitamin A and to a lesser extent vitamins K and E, whereas vitamin D is mainly stored in fat and muscle tissues. Again, because they are stored in the body, large quantities of some of the fat-soluble vitamins, particularly A, can build up to the point of toxicity, causing harmful symptoms and conditions.

Water-Soluble Vitamins Are Not Stored after Absorption

Water-soluble vitamins are absorbed with water and enter the bloodstream directly from the small intestine. Most water-soluble vitamins are absorbed in the duodenum and jejunum, although vitamin B_{12} is absorbed in the ileum. Water-soluble vitamins are not

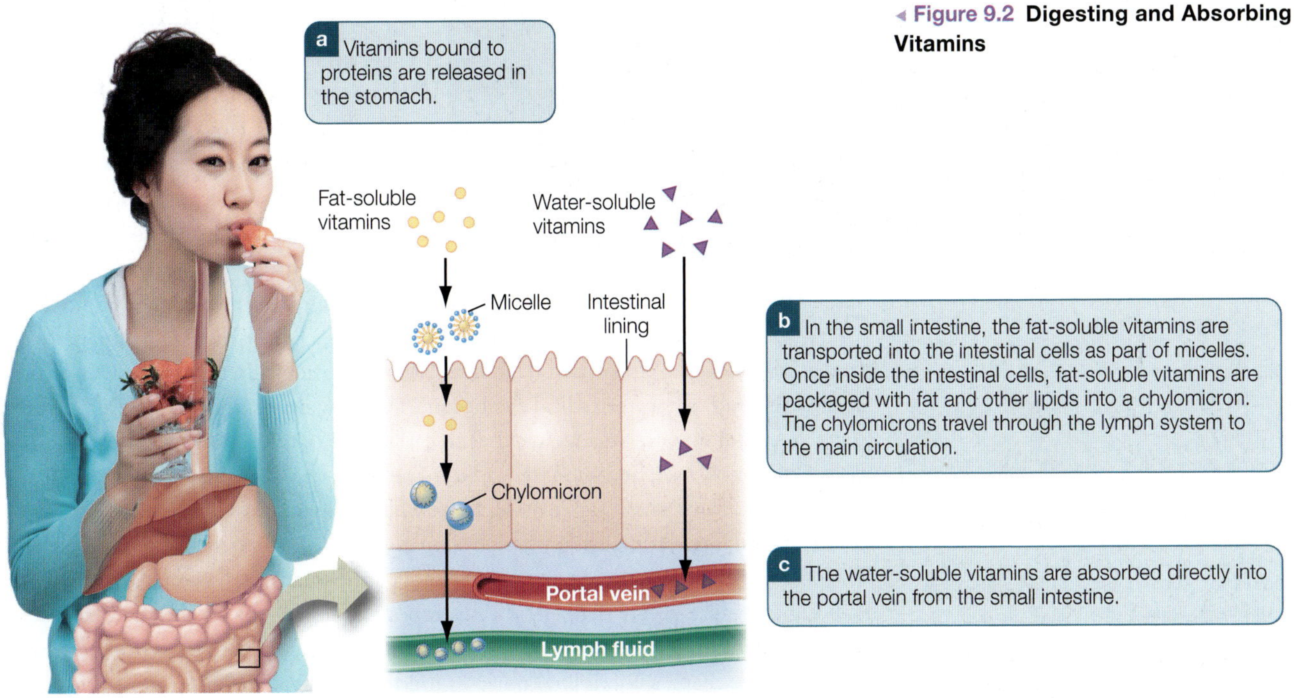

◄ **Figure 9.2 Digesting and Absorbing Vitamins**

a Vitamins bound to proteins are released in the stomach.

Fat-soluble vitamins

Water-soluble vitamins

Micelle

Intestinal lining

Chylomicron

Portal vein

Lymph fluid

b In the small intestine, the fat-soluble vitamins are transported into the intestinal cells as part of micelles. Once inside the intestinal cells, fat-soluble vitamins are packaged with fat and other lipids into a chylomicron. The chylomicrons travel through the lymph system to the main circulation.

c The water-soluble vitamins are absorbed directly into the portal vein from the small intestine.

stored in the body and excess amounts are excreted, so it's important to consume adequate amounts of them every day. Note that even though most water-soluble vitamins aren't stored, megadosing can still be harmful.

> **LO 9.2: THE TAKE-HOME MESSAGE** Bioavailability of individual vitamins varies based on the amount of the vitamin in the food, whether the food is cooked, raw, or refined, the digestibility of the food, an individual's nutrition status, and whether the vitamin is in natural or synthetic form. Fat-soluble vitamins—A, D, E, and K—are not as bioavailable as water-soluble vitamins. They require dietary fat for absorption and are transported in the lymph system. Because they are stored in the liver and other tissues, overconsumption of fat-soluble vitamins can be toxic. The water-soluble vitamins—the B vitamins and vitamin C—are absorbed with water into the portal vein. Excess water-soluble vitamins are excreted through the urine and generally aren't stored.

What Are Antioxidants?

LO 9.3 Define the term *antioxidant* and explain which vitamins perform this function.

Antioxidants (*anti* = against, *oxidants* = oxidizing agents) are a group of compounds that include vitamins E and C, the mineral selenium, and several phytochemicals, including *flavonoids* (colorful pigments found in fruits and vegetables) and *carotenoids* (such as beta-carotene, zeaxanthin, lutein, and lycopene). Just as their name implies, antioxidants counteract oxidation reactions. In Chapter 5, you encountered antioxidants added to foods to prevent the oxidation reactions that cause rancidity. Here, we discuss the role of antioxidants in human health.

As you learned in Chapter 8, oxidation reactions are essential to normal energy metabolism, as oxygen is required for aerobic reactions that result in the production of ATP. However, oxidation reactions release *free radicals,* atoms or molecules with an unpaired electron. Free radicals can also result from exposure to chemicals in the environment (such as cigarette smoke and air pollution) or from the damaging effects of the sun's ultraviolet rays (**Figure 9.3**).

Whatever its source, a free radical is highly unstable. Because it has an unpaired electron, it will "steal" an electron from another atom or molecule. In doing so, it will become stable. Alternatively, a free radical can become stable by depositing its unpaired electron onto another atom or molecule. In either case, the atom or molecule that lost or gained an electron will now itself become a free radical. The chain reaction stops when two free radicals collide to form a new, stable molecule or when antioxidants stabilize the free radical.

Antioxidants accomplish this task by donating an electron to the free radical, thereby stopping the chain reaction in its track. Without antioxidants, the chain reaction of free radicals can cause severe damage to cells, especially to the polyunsaturated fatty acids in lipoproteins and in cell membranes. If free radicals accumulate faster than the body can neutralize them, a condition known as **oxidative stress**, their damaging effects can contribute to various chronic diseases, including cardiovascular disease, cancer, diabetes,

antioxidants Nutrients and phytochemicals that act to neutralize free radicals.

oxidative stress Condition whereby free radicals are being produced in the body faster than they are neutralized.

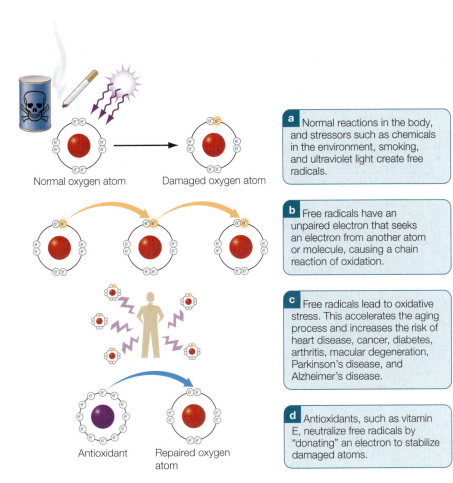

a Normal reactions in the body, and stressors such as chemicals in the environment, smoking, and ultraviolet light create free radicals.

b Free radicals have an unpaired electron that seeks an electron from another atom or molecule, causing a chain reaction of oxidation.

c Free radicals lead to oxidative stress. This accelerates the aging process and increases the risk of heart disease, cancer, diabetes, arthritis, macular degeneration, Parkinson's disease, and Alzheimer's disease.

d Antioxidants, such as vitamin E, neutralize free radicals by "donating" an electron to stabilize damaged atoms.

Normal oxygen atom   Damaged oxygen atom

Antioxidant   Repaired oxygen atom

▲ Figure 9.3 Antioxidants Neutralize Free Radicals

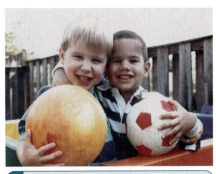

a Normal vision and the ability to clearly see the world around you is often taken for granted.

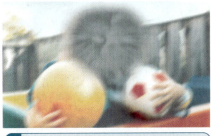

b People with age-related macular degeneration (AMD) have difficulty seeing things directly in front of them.

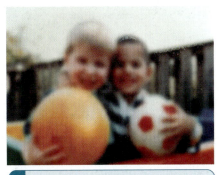

c Cataracts cause vision to become cloudy.

▲ Figure 9.4 Normal and Impaired Vision

Source: National Institutes of Health, National Eye Institute.

arthritis, Parkinson's disease, and Alzheimer's disease.[5] Free radicals can also alter DNA and RNA, cause inflammation, and are thought to contribute to aging.[6]

Free radicals can also damage vision. Two vision disorders linked to oxidative stress are age-related macular degeneration and cataracts.

Age-related macular degeneration (AMD) is the most common cause of permanent impairment for reading and other activities requiring close-up vision in Americans 60 years of age and older.[7] By 2050, the estimated number of people with AMD is expected to more than double, from 2.07 million to 5.44 million.[8] AMD results from damage to the macula, a tiny area of the eye that is needed for central vision—the ability to see things that are directly in front of you. (The macula is shown in the Focus Figure on page 333.) AMD can make activities such as reading, driving, and watching television impossible (**Figure 9.4**). In the early stages of AMD, there are few symptoms of vision loss. As the disease progresses, images become blurred, or a dark, empty area can appear in the center of your vision. While there is no cure for AMD, a number of well-designed studies have indicated that antioxidant supplements containing vitamin A, beta-carotene, vitamin C, and vitamin E, along with the minerals zinc and copper, may be effective in reducing the risk of AMD as well as the progression of the disease in individuals at risk for developing advanced AMD.[9]

Some studies have also suggested that specific antioxidants—namely vitamins C and E and the carotenoids lutein and zeaxanthin—may also help reduce the risk of cataracts.[10] A **cataract** is a common eye condition among older adults in which the lens of the eye becomes cloudy, resulting in blurred vision, as shown in Figure 9.4c. More than 20 million Americans over the age of 40 (17.5 percent) have cataracts in one or both eyes.[11] The National Eye Institute recommends consuming antioxidant- and carotenoid-rich vegetables and fruits, such as citrus fruits, broccoli, and dark green leafy vegetables, for the health of the eyes.[12]

age-related macular degeneration (AMD) Disease that affects the macula of the retina, causing blurry vision and, potentially, blindness.

cataract Common eye disorder that occurs when the lens of the eye becomes cloudy.

TABLE 9.2 The Phytochemical Color Guide

The National Cancer Institute recommends eating a variety of colorful fruits and vegetables daily to provide your body with valuable vitamins, minerals, fiber, and disease-fighting phytochemicals. Whole grains also have phytochemicals and have been added to this list.

Color	Phytochemical	Found in
Red	Anthocyanins	Apples, beets, cabbage, cherries, cranberries, red cabbage, red onions, red beans
Yellow/Orange	Beta-carotene	Apricots, butternut squash, cantaloupe, carrots, mangoes, peaches, pumpkin, sweet potatoes
	Flavonoids	Apricots, clementines, grapefruits, lemons, papaya, pears, pine-apple, yellow raisins
White	Alliums/allicin	Chives, garlic, leeks, onions, scallions
Green	Lutein, zeaxanthin	Broccoli, collard greens, honeydew melon, kale, kiwi, lettuce, mustard greens, peas, spinach
	Indoles	Arugula, broccoli, bok choy, brussels sprouts, cabbage, cauli-flower, kale, Swiss chard, turnips
Blue/Purple	Anthocyanins	Blackberries, black currants, elderberries, purple grapes
	Phenolics	Eggplant, plums, prunes, raisins
Brown	Beta-glucan, lignans, phenols, plant sterols, phytoestrogens, saponins, tocotrienols	Barley, brown rice, oats, oatmeal, whole grains, whole-grain cere-als, whole wheat

Source: Adapted from Fruits & Veggies—More Matters. 2017 Available at www.fruitsandveggiesmorematters.org.

Notice that the antioxidants thought to be beneficial for these vision disorders include vitamins and minerals as well as the carotenoids beta-carotene, lutein, and zeaxanthin and the flavonoids.[13] Some phytochemicals, including carotenoids, are also responsible for the vibrant colors of many fruits and vegetables. **Table 9.2** emphasizes the importance of consuming a colorful diet so as to take in an abundance of phytochemicals.

A question that remains is whether or not antioxidant *supplements* provide the same health protection as antioxidants consumed in foods. Studies are currently under way exploring the role of antioxidant supplements in fighting disease. At this time, the American Heart Association, National Cancer Institute, and United States Preventive Services Task Force do not advocate taking supplements to reduce the risk of specific diseases, but encourage eating a phytochemical- and antioxidant-rich, well-balanced diet.[14] However, the National Eye Institute does advise people at risk for advanced AMD to take a specific formulation of antioxidant supplements in consultation with their physician.[15]

LO 9.3: THE TAKE-HOME MESSAGE Antioxidants, such as vitamins E and C, the mineral selenium, flavonoids, and carotenoids, help counteract the damaging effects of free radicals, atoms or molecules with an unpaired electron. If free radicals accumulate faster than the body can neutralize them, the damaging effects of oxidative stress can contribute to chronic diseases and may accelerate aging. Fruits, vegetables, and whole grains are excellent sources of antioxidant nutrients and phytochemicals.

What's the Best Source of Vitamins?

LO 9.4 Describe the best sources of vitamins and the factors that affect the vitamin content of foods.

Eating whole foods, including fruits, vegetables, and whole grains, remains the best way to meet vitamin needs because these foods are also rich in antioxidant phytochemicals and fiber. The *Dietary Guidelines for Americans* recommends eating a wide variety of foods from

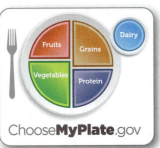

Vegetables	Fruits	Grains	Protein	Dairy
Folate	Folate	Folic acid	Niacin	Riboflavin
Vitamin A	Vitamin C	Niacin	Thiamin	Vitamin A
Vitamin C	Vitamin A	Vitamin B_6	Vitamin B_6	Vitamin B_{12}
Vitamin E		Vitamin B_{12} (if fortified)	Vitamin B_{12}	Vitamin D
Vitamin K		Riboflavin		
		Thiamin		

each food group, with ample amounts of vitamin-rich fruits, vegetables, whole grains, and dairy foods. **Figure 9.5** illustrates each food group and the vitamins it contributes to the diet.

Vitamins Can Be Destroyed during Cooking or Storage

How you prepare and store fresh foods once you obtain them can affect their nutritional content. Water-soluble vitamins can be destroyed by exposure to air, ultraviolet (UV) light, water, changes in pH, or heat. In fact, vegetables and fruits begin to lose their vitamins almost immediately after being harvested, and some preparation and storage methods can accelerate vitamin loss. Though the fat-soluble vitamins tend to be more stable than water-soluble vitamins, some food preparation techniques can cause the loss of these vitamins as well.

Exposure to Oxygen

Air—or, more specifically, exposure to oxygen—can destroy the water-soluble vitamins and the fat-soluble vitamins A, E, and K. Thus, fresh vegetables and fruits should be stored in airtight, covered containers and used soon after being purchased.

Exposure to Light

Light, especially ultraviolet light (UV), can destroy vitamins. For example, up to 80 percent of the riboflavin content of milk stored in clear glass bottles can be destroyed by UV light.[16] For this reason, milk is sold in opaque containers. The traditional methods of sun-drying fruits and vegetables also destroys susceptible vitamins such as beta-carotene and vitamin C. However, new advances in solar drying have shown some promise.[17]

Exposure to Water

Water-soluble vitamins leach out of foods when soaked or cooked in liquids, so cooking foods in as little water as possible is recommended.[18] Water should be boiling before vegetables are added even if you use a steamer basket. Some enzymes naturally found in the food oxidize specific vitamins, changing them to forms that are not metabolically active. Boiling water inactivates these enzymes. For instance, potatoes are a good source of vitamin C but they also contain an enzyme, ascorbic oxidase, that changes the chemical structure of vitamin C to an inactive form. Potatoes added to boiling water retain more vitamin C than if they are added to cold water and brought to a boil.

Changes in Ph

Changes in pH can destroy some vitamins, especially thiamin and vitamin C. Most vitamins are stable in acid, but adding ingredients such as baking soda to foods increases the

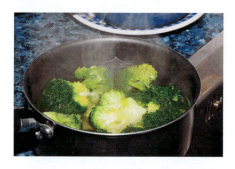

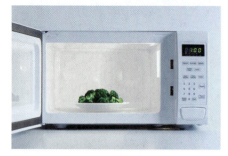

As opposed to boiling, cooking foods in the microwave allows for a shorter cooking time, which means fewer vitamins are lost.

pH and destroys pH-sensitive vitamins. For instance, adding baking soda to shorten the cooking time of beans or other legumes destroys the thiamin content.

Exposure to Heat

Heat, especially prolonged heat from cooking, also destroys water-soluble vitamins, especially vitamin C. Because they are exposed to less heat, vegetables cooked by microwaving, steaming, or stir-frying can have approximately one-and-a-half times more vitamin C after cooking than if they were boiled, which involves longer heat exposure.[19] Whereas heat reduces the vitamin content of foods, cooler temperatures help preserve them. For this reason, produce should be stored in the refrigerator rather than on a counter or in a pantry. A package of fresh spinach left at room temperature loses over half of its folate, a B vitamin, after 4 days. Refrigeration delays that loss to 8 days.[20] See the Table Tips for more ways to preserve the vitamins in foods.

Some Foods Are Fortified with Vitamins

When you pour a glass of orange juice, you know that you are getting a significant intake of vitamin C. However, depending on the brand of orange juice, you may also be meeting the recommendations for vitamin E and vitamin D—two nutrients that are not naturally found in oranges. This is due to a process called *fortification,* the addition of nutrients by manufacturers to enhance the nutrient quality of the food and to prevent or correct dietary deficiencies.

Fortified foods are becoming more popular with the American consumer. For example, worldwide sales of foods fortified with one popular nutrient, omega-3 fatty acids, were projected to exceed $34 billion in 2016.[21] Vitamins and minerals are the most commonly used nutrients in fortified foods, but fiber, amino acids, essential fatty acids, and other bioactive ingredients are also sometimes added. Based on current Food and Drug Administration (FDA) regulations, all 13 vitamins and 20 minerals can be added to foods.[22]

Enrichment of foods is a form of fortification. Foods that are enriched, such as rice, bread, flour, pasta, and other refined grains, have been fortified with a level of nutrients that may bring the nutritional profile closer to its state before the grain was processed. Four water-soluble B vitamins (thiamin, riboflavin, niacin, and folate) and the mineral iron are required by law to be added to refined grains.

Fortified Foods Can Help Ensure Adequate Intake for Some Individuals

Fortified foods can be a valuable option for individuals whose diet falls short of some nutrients. For instance, an adult on a very low-kilocalorie diet may not be getting adequate vitamins and minerals from food and would benefit from fortified cereals. Strict vegans or individuals who are lactose intolerant and do not consume dairy products would benefit from drinking soymilk fortified with vitamins B_{12} and D and calcium. Older adults who are inactive and thus have lower kilocalorie needs may choose fortified foods to add vitamin E to their limited dietary selections. Women in their childbearing years may look to folic acid–fortified cereals to help them meet their daily needs for this B vitamin.

Fortified Foods Can Contribute to Health Risks

Because overconsumption of a vitamin or mineral can result in nutrient toxicity, individuals who consume high amounts of some fortified foods may be at risk for health problems. If a heavily fortified food, like some cereals, snack bars, and beverages, claims to contain "100% of the vitamins needed daily," then eating several servings of the food or a combination of several fortified foods is similar to taking several multivitamin supplements. Individuals are more likely to overconsume vitamins from fortified foods than from whole foods.

Now that we've discussed the general characteristics of vitamins, let's survey the individual fat-soluble vitamins presented in **Table 9.3**. Before we begin, take the Self-Assessment to see if your diet is rich in foods that contain these important nutrients.

TABLE 9.3 Functions, Daily Needs, Food Sources, and Symptoms of Toxicity and Deficiency of the Fat-Soluble Vitamins

Fat-Soluble Vitamin	Metabolic Function	Daily Needs (19 years +)	Food Sources	Toxicity Symptoms/UL	Deficiency Symptoms
Vitamin A	Vision, protein synthesis, growth, immune function, bone health	Males: 900 μg RAE/day Females: 700 μg RAE/day	• Beef liver • Fortified dairy products	Compromised bone health; birth defects during pregnancy UL: 3,000 μg/day	Night blindness, xerophthalmia, keratinization, increased vulnerability to infection
Vitamin D	Calcium balance, bone health, cell differentiation, immune system	Males and females: 15 μg/day (600 IU)	• Fatty fish such as salmon, tuna, sardines • Fortified foods, such as dairy products, orange juice, and cereals	Hypercalcemia UL: 100 μg/day	Rickets and osteomalacia
Vitamin E	Antioxidant, health of cell membranes, heart health	Males and females: 15 mg alpha-tocopherol/ day (22.4 IU)	• Vegetable and seed oils • Nuts, seeds • Fortified cereals • Green leafy vegetables	Nerve problems, muscle weakness, and uncontrolled movement of body parts UL: 1,000 mg/day	Hemolysis of RBCs
Vitamin K	Carboxylation, blood clotting, and bone health	Males: 120 μg/day Females: 90 μg/day	• Green leafy vegetables • Soybeans • Canola and soybean oils • Beef liver	None known UL: none established	Excessive bleeding

LO 9.4: THE TAKE-HOME MESSAGE A well-balanced diet rich in whole foods that provides adequate kilocalories can meet many individuals' daily vitamin needs. Proper handling, storage, and cooking of fresh foods can retain vitamins. Vitamins in foods can be destroyed or lost by exposure to air, water, UV light, changes in pH, and heat. Fortified foods can add nutrients to a low-kilocalorie diet. Fortified foods can also contribute to overconsumption of individual nutrients and may lead to toxicity.

fortified foods Foods with added vitamins and minerals; fortified foods often contain nutrients that are not naturally present in the food or that are in higher amounts than the food contains naturally.

Self-Assessment

Are You Getting Enough Fat-Soluble Vitamins in Your Diet?

Take this brief self-assessment to see if your diet contains enough food sources of the four fat-soluble vitamins.

1. Do you eat at least 1 cup of deep yellow or orange vegetables, such as carrots and sweet potatoes, or dark green vegetables, such as spinach, every day?

   Yes ☐ **No** ☐

2. Do you consume at least two glasses (8 ounces each) of milk daily?

   Yes ☐ **No** ☐

3. Do you eat a tablespoon of vegetable oil, such as corn or olive oil, daily? (*Tip:* Salad dressings, unless they are fat free, count!)

   Yes ☐ **No** ☐

4. Do you eat at least 1 cup of leafy green vegetables in your salad and/or put lettuce in your sandwich every day?

   Yes ☐ **No** ☐

Answers

If you answered yes to all four questions, your diet is close to meeting your fat-soluble vitamin needs! If you answered no to any one of the questions, your diet needs some fine-tuning. Deep orange and dark green vegetables are excellent sources of vitamin A, and milk is an excellent choice for vitamin D. Adding small amounts of vegetable oils to a vitamin K–rich leafy green salad improves the vitamin E content.

EXPLORING Vitamin A

LO 9.5 Describe the functions, recommended intakes, food sources, and deficiency and toxicity effects of vitamin A.

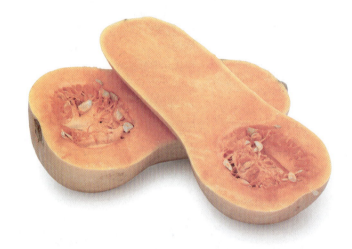

What Is Vitamin A?

The term *vitamin A* refers to a family of fat-soluble **retinoids** that include **retinol**, **retinal**, and **retinoic acid** (**Figure 9.6**). These compounds are similar in their chemical structure. They each contain a ring with a polyunsaturated hydrocarbon chain. Attached at the end of the hydrocarbon chain is either an alcohol group (retinol), an aldehyde group (retinal), or an acid group (retinoic acid). Whereas retinol, retinal, and retinoic acid all participate in essential functions in the body, retinol, the alcohol form, is the most usable. In foods, vitamin A is found as retinol or as a **retinyl ester**, which has an *ester group* (a compound derived from a carboxylic acid) attached at the fatty acid tail. The body also stores vitamin A as a retinyl ester in the liver. Retinol can be reversibly converted to retinal, the aldehyde form. Retinal can be transformed into the acidic form called retinoic acid, but the process is irreversible. Retinoids are preformed vitamin A, which means they are in a form that the body can use immediately without first being activated. Preformed vitamin A is found primarily in animal-based foods.

On the right side of Figure 9.6 is the structure of one of the family of **provitamin-A carotenoids**. These are precursors to retinol. Three such compounds—**beta-carotene** (β-carotene),

---

retinoids Term used to describe the family of preformed vitamin A compounds.

retinol Alcohol form of preformed vitamin A.

retinal Aldehyde form of preformed vitamin A.

retinoic acid Acid form of preformed vitamin A.

retinyl ester Ester form of preformed vitamin A found in foods and stored in the body.

provitamin-A carotenoids Group of yellow, red, and orange plant pigments that act as precursors to vitamin A.

beta-carotene One of the provitamin A carotenoids.

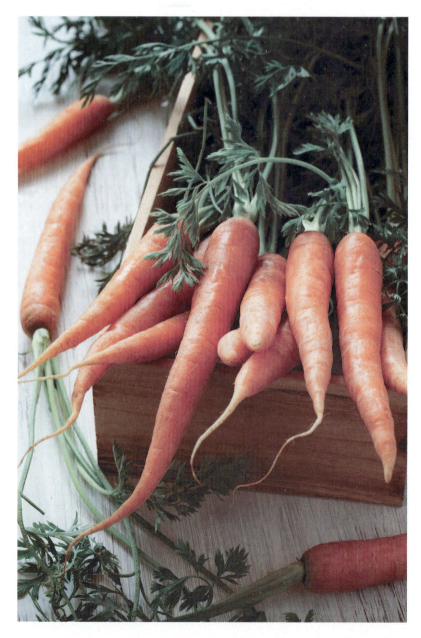

The carotenoid lycopene, found in tomatoes and tomato products, functions as an antioxidant in the body.

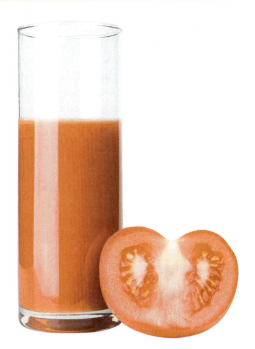

Form found in animal foods and stored in body

Retinyl ester

Form found in plants

Beta-carotene

Splits into 2 retinal

Retinol (alcohol form)
• Reproduction

Retinal (aldehyde form)
• Vision

Retinoic acid
• Regulates growth

▲ **Figure 9.6 The Conversion of the Three Vitamin A Compounds**
Retinyl esters, found in foods and the form of vitamin A stored in the liver, are converted to retinol (alcohol). Retinol can be transformed to retinal (aldehyde) and then to retinoic acid. Beta-carotene is split during digestion to yield two molecules of retinal.

(continued)

beta-cryptoxanthin (β-cryptoxanthin), and alpha-carotene (α-carotene)—are the most common carotenoids, the yellow-red pigments that give carrots, butternut squash, and cantaloupe their vibrant, deep orange color. For vegans, these carotenoids are the only dietary source of vitamin A. Almost 25 to 35 percent of the dietary vitamin A consumed by adults in the United States comes from carotenoids, especially beta-carotene.[23]

Vitamin A Absorption and Transport

All forms of preformed vitamin A are absorbed by active transport in the small intestine with the help of bile and micelles. The rate of absorption of preformed vitamin A is high, ranging from 70 to 90 percent, as long as the diet contains some fat. Beta-carotene, in contrast, is absorbed via passive diffusion at a much lower rate of 5–60 percent.[24] Beta-carotene absorption is reduced with high fiber intakes and improved when foods are cooked. For example, the amount of beta-carotene absorbed from cooked carrots is much higher than that from raw carrots.

Most forms of vitamin A are packaged as chylomicrons along with other dietary lipids and absorbed into the lymph fluid. Retinoic acid doesn't need a chylomicron, but rather is attached to a protein called *albumin* and absorbed into the portal vein.

---

rhodopsin Compound found in the rods of the eye that is needed for night vision; composed of *cis*-retinal and the protein opsin.

iodopsin Compound found in the cones of the eye that is needed for color vision.

rods Light-absorbing cells responsible for black-and-white vision and night vision.

cones Light-absorbing cells responsible for color vision.

bleaching Reaction occurring when light enters the eye and interacts with rhodopsin, splitting it into *trans*-retinal and opsin.

epithelial tissues Tissues that line body cavities or cover body surfaces.

cell division Process of dividing one cell into two separate cells with the same genetic material.

cell differentiation Process of a less specialized immature cell becoming a specialized mature cell.

Carotenes are converted to vitamin A in the intestine before absorption.

Vitamin A is stored in the liver until needed by the body. Retinol-binding protein transports the retinol from storage through the bloodstream to the receptor sites located on the cells.

Vitamin A is difficult to excrete from the body. When the liver becomes saturated with vitamin A, some is excreted through the bile, but vitamin A can accumulate to toxic levels.

Metabolic Functions of Vitamin A

Each form of retinoid plays a specific role in the body. Retinal (the aldehyde form) participates in vision. The hormone-like action of retinoic acid (the acid form) is essential for growth and development of cells, including bone development. Retinol (the alcohol form) supports reproduction and a healthy immune system. In addition to these critical roles, vitamin A may help prevent cancer.

Vitamin A in Vision

One of the best-known functions of vitamin A is to support vision. Light that passes into the eyes and hits the retina is translated into visual images with the help of two vitamin A–dependent proteins, **rhodopsin** and **iodopsin**. These proteins are found in the tips of light-absorbing cells in the retina called **rods** and **cones**, respectively. Rhodopsin, which contains *cis*-retinal (the aldehyde form of vitamin A), absorbs the light entering the rods. The light changes the shape of *cis*-retinal to *trans*-retinal, detaching it from the protein opsin. This change in shape is referred to as **bleaching**. When rhodopsin is bleached, it transmits a signal through the optic nerve to the part of the brain involved in vision.

After rhodopsin is bleached, most of the *trans*-retinal returns to its *cis* shape. This form is now able to bind with opsin, which regenerates rhodopsin and the eye's light-absorbing capabilities. This reaction is illustrated in **Focus Figure 9.7**.

Walking into a dark building after being in the sun without sunglasses may require taking time to adjust to the dimmer light. This adjustment period occurs because the reformation of *trans* to *cis*-retinal takes time. Fortunately, there is a pool of

vitamin A in the retina to help with this conversion.

In order for vitamin A to participate in the visual cycle, it must first be metabolized in the retina. Retinol attaches to retinol-binding protein (RBP) and is transported through the blood to the eye. Once inside the retina, retinol is converted to retinal before moving into the photoreceptor cells of the rods.

Vitamin A Maintains Epithelial Tissues

Vitamin A is important for maintaining the body's **epithelial tissues**. The surface of the skin is a stratified epithelial tissue, whereas the tissue that lines the lungs, nose, eyes, and urinary tract is a columnar epithelium. Columnar epithelial cells are tall, moist, secrete a thick mucus, and are lined with microscopic hair-like structures called *cilia*. The mucus coats the cells and protects them from bacteria and viruses that can infiltrate the body and cause infection. In the respiratory tract, the cilia sweep away dust and germs trapped in the mucus. Vitamin A deficiency can cause these cells to become flattened, hard, and unable to produce mucus (**Figure 9.8**).

Vitamin A stimulates **cell division** and **cell differentiation** of epithelial cells as they grow and develop.[25] Retinoic acid signals genes to make the proteins needed to begin cell division. As cells divide, changes occur that cause them to differentiate from the parent cells. This differentiation determines what cells become in the body; for example, skin cells or bronchial lining cells.

This role of vitamin A is one reason dermatologists prescribe retinoid-based medications for skin conditions, including acne (**Figure 9.9**). Most of these medications are available only by prescription, but the FDA recently approved an over-the-counter (OTC) medication to fight acne called Differin. This new gel contains adapalene, a retinoid, which regulates the turnover of skin cells, inhibits the formation of acne, and reduces inflammation and redness.[26]

Vitamin A in Growth, Reproduction, and Immunity

In addition to its role in cell differentiation, vitamin A plays several critical roles in growth and reproduction. Both retinol

FOCUS Figure 9.7 Retinal and Its Role in Vision

Head to Mastering Nutrition and watch a narrated video tour of this figure by author Joan Salge Blake.

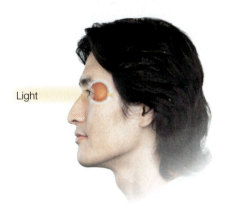

Light

Vitamin A is a component of two light-sensitive proteins, rhodopsin and iodopsin, that are essential for vision. Here we examine rhodopsin's role in vision. Although the breakdown of iodopsin is similar, rhodopsin is more sensitive to light than iodopsin and is more likely to become bleached.

EYE STRUCTURE

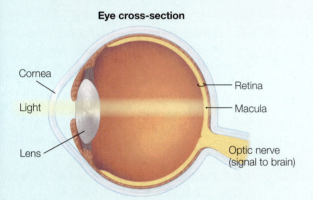

Eye cross-section

Cornea

Light

Lens

Retina

Macula

Optic nerve (signal to brain)

Rod and cone cells in retina

Rod

Cone

Rhodopsin protein in rod cell membrane

Rhodopsin

Opsin

Cis-retinal (Vitamin A)

1 After light enters your eye through the cornea, it travels to the back of your eye to the macula, which is located in the retina. The macula allows you to see fine details and things that are straight in front of you.

2 Inside the retina are two types of light-absorbing cells, rods and cones. Rods are responsible for black-and-white vision and contain the protein rhodopsin. Cones are responsible for color vision and contain the protein iodopsin. Both proteins contain vitamin A in the form of *cis*-retinal.

EFFECT OF LIGHT ON RHODOPSIN

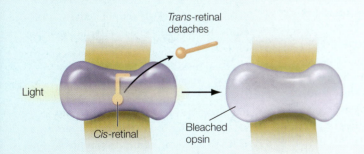

Trans-retinal detaches

Light

Cis-retinal

Bleached opsin

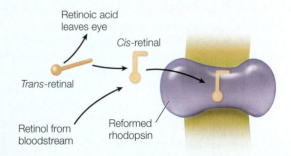

Retinoic acid leaves eye

Cis-retinal

Trans-retinal

Retinol from bloodstream

Reformed rhodopsin

1 As light interacts with rhodopsin, it transforms the *cis*-retinal to *trans*-retinal, separating it from the protein opsin. This process, called bleaching, causes a cascade of events that transmits visual messages through the optic nerve to the brain.

2 *Trans*-retinal is converted back to *cis*-retinal and binds with opsin to reform rhodopsin, regenerating the eye's light-absorbing capabilities. Some *trans*-retinal is irreversibly converted to retinoic acid and leaves the eye tissue. Retinol from the blood is converted to retinal to replenish what is lost.

(continued)

Vitamin A (continued)

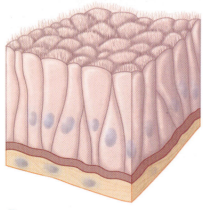

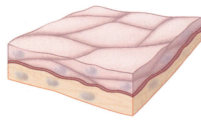

a Healthy columnar epithelial cells are tall, moist, secrete mucus, and are lined with cilia.

b A vitamin A deficiency can lead to flattened epithelial cells that are hard, lacking cilia, and unable to produce mucus.

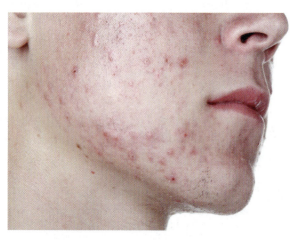

▲ **Figure 9.9 Vitamin A Derivatives Can Help Treat Acne**

and retinoic acid participate in growth, although the mechanism is still unknown. What is known is that without vitamin A, embryonic and fetal development is impaired, especially the development of the limbs, heart, eyes, and ears.[27] Children fail to grow when their diets lack vitamin A, but when either retinol or retinoic acid are given, growth is enhanced.

Retinol, but not retinoic acid, is essential for reproduction. Normal levels of retinol are required for sperm production in males and normal menstrual cycles in females.

Vitamin A also works with the immune system to create white blood cells (*lymphocytes*) and antibodies that fight foreign invaders should they enter the bloodstream. Vitamin A deficiency significantly increases the risk of infectious disease.

Vitamin A and Bone Health

All three forms of vitamin A may help regulate the cells involved in bone growth. Too much vitamin A stimulates bone resorption—breaking down bone—and inhibits bone formation, which can negatively affect healthy bones and may be a risk factor for developing osteoporosis.[28] Both excessive intake and insufficient intake of vitamin A have negative impacts on bone density. Research reports that retinol intakes of less than 510 μg RAE (1,700 IU) and more than 2,030 μg RAE (6,700 IU) per day may increase fracture risk (beta-carotene has no effect).[29] A diet closer to 600–850 μg RAE (2,000–2,800 IU) per day of vitamin A is most likely to improve the bone mineral density of elderly men and women.[30]

Carotenoids as Antioxidants

The carotenoids lycopene, lutein, and zeaxanthin are considered nonprovitamin A compounds because the body does not convert them to vitamin A as it does other carotenoids such as beta-carotene. However, nonprovitamin A compounds are able to stabilize free radicals and protect cells from oxidative damage. Lycopene, which is the form of carotenoid that gives red tomatoes their dark red color, is especially effective in quenching free radicals. Lutein and zeaxanthin (found in corn and dark green leafy vegetables) protect the eyes from free radical damage.[31]

Daily Needs for Vitamin A

The RDA for vitamin A is based on maintaining sufficient storage of the vitamin in the liver. Vitamin A in foods and supplements can be measured in two ways: in micrograms (μg) of **retinol activity equivalents (RAE)** and in **international units (IU)**.

Because retinol is the most usable form of vitamin A and because provitamin A carotenoids can be converted to retinol, the preferred way to measure vitamin A in foods is to include all forms as RAE. However, some vitamin supplements and food labels show the older measure, IU, on their products. (Note: 1 μg RAE is the equivalent of 3.3 IU.) The Calculation Corner provides more detail on the conversion from IU to micrograms RAE.

retinol activity equivalents (RAE) Unit of measure used to describe the total amount of all forms of preformed vitamin A and provitamin A carotenoids in food.

international units (IU) System of measurement of a biologically active ingredient such as a vitamin that produces a certain effect.

Calculation Corner

Converting International Units for Vitamin A

International units (IU) are a system of measurement of the biologic activity or potency of a substance, such as a vitamin, that produces a particular effect. Because each vitamin differs in potency per milligram, the conversion factors from IU to milligrams also differ.

(a) Vitamin A is measured in retinol activity equivalents, or RAE. Use the following conversion factors to determine the micrograms retinol activity equivalents (μg RAE) found in 1 IU:

> 1 IU retinol is the biological equivalent of 0.3 μg retinol or 0.3 μg RAE or 0.6 μg beta-carotene

Example: A vitan misupplement contains 25,000 IU of retinol. How many μg RAE does it contain?

Answer: 0.3 μg $\times$ 25,000 IU
= 7,500 μg RAE

(b) The requirements for vitamin A are expressed as RAE. To determine the amount of RAE in micrograms in a meal, you have to convert the various forms of vitamin A equivalents. For example:

> 1 μg RAE = 1 μg retinol and 12 μg beta-carotene

The first step is to divide the amount of beta-carotene by 12 to convert to RAE. Next, add that number to the preformed vitamin A in the meal.

Example: If a meal contains 500 μg retinol and 1,800 μg beta-carotene, how many μg RAE does the meal contain?

Answer: 500 μg retinol + (1,800 μg beta-carotene $\div$ 12) = 650 μg RAE

Adult females need 700 μg RAE (2,310 IU) of vitamin A daily, whereas adult males need 900 μg RAE (3,000 IU) daily. This is the average amount needed to maintain adequate stores in the liver.[32] A daily recommendation for beta-carotene hasn't been established, but the Institute of Medicine suggests consuming 3–6 milligrams of beta-carotene every day from foods.[33] This can easily be obtained by consuming five or more servings of fruits and vegetables. This amount of beta-carotene also provides about 50 percent of the recommended vitamin A intake. Hence, eating beta-carotene-rich foods adds not only antioxidants to the diet, but also vitamin A.

Vitamin A is provided by both milk and eggs, so vegans need to be especially conscientious about eating carotenoid-rich foods to meet their daily vitamin A needs.

Food Sources of Vitamin A

Milk, cereals, cheese, egg yolks, and organ meats (such as liver) are the most popular sources of preformed vitamin A in the U.S. diet. Liver is especially abundant in vitamin A but can cause toxicity if consumed too often. For example, just 1 ounce of beef liver contains 2 milligrams of retinol, or more than 100 percent of the RDA of vitamin A for adults.

Carrots, spinach, and sweet potatoes are American favorites for provitamin A carotenoids, including beta-carotene. Like vitamin A and other fat-soluble vitamins, carotenoids are absorbed more efficiently when fat is present in the GI tract. Adding as little as 1 tablespoon of vegetable oil, such as in salad dressing, to the diet daily can increase the absorption of carotenoids by as much as 25 percent.[34]

Figure 9.10 shows the vitamin A content in μg RAE, and includes both retinoid- and carotenoid-rich sources.

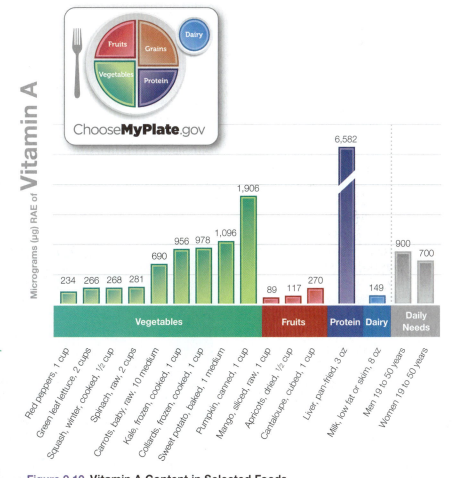

▲ **Figure 9.10** **Vitamin A Content in Selected Foods**

Source: Data from *USDA What's In The Food You Eat?* 2016. Available at https://www.ars.usda.gov. Accessed March 2017.

(continued)

Vitamin A Toxicity

Ingesting too much preformed vitamin A, not carotenoids, causes vitamin A toxicity. Consuming more than 15,000 μg of preformed vitamin A at one time or over a short period of time can lead to nausea and vomiting, headaches, dizziness, and blurred vision. Overconsumption of preformed vitamin A is usually due to taking supplements and is less likely to occur from overeating vitamin A in foods. Vitamin A supplements do not improve acne. Only specially formulated retinoid medications are effective for preventing and treating acne.

Because 90 percent of vitamin A is stored in the liver, chronic daily consumption of more than 30,000 micrograms of preformed vitamin A (more than 300 times the RDA for adults) can lead to **hypervitaminosis A** (*hyper* = over, *osis* = condition), an extremely serious condition in which the liver accumulates toxic levels of vitamin A. Hypervitaminosis A can lead to deterioration and scarring of the liver and even death. To prevent toxicity, the UL of preformed vitamin A for adults has been set at 3,000 μg (10,000 IU) daily.[35]

Higher intake of preformed vitamin A during pregnancy, particularly in the first trimester, can cause birth defects in the face and skull and damage the child's central nervous system. All women of childbearing age who are using retinoids for acne or other skin conditions are required to use an effective form of contraception to avoid becoming pregnant.[36]

Excessive Vitamin A and Osteoporosis

While vitamin A is needed for bone health, some research suggests that consuming too much may lead to osteoporosis, which in turn increases the risk of fractures. Osteoporosis-related hip fractures appear to be prevalent in Swedes and Norwegians, who tend to have high consumption of vitamin A–rich cod-liver oil and specialty dairy products that have been heavily fortified with vitamin A.[37]

Additional studies involving both women and men have shown similar associations between high vitamin A intake and increased risk of fractures. As little as 1,500 micrograms (3,000 IU) of retinol, which is slightly more than twice the RDA recommended for women, can be unhealthy for bones.[38] This amount can be quickly reached when taking a supplement and eating a diet rich in vitamin A–fortified foods.

Overconsuming Carotenoids

The upper levels apply only to preformed vitamin A from foods, fortified foods, and supplements. High levels of provitamin A carotenoids are not toxic. Moreover, if individuals consume more carotenoids than necessary to meet vitamin A needs, the body decreases their conversion to retinol. Extra amounts of carotenoids are stored in the liver and in the subcutaneous fat.

Eating too many carotenoids can, however, cause the nonthreatening condition **carotenodermia** (*carotene* = carotene, *dermia* = skin), which results in orange-tinged skin, particularly in the palms of the hands and soles of the feet (**Figure 9.11**). Because these areas are cushioned with fat, they become more concentrated with the pigments and more visibly orange in color (right hand in photo). Cutting back on carotenoid-rich foods reverses carotenodermia.

Overconsuming Beta-Carotene Supplements

Although a diet abundant in carotenoid-rich foods is not dangerous, carotenoid supplements may be. In a study of adult male smokers, those who consumed beta-carotene supplements were shown to have significantly higher rates of lung cancer than those who didn't take the supplements.[39] While some earlier studies suggested alcohol may contribute to the effects of beta-carotene supplements on lung cancer risk, more recent research shows consistent evidence that beta-carotene supplements alone increase a smoker's risk of lung cancer and mortality.[40]

Vitamin A Deficiency

Vitamin A deficiency is uncommon in the United States but is a serious problem in developing countries. Signs of vitamin A deficiency begin to develop after the liver stores of vitamin A are depleted. To boost your intake of vitamin A, see the Table Tips.

hypervitaminosis A Serious condition in which the liver accumulates toxic levels of vitamin A.

carotenodermia Presence of excess carotene in the blood, resulting in an orange color to the skin due to excessive intake of carrots or other carotene-rich vegetables.

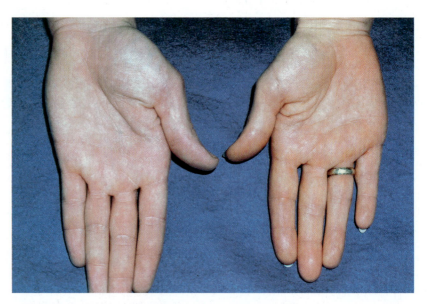

▲ **Figure 9.11 Carotenodermia**
The hand on the right exhibits the orange-tinged skin characteristic of carotenodermia.

TABLE TIPS

Score an A

Dunk baby carrots in a tablespoon of low-fat ranch dressing for a healthy snack.

Keep dried apricots in your backpack for a sweet treat.

Add baby spinach to a lunchtime salad.

Bake sweet potatoes rather than white potatoes at dinner.

Buy frozen mango chunks for a ready-to-thaw beta-carotene-rich addition to cottage cheese or yogurt.

Vitamin A Deficiency and Blindness

If the diet is deficient in vitamin A, an insufficient pool of retinal in the retina can result in **night blindness**, or the inability

night blindness Inability to see in dim light or at night due to a deficiency of retinal in the retina.

xerophthalmia Permanent damage to the cornea causing blindness; due to a prolonged vitamin A deficiency.

keratinization Accumulation of the protein keratin in epithelial cells, forming hard, dry cells unable to secrete mucus; due to vitamin A deficiency.

to see in the dark. Individuals with night blindness have difficulty seeing at dusk because they can't adjust from daylight to dark and may not be able to drive a car during this time of the day. If diagnosed early, taking vitamin A can reverse night blindness.

A prolonged vitamin A deficiency can lead to complete blindness. A severe deficiency of vitamin A results in dryness and permanent damage to the cornea, a condition called **xerophthalmia** (*xero* = dry, *ophthalm* = eye). Up to 10 million children, mostly in developing countries, suffer from xerophthalmia annually, and as many as 500,000 of these children go blind every year because they don't consume enough vitamin A.[41] Vitamin A deficiency is the number-one cause of preventable blindness in children.[42]

Vitamin A Deficiency, Keratinization, and Infection

Keratin is a fibrous protein found in the epithelial cells of the skin, as well as in hair and nails. With vitamin A deficiency, inappropriate **keratinization** of the epithelial tissues occurs throughout the body. In this process, healthy epithelial cells are replaced by hard, dry keratinized cells, which are unable to secrete a protective layer of mucus. Without mucus, the cells are unable to function properly, and they become susceptible to infection, especially in the nasal passages and the urinary and respiratory tracts. Keratinization also occurs in the eyes, contributing to xerophthalmia.

LO 9.5: THE TAKE-HOME MESSAGE

Vitamin A refers to a family of retinoids, which are essential for cell growth and development, reproduction, and a healthy immune system. Retinol is the most usable form of vitamin A in the body; retinal is essential for eye health and vision and retinoic acid regulates growth. Retinyl ester is found in foods and the form of vitamin A stored in the liver. Vitamin A is not excreted. Three carotenoids, including beta-carotene, are provitamins that must be converted to vitamin A to be used in the body. Most of the preformed dietary vitamin A, measured as retinol activity equivalents (RAE), is absorbed. Preformed vitamin A is found in milk, cereals, cheese, egg yolks, and organ meats, especially liver. Provitamin A is found in carrots, spinach, and sweet potatoes. Vitamin A deficiencies can result in vision problems and increased infections. Toxic amounts of vitamin A can compromise bone health and lead to birth defects during pregnancy.

EXPLORING **Vitamin D**

LO 9.6 Describe the functions, recommended intakes, food sources, and deficiency and toxicity effects of vitamin D.

What Is Vitamin D?

Vitamin D (**calciferol**) is called the "sunshine vitamin" because it is derived from the reaction between ultraviolet (UV) rays and a form of cholesterol found in the skin. Exposure to sunlight can enable the synthesis of 100 percent of the vitamin D the body needs.[43] For this reason, vitamin D is often considered a conditionally essential nutrient. However, it still fits the criteria of a vitamin because a deficiency can cause symptoms that are cured once adequate intake is restored.

Vitamin D is found in two forms. **Ergocalciferol (vitamin D$_2$)** is found in plants and dietary supplements. **Cholecalciferol (vitamin D$_3$)** is the form produced in the skin and found in animal foods.

calciferol Family of vitamin D compounds.

ergocalciferol (vitamin D$_2$) Form of vitamin D found in plants and dietary supplements.

cholecalciferol (vitamin D$_3$) Form of vitamin D found in animal foods, supplements, and formed from precalciferol in the skin; absorbed from the skin into the blood.

(continued)

Vitamin D (continued)

Form found in plant foods

Form found in animal foods and made by the body

Vitamin D$_2$ (ergocalciferol)

Vitamin D$_3$ (cholecalciferol)

▲ **Figure 9.12 The Chemical Structure of Vitamin D**
Vitamin D is found in the ergocalciferol (vitamin D$_2$) form in plants and the cholecalciferol (vitamin D$_3$) form in animal foods.

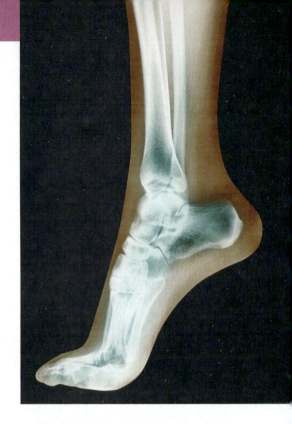

Ergocalciferol and cholecalciferol differ chemically in the structure of their side chains, as illustrated in **Figure 9.12**. Ergocalciferol or D$_2$ contains a double bond in the side chain between carbons 22 and 23 and a methyl group on carbon 24. Cholecalciferol or D$_3$ has a single bond in the place of the double bond and two hydrogens on carbon 24. Even though their structures are different, they both have the same function in the body.

Vitamin D Metabolism

Whether from food or sunlight, vitamin D is obtained in an inactive form. In the skin, a compound called 7-dehydrocholesterol or provitamin D$_3$ (which is made in the liver from cholesterol) is converted to previtamin D$_3$ or precalciferol when UV rays hit the skin (see **Figure 9.13**). Precalciferol is changed to cholecalciferol, which

1,25-dihydroxycholecalciferol (calcitriol) Active form of vitamin D.

parathyroid hormone (PTH) Hormone secreted from the parathyroid glands that activates vitamin D formation in the kidney.

prohormone Physiologically inactive precursor to a hormone.

slowly diffuses from the skin into the blood attached to a protein called vitamin D$_3$ binding protein (DBP). Cholecalciferol is then taken up by the liver to begin the activation process.

Once cholecalciferol reaches the liver, a two-step activation process begins. First, liver enzymes add a hydroxyl group on the 25th carbon of cholecalciferol, forming 25-hydroxycholecalciferol (see step 3 in Figure 9.13). This newly formed compound circulates in the blood transported by DBP. In the kidneys a second hydroxyl group is added on the first carbon, forming **1,25-dihydroxycholecalciferol** (also known as *calcitriol*). This is the active form of vitamin D that leaves the kidney and enters the cells (see step 4 in Figure 9.13).

Vitamin D$_2$ and vitamin D$_3$ consumed in the diet are absorbed into the small intestine as part of a micelle along with other dietary lipids. Each is repackaged into chylomicrons and circulates through the lymph system before arriving at the liver for storage.

Blood calcium levels influence the metabolism of vitamin D (see **Figure 9.14**). When blood calcium levels drop, **parathyroid hormone (PTH)** is secreted from the parathyroid gland and travels to the kidney to activate vitamin D.

This boost in the levels of active vitamin D enhances the intestinal absorption of calcium, increases the amount of calcium reabsorbed through the kidneys, and mobilizes calcium from the bone. The result is that blood calcium levels return to normal.

Metabolic Functions of Vitamin D

Vitamin D regulates two important bone minerals, calcium and phosphorus. Vitamin D also participates in several other functions, including cell differentiation, stimulation of the immune system, blood pressure regulation, and insulin secretion.

Vitamin D Helps Maintain Bone Mass

We just noted that, upon activation by PTH, vitamin D helps regulate blood calcium levels. In this role, it functions as a **prohormone**, an inactive hormone precursor, that is activated inside the body. Vitamin D also functions to maintain a healthy ratio of calcium and phosphorus levels in the blood, which promotes uptake of these two minerals in the bone. As calcium levels in the blood rise, more calcium is deposited in the bone. Vitamin D controls the interaction between *osteoblasts* and *osteoclasts*, specialized bone cells involved in remodeling bone. Because of its role in regulating calcium and

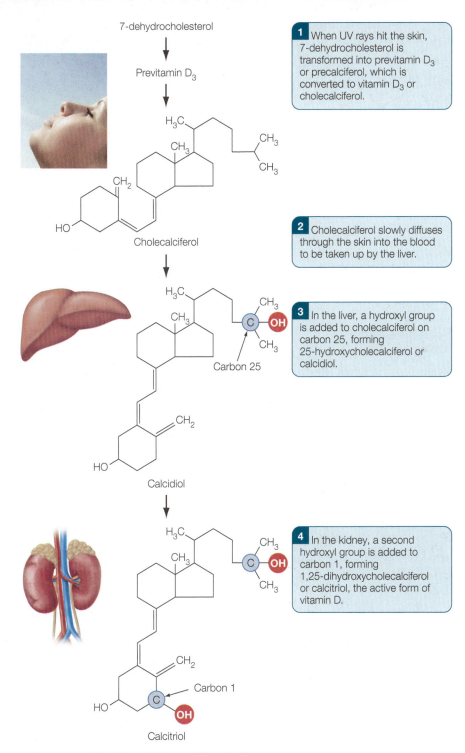

1. When UV rays hit the skin, 7-dehydrocholesterol is transformed into previtamin D_3 or precalciferol, which is converted to vitamin D_3 or cholecalciferol.

2. Cholecalciferol slowly diffuses through the skin into the blood to be taken up by the liver.

3. In the liver, a hydroxyl group is added to cholecalciferol on carbon 25, forming 25-hydroxycholecalciferol or calcidiol.

4. In the kidney, a second hydroxyl group is added to carbon 1, forming 1,25-dihydroxycholecalciferol or calcitriol, the active form of vitamin D.

▲ Figure 9.13 The Metabolism of Vitamin D

phosphorus, vitamin D helps to build and maintain bone mass.

Vitamin D Helps Regulate the Growth of Cells

Research studies have shown that the incidence of breast, colon, and prostate cancers is greater among individuals living in sun-poor areas of the world than among those living in sunny regions.[44] Vitamin D helps regulate the growth and differentiation of certain cells. Researchers speculate that a deficiency of vitamin D in the body may reduce the proliferation of healthy cells and allow cancer cells to flourish.[45]

Vitamin D May Regulate the Immune System

Adequate intake of vitamin D may reduce the risk of developing certain autoimmune disorders, such as inflammatory bowel disease. Most cells in the immune system, such as T cells and macrophages, have a receptor for vitamin D. The role of vitamin D in immune system function is still not understood, but some researchers suggest that it may affect the function of the immune system and inhibit the development of autoimmunity.[46]

Vitamin D may also help reduce the risk of type 1 diabetes (also an autoimmune disease) by up to 50 percent in adults.[47] A large prospective study of military personnel reported that the risk of developing type 1 diabetes was highest when blood levels of 25-hydroxycholecalciferol fell below 20 percent of normal.[48] The researchers proposed that low levels of 25-hydroxycholecalciferol might contribute to the autoimmune process. Low levels of vitamin D have also been reported in individuals who have been diagnosed with type 2 diabetes mellitus, which is not an autoimmune disorder.[49] Another study revealed that insulin resistance was more pronounced in people with low levels of vitamin D in the blood, perhaps reflecting interactions between vitamin D and multiple genes.[50]

Vitamin D May Help Regulate Blood Pressure

Vitamin D reduces hypertension by acting on the gene that regulates the renin-angiotensin system, the system that helps regulate blood pressure.[51] Vitamin D appears to reduce the activity of this gene, which results in less renin being produced. Renin is an enzyme that activates angiotensin, which helps balance sodium and potassium levels in the blood, which affects blood pressure (we discuss the relationship of renin to hypertension in Chapter 11). In addition, blood pressure readings tend to be higher during the winter, when people are exposed to less sunlight, than in the summer. People with mild hypertension may be able to lower their blood pressure by spending a little time in the sun.

(continued)

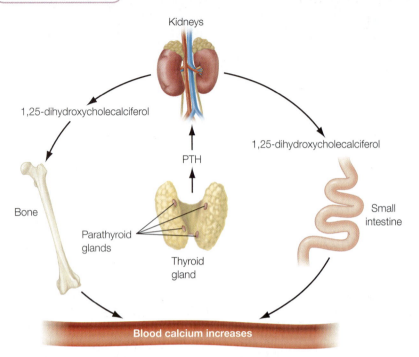

Kidneys

1,25-dihydroxycholecalciferol

1,25-dihydroxycholecalciferol

PTH

Bone

Parathyroid glands

Thyroid gland

Small intestine

Blood calcium increases

▲ **Figure 9.14 The Relationship of Blood Calcium to Parathyroid Hormone and Vitamin D**
Low blood levels of calcium stimulate the parathyroid glands to release parathyroid hormone (PTH). PTH stimulates the kidneys to increase the amount of active vitamin D, which in turn increases calcium absorption from the intestines, stimulates the reabsorption of calcium through the kidneys, and releases calcium from the bone. These actions help raise blood calcium back to normal levels.

Daily Needs for Vitamin D

Not everyone can rely on the sun to meet his or her daily vitamin D needs. There are a number of limiting factors that influence vitamin D synthesis from sun: melanin content of the skin, whether it is cloudy or smoggy, and use of sunscreen. Vitamin D can be synthesized in the skin in adequate amounts at any latitude in the spring, summer, and fall. Because of cloud cover in the winter months, vitamin D synthesis on the skin from the sun can be low.[52]

Individuals with darker skin, such as African Americans, have a higher amount of the skin pigment melanin, which reduces vitamin D production from sunlight. To derive the same amount of vitamin D as people with less melanin, these individuals need a longer period of sun exposure. A cloudy day can reduce the synthesis of vitamin D by 50 percent, and by 60 percent if it is smoggy or you sit in the shade. And the use of sunscreen can block the body's ability to synthesize vitamin

D by more than 95 percent.[53] Because of these variables involving sun exposure, daily vitamin D needs are based on the amount in foods and are not based on the synthesis of vitamin D in the skin from exposure to sunlight.

The RDA for adults is 15–20 micrograms (600–800 IU) of vitamin D daily, depending on your age. These recommendations are listed on supplement labels in both micrograms and international units. Learn how to convert micrograms to IUs in the Calculation Corner.

The RDA for children has been set at 15 micrograms (600 IU) of vitamin D per day for children ages 1–13. Vitamin D supplementation as high as 2,500 IUs is

safe for children ages 1–3 and up to 3,000 IUs for children 4–8 years old.[54]

When reading labels to assess the amount of vitamin D in foods, keep in mind that the %DV on the Nutrition Facts panel is set at 400 IU, a recommendation based on an older DRI for vitamin D. This means that the amount of vitamin D in a serving of a packaged food does not reflect the new, higher recommendations for children and adults.[55]

Food Sources of Vitamin D

One of the easiest ways to get vitamin D from food is to drink fortified milk, which provides 100 IU, or 2.5 micrograms, of vitamin D per 8 fluid ounces. Other than fortified milk and soymilk, breakfast cereals, yogurt, and fatty fish (such as sardines and salmon), very few foods provide ample amounts of vitamin D (see **Figure 9.15**). With this scarcity of naturally occurring food sources, it isn't surprising that many Americans are not meeting their daily vitamin D needs.[56]

Vitamin D Toxicity

The UL for vitamin D has been set at 100 micrograms (4,000 IU) for individuals nine years or older. This upper limit is over six times higher than the recommended daily amount. Consuming too much vitamin D can cause loss of appetite, nausea and vomiting, and constipation.

As with the other fat-soluble vitamins, excess amounts of vitamin D are stored in the adipocytes and an accumulation can reach toxic levels, causing **hypervitaminosis D**. This condition causes overabsorption of calcium from the intestines as well as calcium loss from bones. When both of these symptoms occur, blood calcium levels can become dangerously high.

A chronically high amount of calcium in the blood, or **hypercalcemia** (*hyper* = over, *calc* = calcium, *emia* =

blood), can cause damaging calcium deposits in the tissues of the kidneys, lungs, blood vessels, and heart. Excess vitamin D can also affect the nervous system and cause severe depression.[57]

Hypervitaminosis D rarely occurs as a result of consuming too much vitamin D from foods, even fortified foods. The only exception is fish oils, specifically cod-liver oil, which provides 34 micrograms (1,360 IU) of vitamin D per tablespoon. Luckily, the less-than-pleasant taste of cod-liver oil is a safeguard against overconsumption. A more likely culprit behind hypervitaminosis D is the overuse of vitamin D supplements.

Sun worshippers don't have to worry about hypervitaminosis D from the sun (although they should be concerned about the risk of skin cancer). Overexposing the skin to UV rays eventually destroys the

inactive form of vitamin D in the skin, causing the body to shut down production of vitamin D. It is estimated that about 10–20 minutes of sun exposure two to three times per week is sufficient to obtain adequate vitamin D.[58]

Vitamin D Deficiency

Vitamin D deficiencies are increasing worldwide. Factors contributing to this trend are thought to include individuals' misunderstanding of the critical role of sunshine as a source of vitamin D, as well as poor dietary intake of vitamin D. To boost your intake of vitamin D, see the Table Tips.

Rickets is one of the consequences of a lack of sunshine and insufficient dietary intake of vitamin D in children (**Figure 9.16**). The bones of children with rickets aren't adequately mineralized with calcium and phosphorus, and this causes them to weaken. Because of their "soft bones," these children cannot hold up

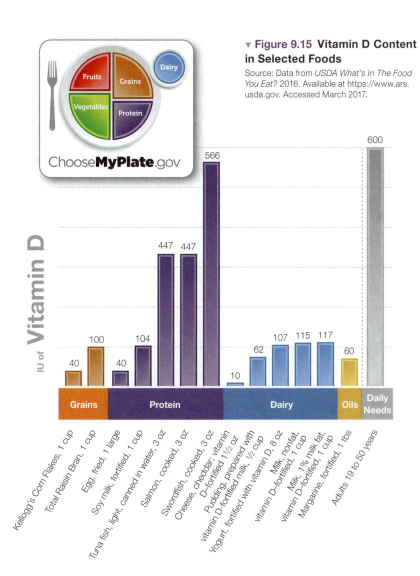

▼ **Figure 9.15 Vitamin D Content in Selected Foods**

Source: Data from *USDA What's In The Food You Eat?* 2016. Available at https://www.ars.usda.gov. Accessed March 2017.

TABLE TIPS

Ways to Get Vitamin D

Use vitamin D–fortified low-fat milk, not cream, in hot or iced coffee.

Buy vitamin D–fortified low-fat yogurts and have one daily as a snack. Top it with a vitamin D–fortified cereal for another boost of D.

Start the morning with vitamin D–fortified cereal and low-fat milk or fortified soymilk.

Flake canned salmon over a lunchtime salad.

Make instant hot cocoa with hot milk rather than water.

Drink vitamin D–fortified orange juice with breakfast.

---

hypervitaminosis D Condition resulting from excessive amounts of vitamin D in the body.

hypercalcemia Chronically high amount of calcium in the blood.

rickets Vitamin D deficiency in children resulting in soft bones.

(continued)

Vitamin D (continued)

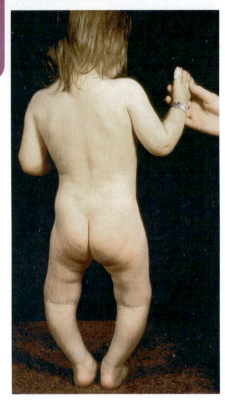

▲ **Figure 9.16 Rickets**
Rickets can cause bowed legs in children.

their own body weight and develop bowed legs.[59] Babies with rickets also have a delayed closure of the anterior fontanel or "soft spot" in the skull.[60, 61]

Since fortification of milk with vitamin D began in the 1930s, rickets has been considered a rare disease among children in the United States. However, the disease has resurfaced as a public health concern, with studies of clinical records in both Georgia and Boston revealing a notable increase in both vitamin D deficiency and rickets.[62] The majority of cases of rickets in the United States have been African American infants who were solely breastfed. In Canada, the incidence of rickets was reported as 2.9 per 100,000 infants, almost all of whom were breastfed.[63] Because the vitamin D content of breast milk is affected by the vitamin D status of the mother, the American Academy

osteomalacia Adult equivalent of rickets, causing muscle and bone weakness and pain.

of Pediatrics recommends that all breastfed infants receive a supplement of 10 micrograms (400 IU) per day until they are also consuming 32 ounces of vitamin D–fortified formula or whole milk daily.[64]

The *2015–2020 Dietary Guidelines for Americans* and the Academy of Pediatrics recommends that all children 2 years and older drink low-fat milk to promote bone health. A National Health and Nutrition Examination Survey (NHANES) of children 2–19 years of age conducted from 2007 to 2008 reported that an average of 70 percent of children are drinking milk daily, most of which was 2 percent milk.[65] Children should be encouraged to drink low-fat milk to lower kilocalorie intake but at the same time consume a good source of vitamin D and calcium.

Increased concern over skin cancer may be a factor in the rise of rickets among American children. Skin cancer is the most common form of cancer in the United States, and childhood sun exposure appears to increase the risk of skin cancer in later years.[66] Because of this, organizations such as the Centers for Disease Control and the American Cancer Society have run campaigns that recommend limiting exposure to ultraviolet light. People are encouraged to use sunscreen, wear protective clothing when outdoors, and minimize activities in the sun. The American Academy of Pediatrics also recommends that infants younger than 6 months not be exposed to direct sunlight. With less exposure to UV light, many children aren't able to synthesize vitamin D in adequate amounts to meet

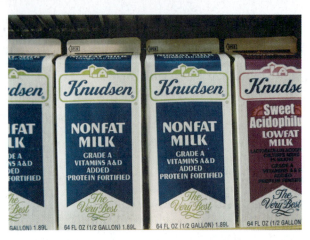

Most milk, such as Knudsen sold in the United States today, has been fortified with vitamin D.

their needs, thereby increasing their risk of developing rickets. The increased use of childcare facilities, which may limit outdoor activities during the day, may also play a role in this increased prevalence of rickets.

Osteomalacia, the adult equivalent of rickets, can cause muscle and bone weakness and pain. The bones can't mineralize properly because there isn't enough calcium and phosphorus available in the blood. Although there may be adequate amounts of these minerals in the diet, the deficiency of vitamin D reduces their absorption. Explore the Nutrition in Practice on page 341. How can Abby's mother improve her vitamin D intake to reduce her risk of osteomalacia?

Vitamin D deficiency and its subsequent effect on decreased calcium absorption can lead to osteoporosis, a condition

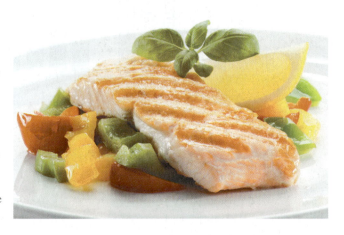

NUTRITION *in* PRACTICE:
Nurse Practitioner

Abby's mom is a cosmetologist, so Abby knows the effect of sunlight exposure and its impact on the aging of skin. Even though Abby grew up in Wisconsin, her mother lathered her up with a SPF 30 sunscreen every day before she left for school or went outside to play, and always dressed Abby in hats and lightweight long-sleeved shirts and pants in the summer. To Abby, putting on sunscreen and covering her skin from hat to toe before leaving the house is as routine as brushing her teeth.

For her college admission, Abby needed to get a complete physical. When the nurse practitioner (NP) was asking about Abby's family history, he uncovered that her mom has osteomalacia. The NP ordered a blood laboratory test. After the laboratory report came back, he called Abby to tell her that her blood level of vitamin D was on the low side of normal and suggested she visit a registered dietitian nutritionist (RDN).

Abby's Stats
- ❏ Age: 17
- ❏ Height: 5 feet 5 inches
- ❏ Weight: 128 pounds

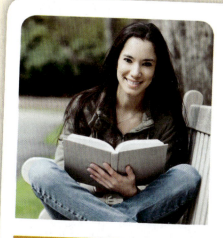

Abby

ABBY'S FOOD LOG

Food/Beverage	Time Consumed	Hunger Rating*	Location
Nothing	6:00 AM	3	
Bagel with cream cheese	9:30 AM	5	High school cafeteria
Turkey and Swiss cheese sandwich, chips, cola	12:30 PM	5	High school cafeteria
Cheese and crackers	3:30 PM	3	Kitchen
Pizza, 2 slices	6:30 PM	4	With friends in a restaurant

* Hunger Rating (1–5): 1 = not hungry; 5 = super hungry.

Critical Thinking Questions

1. What symptoms might Abby expect to have if her levels of vitamin D continue to decline?
2. Why does Abby's avoidance of sunlight increase her potential deficiency of vitamin D?
3. Based on her food record, why do you think that she is deficient in vitamin D?

RDN's Observation and Plan for Abby

- ❏ Discuss the need to add vitamin D–fortified foods to her diet to meet her daily needs. Explain why cheese is a good source of calcium, but it does not contain vitamin D.
- ❏ Confirm that Abby will eat cereal with skim or low-fat milk for breakfast prior to leaving for school, have a vitamin D–fortified yogurt as a daily afternoon snack, and consume a large glass of skim or low-fat milk with dinner.

A month later, Abby returns to the RDN. Because she often eats dinner with her friends at the local pizzeria, she is having a difficult time routinely having a glass of milk with dinner. The dietitian recommends that Abby consume a glass of milk or a mug of hot cocoa made with milk daily when she gets home in the evening.

(continued)

in which a decline in bone density significantly increases the individual's risk of a fracture.

Muscle weakness and pain is also associated with low serum vitamin D concentrations. One study found that a vitamin D supplement of 1,000 IU per day was effective in significantly reducing the number of falls reported by elderly women.[67]

LO 9.6: THE TAKE-HOME MESSAGE Vitamin D can be made in the skin from exposure to ultraviolet rays from the sun. The active form of vitamin D is calcitriol. Vitamin D regulates blood calcium, enhances the absorption of calcium and phosphorus from the small intestine, and maintains healthy bones. It may also help regulate blood pressure and the immune system, and it may play a role in preventing diabetes and some cancers. Fortified dairy products and soymilk are excellent food sources of vitamin D. A deficiency of vitamin D can cause rickets in children and osteomalacia in adults. Hypervitaminosis D can result in hypercalcemia, affect the nervous system, and cause severe depression.

EXPLORING Vitamin E

LO 9.7 Describe the functions, recommended intakes, food sources, and deficiency and toxicity effects of vitamin E.

What Is Vitamin E?

There are eight different forms of naturally occurring vitamin E, but one form, **alpha-tocopherol (α-tocopherol),** is most active in the body. Notice the long side chain of saturated carbons (**Figure 9.17**). The synthetic form of vitamin E found in dietary supplements is only half as active as the natural form. Alpha-tocopherol is the only form of vitamin E that is reflected in the Dietary Reference Intakes.

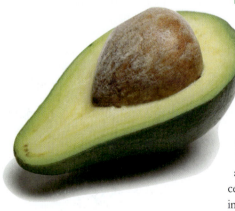

alpha-tocopherol (α-tocopherol) Most active form of vitamin E in the body.

Vitamin E Absorption and Transport

Vitamin E is absorbed with the aid of bile and micelles into the enterocytes. Once absorbed, vitamin E is transported as part of chylomicrons through the lymph fluid into the blood and eventually arrives at the liver. More than 90 percent of stored vitamin E is found in the adipose tissue. Excess vitamin E is excreted through the bile, urine, feces, and the pores in the skin.

Metabolic Functions of Vitamin E

Vitamin E is sometimes referred to as the vitamin in search of a disease to cure. For almost 40 years after its discovery, scientists searched unsuccessfully for a curative role for vitamin E. They now have begun studying the vitamin's roles as an antioxidant and in maintaining healthy cell membranes. Vitamin E also plays an important function in blood clotting. The role of vitamin E in preventing cardiovascular disease is still unclear. Even though vitamin E was thought to show promise in

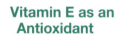

preventing other diseases such as cancer or cataracts, researchers have not been able to provide conclusive evidence supporting this.

Vitamin E as an Antioxidant

Vitamin E's nutritional claim to fame is its role as a powerful antioxidant, particularly in cell membranes. Recall from Chapter 5 that phospholipids are critical components of cell membranes. Many phospholipids contain unsaturated fatty acids, which are vulnerable to the damaging effects of free radicals. Vitamin E is unique in its ability to neutralize free radicals before they can harm cell membranes (**Figure 9.18**). It does this by donating an electron to free radicals, thereby stabilizing them. In doing so, vitamin E is altered and loses its antioxidant abilities.

Oxidation of the LDL cholesterol carrier in the blood is also harmful, as it contributes to the buildup of artery-clogging

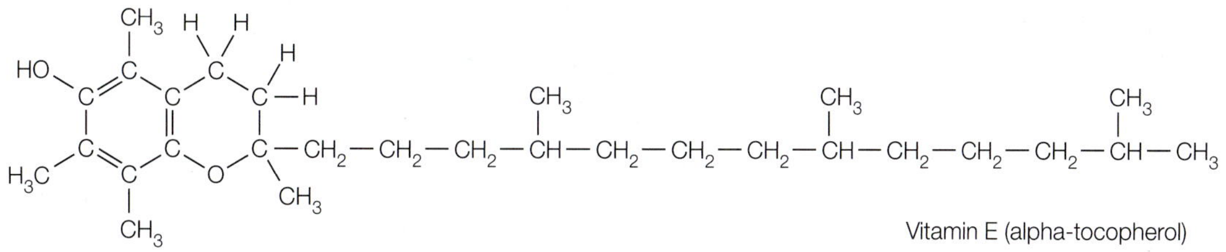

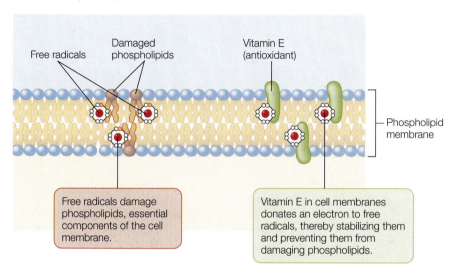

Vitamin E (alpha-tocopherol)

▲ **Figure 9.17 The Structure of Alpha-Tocopherol**
There are eight different types of vitamin E compounds (or tocopherols), but alpha-tocopherol is the most active and is the form reflected in the Dietary Reference Intakes.

Free radicals

Damaged phospholipids

Vitamin E (antioxidant)

Phospholipid membrane

Free radicals damage phospholipids, essential components of the cell membrane.

Vitamin E in cell membranes donates an electron to free radicals, thereby stabilizing them and preventing them from damaging phospholipids.

▲ **Figure 9.18 Vitamin E as an Antioxidant in Cell Membranes**

plaque. Antioxidants, including vitamin E, help protect the LDL cholesterol carrier from being oxidized and reduce the risk of atherosclerosis in the arteries.[68]

Vitamin E as an Anticoagulant

Vitamin E is an *anticoagulant* (*anti* = against, *coagulant* = causes clotting), which means that it inhibits platelets from unnecessarily clumping together and creating a damaging clot in the bloodstream. Vitamin E also lessens the stickiness of the cells that line the blood vessels. This reduces plaque buildup and, in turn, the risk of a heart attack or stroke. Although this function clearly helps maintain the health of the cardiovascular system, studies are still under way to assess if the long-term use of vitamin E supplements could play a protective role against heart disease.

Daily Needs for Vitamin E

For adults, the RDA for vitamin E is 15 milligrams (22.4 IU) daily (see the Calculation Corner to learn how to convert vitamin E in milligrams to international units). Because

alpha-tocopherol is the most active form of vitamin E in the body, vitamin E requirements are presented in alpha-tocopherol equivalents. Researchers speculate that healthy Americans are not consuming adequate amounts of vitamin E.[69]

Food Sources of Vitamin E

Vegetable oils (and foods that contain them), avocados, nuts, and seeds are good food sources of vitamin E. The *Dietary Guidelines for Americans* specifically recommend consuming vegetable oils daily to meet vitamin E needs. Some green leafy vegetables and fortified cereals can also contribute to daily needs (see **Figure 9.19**). For ways to increase your intake of vitamin E, see the accompanying Table Tips.

Vitamin E Toxicity

There isn't any known risk of consuming too much vitamin E from natural food sources. However, overconsumption of the synthetic form that is found in supplements and/or fortified foods could pose risks.

Calculation Corner

Converting International Units for Vitamin E

Vitamin E content in dietary supplements and fortified foods is often listed in international units (IU), while vitamin E found naturally in food is measured in milligrams of alpha-tocopherol (mg α-tocopherol). Use the following conversion factors to determine the alpha-tocopherol equivalents in mg α-tocopherol found in 1 IU.

1 IU of alpha-tocopherol is equivalent to 0.67 mg alpha-tocopherol

1 IU of alpha-tocopherol is equivalent to 0.45 mg of synthetic alpha-tocopherol

Example: A vitamin supplement contains 400 IU of alpha-tocopherol. How many mg α-tocopherol does it contain?

Answer: 0.67 mg × 400 IU
= 268 mg α-tocopherol
or
0.45 mg × 400 IU = 180 mg α-tocopherol (synthetic α-tocopherol)

TABLE TIPS

Enjoying Your Es

Add fresh spinach and broccoli to salad.

Add a slice of avocado or use guacamole as a spread on sandwiches or toast.

Spread peanut butter on apple slices.

Top low-fat yogurt with wheat germ.

Pack a handful of almonds in a zip-closed bag for a snack.

(continued)

▶ **Figure 9.19** **Vitamin E Content in Selected Foods**
Source: Data from *USDA What's In The Food You Eat?* 2016. Available at https://www.ars.usda.gov. Accessed March 2017.

Because vitamin E can act as an anticoagulant and interfere with blood clotting, excess amounts in the body increase the risk of **hemorrhage**. To prevent hemorrhage, the upper limit from supplements and/or fortified foods is 1,000 milligrams for adults. This applies only to healthy individuals consuming adequate amounts of vitamin K. (Vitamin K also plays a role in blood clotting.) A physician should monitor vitamin E intake in individuals who are taking anticoagulant medication to avoid excessive inhibition of blood clotting, which could encourage hemorrhage.

The upper level of 1,000 milligrams may actually be too high. Research has shown that those at risk of heart disease who took 265 milligrams (400 IU) or more of vitamin E daily for at least 1 year had an overall higher risk of dying.[70] One theory is that too much vitamin E may disrupt the balance of other antioxidants in the body, causing more harm than good.

Vitamin E Deficiency

Though rare, a chronic vitamin E deficiency can cause nerve problems, muscle weakness, and uncontrolled movement of body parts and can increase the susceptibility of cell membranes to damage by free radicals. Individuals who can't absorb fat properly may fall short of their vitamin E needs.

hemorrhage Excessive bleeding or loss of blood.

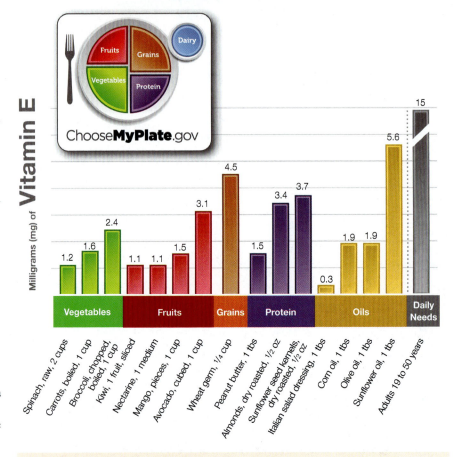

LO 9.7: THE TAKE-HOME MESSAGE There are several forms of naturally occurring vitamin E but alpha-tocopherol is the most active form in the body. Vitamin E is transported via the chylomicron and stored in the adipose tissue. Vitamin E is an antioxidant that protects cell membranes and an anticoagulant that inhibits clot formation. Vitamin E may help prevent the oxidation of LDL cholesterol. Vegetable oils, avocados, nuts, and seeds are good sources of vitamin E. Green leafy vegetables and fortified cereals also contribute to daily intake. The recommended intake for vitamin E is presented in alpha-tocopherol equivalents. Too little vitamin E, although rare, may result in nerve problems and muscle weakness and increase susceptibility to free radical damage. Excess amounts of vitamin E from supplements may cause hemorrhage.

EXPLORING **Vitamin K**

LO 9.8 Describe the functions, recommended intakes, food sources, and deficiency and toxicity effects of vitamin K.

What Is Vitamin K?

Vitamin K is found naturally in two forms. Some plants manufacture **phylloquinone (vitamin K₁)**. Phylloquinone has a long chain of carbons with methyl groups attached at every fourth carbon (**Figure 9.20**). This is the primary source of vitamin K in the diet. In animals, bacteria that reside naturally in the colon synthesize **menaquinone (vitamin K₂)**. A third form of vitamin K, called *menadione*, or *vitamin K₃*, is synthetic and formulated for use in animal feed and vitamin supplements.

Vitamin K Absorption and Transport

About 80 percent of dietary vitamin K is absorbed, mostly in the jejunum. In contrast, only 10 percent of the vitamin K produced by bacteria in the large intestine is absorbed. Both forms of vitamin K are incorporated into chylomicrons and transported to the liver, where they are stored for future use. When the diet is deficient in vitamin K, the storage forms are transported by the lipoproteins VLDL, LDL, and HDL. Excess vitamin K is excreted, mostly bound to bile. It can also be eliminated through the urine once it has been degraded by the liver. Vitamin K is stored in small amounts, mostly in the liver.

Metabolic Functions of Vitamin K

Vitamin K is so named because of its role in *koagulation,* the Danish word for **coagulation**, or blood clotting.[71] It also functions as a cofactor in several key roles in the body and is essential for strengthening the bones.

Vitamin K Promotes Blood Clotting

A series of reactions, referred to as a *cascade,* must happen before the blood coagulates and forms a blood clot. Proteins involved in blood clotting are known as **clotting factors**. Four vitamin K–dependent clotting factors are II (also called *prothrombin*), VII, IX, and X.

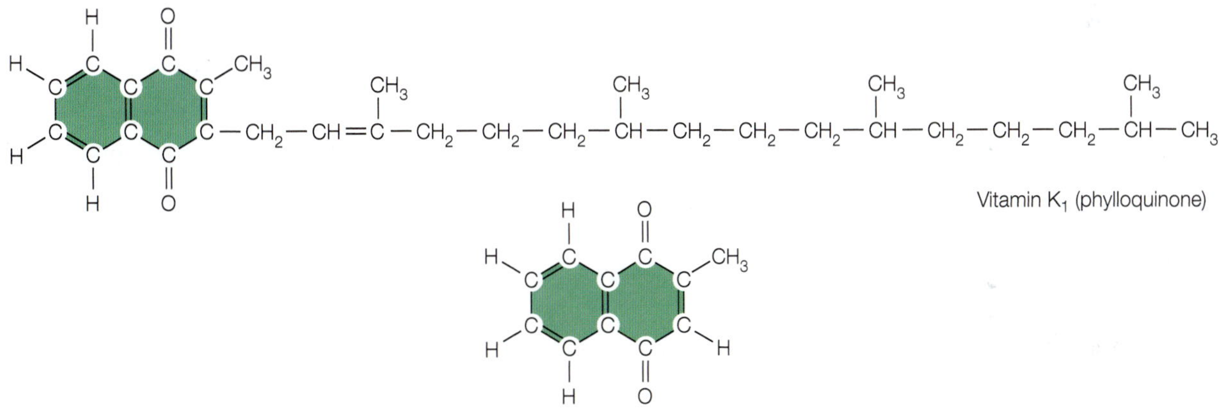

▲ **Figure 9.20 The Structure of Vitamin K**
Vitamin K occurs naturally in plants as phylloquinone. Menadione is the synthetic form of vitamin K.

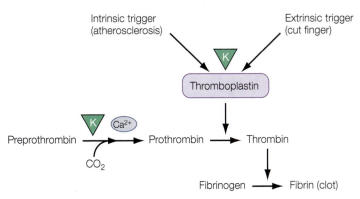

▲ **Figure 9.21 The Role of Vitamin K in Blood Clotting**
Vitamin K is a coenzyme involved in carboxylation reactions of several proteins during blood clotting.

phylloquinone (vitamin K₁) The form of vitamin K found in plants.

menaquinone (vitamin K₂) The form of vitamin K produced by bacteria in the colon.

coagulation The process of blood clotting.

clotting factors Substances involved in the process of blood clotting, such as prothrombin and fibrinogen.

(continued)

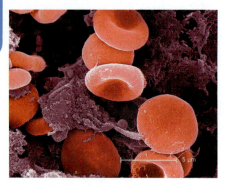

▲ **Figure 9.22 Blood Clot (SEM, magnified 1,900×)**

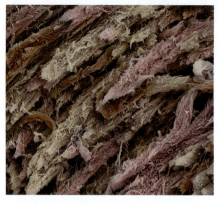

▲ **Figure 9.23 Bone Matrix (colored SEM, magnified 2,000×)**

During a key step in the cascade, a carboxyl group is added to a protein. The reaction, called **carboxylation**, enables the protein to bind calcium ions. (See the Chemistry Boost for an illustration of carboxylation.) A carboxylase enzyme that depends on vitamin K as a coenzyme catalyzes this reaction (**Figure 9.21**). Once calcium is bound to the clotting factors, the clotting process continues with the conversion of prothrombin to thrombin. Thrombin converts fibrinogen to fibrin, which holds together red blood cells to form the actual blood clot (**Figure 9.22**). As soon as vitamin K has completed its role in activating the carboxylase enzyme, it is released and the enzyme must be activated again. Without vitamin K, a simple cut could quickly result in hemorrhage.

Anticoagulants (anticlotting medications) such as Coumadin (or warfarin) decrease vitamin K activity, resulting in thinner blood. Severe liver disease also results in lower blood levels of the vitamin K–dependent clotting factors and increases the risk of hemorrhage.

Vitamin K Promotes Strong Bones

Vitamin K participates in the carboxylation of other proteins. Two of these proteins are essential components in bone formation: *osteocalcin* and *matrix Gla protein*. Osteocalcin is secreted by bone-forming osteoblasts. Matrix Gla protein is found in the bone matrix (**Figure 9.23**), blood vessels, and cartilage. The carboxylation of osteocalcin and matrix Gla protein is necessary for calcium ions to bind to the bone matrix, which strengthens the bone and improves bone mass.[72] Matrix Gla protein may also provide protection against atherosclerosis.[73]

Daily Needs for Vitamin K

Currently, the contribution of vitamin K synthesized by the GI flora to meeting daily needs is not known. Because of this, it is hard to determine an Estimated Average Requirement (EAR), so an Adequate Intake (AI) is reported instead. Therefore, the AI for dietary vitamin K is based on the average amount consumed by healthy Americans.[74] Adult women need 90 micrograms (1,000 IU) of vitamin K per day, and men need 120 micrograms (1,300 IU) daily.

Food Sources of Vitamin K

To meet vitamin K needs, think green. Green vegetables like broccoli, asparagus, spinach, salad greens, brussels sprouts, and green cabbage are all rich in vitamin K. Vegetable oils and margarine are the second largest source of vitamin K in the diet (see **Figure 9.24**). A green salad with oil-and-vinegar dressing at lunch and three-quarters of a cup of broccoli at dinner will meet an individual's vitamin K needs for the entire day.

Vitamin K Toxicity and Deficiency

There are no known adverse effects of consuming too much vitamin K from foods or supplements, so an upper intake level hasn't been set for healthy people.

Individuals taking anticoagulant medications such as Coumadin need to maintain a consistent intake of vitamin K.

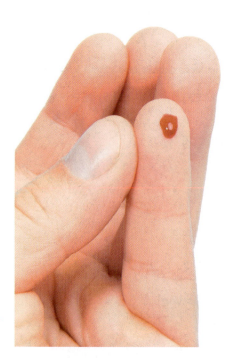

⬡ Chemistry Boost

Reactions

Carboxylation is a chemical reaction that occurs when a carboxyl group (COOH) is added to a protein, such as during the blood-clotting reaction. As illustrated, the glutamic acid molecule is converted to carboxyglutamic acid with the aid of vitamin K. The carboxyl group in this illustration is shown as COO^-.

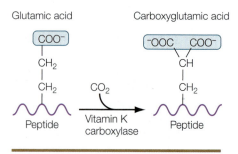

carboxylation Chemical reaction in which a carboxyl group is added to a molecule.

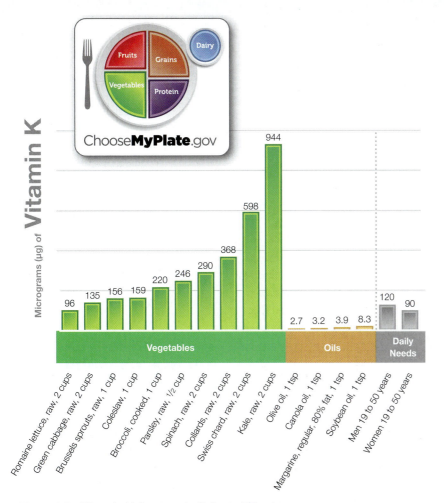

Micrograms (µg) of **Vitamin K**

ChooseMyPlate.gov

Fruits	Grains
Vegetables	Protein
	Dairy

944
598
368
290
246
220
159
156
135
96
120
90
2.7 3.2 3.9 8.3

Vegetables | **Oils** | **Daily Needs**

Romaine lettuce, raw, 2 cups
Green cabbage, raw, 2 cups
Brussels sprouts, raw, 1 cup
Coleslaw, 1 cup
Broccoli, cooked, 1 cup
Parsley, raw, 1/2 cup
Spinach, raw, 2 cups
Collards, raw, 2 cups
Swiss chard, raw, 2 cups
Kale, raw, 2 cups
Olive oil, 1 tsp
Canola oil, 1 tsp
Margarine, regular, 80% fat, 1 tsp
Soybean oil, 1 tsp
Men 19 to 50 years
Women 19 to 50 years

▲ **Figure 9.24 Vitamin K Content in Selected Foods**
Source: Data from *USDA What's In The Food You Eat?* 2016. Available at https://www.ars.usda.gov. Accessed March 2017.

TABLE TIPS
Getting Your Ks

Have a green salad daily.

Cook with soybean oil.

Add shredded green cabbage to salad or top a salad with a scoop of coleslaw.

Add a small amount of margarine to steamed spinach. Both provide some vitamin K.

Dunk raw broccoli florets in salad dressing for two sources of vitamin K.

breast milk is low in vitamin K. For this reason, newborns are routinely given vitamin K soon after birth, either as an injection or by mouth, to enable blood clotting until the bacteria in the intestinal tract can begin to produce it.[76]

A vitamin K deficiency severe enough to affect blood clotting is extremely rare in healthy individuals.[77] People with conditions such as gallbladder disease, which reduces the absorption of fat and fat-soluble vitamins in the intestinal tract, may be at risk for not meeting their vitamin K needs.

Though the exact mechanism is unknown, a chronic dietary deficiency of vitamin K may be a factor in increased hip fractures in older men and women. A diet rich in phylloquinone (vitamin K_1) has been shown to improve bone mineral content in older women.[78]

This medication decreases the activity of vitamin K and prolongs the time it takes for blood to clot. If individuals taking Coumadin suddenly increase the vitamin K in their diets, the vitamin can override the effect of the drug, enabling the blood to clot too quickly. In contrast, a sudden decline in dietary vitamin K can enhance the effectiveness of the drug and increase the risk of bleeding.[75]

Babies are born with low levels of vitamin K. This is because little vitamin K passes through the placenta and newborns have sterile intestinal tracts with few bacteria to produce vitamin K. In addition,

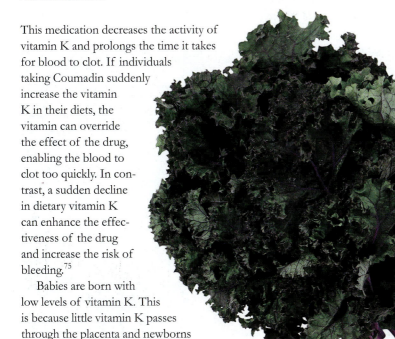

LO 9.8: THE TAKE-HOME MESSAGE
Vitamin K is found in plants as phylloquinone and as menaquinone in the colon manufactured by bacteria. Vitamin K functions as a carboxylation coenzyme active in blood clotting and bone formation. Leafy greens, vegetable oils, and margarine are good dietary sources of vitamin K. While there are no known toxicity problems for vitamin K, a deficiency may result in hemorrhage and bone fractures. Individuals taking anticoagulant medications such as Coumadin should monitor their vitamin K intake.

Are Vitamin Supplements Necessary for Good Health?

LO 9.9 Explain the role of dietary supplements in maintaining a healthy diet.

Sales of dietary supplements in the United States have increased markedly in the last several decades. More than 30 percent of Americans spent over $38 billion in 2015 on dietary supplements as single vitamins or minerals or in the most popular form of a multivitamin and mineral (MVM) combination.[79] One in three Americans reports taking an MVM daily.[80] To encourage supplement use, manufacturers are developing new chewable forms, including chocolate, gummies, and soft gels, alongside the pills, powders, and liquids. Are vitamin supplements worth the money? Are they harmful or essential to be healthy?

Supplements Do Not Reduce Risks for CVD, Cancer, or Cognitive Decline

Concern about aging appears to be one of the forces driving this increase in the use of supplements: Older people may use them in an attempt to mitigate ongoing medical issues or to prevent chronic diseases,[81] especially cardiovascular disease, cancer, and cognitive decline.

A staggering number of studies have examined the association between ingesting specific individual vitamins or combinations of vitamins—including the antioxidant vitamins A, C, E, beta-carotene, and folic acid—to prevent cardiovascular disease and cancer. A recent review found that no single vitamin or combination of vitamins showed any benefit in preventing cardiovascular disease or cancer. In the case of beta-carotene and vitamin E supplements, the risks outweighed any benefits. The researchers concluded that ingesting beta-carotene in supplement form might increase the risk of developing cancer in people who smoke. Vitamin E supplements do not impact the risk of developing cardiovascular disease or cancer,[82] nor does a daily MVM prevent heart attacks, stroke, or death from a cardiovascular event even after 10 years of supplementation.[83]

In addition to cardiovascular disease and cancer, middle-aged Americans are fearful that as they age, cognitive decline will rob them of their independence and quality of life. Does a daily MVM help maintain mental sharpness and prevent cognitive decline? The research says no. In one study, for example, the cognitive decline in men over a 13-year period showed no improvement on four different cognitive skills among participants taking an MVM.[84]

While the idea that taking an MVM daily could ward off cardiovascular disease, cancer, and even cognitive decline is appealing, it's best to save your money.

Vitamin Supplements Are Not a Substitute for Healthy Eating

Consumers often choose supplements because they are unwilling to improve their diets. However, the Academy of Nutrition and Dietetics maintains that an unhealthy diet of non-nutritious foods cannot be transformed into a healthy diet by simply ingesting a daily supplement. There is little scientific evidence to promote the use of dietary supplements in

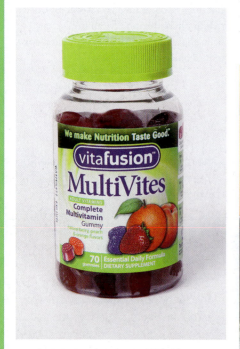

Some of the most popular forms of vitamin supplements sold today are in chewable, candylike forms.

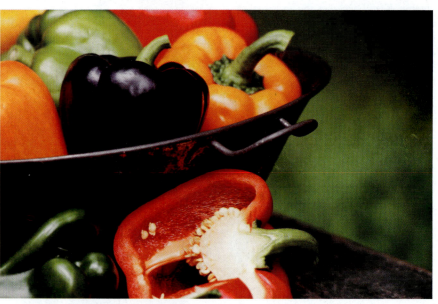

Unlike synthetic supplements, whole fruits and vegetables contain fiber and phytochemicals that provide health benefits beyond those of the micronutrient content.

place of eating a healthy, balanced diet. Remember that disease-fighting phytochemicals, fiber, and other substances that the body needs are all missing from a bottle of supplements.

Furthermore, supplement use may have adverse side effects. In fact, supplement use, not food, is responsible for most of the reported problems associated with vitamin toxicity. Any individual who is considering taking supplements should consult a credible source of nutrition information, such as a registered dietitian nutritionist, before purchasing or consuming supplements.

Supplements May Be Helpful for Some Individuals

Whereas many healthy individuals do not need to consume supplements, some supplements are useful for people who cannot meet their nutrient needs through a regular, varied diet. Others may have been advised by their physician to consume supplements to correct a vitamin or mineral deficiency.

Among those who may benefit from taking a dietary supplement are:[85]

- Women of childbearing age who may become pregnant, as they need to consume adequate synthetic folic acid (a B vitamin) to prevent certain birth defects
- Pregnant and lactating women who can't meet their increased nutrient needs with foods
- Older individuals, who need adequate amounts of synthetic vitamin B_{12}
- Individuals who do not drink enough milk and/or do not have adequate sun exposure to meet their vitamin D needs
- Individuals on low-kilocalorie diets that limit the amount of vitamins and minerals they can consume through food
- Vegans, who have limited dietary options for vitamins D and B_{12} and other nutrients

- Individuals with food allergies or lactose intolerance that limit food choices
- Individuals who abuse alcohol, have medical conditions such as intestinal disorders, or are taking medications that may increase their need for certain vitamins
- Individuals who are food insecure and those who are eliminating food groups from their diet
- Infants who are breastfed should receive 400 IU of vitamin D daily unless they are also consuming at least 1 quart of vitamin D–fortified formula daily. Children age 1 and older should receive 400 IU of vitamin D daily if they consume less than 1 quart of milk per day. Adolescents who consume less than 400 IU of vitamin D daily from their diet would also benefit from a supplement.

Supplements can interact or interfere with certain medications, so individuals should consult a doctor before consuming a supplement if they are taking prescription medications.

Supplements Are Not Regulated Like Drugs

Another factor to keep in mind regarding the use of dietary supplements (including vitamins, minerals, and herbs) is that the FDA does not stringently regulate them. In fact, manufacturers are responsible for ensuring their effectiveness and safety. Unlike drugs, dietary supplements—unless they contain a new ingredient—do not need approval from the FDA before they can be marketed to the public, and the FDA cannot remove a supplement from the marketplace unless it has been shown to be unsafe or harmful to the consumer.[86]

An option exists to help consumers choose among dietary supplements. The **United States Pharmacopeia (USP)** is a nonprofit organization that sets standards for dietary supplements.[87] Though it does not endorse or validate health claims that the supplement manufacturers make, it sets

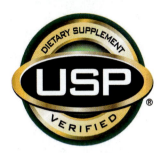

▲ **Figure 9.25 The U.S. Pharmacopeia Verified Mark**
Source: Registered trademark of The United States Pharmacopeial Convention. Used with Permission.

standards for the identity, strength, quality, and purity of dietary supplements. Supplement manufacturers can voluntarily submit their products to the USP's scientists for review. USP verifies supplements through a comprehensive testing and evaluation process and awards its USP Verified mark (**Figure 9.25**) only after rigorous facility audits, product documentation reviews, and product testing have been completed and approved.

For individuals who choose to use supplements, the best place to start when picking a supplement is to carefully read the label. The FDA does have strict guidelines for the information that must appear on any supplement label. For example, the term *high potency* can only be used if at least two-thirds of the nutrients in the supplement contain at least 100 percent of the daily value. The label must also clearly identify the contents of the bottle. While a supplement may have the USP seal of approval for quality and purity, it doesn't have the FDA's approval, even if it makes a claim. Supplements must be labeled with a Supplement Facts panel that lists the serving size, the number of capsules or tablets in the bottle, the amount of the vitamin in each capsule, and the percentage of the daily value (**Figure 9.26**). All the ingredients must also be listed.

United States Pharmacopeial Convention (USP) Nonprofit organization that sets quality standards for dietary supplements.

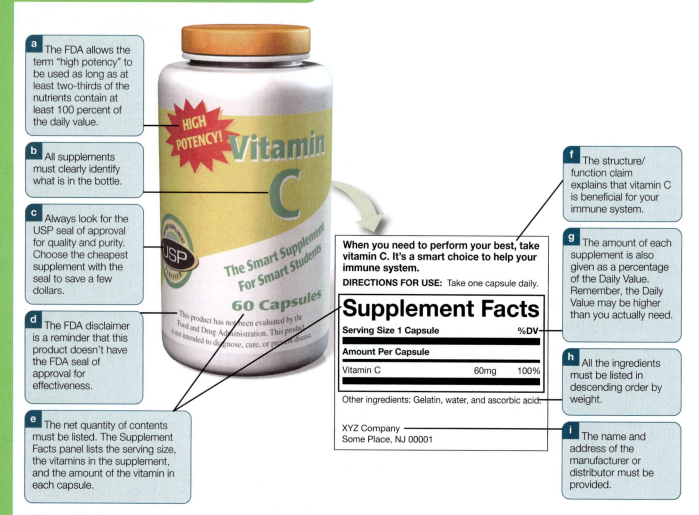

a The FDA allows the term "high potency" to be used as long as at least two-thirds of the nutrients contain at least 100 percent of the daily value.

b All supplements must clearly identify what is in the bottle.

c Always look for the USP seal of approval for quality and purity. Choose the cheapest supplement with the seal to save a few dollars.

d The FDA disclaimer is a reminder that this product doesn't have the FDA seal of approval for effectiveness.

e The net quantity of contents must be listed. The Supplement Facts panel lists the serving size, the vitamins in the supplement, and the amount of the vitamin in each capsule.

f The structure/function claim explains that vitamin C is beneficial for your immune system.

g The amount of each supplement is also given as a percentage of the Daily Value. Remember, the Daily Value may be higher than you actually need.

h All the ingredients must be listed in descending order by weight.

i The name and address of the manufacturer or distributor must be provided.

When you need to perform your best, take vitamin C. It's a smart choice to help your immune system.

DIRECTIONS FOR USE: Take one capsule daily.

Supplement Facts

Serving Size 1 Capsule		%DV
Amount Per Capsule		
Vitamin C	60mg	100%

Other ingredients: Gelatin, water, and ascorbic acid.

XYZ Company
Some Place, NJ 00001

▲ **Figure 9.26 Dietary Supplement Labels**
The FDA has strict guidelines for the information that must appear on any supplement label.

LO 9.9: THE TAKE-HOME MESSAGE The ingestion of a daily multivitamin-mineral supplement is on the rise in the United States, especially among older adults. The research doesn't support dietary supplements as a cure for the chronic diseases that accompany aging, including cardiovascular disease, cancer, or cognitive decline. A well-balanced diet that provides adequate kilocalories can meet most individuals' daily vitamin needs without a supplement; however, supplementation is an option for individuals unable to meet their daily vitamin needs. The FDA does not strictly regulate dietary supplements. If the U.S. Pharmacopoeia (USP) has determined that a supplement meets its criteria for identity, strength, quality, and purity, it will carry the USP Verified mark. Consumers should seek guidance from a qualified health professional before taking a dietary supplement.

Visual Chapter Summary

LO 9.1 Vitamins Are Essential Organic Compounds

Vitamins are essential organic compounds the body requires in small amounts for normal metabolic functions but cannot synthesize in adequate amounts. The 13 different vitamins are classified as either water soluble or fat soluble. The water-soluble vitamins include the B-complex vitamins and vitamin C. The fat-soluble vitamins are vitamins A, D, E, and K. Provitamins, such as the carotenoids, are converted to their active form before they can be directly used in the body. Excesses of water-soluble vitamins are excreted from the body in urine and rarely accumulate to toxic levels. Vitamins A, D, and E are stored in the liver and other body tissues and can build up to toxic levels if taken in megadose amounts.

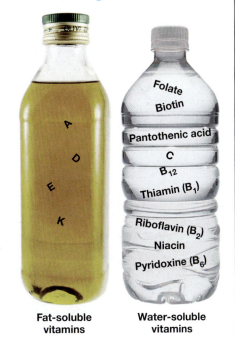

Fat-soluble vitamins — A, D, E, K

Water-soluble vitamins — Folate, Biotin, Pantothenic acid, C, B_{12}, Thiamin (B_1), Riboflavin (B_2), Niacin, Pyridoxine (B_6)

LO 9.2 Vitamins Differ in Their Absorption and Storage

Bioavailability of individual vitamins varies based on the amount of the vitamin in the food, whether the food is cooked, raw, or refined, the food's digestibility, an individual's nutrition status, and whether the vitamin is a natural or synthetic form. Vitamins are often attached to proteins in food and must be released in the stomach to be absorbed. Once freed, fat-soluble vitamins are transported as part of micelles and absorbed through the lymph system as part of chylomicrons. Fat-soluble vitamins require dietary fat to be absorbed. Water-soluble vitamins are absorbed with water and typically aren't stored in the body for extended periods. Fat-soluble vitamins are less bioavailable than water-soluble vitamins.

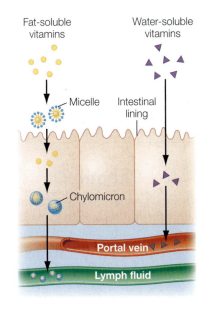

Fat-soluble vitamins   Water-soluble vitamins

Micelle   Intestinal lining

Chylomicron

Portal vein

Lymph fluid

LO 9.3 Antioxidants Stabilize Free Radicals

Free radicals are atoms or molecules with an unpaired electron. They can capture an electron from or donate an electron to other atoms and molecules, thereby destabilizing them. The chain reaction of free radical damage can contribute to chronic diseases such as cancer and cardiovascular disease and accelerate aging. Antioxidants, such as vitamins E and C and the carotenoid and flavonoid phytochemicals, donate an electron to, and thereby neutralize, free radicals. Diets abundant in antioxidant-rich fruits, vegetables, and whole grains are associated with a lower incidence of many diseases.

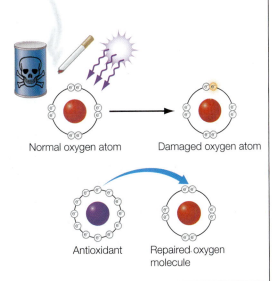

Normal oxygen atom   Damaged oxygen atom

Antioxidant   Repaired oxygen molecule

LO 9.4 Vitamins Are Found in Every Food Group

Whole foods provide phytochemicals and fiber in addition to vitamins. Food handling and preparation techniques that involve exposure to air, water, UV light, changes in pH, and heat can cause the loss of vitamins. Fortified foods and vitamin supplements can help individuals with inadequate diets meet their nutrient needs. However, there are health risks associated with the overconsumption of vitamins in fortified foods and supplements.

Vegetables	Fruits	Grains	Protein	Dairy
Folate	Folate	Folic acid	Niacin	Riboflavin
Vitamin A	Vitamin C	Niacin	Thiamin	Vitamin A
Vitamin C	Vitamin A	Vitamin B_6	Vitamin B_6	Vitamin B_{12}
Vitamin E		Vitamin B_{12} (if fortified)	Vitamin B_{12}	Vitamin D
Vitamin K		Riboflavin		
		Thiamin		

LO 9.5 Vitamin A

Vitamin A refers to a family of retinoids, which include retinol, retinal, and retinoic acid. Retinol is most usable in the body. Vitamin A is essential for vision, cell growth and development, reproduction, and a healthy immune system. Three provitamin A carotenoids, alpha-carotene, beta-carotene, and beta-cryptoxanthin, can be converted to vitamin A in the body; beta-carotene is the most commonly consumed. Vitamin A is stored in the liver until needed and is not easily excreted from the body.

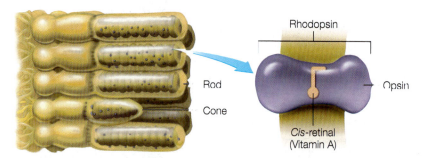

Rod and cone cells in retina

Most of the dietary, preformed vitamin A consumed (70–90 percent) is absorbed; absorption occurs via active transport in the small intestine. Beta-carotene is absorbed at a much lower rate. Vitamin A in foods is measured in retinol activity equivalents (RAE). Preformed vitamin A is found in milk, cereals, cheese, egg yolks, and organ meats, especially liver. Many vegetables are rich sources of provitamin A, including carrots, spinach, and sweet potatoes.

Vitamin A deficiencies can result in vision problems and increased infections. Toxic amounts of vitamin A can compromise bone health and can lead to birth defects during pregnancy.

LO 9.6 Vitamin D

Although vitamin D (the "sunshine vitamin") can be made in the body with the help of ultraviolet rays from the sun, some individuals are not exposed to enough sunlight to meet their needs. The active form of vitamin D, called calcitriol, regulates blood calcium, enhances the absorption of calcium and phosphorus from the small intestine, and maintains healthy bones. It may also help regulate blood pressure and the immune system and it may help prevent diabetes and some cancers.

Fortified milk, yogurts, and soymilk are excellent food sources of vitamin D, as are fatty fish. A deficiency of vitamin D can cause rickets in children and osteomalacia in adults. Hypervitaminosis D can result in hypercalcemia, affect the nervous system, and cause severe depression.

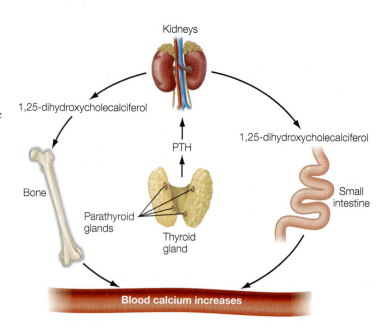

LO 9.7 Vitamin E

Alpha-tocopherol is the most active form of vitamin E in the body. Vitamin E is an antioxidant that protects cell membranes. It plays an important role as an anticoagulant and may help prevent the oxidation of LDL cholesterol.

Vegetable oils, avocados, nuts, and seeds are good sources of vitamin E. Green leafy vegetables and fortified cereals also contribute to daily intake. The recommended intake for vitamin E is presented in alpha-tocopherol equivalents.

Vitamin E deficiencies, although rare, may result in nerve problems, muscle weakness, and increased susceptibility to free radical damage. Excess amounts of vitamin E from supplements may cause hemorrhage.

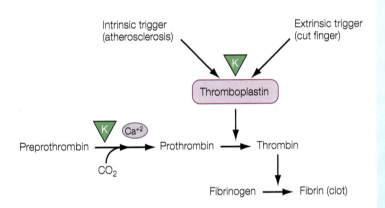

Free radicals   Damaged phospholipids   Vitamin E (antioxidant)

Free radicals damage phospholipids, essential components of the cell membrane.

Vitamin E in cell membranes can neutralize free radicals, preventing them from damaging phospholipids.

LO 9.8 Vitamin K

Vitamin K is a fat-soluble vitamin found naturally as phylloquinone in plants and as menaquinone, the form synthesized by the GI flora. Vitamin K is a coenzyme for the carboxylation of clotting factors and two proteins involved in bone formation. Dietary sources include leafy greens, vegetable oils, and margarine. A deficiency of vitamin K may result in hemorrhage and bone fractures. Individuals taking anticoagulant medications need to carefully monitor their vitamin K intake. There are no known toxicity problems.

Intrinsic trigger (atherosclerosis)   Extrinsic trigger (cut finger)

K → Thromboplastin

Preprothrombin → [K] [Ca^{+2}] → Prothrombin → Thrombin

CO_2

Fibrinogen → Fibrin (clot)

LO 9.9 Vitamin Supplements Are Not a Substitute for Healthy Eating

Individuals often take daily vitamin supplements to prevent chronic disease without scientific research that supports their use. Vitamin supplements should never replace a healthy diet. A vitamin supplement is an option for individuals unable to meet their daily vitamin needs, such as during pregnancy, lactation, solely breastfed infants, older individuals, vegans, people with allergies, or people who are on strict weight-loss diets or who eliminate certain food groups.

The FDA does not regulate dietary supplements, but can remove a supplement from the market if it is found to be harmful. Also, the label of dietary supplements must include a Supplements Facts panel that consumers can use to compare products. The U.S. Pharmacopoeia (USP) Verified mark on a supplement label indicates that the supplement has been tested and meets the criteria for purity and accuracy. It does not ensure safety. Consumers should seek guidance from a qualified health professional before taking a dietary supplement.

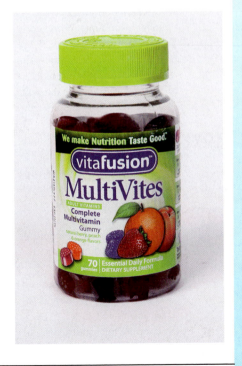

Terms to Know

- vitamins
- provitamins
- preformed vitamins
- toxicity
- hypervitaminosis
- megadose
- bioavailability
- antioxidants
- oxidative stress
- age-related macular degeneration (AMD)
- cataract
- fortified foods
- retinoids
- retinol
- retinal
- retinoic acid
- retinyl ester
- provitamin-A carotenoids
- beta-carotene
- rhodopsin
- iodopsin
- rods
- cones
- bleaching
- epithelial tissues
- cell division
- cell differentiation
- retinol activity equivalents (RAE)
- international units (IU)
- hypervitaminosis A
- carotenodermia
- night blindness
- xeropthalmia
- keratinization
- calciferol
- ergocalciferol (vitamin D₂)
- cholecalciferol (vitamin D₃)
- 1,25-dihydroxycholecaliciferol (calcitriol)
- parathyroid hormone (PTH)
- prohormone
- hypervitaminosis D
- hypercalcemia
- rickets
- osteomalacia
- alpha-tocopherol (α-tocopherol)
- hemorrhage
- phylloquinone (vitamin K₁)
- menaquinone (vitamin K₂)
- coagulation
- clotting factors
- carboxylation
- U.S. Pharmacopoeia (USP)

Mastering Nutrition
Visit the Study Area in Mastering Nutrition to hear an MP3 chapter summary.

Check Your Understanding

LO 9.1 1. Vitamins are
   a. essential nutrients needed in large amounts to prevent disease.
   b. classified as either water-soluble or fat-soluble nutrients.
   c. defined as inorganic nutrients.
   d. easily made by the body from leftover glucose.

LO 9.1 2. Which of the following statements about vitamins is false?
   a. Although the body is capable of synthesizing some vitamins, they are considered essential nutrients.
   b. They are organic compounds present in foods from both animals and plants.
   c. Preformed vitamins must be converted to provitamins to be active.
   d. They are micronutrients.

LO 9.2 3. Which of the following statements about fat-soluble vitamins is true?
   a. They are stored by the body, and thus are not classified as essential nutrients.
   b. After absorption in the enterocytes, they travel via the portal vein to the liver.
   c. They can accumulate to toxic levels in the body.
   d. They are regularly excreted from the body in feces.

LO 9.3 4. Which of the following are considered antioxidants?
   a. Vitamin E and beta-carotene
   b. Vitamin D and vitamin K
   c. Vitamin E and vitamin K
   d. Vitamin A and vitamin D

LO 9.4 5. Vitamins are most likely to be destroyed by
   a. cold.
   b. ultraviolet light.
   c. acid pH.
   d. digestion.

LO 9.5 6. An individual who does not produce enough bile will have difficulty absorbing
   a. thiamin (B₁).
   b. vitamin A.
   c. folate.
   d. pantothenic acid.

LO 9.6 7. Vitamin D
   a. is not toxic even if consumed in amounts greater than the RDA.
   b. is made in the skin from 7-dehydrocholesterol and ultraviolet light.
   c. is found in whole milk, but not in skim milk.
   d. has an AI rather than an RDA.

LO 9.7 8. The primary role of vitamin E in the body is to
   a. prevent oxidative damage to cell membranes.
   b. serve as a coenzyme.
   c. enhance the absorption of calcium and phosphorus.
   d. participate in blood clotting.

LO 9.8 9. Vitamin K is necessary for the synthesis of
   a. glycogen.
   b. rhodopsin.
   c. prothrombin.
   d. cholecalciferol.

LO 9.9 10. On a bottle of multivitamins, the Supplements Facts panel
   a. must include the USP Verified mark.
   b. certifies that the supplement is safe.
   c. certifies that the supplement has been tested and approved by the FDA.
   d. must list the ingredients in descending order by weight.

Answers

1. (b) Vitamins are classified by their solubility, as either fat-soluble or water-soluble nutrients. They are organic nutrients needed in small amounts in the diet because the body cannot synthesize sufficient amounts to maintain health.

2. (c) Vitamins that are already in their active form are called preformed vitamins and do not undergo conversion to their active form. An example is vitamin A. Provitamins are not in an active form and must be converted once they are absorbed. An example is beta-carotene. The remaining three statements are all true.

3. (c) Large quantities of fat-soluble vitamins A, E, and K are stored in the liver and other tissues and can build up to the point of toxicity. All vitamins, whether or not they can be stored by the body, are essential nutrients. After absorption, fat-soluble vitamins travel in the lymphatic system before entering the bloodstream. Fat-soluble vitamins are not readily excreted from the body.

4. (a) Both vitamin E and beta-carotene function as antioxidants in the body. Vitamins A, D, and K perform other essential functions, but are not antioxidants.

5. (b) Some vitamins, especially vitamin B_{12}, are destroyed by exposure to ultraviolet light, heat (such as during cooking), and when prepared in an alkaline pH (adding baking soda, for example). Cold temperatures do not destroy vitamins. Vitamins are not destroyed by digestion; in fact, they are absorbed into the enterocytes intact.

6. (b) Fat-soluble vitamins such as vitamin A are absorbed along with dietary fat, which is emulsified by bile and thereby prepared for digestion. Thiamin, folate, and pantothenic acid are water-soluble vitamins and do not need bile for digestion and absorption.

7. (b) Vitamin D is a fat-soluble vitamin stored in the liver. It can be toxic if ingested in supplemental form in amounts greater than the RDA (not the AI). The form of vitamin D called 7-dehydrocholesterol is the compound in the skin that is converted to vitamin D using energy from sunlight. Both whole and skim milk are usually fortified with vitamin D.

8. (a) Vitamin E functions as an antioxidant to prevent oxidative damage to cell membranes. Water-soluble vitamins usually serve as coenzymes, active vitamin D enhances the absorption of calcium and phosphorus, and vitamin K participates in blood clotting.

9. (c) Vitamin K is necessary for the synthesis of prothrombin, a clotting factor. Rhodopsin is formed with retinal (vitamin A), and cholecalciferol is the active form of vitamin D in the body. Glycogen is the stored form of glucose found in muscles and the liver.

10. (d) The Supplements Facts panel on a bottle of multivitamins must list the ingredients in descending order by weight. All dietary supplements must be labeled with a Supplements Facts panel, but only supplements verified by the USP may be labeled with the USP Verified mark. The FDA does not test and approve dietary supplements.

Answers to True or False?

1. **False.** Although vitamins perform numerous essential functions in the body, they do not provide energy. Only carbohydrates, protein, fat, and alcohol provide kilocalories.

2. **True.** Fat-soluble vitamins are often found in foods that contain fat. For example, vitamin E is found in vegetable oils and vitamin A is found in egg yolks. However, some fat-soluble vitamins are also found in fortified foods that are low in fat, such as fortified cereals.

3. **False.** Overconsumption of vitamin supplements can result in intakes above the UL. Such high intakes can in turn lead to harmful toxicity symptoms.

4. **True.** Healthy individuals can meet their vitamin requirements by consuming an adequate, balanced diet. However, some individuals, such as those with a specific vitamin deficiency, strict vegans, or those with dietary restrictions, may benefit from taking a vitamin supplement.

5. **False.** Cooking foods in a microwave oven helps retain more vitamins because of the reduced cooking time and exposure to heat. Foods prepared in a microwave also require very little cooking water; this prevents leaching of water-soluble vitamins.

6. **True.** Deep orange vegetables and some green vegetables are good sources of the vitamin A precursor beta-carotene, which is converted to vitamin A in the body.

7. **True.** In the skin, a compound called 7-dehydrocholesterol is converted to a vitamin-D precursor when the ultraviolet rays of the sun alter its structure.

8. **False.** Vitamin K actually helps blood clot, as it participates in the synthesis of several proteins involved in the blood-clotting cascade.

9. **False.** The main role of vitamin E is as an antioxidant that helps protect cell membranes. However, the fat-soluble vitamins D and K are involved in bone health.

10. **False.** Antioxidants serve several beneficial functions in the body, but there is no magic pill for aging.

Web Resources

- To learn more about the importance of fruits and vegetables to vitamin intake, visit www.fruitsandveggiesmorematters.org
- To learn more about the role of alternative therapies and dietary supplements in health and disease prevention, visit www.complementarynutrition.org
- To find out the latest recommendations for vitamins, visit http://ods.od.nih.gov

References

1. Rosenfeld, L. 1997. Vitamine-Vitamin: The Early Years of Discovery. *Clinical Chemistry* 43:680–685.
2. Imam, M. H., Y. Ghazzawi, J. A. Murray, and I. Absah. 2014. Is It Necessary to Assess for Fat-soluble Vitamin Deficiences in Pediatric

Patients with Newly Diagnosed Celiac Disease? *Journal of Pediatric Gastroenterology and Nutrition* 59(2):225–228. doi: 10.1097/MPG.0000000000000368.

3. Hubert, G., T. T. Chung, C. Prosser, D. Lien, et al. 2016. Bone Mineral Density and Fat-Soluble Vitamin Status in Adults with Cystic Fibrosis Undergoing Lung Transplantation: A Pilot Study. *Canadian Journal of Dietetic Practice and Research* 77(4):199–202.

4. Siwamogsatham, O., W. Dong, J. Binongo, R. Chowdhury, J. Alvarez, et al. 2014. Relationship Between Fat-soluble Vitamin Supplementation and Blood Concentrations in Adolescent and Adult Patients with Cystic Fibrosis. *Nutrition in Practice and Research* 29(4):491–497.

5. Cristani, M., A. Speciale, A. Saija, S. Gangemi, P. L. Minciullo, and F. Cimino. 2016. Circulating Advanced Oxidation Protein Products as Oxidative Stress Biomarkers and Progression Mediators in Pathological Conditions Related to Inflammation and Immune Dysregulation. *Current Medical Chemistry* 23(34):3862–3882.

6. Ibid.

7. Centers for Disease Control and Prevention. 2013. *Common Eye Disorders*. Available at www.cdc.gov. Accessed February 2017.

8. National Eye Institute. 2017. Age Related Macular Degeneration. Available at https://nei.nih.gov/eyedata/amd#5. Accessed February 2017.

9. Gorusupudi, A., K. Nelson, and P. Bernstein. 2017. The Age-Related Eye Disease Study: Micronutrients in the Treatment of Macular Degeneration. *Advanced Nutrition* 8(1):40–53. doi:10.3945/an.116.013177.

10. AREDS2 Research Group. Lutein/Zeaxanthin and Omega-3 Fatty Acids for Age-Related Macular Degeneration. The Age-Related Eye Disease Study 2 (AREDS2) Controlled Randomized Clinical Trial. 2013.

11. Centers for Disease Control and Prevention. 2013. *Common Eye Disorders*. Available at www.cdc.gov. Accessed February 2017.

12. National Eye Institute. 2013. NIH Study Provides Clarity on Supplements for Protection Against Blinding Eye Disease. Available at www.nei.nih.gov. Accessed March 2017.

13. London, D. S., and B. Beezhold. 2015. A Phytochemical-rich Diet May Explain the Absense of Age-related Decline in Visual Acuity of Amazonian Hunter-gatherers in Ecuador. *Nutrition Research* 35(2):107–117. doi: 10.1016/j.nutres.2014.12.007.

14. Garin, M. 2015. Healthy Eyes — Eating Right For Your Eye's Sake. Available at www.eyehealthweb.com/healthy-eyes. Accessed March 2017.

15. National Eye Institute. 2013. NIH Study Provides Clarity on Supplements for Protection Against Blinding Eye Disease.

16. Ross, A. C., B. Cabellero, R. J. Cousins, K. L. Tucker, and T. R. Ziegler. 2014. *Modern Nutrition in Health and Disease*. 11th ed. Philadelphia: Lippincott Williams & Wilkins.

17. Maqsood, S., I. Omer, and A. K. Eldin. 2015. Quality Attributes, Moisture Sorption Isotherm and Antioxidative Activities of Tomato (Lycopersicon esculentum L.) as Influenced by Method of Drying. *Journal of Food Science and Technology* 52(11):7059–7069.

18. Ross, A. C., B. Cabellero, R. J. Cousins, K. L. Tucker, and T. R. Ziegler. 2014. *Modern Nutrition in Health and Disease*. 11th ed. Philadelphia: Lippincott Williams & Wilkins.

19. Harvard Health Publications. 2015. Microwave Cooking and Health: Is Microwave Food Healthy? Available at www.health.harvard.edu. Accessed March 2017.

20. Pandrangi, S., and L. E. LaBorde. 2004. Retention of Folate, Carotenoid and Other Quality Characteristics in Commercially Packaged Fresh Spinach. *Journal of Food Science* 69:C702–C707.

21. Packaged Facts Projects. 2012. The Global Market for EPA/DHA Omega 3 Products. Available at www.packagedfacts.com. Accessed February 2017.

22. Institute of Medicine, Food and Nutrition Board. 2003. *Dietary Reference Intakes: Guiding Principles for Nutrition Labeling and Fortification*. Washington, DC: National Academies Press.

23. National Institutes of Health. 2013. *Vitamin A Fact Sheet for Health Professionals*. Available at http://ods.od.nih.gov. Accessed February 2017.

24. Institute of Medicine, Food and Nutrition Board. 2001. *Dietary Reference Intakes: Vitamin A, Vitamin K, Arsenic, Boron, Chromium, Copper, Iodine, Iron, Manganese, Molybdenum, Nickel, Silicon, Vanadium, and Zinc*. Washington, DC: National Academies Press.

25. Gropper, S. S., J. L. Smith, and T. P. Carr. 2018. *Advanced Nutrition and Metabolism*. 7th ed. Belmont, CA: Wadsworth/Cengage Learning.

26. Kim, S. Y., and F. R. Ochsendorf. 2016. New Developments in Acne Treatment: Role of Combination Adapalene-benzoylperoxide. *Therapeutics and Clinical Risk Management*. 12:1497–1506.

27. Chien, C. Y., H. S. Lee, C. H. Cho, et al. 2016. Maternal Vitamin A Deficiency During Pregnancy Affects Vascularized Islet Development. *Journal of Nutritional Biochemistry* 36:51–59. doi: 10.1016/j.jnutbio.2016.07.010.

28. Tanumihardjo, A. S. 2013. Vitamin A and Bone Health: The Balancing Act. *Journal of Clinical Densitometry* 16(4):414–419.

29. Fung, T. T., and D. Feskanich. 2016. Dietary Patterns and Risk of Hip Fractures in Postmenopausal Women and Men Over 50 Years. *Osteopros International* 26(6):1825–1830.

30. Tanumihardjo, A. S. 2013. Vitamin A and Bone Health: The Balancing Act. *Journal of Clinical Densitometry* 16(4):414–419.

31. Roberts, R. L., J. Green, and B. Lewis. 2009. Lutein and Zeaxanthin in Eye and Skin Health. *Clinical Dermatology* 27(2):195–201. doi: 10.1016/j.clindermatol.2008.01.011.

32. Institute of Medicine, Food and Nutrition Board. 2001. *Dietary Reference Intakes: Vitamin A, Vitamin K, Arsenic, Boron, Chromium, Copper, Iodine, Iron, Manganese, Molybdenum, Nickel, Silicon, Vanadium, and Zinc*. Washington, DC: National Academies Press.

33. Ibid.

34. WebMD. 2004. A Little Fat Helps the Vegetables Go Down. Available at www.webmd.com. Accessed March 2017.

35. National Institutes of Health. 2016. *Vitamin A Fact Sheet for Health Professionals*. Available at http://ods.od.nih.gov. Accessed February 2017.

36. Ibid.

37. Fung, T. T., and D. Feskanich. 2016. Dietary Patterns and Risk of Hip Fractures in Postmenopausal Women and Men Over 50 Years.

38. Ibid.

39. Virtamo, J., P. R. Tayor, J. Kontto, S. Männistö, M. Utriainen, S. T. Weinstein, J. Huttunen, and D. Albanes. 2014. Effects of α-Tocopherol and β-Carotene Supplementation on Cancer Incidence and Mortality: 18-Year Postintervention Follow-Up of the Alpha-Tocopherol, Beta-Carotene Cancer Prevention Study. *International Journal of Cancer* 135(1):178–185.

40. Ibid.

41. Sommer, A. 2014. Preventing Blindness and Saving Lives: The Centenary of Vitamin A. *Journal of the American Medical Association Ophthalmology* 132(1):115–117.

42. Ibid.

43. Jones, G. 2014. Vitamin D. In A. C. Ross, et al., eds. *Modern Nutrition in Health and Disease*. 11th ed. Philadelphia: Lippincott Williams & Wilkins.

44. Holick, M. F. 2013. Vitamin D, Sunlight, and Cancer Connection. *Anticancer Agents in Medicinal Chemistry* 13(1):70–82.

45. Ibid.

46. Dankers, W., E. M. Colin, J. P. van Hamburg, and E. Lubberts. 2017. Vitamin D in Autoimmunity: Molecular Mechanisms and Therapeutic Potential. *Frontiers in Immunology* 7:697. doi: 10.3389/fimmu.2016.00697.

47. Munger, K. L., L. I. Levin, J. Massa, R. Horst, T. Orban, and A. Ascherio. 2013. Preclinical Serum 25-Hydroxyvitamin D Levels and Risk of Type 1 Diabetes in a Cohort of U.S. Military Personnel. *American Journal of Epidemiology*. doi:10.1093/aje/kws243.

48. Ibid.

49. Mitchell, D.M., B. Z. Leder, E. Cagliero, et al. 2015. Insulin Secretion and Sensitivity in Healthy Adults with Low Vitamin D Are Not Affected by High-Dose Ergocalciferol Administration: A Randomized Controlled Trial. *The American Journal of Clinical Nutrition* 102(2):385–392. doi:10.3945/ajcn.115.111682.

50. Stadlmayr, A., E. Aigner, U. Huber-Schönauer, D. Niederseer, et al. 2014. Relations of Vitamin D Status, Gender and Type 2 Diabetes in Middle-Aged Caucasians. *Acta Diabetologica*. doi.10.1007/s00592-014-0596-9.

51. Min, B. 2013. Effects of Vitamin D on Blood Pressure and Endothelial Function.

Korean Journal of Physiology and Pharmacology 17(5):385–392.

52. Lejnieks, A., A. Slaidina, A. Zvaigzne, et al. 2013. Vitamin D Status and Its Seasonal Variations and Association with Parathyroid Hormone Concentration in Healthy Women in Riga. *Medicina* 49(7):329–334.

53. National Institutes of Health. 2016. *Vitamin D Fact Sheet for Health Professionals.* Available at http://ods.od.nih.gov. Accessed February 2017.

54. Ibid.

55. Institute of Medicine, Food and Nutrition Board. 2010. *Dietary Reference Intakes for Calcium and Vitamin D.* Washington, DC: National Academy Press.

56. Ibid.

57. Ibid.

58. Lejnieks, A., A. Slaidina, A. Zvaigzne, et al. 2013. Vitamin D Status and Its Seasonal Variations and Association with Parathyroid Hormone Concentration in Healthy Women in Riga.

59. Prentice, A. 2013. Nutritional Rickets Around the World. *Journal of Steroid Biochemistry and Molecular Biology* 136:201–206.

60. Pettifor, J. M., and A. Prentice. 2011. The Role of Vitamin D in Paediatric Bone Health. *Best Practice & Research Clinical Endocrinology and Metabolism* 25(4):573–784.

61. Creo, A. L., T. D. Thacher, J. M. Pettifor, M. A. Strand, and P. R. Fischer. 2016. Nutritional Rickets Around the World: An Update. *Paediatrics and International Child Health* 6:1–15.

62. Centers for Disease Control and Prevention. 2001. Severe Malnutrition among Young Children—Georgia, January 1997–1999. *Morbidity and Mortality Weekly Report.* Available at www.cdc.gov. Accessed February 2017.

63. Gallos, S., K. Comeau, C. Vanstone, S. Agellon, et al. 2013. Effect of Different Dosages of Oral Vitamin D Supplementation on Vitamin D Status in Healthy, Breastfed Infants: A Randomized Trial.

Journal of the American Medical Association 309(17):1785–1792.

64. Institute of Medicine, Food and Nutrition Board. 2010. *Dietary Reference Intakes for Calcium and Vitamin D.* Washington, DC: National Academy Press.

65. U.S. Department of Agriculture, U. S. Department of Health and Human Services. 2015. *2015–2020 Dietary Guidelines for Americans.* 8th ed. Washington, DC: U.S. Government Printing Office.

66. Centers for Disease Control and Prevention. 2013. *Skin Cancer Statistics.* Available at www.cdc.gov. Accessed February 2017.

67. Cangussu, L. M., J. Nahas-Neto, C. L. Orsatti, et al. 2016. Effect of Isolated Vitamin D Supplementation on the Rate of Falls and Postural Balance in Postmenopausal Women Fallers: A Randomized, Double-Blind, Placebo-controlled Trial. *Menopause* 23(3):267–274. doi: 10.1097/GME.0000000000000525.

68. National Institutes of Health, Office of Dietary Supplements. 2016. *Vitamin E Fact Sheet for Health Professionals.* Available at http://ods.od.nih.gov. Accessed February 2017.

69. Ibid.

70. Miller, E. R., R. Pator-Barriso, D. Dalal, et al. 2011. Vitamin E Supplementation May Increase All-Cause Mortality. *Annals of Internal Medicine* 142:37–46.

71. Almquist, H. J. 1975. The History of Vitamin K. *American Journal of Clinical Nutrition* 28:656–659.

72. Hamidi, M. S., O. Gajic-Veljanoski, and Cheung, A. M. 2013. Vitamin K and Bone Health. *Journal of Clinical Densitometry* 16(4):409–413.

73. Vossen, L.M., L. J. Schurgers, B. J. van Varik, B. L. Kietselaer, et al. 2015. Menaquinone-7 Supplementation to Reduce Vascular Calcification in Patients with Coronary Artery Disease: Rationale and Study Protocol (VitaK-CAC Trial). *Nutrients* 7(11):8905–8915. doi: 10.3390/nu7115443.

74. National Institutes of Health, Office of Dietary Supplements. 2016. *Vitamin K Fact Sheet for Health Professionals.* Available at http://ods.od.nih.gov. Accessed March 2017.

75. Ambrosi, P., A. Daumas, P. Villani, and R. Giorgi. 2017. Meta-analysis of Major Bleeding Events on Aspirin Versus Vitamin K Antagonists in Randomized Trials. *International Journal of Cardiology* 230:572–576. doi: 10.1016/j.ijcard.2016.12.055.

76. Lippi, G., and M. Franchini. 2011. Vitamin K in Neonates: Facts and Myths. *Blood Transfusion* 9(1):4–9.

77. Shea, M. K., and S. L. Booth. 2016. Concepts and Controversies in Evaluating Vitamin K Status in Population-Based Studies. *Nutrients* 8(1):8. doi: 10.3390/nu8010008.

78. Ibid.

79. *Nutrition Business Journal.* 2016. NBJ's Supplement Business Report 2016. Penton Media, Inc.

80. Ibid.

81. Gahche, J., R. Bailey, B. V. Hughes, E. Yetley, J. Dwyer, et al. 2015. *Dietary Supplement Use among U.S. Adults Has Increased Since NHANES III (1988–1994).* NCHS Data Brief. Available at www.cdc.gov. Accessed February 2017.

82. US Food and Drug Administration. 2016. Dietary Supplements. Available at https://www.fda.gov/Food/DietarySupplements/default.htm

83. Ibid.

84. US Pharmacopeial Convention. 2017. Dietary Supplement Reference Standards. Available at www.usp.org. Accessed March 2017.

85. US Food and Drug Administration. 2016. Dietary Supplements. Available at https://www.fda.gov/Food/DietarySupplements/default.htm. Accessed March 2017.

86. Ibid.

87. Tarken, L. 2016. *What USP Verified and Other Supplement Seals Mean.* Available at www.consumerreports.org. Accessed February 2017.

Water-Soluble Vitamins

Learning Outcomes

After reading this chapter, you will be able to:

10.1 Identify the properties and primary functions of water-soluble vitamins.

10.2 Describe the functions, recommended intakes, food sources, and toxicity and deficiency effects of thiamin.

10.3 Describe the functions, recommended intakes, food sources, and toxicity and deficiency effects of riboflavin.

10.4 Describe the functions, recommended intakes, food sources, and toxicity and deficiency effects of niacin.

10.5 Describe the functions, recommended intakes, food sources, and toxicity and deficiency effects of pantothenic acid.

10.6 Describe the functions, recommended intakes, food sources, and toxicity and deficiency effects of biotin.

10.7 Describe the functions, recommended intakes, food sources, and toxicity and deficiency effects of vitamin B_6.

10.8 Describe the functions, recommended intakes, food sources, and toxicity and deficiency effects of folate.

10.9 Describe the functions, recommended intakes, food sources, and toxicity and deficiency effects of vitamin B_{12}.

10.10 Describe the functions, recommended intakes, food sources, and toxicity and deficiency effects of vitamin C.

10.11 Describe the functions of compounds that have vitamin-like biological roles but are not classified as vitamins.

10.12 Explain the role that a healthy diet and lifestyle plays in cancer risk and progression.

True or False?

1. All water-soluble vitamins are destroyed during cooking. **T**/**F**
2. Biotin and pantothenic acid are lesser-known versions of vitamin C. **T**/**F**
3. The primary role of the B vitamins is to provide energy. **T**/**F**
4. The body can make plenty of niacin from the amino acid tryptophan. **T**/**F**
5. Consuming too much vitamin B_6 can cause nerve damage. **T**/**F**
6. Older adults are likely to absorb less vitamin B_{12} than younger adults. **T**/**F**
7. Folate reduces the risk of certain birth defects. **T**/**F**
8. It is difficult to obtain enough pantothenic acid from foods. **T**/**F**
9. Eating raw egg whites inhibits the absorption of biotin. **T**/**F**
10. Taking vitamin C supplements prevents the common cold. **T**/**F**

See page 402 for the answers.

In the previous chapter you learned that the four fat-soluble vitamins—A, D, E, and K—are vital to health. These micronutrients function to stimulate growth, keep bones strong, maintain sharp vision, clot blood, and protect cells from free-radical damage. This chapter describes the nine water-soluble vitamins, the roles they play in the body, the best food sources, how much you need on a daily basis, and the risks associated with consuming excessive or insufficient amounts. We also look at how these vitamins work together to facilitate metabolism and other body processes. The chapter concludes with a brief look at the role of nutrition in cancer.

What Are Water-Soluble Vitamins?

LO 10.1 Identify the properties and primary functions of water-soluble vitamins.

There are nine water-soluble vitamins: eight of them are B-complex vitamins and the ninth is vitamin C. When initially discovered in the early 1900s, the "water-soluble B" was thought to be one vitamin. After years of research, it became apparent that this was not a single substance but, rather, many vitamins—thiamin, riboflavin, niacin, vitamin B_6, folate, vitamin B_{12}, pantothenic acid, and biotin—known collectively as the B vitamins.

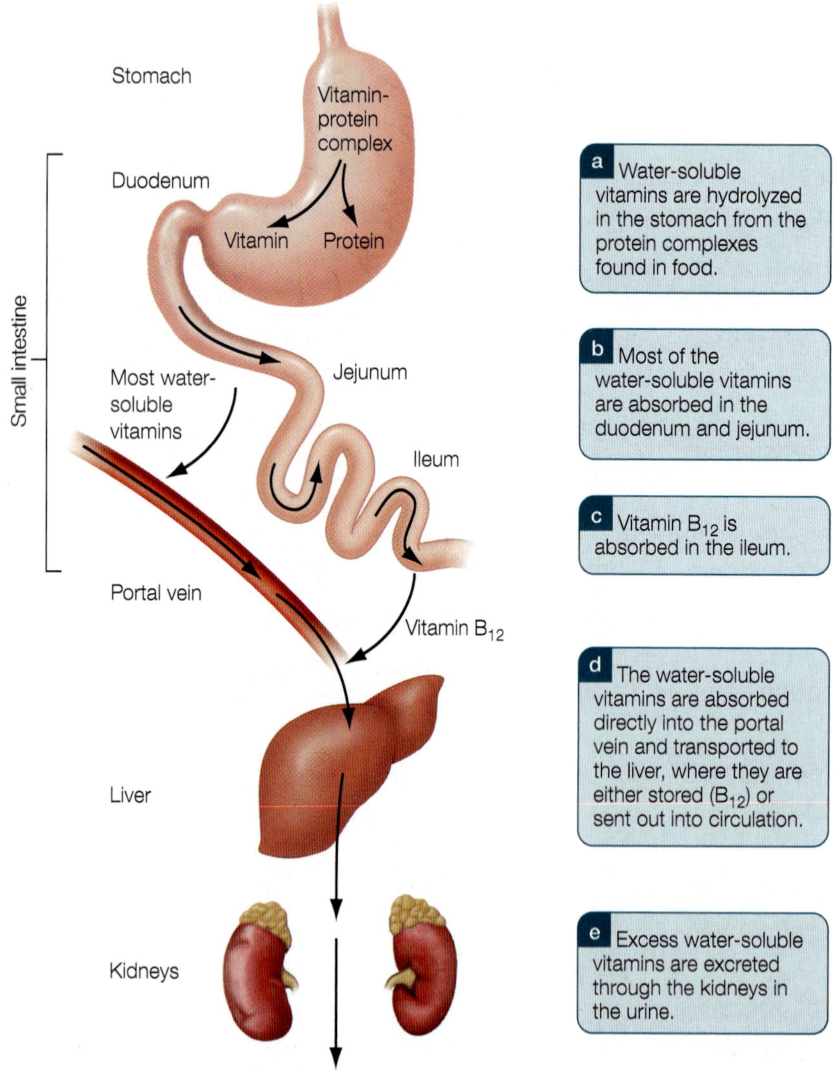

Properties of Water-Soluble Vitamins

Water-soluble vitamins differ from fat-soluble vitamins in that they dissolve in water, are generally not stored in the body, and are often excreted through the urine. Most water-soluble vitamins are also not toxic, though there are exceptions when megadose levels are ingested.

Many water-soluble vitamins leach into water or are easily destroyed by heat, light, pH, or oxidation. Folate deteriorates during cooking; vitamin B_{12} and riboflavin are destroyed by ultraviolet light; thiamin, or B_1, is easily damaged in an alkaline pH, and vitamin C oxidizes when exposed to air and heat. All of the water-soluble vitamins leach when foods are soaked in water. Refer to Chapter 9 on the destruction of water-soluble vitamins.

In general, all water-soluble vitamins are absorbed, transported, and stored in the same way. In foods, water-soluble vitamins are usually attached to proteins and require hydrolysis during digestion to free the vitamin for absorption (**Figure 10.1**). Once digestion has released the vitamins, they pass through the small intestine by passive diffusion when the diet contains large amounts and by active

a. Water-soluble vitamins are hydrolyzed in the stomach from the protein complexes found in food.

b. Most of the water-soluble vitamins are absorbed in the duodenum and jejunum.

c. Vitamin B_{12} is absorbed in the ileum.

d. The water-soluble vitamins are absorbed directly into the portal vein and transported to the liver, where they are either stored (B_{12}) or sent out into circulation.

e. Excess water-soluble vitamins are excreted through the kidneys in the urine.

▲ Figure 10.1 **Digesting and Absorbing Water-Soluble Vitamins**

transport when intakes are low. The absorbed vitamins are then transported through the portal vein to the liver.

The Primary Functions of Water-Soluble Vitamins

Vitamins don't provide kilocalories, and thus aren't a source of energy. The B vitamins do share a role in energy production as **coenzymes** that unlock energy captured in the energy nutrients. Water-soluble vitamins are also involved in blood formation, maintaining a healthy nervous system, and, in the case of vitamin C, act as an antioxidant.

The B Vitamins Act as Coenzymes in Many Metabolic Processes

As coenzymes, vitamins bind to the active site of an enzyme to catalyze the enzyme either to build new compounds or break compounds apart (**Figure 10.2**). In fact, activating enzymes in energy production is the primary function of most water-soluble vitamins. The B vitamins thiamin, riboflavin, niacin, pantothenic acid, biotin, and vitamin B_6 form key coenzymes that assist enzymes to break down carbohydrates, proteins, and fats to ATP. Thiamin activates an enzyme that removes a carbon from pyruvate during glycolysis. Vitamin B_6 acts as a coenzyme in all transamination reactions. Folate and vitamin B_{12} also assist enzymes in producing energy, but in a lesser role. Without the B vitamins, energy production would come to a halt. **Figure 10.3** summarizes their individual roles in energy metabolism.

Water-Soluble Vitamins Play Other Critical Roles

The function of the water-soluble vitamins doesn't end with the B vitamins' roles as coenzymes. Vitamin C acts as an antioxidant and helps neutralize free radicals. Thiamin and vitamin B_{12} are necessary for nerve function, and niacin participates in protein synthesis. Folate and vitamin B_{12} function as coenzymes in the formation of red blood cells, a process called **hemopoiesis**, and the replenishment of cells.

Table 10.1 summarizes the nine water-soluble vitamins, their active coenzyme forms, major functions in the body, major food sources, and the toxicity and deficiency symptoms and diseases that result when the vitamins are consumed in inadequate amounts. Complete the Self-Assessment to see if you are consuming foods that are rich in the B vitamins and vitamin C.

Remember that dietary supplements are not risk free. Many vitamin-mineral supplements contain active ingredients that can have strong biological effects in the body, especially when taken in megadoses. In addition, many foods are fortified with vitamins. These include fortified cereals, flours, and a variety of beverages. Taking too many vitamins from supplements and fortified foods could endanger your health and even be life-threatening. In short, it's best to get vitamins from foods, not supplements.

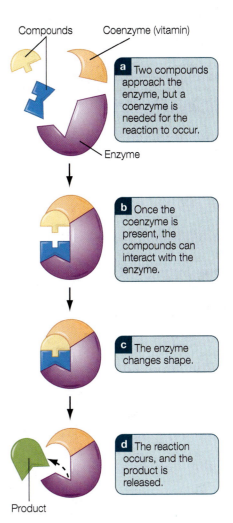

a Two compounds approach the enzyme, but a coenzyme is needed for the reaction to occur.

Compounds   Coenzyme (vitamin)

Enzyme

b Once the coenzyme is present, the compounds can interact with the enzyme.

c The enzyme changes shape.

d The reaction occurs, and the product is released.

Product

▲ **Figure 10.2 B Vitamins Function as Coenzymes**

LO 10.1: THE TAKE-HOME MESSAGE   There are nine water-soluble vitamins: eight B-complex vitamins and vitamin C. All water-soluble vitamins dissolve in water, are absorbed from the small intestine, and travel through the portal vein to the liver. They are generally not stored in the body and are excreted through the urine. Water-soluble vitamins can be lost or destroyed by exposure to air, light, and heat. Most B-complex vitamins function as coenzymes in energy production. Some B vitamins are also involved in nerve health, blood formation, protein synthesis, and heart health. Vitamin C is needed for collagen synthesis and acts as an antioxidant. Consuming dietary supplements is not risk free.

coenzymes Organic substances, often vitamins, that bind to an enzyme to facilitate enzyme activity; unlike enzymes, coenzymes can be altered by the chemical reaction.

hemopoiesis Formation of red blood cells.

Note: TPP, thiamin pyrophosphate; NAD, nicotinamide adenine dinucleotide (niacin); NADP, nicotinamide adenine dinucleotide phosphate (niacin); FAD, flavin adenine dinucleotide (riboflavin); FMN, flavin mononucleotide (riboflavin); PLP, pyridoxal phosphate (B_6); CoA, coenzyme A (pantothenic acid).

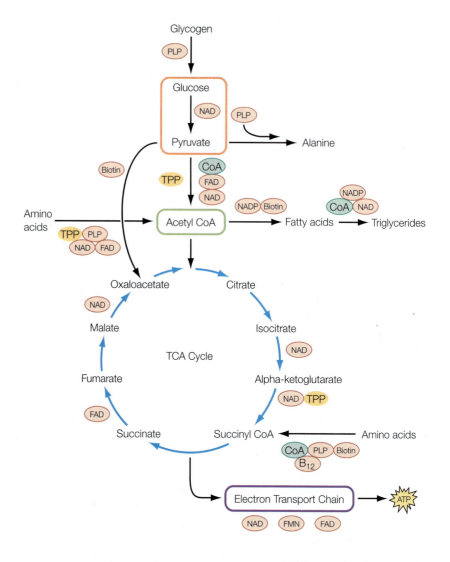

TABLE 10.1 Food Sources, Functions, Symptoms of Deficiencies and Toxicity, and the Recommended Intakes of the Water-Soluble Vitamins

Vitamin	Metabolic Function	Daily Needs (19 years +)	Food Sources	Toxicity Symptoms/UL	Deficiency/ Disease Symptoms	Coenzyme Form
Thiamin (B_1)	Coenzyme in: Carbohydrate metabolism BCAA metabolism	Males: 1.2 mg/day Females: 1.1 mg/day	Pork, enriched and fortified foods, whole grains	None known	Beriberi; characterized by nerve damage	TPP
Riboflavin (B_2)	Coenzyme in oxidation-reduction reactions Energy metabolism Fat metabolism	Males: 1.3 mg/day Females: 1.1 mg/day	Milk, enriched and fortified foods, whole grains	None known	Ariboflavinosis; characterized by inflammation of the mouth and tongue	FAD, FMN
Niacin (B_3)	Coenzyme in oxidation-reduction reactions Energy metabolism Fat metabolism DNA	Males: 16 mg/day Females: 14 mg/day	Lean meats, enriched and fortified grains and cereals	Flushing, blurred vision, liver dysfunction, and glucose intolerance UL: 35 mg/day	Pellagra; characterized by dermatitis, diarrhea, and dementia	NAD, NADP

Vitamin	Metabolic Function	Daily Needs (19 years +)	Food Sources	Toxicity Symptoms/UL	Deficiency/ Disease Symptoms	Coenzyme Form
Pantothenic acid	Part of coenzyme A used in energy metabolism	Males and females: 5 mg/day	Widespread in foods, including whole-grain cereals, nuts and legumes, peanut butter, meat, milk, and eggs	None known	Symptoms include fatigue, nausea and vomiting, numbness, muscle cramps, and difficulty walking	Coenzyme A
Biotin	Energy metabolism Fat synthesis Glycogenesis Amino acid metabolism	Males and females: 30 μg/day	Peanuts, yeast, egg yolks, grains, liver and other organ meats, and fish; also produced by bacteria in the GI tract	None known	Symptoms include dermatitis, conjunctivitis, depression, and hair loss	Biotin
Vitamin B_6	Protein metabolism Homocysteine metabolism Glycogenolysis	Males and females: 1.3 mg/day	Fortified cereals, meat, fish, poultry, many vegetables and fruits, nuts, peanut butter, and other legumes	Sore tongue, dermatitis, depression, confusion, irritability, headaches, and nerve damage UL: 100 mg/day	Microcytic hypochromic anemia; characterized by fatigue, paleness of skin, shortness of breath, dizziness, and lack of appetite	PLP
Folate	DNA and red blood cell formation Homocysteine metabolism	Males and females: 400 μg/day Pregnant women and women of childbearing age who may become pregnant: 600 μg/day	Dark green leafy vegetables, enriched pasta, rice, breads and cereals, legumes	Masks vitamin B_{12} deficiency UL: 1,000 μg/day	Macrocytic anemia; characterized by fatigue, headache, glossitis, and GI tract symptoms such as diarrhea	THF
Vitamin B_{12}	Synthesis of new cells, especially red blood cells Health of nerve tissue Activates folate Catabolism of amino acids and fatty acids in energy metabolism	Males and females: 2.4 μg/day	Animal products, including lean meats, fish, poultry, eggs, and cheese, and fortified foods	None known	Pernicious anemia; characterized by fatigue, glossitis, and nerve damage as indicated by tingling and numbness in the hands and feet	Methyl-cobalamin
Vitamin C	Collagen formation Antioxidant Iron absorption Immune system	Males: 90 mg/day Females: 75 mg/day	Citrus fruit, tomatoes, peppers, potatoes, broccoli, and cantaloupe	Nausea, diarrhea, fatigue, insomnia UL: 2,000 mg/day	Scurvy; characterized by bleeding gums, pinpoint hemorrhages, joint pain	Ascorbic acid

VITAMIN B₁

EXPLORING Thiamin (Vitamin B₁)

LO 10.2 Describe the functions, recommended intakes, food sources, and toxicity and deficiency effects of thiamin.

What Is Thiamin (B₁)?

Thiamin, or vitamin B₁, was the first B vitamin to be discovered. The thiamin molecule (**Figure 10.4**) contains an amine ring, which includes nitrogen, and a thiazole ring that contains sulfur. Dietary forms of thiamin are converted to the active coenzyme form, **thiamin pyrophosphate (TPP)**, in the body by adding two phosphate groups to the molecule.

thiamin pyrophosphate (TPP) Coenzyme form of thiamin with two phosphate groups as part of the molecule.

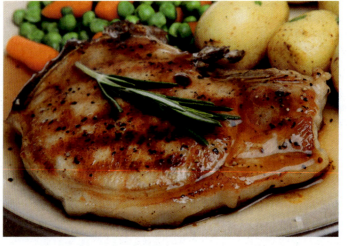

Thiamin is one of the vitamins that are sensitive to changes in pH. The practice of using baking soda during cooking (to cook beans faster, for example) destroys thiamin.

The alkaline solution breaks the bond between the rings and the central carbon. Using more acid-based foods, such as tomatoes, when cooking thiamin-rich foods protects the vitamin from destruction.

Thiamin is absorbed in the small intestine, mostly in the jejunum, primarily by passive diffusion. At lower intakes, thiamin is absorbed by active transport. It is transported through the blood and excreted through the urine.

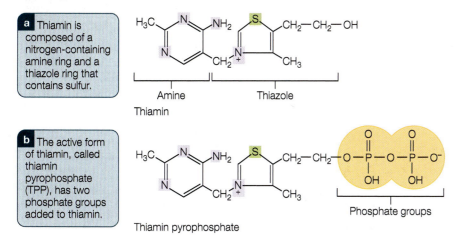

a Thiamin is composed of a nitrogen-containing amine ring and a thiazole ring that contains sulfur.

Amine | Thiazole

Thiamin

b The active form of thiamin, called thiamin pyrophosphate (TPP), has two phosphate groups added to thiamin.

Thiamin pyrophosphate

Phosphate groups

▲ **Figure 10.4 The Structures of Thiamin and Thiamin Pyrophosphate**

Metabolic Functions of Thiamin

Thiamin participates in the production of ATP in several different reactions, most of which involve carbohydrates. The coenzyme TPP activates an enzyme (called a *decarboxylase*) that removes a carbon from pyruvate (a three-carbon molecule) to form acetyl CoA (a two-carbon molecule) and carbon dioxide (**Figure 10.5**). A similar TPP-dependent enzyme converts alpha-ketoglutarate (a five-carbon molecule) to succinyl CoA (a four-carbon molecule) in the TCA cycle.

Thiamin pyrophosphate is also essential for protein metabolism. Thiamin assists in converting three branched-chain amino acids—leucine, isoleucine, and valine—into acetyl CoA to enter the TCA cycle. Without thiamin, energy production from glucose and amino acids would be impossible.

Thiamin is also used to synthesize sugars called *pentoses* that are needed as the starting material for DNA and RNA. This same pathway forms NADPH, a form of niacin needed for fat synthesis.

In addition, thiamin plays a role in the functioning of the nervous system. It does not act as a coenzyme, and the precise mechanism is unclear; however, thiamin may participate in the manufacture of specific chemicals involved in conducting nerve signals.

Daily Needs for Thiamin

The RDA for thiamin for adults is 1.1 milligrams for women and 1.2 milligrams for men. Currently, adult American men consume close to 2 milligrams of thiamin daily, whereas women, on average, consume approximately 1.2 milligrams daily, so both groups are meeting their daily needs.[1] These requirements may be greater for those who ingest more kilocalories, especially from carbohydrates.

Food Sources of Thiamin

Thiamin is present in both unprocessed and enriched foods. Whole-grain and enriched breads, ready-to-eat cereals, and pasta, as well as brown rice, enriched rice, and nuts, are the biggest contributors of thiamin in the American diet. Lean pork is the densest source of naturally occurring thiamin. A medium-sized bowl of thiamin-fortified ready-to-eat cereal in the morning and a ham sandwich on wheat bread at lunch will nearly meet your daily thiamin requirement (see **Figure 10.6**). For more food sources of thiamin, see the nearby Table Tips.

Thiamin Toxicity and Deficiency

There are no known toxicity symptoms from consuming too much thiamin. For this reason no Tolerable Upper Intake Level (UL) has been set.

Glucose
↓
Pyruvate

TPP → CO₂

Acetyl CoA ← BCAA

TCA Cycle

Alpha-ketoglutarate

TPP → CO₂

Succinyl CoA

a Thiamin pyrophosphate (TPP) activates the enzyme decarboxylase that removes a carbon from pyruvate, forming carbon dioxide and acetyl CoA following glycolysis.

b TPP participates in the catabolism of branched-chain amino acids (BCAAs) to acetyl CoA.

c TPP activates the enzyme that removes a carbon from alpha-ketoglutarate, forming carbon dioxide and succinyl CoA in the TCA cycle.

▲ **Figure 10.5 The Function of Thiamin Pyrophosphate in Energy Metabolism**

TABLE TIPS
Thrive with Thiamin
Sprinkle cereal on yogurt.
Toss pasta with peas. Both foods boost thiamin intake.
Add cooked rice to soups.
Have a sandwich made with whole grains and lean meats.
Enjoy oatmeal for breakfast.

(continued)

Vitamin B₁ (continued)

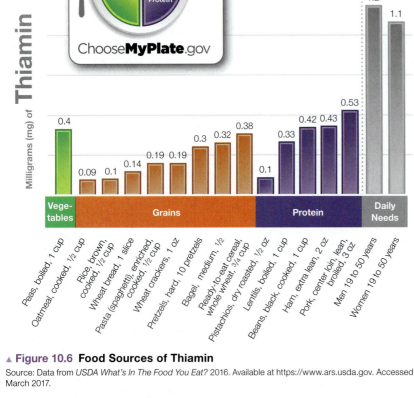

▲ **Figure 10.6 Food Sources of Thiamin**
Source: Data from *USDA What's In The Food You Eat?* 2016. Available at https://www.ars.usda.gov. Accessed March 2017.

Thiamin deficiencies result from insufficient dietary intake, malabsorption, alcoholism, or prolonged diarrhea. A deficiency of thiamin can also occur when there is an increased need, such as during pregnancy and lactation, and insufficient thiamin is consumed.

In the United States, refined grains are enriched with thiamin, so instances of beriberi are rare; however, Americans are not completely immune to thiamin deficiencies. Those who chronically abuse alcohol tend to eat poorly; moreover, chronic alcohol consumption interferes with the absorption of the small amounts of thiamin that may be in the diet, accelerating its loss from the body. Together, these factors commonly lead to an advanced form of thiamin deficiency called *Wernicke-Korsakoff syndrome* (see Chapter 7). This neurological disorder can cause mental confusion and memory loss, impaired vision, low blood pressure, uncontrolled movement of the arms and legs, and even coma. Although some of these symptoms can be reversed after the person is medically treated with thiamin, some of the memory loss may be permanent.[2]

Thiamin-deficiency disease is **beriberi**. The role of thiamin deficiency in beriberi was first confirmed in populations consuming polished white rice—which is depleted of thiamin—as a dietary staple. General symptoms of beriberi include loss of appetite, weight loss, memory loss, confusion, muscle weakness, and **peripheral neuropathy**. *Wet* beriberi is characterized by edema and congestive heart failure, while *dry* beriberi victims show signs of muscle wasting without edema and nerve degeneration.

beriberi Thiamin deficiency that results in weakness; the name translates to "I can not."

peripheral neuropathy Damage to the peripheral nerves causing pain, numbness, and tingling in the feet and hands and muscle weakness.

LO 10.2: THE TAKE-HOME MESSAGE
Thiamin, found abundantly in lean pork and whole-grain foods, is necessary for energy metabolism and plays a role in nerve transmission. Adult females need 1.1 mg and males need 1.2 mg per day of thiamin. There is no known toxicity for thiamin. A thiamin deficiency leads to beriberi.

EXPLORING **Riboflavin (Vitamin B₂)**

LO 10.3 Describe the functions, recommended intakes, food sources, and toxicity and deficiency effects of riboflavin.

flavin mononucleotide (FMN) Coenzyme form of riboflavin, which functions in the electron transport chain.

What Is Riboflavin (B₂)?

Riboflavin, also known as vitamin B₂, is a water-soluble compound composed of a side chain and a ring structure. The structures of riboflavin and its two coenzyme forms are illustrated in **Figure 10.7**. **Flavin mononucleotide (FMN)** is composed of three rings plus a sugar alcohol, shown as a straight chain in Figure 10.7. Attached is one phosphate group. You learned about flavin adenine dinucleotide (FAD) as a hydrogen ion acceptor or donator in oxidation-reduction reactions in Chapter 8. FAD combines FMN plus an additional phosphate group, an adenine and a five-carbon sugar, referred to as *AMP*. Both coenzyme forms are active in the body.

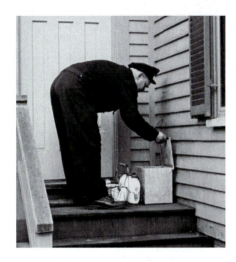

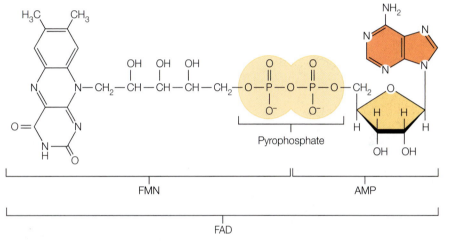

Riboflavin

a Riboflavin contains a 3-ring structure with a side chain attached.

Pyrophosphate

FMN

AMP

FAD

b The two active forms of riboflavin: FMN has one phosphate added to the riboflavin molecule. FAD has FMN plus an AMP molecule a second phosphate.

Riboflavin is fairly stable during cooking, but it degrades in the presence of ultraviolet light. Many decades ago, a milkman delivered milk to households that contained an abundant source of riboflavin. At each delivery, the milkman placed the clear glass milk bottles inside a covered "milk box" outside the home to protect the light-sensitive riboflavin in the milk from being destroyed by sunlight. Today, some dairy farmers sell milk in glass bottles, touting the improved taste and environmental benefits of reusable bottles over opaque plastic or cardboard containers. However, what they don't advertise is that the sunlight that reaches milk in glass containers destroys much of its riboflavin.

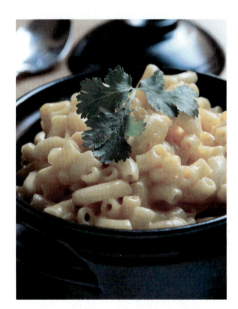

In fact, in just 30 minutes, UV can destroy over 30 percent of the riboflavin in glass-bottled milk.[3] This is the reason that most milk is packaged in opaque containers.

Riboflavin is usually attached to proteins in food and must be released during digestion. Hydrochloric acid denatures the protein, which frees the riboflavin to be absorbed by active transport in the small intestine.

Metabolic Functions of Riboflavin

Riboflavin participates in energy metabolism mostly through oxidation-reduction reactions (see the Chemistry Boost).

Both FMN and FAD are the main carriers of high-energy electrons generated in metabolic reactions. For example, in the conversion of carbohydrates and proteins into energy, high-energy electrons are transferred to FAD in the TCA cycle, which reduces it to FADH$_2$ (see Chapter 8). The FADH$_2$ transports the electrons to the electron transport chain to produce ATP. In addition to riboflavin's function in converting carbohydrates, fats, and proteins into energy, it also participates as FADH$_2$ in beta-oxidation, which converts fatty acids into acetyl CoA. FAD is also involved in oxidation-reduction reactions that protect cells from oxidative stress.[4]

(continued)

Chemistry Boost

The Role of Riboflavin in Redox Reactions

Recall from Chapter 8 that, in a redox reaction, an electron is lost from one molecule in an oxidation reaction and gained by another molecule in a reduction reaction. FAD and FMN are major electron carriers in redox reactions during the TCA cycle. The oxidized form is FAD and the reduced form is $FADH_2$. The redox reaction is illustrated in the example below:

$$succinate + FAD \rightarrow fumarate + FADH_2$$

The oxidized form of flavin mononucleotide is FMN and the reduced form is $FMNH_2$. Other water-soluble vitamins such as niacin (NAD^+) and vitamin C also play important roles in oxidation-reduction reactions.

FAD

FADH₂

During the TCA cycle, compounds release hydrogen ions and their high-energy electrons during oxidation. These are grabbed by FAD to form $FADH_2$.

The reduced form ($FADH_2$) carries the electrons to the electron transport chain, where they are released and FAD is reformed to grab more hydrogen ions. The released hydrogen ions combine with oxygen to form water.

Riboflavin enhances the functions of other B vitamins, such as niacin, folate, and vitamin B_6. For instance, riboflavin as FAD helps convert folate to its active form and aids in the reaction that converts the amino acid tryptophan to niacin, and riboflavin as FMN is essential to convert vitamin B_6 to its coenzyme form. Because riboflavin is involved in the metabolism of several other vitamins, a severe riboflavin deficiency may affect many enzyme systems.

ariboflavinosis Deficiency of riboflavin characterized by stomatitis, glossitis, and cheilosis.

stomatitis Inflammation of the mucous lining of the mouth.

glossitis Inflammation of the tongue.

cheilosis Noninflammatory condition of the lips characterized by chapping and fissuring.

Daily Needs for Riboflavin

The recommended daily intake of riboflavin for adult males is 1.3 milligrams and 1.1 milligrams for females. The average intake of riboflavin in the United States for adult males is about 2 milligrams per day, and adult females consume about 1.5 milligrams per day. This is well above the RDA.

Food Sources of Riboflavin

Milk and yogurt are the most popular sources of riboflavin in the diets of American adults, followed by enriched cereals and grains (see **Figure 10.8**). A breakfast of cereal and milk and a mid-morning yogurt meets riboflavin needs for the day. For those individuals who follow a gluten-free diet, riboflavin needs can

Raise Your Riboflavin

Have a glass of low-fat milk with meals.

A yogurt snack is a riboflavin snack.

Pizza is a good source of riboflavin.

Enriched pasta enriches the meal with riboflavin.

Macaroni and cheese provides a double source of riboflavin—the pasta and the cheese.

Spinach, almonds, Crimini mushrooms, asparagus, and eggs are gluten- and dairy-free sources of riboflavin.

be met by consuming gluten-free grains such as quinoa, rice, or oats. For more food sources of riboflavin, see the nearby Table Tips.

Riboflavin Toxicity and Deficiency

The body tightly controls the metabolism of riboflavin depending on the riboflavin status of the individual. About 95 percent of riboflavin is absorbed, and excessive amounts are excreted in urine. In fact, because riboflavin is a bright yellow compound, consuming large amounts through supplements turns urine as yellow as a school bus. While this isn't dangerous to health, it isn't beneficial either. No UL for riboflavin has been determined.

Ariboflavinosis is the name for riboflavin deficiency (**Figure 10.9**). The term covers a host of symptoms caused by inflammation of the tissues of the mouth and throat. These include a sore throat, irritation of the lining of the inside of the mouth (**stomatitis**), an inflamed tongue (**glossitis**) that may appear shiny and purplish red, and cracked or sore lips (**cheilosis**) with cracks at the corners of the mouth. In older adults, a deficiency of riboflavin reduces the conversion of vitamin B_6 to its active form and is reversed when riboflavin supplements are given. Riboflavin deficiencies also alter iron metabolism and the synthesis of hemoglobin.[5]

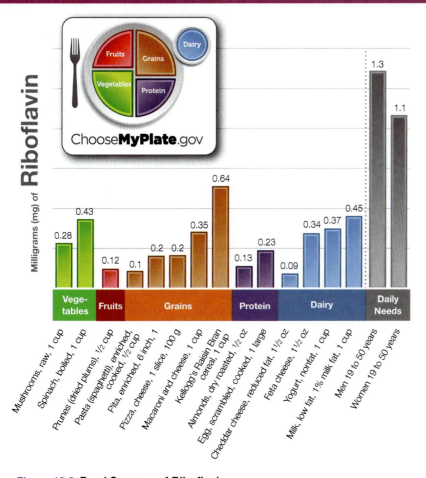

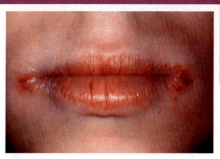

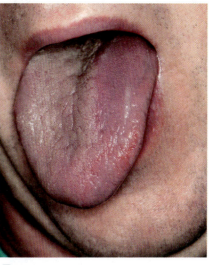

b Glossitis

▲ **Figure 10.8 Food Sources of Riboflavin**
Source: Data from *USDA What's In The Food You Eat?* 2016. Available at https://www.ars.usda.gov. Accessed March 2017.

▲ **Figure 10.9 The Symptoms of Ariboflavinosis**
The symptoms of a deficiency of many of the B vitamins (including ariboflavinosis) include (a) cheilosis and (b) glossitis.

LO 10.3: THE TAKE-HOME MESSAGE Riboflavin, or vitamin B_2, is stable in cooking but is degraded by ultraviolet light. Riboflavin participates in oxidation-reduction reactions. The RDA for adults is 1.3 mg per day for males and 1.1 mg per day for females. Milk and yogurt are the most popular sources of riboflavin. Nondairy sources include enriched grains, leafy green vegetables, eggs, and almonds. Excess amounts are excreted in urine and there are no known toxicity symptoms. A deficiency in riboflavin results in ariboflavinosis.

EXPLORING **Niacin (Vitamin B₃)**

LO 10.4 Describe the functions, recommended intakes, food sources, and toxicity and deficiency effects of niacin.

What Is Niacin (B₃)?

Niacin, or vitamin B_3, is the generic term for nicotinic acid and nicotinamide (not related to nicotine in tobacco), which are the two active forms of niacin derived from food (**Figure 10.10**). Both forms are converted to the active coenzymes **nicotinamide adenine dinucleotide (NAD⁺)** and **nicotinamide adenine dinucleotide phosphate (NADP⁺)** in the liver. These coenzymes play an essential role in energy metabolism.

nicotinamide adenine dinucleotide (NAD⁺) Coenzyme form of niacin that functions as an electron carrier and can be reduced to NADH during metabolism.

nicotinamide adenine dinucleotide phosphate (NADP⁺) Coenzyme form of niacin that functions as an electron carrier and can be reduced to NADPH during metabolism.

(continued)

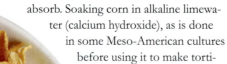
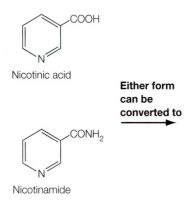

Unlike some B vitamins, niacin is stable in foods and is not destroyed by heat or ultraviolet light. Because niacin is water soluble, it can leach if food is cooked or soaked in water. The niacin found in plant foods, such as wheat or corn, is found complexed with proteins and is much less bioavailable than niacin from meat and dairy products. Niacin in corn, for example, is bound to a protein that is difficult to

niacin equivalents (NE) Measurement that reflects the amount of niacin and tryptophan in foods that can be used to synthesize niacin.

absorb. Soaking corn in alkaline limewater (calcium hydroxide), as is done in some Meso-American cultures before using it to make tortillas, helps release the vitamin and improves its bioavailability.[6] Unfortunately, by increasing the pH, this practice destroys the other B vitamins present in corn.

Most of the niacin in foods is absorbed by a sodium-dependent, carrier-mediated facilitated diffusion in the small intestine. At high concentrations, such as when taking a niacin supplement, niacin is absorbed by passive diffusion. It circulates through the blood to the liver, where it is converted to NAD^+ and $NADP^+$.

Metabolic Functions of Niacin

NAD^+ and $NADP^+$ are key to the metabolism of glucose, protein, fat, and alcohol. These coenzymes both participate in oxidation-reduction reactions but have different roles in the cell. NAD^+ functions mostly in oxidative reactions that are catabolic and produce energy (**Figure 10.11**). In fatty-acid oxidation, for instance,

NAD^+ is reduced to $NADH^+$, which carries electrons to the electron transport chain to produce ATP and water.

$NADP^+$ acts mostly as a reducing agent. In reduction reactions, this coenzyme form of niacin can synthesize compounds such as fat and cholesterol. Niacin also aids in vitamin C and folate metabolism.

Niacin is needed to keep skin cells healthy and the digestive system functioning properly. Niacin in the form of nicotinic acid (not nicotinamide) has been used since 1955 to lower the total amount of cholesterol in the blood by lowering Lp(a) lipoprotein, an LDL cholesterol carrier linked to heart disease. Niacin can also lower high levels of blood triglycerides and simultaneously raise the HDL concentration.[7]

When nicotinic acid is used to treat high blood cholesterol, it is considered a pharmacological dose or drug. The 2–4 grams per day often prescribed by a physician is more than 40 times the UL of 35 milligrams per day for niacin. Individuals should *never* consume high-dose niacin unless a physician prescribes it and monitors them.

Daily Needs for Niacin

Niacin can be synthesized in the body from the amino acid tryptophan. For this reason, daily niacin needs are measured in **niacin equivalents (NE)**. It is estimated

---

a Two forms of niacin found in food.

b NAD^+ is the active coenzyme form of niacin formed in the liver.

c The coenzyme $NADP^+$ is similar to NAD^+ but has a phosphate group in the place of a hydroxyl group.

Nicotinic acid

Nicotinamide

Either form can be converted to

Nicotinamide adenine dinucleotide (NAD^+)

or

Nicotinamide adenine dinucleotide phosphate ($NADP^+$)

▲ **Figure 10.10** **The Structures of Niacin and Its Coenzyme Forms NAD^+ and $NADP^+$**

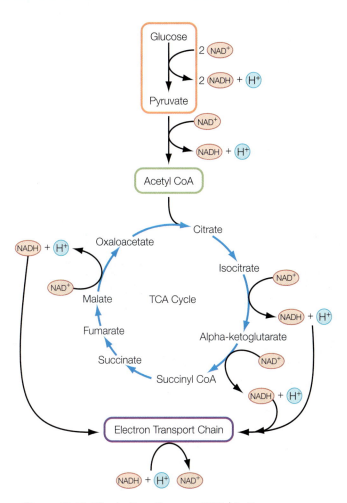

▲ **Figure 10.11 Niacin Functions as NAD⁺ in Energy Metabolism**
The coenzyme form of niacin, NAD⁺, participates in oxidation-reduction reactions in glycolysis, transporting H⁺atoms to the electron transport chain.

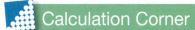
Calculation Corner

Niacin Equivalents

The recommendation for niacin is expressed in milligrams of niacin equivalents (mg NE) that reflect either the amount of preformed niacin in foods or the amount that can be formed from a food's content of the amino acid tryptophan.

Calculating milligrams NE from a meal can be completed by two different methods.

(a) If you know the amount of preformed niacin in milligrams (mg) and the amount of tryptophan in grams (g) in the meal, then use this formula to calculate the total amount of niacin equivalents in the meal:

$$(tryptophan \times 1{,}000 \div 60) + preformed\ niacin = mg\ NE$$

In this formula, the amount of tryptophan must be converted from grams to milligrams (tryptophan × 1,000) and then divided by 60 (60 mg of tryptophan can be converted into 1 mg of niacin). Then add the preformed niacin found in the meal for the total milligrams of niacin.

Example: A breakfast contains 0.02 g of tryptophan and 7.0 mg of preformed niacin. How many mg NE does the meal contain?

Answer: (0.02 g tryptophan × 1,000 ÷ 60) + 7.0 mg niacin = 7.3 mg NE

(b) If you only know the total amount of protein in the meal, but not the tryptophan content, you must estimate the amount of tryptophan. Total protein in a meal is approximately 1.1 percent tryptophan. This formula uses the 1.1 percentage to calculate mg NE:

$$(0.011 \times g\ of\ protein) \times 1{,}000 \div 60 + preformed\ niacin = mg\ NE$$

Example: A breakfast contains 8 g of protein and 3 mg of preformed niacin. How many mg NE does the meal contain?

Answer: (0.011 × 8 g protein) × 1,000 ÷ 60 + 3 mg preformed niacin = 4.5 mg NE

Go to Mastering Nutrition and complete a Math Video activity similar to the problem in this Calculation Corner.

---

that 60 milligrams of tryptophan can be converted to 1 milligram of niacin or 1 milligram NE. This conversion depends on the B vitamins riboflavin and vitamin B₆ and the mineral iron. The Calculation Corner illustrates how to calculate niacin equivalents from tryptophan.

The recommended daily amount of niacin for adults is 14 milligrams NE for women and 16 milligrams NE for men, an amount set to prevent the deficiency disease pellagra. American adults, on average, far exceed their daily niacin needs.[8]

Food Sources of Niacin

Niacin used by the body comes from two sources: preformed niacin found in food and niacin formed from excess amounts of the amino acid tryptophan. Preformed niacin is found in meat, fish, poultry, enriched whole-grain breads and bread products, and fortified cereals (see **Figure 10.12**). Protein-rich foods, particularly animal foods such as meat, are also good sources of tryptophan. However, if an individual is falling short of both dietary protein and niacin, the body first uses tryptophan to make protein, at the expense of niacin needs.[9] For more food sources of niacin, see the nearby Table Tips.

Niacin Toxicity and Deficiency

As with most water-soluble vitamins, there isn't any known danger of consuming too much niacin from foods. However, overconsuming niacin (more than 1 gram per day) by taking supplements can cause *flushing*, a reddish coloring of the face,

---

TABLE TIPS
Need More Niacin?
Have a serving of enriched cereal in the morning.
Dip niacin-rich peppers in hummus.
Enjoy a lean chicken breast at dinner.
Snack on peanuts.
Put tuna fish flakes on salad.

(continued)

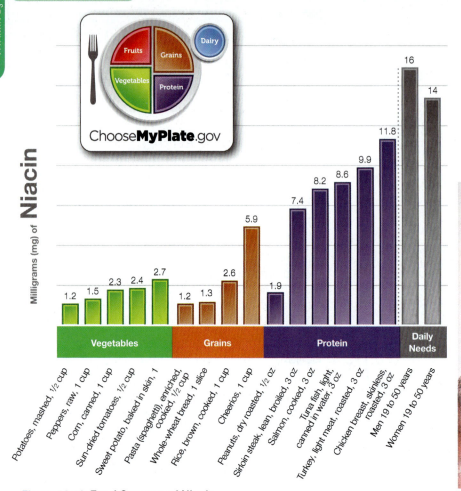

Milligrams (mg) of **Niacin**

ChooseMyPlate.gov — Fruits, Grains, Dairy, Vegetables, Protein

| 16 |
| 14 |
| 11.8 |
| 9.9 |
| 8.6 |
| 8.2 |
| 7.4 |
| 5.9 |
| 2.7 |
| 2.6 |
| 2.4 |
| 2.3 |
| 1.9 |
| 1.5 |
| 1.3 |
| 1.2 |
| 1.2 |

Vegetables | **Grains** | **Protein** | **Daily Needs**

Potatoes, mashed, 1/2 cup; Peppers, raw, 1 cup; Corn, canned, 1 cup; Sun-dried tomatoes, 1/2 cup; Sweet potato, baked in skin, 1; Pasta (spaghetti), enriched, cooked, 1/2 cup; Whole-wheat bread, 1 slice; Rice, brown, cooked, 1 cup; Cheerios, 1 cup; Peanuts, dry roasted, 1/2 oz; Sirloin steak, lean, broiled, 3 oz; Salmon, cooked, 3 oz; Tuna fish, light, canned in water, 3 oz; Turkey, light meat, roasted, 3 oz; Chicken breast, skinless, roasted, 3 oz; Men 19 to 50 years; Women 19 to 50 years

▲ **Figure 10.12** **Food Sources of Niacin**
Source: Data from *USDA What's In The Food You Eat?* 2016. Available at https://www.ars.usda.gov. Accessed March 2017.

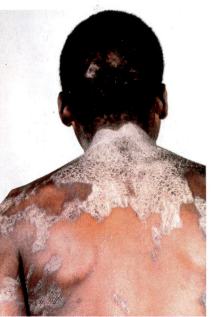

▲ **Figure 10.13** **Pellagra Can Cause Dermatitis**

arms, and chest. Excess niacin can also cause nausea and vomiting and heartburn, be toxic to the liver, and raise blood glucose levels. The UL for niacin for adults is 35 milligrams. This UL applies only to healthy individuals; it may be too high for those with certain medical conditions, such as diabetes mellitus and liver disease.[10]

Too little niacin in the diet can result in the deficiency disease **pellagra** (**Figure 10.13**). In the early 1900s, pellagra was widespread among the poor living in the southern United States, where people relied on corn—which contains little available niacin and no tryptophan—as a dietary staple. The symptoms of pellagra—dermatitis, dementia, and diarrhea—led to its being known as the disease of the three Ds. A fourth D, death, was also often associated with the disease.

Once fortified cereal grains became available, pellagra became rare in the United States. The niacin in fortified grains and protein-rich diets was later identified as the curative factor. Although no longer common in the United States, pellagra does occur among individuals who abuse alcohol and have a very poor diet.

pellagra Disease resulting from a deficiency of niacin or tryptophan.

LO 10.4: THE TAKE-HOME MESSAGE
Niacin functions in the catabolism and anabolism of carbohydrates, fats, and proteins in energy metabolism in oxidation-reduction reactions. The RDA for niacin is 16 NE for males and 14 NE for females. Niacin is found in a variety of foods, including meat, fish, poultry, fortified cereals, and enriched breads. There is no danger of consuming too much niacin, although overconsumption of niacin supplements can cause flushing. A deficiency of niacin results in pellagra.

EXPLORING **Pantothenic Acid**

LO 10.5 Describe the functions, recommended intakes, food sources, and toxicity and deficiency effects of pantothenic acid.

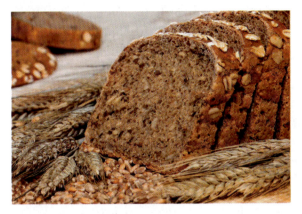

What Is Pantothenic Acid?

Pantothenic acid makes up part of the compound *coenzyme A*, which also contains the amino acid cysteine. Recall from Chapter 8 that coenzyme A combines with a two-carbon acetyl group to become *acetyl CoA*, the gateway molecule in energy metabolism (**Figure 10.14**). The small intestine absorbs this essential B vitamin by active transport when intake is low and by passive diffusion at higher intakes. Once absorbed, pantothenic acid is circulated through the blood to the liver. The vitamin itself is not stored, but high levels of acetyl CoA are found in the liver, kidney, adrenal glands, and brain.[11]

Metabolic Functions of Pantothenic Acid

As part of coenzyme A, pantothenic acid functions in numerous reactions that are essential to metabolism. Coenzyme A is needed in fat metabolism both for lipogenesis to synthesize fatty acids and to convert

them to energy through beta-oxidation. Pantothenic acid participates in the decarboxylation of pyruvate that produces acetyl CoA, the "gateway" molecule for aerobic metabolism. Pantothenic acid as coenzyme A also participates in protein metabolism by converting some amino acids to intermediate substrates in the TCA cycle and in the synthesis of cholesterol, steroid hormones, and the neurotransmitter acetylcholine.[12]

Daily Needs for Pantothenic Acid

The Adequate Intake (AI) for pantothenic acid has been set at 5 milligrams per day for both adult males and females. This recommendation is based on the amount needed to replace the amount excreted in the urine.

Food Sources of Pantothenic Acid

Pantothenic acid gets its name from the Greek word *pantothen,* which means "everywhere," because it is found in almost every food. The highest amounts

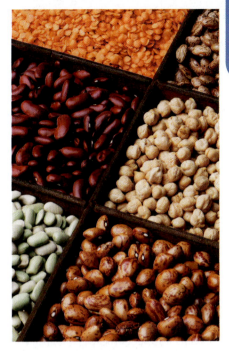

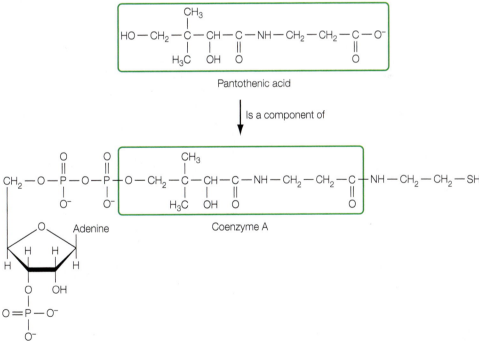

▲ **Figure 10.14 The Structures of Pantothenic Acid and Coenzyme A**
Pantothenic acid combines with the amino acid cysteine to form coenzyme A. To form acetyl CoA, coenzyme A combines with the two-carbon acetyl group. Acetyl CoA is the gateway molecule for all energy nutrients to enter the TCA cycle during energy metabolism.

(continued)

are found in whole-grain cereals, nuts and legumes, peanut butter, meat, milk, and eggs. Pantothenic acid can be destroyed by heat, so refined grains and foods that are processed, such as frozen or canned vegetables, fish, and meat, are lower in pantothenic acid than their fresh counterparts. For more food sources of pantothenic acid, see the nearby Table Tips.

Pantothenic Acid Toxicity and Deficiency

As with many other B vitamins, there are no known adverse effects from consuming too much pantothenic acid, and therefore no UL has been established.

Although a pantothenic acid deficiency is rare, individuals who fall short of their need may experience fatigue, nausea and vomiting, numbness, muscle cramps, and difficulty walking. Sufficient pantothenic acid intakes can prevent these conditions.[13]

TABLE TIPS

A Plethora of Pantothenic Acid

Sprinkle a tablespoon of brewer's yeast on cooked oatmeal in the morning.

Add colorful kale, avocado, and tomatoes to salad greens.

Enjoy a three-bean salad with the midday meal.

Include nuts and seeds, such as peanuts and sunflower seeds, among regular snack foods.

Substitute sweet potatoes for baked potatoes at dinner.

LO 10.5: THE TAKE-HOME MESSAGE

Pantothenic acid, found in whole-grain cereals, nuts and legumes, milk, meat, and eggs, makes up part of the molecule coenzyme A and participates in lipogenesis and beta-oxidation, in the conversion of pyruvate to acetyl CoA, and in converting some amino acids to substrates in the TCA cycle. The AI for panthothenic acid is 5 mg. There are no known adverse effects from consuming too much pantothenic acid and deficiencies are rare.

EXPLORING Biotin

LO 10.6 Describe the functions, recommended intakes, food sources, and toxicity and deficiency effects of biotin.

What Is Biotin?

In 1914, doctors discovered that adding raw egg white to a balanced diet resulted in dermatitis and hair loss, depression, and nausea. The binding of the vitamin biotin with **avidin**, a protein found in egg whites, caused the condition, which they referred to as *egg white injury*. Avidin can bind up to four molecules of biotin, which renders the vitamin unavailable for absorption. The problem only occurs when raw eggs are consumed, as cooking eggs denatures

avidin Protein in raw egg whites that binds biotin.

biotinidase Enzyme in the small intestine that releases biotin from food to allow it to be absorbed.

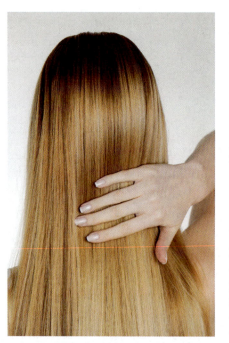

Biotin enhances cell development, promoting the health of hair and nails.

the avidin and prevents it from binding to biotin.

Biotin is made up of sulfur-containing double rings and a side chain (**Figure 10.15**). During digestion, the enzyme **biotinidase** releases biotin from food in the small intestine, allowing the free biotin to be absorbed by active transport. Once absorbed into the portal vein, biotin is taken up by the liver and stored in small amounts.

Metabolic Functions of Biotin

Biotin functions as a coenzyme for enzymes that add carbon dioxide to compounds involved in energy metabolism. As illustrated in **Figure 10.16**, biotin activates enzymes that synthesize fatty acids from acetate formed from acetyl CoA; it replenishes oxaloacetate from pyruvate, which is important in the TCA cycle and in gluconeogenesis; it aids in the metabolism of the amino acid leucine; and helps convert some amino acids into compounds that can be used in the TCA cycle. Thus, without adequate biotin, energy metabolism would be impaired.

Biotin also plays a role in DNA replication; in fact, biotin is required for transcription of over 2,000 genes.[14] It also facilitates cell development and growth. Some people refer to biotin as the "beauty vitamin," for example, because it helps maintain healthy hair and nails. The exact mechanisms of these roles are still unclear.

Daily Needs for Biotin

The AI of biotin has been set at 30 micrograms per day for both adult males and females. However, compared with the other B vitamins, much less data is available on which to base the DRI for biotin. This is one reason that the FDA has set the percent Daily Value for biotin at 300 micrograms, or 10 times the AI.

▲ **Figure 10.15 The Chemical Structure of Biotin**
A molecule of biotin contains both nitrogen and sulfur as part of its structure.

Food Sources of Biotin

Even a small amount of peanuts (¼ cup) provides more than 60 percent of the AI for biotin. Other biotin-rich food sources include yeast, egg yolks, whole grains, liver and other organ meats, and fish. For more food sources of biotin, see the nearby Table Tips.

Biotin Toxicity and Deficiency

There is little evidence that consuming too much biotin can have toxic side effects, even at doses as high as 200 milligrams per day.[15] For this reason, a UL has not been set.

Bacteria in the GI tract synthesize some biotin, which may be a reason deficiencies are rare. However, whether the biotin produced by bacteria is absorbed remains unknown.

An individual would have to eat more than 12 raw eggs or egg whites per day over a prolonged period of time to develop egg white injury. Biotin deficiencies may also occur in patients receiving total nutrition intravenously when the GI tract is not functioning (such as after surgery). Other circumstances in which biotin may be lacking include conditions that impair absorption such as Crohn's disease or ulcerative colitis and in some individuals with rare genetic disorders, such as a lack of biotinidase, the digestive enzyme that hydrolyzes biotin from protein.[16]

Symptoms of a biotin deficiency include dermatitis, especially around the eyes, nose, and mouth; conjunctivitis; hair loss; and alterations in the central nervous system resulting in lethargy, hallucinations, and depression.

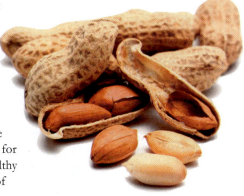

LO 10.6: THE TAKE-HOME MESSAGE
Biotin, found in peanuts, yeast, egg yolks, grains, fish, and liver, is active during energy metabolism, lipogenesis, gluconeogenesis, and the metabolism of amino acids. The AI for biotin is set at 30 micrograms. There is little evidence that excess biotin causes toxicity. Deficiencies of biotin are rare except when large amounts of raw eggs or egg whites are consumed.

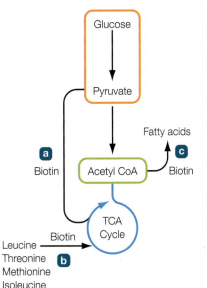

a Biotin helps add a CO_2 to pyruvate to form oxaloacetate, a compound in the TCA cycle. This is a key step in gluconeogenesis.

b Biotin helps break down leucine, threonine, methionine, and isoleucine to be used in the production of energy through the TCA cycle.

c Biotin plays a key role in synthesizing fatty acids from acetyl CoA.

▲ **Figure 10.16 The Role of Biotin as a Coenzyme in Energy Metabolism**

EXPLORING **Vitamin B₆**

LO 10.7 Describe the functions, recommended intakes, food sources, and toxicity and deficiency effects of vitamin B₆.

What Is Vitamin B₆?

Vitamin B₆ is a collective name for several related compounds, including pyridoxine, the major form found in plant foods and used in supplements and fortified foods.[17] Two other forms, pyridoxal and pyridoxamine, are found in animal food sources such as chicken and meat (**Figure 10.17**).

The bioavailability of vitamin B₆ is about 75 percent, and all forms are absorbed in the small intestine by passive diffusion. Once absorbed, the vitamin is attached to albumin and transported to the liver. The liver activates the vitamin by adding a phosphate group to form **pyridoxal phosphate (PLP)**. This active form of B₆ is stored attached to enzymes in the muscle and in smaller amounts in the liver, brain, kidneys, and spleen.

pyridoxal phosphate (PLP) Active coenzyme form of vitamin B₆.

Metabolic Functions of Vitamin B₆

Vitamin B₆ acts as a coenzyme for more than 100 enzymes, most of which are involved in protein metabolism. Vitamin B₆ is also a key player in glucose metabolism and red blood cell synthesis, and it interacts with other nutrients, including riboflavin, niacin, and zinc.

Vitamin B₆ and Amino Acid Metabolism

Almost every amino acid needs PLP for its metabolism. For example, PLP is needed during transamination to create nonessential amino acids (**Figure 10.18**). Thus, without vitamin B₆, all amino acids would become essential. Vitamin B₆ also helps convert the amino acid tryptophan to niacin.[18]

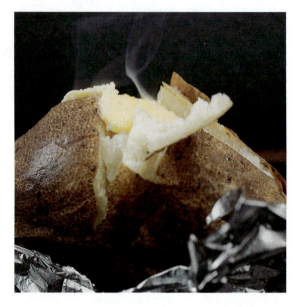

Vitamin B₆ and Carbohydrate Metabolism

Vitamin B₆ has a double role in the metabolism of carbohydrates. The PLP coenzyme participates in glycogenolysis in the muscle, thus enabling the body to tap into its glycogen stores for energy. Its second role is to activate enzymes involved

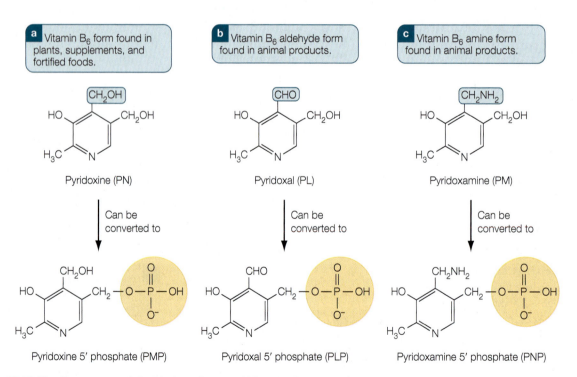

a Vitamin B₆ form found in plants, supplements, and fortified foods.

Pyridoxine (PN)

Can be converted to

Pyridoxine 5′ phosphate (PMP)

b Vitamin B₆ aldehyde form found in animal products.

Pyridoxal (PL)

Can be converted to

Pyridoxal 5′ phosphate (PLP)

c Vitamin B₆ amine form found in animal products.

Pyridoxamine (PM)

Can be converted to

Pyridoxamine 5′ phosphate (PNP)

▲ **Figure 10.17 The Structures of the Various Forms of Vitamin B₆**

$$\text{Pyruvate} + \text{Glutamate} \xrightarrow{\text{PLP}} \text{Alanine} + \alpha\text{-ketoglutarate}$$

▲ **Figure 10.18 Vitamin B$_6$ Assists in Transamination**
PLP helps transfer an amine group to form a new amino acid.

in gluconeogenesis to produce glucose from noncarbohydrate compounds.

Vitamin B$_6$ may also participate in fat metabolism, although the role is still unclear.

Other Functions of Vitamin B$_6$

Vitamin B$_6$ is needed to make the oxygen-carrying protein hemoglobin in the red blood cells.[19] It activates the enzyme responsible for the first step in hemoglobin synthesis and to keep the immune and nervous systems healthy.

As discussed in Chapter 5, research indicates that vitamin B$_6$, along with folate and vitamin B$_{12}$, may help reduce the risk of cardiovascular disease.[20] This reduced risk reflects the role of these B vitamins in converting the amino acid homocysteine to methionine. High homocysteine concentrations are linked to atherosclerosis.

Vitamin B$_6$ is routinely prescribed to reduce nausea and vomiting during pregnancy, although the mechanism is still uncertain. Some double-blind studies have reported that an intake of 30 milligrams of vitamin B$_6$ daily was helpful in reducing morning sickness; other studies have reported no benefit.[21]

Daily Needs for Vitamin B$_6$

Adult women need 1.3–1.5 milligrams and men need 1.3–1.7 milligrams of vitamin B$_6$ daily, depending on their age.

Food Sources of Vitamin B$_6$

Vitamin B$_6$ is found in a wide variety of foods, including fortified ready-to-eat cereals, meat, fish, poultry, many vegetables and fruits, nuts, peanut butter, and other legumes (see **Figure 10.19**). Because of the widespread availability of vitamin B$_6$, Americans on average easily meet their daily needs. For more food sources of vitamin B$_6$, see the nearby Table Tips.

TABLE TIPS

Boost Vitamin B$_6$

Have a stuffed baked potato with steamed broccoli and grilled chicken for lunch.

Grab a banana for a midmorning snack.

Add cooked barley to soup.

Snack on prunes.

Add kidney beans to chili or salad.

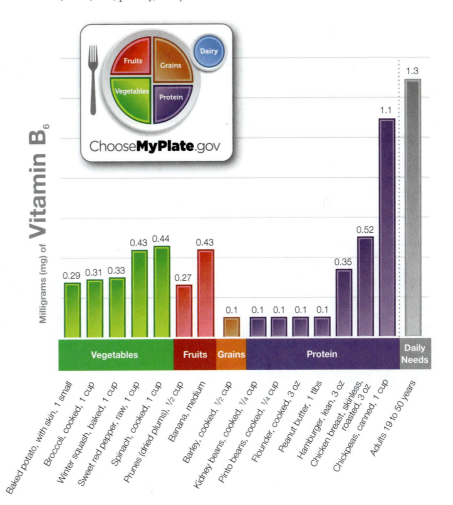

▲ **Figure 10.19 Food Sources of Vitamin B$_6$**
Source: Data from *USDA What's In The Food You Eat?* 2016. Available at https://www.ars.usda.gov. Accessed March 2017.

(continued)

Vitamin B₆ Toxicity and Deficiency

Because vitamin B_6 attaches to enzymes in the muscle and other tissues, it remains in the body, and excess intake can be toxic. To protect against potential nerve damage, a UL of 100 milligrams per day has been set for adults over the age of 18.

Over the years, vitamin B_6 has been touted to aid a variety of ailments, including carpal tunnel syndrome and premenstrual syndrome, and individuals may take a supplement to try to relieve these conditions. However, research studies have failed to show any significant clinical benefit in taking vitamin B_6 supplements for either of these syndromes.[22]

microcytic hypochromic anemia Form of anemia in which red blood cells are small and pale in color due to lack of hemoglobin synthesis.

Taking large amounts of vitamin B_6 through supplements has been associated with a variety of ill effects, including nerve damage. Individuals taking as little as 200 milligrams and as much as 6,000 milligrams of vitamin B_6 daily for 2 months experienced difficulty walking and tingling sensations in their legs and feet.[23] These symptoms subsided once the individuals stopped taking the supplements.

The telltale signs of a vitamin B_6 deficiency are a sore tongue, inflammation of the skin, depression, confusion, and **microcytic hypochromic anemia**. This type of anemia results in small (microcytic) red blood cells that look pale (hypochromic) in comparison with healthy red blood cells.

Those who consume too much alcohol are likely to fall short of their vitamin B_6 needs. Not only does alcohol deplete the body of vitamin B_6, but also those suffering from alcoholism are likely to have an unbalanced, unvaried diet.

LO 10.7: THE TAKE-HOME MESSAGE
Vitamin B_6, found in meat, fish, poultry, legumes, bananas, and fortified cereals, acts as a coenzyme for over 100 enzymes, most of which are involved in protein metabolism, glycogenolysis, and red blood cell synthesis. The RDA for vitamin B_6 is set at 1.3–1.5 mg for females and 1.3–1.7 mg for males depending on age. Excess vitamin B_6 in supplements may cause neurological damage. A deficiency of vitamin B_6 can result in microcytic hypochromic anemia, depression, and inflammation of the skin.

FOLATE

EXPLORING **Folate**

LO 10.8 Describe the functions, recommended intakes, food sources, and toxicity and deficiency effects of folate.

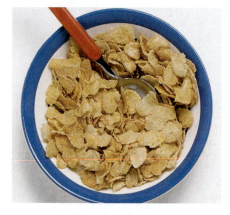

folate The B vitamin that functions as a coenzyme in cell growth and reproduction.

folic acid Form of folate often used in vitamin supplements and fortification of foods.

What Is Folate?

The naturally occurring form of **folate** is found in many foods, while the synthetic form, **folic acid**, is added to foods and found in supplements. (Actually, a very small amount of folic acid can occur naturally in foods. But, for practical purposes, here folic acid refers to the synthetic variety.) Compared with folate, folic acid is a simpler molecule. It is also easier to absorb (more bioavailable) than the natural form, but once absorbed, both forms perform equally well. The synthetic form is more stable and not as easily destroyed as the natural form.[24]

There are three parts to the molecular structure of folate (**Figure 10.20**): *pteridine* (pronounced ter-e-deen), *para-amino-benzoic acid (PABA),* and at least one glutamate. Most folate found in foods is in polyglutamate form, which means it has at least three glutamate molecules.

The synthetic folic acid is in a monoglutamate form.

Before folate can be absorbed, all but one of the glutamates must be

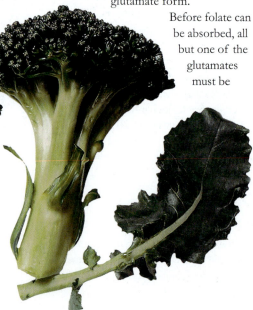

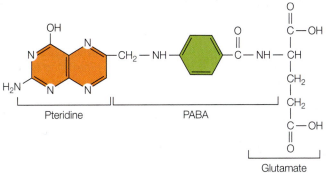

a Folate found in foods is composed of pteridine, PABA, and at least one glutamate molecule.

Pteridine   PABA   Glutamate

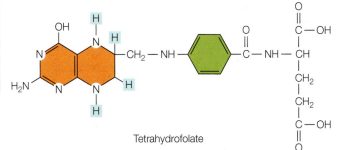

b Folate accepts four hydrogens to become tetrahydrofolate (THF), the active coenzyme form of folate.

Tetrahydrofolate

▲ **Figure 10.20 The Structures of Folate and Its Coenzyme Form**

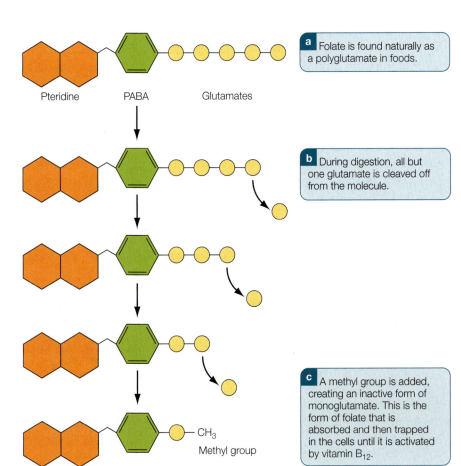

Pteridine   PABA   Glutamates

a Folate is found naturally as a polyglutamate in foods.

b During digestion, all but one glutamate is cleaved off from the molecule.

c A methyl group is added, creating an inactive form of monoglutamate. This is the form of folate that is absorbed and then trapped in the cells until it is activated by vitamin B_{12}.

CH₃
Methyl group

▲ **Figure 10.21 The Digestion of Folate**

removed from the side chain to form monoglutamate (one glutamate) during digestion (**Figure 10.21**). Folic acid is already in the monoglutamate form and thus doesn't need to go through digestion. Once inside the intestinal cell, both folate and folic acid are reduced to dihydrofolate and then further reduced by adding four hydrogen atoms (tetra) and a methyl group (CH_3) to the monoglutamate, creating **5-methyltetrahydrofolate (5-methyl THF)**. This is the form of folate that is transported through the bloodstream to the liver. A small amount of folate is stored in the liver, but the majority is excreted in the urine.

Metabolic Functions of Folate

Vitamin B_{12} is needed to remove the methyl group from 5-methyl THF to form active tetrahydrofolate (THF). Without the interaction with vitamin B_{12}, folate would be trapped in the cell and unable to perform its functions (see **Figure 10.27** on page 386).

The active form of folate acts as a coenzyme in the transfer of single-carbon compounds, such as a methyl group (CH_3), to other compounds. Folate accepts single-carbon compounds on the pteridine ring of THF and then donates the single-carbon compounds to other structures. This function is necessary to form new compounds.

DNA and Amino Acid Synthesis

The transfer of single-carbon compounds is essential for DNA metabolism and amino acid synthesis. To convert homocysteine to methionine requires both 5-methyl folate and vitamin B_{12}–dependent coenzymes. Methionine, in turn, provides the methyl group used in DNA and RNA synthesis.

If the synthesis of DNA is disrupted, the body's ability to create and maintain new cells is impaired. For this reason, folate plays many important roles, from preventing birth defects to fighting cancer and heart disease. Folate also helps the

5-methyltetrahydrofolate (5-methyl THF) Most active form of folate.

(continued)

Folate (continued)

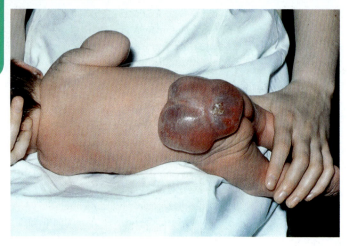

▲ **Figure 10.22 An Infant with Spina Bifida**

body use amino acids and is needed to help red blood cells divide and increase in adequate numbers.

Neural Tube Development

Because of its participation in DNA synthesis, folate plays an extremely important role during pregnancy, particularly in the first few weeks after conception. Cells divide rapidly during the embryonic period, and a folate deficiency at this time can result in a **neural tube defect**. The neural tube is the primitive form of the spinal cord and brain. If it doesn't develop properly, either of two neural tube defects can occur. In **anencephaly**, the brain doesn't completely form, and the newborn dies soon after birth. In **spina bifida**, the baby's spinal cord and vertebral column aren't properly developed (**Figure 10.22**). Spina bifida can cause both learning and physical disabilities, such as the inability to walk.[25]

Neural tube defects occur during the early stages of embryonic development, at a point when the mother may not even

neural tube defects Any major birth defect of the central nervous system, including the brain, caused by failure of the neural tube to properly close during embryonic development.

anencephaly Neural tube defect that results in the absence of major parts of the brain.

spina bifida Serious birth defect in which a portion of the spinal cord and its protective membranes (meninges) protrude from the vertebral column.

dietary folate equivalents (DFE) Measurement used to express the amount of folate in a food or supplement.

know she is pregnant. Increased folic acid consumption by the mother reduces the risk of these birth defects by 50–70 percent if begun at least a month prior to conception and continued during the early part of pregnancy.[26] Research studies to date suggest that synthetic folic acid has a stronger protective effect than food folate.[27] Since 1998, the FDA has mandated that folic acid be added to all enriched grains and cereal products. This enrichment program has reduced the incidence of neural tube defects by over 25 percent.[28]

Folate and Cancer Risk

Inadequate amounts of folate in the body can disrupt the cell's DNA and prevent repair, potentially triggering the development of cancer.[29] In particular, folate has been shown to help reduce the risk of colon cancer, and adults who are deficient in dietary folate have a higher risk of developing colon cancer.[30] Other studies report an association between diets low in folate and an increased risk of breast[31] and pancreatic cancers.[32]

Daily Needs for Folate

Synthetic folic acid is absorbed 1.7 times more efficiently than folate that is found naturally in foods.[33] Because of this, folate needs are measured in **dietary folate equivalents (DFE)**. Most adults should consume 400 micrograms DFE of folate daily.

The Nutrition Facts panel on food labels doesn't make a distinction between folate and dietary folate equivalents. Some manufacturers use folate while others use folic acid, depending on the form used in the product. The Calculation Corner describes how to convert folic acid measurements on food labels to DFE.

Calculation Corner

Dietary Folate Equivalents

The RDA for folate is expressed in dietary folate equivalents (DFE) to account for the differences between the absorption of naturally occurring folate and the synthetic folate used in fortified foods and supplements. Folate found naturally in foods is only half as bioavailable as folate found in supplements or fortified foods. To adjust for this difference in bioavailability, one DFE is equal to 1 microgram (μg) of naturally occurring folate or 0.6 μg of folic acid. To convert the micrograms of folic acid found on a food label to DFE, multiply the amount listed on the label by the constant 1.7.

Example: A ready-to-eat cereal label shows that a serving contains 25 percent of the Daily Value for folate. The Daily Value uses 400 μg as the standard value. To find the folate in micrograms in a serving of cereal, multiply 400 μg $\times$ 0.25 = 100 μg of folate.

Next, multiply 100 μg of folate $\times$ 1.7 to determine the dietary folate equivalents:

Answer: 100 μg $\times$ 1.7 = 170 μg DFE

Remember, the RDA for folate is 400 μg DFE.

Women who are planning to become pregnant should consume 600 micrograms of folic acid daily from fortified foods or supplements, along with a diet high in naturally occurring folate. Women with a family history of neural tube defects should, under the guidance of their physicians, take even larger amounts.[34] Because 50 percent of pregnancies in the United States are unplanned, any woman who may become pregnant is advised to follow these same recommendations.

Food Sources of Folate

Folate-rich foods can lose folate when exposed to heat and light, making raw foods more abundant in folate than cooked foods. Folic acid found in fortified foods is stable in heat but unstable in light. The bioavailability of folate can vary, and some foods, including beans, legumes, and cabbage, contain inhibitors of the enzymes that remove the glutamates during digestion. This reduces the absorption of folate.[35] Folic acid from supplements is

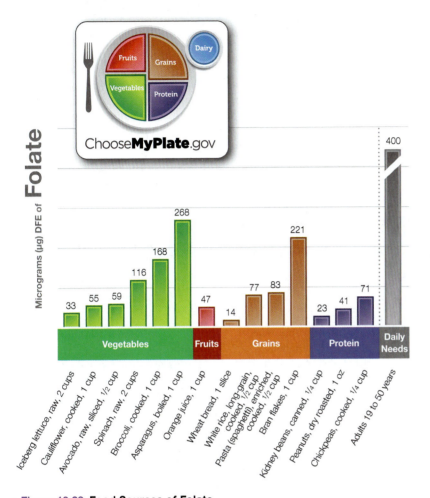

▲ Figure 10.23 Food Sources of Folate
Source: Data from *USDA What's In The Food You Eat?* 2016. Available at https://www.ars.usda.gov. Accessed March 2017.

those who may be unknowingly deficient in vitamin B_{12}. Over-the-counter prenatal vitamins can contain as much as 800 micrograms of folic acid.

A folate deficiency interferes with normal red blood cell division and results in abnormally large and immature red blood cells known as *megaloblasts* (*megalo* = large). These cells develop into abnormally large red blood cells called *macrocytes*, which have a diminished oxygen-carrying capacity. Eventually, macrocytic anemia causes a person to feel tired, weak, and irritable and to experience shortness of breath. Because folate needs vitamin B_{12} to participate in cell division and produce healthy red blood cells, a deficiency of either vitamin can lead to macrocytic anemia (**Figure 10.24**).

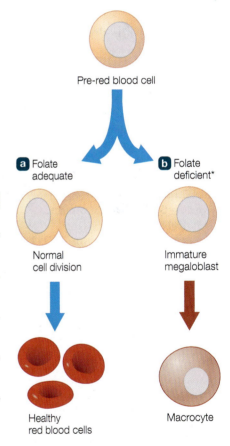

*A vitamin B_{12} deficiency can also cause the formation of macrocytes.

▲ Figure 10.24 Altered Red Blood Cells with Folate Deficiency
Folate is required for normal cell division. If the diet is deficient in folate, macrocytes are formed.

almost entirely all absorbed, especially on an empty stomach.[36]

Folic acid is required by law to be added to enriched cereals and grains, pastas, breads, rice, and flours. The best natural food sources of folate are dark green leafy vegetables such as spinach, broccoli, and asparagus. (This is easy to remember if you know that the term *folate* is derived from the Latin name *folium,* or foliage). In addition, legumes (dried peas and beans), seeds, and liver are all good sources of this vitamin (see **Figure 10.23**). For more food sources of folate, see the nearby Table Tips.

Folate Toxicity and Deficiency

There is no danger in consuming excessive amounts of naturally occurring folate in foods. However, consuming too much folic acid, either through supplements or

TABLE TIPS
Fulfill Folate Needs

Have a bowl of fortified cereal in the morning.

Add chickpeas to a tossed green salad at lunch.

Add layers of fresh spinach leaves to your sandwich.

Have a handful of enriched crackers as a late-afternoon snack.

fortified foods, can be harmful for individuals who are deficient in vitamin B_{12} because excessive folate masks the symptoms of B_{12} deficiency.

An UL of 1,000 micrograms has been set for folic acid from enriched and fortified foods and supplements (not naturally occurring folate in foods) to safeguard

(continued)

Folate (continued)

LO 10.8: THE TAKE-HOME MESSAGE Folate coenzymes function to accept and donate one-carbon compounds in a number of metabolic reactions, including DNA and amino acid synthesis. Adults need 400 micrograms DFE of folate per day. Folic acid is found in fortified foods such as enriched pasta, breads, and cereals. Leafy green vegetables, asparagus, oranges, and rice are excellent sources of folate. Consuming too much folic acid from supplements can obscure a vitamin B_{12} deficiency. Babies born to mothers who are deficient in folate have a higher risk of neural tube defects such as anencephaly and spina bifida. A deficiency of folate results in macrocytic anemia.

EXPLORING Vitamin B₁₂

LO 10.9 Describe the functions, recommended intakes, food sources, and toxicity and deficiency effects of vitamin B_{12}.

What Is Vitamin B₁₂?

The family of compounds referred to as vitamin B_{12} is also called **cobalamin** because it contains the mineral cobalt. In **Figure 10.25**, two forms of vitamin B_{12} are illustrated: cyanocobalamin, the form of vitamin B_{12} found in foods, and methylcobalamin, the active form of vitamin B_{12}. Both forms contain cobalt (highlighted in orange in **Figure 10.27**), but cyanocobalamin also contains a cyanide, illustrated as CN.[37] Methylcobalamin is similar in structure, except the cyanide is replaced with a methyl group.

In the stomach, vitamin B_{12} is released from food by the action of pepsin and

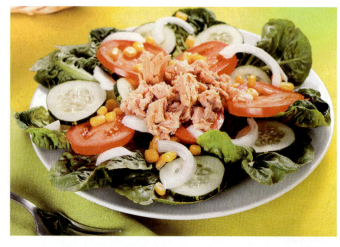

hydrochloric acid during digestion, and then attaches to a transport protein secreted from the salivary glands called **R protein**, which carries vitamin B_{12} into the small intestine. Another protein called **intrinsic factor (IF)** is secreted from the parietal cells in the stomach (**Figure 10.26**) and travels in the chyme into the intestine. Pancreatic proteases hydrolyze the vitamin B_{12}–R protein complex, releasing vitamin B_{12} to bind with intrinsic factor. This newly formed complex travels to the ileum, where a specific receptor site recognizes the intrinsic factor and absorbs the vitamin B_{12}–IF complex by endocytosis into the cell. Inside the intestinal cell, IF is degraded, releasing B_{12} to bind to another protein carrier

called *transcobalamin* for transport throughout the blood.

Excess amounts of vitamin B_{12} are excreted through the bile and urine. Unlike the other water-soluble vitamins, vitamin B_{12} is stored in the body, mostly in the liver, so symptoms of a deficiency can take years to develop.[38]

Metabolic Functions of Vitamin B₁₂

Vitamin B_{12} functions as two coenzymes. **Methylcobalamin** is used to convert homocysteine

cobalamin Vitamin involved in energy metabolism and the conversion of homocysteine to methionine; another name for vitamin B_{12}.

R protein Protein secreted from the salivary glands that binds vitamin B_{12} in the stomach and transports it into the small intestine during digestion.

intrinsic factor (IF) Glycoprotein secreted by the stomach that facilitates the absorption of vitamin B_{12}.

methylcobalamin Coenzyme form of vitamin B_{12} that converts homocysteine to methionine.

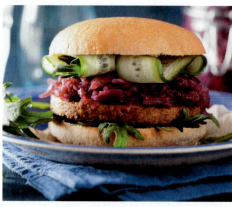

Vitamin B_{12} is naturally found in animal products, but vegans can meet their daily needs by consuming fortified products, such as soy burgers or veggie burgers.

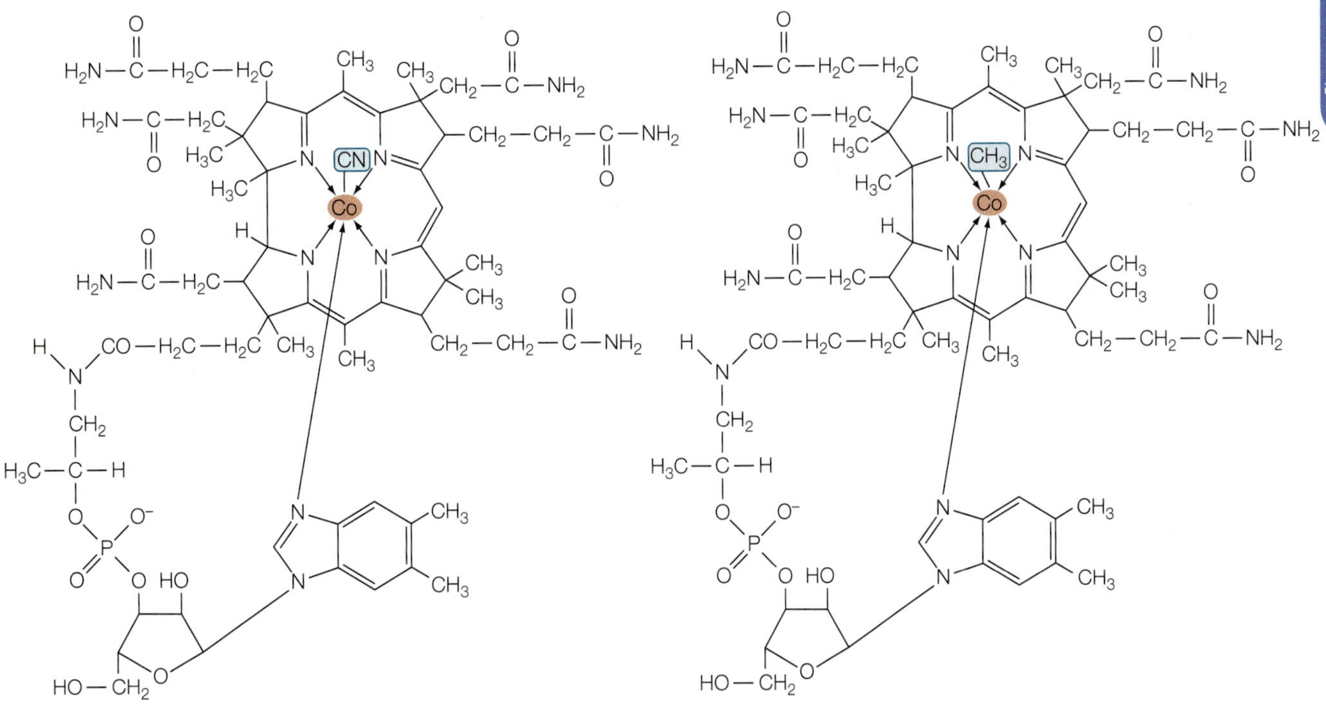

a **Cyanocobalamin** is the form of vitamin B$_{12}$ found in foods. It contains an atom of cobalt and an atom of cyanide (shaded blue).

b **Methylcobalamin** is the active form of vitamin B$_{12}$. The cyanide has been replaced with a methyl group (shaded blue).

▲ **Figure 10.25 The Structure of Vitamin B$_{12}$**

to the amino acid methionine, which, as noted in the discussion of folate, provides the methyl group used in DNA and RNA synthesis. Without adequate vitamin B$_{12}$, homocysteine levels accumulate. As noted earlier, a high concentration of homocysteine is considered a risk factor for atherosclerosis. Vitamin B$_{12}$ deficiency also slows DNA synthesis, causing macrocytic anemia. **Deoxyadenosylcobalamin** helps form succinyl CoA during the TCA cycle, thereby playing an essential role in energy metabolism.

The relationship between vitamin B$_{12}$ and folate is important to emphasize: Vitamin B$_{12}$ activates folate and in turn becomes activated (see **Figure 10.27**). Recall in the discussion on folate that for folate to be converted from the inactive 5-methyl THF, vitamin B$_{12}$ must first

cleave off the methyl group. The vitamin B$_{12}$-plus-methyl group is now active itself.

Like folate, vitamin B$_{12}$ plays an important role in keeping cells, particularly red blood cells, healthy. The maintenance of the **myelin sheath** that protects nerve fibers and speeds the transmission of neural messages also depends on vitamin B$_{12}$. Finally, vitamin B$_{12}$ stimulates osteoblast activity for healthy bone.[39]

Daily Needs for Vitamin B$_{12}$

Adults need 2.4 micrograms of vitamin B$_{12}$ daily. Nonvegetarian American adults, on average, consume over 4 micrograms daily through animal foods.

The body's ability to absorb naturally occurring vitamin B$_{12}$ diminishes with age. This decline appears to be due to a reduction in hydrochloric acid in the stomach, which is needed to activate pepsinogen to pepsin. Pepsin is the enzyme that hydrolyzes the bonds that bind the B$_{12}$ to the proteins in food. If the bonds aren't broken, the vitamin can't be released. This condition, called **atrophic gastritis**, is experienced by up to 30 percent of

deoxyadenosylcobalamin Coenzyme form of vitamin B$_{12}$ that converts intermediate substances in the TCA cycle.

myelin sheath Tissue that surrounds nerves and speeds the transmission of nerve impulses.

atrophic gastritis Chronic inflammation of the stomach.

(continued)

B_{12}
Proteins
R proteins
Salivary fluid
Gastric cells
Pepsin
HCl
B_{12}-R complex
Intrinsic factor
Pancreas
Proteases
Splitting of B_{12}-R complex
B_{12}-IF complex
Ileal cell
IF receptor
Ileum
a The salivary glands produce R protein that will travel to the stomach and bind with vitamin B_{12} there.
b Cells lining the stomach wall secrete HCl and pepsin, which release B_{12} from proteins in the food, and intrinsic factor (IF), which travels with the chyme into the small intestine.
c After vitamin B_{12} has been released from food proteins, it binds with R protein and moves into the small intestine.
d In the small intestine, pancreatic proteases release vitamin B_{12} from the R protein. Vitamin B_{12} then binds with IF and travels to the ileum.
e IF binds to a receptor site on an intestinal cell in the ileum and releases vitamin B_{12} into the cell.

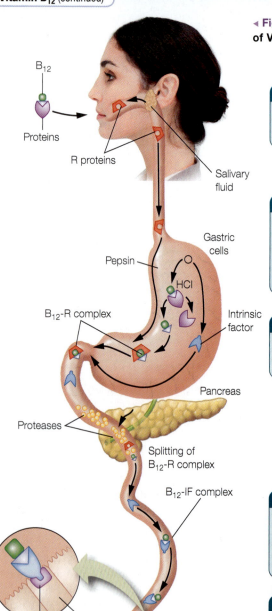

◂ **Figure 10.26 The Absorption of Vitamin B_{12}**

individuals over the age of 50. Luckily, the synthetic form of vitamin B_{12} used in fortified foods and supplements isn't bound to a protein and doesn't depend on hydrochloric acid secretions to be absorbed. Because the synthetic variety is a more reliable source, individuals over the age of 50 should meet their vitamin B_{12} needs primarily from fortified foods or a supplement.

Hydrochloric acid is also important to keep an appropriate ratio of healthy bacteria to pathogenic bacteria in the intestine. With less acid present, the pathogenic bacteria normally found in the intestines aren't properly destroyed and so tend to overgrow. These abundant bacteria feed on unabsorbed vitamin B_{12}, diminishing the amount of the vitamin that may be available for absorption.

Inactive Folate
B_{12}
CH_3
+ B_{12}—CH_3
Active Folate
a Vitamin B_{12} activates folate by removing the methyl group.
b Both folate and vitamin B_{12} are now active and able to synthesize DNA.

▴ **Figure 10.27 Vitamin B_{12} Activates Folate**

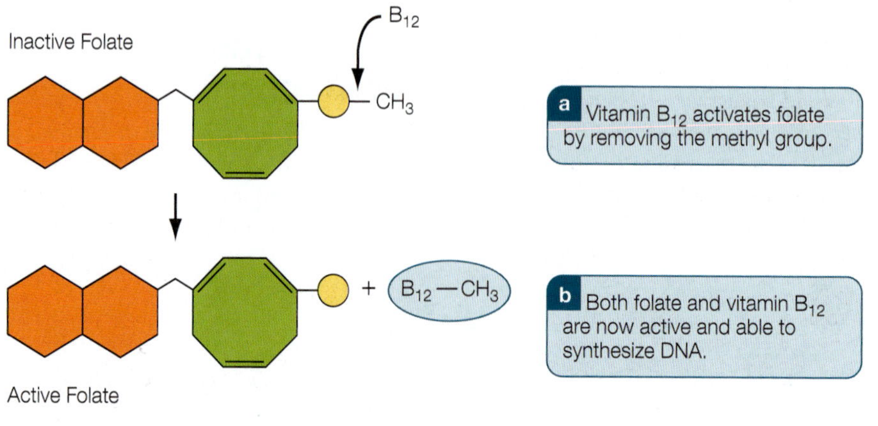

Food Sources of Vitamin B_{12}

Naturally occurring vitamin B_{12} is found only in foods from animal sources, such as meat, fish, poultry, eggs, and dairy products. A varied diet that includes the minimum recommended servings of these food groups would easily meet daily needs (see **Figure 10.28**).

Using a microwave to cook vitamin B_{12}–rich foods may convert the active form of vitamin B_{12} in the food to an inactive form, thus reducing the amount of the active vitamin by as much as 30–40 percent.[40] It appears that vitamin B_{12} is the one exception when it comes to using a microwave to retain vitamins.

Synthetic vitamin B_{12} is found in fortified soymilk and some ready-to-eat cereals, which are ideal sources for older adults and vegans. For more food sources of vitamin B_{12}, see the nearby Table Tips.

TABLE TIPS

Bolster Vitamin B_{12}

- Enjoy heart-healthy fish at least twice a week.
- Sprinkle steamed vegetables with reduced-fat shredded cheese.
- Drink milk or fortified soymilk.
- Try a snack of cottage cheese and fruit in the afternoon.
- Enjoy a grilled chicken breast on a bun for lunch.

THF and can't be used properly. Thus, DNA synthesis slows down. In fact, in most cases of macrocytic anemia, the true cause is a B$_{12}$ deficiency, not a folate deficiency. If folate supplements are given, rather than vitamin B$_{12}$ supplements, the anemia may clear up but the overabundance of folate masks the B$_{12}$ deficiency and allows other B$_{12}$ deficiency problems to continue. This delays a proper diagnosis and corrective therapy with regular injections of vitamin B$_{12}$, which deliver the vitamin directly into the muscle and blood.

Because vitamin B$_{12}$ is also needed to protect the myelin sheath covering nerves, including those in the brain and spinal cord, one long-term consequence of a vitamin B$_{12}$ deficiency is nerve damage, indicated by tingling and numbness in the arms and legs, problems walking, and dementia. If diagnosed early enough, these symptoms can be reversed with treatments of vitamin B$_{12}$. If the diagnosis is delayed, more dangerous, crippling, and irreversible nerve damage can occur.

Review the case of Leland, who was diagnosed with a vitamin B$_{12}$ deficiency, in the Nutrition in Practice feature on page 388.

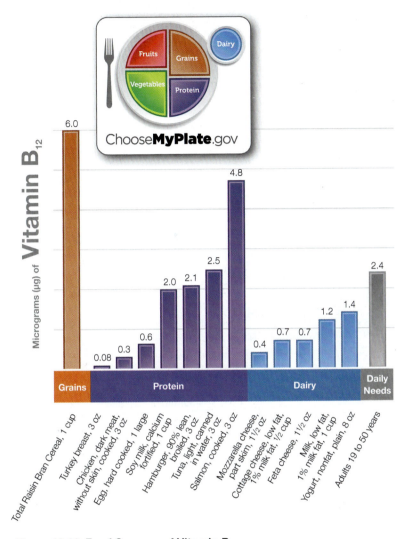

▲ Figure 10.28 Food Sources of Vitamin B$_{12}$
Source: Data from USDA What's In The Food You Eat? 2016. Available at https://www.ars.usda.gov. Accessed March 2017.

Vitamin B$_{12}$ Toxicity and Deficiency

At present, there are no known risks of consuming too much vitamin B$_{12}$ from foods, fortified foods, or supplements, and no UL has been set. This may be due to reduced absorption of the vitamin at higher intakes. For healthy individuals under age 50, there is no known benefit from taking B$_{12}$ supplements if the diet provides adequate amounts of the vitamin.

Vitamin B$_{12}$ deficiency results either from a lack of adequate intake, such as in people following a vegan diet who don't consume vitamin B$_{12}$–fortified foods or supplements, or from malabsorption. Four factors can lead to malabsorption. These include a lack of adequate HCl, which

impairs the body's ability to begin breaking apart the vitamin B$_{12}$–protein complex in the stomach; insufficient pancreatic enzymes to hydrolyze the B$_{12}$–R protein complex in the small intestine; gastric bypass surgery; and **pernicious anemia** (*pernicious* = harmful), which is a form of macrocytic anemia characterized by a lack of sufficient intrinsic factor to release the B$_{12}$ in foods. Inadequate intrinsic factor is often caused by either gastritis or an autoimmune reaction in which the body's immune system attacks the parietal cells.[41] Pernicious anemia develops in about 10 percent of individuals over the age of 60.[42]

When macrocytic anemia is due to a vitamin B$_{12}$ deficiency, there is enough folate available for red blood cells to divide, but the folate is trapped as 5-methyl

pernicious anemia Form of anemia caused by a lack of intrinsic factor needed for absorption of vitamin B$_{12}$, forming large, immature red blood cells.

(continued)

NUTRITION *in* PRACTICE:
Physician's Assistant

David has been a lacto-vegetarian for over 10 years. At 62 years of age, he attributes his low blood pressure and healthy weight to his vegetarian lifestyle. The only animal food he eats is cheese. However, lately he has been experiencing shortness of breath when he climbs the stairs at work and has had bouts of numbness and "pins and needles" feeling in his hand and feet. Sometimes, it feels as though his toes "fall asleep" when he is at his desk at work. David made an appointment at his doctor's office and met with the physician's assistant (PA). After listening to David's symptoms, the PA ordered blood tests and uncovered that David was deficient in vitamin B$_{12}$, which is essential for a red blood cells and a healthy nervous system. The PA gave David a vitamin B$_{12}$ shot, recommended that he take a vitamin B$_{12}$ supplement, and also meet with a registered dietitian nutritionist (RDN) to have his diet assessed.

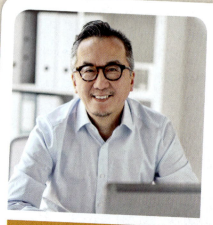

David

David's Stats:
- ❑ Age: 62
- ❑ Height: 5 feet 10 inches
- ❑ Weight: 150 pounds
  BMI: 22.3

DAVID'S FOOD LOG

Food/Beverage	Time Consumed	Hunger Rating*	Location
Whole-wheat bread with almond butter, orange juice fortified with calcium.	5:30 A.M.	5	Kitchen
Handful of peanuts and raisins	10:00 A.M.	3	Office
Mozzarella cheese, tomato, and basil roll-up with lettuce and olive oil.	12:30 P.M.	5	Office at his desk
Banana and peanut butter	3:00 P.M.	3	Office at his desk
Soy burger on whole wheat bun, broccoli, cookies, and orange juice fortified with calcium.	6:30 P.M.	5	Kitchen

* Hunger Rating (1–5): 1 = not hungry; 5 = super hungry.

Critical Thinking Questions

1. Which of David's symptoms were clues that he had a vitamin B$_{12}$ deficiency?
2. Even though David was a lacto-vegetarian, why do you think he was deficient in vitamin B$_{12}$.
3. What changes should David make based on his age to meet his daily need of this vitamin?

RDN's Observation and Plan for David:
- ❑ Discuss the need to add sufficient amounts of dairy foods to increase his consumption of vitamin B$_{12}$ to his diet. His one serving of cheese daily did not provide adequate amounts of vitamin B$_{12}$ to meet his daily needs.
- ❑ Add a food source that contain synthetic vitamin B$_{12}$ to his diet as he is over the age of 50. Advised adding a serving of a whole-grain cereal that is fortified with vitamin B$_{12}$, either at breakfast or as a snack along with his afternoon.

Two weeks later, David returned for a follow-up visit with the RDN. Every afternoon, he tops a soy yogurt with a fortified cereal as a snack. The RDN recommended that he continue taking the vitamin B$_{12}$ supplement that was recommended by the PA as well as continue with a healthy, well-balanced diet.

EXPLORING Vitamin C

Describe the functions, recommended intakes, food sources, and toxicity and deficiency effects of vitamin C.

What Is Vitamin C?

Vitamin C, also known as **ascorbic acid**, is probably better known to the public than any other vitamin. Whereas almost

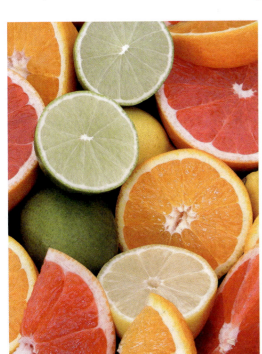

all other mammals can synthesize vitamin C, humans lack the necessary enzyme to convert glucose to vitamin C in the cells, and must rely on food to meet their daily needs.[43] The structure of vitamin C is similar to glucose in that it's a six-carbon molecule (**Figure 10.29**).

Vitamin C is absorbed all along the small intestine, mostly by active transport. Higher intakes are absorbed by simple diffusion in the stomach and small intestine. As the intake of vitamin C increases, the amount absorbed decreases. In fact, the body absorbs less than 50 percent of vitamin C when the intake is 1 gram or greater, whereas almost 98 percent is absorbed from intakes of less than 20 milligrams. Additionally, more vitamin C is excreted through the kidneys when intake is high.

Once absorbed into the portal vein, vitamin C is transported to the liver. The cells take up vitamin C assisted by glucose transport proteins. Vitamin C is not stored.

Metabolic Functions of Vitamin C

Vitamin C plays a complex role in most of the biological systems in the body. For instance, it is necessary for the synthesis of certain tissues, neurotransmitters, and hormones; it acts as an antioxidant; and it assists the absorption of iron. It differs from the B vitamins in that it does not act as a coenzyme in energy metabolism.

Vitamin C and Collagen Synthesis

Vitamin C is essential to the formation of the fibrous protein **collagen**, the most abundant protein in the body. Because collagen gives strength to connective tissue and acts as a glue that keeps cells together (including in the skin, bones, teeth, cartilage, tendons, and blood vessels),[44] a vitamin C–deficient diet affects the entire body.

Collagen formation happens in several steps. First, three chains of amino acids are assembled and twisted together to form a ropelike structure called *procollagen*. Next, vitamin C activates an iron-containing enzyme essential for collagen formation. This enzyme must be reduced for activation (**Figure 10.30**). Vitamin C acts as the reducing agent, changing the iron (Fe^{+3}) cofactor back to its reduced form (Fe^{+2}). By donating the hydrogen to the inactive iron–enzyme complex, vitamin C is destroyed and can't be reused in the next reaction.

Vitamin C as an Antioxidant

Like beta-carotene and vitamin E, vitamin C acts as an antioxidant that may help reduce the risk of chronic diseases such as heart disease and cancer. Vitamin C can donate or accept an electron to stabilize a free radical or change the charge in oxidation-reduction reactions.[45] For example, vitamin C restores vitamin E after it has donated an electron to a free radical.

Vitamin C and Iron Absorption

Vitamin C enhances the absorption of nonheme iron. Plants and iron-fortified foods contain nonheme iron only, while meats, poultry, and fish contain both heme (found in red blood cells) and nonheme iron. When individuals consume vitamin C with foods that contain nonheme iron, it acts as a reducing agent, which improves the absorption of that form of iron.[46] It also boosts the absorption of other minerals such as copper and chromium.

Ascorbic acid

▲ **Figure 10.29 The Structure of Ascorbic Acid**
The hydrogen atoms of ascorbic acid are easily donated to free radicals.

ascorbic acid Active form of vitamin C.

collagen Protein found in connective tissue, including bones, teeth, skin, cartilage, and tendons.

(continued)

Vitamin C (continued)

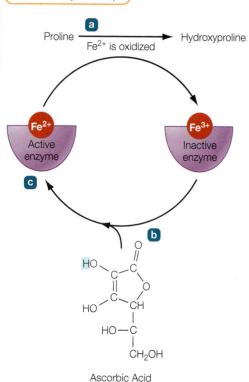

Proline $\xrightarrow[\text{Fe}^{2+} \text{ is oxidized}]{\textbf{a}}$ Hydroxyproline

Fe^{2+} Active enzyme

Fe^{3+} Inactive enzyme

a When the iron enzyme complex converts proline to hydroxyproline, the iron becomes oxidized and the enzyme becomes inactive.

b Vitamin C (ascorbic acid) donates a hydrogen with its electron to the inactive iron enzyme complex, reducing the Fe^{3+} to Fe^{2+}.

c The enzyme is now reactivated.

Ascorbic Acid

▲ **Figure 10.30 The Role of Vitamin C in Collagen Formation**

Vitamin C and the Immune System

Vitamin C helps maintain a healthy immune system by enabling the body to make white blood cells, like the ones shown in the photo. These blood cells fight infections. This immune-boosting role has fostered the belief that high doses of vitamin C can cure the common cold.

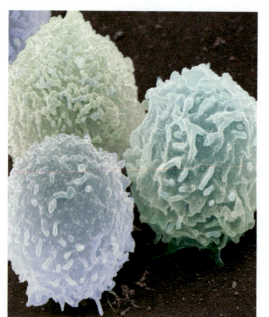

Examining the Evidence: Does Vitamin C Prevent the Common Cold? on page 392 takes a look at this theory.

Vitamin C and Stress

Vitamin C may reduce the body's response to stress, although the mechanism is unclear. When the body responds to a stressful situation, the hypothalamus begins a cascade of reactions, starting with stimulating the pituitary gland to secrete stress hormones. In turn, the pituitary hormones direct the adrenal glands to synthesize and secrete cortisol into the blood. The cells of the adrenal glands contain high levels of vitamin C, which is released after cortisol during a response to stress.[47] The relationship between the stress response and vitamin C has prompted researchers to study the possibility of a link in humans, despite a lack of direct evidence for such a link.

Other Functions of Vitamin C

Vitamin C also participates in other important reactions in the body. It donates an electron in the conversion of tryptophan and tyrosine to two neurotransmitters, *serotonin* and *norepinephrine*. Vitamin C is also essential in the synthesis of *thyroxine* (the hormone produced by the thyroid gland). It also helps convert cholesterol to bile and helps break down *histamine,* the component behind the inflammation seen in many allergic reactions.[48]

Daily Needs for Vitamin C

Women need to consume 75 milligrams of vitamin C daily and men need to consume 90 milligrams daily to meet their needs. Smoking accelerates the breakdown and elimination of vitamin C from the body, so all individuals who smoke need to consume an additional 35 milligrams of vitamin C every day to make up for these losses.[49]

Food Sources of Vitamin C

Americans meet about 90 percent of their vitamin C needs by consuming fruits and vegetables, with orange juice and grapefruit juice being the most popular sources in the diet. One serving of either juice just about meets an adult's daily needs. Tomatoes, peppers, potatoes, broccoli, oranges, and cantaloupe are also excellent sources (see **Figure 10.31**). Meats, dairy, grains, and legumes are considered poor sources of the vitamin. For more food sources of vitamin C, see the nearby Table Tips.

TABLE TIPS

Juicy Ways to Get Vitamin C

Have at least one citrus fruit (such as an orange or grapefruit) daily.

Put sliced tomatoes on sandwiches.

Enjoy a fruit cup for dessert.

Drink low-sodium vegetable juice for an afternoon refresher.

Add strawberries to low-fat frozen yogurt.

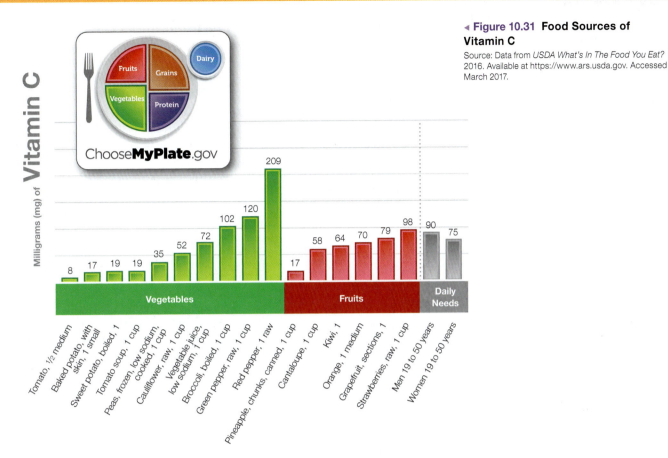

◄ **Figure 10.31** Food Sources of Vitamin C

Source: Data from *USDA What's In The Food You Eat?* 2016. Available at https://www.ars.usda.gov. Accessed March 2017.

Vitamin C Toxicity and Deficiency

Although excessive amounts of vitamin C aren't known to be toxic, consuming over 3,000 milligrams daily through the use of supplements has been shown to cause nausea, stomach cramps, and diarrhea. The UL for vitamin C for adults is set at 2,000 milligrams. Too much vitamin C can also lead to the formation of kidney stones in individuals with a history of kidney disease or gout. In addition, vitamin C supplementation can result in false positives or false negatives in some medical tests.

Because vitamin C helps to absorb the form of iron found in plant foods, those with a rare disorder called **hemochromatosis**, which causes the body to store too much iron, should avoid excessive amounts of vitamin C. Iron toxicity can damage many organs, including the liver and heart.

For centuries, **scurvy**, the disease of vitamin C deficiency, was the affliction of sailors on long voyages. Without access to vitamin C–rich produce, sailors would develop the telltale signs of failure of

collagen synthesis: swollen and bleeding gums (**Figure 10.32**), a rough rash on the skin, wounds that wouldn't heal, and internal bleeding.

Although rare, scurvy in the twenty-first century is associated with poverty, especially in young children.[50] Adult males are more susceptible than adult females, possibly due to lack of knowledge, lower intakes of fruits and vegetables, poor access to groceries, reclusiveness, or alcoholism.[51]

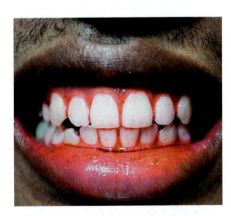

▲ **Figure 10.32** Gum Disease Can Result from Scurvy

Scurvy can be prevented by as little as 10 milligrams of vitamin C per day, or the amount found in a single slice of a fresh orange.

LO 10.10: THE TAKE-HOME MESSAGE

Vitamin C, found in a variety of fruits and vegetables, assists in the formation of collagen, acts as an antioxidant, supports the immune system, and improves the absorption of nonheme iron. The RDA for vitamin C is 75 mg for women and 90 mg for men per day. Excessive amounts of vitamin C from supplements can cause intestinal discomfort. A deficiency of vitamin C results in scurvy.

---

hemochromatosis Blood disorder characterized by the retention of an excessive amount of iron.

scurvy Disease caused by a deficiency of vitamin C and characterized by bleeding gums and a skin rash.

Does Vitamin C Prevent the Common Cold?

More than 200 viruses can cause the common cold, and colds are the leading cause of doctor visits in the United States. Americans will suffer a billion colds this year alone.[1] Symptoms often last for up to 2 weeks, and children and adolescents miss over 22 million school days every year battling the common cold.[2]

The Truth about Catching a Cold

Contrary to popular belief, you can't catch a cold from being outside without a coat or hat on a cold day. Rather, the only way to catch a cold is to come into contact with a cold virus. Contact can be direct, such as by hugging or shaking hands with someone who is carrying the virus, or indirect, such as by touching an object like a keyboard or telephone contaminated with a cold virus. After you touch a contaminated object, the next time you touch your nose or rub your eyes, you transfer these germs from your hands into your body. You can also catch a cold virus by inhaling virus-carrying droplets from a cough or sneeze of someone with the cold.

The increased frequency of colds during the fall and winter is likely due to people spending more time indoors

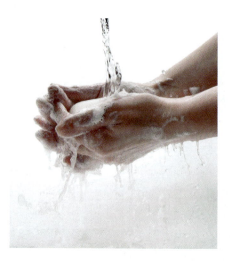

in the close quarters of classrooms, dorm rooms, and the workplace, which makes the sharing of germs easier. The low humidity of the winter air can also cause mucous membranes to be drier and more permeable to the invasion of these viruses. In addition, the most common cold viruses survive longer when the weather is colder and the humidity is low.

Vitamin C and the Common Cold

In the 1970s, a scientist named Linus Pauling theorized that consuming at least 1,000 milligrams of vitamin C daily would prevent the common cold.[3] Since that initial theory was published, there have been a number of double-blind studies to test whether vitamin C prevents the common cold or can be an effective treatment to reduce the duration and severity of the cold once it is contracted. A meta-analysis reported that supplementing with vitamin C did not affect the incidence of the common cold.[4] The same study did note that vitamin C supplements can modestly reduce the duration of the cold. In special circumstances, such as marathon athletes using vitamin C prior to extreme exercise[5] or in people with other illnesses,[6] vitamin C supplementation may have some benefit in preventing upper respiratory infections, especially for people who have a low intake of dietary vitamin C or are under severe acute stress.

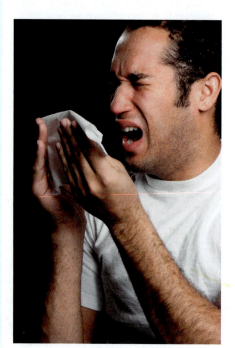

Other Cold Remedies: The Jury Is Still Out

Recently, other dietary substances, such as the herb echinacea and the mineral zinc, have emerged as popular treatment strategies for the common cold. The results of a recent review of studies testing echinacea found no benefit of using it to either prevent or cure the common cold.[7] Studies of zinc have had mixed results. In a randomized, double-blind, placebo-controlled study, individuals who received 13 milligrams of zinc gluconate in lozenge form had fewer days of cold symptoms than the placebo group.[8] Similar results have been reported with zinc acetate.[9] A recent review reported that zinc lozenges, not pills or syrup, taken within 24 hours of the first sign of a cold, reduced the duration of the cold in otherwise healthy people.[10] Caution should be exercised, however, because chronic intake of zinc supplements can actually suppress the immune system.[11] We cover zinc and its role in the immune system in the chapter on trace minerals.

What You Can Do to Reduce Your Risk for a Cold

One of the best ways to reduce your chances of catching a cold is to wash your hands frequently with soap and water. This lowers the likelihood of transmitting germs from hands to mouth, nose, or eyes. One study found that children who washed their hands four times a day had over 20 percent fewer sick days from school than those who washed their hands less frequently.[12] When soap and water aren't available, gel sanitizers or disposable alcohol-containing hand wipes can be an effective alternative.[13] Covering the mouth and nose during coughing or sneezing and then immediately washing the hands helps prevent the spread of germs to other people and objects.

The Centers for Disease Control recommends the following steps to take if you do get a cold:[14]

- Get plenty of rest.
- Drink plenty of fluids. (Soups and juices are considered fluids.)

- Gargle with warm salt water or use throat lozenges for a sore throat.
- Dab petroleum jelly on a raw nose to relieve irritation.
- Take aspirin or acetaminophen (Tylenol) for headache or fever.

References

1. Doerr, S. 2017. *Common Cold*. Available at www.medicinenet.com. Accessed February 2017.
2. Centers for Disease Control. 2015. *Stopping Germs at Home, Work and School*. Available at www.cdc.gov. Accessed February 2017.
3. Pauling, L. 1971. The Significance of the Evidence about Ascorbic Acid and the Common Cold. *Proceedings from the National Academy of Science* 68:2678–2681.
4. Hemilä, H., and E. Chalker. 2013. Vitamin C for Preventing and Treating the Common Cold. *Cochrane Database of Systematic Reviews* 1, Art. No.: CD000980. doi: 10.1002/14651858. CD000980.pub4.
5. Hemilä, H. 2014. The Effect of Vitamin C on Bronchoconstriction and Respiratory Symptoms Caused By Exercise: A Review and Statistical Analysis. *Allergy, Asthma, and Clinical Immunology* 10(1):58. doi: 10.1186/1710-1492-10-58.
6. Hemilä, H. 2013. Vitamin C and Common Cold-Induced Asthma: A Systematic Review and Statistical Analysis. *Allergy, Asthma, and Clinical Immunology* 9(1):46. doi: 10.1186/1710-1492-9-46.
7. Karsch-Volk, M., B. Barrett, et al. 2014. Echinacea for Preventing and Treating the Common Cold. *Cochrane Database of Systematic Review* 2:CD000530.
8. Singh, M., and R. R. Das, 2013. Zinc for the Common Cold. *Cochrane Database of Systematic Reviews* 6, Art. No.: CD001364. doi: 10.1002/14651858.CD001364.pub4.
9. Hemilä, H., E. J. Petrus, et al. 2016. Zinc Acetate Lozenges for Treating the Common Cold: An Individual Patient Data Meta-analysis. *British Journal of Clinical Pharmacology* 82(5):1393–1398. doi: 10.1111/bcp.13057.
10. Singh, M., and R. R. Das. 2013. Zinc for the Common Cold.
11. Institute of Medicine. 2006. *Dietary Reference Intakes: The Essential Guide to Nutrient Requirements*. Washington, DC: National Academies Press.
12. Education World. 2015. *School-Wide Handwashing Campaigns Cut Germs, Absenteeism*. Available at www.educationworld.com. Accessed March 2017.
13. National Institute of Allergy and Infectious Diseases, National Institutes of Health. 2016. *Omalizumab Decreases Colds in Inner-City Children with Asthma, NIH Study Reports*. Available at https://www.niaid.nih.gov. Accessed March 2017.
14. Centers for Disease Control. 2015. *Stopping Germs at Home, Work and School*. Available at www.cdc.gov. Accessed February 2017.

What Are Other Vitamin-Like Compounds?

LO 10.11 Describe the functions of compounds that have vitamin-like biological roles but are not classified as vitamins.

Some organic compounds may not be classified as a vitamin by strict definition but are still essential to overall health. These compounds are often synthesized in adequate amounts in the body but may become essential in the diet under certain circumstances, such as during illness or chronic disease. The vitamin-like compounds include choline, carnitine, lipoic acid, and inositol.

Choline Helps Protect the Liver

Choline is a conditionally essential nutrient that the body needs for healthy cells and nerves. Choline is a nitrogen-containing compound that is often grouped with the family of B vitamins but by strict definition is not classified as a vitamin. Although the body can synthesize choline from the amino acid methionine, it isn't able to synthesize enough of it to meet the body's needs.[52]

Choline serves a number of uses in the body. It is part of the phospholipid that makes up cell membranes; it functions in liver metabolism; it is a precursor for the neurotransmitter acetylcholine and thus participates in nerve transmission; it assists in the transport of lipids as part of the VLDL; and it plays a key role in fetal development.[53]

The current recommendation of 425 milligrams for women and 550 milligrams for men is based on the amount of choline needed to guard against liver damage. Choline is so widely available in foods, especially milk, liver, eggs, and peanuts, that it is unlikely intake would ever fall short. However, too much choline from supplements can cause sweating and vomiting as well as hypotension (*hypo* = low), or low blood pressure. It can also cause the body to emit an unpleasant fishy odor as it tries to excrete the excess. The UL of 3,500 milligrams for choline has been set to prevent hypotension.

choline Vitamin-like substance that is a precursor for the neurotransmitter acetylcholine, which is essential for healthy nerves.

Carnitine, Lipoic Acid, and Inositol Are Needed for Overall Health

Carnitine, lipoic acid, and inositol, all vitamin-like substances, are needed for overall health and important body functions. Unlike choline, however, they are not essential nutrients because the body can synthesize them in adequate amounts. Deficiency symptoms are not known to occur in humans.

Carnitine (*carnus* = flesh), which is synthesized from the amino acids lysine and methionine, is needed to properly utilize fat. It is abundant in foods from animal sources, such as meat and dairy products. Although there is no research to support the claim, carnitine supplements are sometimes advertised to promote weight loss and help athletes improve their performance.[54]

Lipoic acid is an organic compound that contains sulfur. Similar to many B vitamins, it helps cells generate energy. In fact, when it was discovered, it was initially thought to be a vitamin.[55] The body synthesizes adequate amounts of lipoic acid from short-chain fatty acids, so it is not necessary to consume lipoic acid in the diet; however, it is found in a variety of plant and animal foods. In addition to its role in energy metabolism, lipoic acid is being studied for its potential role as an antioxidant that could help reduce the risk of diabetes and cataracts.[56]

Lastly, **inositol** is an organic compound classified as an alcohol. It is needed to keep cell membranes healthy. Healthy individuals can synthesize enough inositol from glucose to meet their needs. Inositol is also abundant in plant-based foods. Thus, supplements are not necessary.

carnitine Vitamin-like substance used to transport fatty acids across the mitochondrial membrane to properly utilize fat.

lipoic acid Vitamin-like substance used in energy production; may also act as an antioxidant.

inositol Water-soluble compound synthesized in the body that maintains healthy cell membranes.

LO 10.11: THE TAKE-HOME MESSAGE Choline is a conditionally essential nutrient that is needed for the integrity of cell membranes, nerve transmission, lipid transport, and liver health. Carnitine, lipoic acid, and inositol are needed for important body functions and overall health, but are not essential nutrients because the body is able to synthesize them in sufficient amounts.

HEALTH**CONNECTION**

Do Antioxidant Nutrients and Phytochemicals Reduce the Risk of Cancer?

LO 10.12 Explain the role that a healthy diet and lifestyle plays in cancer risk and progression.

The term **cancer** describes a group of more than 100 diseases characterized by

cancer General term for a large group of diseases characterized by uncontrolled growth of abnormal cells.

uncontrolled growth and spread of abnormal cells.[57] The most common type for both men and women is lung cancer, with skin, breast, prostate, and colorectal cancers also occurring in large numbers. The types differ not only in where they occur in the body (see **Table 10.2**), but also in their causes, treatments, and prognoses. *Carcinomas*—cancers of epithelial cells—represent almost 80–90 percent of all cancers in adults. *Sarcomas*, cancers of the connective tissue, occur in bone and muscle. *Lymphomas*, including both Hodgkin's disease and non-Hodgkin's lymphoma, are cancers of the lymphatic tissues

TABLE 10.2	Types of Cancer
Type of Cancer	**Description**
Carcinoma	Cancer of the epithelial cells; includes cancers of various glandular tissue, including breast, thyroid, and skin
Sarcoma	Cancer of connective tissue, such as bone or muscle
Leukemia	Cancer associated with proliferation of immature white blood cells
Lymphoma	Cancer of the lymph tissues and lymphocytes

characterized by uncontrolled growth of lymphocytes, a type of white blood cell. Closely related are *leukemias,* which feature uncontrolled growth of immature white blood cells—called *leukemia cells*—in the bone marrow.

Cancer is responsible for almost 25 percent of all deaths in the United States, making it the second leading cause of death, behind heart disease.[58] Even though the death rate from cancer has declined slightly since 2004, an estimated 600,920 Americans will die of cancer in 2017, or 1,650 per day. About one-third of these cancer deaths in 2014 were related to overweight or obesity, physical inactivity, and poor diet.[59]

Carcinogenesis: The Cancer Process

Normal cell growth is regulated by two types of genes: *proto-oncogenes* turn the cell replication cycle on and off, and *tumor suppressor genes* stop any cells with DNA mutations from replicating. Mutated proto-oncogenes are known as *oncogenes* (*onco-* means "tumor"). Together, oncogenes and mutated tumor suppressor genes promote uncontrolled cell growth, failure of cell differentiation, and a decrease in normal cell death (called *apoptosis*). These three mechanisms underlie the process of cancer development, or **carcinogenesis**, which generally takes years or even decades from the initial mutations to patient symptoms.

Carcinogenesis generally occurs in three stages: initiation, promotion, and progression. Normally, cell damage is repaired before abnormal cells begin to accumulate. Alternatively, the cell dies before it proliferates, as checkpoints along the various stages of cell division help maintain the integrity of DNA. The initiation stage begins when a cell is exposed to a **carcinogen**, or cancer-causing agent, that damages the DNA (see **Figure 10.33**). Carcinogens include a variety of environmental factors such as hormones, viruses, ultraviolet light, or smoke, or dietary factors such as alcohol, excess kilocalories, and excess dietary fat.

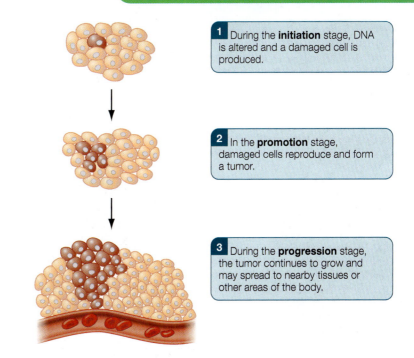

1. During the **initiation** stage, DNA is altered and a damaged cell is produced.

2. In the **promotion** stage, damaged cells reproduce and form a tumor.

3. During the **progression** stage, the tumor continues to grow and may spread to nearby tissues or other areas of the body.

▲ Figure 10.33 **The Stages of Carcinogenesis**

This stage of cancer development is usually short-lived because the damaged DNA is either repaired quickly or carcinogenesis progresses to the next stage, promotion.

Once the mutation is initiated, a cancer promoter, such as the hormone estrogen or alcohol, stimulates the damaged cells to divide and multiply. Left unchecked by mutated tumor suppressor genes, the mass of cells, or *tumor,* grows. In the third stage, progression, the tumor can invade surrounding tissues, develop its own network of blood vessels to obtain nutrients, and release *malignant* (cancerous) cells into the blood and lymph. These cells can spread—or *metastasize*—to other regions of the body and eventually form new tumors.

Physical Activity, Obesity, and Cancer Risk

Maintaining a healthy weight throughout life may be one of the most important ways to protect against cancer. Among U.S. adults 50 years of age or older, it is estimated that 25–33 percent of all cancers are related to physical inactivity and obesity.[60] A healthy weight and physical activity reduce the risk of developing breast, colon, rectal, endometrial, esophageal, and kidney cancer.[61]

Routine physical activity reduces the risk of several types of cancer, in part by helping individuals maintain a healthy weight. The exercise does not have to be intense to be effective. In one study, women who participated in moderate exercise had a greater reduction in colon cancer risk than women who reported more strenuous physical activity.[62] The reason exercise reduces cancer risk is still not clear. However, the benefits may be due to reducing chronic inflammation, stimulating the immune system, or reducing obesity.[63]

Overconsumption of energy-dense foods can increase risk of obesity and thus cancer risk. An energy-dense diet, especially one high in dietary fat, may contribute to obesity, especially in sedentary individuals. Dietary fat intake does not cause breast cancer, but weight gain later in life may.[64]

carcinogenesis Process of cancer development.

carcinogen Cancer-causing substance, including tobacco smoke, air and water pollution, ultraviolet radiation, and various chemicals.

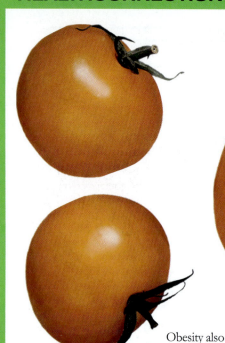

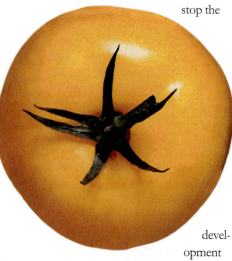

Obesity also increases the risk for thyroid, cervical, and prostate cancers.[65]

(vitamin A), vitamin D, folate, and the mineral selenium help repair DNA in the initiation stage and can stop the development of cancer by inhibiting the progression of damaged cells (**Figure 10.34**). Vitamins C and E and selenium may prevent cancer from spreading to nearby tissues. Omega-3 fatty acids may help to reduce cancer cell growth. Vitamin D may inhibit the proliferation of cancer cells and stimulate cell differentiation.[69] This research is in the early stages, however, and no conclusive cause-and-effect evidence has been presented.

Dietary fiber helps dilute potentially carcinogenic chemicals in feces and moves them more quickly out of the body, reducing your exposure. Also, the healthy bacteria that live in the colon feast on the fiber, creating butyrate, a by-product that may also help in the fight against colorectal cancer. Fiber-containing fruits and vegetables are also low in kilocalories and high in bulk, so they improve satiety. Thus, a fiber-rich diet can help individuals maintain a healthy body weight.

The Role of Diet in Cancer Risk and Progression

Dietary factors can influence the development of cancer cells at the initiation, promotion, and progression stages.

Foods That Can Lower Cancer Risk

Research suggests that consuming a plant-based diet may modestly reduce cancer risk.[66] For example, consumption of nonstarchy vegetables and fruits is associated in some studies with reductions in lung, mouth and esophageal, stomach, and colon cancer.[67] The risk for bladder cancer in men has been reduced in some studies with a higher intake of cruciferous vegetables, such as cauliflower, broccoli, and brussels sprouts. Eating more tomatoes and tomato products such as pasta sauce may reduce the risk of developing prostate cancer.[68] These foods are high in antioxidant nutrients, phytochemicals, and dietary fiber and low in energy density.

Some specific vitamins and minerals may help lower cancer risk. Retinoids

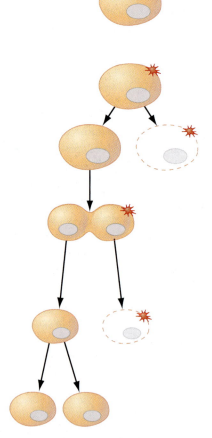

1 Hormones and growth factors stimulate the cell to grow. Nutrients are needed for parts of the cell to develop.

2 The cycle stops if DNA is damaged. Vitamin A can arrest the cell cycle at this time. The cell is either repaired or dies.

3 DNA is replicated. Folate is required at this step.

4 A second checkpoint stops the cell cycle if the DNA is damaged. The cell is either repaired or dies. DNA repair is stimulated by vitamin A, vitamin D, folate, and selenium.

5 A final checkpoint before the cell divides into two identical daughter cells ensures each daughter cell has the correct DNA.

▲ **Figure 10.34 Micronutrient Roles in Normal Cell Growth and Division** Normally, damaged or mutated cells are repaired or die off to prevent them from producing more damaged cells. Various micronutrients are involved in different stages of the process.

There is epidemiological evidence that some nutrients, including vitamins A, C, and E, may protect DNA from damage, thereby reducing the initiation of cancer. The exact mechanism that might confer this protection is still unknown.[70]

Foods That Can Raise Cancer Risk

Some foods may increase the risk of developing cancer. For example, red meat, especially when grilled, is associated with an increased risk of stomach, pancreatic, colon, and kidney cancer.[71] When the saturated fat in meat hits a hot surface below the meat, such as a frying pan or charcoal grill, it forms benzopyrene, a probable carcinogen, which

is absorbed back into the meat. Nitrates and nitrites, used as preservatives in processed meats such as deli meats and hotdogs, can be converted to another class of carcinogens known as nitrosamines. Evidence also suggests that excessive alcohol consumption increases liver, mouth and esophageal, breast, and colon cancer.[72]

Dietary and Lifestyle Recommendations for Cancer Prevention

The American Institute of Cancer Research continually updates a report identifying nutritional and lifestyle factors that may reduce the risk of

developing cancer. Their current recommendations are summarized in **Table 10.3**.

Several promising areas of research are exploring the relationship between nutrition and cancer. For example, consuming specific nutrients might, via epigenetic mechanisms, turn on and off cancer genes.[73] Certain nutrients that contribute to healthy GI flora are being investigated for their potential in reducing colon cancer risk.[74] The effect on cancer risk of a high BMI in childhood is also on the research agenda.

For now, the best advice for reducing the risk of cancer is to consume a varied, healthy, plant-based diet; limit saturated fat and sugar intake; maintain a healthy weight; avoid tobacco; limit alcohol intake; and lead an active lifestyle.[75] Because many cancers take years, if not decades, to develop after the initial DNA damage, the sooner healthy changes are made, the more likely they are to help individuals avoid cancer later in life.

TABLE 10.3 Recommendations for Reducing Cancer Risk

Recommendations	Personal Health Goals
Be as lean as possible within the normal range of body weight	• Ensure that body weight through childhood and adolescent growth projects toward the lower end of the normal BMI range at age 21 • Maintain body weight within the normal range from age 21 • Avoid weight gain and increases in waist circumference throughout adulthood
Be physically active for 30 minutes every day	• Be moderately physically active, equivalent to brisk walking, for at least 30 minutes every day • As fitness improves, aim for 60 minutes or more of moderate, or 30 minutes or more of vigorous, physical activity every day • Limit sedentary habits such as watching television
Limit consumption of energy-dense foods and avoid sugary drinks	• Consume energy-dense foods sparingly • Avoid sugary drinks • Avoid fast foods or consume only sparingly
Eat more of a variety of vegetables, fruits, whole grains, and legumes such as beans	• Eat at least five portions/servings (at least 400 g or 14 oz) of a variety of fruits and nonstarchy vegetables every day • Eat relatively unprocessed cereals (grains) and/or legumes with every meal • Limit refined starch foods • People who consume starchy roots or tubers as staples need to also consume sufficient nonstarchy vegetables, fruits, and legumes
Limit intake of red meat and avoid processed meat	• People who eat red meat should consume less than 500 g (18 oz) a week and avoid processed meats
Limit alcoholic drinks	• If alcoholic drinks are consumed, limit consumption to no more than two drinks a day for men and one drink a day for women
Limit consumption of salty foods and foods processed with salt	• Avoid salt-preserved, salted, or salty foods; preserve foods without using salt • Limit consumption of processed foods with added salt to ensure an intake of less than 6 g (2.4 g sodium) a day
Aim to meet nutritional needs through diet alone	• Dietary supplements are not recommended for cancer prevention

Source: Adapted from the American Institute of Cancer Research. 2017. *Recommendations for Cancer Prevention.* Available at www.aicr.org. Accessed March 2017.

LO 10.12: THE TAKE-HOME MESSAGE

Cancer is a disease caused by the uncontrolled reproduction of damaged cells. Carcinogens, or cancer-causing substances, damage cells by altering their DNA. Genetic, environmental, and lifestyle factors all play a role in cancer risk. Some research suggests that certain dietary factors may reduce the risk for cancer. These include consumption of abundant amounts of fruits, vegetables, and whole grains, which provide antioxidant nutrients and phytochemicals, as well as dietary fiber, and limiting your consumption of red and processed meats and alcohol. Staying physically active and maintaining a healthy body weight are key to reducing cancer risk.

Visual Chapter Summary

LO 10.1 Water-Soluble Vitamins Act as Coenzymes and Play Other Metabolic Roles

The nine water-soluble vitamins are absorbed after hydrolysis releases them from protein complexes. When consumed in excess, most are excreted in the urine and not stored, with the exception of vitamin B_6 and vitamin B_{12}. Most of these vitamins leach into water or are easily destroyed by heat, light, pH, or oxidation.

The B-complex vitamins thiamin, riboflavin, niacin, vitamin B_6, pantothenic acid, and biotin function primarily as coenzymes in energy metabolism. As coenzymes, they catalyze enzyme activity when they bind to the active site of an enzyme. Folate and vitamin B_{12} form coenzymes that participate in the formation of red blood cells and are required for several other body functions. Vitamin C acts as an antioxidant to neutralize free radicals, stimulates collagen synthesis, and plays many other roles.

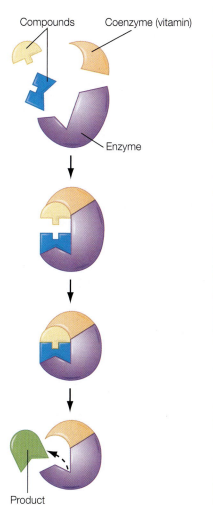

Compounds   Coenzyme (vitamin)

Enzyme

Product

LO 10.2 Thiamin (B₁)

Thiamin in the active form of TPP functions in glycolysis and the TCA cycle. Thiamin also participates in nerve impulse transmission. The best sources of thiamin are lean pork, enriched and whole-grain foods, ready-to-eat cereals, pasta, rice, and nuts. The thiamin RDA for adults is 1.1 milligrams for women and 1.2 milligrams for men. There are no known toxicity problems for thiamin. A deficiency of thiamin can result in beriberi. Chronic alcohol abuse can lead to an advanced form of thiamin deficiency called Wernicke-Korsakoff syndrome.

Phosphate groups

Thiamin pyrophosphate

LO 10.3 Riboflavin (B₂)

Riboflavin, or vitamin B_2, functions as two coenzymes, FMN and FAD, to transfer electrons in oxidation-reduction reactions. Riboflavin participates in the conversion of folate to its active form, vitamin B_6 to its coenzyme form, and the conversion of tryptophan to niacin. Milk and yogurt are the most popular sources of riboflavin. Riboflavin is stable in cooking but is degraded in ultraviolet light. The riboflavin RDA for adults is 1.1 milligrams for women and 1.3 milligrams for men. There are no known riboflavin toxicity symptoms. A deficiency in riboflavin results in ariboflavinosis.

$2\,H^+, 2\,e^-$

FAD

FADH₂

LO 10.4 Niacin (B₃)

Niacin, also called nicotinic acid and nicotinamide, functions as the active coenzyme forms, nicotinamide adenine dinucleotide (NAD^+) and nicotinamide adenine dinucleotide phosphate ($NADP^+$). These two coenzymes are involved in the metabolism of carbohydrates, fats, and proteins, maintenance of healthy skin, and promotion of a functional GI tract. Niacin is found in a variety of foods, including meat, fish, poultry, fortified cereals, and enriched breads. The niacin RDA for adults is 14 milligrams NE for women and 16 milligrams NE for men. Megadoses of niacin supplements can cause flushing. A deficiency of niacin results in pellagra.

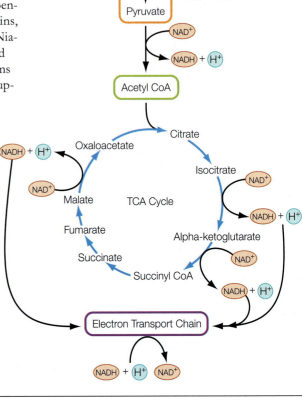

LO 10.5 Pantothenic Acid

Pantothenic acid makes up part of the molecule coenzyme A and participates in lipogenesis and beta-oxidation, in the conversion of pyruvate to acetyl CoA, and in converting some amino acids to substrates in the TCA cycle. The AI of pantothenic acid for adult males and females is 5 milligrams. Pantothenic acid is found in a number of foods, including whole-grain cereals, nuts and legumes, milk, meat, and eggs. There are no known adverse effects from consuming too much pantothenic acid and deficiencies are rare.

Pantothenic acid

Is a component of

Coenzyme A

Adenine

LO 10.6 Biotin

Biotin is a coenzyme for enzymes that add carbon dioxide to compounds during energy metabolism, and for enzymes that participate in lipogenesis, gluconeogenesis, and the metabolism of amino acids. Biotin also plays a role in DNA replication and the transcription of genes. The AI of biotin for adult males and females is 30 micrograms. Biotin is found in peanuts, yeast, egg yolks, grains, fish, and liver. There is little evidence that excess biotin causes toxicity. Deficiencies of biotin are rare except when large amounts of raw eggs or egg whites are consumed.

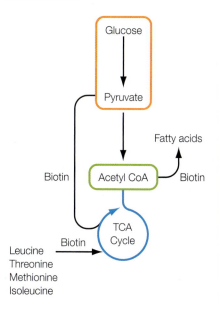

LO 10.7 Vitamin B6

Vitamin B_6, also known as pyridoxine, pyridoxal, and pyridoxamine, acts as a coenzyme for over 100 enzymes involved in protein metabolism and red blood cell synthesis. Vitamin B_6 is also a key player in glycogenolysis, and interacts with other nutrients including riboflavin, niacin, and zinc. The active form of vitamin B_6 is pyridoxal phosphate (PLP). Vitamin B_6 is found in meat, fish, poultry, legumes, bananas, and fortified cereals. Adult women need 1.3–1.5 milligrams and adult men need 1.3–1.7 milligrams of B_6, depending on their age. In high supplement doses, PLP may cause neurological damage. A deficiency of vitamin B_6 can result in microcytic hypochromic anemia, depression, and inflammation of the skin. Drinking too much alcohol can deplete the body of vitamin B_6.

Pyruvate Glutamate   Alanine α-ketoglutarate

Transamination

LO 10.8 Folate

Folate is naturally found in foods, but is more easily absorbed as the synthetic form, folic acid, found mostly in fortified foods and supplements. The active form of folate is called tetrahydrofolate, or THF. Its role in metabolism is transferring single-carbon compounds, such as a methyl group, to other compounds. This function of folate is critical to DNA and amino acid synthesis and cell division. Folate is found in fortified foods, leafy green vegetables, enriched pasta, rice, breads, and cereals. Adults should consume 400 micrograms DFE of folate daily. Consuming too much folate can obscure a vitamin B_{12} deficiency. A deficiency of folate results in macrocytic anemia. Babies born to mothers who are deficient in folate have a higher risk of neural tube defects such as spina bifida.

Tetrahydrofolate

LO 10.9 Vitamin B12

Vitamin B_{12} is a family of compounds also referred to as cobalamin. To be absorbed, vitamin B_{12} requires the aid of R protein from the salivary glands and hydrocholoric acid and intrinsic factor from the stomach. Vitamin B_{12} functions as two different coenzymes involved in DNA and RNA synthesis, the conversion of homocysteine to methionine, the utilization of fats and proteins for energy, and the maintenance of the myelin sheath surrounding nerves. Vitamin B_{12} also activates folate by removing the methyl group from folate, which in turn activates vitamin B_{12}. Vitamin B_{12} is found naturally only in animal-based foods. The synthetic form is used in fortified soymilk and some cereals. Adults need 2.4 micrograms daily. There are no known toxicity risks of consuming too much vitamin B_{12}. A deficiency of vitamin B_{12} causes macrocytic anemia. Pernicious anemia is due to insufficient production of intrinsic factor for adequate B_{12} absorption. A prolonged vitamin B_{12} deficiency can cause nerve damage.

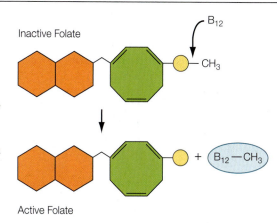

Inactive Folate

Active Folate

LO 10.10 Vitamin C

Ascorbic acid

Vitamin C, also known as ascorbic acid, assists in the formation of collagen necessary for healthy bones, teeth, skin, and blood vessels. As an antioxidant, vitamin C reduces free radical damage and supports a healthy immune system. Vitamin C also improves the absorption of nonheme iron. Vitamin C is found in a wide variety of fruits and vegetables. Adult women need 75 milligrams and men need 90 milligrams of vitamin C daily. Smokers need to increase their daily intake by 35 mg. The UL is set at 2,000 milligrams per day. Vitamin C doesn't prevent the common cold but may reduce the duration of a cold in some people. A deficiency of vitamin C results in scurvy.

LO 10.11 Other Vitamin-Like Compounds Are Not Essential

Choline is a conditionally essential nutrient that the body needs for healthy cells and nerves. Carnitine, lipoic acid, and inositol are vitamin-like compounds that are used for important body functions and overall health. They are not considered essential because they can be synthesized in sufficient amounts in the body.

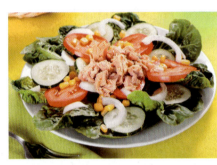

LO 10.12 A Healthy Diet and Lifestyle May Reduce Cancer Risk

Cancer, the second leading cause of death in the United States, is a disease of uncontrolled replication of abnormal cells. Cancer develops in three stages: initiation, promotion, and progression. Carcinogens, or cancer-causing substances, damage cells by altering their DNA. Genetic, environmental, and lifestyle factors all play a role in cancer risk, but lifestyle factors, including diet, have the most influence. Plant-based foods high in fiber and vitamins A, D, E, C, and folate reduce the risk of cancer, whereas red and processed meats as well as alcohol can increase risk. Avoiding tobacco, keeping physically active, and maintaining a healthy body weight may also reduce the risk of cancer.

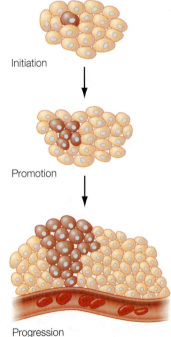

Initiation

Promotion

Progression

Terms to Know

- coenzymes
- hemopoiesis
- thiamin pyrophosphate (TPP)
- beriberi
- peripheral neuropathy
- flavin mononucleotide (FMN)
- ariboflavinosis
- stomatitis
- glossitis
- cheilosis
- nicotinamide adenine dinucleotide (NAD^+)
- nicotinamide adenine dinucleotide phosphate ($NADP^+$)
- niacin equivalents (NE)
- pellagra
- avidin
- biotinidase
- pyridoxal phosphate (PLP)
- microcytic hypochromic anemia
- folate
- folic acid
- 5-methyltetrahydrofolate (5-methyl THF)
- neural tube defects
- anencephaly
- spinal bifida
- dietary folate equivalents (DFE)
- cobalamin
- R protein
- intrinsic factor (IF)
- methylcobalamin
- deoxyadenosylcobalamin
- myelin sheath
- atrophic gastritis
- pernicious anemia
- ascorbic acid
- collagen
- hemochromatosis
- scurvy
- choline
- carnitine
- lipoic acid
- inositol
- cancer
- carcinogenesis
- carcinogen

Check Your Understanding

1. **LO 10.1** The primary function of the B-complex vitamins is to act as
   a. sources of energy.
   b. coenzymes.
   c. antioxidants.
   d. epigenetic factors.

2. **LO 10.2** A deficiency of thiamin can cause
   a. rickets.
   b. beriberi.
   c. scurvy.
   d. osteomalacia.

3. **LO 10.3** The coenzyme that functions in the transfer of hydrogen atoms is
   a. pantothenic acid.
   b. vitamin B_6.
   c. riboflavin.
   d. biotin.

4. **LO 10.4** The body requires more of this water-soluble vitamin than any other.
   a. Vitamin B_6
   b. Niacin
   c. Riboflavin
   d. Vitamin B_{12}

5. **LO 10.5** The vitamin that is part of the structure of acetyl CoA is
   a. biotin.
   b. thiamin.
   c. pantothenic acid.
   d. niacin.

6. **LO 10.6** Which of the following is a function of biotin?
   a. It helps prevent scurvy.
   b. It helps to reduce cholesterol.
   c. It has an antioxidant effect on free radicals.
   d. It acts as a coenzyme in fatty-acid synthesis.

7. **LO 10.7** The vitamin involved as a coenzyme in more than 100 enzymes, most of which are amino acid reactions, is
   a. riboflavin.
   b. pantothenic acid.
   c. vitamin B_6.
   d. biotin.

8. **LO 10.8** Folic acid can reduce the risk of
   a. acne.
   b. neural tube defects.
   c. night blindness.
   d. pellagra.

9. **LO 10.9** Vitamin B_{12} is essential for the health and function of
   a. nerves.
   b. epithelial cells.
   c. eye tissue.
   d. collagen.

10. **LO 10.10** You are enjoying a breakfast of raisin bran cereal in skim milk accompanied by a glass of orange juice. The vitamin C in the orange juice will enhance the absorption of
    a. the calcium in the milk.
    b. the vitamin D in fortified milk.
    c. the iron in the cereal.
    d. the fiber in the cereal.

11. **LO 10.11** All of the following are classified as B vitamins *except*
    a. choline.
    b. niacin.
    c. pantothenic acid.
    d. pyridoxine.

12. **LO 10.12** By what mechanism do carcinogens damage cells?
    a. Gene transfer
    b. Acid–base imbalances
    c. DNA mutation
    d. Carboxylation

Answers

1. (b) The primary function of the B-complex vitamins is to activate enzymes involved in a variety of chemical reactions. B-complex vitamins are not a source of energy but do act as coenzymes in energy metabolism. Unlike vitamin C, the B-complex vitamins are not antioxidants. Even though some of the B-complex vitamins are involved in DNA synthesis, their primary function is not to act as epigenetic factors.

2. (b) A thiamin deficiency results in beriberi. Rickets and osteomalacia are caused by a lack of vitamin D and scurvy results from a vitamin C deficiency.

3. (c) Riboflavin, in the form of FAD and FMN, transfers hydrogen atoms during energy metabolism.

Pantothenic acid is part of coenzyme A, which forms acetyl CoA; vitamin B_6 is a coenzyme for protein metabolism; and biotin is a coenzyme for carboxylase enzymes.

4. (b) The dietary requirement for niacin is 16 milligrams per day for males and 14 milligrams for females, compared with 1.3 milligrams of vitamin B_6 for males and females, 1.3 milligrams or 1.1 milligrams of riboflavin for males or females, respectively, and 2.4 micrograms per day of vitamin B_{12} for both genders.

5. (c) Pantothenic acid is part of coenzyme A, which forms acetyl CoA. Biotin, thiamin, and niacin all function as coenzymes.

6. (d) Biotin activates enzymes involved in fatty acid synthesis. Ascorbic acid or vitamin C prevents scurvy and functions as an antioxidant to reduce free radicals. Niacin lowers LDL-cholesterol in the blood.

7. (c) Vitamin B_6 activates more than 100 enzymes involved in protein metabolism. Riboflavin, pantothenic acid, and biotin are all involved in energy metabolism.

8. (b) Folic acid reduces the risk of neural tube defects. Vitamin A can reduce acne and night blindness, whereas niacin can prevent pellagra.

9. (a) Vitamin B_{12} maintains the myelin sheath that covers nerves, and thus is essential for their health and function. Vitamin A is essential for epithelial cells and eye tissue. Vitamin C participates in collagen formation.

10. (c) Vitamin C will increase the absorption of iron in grain products and cereals but does not affect the absorption of calcium or vitamin D. Fiber passes through the GI tract and is not absorbed.

11. (a) Choline is not considered a B vitamin because it is only conditionally essential. Niacin, pantothenic acid, and pyridoxine are B vitamins.

12. (c) Carcinogens, or cancer-causing agents, cause mutations in the DNA of body cells. If the damage is not repaired or the cell does not die, it can replicate and eventually form a tumor.

Answers to True or False?

1. **False.** Some water-soluble vitamins, such as vitamin C and folate, are easily destroyed by heat while niacin and vitamin B_6 are stable in cooking. However, all water-soluble vitamins leach into water, so drier cooking methods help retain more of these vitamins.

2. **False.** Biotin and pantothenic acid are both B vitamins involved in energy production, not forms of vitamin C.

3. **False.** Vitamins do not provide energy. However, the B-complex vitamins are essential to energy metabolism.

4. **False.** Niacin can be made from excess tryptophan, but the amount of niacin synthesized is insufficient to meet the body's needs.

5. **True.** Very large doses of vitamin B_6 (from as low as 500 milligrams) can cause sensory neuropathy, which causes pain, numbness, and tingling in the feet and hands.

6. **True.** Older adults may produce less hydrochloric acid and intrinsic factor than younger adults, which can hinder their ability to absorb adequate amounts of vitamin B_{12}.

7. **True.** Adequate folate intake before and during the early months of pregnancy can lower the risk of neural tube defects, including spina bifida and anencephaly.

8. **False.** A dietary deficiency of pantothenic acid is rare because this B vitamin is widespread throughout the food supply. Excellent sources include chicken, beef, egg yolk, and vegetables such as broccoli, tomatoes, and mushrooms.

9. **True.** The protein avidin, found in egg whites, can bind biotin and prevent it from being absorbed. Cooking the egg denatures the avidin and prevents this problem.

10. **False.** There is no clear evidence that vitamin C supplements prevent the common cold, though they may reduce the severity of cold symptoms in some people.

Web Resources

- To learn more about vitamin and mineral supplements, visit http://ods.od.nih.gov
- For tips on how to include more fruits and vegetables in your diet, visit www.cdc.gov/nccdphp/dnpao
- For more information on cooking with microwave ovens to preserve vitamins, visit www.foodscience.csiro.au/micwave1.htm

References

1. Institute of Medicine, Food and Nutrition Board. 1998. *Dietary Reference Intakes: Thiamin, Riboflavin, Niacin, Vitamin B₆, Folate, Vitamin B₁₂, Pantothenic Acid, Biotin, and Choline.* Washington, DC: National Academies Press.
2. Wijnia, J. W., E. Oudman, et al. 2016. Severe Infections Are Common in Thiamine Deficiency and May Be Related to Cognitive Outcomes: A Cohort Study of 68 Patients With Wernicke-Korsakoff Syndrome. *Psychosomatics* 57(6):624–633. doi: 10.1016/j.psym.2016.06.004.
3. Herreid, E. O., B. Ruskin, et al. 1952. Ascorbic Acid and Riboflavin Destruction and Flavor Development in Milk Exposed to the Sun in Amber, Clear, Paper, and Ruby Bottles. *Journal of Dairy Science* 35:772–778.
4. Institute of Medicine. 2006. *Dietary Reference Intakes: The Essential Guide to Nutrient Requirements.* Washington, DC: National Academies Press.
5. Barile, M., T. A. Giancaspero, et al. 2016. Riboflavin Transport and Metabolism in Humans. *Journal of Inherited Metabolic Disease* 39(4):545–557. doi: 10.1007/s10545-016-9950-0.
6. Squibb, R. L., J. E. Braham, et al. 1958. A Comparison of the Effect of Raw Corn and Tortillas (Lime-Treated Corn) with Niacin, Tryptophan or Beans on the Growth and Muscle Niacin of Rats. *Journal of Nutrition* 67:351–361.
7. La Paz, S. M., B. Bermudez, et al. 2016. Pharmacological Effects of Niacin on Acute Hyperlipemia. *Current Medicinal Chemistry* 23(25):2826–2835.
8. Institute of Medicine, Foods and Nutrition Board. 1998. *Dietary Reference Intakes: Thiamin, Riboflavin, Niacin, Vitamin B₆, Folate, Vitamin B₁₂, Pantothenic Acid, Biotin, and Choline.*
9. Kirkland, J. 2014. Niacin. In A. C. Ross, B. Caballero, et al. *Modern Nutrition in Health and Disease.* 11th ed. Baltimore: Lippincott Williams & Wilkins.
10. Institute of Medicine, Food and Nutrition Board. 1998. *Dietary Reference Intakes: Thiamin, Riboflavin, Niacin, Vitamin B₆, Folate, Vitamin B₁₂, Pantothenic Acid, Biotin, and Choline.*
11. Trumbo, P. R. 2014. Pantothenic Acid. In A. C. Ross, B. Caballero, et al. eds. *Modern Nutrition in Health and Disease.* 11th ed. Baltimore: Lippincott Williams & Wilkins.
12. Said, H. M. 2011. Intestinal Absorption of Water-soluble Vitamins in Health and Disease. *Biochemistry Journal* 437(3):357–372. doi: 10.1042/BJ20110326.
13. Glusman, M. 1947. The Syndrome of "Burning Feet" (Nutritional Melagia) as a Manifestation of Nutritional Deficiency. *American Journal of Medicine* 3:211–223.
14. Gropper, S. S., and J. L. Smith. 2018. *Advanced Nutrition and Human Metabolism.* 7th ed. Belmont, CA: Wadsworth, Cengage Learning.
15. Institute of Medicine. 2006. *Dietary Reference Intakes: The Essential Guide to Nutrient Requirements.*
16. U. S. National Library of Medicine. 2017. *Biotinidase Deficiency.* Available at http://ghr.nlm.nih.gov. Accessed February 2017.
17. Institute of Medicine, Food and Nutrition Board. 1998. *Dietary Reference Intakes: Thiamin, Riboflavin, Niacin, Vitamin B₆, Folate, Vitamin B₁₂, Pantothenic Acid, Biotin, and Choline.*
18. Da Silvia, V. R., A. D. Mackey, et al. 2014. Vitamin B₆. In A. C. Ross, B. Caballero, et al. eds. *Modern Nutrition in Health and Disease.* 11th ed. Baltimore: Lippincott Williams & Wilkins.
19. Ibid.
20. Qin, X., F. Fan, et al. 2014. Folic Acid Supplementation with and without Vitamin B₆ and Revascularization Risk: A Meta-Analysis of Randomized Controlled Trials. *Clinical Nutrition* doi:10.1016/j.clnu.2014.01.006.
21. O'Donnell, A., McParlin, C., Robson, S.C., et al. 2016. Treatments for Hyperemesis Gravidarum and Nausea and Vomiting in Pregnancy: a Systematic Review and Economic Assessment. *Health Technology Assessment* 20(74):1–268.
22. Masoumi, S. Z., M. Ataollahi, et al. 2016. Effect of Combined Use of Calcium and Vitamin B6 on Premenstrual Syndrome Symptoms: a Randomized Clinical Trial. *Journal of Caring Sciences* 5(1):67–73. doi: 10.15171/jcs.2016.007.
23. Kulkantrakorn, K. 2014. Pyridoxine-induced Sensory Ataxic Neuronopathy and Neuropathy: Revisited. *Neurological Sciences* 35(11):1827–1830. doi: 10.1007/s10072-014-1902-6.
24. Marchetta, C. M., O. J. Devine, et al. 2015. Assessing the Association Between Natural Food Folate Intake and Blood Folate Concentrations: a Systematic Review and Bayesian Meta-analysis of Trials and Observational Studies. *Nutrients* 7(4):2663–2686. doi: 10.3390/nu7042663.
25. Centers for Disease Control and Prevention. 2014. *Folic Acid.* Available at www.cdc.gov. Accessed February 2017.
26. Ibid.
27. Rosenthal, J., J. Casas, et al. 2014. Neural Tube Defects in Latin American and the Impact of Fortification: A Literature Review. *Public Health Nutrition* 17(3):537–550. doi: 10.1017/S1368980013000256.

28. Centers for Disease Control and Prevention. 2014. *Folic Acid.* Available at www.cdc.gov. Accessed February 2017.

29. Mason, J. B., and S. Y. Tang. 2017. Folate Status and Colorectal Cancer Risk: A 2016 Update. *Molecular Aspects of Medicine* 53:73–79. doi: 10.1016/j.mam.2016.11.010.

30. Nitter, M., B. Norgård, et al. 2014. Plasma Methionine, Choline, Betaine, and Dimethylglycine in Relation to Colorectal Cancer Risk in the European Prospective Investigation into Cancer and Nutrition (EPIC). *Annals of Oncology* doi: 10.1093/annonc/mdu185.

31. Li, B., Y. Lu, et al. 2014. Folate Intake and Breast Cancer Prognosis: A Meta-Analysis of Prospective Observational Studies. *European Journal of Cancer Prevention.* doi: 10.1097/CEJ.0000000000000028.

32. Lin, H. L., An, Q. Z., Wang, Q. Z., and Liu, C. X. 2013. Folate Intake and Pancreatic Cancer Risk: An Overall and Dose-response Meta-Analysis. *Public Health* 127(7):607–613. doi: 10.1016/j.puhe.2013.04.008.

33. Institute of Medicine, Food and Nutrition Board. 1998. *Dietary Reference Intakes: Thiamin, Riboflavin, Niacin, Vitamin B₆, Folate, Vitamin B₁₂, Pantothenic Acid, Biotin, and Choline.*

34. National Institutes of Health, Office of Dietary Supplements. 2016. *Dietary Supplement Fact Sheet: Folate.* Available at http://ods.od.nih.gov. Accessed February 2017.

35. Ibid.

36. Ibid.

37. Institute of Medicine, Food and Nutrition Board. 1998. *Dietary Reference Intakes: Thiamin, Riboflavin, Niacin, Vitamin B₆, Folate, Vitamin B₁₂, Pantothenic Acid, Biotin, and Choline.*

38. Ibid.

39. Bailey, R. L., and J. P. van Wijngaarden. 2015. The Role of B-Vitamins in Bone Health and Disease in Older Adults. *Current Osteoporosis Report* 13(4):256–261. doi: 10.1007/s11914-015-0273-0.

40. Watanabe, F., K. Abe, et al. 1998. Effects of Microwave Heating on the Loss of Vitamin B₁₂ in Foods. *Journal of Agricultural Food Chemistry* 46:206–210.

41. Abdulmanea, A. A., A.H. Alsaeed, et al. 2014. Prevalence of Pernicious Anemia in Patients with Macrocytic Anemia and Low Serum B12. *Pakistan Journal of Medical Sciences* 30(6):1218–1222. doi: 10.12669/pjms.306.5413.

42. Mendonça, N., J. C. Mathers, et al. 2016. Intakes of Folate and Vitamin B12 and Biomarkers of Status in the Very Old: The Newcastle 85+ Study. *Nutrients* 8(10). pii: E604.

43. Covarrubias-Pinto, A., A. I. Acuña, et al. 2015. Old Things New View: Ascorbic Acid Protects the Brain in Neurodegenerative

Disorders. *International Journal of Molecular Science* 16(12): 28194–28217.

44. Gropper, S. S., and J. L. Smith. 2018. *Advanced Nutrition and Human Metabolism.*

45. Ibid.

46. Singh, A., K. Bains, et al. 2016. Relationship of Dietary Factors with Dialyzable Iron and In Vitro Iron Bioavailability in the Meals of Farm Women. *Journal of Food Science Technology* 53(4):2001–2008. doi: 10.1007/s13197-015-2153-0.

47. Padayatty, S., J. Doppman, et al. 2007. Human Adrenal Glands Secrete Vitamin C in Response to Adrenocorticotropic Hormone. *American Journal of Clinical Nutrition* 86:145–149.

48. Gropper, S. S., and J. L. Smith. 2018. *Advanced Nutrition and Human Metabolism.*

49. National Institutes of Health, Office of Dietary Supplements. 2016. *Dietary Supplement Fact Sheet: Vitamin C.* Available at http://ods.od.nih.gov. Accessed March 2017.

50. Shaath, T., R. Fischer, et al. 2016. Scurvy in the Present Times: Vitamin C Allergy Leading to Strict Fast Food Diet. *Dermatology Online Journal* 22(1). pii: 13030/qt50b8w28b.

51. English, J. 2013. *Vitamin C, Colds, and Acute Induced Scurvy.* Available at www.nutritionreview.org. Accessed March 2017.

52. Sherriff, J. L., T. A. O'Sullivan, et al. 2016. Choline, Its Potential Role in Nonalcholic Fatty Liver Disease and the Case for Human and Bacterial Genes. *Advanced Nutrition* (1):5–13. doi: 10.3945/an.114.007955.

53. Ziesel, S. H. 2014. Choline. In A. C. Ross, B. Caballero, R. J. Cousins, K. L. Tucker, and T. R. Ziegler, eds. *Modern Nutrition in Health and Disease.* 11th ed. Baltimore: Lippincott Williams & Wilkins.

54. National Institutes of Health, Office of Dietary Supplements. 2013. *Carnitine.* Available at http://ods.od.nih.gov. Accessed March 2014.

55. Hu, H., C. Wang, Y. Jin, Q. Meng, Q. Liu, K. Liu, and H. Sun. 2016. Alpha-lipoic Acid Defends Homocysteine-induced Endoplasmic Reticulum and Oxidative Stress in HAECs. *Biomedical Pharmacotherapy* 80:63–72. doi: 10.1016/j.biopha.2016.02.022.

56. Román-Pintos, L. M., G. Villegas-Rivera, et al. 2016. Polyneuropathy in Type 2 Diabetes Mellitus: Inflammation, Oxidative Stress, and Mitochondrial Function. *Journal of Diabetes Research* 2016:3425617. doi: 10.1155/2016/3425617.

57. World Cancer Research Fund. 2014. *Stopping Cancer before It Starts.* Available at www.wcrf.org. Accessed March 2017.

58. American Cancer Society. 2017. *Cancer Facts and Figures 2017.* Available at www.cancer.org. Accessed March 2017.

59. Ibid.

60. American Cancer Action Network. 2017. *Cancer Prevention and Early Detection Facts and Figures.* Available at www.cancer.org. Accessed March 2017

61. Ibid.

62. Boyle, T., T. Keegle, et al. 2012. Physical Activity and Risks of Proximal and Distal Colon Cancers: A Systematic Review and Meta-Analysis. *Journal of the National Cancer Institute* 104(20):1548–1561.

63. Ibid.

64. van den Brandt, P. A., and M. Schulpen. 2017. Mediterranean Diet Adherence and Risk of Postmenopausal Breast Cancer: Results of a Cohort Study and Meta-analysis. *International Journal of Cancer* doi: 10.1002/ijc.30654.

65. Kyrgiou, M., I. Kalliala, et al. 2017. Adiposity and Cancer at Major Anatomical Sites: Umbrella Review of the Literature. *BMJ* 356:j477. doi: 10.1136/bmj.j477.

66. Lavender, N., D. W. Hein, et al. 2015. Evaluation of Oxidative Stress Response Related Genetic Variants, Prooxidants, Antioxidants and Prostate Cancer. *AIMS Medical Science* 2(4):271–294.

67. Parsons, J. K., J. P. Pierce, et al. 2013. A Randomized Pilot Trial of Dietary Modification for the Chemoprevention of Noninvasive Bladder Cancer: The Dietary Intervention in Bladder Cancer Study. *Cancer Prevention Research* 6:971–978.

68. Ibid.

69. Schwingshackl, L., H. Boeing, et al. 2017. Dietary Supplements and Risk of Cause-Specific Death, Cardiovascular Disease, and Cancer: A Systematic Review and Meta-analysis of Primary Prevention Trials. *Advanced Nutrition* 8(1):27–39. doi: 10.3945/an.116.013516.

70. Ibid.

71. American Cancer Society. 2017. *10 Facts About What Really Causes Cancer.* Available at www.cancer.org. Accessed March 2017.

72. Álvarez-Avellón, S. M., A. Fernández-Somoano, et al. 2017. Effect of Alcohol and Its Metabolites in Lung Cancer: CAPUA Study. *Medicina Clinica* pii: S0025-7753(17)30036-2. doi: 10.1016/j.medcli.2016.12.033.

73. Bouchard-Mercier, A., A. M. Paradis, et al. 2013. Associations between Dietary Patterns and Gene Expression Profiles of Healthy Men and Women: A Cross-Sectional Study. *Nutrition Journal* doi: 10.1186/1475-2891-12-24.

74. Underwood, M. A. 2014. Intestinal Dysbiosis: Novel Mechanisms by Which Gut Microbes Trigger and Prevent Disease. *Preventive Medicine* doi: 10.1016/j.ypmed.2014.05.010.

75. World Cancer Research Fund. 2014. *Stopping Cancer before It Starts.*

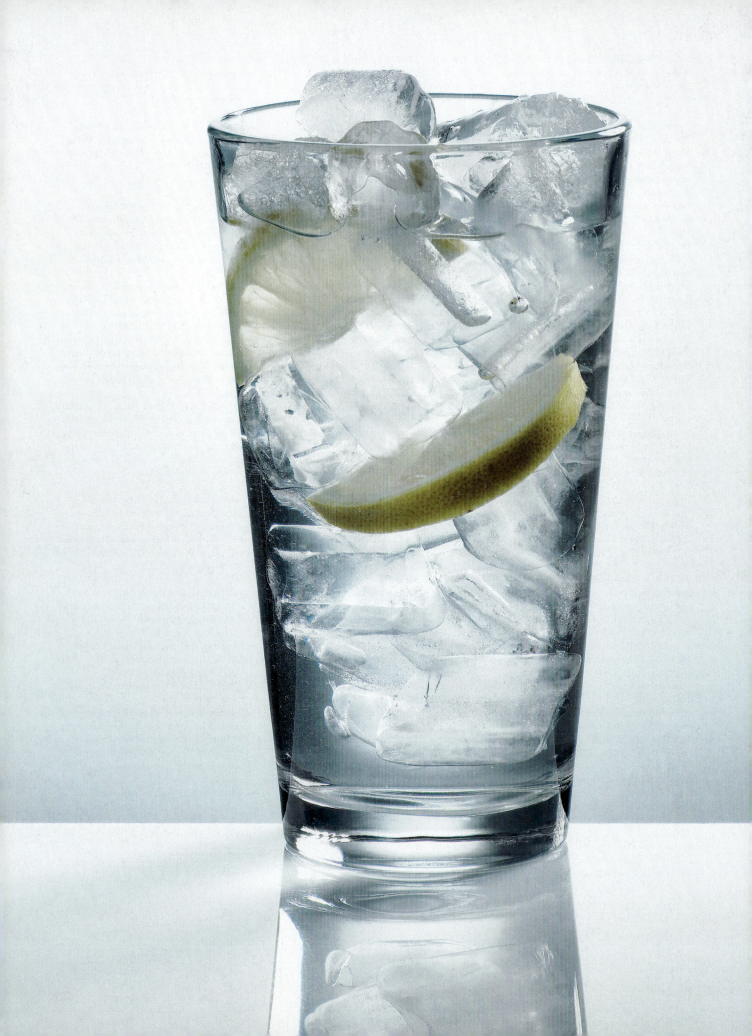

Water

Learning Outcomes

After reading this chapter, you will be able to:

11.1 Explain why water is essential to life.

11.2 Describe the various processes that maintain water balance in the body.

11.3 Describe the roles of water, sodium, hormones, and enzymes in the development of hypertension.

11.4 Identify the Dietary Reference Intake for water.

11.5 Explain the effects of diuretics, such as caffeine and alcohol, on fluid balance.

11.6 Differentiate between dehydration and water intoxication, and describe the signs and symptoms of each.

True or False?

1. The body can survive for weeks without food and water. **T**/**F**

2. A morning mug of coffee counts toward daily water needs. **T**/**F**

3. Daily consumption of at least 8 cups of fluids is essential for health. **T**/**F**

4. Drinking large amounts of water helps flush waste from the body. **T**/**F**

5. Drinking extra water leads to weight loss. **T**/**F**

6. Exercise often leads to dehydration. **T**/**F**

7. Sodium should be eliminated from the diet to prevent fluid retention. **T**/**F**

8. Eating bananas reduces hypertension. **T**/**F**

9. Drinking alcohol causes dehydration. **T**/**F**

10. Enhanced waters are healthier than plain water. **T**/**F**

See Page 429 for the answers.

veryone needs water to live. But exactly why is this the case, and how much water do you really need? In this chapter, we explore the essential functions that water plays in the body, as well as the mechanisms that keep fluids and other substances in a healthy balance. We also explain how to make sure that you are meeting your daily needs and, equally important, how to avoid consuming toxic amounts of water.

Why Is Water Essential to Life?

LO 11.1 Explain why water is essential to life.

Water (H_2O) is the most abundant substance in the body and, as such, is the most important. You could survive for weeks without food, but only for a few days without water.

The average healthy adult body is composed of about 45–75 percent water. The distribution of this water depends on an individual's age, gender, and the composition of fat and muscle in the body (**Figure 11.1**). Because lean muscle tissue is approximately 75 percent water, while fat tissue contains very little water (up to 20 percent), some individuals have less body water than others.[1] In general, males have a higher percentage of muscle mass and a lower percentage of fat tissue than females of the same age, and therefore males have more body water. For the same reason, muscular athletes have a higher percentage of body water than sedentary individuals. Body water also decreases with age. A newborn averages about 73 percent of body weight as water, while an older adult only has about 45 percent.[2]

Water is a polar molecule, which means it has an unbalanced charge from the positive charge on the hydrogen atoms and the negative charge on the oxygen atoms. This is possible because water, unlike carbon dioxide, is not linear but bent in shape (see the left side of **Figure 11.2**). Its polarity allows water to attract other charged molecules and help maintain acid–base balance in the body.

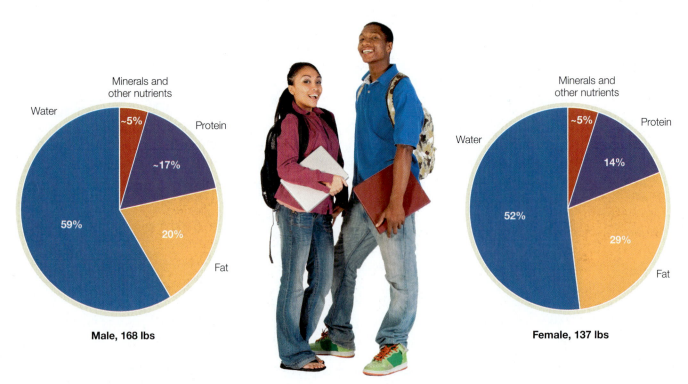

Male, 168 lbs

Water 59%

Minerals and other nutrients ~5%

Protein ~17%

Fat 20%

Female, 137 lbs

Water 52%

Minerals and other nutrients ~5%

Protein 14%

Fat 29%

▲ Figure 11.1 **The Composition of the Body**
Water is the predominant body component for both men and women.

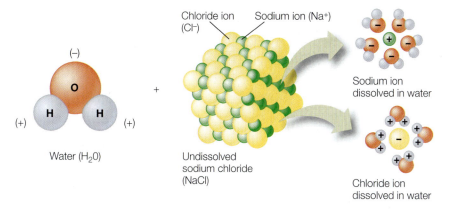

Chloride ion (Cl⁻) Sodium ion (Na⁺)

(−)
O
H   H
(+)   (+)

Water (H₂O)

+

Undissolved sodium chloride (NaCl)

Sodium ion dissolved in water

Chloride ion dissolved in water

◀ **Figure 11.2 Water Is a Universal Solvent**
The oxygen atom of water has a partial negative charge and the hydrogen atoms have a partial positive charge. This property makes water a universal solvent that can dissolve polar molecules such as sodium chloride (NaCl). The negatively charged Cl⁻ is attracted to the positive charge of the hydrogen ions (H⁺) and the positive charge of Na⁺ is attracted to the negative charge of oxygen (O⁻). Thus, the water slowly dissolves the salt.

Water's polar quality enables it to play a role as a medium in which other substances can dissolve. As part of blood and other fluids, water transports nutrients, waste products, and other substances between cells and tissues. Water also helps maintain a constant body temperature; lubricates and protects joints and other areas; triggers chemical reactions, including those that provide the body with energy; and enables acid–base balance to take place within the cells. Without water, metabolism would grind to a halt.

Water Is a Universal Solvent and Transport Medium

Water is commonly known as a universal **solvent** because it dissolves more substances than any other liquid. Its polarity allows it to attract charged particles into a solution and dissolve a variety of other polar substances, including proteins, glucose, and some minerals. As illustrated in **Figure 11.2**, the positive and negative charges of water attract the positive and negative charges of table salt, called sodium chloride (Na⁺Cl⁻). The result is that salt dissolves in water. Compounds that are not polar, such as lipids, are not attracted to water and thus do not dissolve.

Water's function as a solvent is critically important in digestion and transport. For example, about 7,000 milliliters of watery gastric juices dissolve digested nutrients. About 83 percent of blood is water, which enables it to transport oxygen-carrying red blood cells, white blood cells, nutrients, hormones, and other substances to the cells. Water also helps transport waste products away from cells to be excreted in urine and stool.

Water Helps Maintain Body Temperature

Water is a heat buffer similar to the coolant fluid in a car. It absorbs heat from the body's internal core and carries it to the skin for release. Water works well as a coolant because it has a high **specific heat**, the amount of energy required to raise 1 gram of water 1 degree Celsius (1°C). Thus, with only a small rise in body temperature, water can absorb, hold onto, and release heat to return the body to a safe temperature.

A jog on a hot summer day, for example, can generate an enormous amount of internal heat. As the core temperature increases, temperature receptors in the hypothalamus trigger blood vessel dilation, increasing the flow of warmed blood to the skin's surface. At the same time, the rising skin temperature activates the 3 million sweat glands to release additional water and salts through the pores of the skin. The increasing heat breaks apart the hydrogen bonds of the water and transforms it from a liquid (*sweat*) to a vapor. Heat dissipates as the sweat evaporates from the surface of the skin, thus cooling the skin (**Figure 11.3**), leaving the salt behind. The cooled blood returns to the muscle. The water in sweat that drips off your body releases very little heat.

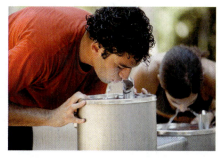

Water is vital for many body functions, but it is not stored in the body, so adequate amounts must be consumed daily.

solvent Liquid in which substances dissolve to form a new solution. Water is called the universal solvent because it can dissolve a variety of substances, including minerals and glucose.

specific heat Measurement of the energy required to raise a gram of a substance, such as water, 1 degree Celsius.

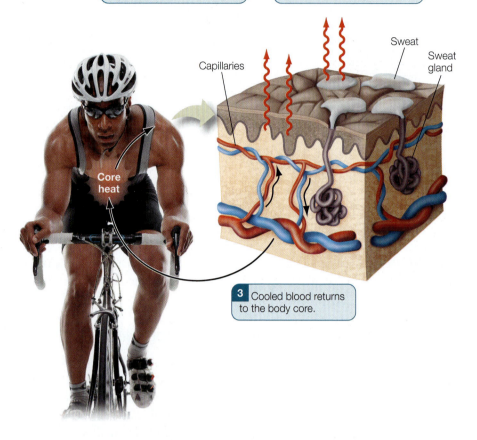

1 The water in blood carries heat to the capillaries at the skin surface.

2 The heat is released at the skin surface. Evaporation of sweat cools the skin.

Capillaries

Sweat

Sweat gland

Core heat

3 Cooled blood returns to the body core.

Water Is a Lubricant and a Protective Cushion and Provides Structure to Muscle Cells

Water acts as a lubricant for joints and sensitive eye tissue. It lubricates and moistens food in the mouth as part of saliva and is part of the mucus that lubricates the intestinal tract. Water is the main component of the fluid that bathes certain organs, including the brain. It thus acts as a cushion to protect organs from injury during a fall or other trauma. During pregnancy, a sac of protective amniotic fluid surrounds a developing fetus.

Water also provides a structural component to cells, much like air in a balloon. Without water, a cell would be limp and shriveled. Athletes experience the structural features of water when the muscle feels full following a carbohydrate-loading diet. This is because glycogen is surrounded by water when it is stored in muscle cells. Every molecule of glucose within the glycogen structure has 2.7 grams of water associated with it, adding bulk and structure to the muscle cells.[3]

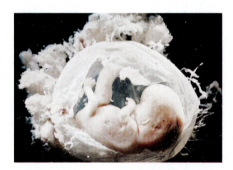

A developing fetus is cushioned in a sac of watery amniotic fluid to protect it from physical harm during pregnancy.

Water Participates in Hydrolysis and Condensation Reactions

Water is essential for most chemical reactions in the body. During digestion water hydrolyzes the bonds that hold carbohydrate, protein, and fat molecules together. For example, when sucrose is digested (refer to Chapter 4), hydrolysis adds a hydrogen ion to fructose and a hydroxyl group to glucose; then each monosaccharide is absorbed. When smaller molecules are combined through condensation, such as when excess glucose is stored as glycogen in the liver and muscle, the opposite occurs. In this case, a water molecule is released for every bond that is formed.

Water Plays a Role in Acid–Base Balance

Acid–base balance is essential to maintain homeostasis in the body. As you learned in Chapter 3, a normal pH in human blood ranges from 7.35 to 7.45, which reflects the amount of hydrogen ions present—more hydrogen ions means a lower, more acidic pH. Because water is polar, it can function to reduce or increase the pH levels by either breaking down or forming carbonic acid. In other words, water can act as either an acid or a base. These reactions are described in the Chemistry Boost.

> **LO 11.1: THE TAKE-HOME MESSAGE** The body is 45–75 percent water. Muscle tissue has more water than fat tissue; therefore, men have more body water than women and younger individuals have more body water than older individuals. Water is polar, interacts with other nutrients, serves as an acid–base buffer, transports oxygen and nutrients throughout the body, regulates body temperature, is a lubricant, adds structure to cells, participates in hydrolysis and condensation, and provides a protective cushion for the brain and other organs.

Chemistry Boost

Water and Acid–Base Balance

When water dissociates, one hydrogen atom breaks its bond with oxygen, leaving behind its electron and becoming a positively charged hydrogen ion (H^+). The other hydrogen remains attached to the oxygen atom. Oxygen retains both of its original electrons but also has the extra electron left from the hydrogen, which gives the molecule a negative charge. The OH^- molecule is called a hydroxide ion.

$$H_2O \leftrightarrow H^+ + OH^-$$

When a solution has more H^+ than OH^- ions, it is acidic. When the solution has more OH^- than H^+ ions, it is basic (refer to the pH scale in Chapter 3).

Water can regulate acid–base balance by forming or breaking down carbonic acid (H_2CO_3). This buffering action is reversible, as illustrated in the following two reactions:

a. During exercise, carbon dioxide is produced as a by-product of energy metabolism. Carbon dioxide is a gas that quickly dissolves in water, forming carbonic acid (H_2CO_3). If the reaction continues, carbonic acid can be further reduced to hydrogen (H^+) and bicarbonate ions (HCO_3^-). The increase in H^+ results in a decrease in pH and makes the environment more acidic.

$$H_2O + CO_2 \rightarrow H_2CO_3 \rightarrow H^+ + HCO_3^-$$

b. The reaction can be reversed and act as a buffer to neutralize excess hydrogen ions. In this reaction, H^+ ions formed during energy metabolism (recall from Chapter 8 that H^+ are formed during glycolysis and the TCA cycle) combine with bicarbonate (HCO_3^-) to form water and carbon dioxide. This increases the pH and makes the environment more alkaline.

$$H^+ + HCO_3^- \rightarrow H_2CO_3 \rightarrow H_2O + CO_2$$

How Is Water Balance Maintained?

LO 11.2 Describe the various processes that maintain water balance in the body.

The amount of water in the body is tightly regulated because fluid homeostasis is necessary for normal chemical reactions to take place within cells. The body maintains this delicate balance by adapting to changes in water intake and water loss. When the amount of water consumed is equal to the amount excreted, the body is in **water balance**.

acid–base balance Mechanisms used to maintain body fluids close to a neutral pH so the body can function properly.

water balance State of equilibrium when the intake of water equals the amount of water excreted.

Sources of Body Water Include Beverages and Food

The body's largest source of water is the beverages we consume, including tap or bottled water, milk, juices, coffee, and soft drinks. An additional source of water is foods, especially fruits and vegetables, which contain more water by weight than do grains or meats. Most foods contain some water.

In addition to the water consumed through beverages and foods, water is generated during metabolism. This source is referred to as **metabolic water**. For example, condensation reactions, such as those that occur during energy metabolism, yield a small amount of water. One hundred grams of carbohydrate can yield almost 55 grams of metabolic water by the time it has been catabolized to ATP. In addition, the water that was joined with glucose during glycogenesis is later released when glycogen is hydrolyzed to produce glucose.

The intake of water from fluids, food, and metabolism contributes to the total average intake of 2,550 milliliters daily (about 2 quarts). **Figure 11.4** illustrates the sources of water in the body and the routes of excretion.

Water Is Excreted through the Kidneys, Large Intestine, Lungs, and Skin

To maintain water balance, water is excreted through urine and sweat, stool, and as water vapor through the lungs. The kidneys play the primary role in fluid excretion.

Every day the kidneys filter nearly 200 liters of blood; thus, the body's entire blood volume is filtered 20 or more times each day. Filtration allows toxins, metabolic wastes, and excess ions to leave the body in urine while returning needed substances to the blood. Much like a water purification plant that keeps a city's water drinkable and disposes of its wastes, the kidneys are usually unappreciated until they malfunction and body fluids become contaminated.

The kidneys excrete metabolic wastes and other substances in urine, producing approximately 1,500 milliliters of urine each day. The more water consumed, the more urine produced. The opposite is also true. The less water an individual consumes, the less urine is produced. High water losses, for example via sweat, also reduce urine output.

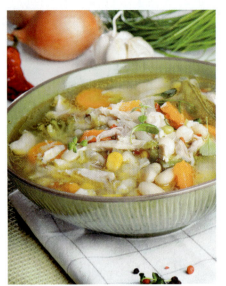

Food and beverages are a source of water for the body.

metabolic water Water that is formed in the body as a result of metabolic reactions. Condensation reactions are an example of a chemical reaction that results in the production of water.

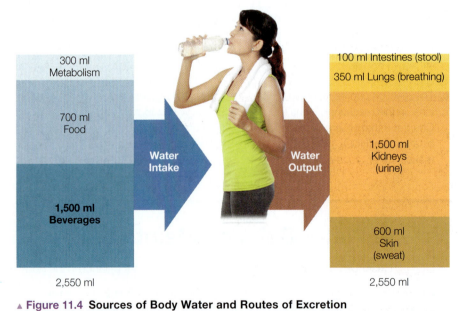

▲ **Figure 11.4 Sources of Body Water and Routes of Excretion**
Most of the body's water comes from foods and beverages and a small amount is generated during metabolism. Water is lost from the body through urine, stool, sweat, and exhaled breath. The amount of water consumed and generated is balanced with the amount excreted each day.

About 100 milliliters of water is also lost through intestinal fluids in the stool. This amount can vary depending on the dietary intake of plant fibers and whether an individual is experiencing diarrhea or vomiting. Excess water loss through diarrhea and vomiting can amount to as much as 1,500–5,000 milliliters and can result in dehydration. (We discuss dehydration in detail later in the chapter.)

Water that evaporates during exhalation and water lost through the skin as the body releases heat constitute **insensible water loss**, which takes place throughout the day, generally without being noticed. Exhaled air, which contains small water droplets, releases about 200–400 milliliters of water per day. This amount increases in an arid climate and with the heavier breathing that occurs during physical activity.

Insensible water loss doesn't include the water lost in sweat. The amount of water lost during sweating varies greatly and depends on many environmental factors, such as the temperature, humidity, wind, sun's intensity, clothing worn, and amount of physical activity. If you jump rope in the noontime sun on a summer day wearing a heavy coat, you could lose almost 2,000–3,000 milliliters of water per hour as sweat.[4] In contrast, you would lose only about 50 milliliters of water per hour as sweat if you sat under a shady tree on a dry, cool day wearing a light tee shirt and slacks.

Body Water Is Balanced between Fluid Compartments

Two-thirds of the body's fluids are located within cells; this is called **intracellular fluid (ICF)**. The remaining one-third is located outside the cells and is called **extracellular fluid (ECF)**. This balance of body water between compartments is critical for optimal health of the cell. Each fluid contains specific components. ICF contains high levels of potassium and phosphate and low levels of sodium and chloride. ECF has high levels of sodium and chloride and low levels of potassium and phosphate. Both compartments have varying levels of calcium and magnesium, proteins, bicarbonate, and other substances.

There are two types of ECF: intravascular fluid and interstitial fluid. **Intravascular fluid** is the fluid portion of blood—called *plasma*—and lymph and circulates throughout the body. **Interstitial fluid** bathes the outside of cells, but does not circulate throughout the body. It makes up about 75 percent of the ECF and acts as an area of exchange between the blood and the cells (**Figure 11.5**).

Electrolytes Participate in Fluid Balance

The fluids in the ECF and ICF are not static—they move between compartments easily. Water flows passively across cell membranes based on the concentration of dissolved minerals inside or outside the cell. A change in the concentration of these minerals on either side of the cell membrane will cause a shift in water flow from a low concentration to a high concentration.

The minerals that participate in fluid balance are known as **electrolytes** (*electro* = electricity, *lytes* = soluble) because, in solution, they exist as charged ions capable of conducting an electrical current. Ions with a positive charge are classified as **cations**, whereas negatively charged ions are called **anions**. Sodium (Na^+) and chloride (Cl^-) are the main electrolytes in the ECF, while potassium (K^+) and phosphate (HPO_4^{-2}) are the major electrolytes in the ICF. Electrolytes help maintain water balance between compartments by "pulling" water into and out of blood and cells, a process referred to as **osmosis**.

Osmosis

Shifts in fluid from the ICF to the ECF are solely due to osmosis (*osmos* = pushing). *Solutes*—dissolved substances such as electrolytes, glucose, and proteins—attract water. Cell membranes are **selectively permeable**, which means they allow some substances,

insensible water loss Loss of body water that goes unnoticed, such as by exhalation during breathing and the evaporation of water through the skin.

intracellular fluid (ICF) Fluid found in the cytoplasm within cells.

extracellular fluid (ECF) Water found outside the cell, including the intravascular fluid and the interstitial fluid.

intravascular fluid Fluid found inside the blood and lymphatic vessels.

interstitial fluid Tissue fluid; the fluid that surrounds cells.

electrolytes Ions such as sodium, potassium, chloride, and calcium that are able to conduct electrical current when they are dissolved in body water.

cations Positively charged ions.

anions Negatively charged ions.

osmosis Diffusion of water or any solvent across a semipermeable membrane from an area of lower solute concentration to an area of higher solute concentration.

selectively permeable Characteristic of cell membranes that allows some substances to cross more easily than others.

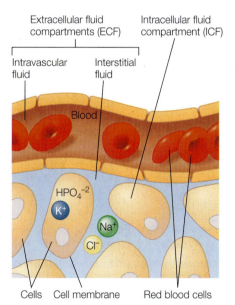

▲ **Figure 11.5 Intracellular and Extracellular Fluid Compartments** Water is a key component of the fluid both inside (intracellular) and outside (extracellular) of cells. Potassium (K^+) is the major electrolyte found in the ICF and sodium (Na^+) is the major electrolyte located in the ECF.

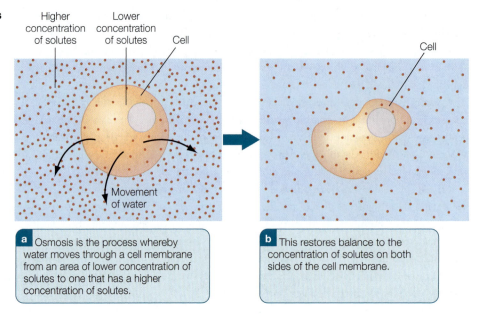

Higher concentration of solutes   Lower concentration of solutes   Cell

Cell

Movement of water

a Osmosis is the process whereby water moves through a cell membrane from an area of lower concentration of solutes to one that has a higher concentration of solutes.

b This restores balance to the concentration of solutes on both sides of the cell membrane.

such as water, to pass freely while most solutes are restricted. Water diffuses by osmosis through cell membranes, moving from a dilute or lower concentration of solutes on one side of the membrane to a higher concentration of solutes on the other side of the membrane. That is, the **osmolality**, or concentration of solutes in a solution, controls the directional flow of water. The difference between the osmolality on each side of the permeable membrane is called the **osmotic gradient**. As the osmolality on one side of the membrane increases, the osmotic gradient increases, and water is drawn across the membrane to the solutes (**Figure 11.6**).

The pressure exerted by the flow of water toward either side of a semipermeable membrane is known as the **osmotic pressure**. An increase in osmotic pressure prevents water from flowing away from the concentrated side of the membrane until balance has been restored between the fluid compartments. For example, heavy sweating during work or exercise outdoors results in a greater loss of water than electrolytes from the blood plasma (sweat is 75 percent water), which increases the osmolality of the ECF and creates an osmotic gradient relative to the ICF. As the osmolality increases in the ECF, water is drawn from the ICF into the ECF, which increases the osmotic pressure in the ECF until balance is achieved. The opposite is also true. If you drink a large amount of water quickly, that increased water in the ECF dilutes the concentration of the solutes there as compared with the solute concentration in the ICF. The reduced osmotic pressure in the ECF allows the flow of water from the ECF into the ICF. If the concentration of solutes to water is similar on either side of the membrane, water reaches equilibrium (see Figure 11.6).

Notice that osmosis affects the movement between compartments of water only, not of the electrolytes themselves. Electrolytes are moved between the two fluid compartments by the mechanism referred to as the sodium-potassium pump.

osmolality Measurement of the concentration of solutes per kilogram of solvent in a solution.

osmotic gradient Difference in concentration between two solutions on either side of the cell membrane.

osmotic pressure Pressure that prevents the solutes in a solution from drawing water across a semipermeable membrane.

sodium-potassium pump Protein located in the cell membrane that actively transports sodium ions out of the cell and potassium ions into the cell.

The Sodium-Potassium Pump

Although the minerals sodium, potassium, phosphate, magnesium, calcium, and chloride all function as electrolytes in the body, sodium has the greatest effect on fluid balance. Sodium and potassium influence fluid balance through the action of the **sodium-potassium pump**, which is the mechanism that maintains the normal electrolyte concentrations within the cell (**Figure 11.7**). Recall from Chapter 3 that the absorption of nutrients against a concentration gradient requires a carrier molecule and ATP for active transport. The sodium-potassium pump is a prime example of an active transport system in which an enzyme called Na^+-$K^+ATPase$ acts as the carrier molecule to "pump" sodium ions out of, and potassium ions into, the ICF.

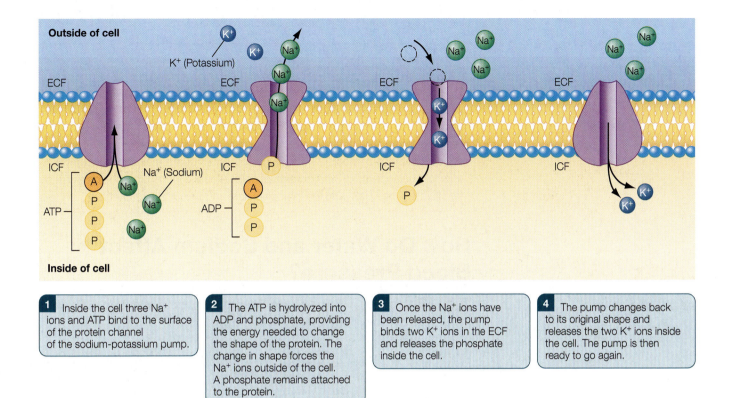

Outside of cell

ECF

K⁺ (Potassium)

Na⁺ (Sodium)

ATP

ADP

ICF

P

Inside of cell

1	Inside the cell three Na⁺ ions and ATP bind to the surface of the protein channel of the sodium-potassium pump.
2	The ATP is hydrolyzed into ADP and phosphate, providing the energy needed to change the shape of the protein. The change in shape forces the Na⁺ ions outside of the cell. A phosphate remains attached to the protein.
3	Once the Na⁺ ions have been released, the pump binds two K⁺ ions in the ECF and releases the phosphate inside the cell.
4	The pump changes back to its original shape and releases the two K⁺ ions inside the cell. The pump is then ready to go again.

▲ Figure 11.7 **The Sodium-Potassium Pump**
The sodium-potassium pump is a protein in the cell membrane that transports sodium ions out of a cell while moving potassium ions inside the cell. This active transport of Na⁺ and K⁺ ions requires energy. For every three sodium ions pumped out of the cell, two potassium ions are transported into the cell.

Sodium is normally more concentrated in the ECF than the ICF, and sodium tends to leak into the cell, whereas potassium leaks out of the cell. As sodium enters the ICF, water diffuses across the cell membrane to follow the sodium ions. As water moves into the cell, the cell swells, and osmotic pressure increases. Healthy cells do not burst, however, because the sodium-potassium pump transports three sodium (Na^+) ions out of the cell and exchanges them for two potassium (K^+) ions that move inside the cell. In other words, both Na^+ and K^+ ions are moving against their concentration gradients. The pump causes a net loss of intracellular ions, which creates an electrical and chemical gradient that drives water out of the cell and reduces the swelling.

The sodium-potassium pump is found in every cell, but plays an especially important role in electrical conduction in nerve and muscle cells, its ion transport changing the electrical charge that causes the nerve to transmit a signal or the muscle to contract. The sodium-potassium pump is also the driving force behind the absorption of as much as 2 liters of consumed fluid each day, plus the water secreted into the GI tract in gastric juices. It also drives the absorption of other nutrients, including glucose and amino acids. For example, as sodium ions move back inside the cell and across the cell membrane, they *drag* glucose along with them by binding to the same carrier protein. This allows glucose to move from a lower concentration in the ECF to a higher concentration in the ICF. The sodium is then pumped back out of the cell to begin again.

Proteins Help Regulate Fluid Balance

Proteins play a major role in keeping water dispersed evenly between the interstitial and the intravascular fluid compartments (refer to Chapter 6). This is especially true for the protein albumin. As the concentration of albumin rises in the blood, water is drawn out of the interstitial fluid into the blood plasma by osmosis. If your diet is severely low in protein, the blood levels of albumin drop, causing an accumulation of water in the interstitial spaces and swelling of the body tissues. Adequate protein intake is essential to fluid balance.

> **LO 11.2: THE TAKE-HOME MESSAGE** When the amount of water consumed in foods and beverages, and produced as metabolic water, is equal to the amount excreted through urine, stool, skin, sweat, and water vapor, the body is in water balance. Two-thirds of body water is in the ICF and one-third in the ECF. Water moves from an area of higher solute concentration to an area of lower solute concentration by osmosis. The sodium-potassium pump maintains electrolyte and fluid balance inside and outside of cells. Albumin in the blood helps maintain fluid balance between the interstitial fluid and the intravascular fluid.

How Do Water and Sodium Affect Blood Pressure?

LO 11.3 Describe the roles of water, sodium, hormones, and enzymes in the development of hypertension.

If the body retains too much fluid, blood volume—and therefore blood pressure—is likely to rise. The kidneys play a key role in regulating blood volume, as well as electrolyte balance, through tightly controlled hormonal signals. Three hormones, including antidiuretic hormone (also called *vasopressin*), angiotensin, and aldosterone, plus an enzyme called *renin*, together orchestrate the retention and excretion of water and electrolytes based on blood volume (**Figure 11.8**).

ADH Helps Stimulate Fluid Intake and Reduce Urine Output

When blood volume drops, the hypothalamus detects a decrease in blood pressure and an increase in the concentration of electrolytes (osmolality). This stimulates the thirst mechanism and fluid intake. At the same time you begin to feel thirsty, the hypothalamus stimulates the pituitary gland to release **antidiuretic hormone (ADH)**. ADH travels through the blood to the kidneys and stimulates the reabsorption of water, which reduces urine production. Together, the intake of water and the reduced urine output restore blood volume and return osmolality to normal levels.

Renin Helps the Body Reabsorb Water and Salts

The enzyme **renin**, secreted by the kidneys, is released when blood pressure falls or plasma sodium concentration decreases. This enzyme splits off a protein called *angiotensin I* from a precursor protein called *angiotensinogen* that is produced by the liver and found in the blood. As the blood flows into the lungs, angiotensin I is swiftly converted into **angiotensin II**, which has both short-term and long-term effects on blood pressure.

Angiotensin II is a powerful *vasoconstrictor* (*vaso* = vessel, *constrictor* = tightening) that narrows the blood vessels and raises blood pressure. This short-term reaction can prevent severe blood loss from hemorrhage or after an injury.

The long-term blood pressure control of angiotensin II relates to its action on the kidneys. First, it directly stimulates the kidneys to reabsorb water and electrolytes to increase blood volume and blood pressure. Second, angiotensin II stimulates the adrenal glands to release aldosterone. These long-term effects take hours or days to affect blood pressure.

Aldosterone Stimulates Sodium Reabsorption

The renin-angiotensin system adapts to changes in dietary sodium intake. If you consume very little sodium, osmolality drops in the ECF. Fluid automatically shifts from the

antidiuretic hormone (ADH) Pituitary hormone secreted in response to low blood volume; acts to reduce renal excretion of water, constrict blood vessels, and raise blood pressure; also known as *vasopressin*.

renin Enzyme secreted by the kidneys that increases blood volume, vasoconstriction, and blood pressure.

angiotensin II Blood protein that causes vasoconstriction and triggers the release of aldosterone from the adrenal glands, which raises blood pressure.

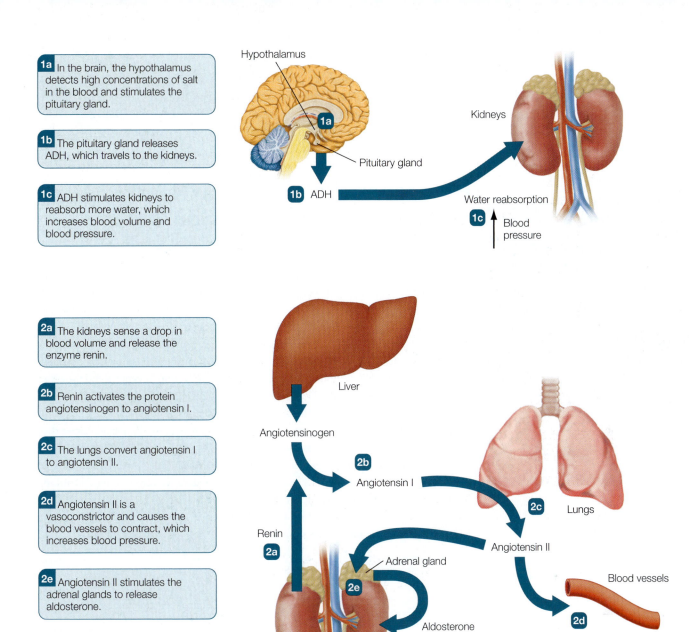

1a In the brain, the hypothalamus detects high concentrations of salt in the blood and stimulates the pituitary gland.

1b The pituitary gland releases ADH, which travels to the kidneys.

1c ADH stimulates kidneys to reabsorb more water, which increases blood volume and blood pressure.

2a The kidneys sense a drop in blood volume and release the enzyme renin.

2b Renin activates the protein angiotensinogen to angiotensin I.

2c The lungs convert angiotensin I to angiotensin II.

2d Angiotensin II is a vasoconstrictor and causes the blood vessels to contract, which increases blood pressure.

2e Angiotensin II stimulates the adrenal glands to release aldosterone.

2f Aldosterone signals the kidneys to reabsorb more sodium, which increases blood volume and blood pressure.

Hypothalamus

1a

Pituitary gland

1b ADH

Kidneys

Water reabsorption

1c Blood pressure

Liver

Angiotensinogen

2b

Angiotensin I

Renin

2a

2e Adrenal gland

Kidneys

Aldosterone

Sodium reabsorption

2f Blood pressure

Lungs

2c

Angiotensin II

Blood vessels

2d

▲ **Figure 11.8 Blood Volume Regulates Blood Pressure**
Blood volume and blood pressure are regulated by three hormones: antidiuretic hormone (ADH) secreted from the pituitary gland (1a–1c); angiotensin activated in the blood by renin (2a–2d); and aldosterone released from the adrenal glands (2e–2f).

plasma to the interstitial fluid, causing a decrease in blood volume and blood pressure. Under these circumstances, angiotensin II would trigger the adrenal glands to release **aldosterone**, which signals the kidney to retain more sodium; this indirectly leads to water being retained. The opposite would be true if you consumed a very large amount of sodium: The renin-angiotensin system would cause the kidneys to excrete the excess.

The mechanisms involved in controlling blood pressure are directly related to blood volume and sodium concentrations in the ECF. This explains the need for controlling dietary sodium and remaining hydrated, especially for individuals with high blood pressure. Any factors that interfere with these control mechanisms can lead to chronic high blood pressure, or hypertension.

aldosterone Hormone secreted from the adrenal glands in response to reduced blood volume; signals the kidneys to reabsorb sodium, which increases blood volume and blood pressure.

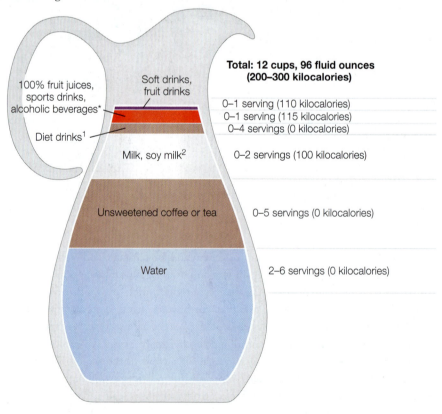

LO 11.3: The Take-Home Message In response to changes in blood volume and osmolality, the body takes action to maintain homeostasis and return blood pressure to normal. The hormones antidiuretic hormone and aldosterone direct the kidneys to reabsorb water and sodium. The enzyme renin increases sodium retention, and angiotensin II is a vasoconstrictor. These control mechanisms adjust to changes in dietary sodium and fluid intake to prevent hypertension.

How Much Water Do You Need and What Are the Best Sources?

LO 11.4 Identify the Dietary Reference Intake for water.

Your daily water requirements may be different from those of your grandparents, parents, siblings, and even the classmate sitting next to you. The amount of water a person needs depends on physical activity, diet, and environmental factors such as air temperature and humidity.

The current Adequate Intake (AI) for water is based on the reported total water intake (from both beverages and food) of healthy Americans.[5] Currently, healthy female adults consume the equivalent of 12 cups of water daily, whereas men consume the equivalent of 16 cups of water daily. About 80 percent of this intake is from beverages and the other 20 percent comes from foods. Therefore, adult women should drink about 9 cups (~80 percent of 12 cups) and adult males approximately 13 cups (~80 percent of 16 cups) of beverages daily. People who are very active have higher water requirements because they lose more water by sweating. These beverage guidelines are illustrated in **Figure 11.9**.

If that sounds like a lot, keep in mind that a well-balanced, 2,200–kilocalorie diet that includes beverages at all meals and snacks provides about 12 cups of water.[6] Drinking bottled or tap water, milk, and juices throughout the day can help meet the body's needs. Are there benefits to drinking bottled water? What about enhanced waters? See the Examining the Evidence box for some answers.

Physically active people and other individuals who lose a lot of water through sweating have higher water requirements.

Total: 12 cups, 96 fluid ounces (200–300 kilocalories)

100% fruit juices, sports drinks, alcoholic beverages*

Soft drinks, fruit drinks

Diet drinks[1]

0–1 serving (110 kilocalories)
0–1 serving (115 kilocalories)
0–4 servings (0 kilocalories)

Milk, soy milk[2] — 0–2 servings (100 kilocalories)

Unsweetened coffee or tea — 0–5 servings (0 kilocalories)

Water — 2–6 servings (0 kilocalories)

▶ **Figure 11.9 Daily Beverage Recommendations**
The acceptable beverage patterns for an adult female on a 2,200-kilocalorie daily intake.
Source: B. M. Popkin, L. E. Armstrong, G. M. Bray, B. Caballero, B. Frei, and W. C. Willett. 2006. A New Proposed Guidance System for Beverage Consumption in the United States. *American Journal of Clinical Nutrition* 83:529–542.

[1] Includes diet soft drinks and tea or coffee with sugar substitutes.
[2] Includes fat-free or 1% milk and unsweetened fortified soy milk.
* 0–2 servings of alcohol are okay for men.

Is Bottled Water—Plain or Enhanced—Healthier than Tap?

Bottled water has recently overtaken carbonated soft drinks as the number-one beverage sold in the United States. Americans drank an average of 39.3 gallons of bottled water in 2016 compared to 38.5 gallons of soft drinks.[1] Environmental concerns about lead contamination of tap water and the growing evidence of the contribution of sugary beverages to obesity and tooth decay appear to be responsible for the shift to bottled water.[2] If you buy bottled water—plain or enhanced—you're certainly not alone. But is it really healthier than tap water?

The EPA Regulates the Quality of Tap Water

Tap water in the United States is clean and safe. Most Americans obtain their drinking water from a community water system. The source of this municipal water can be underground wells or springs, rivers, lakes, or reservoirs. Regardless of the source, all municipal water is sent to a treatment plant where dirt and debris are filtered out, bacteria are killed, and other contaminants are removed. Hundreds of billions of dollars have been invested in these treatment systems to ensure that public water is safe to drink.[3] The Environmental Protection Agency (EPA) sets national standards for drinking water quality that establish limits for more than 80 contaminants. Each year, community water suppliers must provide an annual report about the quality and source of tap water. Many of these regional reports can be accessed online at *www.epa.gov*.

Tap water is not only safe but also provides minerals. You may have heard the terms "hard" or "soft" water used to describe tap water. The "hardness" refers to the amount of minerals—specifically, calcium and magnesium—in the water. The more minerals in the water, the harder the water. There aren't any health concerns from drinking hard water. In fact, there may be a benefit, as hard water may contribute small amounts of these minerals to your daily diet. About two-thirds of Americans who drink from community water systems are also getting the trace mineral fluoride in their water.[4] Fluoridation of water has been shown to reduce the incidence of dental caries by strengthening tooth enamel.[5] Many bottled waters are not fluoridated, so relying on bottled water as a primary water source can shortchange your dental health.[6]

The FDA Regulates the Quality of Bottled Water

The U.S. Food and Drug Administration (FDA) regulates bottled water that is sold through interstate commerce. Manufacturers must adhere to specific FDA standards of identity. In other words, if the label on the bottle states that it contains "spring water," the manufacturer must derive the water from a very specific source (see Table 1). Interestingly, some

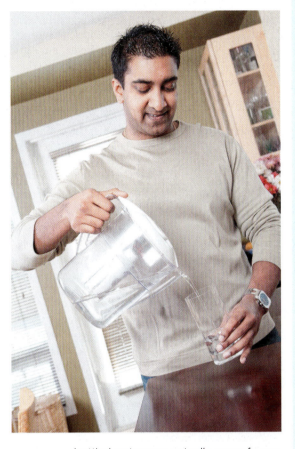

bottled water may actually come from a municipal water source!

Bottled water must also adhere to FDA standards of quality, which specify the maximum amount of contaminants that can be in the water for it still to be considered safe for consumption. The FDA bases its standards for bottled water on the EPA's standards for public drinking water.[7] Although many people drink bottled water in the belief that it is "pure," drinking 100 percent *pure* water is unlikely. Only sterile water is entirely free from impurities. However, these impurities do not make the water unsafe for most individuals to drink. (Note that individuals with a weakened immune system, such as those with HIV/AIDS, undergoing chemotherapy, and/or taking steroids, should speak with their health care provider about water consumption. These individuals may need to take precautions such as boiling their water—no matter the source—before consuming it.[8])

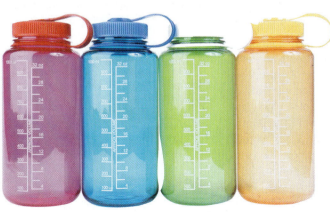

TABLE 1   Sources of Bottled Water

Bottled water is labeled according to its source or how it is treated prior to bottling.

Mineral water	Water that is derived from an underground source that contains a specific amount of naturally occurring minerals and trace elements. These minerals and elements cannot be added to the water after it has been bottled.
Spring water	Water that is obtained from underground water that flows naturally to the surface. The water is collected at the spring or at the site of a well purposefully drilled to obtain this water.
Sparkling water	Spring water that has carbon dioxide gas added before it is bottled. Also called seltzer water or club soda. *Note:* This is technically considered a soft drink, not a bottled water. Sparkling water does not have to adhere to FDA regulations for bottled water.
Distilled water	Water that has been boiled and processed to remove most, but not all, contaminants.
Flavored water	Water that has a flavor such as lemon or lime added. It may also contain added sugars and kilocalories.
Enhanced water	Water that has micronutrients, caffeine, herbs, or other additives. Such water may also contain added sugars and kilocalories.

Source: Do You Know Where Your Bottled Water Comes From? *Consumer Reports* (2015).

The Benefits of Enhanced Waters Are Not Clear

Sales of plain bottled water seem to be losing ground to sales of enhanced waters, which often advertise health benefits beyond hydration. The name "enhanced water" generally refers to any type of bottled water that has added ingredients to improve its taste and increase its nutrient content. These beverages, which are sold under brand names such as VitaminWater, Aquafina Alive, and others, are typically fortified with vitamins, minerals, fiber, caffeine, herbs, protein, and sometimes even oxygen. Some contain as many kilocalories as a soft drink, or as much as 13 teaspoons of sugar. Some claim to boost energy—because they contain caffeine—whereas others claim to relax nerves, improve mental acuity, or elevate mood.

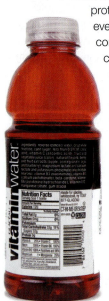

Do enhanced waters provide any health benefits? One recent review study suggests that the answer is no. Most of the waters reviewed had two to four nutrients added per product, with vitamins B_6, B_{12}, C, and niacin most commonly added in *excess* of daily requirements.[9] Results from another study suggest that the use of multivitamin supplements, which includes vitamins found in enhanced waters, increases total mortality risk.[10] These results raise concerns. Although some studies have suggested benefits for consuming enhanced waters, the bottom line is that the benefits claimed for these products are not clear. Adding vitamins to a sugary drink does not make it a healthy choice.[11]

Bottled Waters Have Financial and Environmental Costs

Tap water costs less than a penny a gallon, making it a very affordable way to stay hydrated. Moreover, a generic multivitamin-mineral pill costs approximately 10 cents a day for 100 percent or more of 13 vitamins and minerals.

In contrast, the price of bottled water can be hefty, ranging from $1 to $4 a gallon. Some enhanced waters can cost as much as $3.00 for a single 20-ounce bottle. An individual who spends $1.50 per bottle of water and buys one bottle daily would spend more than $10 per week and more than $40 per month buying bottled water. Over the course of an academic school year, that amounts to almost $400 for a beverage that you can get for free from a water fountain. But bottled water has significant hidden costs as well—to the environment.

Almost 30 billion plastic bottles are sold each year in the United States, but only two out of every 10 of these bottles are recycled[12]; the rest end up in landfills. Not only that, researchers estimate that the energy equivalent of more than 17 million barrels of oil are used to produce the plastic water bottles Americans use each year—enough energy to fuel a million cars for a year.[13]

Although refilling and reusing the bottles from bottled water may seem like an environmentally friendly and cost-effective idea, the practice is not advised. The plastic containers cannot withstand repeated washing and the plastic can actually break down, causing chemicals to leach into the water. Sturdier water bottles that are designed for reuse must be thoroughly cleaned with hot soapy water after each use to kill germs.

The bottom line? Tap water, plain bottled water, and enhanced water can all be safe to drink. Nonetheless, tap water won't strain your budget and is the best choice for the environment.

References

1. CBS News. 2017. Bottled Water Sales Outpace Soda for the First Time in U.S. Available at www.cbsnews.com. Accessed March 2017.
2. Ibid.
3. U. S. Environmental Protection Agency. 2017. Basic Information About Your Drinking Water. Available at www.epa.gov. Accessed April 2017.
4. ThoughtCo. 2017. How Safe Is Tap Water? Available at https://www.thoughtco.com. Accessed March 2017.
5. Shetty, S., M. N. Hedge, et al. 2014. Enamel Remineralization Assessment After Treatment with Three Different Remineralizing Agents Using Surface Microhardness: An In Vitro Study. *Journal of Conservative Dentistry* 17(1):49–52.
6. Marieb, E. N., and K. Hoehn. *Human Anatomy and Physiology*. 10th ed. (San Francisco: Pearson/Benjamin Cummings, 2016).
7. U. S. Environmental Protection Agency. 2017. *Drinking Water Contaminants: Standards and Regulations*. Available at http://water.epa.gov. Accessed March 2017.

8. Center for Disease Control and Prevention. 2016. *FDA Regulates the Safety of Bottled Water Beverages Including Flavored Water and Nutrient-Added Water Beverages.* Available at https://www.cdc.gov. Accessed March 2017.

9. Dachner, N., R. Mendelson, et al. 2015. Examination of the Nutrient Content and On-package Marketing of Novel Beverages. *Applied Physiology, Nutrition, and Metabolism* 40(2):191–198.

10. Elia, M., C. Normand, et al. 2016. A Systematic Review of the Cost and Cost Effectiveness of Using Standard Oral Nutritional Supplements in the Hospital Setting. *Clinical Nutrition* 33(2):370–380. doi:10.1016/j.clnu.2015.05.010.

11. Harvard School of Public Health. 2012. Enhanced Water "Unequivocally Harmful to Health," Says HSPH Nutrition Expert. Available at www.hsph.harvard.edu. Accessed March 2017.

12. Earth 911.com. 2016. How to Recycle Plastic Jugs. Available at http://earth911.com. Accessed March 2017.

13. International Bottled Water Association. 2017. Types of Water—Municipal. Available at www.bottledwater.org/types/tap-water. Accessed March 2017.

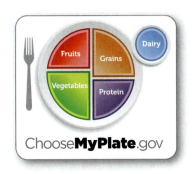

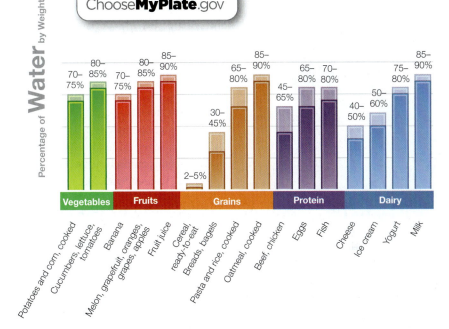

▲ Figure 11.10 **Water Content of Foods**

Source: A. Grandjean and S. Campbell, *Hydration: Fluids for Life* (Washington, DC: ILSI Press, 2004). Available at www.ilsi.org.

Most foods can also contribute to daily water needs (**Figure 11.10**). Fruits and vegetables, such as watermelon, grapes, and lettuce, which can be more than 70 percent water by weight, rank as the best food sources of water. Even grain products, like bagels and bread, provide some water. For more ideas, see the nearby Table Tips.

LO 11.4: The Take-Home Message Daily water needs vary according to an individual's physical activity level, environment, and diet. Adult women should consume about 12 cups of water (9 cups from beverages; 3 cups from foods) daily, whereas adult men should consume about 16 cups (13 cups from beverages; 3 cups from foods) daily. Those who are very active need more water to avoid dehydration.

TABLE TIPS

Bottoms Up

Drink low-fat or skim milk with each meal to help meet both calcium and fluid needs.

Freeze grapes for a juicy and refreshing snack.

Add a vegetable soup to lunch for a fluid-packed meal.

Spoon slightly thawed frozen strawberries onto low-fat vanilla ice cream for a cool sweet treat. Look for packaged berries in the frozen food section of the supermarket.

Add a slice of fresh lemon or lime to a glass of water to make it even more refreshing.

Do Diuretics Like Caffeine and Alcohol Affect Fluid Balance?

LO 11.5 Explain the effects of diuretics, such as caffeine and alcohol, on fluid balance.

Alcoholic beverages, regular coffee, and tea contribute significantly to total water intake, but alcohol and caffeine are also considered **diuretics**, and contribute to water loss. Overconsumption of some of these substances can upset fluid balance.

Caffeine Does Not Cause Significant Loss of Body Water

Caffeine is a mild diuretic that blocks the action of ADH in the kidneys. However, researchers have not found that this mild diuretic actually results in dehydration. In fact, caffeine doesn't cause a significant loss of body water over the course of a day compared with noncaffeinated beverages. Individuals who routinely consume caffeinated beverages actually develop a tolerance for their diuretic effect and experience less water loss over time.[7] Although caffeine may have other detrimental effects on the body, such as jitteriness and insomnia, moderate intakes of caffeinated beverages don't appear to have a significant negative effect on hydration.

Alcohol Can Be Dehydrating

Like caffeine, alcohol interferes with water balance by inhibiting ADH. This effect can induce urination as quickly as 20 minutes after alcohol is consumed. However, unlike caffeine, alcohol can be dehydrating. The water lost affects the concentrations of electrolytes in the body, especially potassium, which affects metabolism. This may at least partly explain the thirst, lightheadedness, and dry mouth that are often part of a hangover. Older drinkers appear to overcome this suppression of ADH faster and resist dehydration better than do younger drinkers. Reducing the amount of alcohol consumed and drinking water after an alcoholic beverage can help prevent dehydration. (For more on alcohol, see Chapter 7.)

Diuretic Medications Can Help Treat Hypertension

Pharmaceutical diuretics are often prescribed as a first line of treatment for hypertension. These drugs promote diuresis (increased excretion of urine) by inhibiting the reabsorption of sodium. As you've already learned, if the kidney excretes more sodium, water loss also increases. This action reduces blood volume, which lowers blood pressure.

Some types of diuretics also increase potassium loss. This is because the increase in sodium loss from the ECF into the urine stimulates aldosterone and the sodium-potassium pump, which increases sodium reabsorption in exchange for potassium. This potassium loss raises the risk of **hypokalemia**. A small drop in potassium levels usually doesn't cause symptoms, but moderate potassium loss can cause lower blood pressure, muscle weakness and cramps, and constipation. Doctors closely monitor patients taking diuretics to prevent electrolyte imbalances. Patients are encouraged to eat potassium-rich foods such as bananas, peanut butter, and tomatoes. In some cases, potassium supplements or potassium-sparing diuretics may be prescribed.

LO 11.5: THE TAKE-HOME MESSAGE Both caffeine and alcohol reduce the activity of ADH, but moderate caffeine intake does not appear to cause dehydration. Alcohol affects metabolism in a way that can lead to dehydration. Pharmaceutical diuretics are prescribed to treat hypertension but may cause electrolyte imbalances.

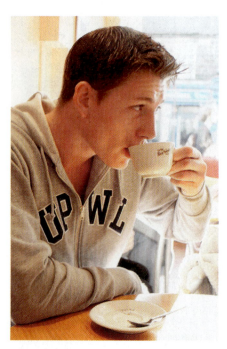

A cup of coffee gives you a "pick me up" without causing dehydration.

diuretics Substances that increase the production of urine; often used as antihypertensive drugs.

hypokalemia Dangerously low level of blood potassium.

What Are the Effects of Too Much or Too Little Water?

LO 11.6 Differentiate between dehydration and water intoxication, and describe the signs and symptoms of each.

Although water is an essential nutrient, it can be harmful if consumed in excess. And, just as with other nutrients, consuming too little can be dangerous as well.

Consuming Too Much Water Can Cause Hyponatremia

Water intoxication is rare because healthy individuals who consume a balanced diet simply produce more urine to eliminate excess water. However, drinking fluids too quickly without adequate sodium replacement—especially during strenuous exercise—dilutes sodium in the ECF (see **Focus Figure 11.11**, middle panel). As the electrolyte concentration inside the cells rises above the concentration in the ECF, water flows by osmosis into the cells, which swell with the excess fluid. Excessive dilution or depletion of blood sodium is known as **hyponatremia** (*hypo* = under, *natrium* = sodium, *emia* = blood). It can also be caused by heart failure, kidney disease, diarrhea, and other disorders.

In 2015, a 30-year-old British triathlete collapsed at the finish line of the Ironman European Championship in Frankfort, Germany, and died a few days later. The cause of death was hyponatremia. The athlete had consumed too much plain water and insufficient salt during the race. Such deaths don't only occur among endurance athletes. In 2014, an American high school football player died after collapsing on the field during practice.

The cause of death for both of these individuals was swelling in the brain. Again,

when too much water enters the ICF, the cells swell to the point of bursting. If such swelling occurs in brain cells, it may be fatal. Treatment includes restriction of water intake and administration of a saline (salt) solution to restore appropriate electrolyte levels in the ECF.

Symptoms of water intoxication include fatigue, confusion, and disorientation.[8] Mistakenly treating these symptoms by consuming more fluids only makes matters worse. Anyone who is sweating heavily during physical activity lasting 1 hour or more is advised to consume a sports beverage with added Na^+ instead of plain water to replenish both fluid and electrolytes.[9] A recent meta-analysis on hydration during exercise found that drinking enough to satisfy thirst resulted in a 90 percent performance advantage compared to drinking below thirst and a 63 percent performance advantage over drinking more than your thirst required.[10]

Consuming Too Little Water Can Cause Dehydration

While overhydration can have dire effects on the body, **dehydration**, a depletion of body fluids, occurs much more frequently and can be just as harmful. Dehydration can result from inadequate fluid consumption, strenuous exercise in the heat, or losing excessive amounts of water as a result of diarrhea, vomiting, high fever, or the use of diuretics. As little as a 2 percent loss of body water can trigger a loss

of short-term and long-term memory, lower attention span and cognition, fatigue, and reduced ability to maintain core temperature.

For some populations, such as children, older adults, and athletes, the consequences of dehydration can be severe. In older adults, for example, dehydration has been misdiagnosed as dementia.[11] Even a 1–2 percent loss of body water can impair an athlete's cardiovascular and thermoregulatory response and reduce the athlete's capacity for exercise. See **Table 11.1** for common signs and symptoms of dehydration. Apply what you've learned about fluid balance in the nearby Nutrition in Practice.

The Thirst Mechanism Signals Dehydration

Have you ever been outside for a while on a hot day and noticed that your mouth was as dry as the Sahara Desert? The dry mouth is part of your **thirst mechanism**, which is controlled by a cluster of cells,

water intoxication Potentially dangerous medical condition that results from drinking too much water too quickly, also known as *hyperhydration*; can lead to hyponatremia and possible death.

hyponatremia Dangerously low level of sodium in the blood that can result from dilution or depletion of sodium.

dehydration Excessive loss of body fluids; usually caused by inadequate fluid intake, diarrhea, vomiting, or excessive sweating.

thirst mechanism Complex interaction between the brain and the hypothalamus triggered by a depletion of body water; the interaction leads to a feeling of thirst.

TABLE 11.1 Signs and Symptoms of Dehydration		
Mild Dehydration	**Moderate Dehydration**	**Severe Dehydration**
Dry lips and mouth	Thirst	All signs of moderate dehydration
Thirst	Very dry mouth	Rapid and weak pulse
Inside of mouth slightly dry	Sunken eyes	Cold hands and feet
Low urine output; concentrated urine appears dark yellow	Sunken fontanelles (the soft spots on an infant's head)	Rapid breathing
	Tenting (skin doesn't bounce back readily when pinched and lifted slightly)	Blue lips
		Lethargic, comatose

Head to Mastering Nutrition and watch a narrated video tour of this figure by author Joan Salge Blake.

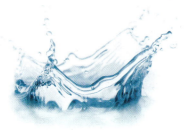

The health of our body's cells depends on maintaining the proper balance of fluids and electrolytes on both sides of the cell membrane, both at rest and during exercise. Let's examine how this balance can be altered under various conditions of exercise and fluid intake.

MODERATE EXERCISE

When you are appropriately hydrated, engaged in moderate exercise, and not too hot, the concentration of electrolytes is likely to be the same on both sides of cell membranes. You will be in fluid balance.

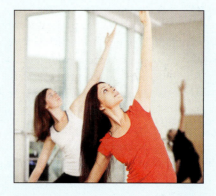

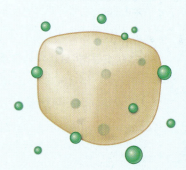

Concentration of electrolytes about equal inside and outside cell

STRENUOUS EXERCISE WITH RAPID AND HIGH WATER INTAKE

If a person drinks a great deal of water quickly during intense, prolonged exercise, the extracellular fluid becomes diluted. This results in the concentration of electrolytes being greater inside the cells, which causes water to enter the cells, making them swell. Drinking moderate amounts of water or sports drinks more slowly will replace lost fluids and restore fluid balance.

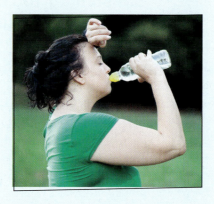

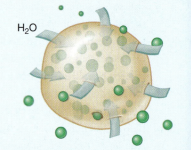

Lower concentration of electrolytes outside

H_2O

Higher concentration of electrolytes inside

STRENUOUS EXERCISE WITH INADEQUATE FLUID INTAKE

If a person does not consume adequate amounts of fluid during strenuous exercise of long duration, the concentration of electrolytes becomes greater outside the cells, drawing water away from the inside of the cells and making them shrink. Consuming sports drinks will replace lost fluids and electrolytes.

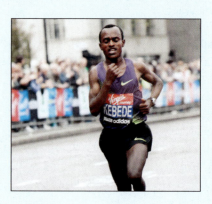

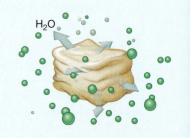

Higher concentration of electrolytes outside

H_2O

Lower concentration of electrolytes inside

NUTRITION *in* PRACTICE:
Athletic Trainer

College freshman Jim is a running back on his university's football team. He was excited to be recruited to one of the best Division 1 teams in the South on a full scholarship. Jim arrived at his school in steamy August, two weeks before classes started, in order to begin training with the team. He was to participate in all-day outdoor practices in temperatures over 90 degrees Fahrenheit.

Jim was sick the entire weekend before the first day of practice, vomiting from a "stomach bug." Being a freshman and eager to impress the coach, Jim did not want to miss the first day of football practice. Fearing that if he ate or drank anything he would get sick on the field, Jim skipped breakfast. After several hours of running drills in the hot sun, he started to feel dizzy and nauseated. Muscle cramps prevented him from completing the required drills at the level that he was able to do in a typical practice. In between plays, a team member standing next to Jim on the sideline noticed he was sweating profusely and called over the athletic trainer. The athletic trainer (AT) took one look at Jim and diagnosed heat illness. He removed him from practice, then questioned Jim on what he had eaten and drunk previous to the practice and throughout the practice. Jim explained that his weekend illness had prevented him from eating or drinking anything that day. He removed him from practice, then recommended that Jim consult with a registered dietitian nutritionist (RDN) to develop a balanced meal plan that provides adequate fluid and kilocalories.

Jim's Stats:
- Age: 18
- Height: 6 feet 0 inches
- Weight: 210 pounds (typically)
- Weight: 204 pounds (Monday morning weigh in)
- BMI: 28.5 (typically)
- BMI: 27.7 (Monday morning weigh in)

Critical Thinking Questions
1. Why was Jim at risk for dehydration during Monday's practice?

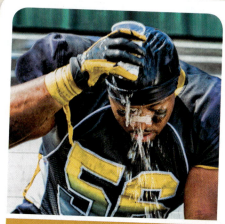

Jim

JIM'S FOOD LOG

Food/Beverage	Time Consumed	Hunger Rating*	Location
Nothing	6 AM	1	Dorm room
Nothing, feeling nauseated	7:30 AM	1	On the practice field
Nothing, feeling tired	11 AM	1	On the practice field

* Hunger Rating (1–5): 1 = not hungry; 5 = super hungry.

2. What are three physical changes brought about by dehydration that Jim might have experienced?
3. How could his dehydration have been prevented?

AT's Observation and Plan for Jim:
- ❏ Monitor body weight before and after practice or an event. Consume 8 fluid ounces for each pound of body weight lost.
- ❏ To replace fluid lost during exercise, especially in the heat, athletes can meet their fluid requirements by drinking during each hour 625 to 1250 mL (average about 250 mL every 15 min).

RDN's Observation and Plan for Jim:
- ❏ Add sufficient amounts of fluids in addition to water and sports drinks to increase his fluid consumption, including other beverages, soups, dairy, whole fruits and vegetables.
- ❏ Avoid drinking concentrated sugar-containing beverages. They can slow the gastric emptying rate, which can upset fluid balance during exercise and heat stress. Choose a beverage that contains 4 to 8 percent carbohydrates, such as Gatorade or Exceed.

The next day Jim met with the RDN to discuss his weight, diet, and fluid intake. The RDN recommended including foods that contain other fluids including soups, dairy, other beverages, and fresh fruits and vegetables. Both the AT and the RDN advised Jim that he needs to drink 8 ounces of fluid for every pound of weight he has lost. Since he lost 6 pounds, he will need to drink an additional 48 ounces of fluid. The RDN also reminded Jim not to skip meals before or after practice. Finally, the AT suggested Jim invest in a large reusable water bottle, to be sure he is drinking adequate amounts of fluids throughout the day. One week later, Jim feels much better during the all-day practices. He has been eating before and after practice and drinking enough fluids to avoid dehydration.

collectively called the *thirst center*, in the hypothalamus. Activation of the thirst center results in the urge to drink, and thereby plays an important role in preventing further dehydration and restoring water balance in the body. **Figure 11.12** illustrates the factors that prompt the thirst mechanism and the reactions that follow.

Dehydration Depletes ECF and ICF

When you are dehydrated, water is depleted from the ECF and the ICF, but not necessarily in equal proportions. Initially, water loss is from the ECF, which becomes more concentrated in electrolytes. This increase in osmolality activates osmoreceptors in the hypothalamic thirst center and prompts the sensation of thirst.

The dry mouth that makes you feel thirsty can also be explained by an increased ECF osmolality. As the concentration of blood electrolytes increases, less water is available to your salivary glands to make saliva, making your mouth feel dry. This state also contributes to activation of the hypothalamic thirst center.

When fluid is lost from the ECF, reduced blood volume (called **hypovolemia**; *hypo* = reduced, *vol* = volume, *emia* = blood) can occur. Less circulating blood reduces blood pressure, and signals the hypothalamic thirst center to stimulate thirst and fluid intake. The hypothalamus also triggers the pituitary gland to release ADH (see Figure 11.8). Both actions help bring blood volume back to normal. If thirst is ignored and fluid is not replaced, hypovolemia and hypotension can reduce cardiac output and may cause fainting.

In addition, as solute concentration in the ECF increases, water is drawn from the ICF, causing the cells to *shrink* (see Focus Figure 11.11, bottom panel). In response, the hypothalamus triggers the

hypovolemia Low blood volume.

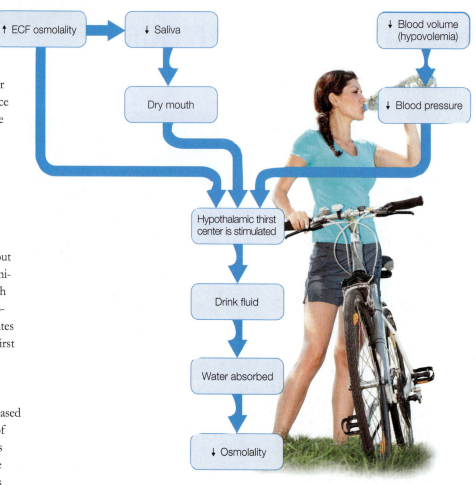

▲ **Figure 11.12 The Thirst Mechanism**
The thirst mechanism is stimulated when solutes in the blood become more concentrated; saliva production decreases and the mouth dries; or blood volume significantly drops. The thirst center in the hypothalamus stimulates a sensation of thirst, which in turn stimulates water consumption and returns the blood osmolality to normal.

renin-angiotensin system (see Figure 11.8) and stimulates thirst and an appetite for salt. Antidiuretic hormone is also triggered, reducing the amount of water excreted through the skin, lungs, and kidneys. These adaptations are important to preserve blood volume, but they do not return fluid levels to normal. Fluids must be consumed to restore blood volume and adequate hydration of body cells.

For healthy, moderately active individuals eating a balanced diet, fluids from beverages and foods throughout the day will prevent dehydration.[12] However, older adults and individuals who are very physically active, such as athletes and laborers,

are at risk of dehydration if they don't take in enough fluid, or they lose body water copiously through sweating. These individuals need to take additional steps to ensure that they are properly hydrated.

Monitor Water Intake to Avoid Overhydration and Dehydration

One way to monitor hydration is the cornerstone method, which involves measuring body weight before and after long bouts of vigorous physical activity or labor and noting changes. If a person weighs less after an activity than before, the weight change is due to loss of body water, and that water must be replenished. The American College of Sports Medicine generally recommends that for every pound of weight lost in water, 20–25 fluid ounces (about 2.5–4 cups) of water should be consumed.[13] Alternatively, if a weight gain is noted, overhydration is likely; that is, the athlete drank too much fluid during the game or practice. Less fluid should be consumed before the next activity.

Urine color can also be used to assess hydration. Individuals who are dehydrated produce less urine—one of the effects of the release of ADH. The urine that is produced is more concentrated, as it contains a higher proportion of solutes to the smaller volume of water. This causes the urine to be darker in color.[14] The National Athletic Trainers Association has created a chart to help individuals assess if they are drinking enough fluids to offset the amount of water lost through sweating (see **Figure 11.13**).[15] Individuals who are very physically active and who notice that the color of their urine darkens during the day, to the point where it resembles the shade of a yield sign or darker, likely need to increase their fluid intake. (*Note:* Other factors, such as consuming excessive amounts of the B vitamin riboflavin, and certain medications, can also affect the color of urine.)

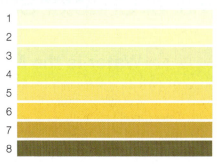

▲ **Figure 11.13 Urine Color Guide**
Clear or light yellow urine indicates adequate hydration. Dark urine (color 7 or darker) indicates dehydration and the need to consume more fluids.

LO 11.6: The Take-Home Message

Excess water ingestion can result in water intoxication. Dehydration occurs when water consumed is less than water lost. The thirst mechanism is stimulated by increased ECF osmolality, dry mouth, and hypovolemia. Monitor your weight loss to ensure proper hydration during exercise. For every pound of weight lost during exercise, drink at least two and a half cups of water to rehydrate. Clear or light-colored urine signals hydration.

Visual Chapter Summary

LO 11.1 Water Is the Most Abundant Nutrient in the Body

Water (H_2O) is the most abundant substance in the body and makes up about 45–75 percent of body weight. A polar molecule, water makes an excellent solvent. It is a key component of all body fluids, including blood, lymph, and the fluid inside and around cells. Water contributes to digestive juices; transports oxygen, nutrients, and hormones to the cells; and transports waste products to be excreted in urine and stool. Water helps maintain body temperature, acts as a lubricant, moistens food through the action of saliva, and bathes organs, including the brain. Water is essential for most chemical reactions in the body.

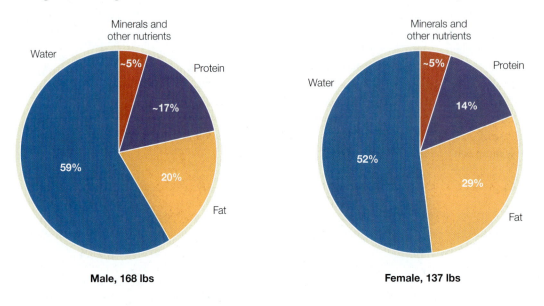

Male, 168 lbs   Female, 137 lbs

LO 11.2 Water Balance Is Maintained through Ingestion and Excretion and between Fluid Compartments

Water balance is achieved when the amount of water consumed and produced by the body via food, beverages, and metabolism equals the amount excreted through the kidneys, skin, lungs, and feces. The majority of water intake comes from beverages (about 1,500 milliliters) and food (700 milliliters). Metabolic water produces about 300 milliliters per day. Water is lost through the urine (1,500 milliliters), the lungs as water vapor (350 milliliters), the feces (100 milliliters), and sweat (600 milliliters).

Two-thirds of body water is contained in the intracellular fluid found inside the cell and one-third in the extracellular fluid compartments. These include interstitial fluid, found immediately outside and between the cells, and intravascular fluid, found in blood and lymph. Osmosis and the sodium-potassium pump influence water balance between the ICF and the ECF. Blood levels of the protein albumin help maintain fluid balance between the blood and interstitial fluid.

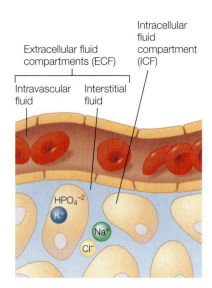

LO 11.3 Water, Sodium, and Hormones Affect Blood Pressure

The kidneys, hypothalamus, pituitary gland, lungs, adrenal glands, and liver all play a role in maintaining blood volume. The hypothalamus detects a drop in blood volume and signals the pituitary gland to release ADH, which increases the absorption of water through the kidneys. The kidneys also respond to the reduction in blood volume by releasing the enzyme renin to convert a liver protein to angiotensin. This protein stimulates the adrenal gland to release the hormone aldosterone, which stimulates the kidneys to reabsorb sodium. The result is a return of blood volume and blood pressure to normal.

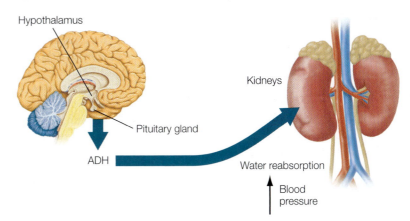

The mechanisms involved in blood pressure regulation directly relate to the sodium concentrations in the ECF. Low intakes of sodium cause decreased ECF osmolality, which stimulates the renin-angiotensin system. If sodium intake is high, the renin-angiotensin system is reduced and more sodium is excreted. Any factors that alter this control mechanism can result in chronic hypertension.

LO 11.4 Daily Water Recommendations Are Based on Water Balance

The Adequate Intake (AI) for water is based on the reported total water intake (from both beverages and food) of healthy Americans. Women should drink about 9 cups (~80 percent of 12 total cups) of water and other beverages daily and men approximately 13 cups (~80 percent of 16 total cups). People who are very active and sweat a lot have higher water requirements. All foods contain some water. Cooked hot cereals and fruits and vegetables are robust sources of water.

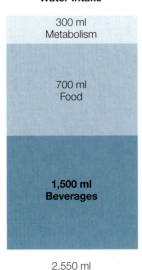
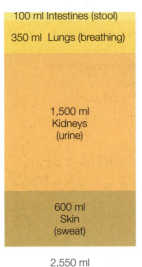

Water Intake

300 ml Metabolism

700 ml Food

1,500 ml Beverages

2,550 ml

Water Output

100 ml Intestines (stool)

350 ml Lungs (breathing)

1,500 ml Kidneys (urine)

600 ml Skin (sweat)

2,550 ml

LO 11.5 Diuretics Can Cause Dehydration

Caffeinated beverages such as coffee, tea, and soft drinks contribute to daily water needs. Caffeine is a mild diuretic but doesn't cause a significant loss of body water. Individuals who routinely consume caffeine develop a tolerance to its diuretic effect and experience less water loss over time. Alcohol is also a diuretic. It interferes with water balance by inhibiting ADH and can cause dehydration.

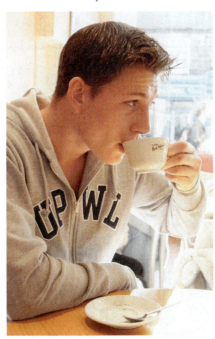

LO 11.6 Consuming Too Much or Too Little Water Can Be Dangerous

Consuming too much water too quickly can result in water intoxication, which in turn leads to an excessive dilution of blood sodium levels known as hyponatremia. This condition can cause fatigue, muscle weakness, confusion, convulsions, and even death.

Dehydration occurs when there is an insufficient amount of water in the body due to reduced fluid intake or to excessive loss due to diarrhea, vomiting, high fever, or the use of diuretics. Dehydration can trigger memory loss, fatigue, reduced ability to maintain core temperature, and other health problems.

Thirst is often the first sign of dehydration. When water is lost from the body, increased blood osmolality, dry mouth, and hypovolemia trigger the thirst mechanism, which is governed by the thirst center in the hypothalamus. The thirst mechanism stimulates fluid consumption. Urine color can be used to monitor hydration.

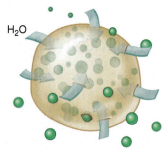

Lower concentration of electrolytes outside

Higher concentration of electrolytes inside

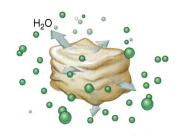

Higher concentration of electrolytes outside

Lower concentration of electrolytes inside

Terms to Know

- solvent
- specific heat
- acid–base balance
- water balance
- metabolic water
- insensible water loss
- intracellular fluid (ICF)
- extracellular fluid (ECF)
- intravascular fluid
- interstitial fluid
- electrolytes
- cations
- anions
- osmosis
- selectively permeable
- osmolality
- osmotic gradient
- osmotic pressure
- sodium-potassium pump
- antidiuretic hormone (ADH)
- renin
- angiotensin II
- aldosterone
- diuretics
- hypokalemia
- water intoxication
- hyponatremia
- dehydration
- thirst mechanism
- hypovolemia

Mastering Nutrition

Visit the Study Area in Mastering Nutrition to hear an MP3 chapter summary.

Check Your Understanding

LO 11.1 1. Which of the following is a function that water performs in the body?
   a. Provides energy to the muscles
   b. Helps transport waste products for excretion
   c. Acts as an antioxidant
   d. Participates in the synthesis of proteins

LO 11.2 2. Under normal conditions, which of the following contributes most significantly to loss of body water?
   a. Exhaled water vapor
   b. Fecal matter
   c. Urine
   d. Sweat

LO 11.2 3. The fluid in the blood is an example of
   a. intracellular fluid.
   b. extracellular fluid.
   c. interstitial fluid.
   d. both b and c.

LO 11.3 4. The sodium-potassium pump functions to pump
   a. sodium ions out of the cell and potassium ions into the cell.
   b. sodium ions into the cell and potassium ions out of the cell.
   c. sodium and potassium ions into the cell.
   d. sodium and potassium ions in both directions in and out of the cell.

LO 11.3 5. The hormone that signals the kidneys to reabsorb sodium is called
   a. antidiuretic hormone.
   b. aldosterone.
   c. angiotensin II.
   d. renin.

LO 11.4 6. Which of the following foods has the highest percentage of water content?
  a. Beef
  b. Cucumber
  c. Ice cream
  d. Bagels

LO 11.4 7. On average, how many cups of water does a well-balanced 2,200-kilocalorie diet provide?
  a. 8 cups
  b. 10 cups
  c. 12 cups
  d. 16 cups

LO 11.5 8. The consumption of pharmaceutical diuretics increases the risk of
  a. increased sodium reabsorption.
  b. increased calcium reabsorption.
  c. loss of potassium.
  d. loss of magnesium.

LO 11.6 9. The hypothalamic thirst center is stimulated by
  a. hypertension.
  b. decreased blood albumin.
  c. consumption of dry foods such as nuts and crackers.
  d. increased ECF osmolality.

LO 11.6 10. Consuming too much ___ can cause hyponatremia.
  a. salt
  b. water
  c. alcohol
  d. potassium

Answers

1. (b) Water picks up waste products from cells and transports them to the kidneys to be excreted in the urine. Water participates in chemical reactions that provide energy but does not provide energy itself, nor does it act as an antioxidant or help synthesize proteins.

2. (c) The majority of fluid lost is through the kidneys, which produce approximately 1,500 milliliters of urine each day. Exhaled air and lung vapor excrete about 200 to 400 milliliters of water per day, and about 100 milliliters of water is lost through intestinal fluids in the stool. The amount of water lost through the skin as sweat varies depending on environmental temperatures and physical activity.

3. (b) Extracellular fluid is the fluid outside cells. It includes the blood plasma (the intravascular fluid) and interstitial fluid, found in tissue spaces between the cells. Intracellular fluid is located inside the cells.

4. (a) The sodium-potassium pump moves sodium ions out of the cell and potassium ions into the cell. This helps the body maintain fluid and electrolyte balance.

5. (b) The hormone aldosterone signals the kidneys to reabsorb sodium, increasing blood volume. Antidiuretic hormone signals the kidneys to reabsorb water. Angiotensin II is a vasoconstrictor and renin is an enzyme.

6. (b) Most vegetables and fruits can be more than 70 percent water by weight. Cucumbers contain 80–85 percent water by weight. Even grain products such as bagels contain some water. Beef contains less than 65 percent water.

7. (c) A normal mixed diet of 2,200 kilocalories that includes both beverages and foods generally contains about 12 cups of water.

8. (c) Using pharmaceutical diuretics increases the risk of excreting excessive potassium through the urine. This can lead to hypokalemia (abnormally low blood potassium).

9. (d) The hypothalamic thirst center is stimulated by increased ECF osmolality. Hypotension—not hypertension—also triggers the thirst mechanism. Decreased blood albumin, which is likely to occur with malnutrition, promotes excessive interstitial fluid, but does not trigger the thirst center. Food intake does not stimulate the thirst center.

10. (b) Consuming too much water can result in excessive dilution of blood sodium, which is referred to as hyponatremia.

Answers to True or False?

1. **False.** You may be able to survive weeks without food but you can't live for more than a few days without water.

2. **True.** Your morning cup of java does contribute to daily water needs, even though it may contain caffeine, a diuretic.

3. **True.** Depending on age, gender, and body composition, a minimum of eight glasses of water or other fluids per day may be necessary to maintain a healthy level of body water. The recommended intake for adult women is 9 cups per day and for men 13 cups per day.

4. **False.** Water does transport waste products for excretion from the body, but drinking large amounts will not increase that function and may cause overhydration and hyponatremia, which is a dangerous condition.

5. **False.** Water participates in energy metabolism but does not directly contribute to weight loss.

6. **True.** It is easy to become dehydrated during exercise because of excess sweating, especially in warm, humid environments. Drinking adequate fluid before, during, and after a workout is key to maintaining hydration.

7. **False.** Sodium is an essential nutrient and should never be eliminated from the diet. A balanced diet and adequate fluid intake prevent fluid retention.

8. **True.** Potassium-rich foods such as bananas can play a role in reducing hypertension. Potassium works together with sodium to regulate fluid balance and reduce blood pressure.

9. **True.** Alcohol is a diuretic and excess consumption can cause dehydration.

10. **False.** Enhanced waters such as vitamin waters typically contain additional kilocalories. To maintain hydration, plain water is just as healthy and much cheaper.

Web Resources

■ For more information on high blood pressure, visit Your Guide to Lowering High Blood Pressure at www.nhlbi.nih.gov

■ For more information on current research related to hydration during exercise, visit the Gatorade Sports Science Institute at www.gssiweb.com

■ For more information on FDA regulations and bottled water, visit www.fda.gov

References

1. Dunford, M., and J. A. Doyle. 2014. *Nutrition for Sport and Exercise*. 3rd ed. Belmont, CA: Wadsworth/Cengage Learning.
2. Marieb, E. N., and K. Hoehn. 2016. *Human Anatomy and Physiology*. 10th ed. San Francisco: Pearson/Benjamin Cummings.
3. McArdle, W. D., F. I. Katch, et al. 2016. *Sports and Exercise Nutrition*. 5th ed. Baltimore: Lippincott Williams & Wilkins.
4. Ibid.
5. Maughan, R. J., P. Watson, and S. Shirreffs. 2015. Implications of Active Lifestyles and Environmental Factors for Water Needs and Consequences of Failure to Meet Those Needs. *Nutriton Reviews* 73(Suppl. 2): 130–140.
6. Institute of Medicine. 2004. *Dietary Reference Intakes: Water, Potassium, Sodium, Chloride, and Sulfate*. Washington, DC: National Academies Press.
7. Killer, S. C., A. K. Blannin, et al. 2014. No Evidence of Dehydration with Moderate Daily Coffee Intake: A Counterbalanced Cross-Over Study in a Free-Living Population. *PLoS One* 9(1):e84154. doi: 10.1371/journal.pone.0084154.
8. Thompson, D. 2016. Water: Can It Be Too Much of a Good Thing? Available at www.webmd.com. Accessed March 2017.
9. Quinn, E. 2016. ACSM Clarifies Hydration Recommendations for Athletes. Available at

https://www.verywell.com/acsm-clarifies-hydration-recommendations-for-athletes-3119234. Accessed April 2017.

10. Goulet, E. D. 2012. Effect of Exercise-Induced Dehydration on Endurance Performance: Evaluating the Impact of Exercise Protocols on Outcomes Using a Meta-analytic Procedure. *British Journal of Sports Medicine*. Available at http://running.competitor.com/2014/05/nutrition/the-truth-about-dehydration-and-performance_76027#BldmTRLRYSXTKTx0.99. Accessed March 2017.

11. Ibid.

12. Binder, H. J., I. Brown, et al. 2014. Oral Rehydration Therapy in the Second Decade of the Twenty-first Century. *Current Gastroenterology Reports* 16(3):376. http://doi.org/10.1007/s11894-014-0376-2.

13. Sawka, M. N., L. M. Burke, et al. 2007. American College of Sports Medicine Position Stand: Exercise and Fluid Replacement. *Medicine and Science in Sports and Exercise* 39:377–390.

14. Ibid.

15. Casa, D. J., L. E. Armstrong, et al. 2000. National Athletic Trainers Association Position Statement: Fluid Replacement for Athletes. *Journal of Athletic Training* 35:212–224.

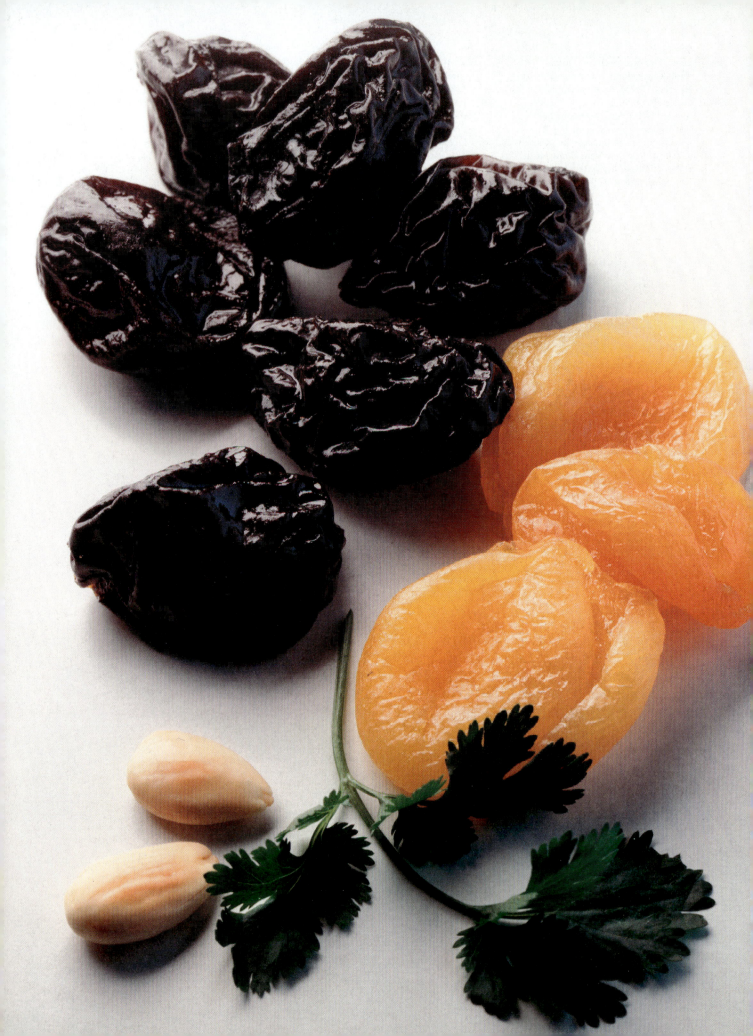

Major Minerals

Learning Outcomes

After reading this chapter, you will be able to:

12.1 Distinguish between the major and trace minerals and identify the factors that affect their bioavailability.

12.2 Describe the functions, food sources, and toxicity and deficiency effects of sodium.

12.3 Describe the functions, food sources, and toxicity and deficiency effects of chloride.

12.4 Describe the functions, food sources, and toxicity and deficiency effects of potassium.

12.5 Describe the functions, food sources, and toxicity and deficiency effects of calcium.

12.6 Describe the functions, food sources, and toxicity and deficiency effects of phosphorus.

12.7 Describe the functions, food sources, and toxicity and deficiency effects of magnesium.

12.8 Describe the functions and food sources of sulfate.

12.9 Discuss the roles of minerals in the development of healthy bone tissue and the factors that influence the risk of developing osteoporosis.

True or False?

1. The very best way to ensure an adequate intake of minerals is to take supplements. **T**/**F**

2. Minerals are simple molecules. **T**/**F**

3. For most people, hypertension is a preventable condition. **T**/**F**

4. Minerals are more bioavailable from plant-based foods than from animal-based foods. **T**/**F**

5. Eating more fruit can improve bone density. **T**/**F**

6. A diet rich in potassium can help lower blood pressure. **T**/**F**

7. Most dietary sodium comes from salt added to foods during cooking. **T**/**F**

8. A serving of milk provides almost a third of an adult's daily calcium needs. **T**/**F**

9. Sulfate is not an essential nutrient. **T**/**F**

10. Alcohol consumption in any amount increases the risk of developing osteoporosis. **T**/**F**

See page 464 for the answers.

What do a cast-iron skillet, the salt on an icy road, and the copper pipes used in plumbing all have in common? They contain one or more of the same minerals that play essential roles in the body.

In this chapter, we explore the roles that the major minerals play in fluid balance, metabolism, and bone building. We discuss the average person's daily needs for each mineral and, equally important, how to avoid consuming toxic amounts. We cover the trace minerals in Chapter 13.

What Are Minerals?

LO 12.1 Distinguish between the major and trace minerals and identify the factors that affect their bioavailability.

Like vitamins, **minerals** are essential to overall health and well-being. Although the body can synthesize small amounts of a few vitamins, the body cannot synthesize minerals. They must be consumed in the diet.

Minerals Are Inorganic Elements

Minerals do not contain carbon and are therefore classified as inorganic. Unlike vitamins, which are compounds, minerals are elements, containing only one kind of atom, such as calcium (Ca) or iron (Fe) or sodium (Na^+) (**Figure 12.1**). In nature, minerals often exist in compounds; for example, in the form of mineral salts such as sodium chloride (NaCl). When mineral salts dissolve in body water, they separate (or *dissociate*) into individually charged particles, or ions. Thus, minerals in the body are most often found as individual ions. They are also found as components of compounds such as the calcium in hydroxyapatite crystals in bone, the iron in hemoglobin, or the phosphorus in ATP.

Like all elements, minerals cannot be broken down by natural processes. Thus, unlike vitamins, they are not destroyed by heat, acid, oxygen, or ultraviolet light.[1] Most minerals are similar to water-soluble vitamins, however, in that they can leach out of foods. Minerals also remain intact during digestion and generally don't change their shape or structure when performing their biological functions. The potassium in bananas, for example, has the same structure and ionic charge as the potassium inside muscle cells.

Minerals are classified into two groups. The **major minerals,** or *macrominerals,* are *major* because humans need to consume them in amounts greater than 100 milligrams per day (daily needs for some major minerals exceed 1,000 milligrams per day), and there are at least 5 grams of the mineral in the body (**Figure 12.2**). The major minerals are sodium, chloride, potassium, phosphorus, calcium, magnesium, and sulfur.

The second group, the **trace minerals,** or *microminerals,* are needed in amounts less than 20 milligrams per day, and the body contains less than 5 grams total. Iron is an example of a trace mineral; the average adult male needs about 8 milligrams of iron per day and has a total of about 3–4 grams in his body. The other trace minerals are zinc, copper, selenium, chromium, iodide, manganese, molybdenum, and fluoride.

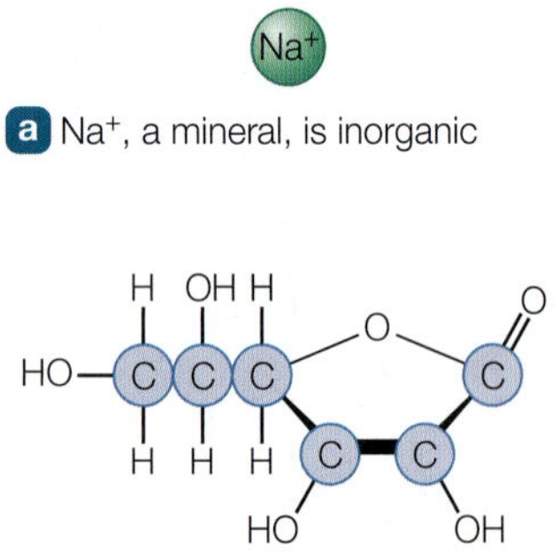

Minerals Vary in Their Bioavailability

The degree to which a nutrient is absorbed and ultimately available to be used in the body is called its *bioavailability*. The bioavailability of minerals is affected by several factors, including your nutritional status and the other contents in the GI tract. Nutritional status, or the amount of the mineral stored in the body, influences how much is absorbed. If you are deficient in a mineral, such as calcium, you absorb a greater percentage of that mineral from food. Similarly, if your body has an adequate amount of a mineral, it absorbs less of it from food. Because some minerals can be toxic in high amounts, this ability to adjust the

minerals Inorganic elements essential to the nutrition of humans.

major minerals Minerals needed in amounts greater than 100 milligrams per day. These include sodium, chloride, potassium, calcium, phosphorus, magnesium, and sulfur.

trace minerals Minerals needed in amounts less than 20 milligrams daily. These include iron, zinc, selenium, fluoride, chromium, copper, manganese, and molybdenum.

a Na^+, a mineral, is inorganic

b Vitamin C is an organic nutrient

▲ **Figure 12.1 The Structure of a Mineral versus a Vitamin**
(a) Minerals are elements. Although in nature minerals often occur in combinations such as salts, their fundamental structure consists solely of the element itself. Thus, they are inorganic: they do not "contain" any additional elements, including carbon. **(b)** Organic nutrients, including carbohydrates, proteins, lipids, and vitamins, contain carbon, hydrogen, and oxygen and sometimes nitrogen.

amount absorbed helps prevent the body from accumulating harmful amounts.

Eating a meal that contains a food high in a particular mineral does not necessarily mean the body will absorb that mineral because minerals often compete with each other for absorption in the GI tract. Some minerals, such as calcium, magnesium, iron, copper, and zinc, are absorbed in their ionic state. These minerals have the same ionic charge, so they vie for the same protein carriers during absorption. Too much of one mineral, such as calcium, Ca^{2+}, can cause a decrease in the absorption and metabolism of another mineral, such as magnesium, Mg^{2+}, leading to an imbalance.[2,3] Thus, bioavailability of each mineral depends on the amount of both minerals in the GI tract at the time of absorption.[4] This is one reason why most people should avoid taking single-mineral supplements.

The bioavailability of minerals can also be reduced if the minerals are attached to **binders** such as *oxalates* (acids found in certain fruits and vegetables, chocolate, tea, coffee, beer, and nuts) or *phytates* (acids found in nuts, whole grains, and legumes). The acid–mineral complex passes through the GI tract unabsorbed. Spinach, for example, is technically high in calcium, but the vegetable is actually a poor calcium source because its oxalates render most of the mineral unavailable for absorption. In fact, an individual absorbs only about one-tenth as much calcium from spinach as from milk.[5] In some cases, cooking a food, such as legumes that contain phytates, can help increase the bioavailability of its minerals by breaking the bonds between the minerals and the binders.[6]

Polyphenols as well as oxalates in tea and coffee also bind and inhibit the body's absorption of minerals, such as iron, reducing bioavailability.[7] Juice, milk, or water are better choices for aiding mineral absorption than are coffee or tea.

Some nutrients improve the bioavailability of minerals.[8] Vitamin C enhances the absorption of iron from plant foods. Animal protein from meat, fish, and poultry enhances zinc absorption, and vitamin D enhances calcium, phosphorus, and magnesium absorption. **Table 12.1** presents a summary of the factors that affect the bioavailability of minerals.

The body maintains a tight control over mineral balance. Recall from Chapter 11 that the GI tract and the kidneys help to closely regulate electrolyte balance. The GI tract exerts another control on mineral homeostasis: Minerals in gastric juices and in sloughed-off intestinal cells are either excreted through the feces or reabsorbed in the large intestine. Moreover, the kidneys respond to changing levels of minerals in the blood by either excreting the excess minerals through the urine or reabsorbing them back into the blood when levels are low. These controls ensure that excessive minerals are excreted, while sufficient amounts are available to perform normal muscle contraction, transmit nerve impulses, sustain heart function, and maintain healthy blood.

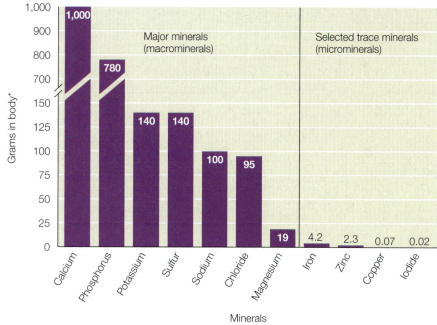

* Based on a 154-pound person

▲ **Figure 12.2 The Minerals in Your Body**
Major minerals are present in larger amounts than are trace minerals in the human body. However, all are equally important to health.

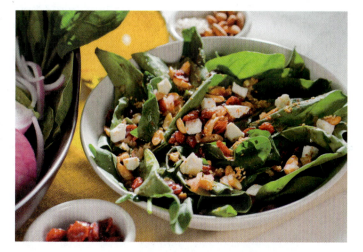

Oxalates found in spinach bind to calcium, reducing the amount of calcium the body is able to absorb.

binders Compounds such as oxalates and phytates that bind to minerals in foods and reduce their bioavailability.

TABLE 12.1 Factors That Affect the Bioavailability of Minerals	
Factors That Increase Bioavailability	**Factors That Reduce Bioavailability**
Deficiency in a mineral increases absorption	Binders, such as oxalates found in many foods
Cooking increases the bioavailability of minerals in legumes	Phytates found in nuts, whole grains, and many legumes
Vitamin C increases the absorption of some minerals such as iron	Polyphenols in tea and coffee
Vitamin D increases the absorption of calcium, phosphorus, and magnesium	Supplementation of single minerals affects absorption of competing minerals

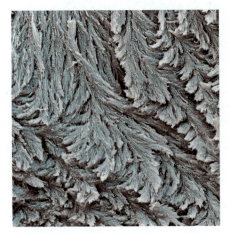

Hydroxyapatite crystals in the outer layer of bone.

cofactor Substance that binds to an enzyme to help catalyze a reaction; generally refers to a metal ion, whereas a coenzyme is usually an organic compound such as a vitamin.

hydroxyapatite Crystalline salt structure that provides strength in bones and teeth. Calcium and phosphorus are the main minerals found in the structure.

mineralization Process of adding minerals, including calcium and phosphorus, to the collagen matrix in the bone, which makes the bone strong and rigid.

Minerals Serve Numerous Functions

Minerals play roles in fluid and electrolyte balance, form blood cells (iron and copper), build healthy bones (calcium, phosphorus, magnesium, and fluoride), and maintain a healthy immune system (zinc).[9] Minerals can also be part of enzyme complexes, participate in energy metabolism, and play an invaluable role in structural growth.

Fluid and Electrolyte Balance

As discussed in Chapter 11, mineral ions are essential to balance extracellular fluid (ECF) with intracellular fluid (ICF). The sodium and chloride located mainly outside of cells, and the potassium (with the help of calcium, phosphorus, magnesium, and sulfur) located mainly inside cells, all play key roles in maintaining fluid balance. Without these electrolytes, cells could swell and burst from taking in too much fluid or shrink from dehydration.

A balance of electrolytes is also essential for transmission of nerve impulses and contraction of muscles. Electrolyte imbalances can lead to confusion, seizures, muscle spasms, and convulsions.

Cofactors in Enzyme Systems

Minerals are similar to many vitamins in that they can act as **cofactors** in important enzyme systems. Mineral cofactors may be loosely or tightly bound to an enzyme, and once a reaction is complete, the mineral is released. For example, the mineral selenium acts as a cofactor for the complex antioxidant enzyme system glutathione peroxidase. This system reduces free-radical formation and repairs the damage already done by free radicals. Without the mineral selenium, glutathione peroxidase would be unable to convert free radicals to less harmful substances. The resulting oxidative stress could lead to cardiovascular disease and cancer. Energy metabolism also requires minerals as cofactors.

Mineralization of Bones and Teeth

The major minerals calcium, phosphorus, and magnesium, along with the trace mineral fluoride, make up the crystalline structure that gives strength to bones and teeth. In fact, **hydroxyapatite** crystals make up about 60 percent of bone mass. The hydroxyapatite minerals attach to the protein collagen in the process of **mineralization.** Inadequate buildup of hydroxyapatite crystals during bone formation, or too much withdrawal of the minerals during adulthood, leads to weakened and brittle bones.

Minerals Can Be Toxic

Like some fat-soluble vitamins, minerals can be toxic if ingested in high amounts. However, mineral toxicity from an excess dietary intake is rare in healthy individuals because the amounts found in foods is not that high, and most Americans do not generally exceed the UL for minerals. Also, as just discussed, the body can adapt its absorption or excretion of many minerals according to its needs.

However, ingesting more than the UL of a mineral, such as by taking large amounts of supplements, may lead to illness and even death. Excessive levels of magnesium in the blood can result in heart problems or an inability to breathe, while excessive amounts of calcium may cause nausea and vomiting, loss of appetite, constipation, increased urination, kidney toxicity, confusion, and irregular heart rhythm.[10] Although mineral toxicity is more likely to occur in individuals with certain conditions, such as kidney failure, even healthy people ingesting excessive amounts of minerals may experience unwanted side effects.

Though minerals have much in common with each other and work together to support numerous body functions, they are each important for individual reasons, and we explore these in greater detail. In the following pages, we discuss the metabolic functions, daily needs, food sources, and toxicity and deficiency symptoms for each of the major minerals. An overview of each of these major minerals is presented in **Table 12.2.**

TABLE 12.2	Metabolic Function, Daily Needs, Food Sources, and Symptoms of Toxicity and Deficiency of the Major Minerals				
Major Mineral	**Metabolic Function**	**Daily Needs (19 years +)**	**Food Sources**	**Toxicity Symptoms**	**Deficiency Symptoms**
Sodium (Na^+)	▪ Major cation outside the cell ▪ Regulates body water and blood pressure	1,500 mg/day	Processed foods, seaweed, table salt	▪ Edema ▪ Hypertension UL: 2,300 mg/day	▪ Headache ▪ Nausea and vomiting ▪ Fatigue ▪ Disorientation
Chloride (Cl^-)	▪ Major anion outside the cell ▪ Part of HCl ▪ Participates in acid–base balance	2,300 mg/day	Processed foods, seaweed, table salt, and rye	▪ Vomiting UL: 3,600 mg/day	▪ Rare that symptoms occur unless related to loss of sodium
Potassium (K^+)	▪ Major cation inside the cell ▪ Regulates body water and blood pressure	4,700 mg/day	Unprocessed foods, fruits and vegetables, meat, dairy, and nuts	▪ Irregular heartbeat and heart damage UL: None established	▪ Muscle weakness and cramps ▪ Glucose intolerance ▪ Irregular heartbeat and paralysis
Calcium (Ca^{+2})	▪ Formation of bones and teeth ▪ Muscle contraction and relaxation ▪ Blood clotting ▪ Heart and nerve function	1,000 mg/day	Milk and dairy products, leafy greens, broccoli, salmon, sardines, legumes, calcium-fortified soymilk and juices	▪ Constipation ▪ Impaired kidneys ▪ Calcium deposits in tissues UL: 2,500 mg/day	▪ Bone loss (osteoporosis) ▪ Bone fractures
Phosphorus (PO_4^{-3})	▪ Formation of bones and teeth ▪ Part of DNA, RNA, coenzymes, and the ATP energy molecule ▪ Transport of lipids ▪ Acid–base balance	700 mg/day	Meat, fish, poultry, eggs, cereals	▪ Decrease in bone mass ▪ Calcium deposits in tissues UL: 4,000 mg/day	▪ Muscle weakness ▪ Bone pain
Magnesium (Mg^{+2})	▪ Participates as a cofactor in many biochemical reactions including muscle contraction and nerve conduction	Women: 310 mg/day Men: 400 mg/day	Green leafy vegetables, whole grains, nuts, legumes, dairy, and fruits	▪ Diarrhea, cramps, and nausea (from supplements, not food) UL: 350 mg/day (from supplements only; all adults)	▪ Weakness and fatigue ▪ Confusion and seizures ▪ Depression ▪ Irregular heartbeat
Sulfate (SO_4^{-2})	▪ Part of keratin found in hair and skin ▪ Formation of collagen ▪ Participates in acid–base balance and cellular respiration	None established	All protein-containing foods such as meat, fish, poultry, eggs, legumes, nuts, and dairy	▪ May promote ulcerative colitis UL: None established	▪ None known

LO 12.1: THE TAKE-HOME MESSAGE Minerals are chemical elements essential to body function. Like all elements, minerals can neither be created nor destroyed by ordinary processes. Major and trace minerals are classified based on the amount found in the body and the amount needed daily. The bioavailability of minerals varies based on nutrient status and whether the mineral is bound with other substances in food or ingested together. Minerals play a vital role in bone and blood health, fluid balance, energy metabolism, nerve impulse transmission, and muscle contraction. Mineral toxicity is rare in healthy individuals but can occur by ingesting high doses of minerals through supplementation.

EXPLORING **Sodium**

LO 12.2 Describe the functions, food sources, and toxicity and deficiency effects of sodium.

What Is Sodium?

In the body, **sodium (Na$^+$)** is a major electrolyte and cation found primarily in the blood and interstitial fluid. In the form of sodium chloride (NaCl), or table salt, sodium has been part of our diet since the earliest recorded history when it was used to preserve and flavor food. In breads, sodium serves multiple functions beyond enhancing flavor: It is added to yeast breads to prevent the yeast from overexpanding the dough. It is also used to reduce the growth of bacteria and mold in many bread products and luncheon meats. Sodium chloride accounts for about 90 percent of the sodium you consume. It is approximately 40 percent sodium; thus, 6 grams (1 teaspoon) of table salt contains approximately 2.4 grams of sodium. Sodium in other forms, such as sodium phosphate, sodium carbonate, and sodium bicarbonate (baking soda), are food additives and preservatives.

Monosodium glutamate (MSG) is a form of sodium commonly added to Asian cuisines to intensify the flavor of foods.

Absorption, Transport, and Excretion of Sodium

When you consume table salt, gastric juices from the lining of the stomach break the bonds between the sodium and chloride ions. Once the two ions dissociate, they are ready for absorption.

Most sodium (95–100 percent) is absorbed throughout the small intestine. A small amount (up to 5 percent) passes through the GI tract and is excreted in the feces. Once absorbed, sodium moves freely throughout the blood until it is filtered by the kidneys and excreted through the urine.

The kidneys maintain the amount of sodium in the blood at a precise level. To maintain sodium balance, the amount eaten must equal the amount lost. If blood sodium levels drop, the hormone angiotensin II stimulates the adrenal glands to secrete the hormone aldosterone, which in turn stimulates the kidneys to reabsorb more

sodium, returning the blood levels to normal (see Chapter 11 to review this process). Likewise, when the blood levels of sodium are too high, angiotensin II is reduced and the adrenal glands stop releasing aldosterone, allowing the kidneys to excrete the excess sodium in the urine (**Figure 12.3**). The kidneys also reabsorb sodium in exchange for H$^+$ when the pH is too acidic, thereby restoring acid–base balance.

A small amount of sodium is also lost through daily perspiration. The amount of sodium lost through the skin depends on the rate of sweating, the amount of sodium consumed (the more sodium in the diet, the higher the loss through sweat), and the intensity of heat in the environment. As you become more acclimated to environmental heat, you lose less sodium over time.

Metabolic Functions of Sodium

Sodium plays an important role in regulating fluid balance, transmission of nerve impulses, muscle contractions, and transport of nutrients.

When Sodium Levels Are Low

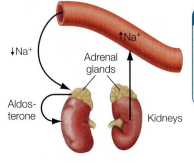

a When sodium levels in the blood are low, aldosterone is released from the adrenal glands. Aldosterone triggers the kidneys to reabsorb sodium into the blood.

When Sodium Levels Are High

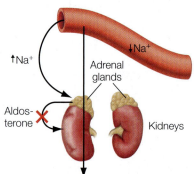

b When sodium levels in the blood are high, the adrenal glands stop secreting aldosterone, and the kidneys excrete the excess sodium through the urine. This lowers the levels of sodium in the blood.

▲ **Figure 12.3 Sodium Balance Is Maintained by the Kidneys**

sodium (Na$^+$) Major cation in the extracellular fluid.

Sodium Helps Regulate Fluid Balance

The volume of fluid in any fluid compartment is determined by the concentration of electrolytes, including sodium, that are present. Any shift in the electrolyte concentration in any fluid compartment affects the amount of fluid present.

As soon as dietary sodium is absorbed, it is quickly distributed throughout the circulation, increasing the concentration of Na^+ in the blood. This increased blood osmolality, in turn, stimulates the hypothalamic thirst center, which activates the thirst mechanism and triggers the release of ADH from the pituitary gland. The result is that you drink more water and excrete less urine, thereby diluting the sodium and restoring the balance between sodium and fluid in the blood.

Sodium Transmits Nerve Impulses and Participates in Muscle Contraction

Sodium works with potassium to help transmit all nerve impulses, including those that signal muscles to contract. Recall that sodium is a cation in higher concentration outside the cell. In response to a stimulus, such as a touch or the sound of your cell phone, the sodium-potassium pump transports ECF sodium across the nerve cell membrane. As a result, the nerve cell interior becomes more positively charged. This weak positive charge opens more sodium channels, generating a stronger positive charge that triggers a nerve impulse (called an *action potential*) that is transmitted along the length of the nerve cell. At the end of the nerve cell, the impulse may cross a gap (synapse) and continue along another nerve cell—for example, in the brain or spinal cord. Alternatively, an impulse may cross from a nerve cell to a muscle fiber (muscle cell), where it

will generate a release of calcium ions, which in turn stimulate muscle contraction.

Sodium Helps Transport Glucose and Amino Acids

As you learned in Chapter 11, sodium and potassium cross the cell membrane via the sodium-potassium pump, which moves three sodium ions out of the cell for every two potassium ions pumped into the cell. This movement of ions creates a gradient in which the electrolyte concentration is higher in the ECF than in the ICF.

In contrast, in both enterocytes and certain kidney cells, the concentration of glucose is higher in the ICF. Thus, any movement of glucose into these cells must occur against its concentration gradient. This "upstream" movement of glucose is facilitated by sodium-dependent glucose transport proteins located in the cell membrane (**Figure 12.4**). Sodium and glucose simultaneously bind to these membrane proteins, which release them into the cell interior. Sodium-dependent amino acid transporters act in a similar way to shuttle amino acids into enterocytes and kidney cells.

Daily Needs for Sodium

The daily minimum amount of sodium needed for normal body function is 180 milligrams— about enough to cover the face of a penny (less than 1/16th of a teaspoon).[11] However, planning a balanced diet with such a small amount of sodium is virtually impossible, so the DRI committee set an AI recommendation at a more realistic level: 1,500 milligrams daily (about $^3/_4$ of a teaspoon) for adults up to 51 years of age (see **Figure 12.5**).[12] This sodium recommendation, which is about eight times the minimum amount needed, is set

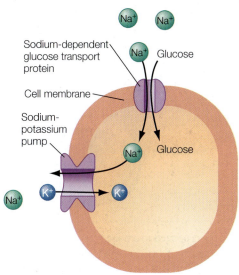

▲ **Figure 12.4 Sodium Helps Transport Glucose**

A sodium-dependent glucose transport protein in the membrane of enterocytes and certain kidney cells transports sodium (Na^+) and glucose simultaneously into the cell interior. Na^+ moves down its concentration gradient as glucose is transported up its concentration gradient. Similar sodium-dependent transport proteins shuttle amino acids. Once inside the cell, Na^+ is pumped back out of the cell in exchange for K^+ through the sodium-potassium pump.

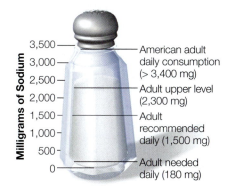

▲ **Figure 12.5 Recommended Intake of Sodium**

(continued)

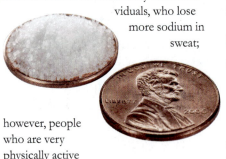

to accommodate a variety of foods from all the food groups so individuals can meet all their other nutrient needs. It also allows for increased needs of moderately active individuals, who lose more sodium in sweat; however, people who are very physically active or not acclimated to a hot environment likely need to consume a higher amount of sodium. Americans currently consume more than double the recommended amount, or over 3,400 milligrams, of sodium (about $1\frac{1}{2}$ teaspoons) daily, on average.[13]

Food Sources of Sodium

The vast majority of dietary sodium, a hefty 77 percent in American diets, comes from salt used in processed foods such as canned goods (particularly soups), cured meats, and frozen or packaged meals.[14] Comparing the amount of sodium in a fresh tomato (11 milligrams) to the amount found in a cup of canned tomatoes (355 milligrams) quickly illustrates just how much sodium is added by manufacturers during processing. Some sauces and condiments, such as soy sauce (900 milligrams/tablespoon) or ketchup (190 milligrams/tablespoon), also contribute hefty amounts of sodium.[15] Typically, as the sodium in processed foods increases, the amount of potassium—a mineral protective of cardiovascular health—decreases (see **Table 12.3**).

About 12 percent of Americans' sodium consumption is from eating foods that naturally contain sodium (see **Figure 12.6**). For example, sushi made with seaweed is naturally high in sodium (240 milligrams per serving) because of the high salt concentration in the seaweed. Another 5 percent of sodium intake is from salt that's added during cooking, and 6 percent is from salt used to season foods at the table.

Sodium Excess

Given that the body excretes excess dietary sodium, do you need to worry about eating too much? Yes. Researchers have established that there is a direct relationship between excessive sodium intake from salt (sodium chloride) and hypertension (defined in Chapter 5), particularly in individuals who are *salt sensitive* (show a rise in blood pressure after eating salt).

Certain segments of the population are more likely to be salt sensitive, including older adults, people with diabetes or chronic kidney disease, and African Americans.[16] Whereas about 35 percent of Caucasians appear to be salt sensitive, African Americans have a much higher rate of 75 percent. Overall, about 50 percent of individuals with hypertension are salt sensitive. However, in general, even if you are not salt sensitive, as a person's intake of sodium increases, so does his or her blood pressure,[17] and reducing dietary sodium may improve blood pressure.

High blood pressure increases the risk for heart disease, stroke, and kidney disease. Unfortunately, many Americans will develop hypertension sometime during their life. The Tolerable Upper Intake Level (UL) for sodium for adults is set at 2,300 milligrams, or about 1 teaspoon of table salt, in order to help reduce the risk. The current *Dietary Guidelines for Americans* also recommend that sodium intake should be limited (see Chapter 2).

Hypernatremia

Hypernatremia (*hyper* = too much, *natrium* = sodium, *emia* = blood) is excessive blood sodium. The most common reason for hypernatremia to develop is a failure to adequately replace water that is lost due to vomiting or diarrhea, which causes blood levels of Na^+ to become too concentrated. This can also occur if too much Na^+ is ingested without sufficient water intake, such as can occur among athletes using salt tablets.

As the ECF becomes **hypertonic** (too concentrated in solutes), water is drawn from the ICF via osmosis until a balance of concentrated ions to fluid is restored. This water loss from the cells can cause dehydration. The thirst mechanism will be stimulated, and the kidneys will conserve water and excrete less urine. Signs and symptoms of hypernatremia therefore include thirst, dry mouth, decreased urination, dark urine, and lightheadedness.

hypernatremia Excessive amounts of sodium in the blood.

hypertonic Having a high solute concentration.

TABLE 12.3	Sodium and Potassium Content in Whole and Processed Foods		
Whole Food	**Mineral Content**	**Processed Food**	**Mineral Content**
Baked potato, medium	10 mg Na^+; 870 mg K^+	Hash browns, one serving	746 mg Na^+; 513 mg K^+
Orange juice, 1 cup	2.5 mg Na^+; 498 mg K^+	Orange soda, 1 cup	30 mg Na^+; 5 mg K^+
Milk, 1 cup	107 mg Na^+; 366 mg K^+	Vanilla pudding, 1 cup	156 mg Na^+; 71 mg K^+
Tri-tip, 3 oz.	141 mg Na^+; 869 mg K^+	Beef jerky, 3 oz	443 mg Na^+; 119 mg K^+
Strawberries, 1 cup	1.5 mg Na^+; 233 mg K^+	Strawberry pie, 1 serving	284 mg Na^+; 118 mg K^+
Green beans, 1 cup	6.6 mg Na^+; 230 mg K^+	Green beans, canned, 1 cup	382 mg Na^+; 169 mg K^+
Oatmeal, 1 cup	3.1 mg Na^+; 166 mg K^+	Oat cereal, 1 cup	864 mg Na^+; 184 mg K^+

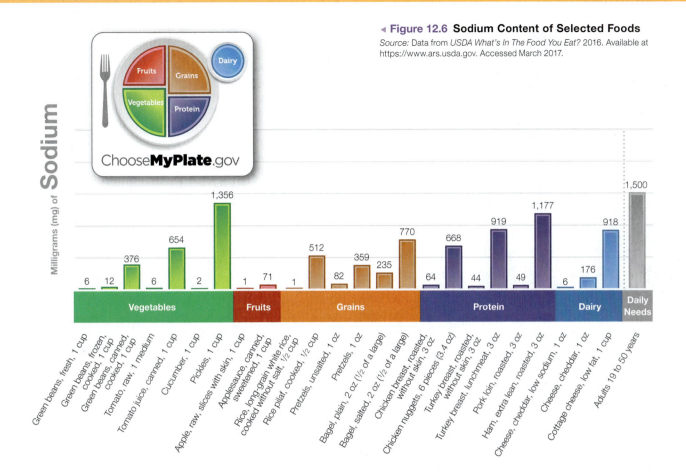

Osteoporosis and Other Disorders

Consuming too much sodium may also contribute to calcium-deficiency osteoporosis.[18,19] In both human and animal studies, research has shown that sodium in the urine correlates to reduced reabsorption of calcium by the kidneys. This lack of reabsorption leads to greater calcium loss in the urine and may contribute to bone loss, especially in postmenopausal women.[20] Consuming too much sodium can also contribute to fluid retention, weight gain, stomach ulcers, and stomach cancer.[21]

Reducing Sodium Intake

The Mediterranean diet (described in the Spotlight in Chapter 5) and the DASH (Dietary Approaches to Stop Hypertension) diet have both been shown to reduce hypertension.[22] The DASH diet is a flexible and balanced eating plan low in sodium. Both plans focus on consuming fruits, legumes and other vegetables, low-fat or nonfat dairy products, fish, lean meats, whole grains, and plant oils.

Because the majority of sodium comes from sodium chloride in processed foods and a fair amount comes from the salt that you add to your foods, cutting back on these two sources is the best way to lower dietary intake. One way to scale back sodium intake in processed foods is to read labels carefully. However, this can be a challenge if you're not well versed in label terms.

"Low sodium," for instance, means there is less than 140 milligrams of sodium per serving, while "sodium free" means the product may contain up to 5 milligrams per serving. "Reduced sodium" means only that the sodium content of the "regular" version has been reduced by 25 percent, and "light in sodium" means it has been reduced by 50 percent. A regular version of a product like soy sauce may have 1,000 milligrams of sodium in 1 tablespoon, while 1 tablespoon of light soy sauce contains 500 milligrams, or 33 percent of the AI. Note that even

though this product's sodium has been reduced, it is still considered high in sodium.

Reading nutrition labels is helpful in controlling sodium intake; however, the FDA's Daily Value for sodium is less than 2,400 milligrams of sodium per day, an amount that is higher than either the AI (1,500 milligrams) or the UL (2,300 milligrams). For example, the sodium content for a beef hot dog with a bun is approximately 1,400 milligrams, an amount that would nearly satisfy the AI for sodium for the day. If you ate two hot dogs, your sodium intake would be 2,800 milligrams, which is greater than the UL or the FDA's Daily Value.[23]

The best way to reduce sodium intake is to limit consumption of processed foods and bypass the salt shaker at the table. If you do purchase processed foods, buy only products labeled as "low sodium" or "sodium free." When cooking, season foods with a variety of herbs or other flavorings such as black pepper, Tabasco sauce, lemon juice, or a no-salt seasoning

(continued)

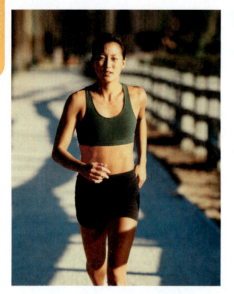

blend instead of salt. For more information on reducing your sodium intake, see the Table Tips.

Sodium Deficiency

Dietary sodium deficiency is rare in healthy individuals who consume a balanced diet.

hypotonic Having a low solute concentration.

Shake the Salt Habit

Dilute canned soups by combining a can of regular vegetable soup and a can of low-sodium vegetable soup for soup with less sodium. Add cooked, frozen vegetables for an even healthier meal.

Limit deli meats to no more than 3 ounces on your sandwich, and pile on naturally low-sodium tomatoes, lettuce, cucumbers, and shredded cabbage.

Choose low-sodium dried fruits (apricots and raisins) and unsalted walnut pieces or almonds for a sweet or crunchy snack.

Skip salty french fries and enjoy a sodium-free baked potato instead.

Use olive oil and vinegar instead of salad dressing on your salad, or choose low-sodium salad dressing.

However, individuals who consume too much water in a short amount of time, such as marathon runners or military trainees, risk diluting sodium and other electrolytes in the excessive volume of body fluid (referred to as **hypotonic**), which can result in hyponatremia. As discussed in Chapter 11, hyponatremia can be fatal. Symptoms include headache, muscle weakness, fatigue, and seizures that can eventually lead to coma and death. Too little sodium can also result when excessive amounts of the mineral are lost through the kidneys, such as with the use of diuretics.[24]

LO 12.2: THE TAKE-HOME MESSAGE
Sodium helps maintain fluid balance, transmits nerve impulses, participates in muscle contraction, and helps transport some nutrients across cell membranes. Adults need about 1,500 milligrams of sodium daily but consume more than double that amount, predominantly as sodium chloride. Processed foods are the major source of sodium in the diet. Excess sodium in the blood can cause hypertension, hypernatremia, and bone loss. Low sodium levels in the blood result in hyponatremia.

CHLORIDE

EXPLORING **Chloride**

LO 12.3 Describe the functions, food sources, and toxicity and deficiency effects of chloride.

What Is Chloride?

Chloride (Cl⁻) is an anion almost always found bonded to sodium as sodium chloride in foods. Within the body, this major electrolyte is found mostly in the blood (approximately 88 percent), with the remainder (approximately 12 percent) found in the interstitial fluid and as part of hydrochloric acid in the stomach. Chloride is the ionic form of chlorine and should not be confused with the powerful disinfectant that is toxic when inhaled or ingested.

chloride (Cl⁻) Major anion in the extracellular fluid.

When table salt is consumed (**Figure 12.7**), it dissociates in the stomach into sodium and chloride ions, which mix with the gastric juices. Chloride ions are absorbed through the small intestine. Excess chloride is excreted through the urine, although small amounts of chloride can be lost in the feces and through the skin.

Metabolic Functions of Chloride

The negative charge of Cl^- balances the positive charge of Na^+ in the ECF to maintain fluid balance. Chloride assists in the removal of CO_2 from the blood, helping maintain a normal pH range, and participates in digestion as part of hydrochloric acid (HCl).

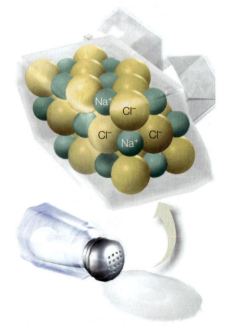

▲ **Figure 12.7 Sodium Chloride**
Sodium chloride, or table salt, is 60 percent chloride and 40 percent sodium.

Daily Needs for Chloride

The AI for chloride is set at about 2,300 milligrams a day for adults age 19–50. Americans in general consume well above this requirement. In fact, on average, Americans consume an estimated 3,400 milligrams to just over 7,000 milligrams of dietary chloride daily.[25]

Food Sources of Chloride

Table salt accounts for almost all the chloride you ingest daily. Approximately 60 percent of the weight of table salt is chloride. Thus, in 6 grams (1 teaspoon) of table salt, approximately 3.6 grams are chloride. In addition to processed foods that contain sodium chloride, chloride is found naturally in seaweed, tomatoes, olives, lettuce, celery, and rye. Chloride is also part of potassium chloride, the main ingredient in salt substitutes.

Chloride Toxicity and Deficiency

Because sodium chloride is the major source of chloride in the diet, the UL for adults for chloride is set at 3,600 milligrams to coincide with the UL for sodium.[26]

Chloride toxicity is rare and produces no symptoms. However, athletes who become extremely dehydrated from prolonged sweating may experience **hyperchloremia,** an abnormally high concentration of chloride in the blood. The best way to avoid this condition is to drink sufficient fluid and electrolytes when exercising in extreme heat.

Though chloride deficiency rarely occurs in healthy individuals, a serious bout of vomiting and/or diarrhea can cause excessive loss of chloride as part of hydrochloric acid. Some diuretics can cause an increase in chloride excretion in the urine, resulting in low chloride levels in the blood, or **hypochloremia.** The symptoms of hypochloremia include shallow breathing, muscle weakness, muscle spasms, and twitching.

LO 12.3: THE TAKE-HOME MESSAGE
Chloride helps maintain fluid balance, helps remove CO_2 from the blood, helps maintain pH balance, and participates in digestion as part of HCl in the stomach. Adults need 2,300 milligrams per day. Almost all the chloride ingested comes from sodium chloride (table salt). Hyperchloremia and hypochloremia are rare.

---

hyperchloremia Abnormally high level of chloride in the blood.

hypochloremia Abnormally low level of chloride in the blood.

EXPLORING Potassium

LO 12.4 Describe the functions, food sources, and toxicity and deficiency effects of potassium.

What Is Potassium?

Potassium (K^+) is the major cation found in the ICF. About 85 percent of consumed potassium is absorbed throughout the small intestine and colon. The kidney maintains potassium balance by excreting excess potassium through the urine and minor amounts through the sweat.

Potassium Balance in the Body

After it enters the blood, dietary potassium is quickly taken up into the cells. When there is excess potassium in the blood, the kidneys excrete more potassium in the urine. The kidneys control the level of potassium in the same way that they control sodium.

When the blood levels of potassium are low, the kidneys reabsorb potassium and return the blood levels to normal. The difference between the maintenance of potassium and sodium blood levels is that the hormone aldosterone is stimulated when blood K^+ is high and Na^+ is low, resulting in potassium excretion and sodium reabsorption. In other words, the release of aldosterone causes potassium to be lost from the body, while sodium is retained.

Metabolic Functions of Potassium

Potassium is essential for cellular and electrical function of all cells, tissues, and organs in the human

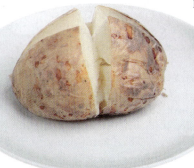

potassium (K^+) Main cation in the intracellular fluid.

(continued)

Potassium (continued)

body. Together with other minerals, potassium participates in fluid and pH balance, conducts electrical impulses in the body (which helps maintain a regular heartbeat), and plays a key role in skeletal and smooth muscle contraction, making it important for normal digestive and muscular function.

Potassium Helps Maintain Fluid Balance

Over 95 percent of the potassium in the body is found within cells. Potassium is part of the sodium-potassium pump described in Chapter 11 in which three sodium ions are exchanged for two potassium ions, maintaining fluid and electrolyte balance between the ECF and ICF.

Potassium Helps with Nerve Impulse Conduction and Muscle Contraction

As mentioned earlier, potassium, together with sodium, plays a key role in the conduction of nerve impulses and the contraction of muscles, including the heart. The exchange of potassium for sodium in the sodium-potassium pump generates an electrical current that travels as a wave along nerve cells and to muscle fibers, triggering the influx of calcium ions that causes the muscle to contract.

Potassium Can Help Lower High Blood Pressure

A diet that is plentiful in potassium has been shown to help lower blood pressure, especially in salt-sensitive individuals who respond more intensely to sodium's blood pressure–raising capabilities. As potassium in the blood is filtered through the kidneys, it causes the kidneys to excrete excess sodium from the body, and keeping sodium levels low can help lower blood pressure. The DASH diet that was discussed earlier in relation to reducing hypertension is abundant in potassium-rich fruits and vegetables. Furthermore, substituting potassium chloride for sodium chloride when seasoning foods during cooking or at the table has been found to reduce blood pressure.[27]

Potassium Plays a Role in Bone Health and Reduces Kidney Stones

Because potassium acts as a buffer in the blood, it helps keep the bone-strengthening minerals calcium and phosphorus from being used for this purpose and therefore lost from the bones. Numerous studies suggest that having plenty of potassium in the diet helps increase bone density, and thus bone strength.[28] Consuming potassium-rich foods may reduce the amount of calcium excreted and improve bone health.[29]

Potassium may also be beneficial in reducing kidney stones. Individuals with unusually high levels of calcium in the urine are at a higher risk of developing kidney stones. Increasing dietary potassium through fruits and vegetables or potassium supplements, such as potassium citrate, reduces the amount of calcium excreted in the urine. Potassium attaches to the calcium and prevents the formation of mineral crystals that can form kidney stones (**Figure 12.8**).[30]

Daily Needs for Potassium

An AI of 4,700 milligrams has been established for potassium for all adults. This amount is recommended to help those with sodium sensitivity reduce their risk of high blood pressure. This AI also lowers the risk of developing kidney stones and preserves bone health. A UL for potassium has not been established because there is no evidence that high levels of dietary potassium cause detrimental effects.

Because Americans fall short on recommended servings of fruits and vegetables, adult females consume only about 2,200–2,500 milligrams of potassium daily, and adult males consume only 3,300–3,400 milligrams daily.[31]

Food Sources of Potassium

Fruits and vegetables, especially bananas, watermelon, potatoes, leafy green vegetables, and sweet potatoes, are excellent sources of potassium. The *Dietary Guidelines for Americans* recommend consuming an abundance of fruits and vegetables to meet potassium needs. Seven servings, or about 4 cups, of fruits and vegetables is the minimum amount recommended daily for adults age 19 and older. Lean meat, low-fat dairy products, and nuts are also good sources of potassium in the diet (**Figure 12.9**). For more information on boosting your potassium intake, see the Table Tips.

Potassium Toxicity and Deficiency

There is little danger of consuming too much potassium from foods, and excess amounts are excreted in the urine. However, consuming too much potassium from supplements or salt substitutes can cause **hyperkalemia** (*kalemia* = potassium in blood) for some people. Hyperkalemia can cause an irregular heartbeat and damage the heart and can even be life-threatening. The symptoms of hyperkalemia include nausea, fatigue, muscle weakness, and tingling in feet and hands.

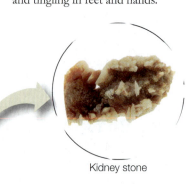

Kidney stone

▲ **Figure 12.8 Kidney Stones**
A potassium-rich diet may reduce the risk of developing kidney stones.

hyperkalemia Abnormally high levels of potassium in the blood.

TABLE TIPS

Potassium Pointers

Enjoy a 6-ounce glass of a citrus juice, such as orange or grapefruit, at breakfast to boost potassium intake.

Add leafy greens, such as spinach, to your lunchtime sandwich.

Add a spoonful of chopped nuts, such as walnuts or almonds, to yogurt.

Choose bean soup to go with a sandwich.

Bake a regular or sweet potato to increase potassium at dinner.

Those at a higher risk for hyperkalemia include individuals with impaired kidneys, such as people with type 1 diabetes mellitus, those with kidney disease, and individuals taking medications for heart disease or diuretics that cause the kidneys to block the excretion of potassium. These individuals may also need to consume less dietary potassium than the recommended daily amount as advised by their health care professional.

Hypokalemia is rare except—as discussed in Chapter 11—among individuals taking certain prescription diuretics. It sometimes results from vomiting and/or diarrhea, and has been observed in individuals who suffer with anorexia nervosa or bulimia nervosa. Hypokalemia can cause muscle weakness, cramps, glucose intolerance, and, in severe situations, irregular heartbeat and paralysis.[32] Even a moderately low intake of potassium can increase the risk of developing hypertension, kidney stones, and loss of bone mass. Signs and symptoms of hypokalemia include nausea, heart palpitations, weakness or tiredness, and fainting.

LO 12.4: THE TAKE-HOME MESSAGE

Potassium functions in muscle contraction and nerve conduction, maintains fluid and pH balance, preserves bone health, lowers blood pressure, and may prevent kidney stones. Adults need 4,700 milligrams of potassium per day. Fruits, vegetables, lean meats, low-fat dairy, and nuts are good food sources of potassium. Toxicity is rare from food but can cause hyperkalemia when taking supplements. Potassium deficiency, called hypokalemia, is rare.

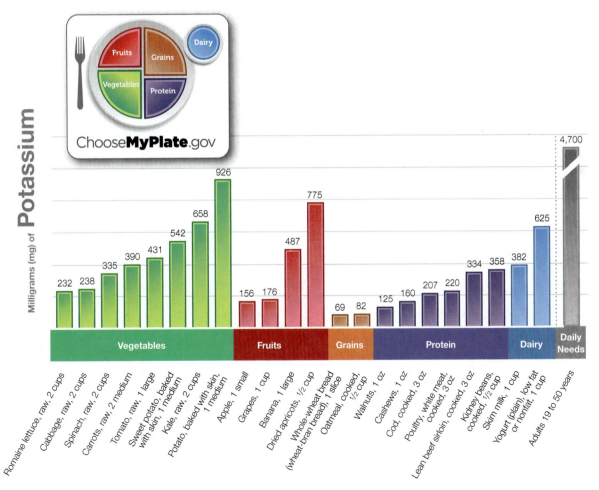

▲ Figure 12.9 **Potassium Content of Selected Foods**
Source: Data from *USDA What's In The Food You Eat?* 2016. Available at https://www.ars.usda.gov. Accessed March 2017.

EXPLORING **Calcium**

LO 12.5 Describe the functions, food sources, and toxicity and deficiency effects of calcium.

What Is Calcium?

Calcium (Ca^{+2}) is one of the most abundant divalent (two positive charges) cations in nature. Calcium is also the most abundant mineral in the body. Over 99 percent of the body's calcium is in the bones and teeth.

Bioavailability and Absorption of Calcium

The bioavailability of calcium in various foods can be influenced by other food components. For example, vitamin D and lactose each improve the absorption of calcium, so vitamin D–fortified milk is a good source of absorbable calcium. Protein intake may also influence the absorption of calcium from a meal. Low protein intake reduces the amount of calcium absorbed through the intestines, and high protein intake may increase the amount of calcium excreted in the urine.[33,34] On the other hand, oxalates and phytates found in foods that contain calcium, such as spinach (contains oxalates) or whole-wheat bread (contains phytates), reduce the bioavailability of calcium (**Figure 12.10**).[35]

A person who is deficient in calcium absorbs more of the mineral from foods than someone whose body has an adequate amount. However, the more calcium consumed at one time, the lower the rate of absorption. Therefore, consuming a calcium-containing food in smaller and more frequent portions—such as one 8-ounce glass of milk with breakfast and another with lunch, rather than a 16-ounce glass with dinner—increases the amount of calcium you absorb overall.

calcium (Ca^{2+}) One of the most abundant divalent cations found in nature and in the body.

calcitonin Hormone secreted by the thyroid gland that lowers blood calcium levels.

cortical bone Hard outer layer of bone.

trabecular bone Inner structure of bone, also known as *spongy bone* because of its appearance. This portion of bone is often lost in osteoporosis.

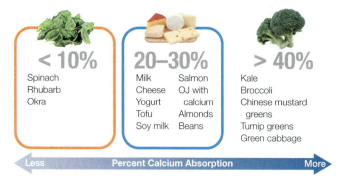

< 10%	20–30%		> 40%
Spinach	Milk	Salmon	Kale
Rhubarb	Cheese	OJ with	Broccoli
Okra	Yogurt	calcium	Chinese mustard
	Tofu	Almonds	greens
	Soy milk	Beans	Turnip greens
			Green cabbage

Less ◄ Percent Calcium Absorption ► More

▲ **Figure 12.10**   **Bioavailability of Calcium**

Hormones Regulate Calcium Balance

Hormones that respond to changes in blood calcium levels tightly control the amount of calcium in the body. When blood calcium levels are low (see **Focus Figure 12.11**), the parathyroid gland releases parathyroid hormone (PTH), which responds by stimulating the kidneys to convert more vitamin D to its active form, calcitriol. Together, calcitriol and PTH increase blood levels of calcium by increasing the amount of calcium absorbed through the GI tract, reducing the amount of calcium excreted through the kidneys, and releasing calcium from bone.

Another hormone, **calcitonin**, decreases blood calcium levels after a calcium-rich meal by stimulating the uptake of calcium into the bone. Calcitonin may also reduce the activation of vitamin D, thus reducing the amount of calcium absorbed through the small intestine. The action of calcitonin results in less calcium being absorbed, more calcium being deposited into the bone, and more calcium being excreted through the urine. The end result is normal levels of calcium in the blood and increased calcium levels in bones.[36]

Metabolic Functions of Calcium

Most people are probably aware that calcium is essential for building strong bones and teeth. But an optimal level of dietary intake of calcium is also essential for many other body functions.

Calcium Helps Build Strong Bones and Teeth

Calcium is the primary mineral in the hydroxyapatite crystals that, along with collagen, provide strength and structure to the bones and the enamel on teeth.[37]

The skeleton is made up of two types of bone (**Figure 12.12**): **cortical bone,** which is the compact, dense bone that makes up the surface of bone tissue, and **trabecular bone,** which is the spongy interior portion. The trabecular bone has a high rate of turnover and is sensitive to changes in dietary calcium intake. It provides a reserve of calcium that can be used to raise blood levels when the diet is deficient in calcium.

Calcium Plays a Role in Muscles, Nerves, and Blood

The 1 percent of calcium that's not in the bones or teeth is in the ECF and the ICF, including in muscle fibers. When a muscle fiber is stimulated by a nerve impulse, calcium ions flow into the cell through a calcium channel and bind to proteins in the cell. This binding initiates a chain of events that results in muscle contraction.

Calcium in the blood stimulates the release of hormones, activates enzymes, and helps the nervous system transmit messages. For example, calcium activates the enzyme that breaks down glycogen to provide energy for muscles to contract. Blood calcium must be maintained at a constant level for the body to function properly.

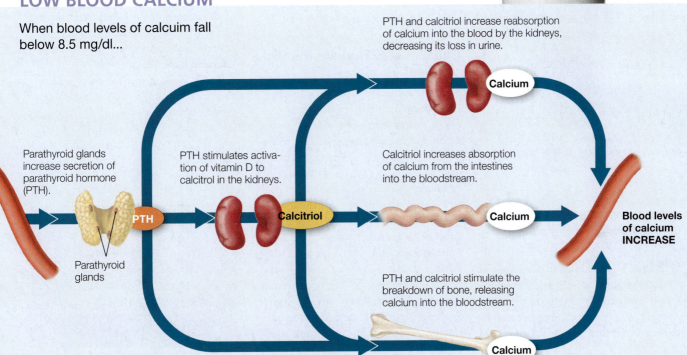

FOCUS Figure 12.11 Hormones Maintain Calcium Homeostasis

Head to Mastering Nutrition and watch a narrated video tour of this figure by author Joan Salge Blake.

CHLORIDE

Calcium homeostasis is tightly controlled to maintain a normal blood level of 8.5 to 11 mg per deciliter. Parathyroid hormone, calcitriol (activated vitamin D), and calcitonin are the three hormones involved in regulating blood calcium levels.

LOW BLOOD CALCIUM

When blood levels of calcuim fall below 8.5 mg/dl...

PTH and calcitriol increase reabsorption of calcium into the blood by the kidneys, decreasing its loss in urine.

Parathyroid glands increase secretion of parathyroid hormone (PTH).

Parathyroid glands

PTH

PTH stimulates activation of vitamin D to calcitrol in the kidneys.

Calcitriol

Calcitriol increases absorption of calcium from the intestines into the bloodstream.

Calcium

Calcium

Calcium

Blood levels of calcium INCREASE

PTH and calcitriol stimulate the breakdown of bone, releasing calcium into the bloodstream.

Calcium

HIGH BLOOD CALCIUM

When blood levels of calcium rise above 11 mg/dl...

Calcitonin reduces reabsorption of calcium by the kidneys, increasing its loss of urine.

Less Calcium

Thyroid gland releases calcitonin.

Calcitonin

Calcium

Less Calcium

Calcitonin stimulates bone building, removing calcium from the bloodstream.

Blood levels of calcium DECREASE

Parathyroid glands decrease secretion of parathyroid hormone (PTH), which in turn suppresses activation of vitamin D to calcitriol.

Less PTH

Less Calcitriol

Suppression of PTH and calcitriol decreases reabsorption of calcium by the kidneys, decreases absorption of calcium from the intestines, and inhibits release of calcium from bone.

Less Calcium

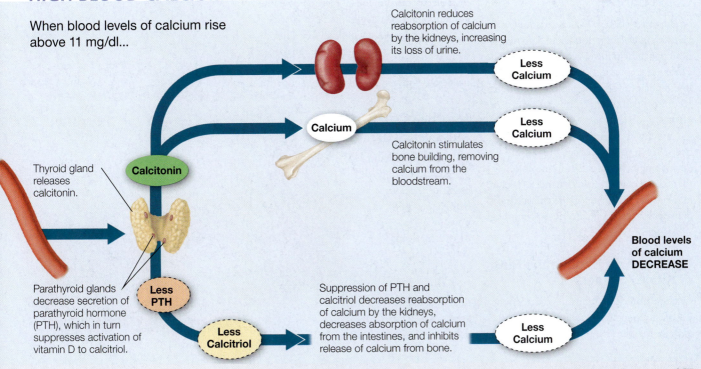

Calcium (continued)

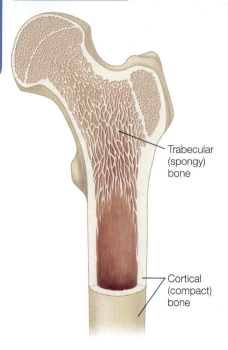

▲ **Figure 12.12 Trabecular and Cortical Bone**

Calcium is also needed to dilate and contract the blood vessels and help blood to clot. Calcium ions bind to the seven vitamin K–dependent clotting factors, resulting in the formation of blood clots after an injury.

Calcium May Help Lower High Blood Pressure and Prevent Colon Cancer

Studies have shown that a heart-healthy diet rich in calcium, potassium, and magnesium can help lower blood pressure. The DASH diet contains three daily servings of low-fat dairy foods, the minimum amount recommended to obtain this protective effect.[38,39]

A diet with plenty of calcium has also been shown to help reduce the risk of developing benign tumors in the colon that may eventually lead to cancer. Calcium may protect the lining of the colon from damaging bile acids and cancer-promoting substances.[40]

Calcium May Reduce the Risk of Kidney Stones

Calcium from food binds to oxalate in the GI tract, reducing the ability of oxalate to enter the blood and pass through the filtration vessels in the interior of the kidney. With less oxalate filtering through the kidneys, fewer stones are formed. Thus, even though the majority of the more than 2 million kidney stones that Americans suffer every year consist mainly of calcium oxalate, dietary calcium is not the culprit. Research has shown that a balanced diet, along with adequate (but not excessive) amounts of calcium, may actually reduce the risk of developing kidney stones.[41]

Calcium May Reduce the Risk of Obesity

Some preliminary research suggests that low-calcium diets may trigger several responses that increase the risk for obesity, at least in those who are genetically predisposed to obesity.[42,43] When calcium intake is inadequate, PTH is increased to reduce the amount of calcium lost through the urine. At the same time, the active form of vitamin D, calcitriol, increases in the body to enhance dietary calcium absorption. These hormonal responses also cause a shift of calcium into fat cells, which stimulates fat production and storage. The opposite also appears to be true: When the diet is high in calcium, less PTH and calcitriol are produced, resulting in more calcium excreted in the urine to maintain calcium balance in the blood, less calcium stored in fat cells, and more fat being burned for energy. In addition, preliminary results suggest that high dietary calcium intake may increase the amount of fat excreted in the feces as well as increase core body temperature.[44] However, calcium is not a magic pill in the battle against obesity and clearly more research is needed to confirm this relationship.

Daily Needs for Calcium

The RDA for calcium is 1,000–1,200 milligrams of calcium daily, depending on your age. Most Americans 20 years of age and older are consuming less than 800 milligrams of calcium daily.[45]

Food Sources of Calcium

Americans get the majority of their calcium from dairy products, with an average of 55 percent of their intake coming from these sources. An 8-ounce glass of milk, 1 cup of yogurt, or $1\frac{1}{2}$ ounces of hard cheese each provides 300 milligrams of calcium. Three servings (or about 3 cups) of dairy foods will just about meet many adults' daily needs. Selecting low-fat and nonfat dairy products will help minimize saturated fat intake.

Dairy foods are not the only excellent source of calcium. Bok choy, broccoli, canned salmon with bones (the calcium is in the bones), and tofu that is processed with calcium can also add calcium to the diet. Calcium-fortified foods, such as juices

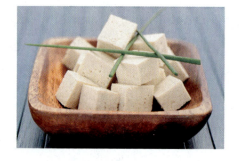

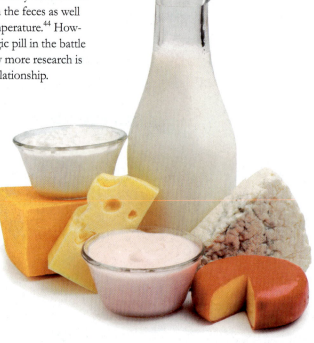

TABLE TIPS

Calcium Counts

Use skim or low-fat milk on your morning cereal.

Spoon a few chunks of tofu onto a salad bar lunch for extra calcium.

Use low-fat pudding or yogurt to satisfy a sweet tooth.

Top calcium-rich pizza with more calcium from vegetables such as broccoli and raw leafy greens.

Spread nonfat or low-fat ricotta cheese on toast for a snack.

Drink calcium-fortified orange juice with your morning cereal.

and cereals, are also excellent sources (**Figure 12.13**). For more information on increasing your calcium intake, see the Table Tips.

Calcium Toxicity and Deficiency

The UL for calcium is 2,500 milligrams daily to avoid **hypercalcemia,** or too much calcium in the blood, subsequent impaired kidneys, and calcium deposits in the body. Too much dietary calcium can also cause stomach upset, nausea, constipation, bone pain, muscle weakness, and mental confusion. Excess calcium can interfere with the absorption of other minerals, such as iron, zinc, magnesium, and phosphorus.

If the diet is low in calcium, the mineral will be pulled from bone for the sake of maintaining a constant level in the blood. When blood calcium levels fall below normal, **hypocalcemia** results. A chronic deficiency of dietary calcium may not show any symptoms but can lead to less dense, weakened, and brittle bones (**Figure 12.14**) and increased risk for osteoporosis, osteomalacia, rickets (in children), and bone fractures. Acute calcium deficiencies can cause memory loss, muscle spasms, and numbness or tingling in your feet and hands. See Health Connection: What Is Osteoporosis? on page 455 for more about this common disorder.

Calcium Supplements

Some individuals, because of their diet, medical history, or both, are advised by their health care provider to take a calcium supplement. The calcium in supplements is part of a compound, typically either calcium carbonate or calcium citrate. Calcium carbonate tends to be the least expensive and the most common form of calcium purchased. It is most effective when consumed with a meal, as the acidic gastric juices help with its absorption.[46] Calcium citrate can be taken anytime throughout the day, as it doesn't need the help of acidic juices to be absorbed. Calcium citrate usually works best for those age 50 and older who may produce less stomach acid as they age.[47]

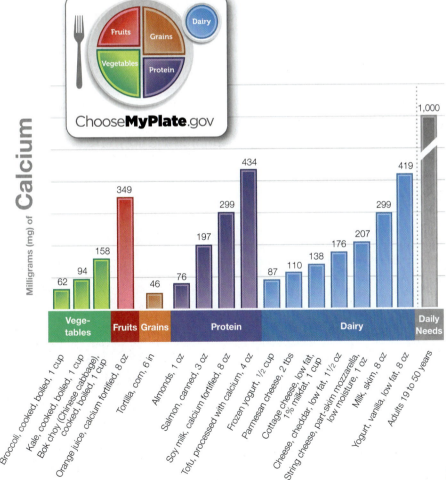

▲ **Figure 12.13 Calcium Content of Selected Foods**
Source: Data from *USDA What's In The Food You Eat?* 2016. Available at https://www.ars.usda.gov. Accessed March 2017.

hypercalcemia Abnormally high levels of calcium in the blood.

hypocalcemia Abnormally low levels of calcium in the blood.

(continued)

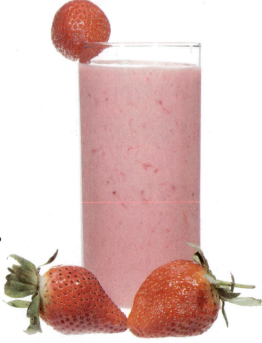

▲ **Figure 12.14** **Normal and Abnormal Bone**
Healthy bone (left) versus weakened bone (right).

Calcium from unrefined oyster shell, bone meal, or dolomite (a rock rich in calcium) may contain lead and other toxic metals. Supplements from these sources should state on the label that they are "purified" or carry the USP Verified mark.

Regardless of the form, all calcium, whether from supplements or from fortified or naturally occurring foods, should be consumed in doses of 500 milligrams or less, as this is the maximum that the body can absorb efficiently at

one time. In other words, if a person has been advised to take 1,000 milligrams of calcium daily, 500 milligrams should be consumed in the morning and the other 500 milligrams in the afternoon or evening.[48] Because calcium can interfere with and reduce the absorption of iron, a calcium supplement shouldn't be taken at the same time of day as an iron supplement.

Calcium supplements can sometimes cause constipation and flatulence (gas), especially when taken in large amounts.

Increasing the amount of fiber in the diet helps avoid these side effects. As with any mineral supplement, be cautious about adding a calcium supplement to your diet if you are already consuming plenty of low-fat dairy foods and/or calcium-fortified foods.

LO 12.5: THE TAKE-HOME MESSAGE
Calcium provides strength and structure to bones and teeth, is critical for muscle contraction, helps maintain a normal heartbeat, participates in blood clotting, and may reduce the risk for hypertension, colon cancer, kidney stones, and obesity. The RDA for calcium for adults is 1,000–1,200 milligrams per day. Dairy products, green vegetables, canned salmon, tofu, and calcium-fortified foods are good sources of calcium. Toxicity of calcium is called hypercalcemia. Calcium deficiency or hypocalcemia can increase risk of osteoporosis and bone fractures.

EXPLORING **Phosphorus**

LO 12.6 Describe the functions, food sources, and toxicity and deficiency effects of phosphorus.

What Is Phosphorus?

Phosphorus (P) is the second most abundant mineral in the body. The majority of phosphorus—about 85 percent—is found in bone tissue and teeth bound with calcium. The remainder is in the muscle, cell membranes, and intracellular fluids. Phosphorus differs from phosphate (PO_4^{-3}), which is a salt containing the mineral phosphorus.

phosphorus (P) Second most abundant mineral in the body.

About 70 percent of the phosphorus in the diet is absorbed through the small intestine. Foods that contain the binder phytate reduce the absorption of phosphorus, whereas vitamin D enhances its absorption. Phosphorus absorption is decreased by magnesium, calcium, and aluminum. These three minerals are often found in antacids and can be used to reduce high blood levels of phosphorus.[49]

Parathyroid hormone (PTH) controls phosphorus metabolism in a way similar to that in which it regulates calcium metabolism. When blood levels of phosphorus are low, PTH stimulates the resorption of the mineral from the bone to raise blood levels. PTH also stimulates the kidneys

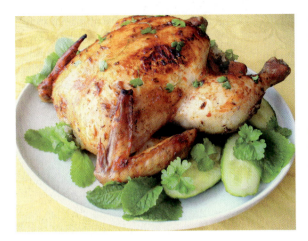

is found in muscle, can be provided to ADP to form ATP when cells require more energy. Phosphorus is also a part of several coenzymes.

If the blood or the ICF becomes too acidic or too basic, phosphorus can act as a buffer, binding or releasing hydrogen ions. Phosphorus is also a component of the backbone of DNA and RNA molecules.

Daily Needs for Phosphorus

The RDA for adult males and females is 700 milligrams of phosphorus daily. Americans, on average, consume more than 1,000 milligrams of phosphorus daily.

Food Sources of Phosphorus

A balanced, varied diet easily provides an adequate amount of phosphorus (**Figure 12.16**). Foods from animal sources such as meat, fish, poultry, and dairy products are excellent sources. Plant seeds such as beans, peas, nuts, and cereal grains contain phosphorus in the form of phytates, which are only about 50 percent bioavailable. Soft drinks, which contain the additive phosphoric acid, are another common food source of phosphorus. However, soft drinks containing added sugars should be limited in the diet. For information on balancing your phosphorus intake with calcium, see the Table Tips.

to excrete phosphorus through the urine. Most phosphorus excess is excreted in the urine and the rest is lost in the feces.

Metabolic Functions of Phosphorus

Together with calcium, phosphorus plays a key role in the formation of the hydroxyapatite crystalline structure of bones and teeth. There is about half as much total phosphorus in the bone as there is calcium. Some of the body's phosphorus is found in the cells as part of phospholipids (**Figure 12.15**), which give cell membranes their structure. Phospholipids act as a barrier to keep specific substances out of the cells while letting others in.

Phosphorus is also part of adenosine triphosphate (ATP) and thus helps store energy generated from the catabolism of carbohydrates, protein, and fat. The phosphorus in creatine phosphate, which

▲ **Figure 12.15 Phosphorus Forms Phospholipids**
Phosphorus makes up part of the phospholipids found in cell membranes.

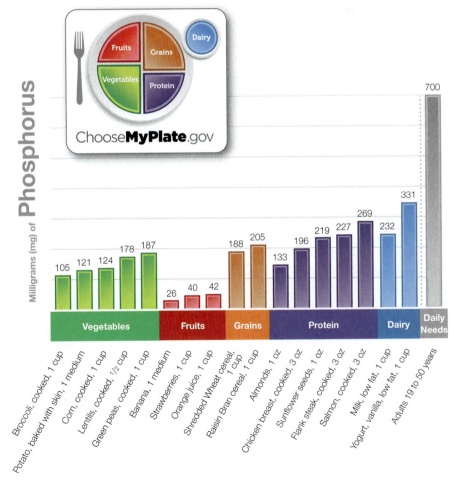

▲ **Figure 12.16 Phosphorus Content of Selected Foods**
Source: Data from USDA *What's In The Food You Eat?* 2016. Available at https://www.ars.usda.gov. Accessed March 2017.

(continued)

TABLE TIPS

Balance Phosphorus with Calcium

Substitute sodas with refreshing lemonade to quench your thirst.

Blend together calcium-fortified orange juice and slightly thawed frozen strawberries for a refreshing smoothie.

Skip the butter and sprinkle chopped unsalted peanuts over calcium-rich steamed vegetables for a crunchy topping.

Dip raw broccoli florets into a nonfat sour cream–based dip for a snack.

Stir-fry chicken breast with calcium-rich vegetables for a balanced ratio of phosphorus to calcium.

hyperphosphatemia Abnormally high level of phosphorus in the blood.

hypophosphatemia Abnormally low level of phosphorus in the blood.

Phosphorus Toxicity and Deficiency

Typically, consuming too much dietary phosphorus and its subsequent effect, **hyperphosphatemia,** is only an issue for individuals with kidney problems who cannot excrete excess phosphorus. Consistently high phosphorus and low calcium intake can cause the loss of calcium from bones and a subsequent decrease in bone mass. Loss of bone mass increases the risk of osteoporosis. Hyperphosphatemia can also lead to depositing calcium (also known as *calcification*) in soft tissues such as the arteries and kidneys. To protect against this, the UL for phosphorus has been set at 4,000 milligrams daily for adults age 19–50 and 3,000 milligrams for those 50 years of age and older. Symptoms of hyperphosphatemia may include muscle cramps and spasms and numbness or tingling in the feet and hands.

Too little phosphorus in the diet can cause dangerously low blood levels, a condition called **hypophosphatemia,**
and result in muscle weakness, bone pain, rickets in children, confusion, and, at the extreme, death. Because phosphorus is so abundant in the diet, however, a deficiency is very rare. In fact, a person would have to be in a state of near starvation before experiencing a phosphorus deficiency.

LO 12.6: THE TAKE-HOME MESSAGE

Phosphorus is a structural component of bones and teeth, provides energy as part of ATP, acts as an acid–base buffer, and is part of DNA and RNA. Adults need 700 milligrams daily of phosphorus, which can be found in meat, fish, poultry, dairy, legumes, nuts, and cereal grains. Toxicity of phosphorus, hyperphosphatemia, occurs when the kidney can't excrete excess phosphorus. A dietary deficiency of phosphorus causes hypophosphatemia.

EXPLORING **Magnesium**

LO 12.7 Describe the functions, food sources, and toxicity and deficiency effects of magnesium.

What Is Magnesium?

Magnesium (Mg^{+2}) is the fourth most abundant cation in the body after calcium (Ca^{+2}), potassium (K^+), and sodium (Na^+). About 60 percent of the body's magnesium is found in bones, 25 percent in muscle, and the remainder inside various other cells. A mere 1 percent is found in the blood—though, as with blood calcium, this amount must be maintained at a constant level.

The bioavailability of magnesium in a typical diet is about 50 percent. Diets that

magnesium (Mg^{+2}) Major divalent cation in the body.

are high in fiber and whole grains, which are high in phytates, lower magnesium absorption.

The intestines and kidneys control the levels of magnesium in the body. When dietary intake is low, absorption of magnesium through the small intestine increases and the kidneys excrete less.

Metabolic Functions of Magnesium

Magnesium participates in more than 300 enzymatic reactions in the body, including many associated with the metabolism of carbohydrates, proteins, and fats, and the phosphorylation of ADP to ATP. It is also

used in the synthesis of DNA, RNA, body proteins, and the cell membrane. Magnesium also plays a vital role in bone metabolism and maintenance of bone tissue and helps nerves and muscles, including the heart muscle, to function properly. Some studies suggest that a diet abundant in magnesium may help decrease the risk of type 2 diabetes.[50] Low blood levels of magnesium, which often occur in individuals with type 2 diabetes, may impair the release of insulin, one of the hormones that regulate blood glucose. This may lead

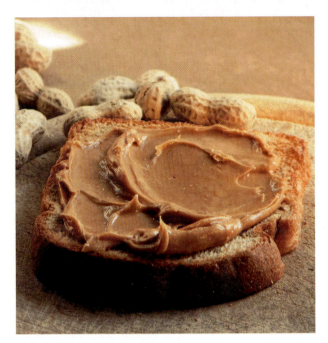

200 milligrams, or about half of an adult's daily needs. Because the majority of the magnesium in bread products is in the bran and germ of the grain kernel, products made with refined grains such as white flour are poor magnesium sources. Finally, beverages such as coffee, tea, and cocoa also contain some magnesium. For more information on boosting your magnesium intake, see the Table Tips.

to elevated blood glucose levels in those with preexisting diabetes and those at risk for type 2 diabetes.[51]

Daily Needs for Magnesium

The RDA for adult females age 19 and older ranges from 310 milligrams to 320 milligrams of magnesium, whereas men of the same age need 400 milligrams to 420 milligrams of magnesium daily.

Currently, many Americans fall short of the recommended intake of magnesium. Females consume only about 70 percent of their RDA and males approximately 80 percent. Because older adults tend to consume fewer kilocalories, and thus less dietary magnesium, they are at an even higher risk of falling short of their needs.

Food Sources of Magnesium

The biggest contributors of magnesium in Americans' diets are green leafy vegetables, whole grains, nuts, legumes, and fruits. Milk, yogurt, meat, and eggs are also good sources (see **Figure 12.17**). A peanut butter sandwich on whole-wheat bread, along with a glass of low-fat milk and a banana, provides more than

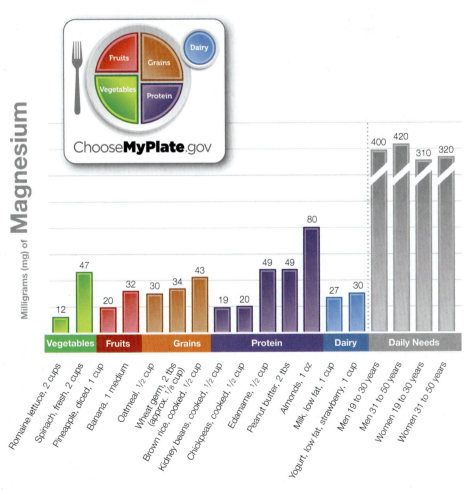

▲ **Figure 12.17** **Magnesium Content of Selected Foods**
Source: Data from *USDA What's In The Food You Eat?* 2016. Available at https://www.ars.usda.gov. Accessed March 2017.

(continued)

Magnesium (continued)

Magnesium Toxicity and Deficiency

There is no known risk in consuming too much magnesium from food sources. However, consuming large amounts from supplements has been shown to cause intestinal problems such as diarrhea, cramps, and nausea. In fact, some laxatives (such as milk of magnesia) contain magnesium because of its known cathartic effect. The upper level for magnesium from supplements, not foods, is set at 350 milligrams for adults.[52] This level is to prevent diarrhea, the first symptom that typically arises when too much magnesium is consumed.

Even though many Americans don't meet their dietary magnesium needs, deficiencies are rare in healthy individuals because the kidneys compensate for low magnesium intake by excreting less of it. However, some medications may cause magnesium deficiency. Certain diuretics can cause the body to lose too much magnesium, and some antibiotics, such as tetracycline, can inhibit the absorption of magnesium, both of which can lead to a deficiency. Individuals with poorly controlled diabetes or who abuse alcohol can experience excessive losses of magnesium in the urine, which could also cause a deficiency. A severe magnesium deficiency can cause muscle weakness, seizures, fatigue, depression, and irregular heartbeat.

LO 12.7: THE TAKE-HOME MESSAGE
Magnesium participates in metabolism; the synthesis of DNA, RNA, and proteins; and nerve impulse transmission and muscle contraction. Magnesium also contributes to bone metabolism and neuromuscular function. The RDA for magnesium for adult females ranges from 310 milligrams to 320 milligrams, whereas men need 400 milligrams to 420 milligrams of magnesium daily. Magnesium is abundant in leafy green vegetables, legumes, and beverages such as coffee and tea. Magnesium toxicity only occurs with supplements. Deficiencies of magnesium are rare.

EXPLORING **Sulfate**

LO 12.8 Describe the functions and food sources of sulfate.

What Is Sulfate?

Sulfate (SO_4^{2-}) is the oxidized form of the mineral sulfur that is found in plants and occurs naturally in drinking water. In the body, sulfur is usually found as part of other compounds, mostly proteins. It is also part of two important B vitamins, thiamin and biotin.

Sulfate is absorbed throughout the GI tract, including the stomach, small intestine, and colon. About 80 percent of the sulfate you eat is absorbed, and the excess excreted in the urine. Sulfate is found in the body's tissues as part of keratin, especially in hair, skin, and nails.

Metabolic Functions of Sulfate

The amino acids methionine and cysteine both contain sulfur. These two amino acids are incorporated into body proteins

sulfate (SO₄) Oxidized form of the mineral sulfur.

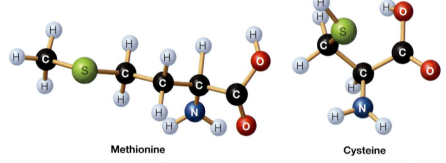

Methionine   Cysteine

▲ **Figure 12.18 Sulfur Is Part of Some Amino Acids**

and help give proteins their three-dimensional shape (**Figure 12.18**). This enables the proteins to perform effectively as enzymes and hormones and provide structure to the body.

Food manufacturers use sulfur-based substances, called *sulfites*, as preservatives. They help prevent food spoilage and discoloration in

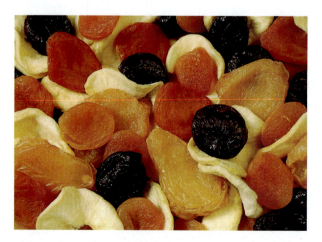

foods such as dried fruits. Sulfites occur naturally in wine due to the fermentation process and are added to prevent oxidation. People who are sensitive to sulfites may experience headache, sneezing, swelling of the throat, or hives and should avoid sulfite-containing foods and beverages.

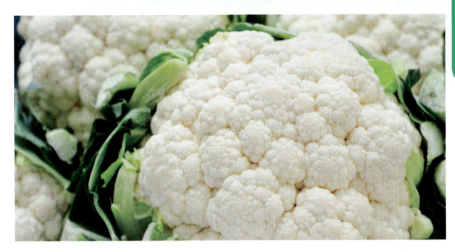

Daily Needs for Sulfate

There is insufficient data to determine an EAR, an RDA, an AI, or even a UL for sulfate. The amount of sulfate most Americans consume has been estimated from consumption data on the sulfur-containing amino acids.

Food Sources of Sulfate

About 65 percent of dietary sulfate comes from foods that contain methionine, cysteine, glutathione, and taurine. A varied diet that contains meat, poultry, fish, eggs, legumes, dairy foods, and fruits and vegetables provides good sources of sulfate.

Beverages including beer, wine, and some juices that are made from municipal water supplies also contain sulfate. As much as 1.3 grams of sulfate per day may come from drinking water due to contamination from groundwater, pipes, and harmless bacteria.[53] Some dietary supplements may also add to total sulfate intake. For example, chondroitin sulfate and glucosamine are popular supplements for osteoarthritis and joint problems.

Sulfate Toxicity and Deficiency

Although a UL has not been established, a possible link has been suggested between high levels of sulfate and ulcerative colitis. Bacteria in the colons of people with this condition appear to convert some of the sulfite-containing compounds into by-products that promote the disease.[54]

Most people eat sufficient protein to provide adequate amounts of sulfur-containing amino acids. There are no known toxicity or deficiency symptoms for sulfate.

LO 12.8: THE TAKE-HOME MESSAGE
Sulfur provides shape to proteins and is part of the vitamins thiamin and biotin and the amino acids cysteine and methionine. There is insufficient data to establish an EAR, RDA, AI, or UL for sulfate. Sulfur is consumed in its oxidized form, sulfate, and is found in meat, poultry, fish, eggs, legumes, dairy foods, fruits and vegetables, and also beer and wine. Excess sulfate may contribute to ulcerative colitis. There are no known deficiency symptoms for sulfate.

HEALTH**CONNECTION**

What Is Osteoporosis?

LO 12.9 Discuss the roles of minerals in the development of healthy bone tissue and the factors that influence the risk of developing osteoporosis.

If you are fortunate enough to have elders, such as grandparents, in your life, you may have heard them comment that they are "shrinking" as they age. Of course, they aren't really shrinking, but they may be losing height as the tissues supporting their spine lose mass and elasticity and the joint capsules between the vertebrae of the spine lose their cushion of fluid.[55] This is a normal age-related change in many older adults. In some older adults, however, the vertebrae themselves lose mass and begin to collapse, so that it becomes more difficult for the spine to hold the weight of the head and upper body. This leads to a gradual curvature of the spine, which affects posture (**Figure 12.19**).[55]

Strong, healthy bones have a high **bone mineral density (BMD)**. BMD is the density of hydroxyapatite crystals within the trabecular bone and cortical bone.

Low BMD is a hallmark of **osteoporosis** (*osteo* = bone, *porosis* = porous), one of the most common disorders experienced by older adults in the United States. Older adults with osteoporosis experience a myriad of health problems, from bone breaks and fractures to reduced mobility and diminished quality of life. Unfortunately, by

bone mineral density (BMD) Amount of minerals, in particular calcium, per volume in an individual's bone.

osteoporosis Disorder characterized by low bone mineral density, which increases the individual's risk of fractures.

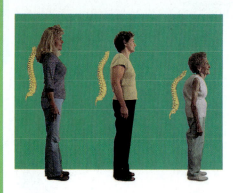

▲ **Figure 12.19 Deterioration of the Vertebrae**
Weakened bones in the vertebrae cause the spine to collapse over time, resulting in the "shrinking" effect experienced by some older adults.

the time an older adult finds out he or she has the condition, little can be done because an individual's lifelong bone health is largely determined during childhood, adolescence, and early adulthood, when the person is accumulating **peak bone mass.** This means that, during your college years, you are building up the bone health you'll need for a healthy older age.

You can think of BMD as being like a retirement account. The more you build and preserve while you're young, the more you'll have for your later years. If an adult doesn't have a healthy diet and a lifestyle that includes regular exercise, he or she may experience accelerated bone loss after age 30.

Most Bone Growth Occurs Early in Life

Bones are dynamic, living tissues that are constantly being broken down and reformed. Specialized cells called

peak bone mass Genetically determined maximum amount of bone mass an individual can build up.

Type I osteoporosis Form of osteoporosis that results from reduced estrogen levels and is characterized by rapid loss of bone mass.

Type II osteoporosis Form of osteoporosis that results from aging and is characterized by the slow loss of bone mass over time.

osteoclasts work to remove older layers of bones, while *osteoblasts* continuously form new bone. Although this process occurs throughout the lifespan, the majority of bone growth and buildup of BMD occurs during childhood, adolescence, and early adulthood, when the osteoblasts are more active than the osteoclasts. During these life stages, more bone mass is added than is lost. Adults typically reach peak bone mass sometime in their 20s. Some additional bone mass can be added when an individual is in his or her 30s.

After peak bone mass is reached, the loss of bone mass begins to slowly exceed the rate at which new bone is added.[57] Starting in their mid-30s, women begin to slowly lose bone mass until menopause, when the rate of loss accelerates for several years (**Figure 12.20**). Bone loss continues in women after age 60, but at a slower rate. Bone loss also occurs in men as they age.[58]

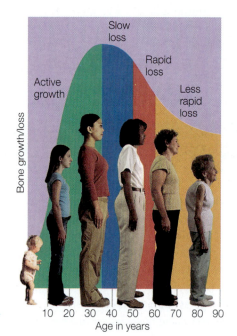

▲ **Figure 12.20 Change in Bone Mass As You Age**
In your early years, more bone is added than lost in your body. In their mid-30s, women begin to slowly lose bone mass until menopause, when the rate of loss is accelerated for several years. Bone loss continues after age 60 but at a slower rate.

Osteoporosis Is a Disease of Progressive Bone Loss

There are two main classifications of osteoporosis. **Type I osteoporosis** is associated with a decrease in estrogen levels during menopause and is present in 5–20 percent of American women age 50–75.[59] The lower levels of estrogen in a postmenopausal woman's body cause a reduction in BMD. This, in turn, leads to weak and brittle bones. Type I osteoporosis is often associated with fractures of the spine, hip, wrist, or forearm.

Type II osteoporosis, or age-related osteoporosis, occurs when the breakdown of bone outpaces the rebuilding of bone over time. Type II osteoporosis is mostly associated with leg and spinal fractures and occurs in both men and women, although it is more common in women. Note that older women can have both types of osteoporosis simultaneously.[60]

The weakened, fragile bones associated with both types of osteoporosis are prone to fractures. A minor stumble while walking can result in a fall that breaks a hip, ankle, or arm. Hip fractures can be devastating because they often render a person immobile. Feelings of helplessness and depression often ensue. Up to two-thirds of all individuals with hip fractures are never able to regain the quality of life they had prior to the injury, and about 20 percent will die within a year due to complications from the injury.[61] By the year 2020, it is estimated that more than 61 million Americans will either have or be at risk for hip fractures due to osteoporosis, and even more will be at risk for fractures of other bones.[62]

Bone Density Can Be Measured by DEXA

Bone density tests for adults compare an individual's BMD with that of a healthy 30-year-old. The most accurate tool is a dual-energy X-ray absorptiometry (DEXA) test, which is a fast and easy scan that uses two beams of low-energy X-ray radiation (**Figure 12.21**). DEXA

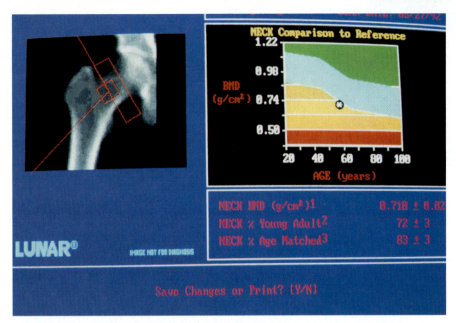

▲ Figure 12.21 **Dual-Energy X-Ray Absorptiometry**
A DEXA scan is the most accurate way to measure bone mineral density.

can measure bone loss of as little as 2 percent per year. In a DEXA scan, dense bone allows less of the X-ray beam to pass through than porous bone. The data from a DEXA is presented as a T-score, which is compared with the ideal BMD of a healthy 30-year-old adult. A normal T-score is +1 to −1, whereas a low T-score between −1 and −2.5 indicates **osteopenia** (*penia* = poverty), signaling low bone mass. A very low score, less than −2.5, indicates osteoporosis.

Several Lifestyle Factors Influence Bone Mass

As with hypertension, diabetes, and other chronic conditions, there are choices you can make today to lessen your likelihood of developing osteoporosis in the future. Among the factors that matter most are diet, exercise, and the use of drugs (including nicotine) and alcohol.

The Role of Diet

Calcium intake during childhood and adolescence is strongly related to higher BMD in older men and women. Adequate vitamin D intake is also important,

as vitamin D promotes the absorption of calcium and is essential to attain peak bone mass.

Sufficient intake of the minerals magnesium and potassium has also been associated with increased bone health. One study found that the BMD in the neck of the femur (or thigh bone) was higher in women who had consumed high amounts of fruit (a good source of both magnesium and potassium) in their childhood than in women who had consumed medium or low amounts.[63] Although vitamin K doesn't appear to improve BMD, diets rich in vitamin K may reduce the risk of hip fractures, probably because of a reduction in bone turnover.[64] Consuming adequate levels of omega-3 fatty acids also has a positive effect in achieving peak bone mass.[65] Consuming too much sodium may contribute to osteoporosis because it increases excretion of calcium in the urine. A healthy diet that meets the current recommendations for calcium and sodium is adequate for the health and maintenance of bone.

One dietary habit that may have a negative impact on BMD is the regular consumption of carbonated beverages. Several observational studies have shown a relationship between low BMD and an

increase in fracture rates in teenagers who consume higher amounts of soda and other carbonated beverages. In one study, the BMD in the heels of females age 12–15 was inversely related to the amount of carbonated beverages they consumed; however, no relationship was observed in boys the same age.[66] A similar study reported a relationship between carbonated beverage intake and risk of fracture.[67] However, this relationship has not been substantiated with experimental studies.[68] Researchers theorize that the correlation between carbonated beverage intake and poor bone health may have more to do with the displacement of milk in the diet than with the carbonated beverages themselves.

Adequate protein intake positively correlates with an increase in bone density, but high protein intakes combined with lower intakes of calcium increase urinary calcium loss. It appears that protein is not detrimental to bone density if both protein and calcium are present in the recommended levels.

Food is the best source of nutrients to develop and maintain healthy bones. Some individuals are advised to take a supplement by their health care provider. However, supplements that contain high doses of nutrients other than calcium have been shown to have adverse effects on bone health.[69]

Maintaining adequate vitamin C intake may boost bone health. In some studies, vitamin C intakes of 100–125 milligrams have improved BMD and reduced the risk of hip fractures in postmenopausal women.[70] However, megadoses of vitamin C (greater than 2,000 milligrams) may increase the risk of fracture, as well as the risk of developing kidney stones, although more research is required to support these findings.

Complete the Self-Assessment "Estimating Your Calcium Intake" to see whether you consume sufficient calcium.

---

osteopenia Condition in which the bone mineral density is lower than normal but not low enough to be classified as osteoporosis.

Self-Assessment

Estimating Your Calcium Intake

Complete the table below to estimate the total amount of calcium you consumed yesterday. How does your calcium intake compare to the RDA of 1,000 mg per day? Are you meeting your calcium needs?

Product	Number of Servings	Calcium Content per Serving	Total Amount of Calcium (mg)
Milk or fortified soymilk, 8 oz		300 mg	
Fortified orange juice, 8 oz		300 mg	
Fortified cereals, snacks (no milk added)		100 mg	
Fortified cereal with 4 oz milk or soymilk		250 mg	
Yogurt, 8 oz		400 mg	
Cheese, 1 oz		200 mg	
Legumes, 1 cup		225 mg	
Leafy green vegetables, 1 cup cooked (low-oxalate vegetables such as kale and collard greens)		185 mg	
Total mg calcium			

Source: Adapted from the International Osteoporosis Foundation, 2014. www.iofbonehealth.org.

The Role of Exercise

Weight-bearing exercises, including walking, hiking, jumping rope, and weight-training, appropriately stress bone and thereby increase bone mass. The stress of muscle pulling on bone stimulates the osteoblasts to build more bone. When exercising for bone health, impact, body region involved, and intensity are important considerations.

High-impact physical activity has been shown to increase the growth and the mineral content of the bones in girls and adolescent females.[71,72] Similar increases in bone mass with high-impact activity are reported in premenopausal women over the age of 18 who have stopped growing in height but can still improve BMD.[73] Even after menopause, high-impact exercise appears to increase not only BMD but also overall muscle strength.[74] Low-impact activities, such as swimming, can help increase cardiorespiratory health and muscle strength, but have only minimal benefits for bone.[75]

Exercise only improves BMD in the bones that are involved.[76] For example, weight-training the lower body will not improve the upper arms or bones of the wrist, where many older women sustain fractures.

Intensity is also important to consider when choosing an exercise to improve BMD. For example, relative to a leisurely stroll, moderate- to high-intensity walking at a pace of more than 4 miles per hour

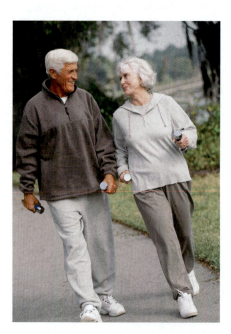

increases the stress on the muscle and bone and results in an increase in the BMD of the hip.[77] The bottom line? Choose a variety of exercises that you enjoy, but make sure that some of your choices appropriately stress your bones.

The Impact of Body Weight

Body weight also has an impact on achieving peak bone mass. Women who are slightly heavier than their normal-weight counterparts have higher BMD, especially in the spine and the hip. However, when an individual loses weight, the effect may be detrimental to their bone. During moderate weight loss, bones appear to maintain mineral density, especially when there is adequate calcium in the diet.[78] However, when the weight loss is severe, such as in young women diagnosed with anorexia nervosa, the loss of BMD is significant.[79] The key to maintaining healthy bone mass appears to be losing weight slowly and eating adequate amounts of calcium and kilocalories.

The Effects of Smoking

Bone mineral density is significantly reduced in people who smoke.[80] Postmenopausal women who reportedly smoked prior to menopause were found to have significantly lower DEXA scores than women who never smoked.[81] Though the mechanism by which smoking has an impact on BMD and fracture risk is not completely understood, several theories have been suggested. First, smokers have lower levels of parathyroid hormone and calcitriol, suggesting that smoking increases calcium removal from the bone. Women who smoke also have lower body weights, on average, which could account for less estrogen, less protective body fat (important during a fall), and reduced load on bones (load improves bone density). Regardless of the mechanism, the risk of fracture in smokers has been reported to be 35 percent higher compared with nonsmokers.[82] Similar effects of smoking have also been reported in men.[83] The good news is that stopping smoking improves BMD.[84]

The Impact of Alcohol

Excessive alcohol intake has been associated with osteoporosis[85] and related fractures. This is due in part to the malnourishment often seen in chronic alcoholics, which may include insufficient calcium intake. In addition, alcohol may reduce vitamin D metabolism and alter osteoblast activity, thereby interfering with calcium absorption and bone formation, and produce a hormonal imbalance affecting parathyroid hormone, estrogen, and testosterone.

In contrast to heavy drinking, moderate alcohol intake may contribute to bone health.[86] Researchers reported that alcohol intake of about one to three glasses of wine per day in elderly women correlated with higher BMD. Two possible

mechanisms have been proposed for this effect. First, calcitonin production may be stimulated, which has been shown to improve BMD in the spine. Second, moderate alcohol intake may stimulate higher estrogen levels. More research is needed to clarify the impact of alcohol consumption on bone health.

Strategies to Prevent Osteoporosis

Osteoporosis has a strong genetic component, with multiple genes thought to influence the risk.[87] However, the disorder is not inevitable as you age. To preserve bone mass, consume a diet rich in calcium and vitamin D, maintain a healthy body weight, participate in regular exercise, don't smoke, and if you drink alcohol, do so in moderation. Apply the concepts of an adequate diet, healthy

lifestyle, and exercise in the Nutrition in Practice to help Kathy improve her bone density.

LO 12.9: THE TAKE-HOME MESSAGE
Bone mineral density increases during childhood and adolescence, and peaks in early adulthood. Decreased bone mineral density is the hallmark of osteoporosis, a disorder of bones that increases the risk of fracture. To improve and maintain bone mineral density, consume a diet adequate in calcium, magnesium, and potassium, vitamins D and K, omega-3 fatty acids, protein, and kilocalories. Maintain a healthy body weight, participate in weight-bearing exercise, don't smoke, and, if you drink alcohol, do so only in moderation.

NUTRITION *in* PRACTICE:

Physical Therapist and Nurse Practitioner

Kathy is postmenopausal, so her doctor did a bone density scan at her last annual physical. Approximately two weeks after the test the nurse practitioner (NP) called and told Kathy that her T-score was lower than it should be. Kathy was surprised to hear this, as she walks 4 miles daily and considers herself to be in good shape. The NP recommended that she start lifting weights to help increase her bone mineral density as well as her muscle strength. Kathy was reluctant to follow the NP's recommendation as she injured her back in the past when she attempted to lift weights. The NP referred Kathy to a physical therapist (PT) to provide guidance on how to safely add weight lifting to her exercise regimen. The NP also asked Kathy if she drinks milk daily. Because she doesn't, the NP recommended that she take a calcium supplement to make sure that she is consuming adequate amounts of this mineral in her diet. Unfortunately, Kathy once choked when trying to swallow a calcium supplement, and so is scared to try consuming them again. The NP convinces Kathy to make an appointment with a Registered Dietitian Nutritionist (RDN) for dietary guidance.

Kathy's Stats
- Age: 57
- Height: 5 feet 6 inches
- Weight: 155 pounds
- BMI: 25

Critical Thinking Questions

1. Based on her food log, approximately how much calcium is Kathy consuming daily? How much does she need based on her age?

2. How can Kathy add more calcium-rich dairy foods at her meals and snacks to meet her daily needs?

3. What other foods or beverages can she add to her diet to bump up her calcium intake?

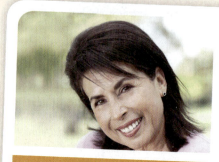

Kathy

KATHY'S FOOD LOG

Food/Beverage	Time Consumed	Hunger Rating*	Location
Coffee with cream (before her morning walk)	6:00 A.M.	4	Kitchen
Oatmeal made with water, orange juice, and coffee with cream	7:30 A.M.	5	Kitchen
Roast beef sandwich with lettuce, a piece of fruit	12:00 P.M.	5	At her desk at work
Baked chicken, small baked potato, and sautéed kale	6:30 P.M.	5	Kitchen
½ pint of sorbet	8:00 P.M.	3	Watching TV

* Hunger Rating (1–5): 1 = not hungry 5 = super hungry.

PT's Observation and Plan for Kathy

- Observe Kathy's weight lifting posture. The PT notices Kathy is using improper form and corrects her technique.
- Recommend Kathy reduce the amount of weight she lifts during her exercises. The PT noticed that some of the problems with Kathy's form were due to selecting weights that were too heavy.
- Create an exercise plan that gradually progresses to more difficult strengthening exercises using heavier weights.

RDN's Observation and Plan for Kathy

- Discuss the need to consume at least 3 servings of low-fat dairy plus a serving of a calcium-fortified food to meet the 1,200 mg of calcium needed daily. Additionally, discuss the need to consume adequate vitamin D in order to use the calcium.
- Replace cream with milk in her morning coffees.

- Prepare her morning oatmeal with skim milk rather than water and switch to calcium-fortified orange juice in the am for another serving of calcium.
- Swap out an ounce of roast beef for 1.5 ounces of low-fat Cheddar cheese to her lunchtime sandwich to add more calcium at the meal.
- Replace her evening snack with a blender smoothie made with 8 ounces of yogurt, ½ cup of frozen berries, and a splash of milk.

Two weeks later, Kathy returns for a follow-up visit with the RDN. She has made all of the changes that the RDN recommended, but doesn't like the evening smoothie. She complains that the smoothie is "too watery." The RDN recommends that she add a half of a banana to the smoothie to thicken it up. Kathy also returns to the PT. After lifting weights three times a week for two weeks, she is ecstatic to be pain free. Kathy is feeling stronger with her new weight training program and plans to continue it for the foreseeable future.

Visual Chapter Summary

LO 12.1 Major and Trace Minerals Are Essential Inorganic Nutrients

Major and trace minerals are chemical elements classified as nutrients because they are essential to human health and must be consumed in the diet. Minerals act as cofactors for enzymes; help maintain fluid and acid–base balance; play a role in energy metabolism, nerve impulse transmission, and muscle contraction; help strengthen bones and teeth; support the immune system; and are involved in growth. The major minerals include sodium, chloride, calcium, phosphorus, potassium, magnesium, and sulfur. The trace minerals include iron, zinc, copper, selenium, chromium, iodide, manganese, molybdenum, and fluoride.

Minerals are found in both plant and animal foods. They vary in their bioavailability. Mineral absorption can be influenced by binding agents in foods, the individual's current mineral status, the amount of the mineral consumed at one time, and competition with other minerals in the GI tract. The kidney regulates mineral levels in the blood by excreting more or less of the mineral as needed, so mineral toxicity is generally rare except through ingesting high doses of supplements.

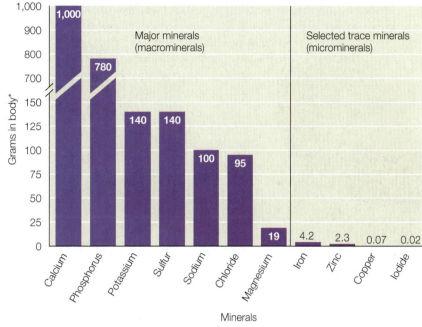

* Based on a 154-pound person

LO 12.2 Sodium

Sodium is a cation that plays important roles in balancing the fluid between the ECF and ICF, transmitting nerve impulses, triggering muscle contractions, and transporting some nutrients across cell membranes. Sodium is also used to preserve food and enhance food flavors. Adults need about 1,500 milligrams of sodium daily but consume more than double that amount, predominantly as sodium chloride (table salt). Processed foods are the major source of sodium in the diet. Too much sodium can contribute to hypertension, hypernatremia, and possibly bone loss. Hypernatremia causes thirst, dry mouth, decreased urination, and lightheadedness. Too little sodium results in hyponatremia, which is characterized by headache, muscle weakness, fatigue, and even seizures and coma.

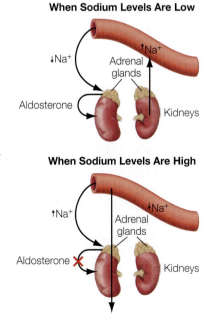

When Sodium Levels Are Low

When Sodium Levels Are High

LO 12.3 Chloride

The anion chloride works with sodium to help maintain fluid balance. Chloride also assists in maintaining pH balance in the blood and is part of hydrochloric acid in the stomach. Adults need 2,300 milligrams per day. Table salt accounts for almost all the chloride you consume. Chloride toxicity is rare and often goes unnoticed, but hyperchloremia can occur due to extreme dehydration. Deficiencies are also rare and are generally caused by extreme vomiting and diarrhea, resulting in hypochloremia, which causes shallow breathing, muscle weakness, spasms, and twitching.

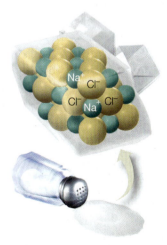

LO 12.4 Potassium

Potassium is a cation that functions in muscle contraction and nerve impulse conduction; it can lower blood pressure, help maintain bone health and fluid balance, act as a blood buffer, and may prevent kidney stones. Adults need 4,700 milligrams of potassium per day. The current recommendations to increase fruits and vegetables in the diet will help meet potassium needs. Excess potassium from dietary supplements results in hyperkalemia, whereas a potassium deficiency causes hypokalemia. Either disorder can cause an irregular heartbeat, nausea, fatigue, and muscle weakness.

Kidney stone

LO 12.6 Phosphorus

Phosphorus is a major component of bones and teeth and cell membranes. It functions as a component of ATP, as part of phospholipids, as an acid–base buffer, and as part of DNA and RNA. Phosphorus is abundant in meat, fish, poultry, and dairy products. The RDA for adults is 700 milligrams of phosphorus daily. Consuming too much phosphorus results in hyperphosphatemia, which can cause calcification of the soft tissues. Symptoms may include muscle cramps and spasms and numbness or tingling. Too little phosphorus causes hypophosphatemia and results in muscle weakness, bone pain, and confusion. In children, rickets can develop.

Phosphorus in phospholipid head — Outside of cell
— Cell membrane
Phospholipid — Inside of cell

LO 12.5 Calcium

Calcium, along with phosphorus, forms hydroxyapatite crystals, which along with collagen provide bones and teeth with strength and structure. Calcium also participates in muscle contraction, the transmission of nerve impulses, blood clotting, and maintaining a normal heartbeat. It may also help to prevent colon cancer and reduce the risk of kidney stones. The RDA for adults is 1,000–1,200 milligrams of calcium per day. Dairy foods can be a good source of both calcium and phosphorus. An excess of calcium causes hypercalcemia, which may result in stomach upset, nausea, bone pain, muscle weakness, kidney stones, or constipation. It may also interfere with the absorption of iron, zinc, magnesium, and phosphorus. A deficiency of calcium causes hypocalcemia and may lead to osteoporosis and bone fractures.

LO 12.7 Magnesium

Magnesium is part of more than 300 enzymes needed for metabolism and to maintain healthy muscles, nerves, heart function, and bone structure. The RDA for adult females ranges from 310 milligrams to 320 milligrams daily, whereas men need 400–420 milligrams. Magnesium is abundant in leafy green vegetables, legumes, and beverages such as coffee and tea. Too much magnesium from taking supplements can cause intestinal problems such as diarrhea, cramps, and nausea. Deficiencies of magnesium are rare but can result from the use of certain medications and cause muscle weakness, seizures, fatigue, depression, and irregular heartbeat.

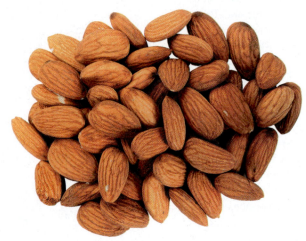

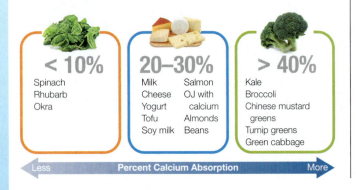

< 10%	20–30%		> 40%
Spinach	Milk	Salmon	Kale
Rhubarb	Cheese	OJ with	Broccoli
Okra	Yogurt	calcium	Chinese mustard
	Tofu	Almonds	greens
	Soy milk	Beans	Turnip greens
			Green cabbage

Less ← Percent Calcium Absorption → More

LO 12.8 Sulfate

Sulfate is the oxidized form of the mineral sulfur found in plants and water. In the body, sulfur provides shape to proteins and is part of the vitamins thiamin and biotin. Sulfur is part of some amino acids and is used as a preservative in processed foods. There is insufficient data to establish an EAR, RDA, AI, or UL for sulfate. The best food sources of sulfate are meats, chicken, and fish, and it can also be found in beverages such as beer and wine. Too much sulfate may contribute to ulcerative colitis. There are no known deficiency symptoms of sulfate.

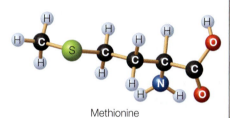

Methionine

LO 12.9 Mineral Intake Influences Bone Health

Osteoporosis is a progressive disorder that results in weak, porous bones that are prone to fracture. Bone growth and buildup of bone mineral density occurs during childhood, adolescence, and early adulthood, when the osteoblasts are more active than the osteoclasts and more bone mass is added than lost. Peak bone mass usually occurs in your 20s. Some additional bone mass can be deposited in your early 30s. The loss of bone mass begins by the mid-30s and continues as you age. Chronic deficiency of dietary calcium and/or vitamin D, excess alcohol consumption, and smoking contribute to an increased risk of osteoporosis. Exercise can help slow the loss of bone mineral density. Other strategies for preserving bone mass include maintaining a healthy body weight, participating in weight-bearing exercise, not smoking, and drinking alcohol only in moderation, if at all.

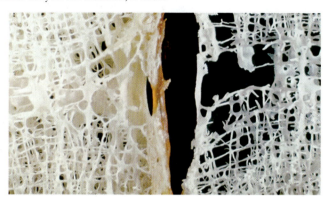

Terms to Know

- minerals
- major minerals
- trace minerals
- binders
- cofactor
- hydroxyapatite
- mineralization
- sodium (Na^+)
- hypernatremia
- hypertonic

- hypotonic
- chloride (Cl^-)
- hyperchloremia
- hypochloremia
- potassium (K^+)
- hyperkalemia
- calcium (Ca^{+2})
- calcitonin
- cortical bone
- trabecular bone
- hypercalcemia
- hypocalcemia

- phosphorus (P)
- hyperphosphatemia
- hypophosphatemia
- magnesium (Mg^{+2})
- sulfate (SO_4)
- bone mineral density (BMD)
- osteoporosis
- peak bone mass
- Type I osteoporosis
- Type II osteoporosis
- osteopenia

Mastering Nutrition
Visit the Study Area in Mastering Nutrition to hear an MP3 chapter summary.

Check Your Understanding

LO 12.1 1. The bioavailability of minerals is reduced by
   a. phytates.
   b. ascorbic acid.
   c. having a deficiency in the mineral.
   d. vitamin D.

LO 12.1 2. Which of the following statements about minerals is true?
   a. Minerals are absorbed in the small intestine in the form of mineral salts.
   b. Like water, minerals are inorganic molecules.
   c. Many minerals in foods are susceptible to destruction by heat.
   d. Abnormally high or abnormally low levels of certain minerals can lead to seizures or convulsions.

LO 12.2 3. The AI for sodium intake for adults up to age 51 is
   a. 3,400 milligrams.
   b. 2,300 milligrams.
   c. 1,500 milligrams.
   d. 180 milligrams.

LO 12.3 4. The major anion found in the extracellular fluid is
   a. potassium.
   b. phosphorus.
   c. sulfate.
   d. chloride.

LO 12.4 5. Hypokalemia is an abnormally low level of _____ in the blood.
a. potassium
b. phosphorus
c. calcium
d. sodium

LO 12.5 6. Blood levels of calcium can be increased by
a. increased excretion of calcium in the urine.
b. increased absorption of calcium through the small intestine.
c. suppression of PTH.
d. high dietary intake of oxalates.

LO 12.6 7. Phosphorus is necessary
a. to maintain magnesium balance.
b. to promote blood clotting.
c. to provide energy as part of ATP.
d. to transmit nerve impulses.

LO 12.7 8. The majority of magnesium is in the
a. blood.
b. bones.
c. muscle cells.
d. extracellular fluid.

LO 12.8 9. Which of the following nutrients does not have an EAR, RDA, AI, or UL?
a. Sulfate
b. Magnesium
c. Calcium
d. Sodium

LO 12.9 10. Which of the following statements about bone mineral density is true?
a. On average, women who are heavier than normal weight have a higher bone mineral density than women who are normal weight or underweight.
b. Most people reach peak bone mass in their mid-30s.
c. DEXA tests compare an individual's bone mineral density with the ideal bone density of a healthy 65-year-old.
d. Moderate alcohol consumption is associated with a decreased bone mineral density.

Answers

1. (a) The bioavailability of minerals is reduced by binders in food, including phytates found in grains. Ascorbic acid (vitamin C) actually increases absorption of certain minerals, as would a deficiency in the mineral.

2. (d) Although you need only small amounts of minerals in your diet, they play enormously important roles in the body, including in fluid and electrolyte balance, nerve impulse transmission, and muscle contraction. Abnormally high or abnormally low levels of electrolytes can lead to seizures or convulsions. Mineral salts in foods dissociate in the stomach and the minerals are absorbed as individual ions in the small intestine. Minerals, which are elements not molecules, are not destroyed by heat.

3. (c) The AI for sodium for adults up to 51 years of age is 1,500 milligrams. The UL for sodium daily is 2,300 milligrams, whereas the absolute minimum is 180 milligrams per day.

4. (d) Chloride is the major anion in the extracellular fluid. Potassium is a major cation inside cells. Phosphorus is a major component of bones and teeth, and sulfate is the oxidized form of sulfur that helps give shape to proteins.

5. (a) Hypokalemia is an abnormally low level of potassium in the blood. The term for low blood phosphorus is hypophosphatemia; hypocalcemia is a low level of calcium; hyponatremia is a low level of sodium in the blood.

6. (b) Calcium blood levels can be raised by increasing the amount absorbed through the small intestine. Suppression of parathyroid hormone (PTH) lowers the level of calcium in the blood by stimulating the kidney to excrete more calcium in the urine. Dietary oxalates reduce the bioavailability of calcium.

7. (c) Phosphorus is a necessary mineral because it is part of the energy molecule ATP.

8. (b) More than half of the magnesium in the body is found in bone. Less than 1 percent is found in the extracellular fluid or the blood. Twenty-five percent of magnesium is found in the muscle.

9. (a) There is not enough data to determine an EAR, RDA, AI, or UL for sulfate. Sodium has an AI, while calcium and magnesium have enough data for an RDA.

10. (a) On average, women who are heavier than normal weight have higher bone mineral density compared to women who are lighter in body weight. Most people reach peak bone mass in their 20s. DEXA tests compare an individual's bone mineral density with that of a healthy 30-year-old. Heavy—not moderate—alcohol consumption is associated with a decreased bone mineral density.

Answers to True or False?

1. **False.** Consuming a diet rich in fruits and vegetables, lean meats, and low-fat dairy products provides ample intake of minerals without the need to take a supplement.

2. **False.** Minerals are not molecules. They are single elements. They are often found either chemically bonded in salts such as sodium chloride or as electrically charged ions such as the electrolytes that contribute to fluid balance.

3. **True.** For most people, following a diet rich in fruits and vegetables, maintaining a healthy weight, avoiding smoking, moderating alcohol intake, and participating in aerobic exercise can reduce the risk of developing hypertension. However, some people who follow these lifestyle choices still develop hypertension.

4. **False.** Foods from both plants and animals are sources of bioavailable minerals.

5. **False.** Eating foods abundant in bioavailable calcium will improve bone density. Fruits are typically not high in calcium.

6. **True.** The DASH diet, which is high in potassium-rich fruits and vegetables, has been shown to lower blood pressure.

7. **False.** Most of the sodium Americans eat is from processed foods.

8. **True.** One serving of milk contains about 300 milligrams of calcium. The RDA for adults age 19–50 is 1,000 milligrams of calcium daily.

9. **False.** Sulfate plays a key role in shaping proteins and in the vitamins thiamin and biotin and is essential to overall health. It is therefore an essential nutrient consumed in the oxidized form.

10. **False.** Excessive alcohol consumption increases the risk of developing osteoporosis. However, moderate alcohol consumption may contribute to bone health.

Web Resources

- For more on the DASH diet, visit DASH for Health at www.dashforhealth.com
- For more on osteoporosis, visit the National Osteoporosis Foundation at www.nof.org
- For more on high blood pressure, visit www.nhlbi.nih.gov

References

1. Nkundabombi, M. G., D. Nakimbugwe, et al. 2016. Effect of Processing Methods on Nutritional, Sensory, and Physicochemical Characteristics of Biofortified Bean Flour. *Food Science and Nutrition* 4(3):384–397. doi: 10.1002/fsn3.301.

2. de Figueiredo, M. A., P. F. Boldrin, et al. 2017. Zinc and Selenium Accumulation and Their Effect on Iron Bioavailability in Common Bean Seeds. *Plant Physiology Biochemistry* 111:193–202. doi: 10.1016/j.plaphy.2016.11.019.

3. Espinoza, A., S. La Blanc, et al. 2012. Iron, Copper, and Zinc Transport: Inhibition of Divalent Metal Transporter 1 (DMT1) and Human Copper Transporter 1 (hCTR1) by shRNA. *Biological Trace Element Research* 146(2):281–286.

4. de Figueiredo, M. A., P. F. Boldrin, et al. 2017. Zinc and Selenium Accumulation and Their Effect on Iron Bioavailability in Common Bean Seeds.

5. Institute of Medicine. 2006. *Dietary Reference Intakes: The Essential Guide to Nutrient Requirements.* J. Otten, J. Hellwig, and L. Meyers, eds. Washington, DC: National Academies Press.

6. Nkundabombi, M. G., D. Nakimbugwe, et al. 2016. Effect of Processing Methods on Nutritional, Sensory, and Physicochemical Characteristics of Biofortified Bean Flour.

7. Dainty, J. R., R. Berry, et al. 2014. Estimation of Dietary Iron Bioavailability from Food Iron Intake and Iron Status. *PloS One* 9(10):e111824. doi: 10.1371/journal.pone.0111824.

8. Gropper, S. S., and J. L. Smith. 2018. *Advanced Nutrition and Human Metabolism.* 7th ed. Belmont, CA: Thomson Wadsworth.

9. Stipanuk, M. H., and M. A. Caudill. 2013. *Biochemical, Physiological, and Molecular Aspects of Human Nutrition.* 3rd ed. Philadelphia: W. B. Saunders.

10. Institute of Medicine. 2006. *Dietary Reference Intakes.*

11. Stipanuk. 2013. *Biochemical, Physiological, and Molecular Aspects of Human Nutrition.*

12. Ibid.

13. Institute of Medicine. 2006. *Dietary Reference Intakes.*

14. Ibid.

15. Ibid.

16. Ibid.

17. American Heart Association. 2017. *The Facts About High Blood Pressure.* Available from www.heart.org. Accessed March 2017.

18. Ibid.

19. Jones, G., T. Beard, et al. 2017. A Population-Based Study of the Relationship between Salt Intake, Bone Resorption, and Bone Mass. *European Journal of Clinical Nutrition* 51:561–565.

20. Kwon, S. J., Y. C. Ha, et al. 2017. High Dietary Sodium Intake Is Associated with Low Bone Mass in Postmenopausal Women: Korea National Health and Nutrition Examination Survey, 2008–2011. *Osteoporosis International* 28(4):1445–1452. doi: 10.1007/s00198-017-3904-8.

21. Shin, J. Y., J. Kim, et al. 2015. Relationship Between Salt Preference and Gastric Cancer Screeing: An Analysis of a Nationwide Survey in Korea. *Cancer Research and Treatment* 48(3):1037–1044. doi: 10.4143/crt.2015.333.

22. The DASH Diet Eating Plan. 2017. Available at http://dashdiet.org. Accessed April 2017.

23. U.S. Food and Drug Administration. 2016. Sodium in Your Diet: Use the Nutrition Facts Label and Reduce Your Intake. Available at https://www.fda.gov/Food/ResourcesForYou/Consumers/ucm315393.htm Accessed March 2017.

24. Institute of Medicine. 2006. *Dietary Reference Intakes.*

25. Ibid.

26. Institute of Medicine. 2005. *Dietary Reference Intakes for Water, Potassium, Sodium, Chloride, and Sulfate.*

27. Moseley, K. F., C. M. Weaver, et al. 2013. Potassium Citrate Supplementation Results in Sustained Improvement in Calcium Balance in Older Men and Women. *Journal of Bone and Mineral Research* 28(3):497–504.

28. Sacco, S. M., M. N. Horcajada, et al. 2013. Phytonutrients for Bone Health during Ageing. *British Journal of Clinical Pharmacology* 75(3):697–707.

29. Areco, V., M. A. Rivoira, et al. 2015. Dietary and Pharmacological Compounds Altering Intestinal Calcium Absorption in Humans and Animals. *Nutrition Research Reviews* 28(2):83–99.

30. Cunningham, P., H. Noble, et al. 2016. Kidney Stones: Pathophysiology, Diagnosis, and Management. *British Journal of Nursing* 25(20):1112–1116.

31. Institute of Medicine. 2006. *Dietary Reference Intakes.*

32. Liu, G. H., and J. S. Zhao. 2017. Truth Behind Hypokalemia. *Annals of Translational Medicine* 5(5):124. doi: 10.21037/atm.2017.03.07.

33. Sheng, P. H. 2013. Body Fluids and Water Balance. In *Biochemical, Physiological, and Molecular Aspects of Human Nutrition.* 3rd ed. Philadelphia: W. B. Saunders.

34. Bihuniak, J. D., R. R. Sullivan, et al. 2014. Supplementing a Low-Protein Diet with Dibasic Amino Acids Increases Urinary Calcium Excretion in Young Women. *Journal of Nutrition* 144(3):282–288.

35. Krupa-Kozak, U., and N. Drabińska. 2016. Calcium in Gluten-Free Life: Health-Related and Nutritional Implications. *Foods* 5(3):51. doi: 10.3390/foods5030051.

36. Stipanuk, M. H. 2013. *Biochemical, Physiological, and Molecular Aspects of Human Nutrition.*

37. Ibid.

38. Da Silva, M. S., and I. Rudkoska. 2014. Dairy Products on Metabolic Health: Current Research and Clinical Implications. *Maturitas* 77(3):221–228.

39. Bertoia, M. L., E. W. Triche, et al. 2014. Mediterranean and Dietary Approaches to Stop Hypertension Dietary Patterns and Risk of Sudden Cardiac Death in Postmenopausal Women. *American Journal of Clinical Nutrition* 99(2):344–351.

40. Heine-Bröring, R. C., R. M. Winkels, et al. 2015. Dietary Supplement Use and Colorectal Cancer Risk: A Systematic Review and Meta-analyses of Prospective Cohort Studies. *International Journal of Cancer* 136(10):2388–2401. doi: 10.1002/ijc.29277.

41. Manson, J. E., and S. S. Bassuk. 2014. Calcium Supplements: Do They Help or Harm? *Menopause* 21(1):106–108.

42. Li, P., C. Fan, et al. 2016. Effects of Calcium Supplementation on Body Weight: A Meta-analysis. *American Journal of Clinical Nutrition* 104(5):1263–1273.

43. Larsen, S. C., L. Angquist, et al. 2014. Interaction between Genetic Predisposition to Obesity and Dietary Calcium in Relation to Subsequent Change in Body Weight and Waist Circumference. *American Journal of Clinical Nutrition* 99(4):957–965.

44. Boon, N., G. B. J. Hul, et al. 2007. An Intervention Study of the Effects of Calcium Intake on Faecal Fat Excretion, Energy Metabolism, and Adipose Tissue mRNA Expression of Lipid Metabolism-Related Proteins. *International Journal of Obesity* 31:1704–1712.

45. Institute of Medicine. 2006. *Dietary Reference Intakes.*

46. NIH Medline Plus. 2011. New Recommended Daily Amounts for Calcium and

Vitamin D. Available at https://medlineplus.gov/magazine/issues/winter11/articles/winter11pg12.html. Accessed March 2017.

47. Stipanuk, M. H. 2013. *Biochemical, Physiological, and Molecular Aspects of Human Nutrition.*

48. Straub, D. 2007. Calcium Supplementation in Clinical Practice: A Review of Forms, Doses, and Indications. *Nutrition in Clinical Practice: Official Publication of the American Society for Parenteral and Enteral Nutrition* 22:286–296.

49. Gropper, S. S., and J. L. Smith. 2018. *Advanced Nutrition and Human Metabolism.* 7th ed. Belmont, CA: Thomson Wadsworth.

50. Ibid.

51. Fang, X., K. Wang, et al. 2016. Dietary Magnesium Intake and the Risk of Cardiovascular Disease, Type 2 Diabetes, and All-Cause Mortality: A Dose Response Meta-Analysis of Prospective Cohort Studies. *BMC Medicine* 14:210. doi: 10.1186/s12916-016-0742-z.

52. Verma, H., and R. Garg. 2017. Effect of Magnesium Supplementation on Type 2 Diabetes Associated Cardiovascular Risk Factors: A Systematic Review and Meta-analysis. *Journal of Human Nutrition and Dietetics.* doi: 10.1111/jhn.12454.

53. Sun, H., B. Shi, et al. 2017. Effects of Sulfate on Heavy Metal Release from Iron Corrosion Scales in Drinking Water Distrubution System. *Water Research* 114:69–77. doi: 10.1016/j.watres.2017.02.021.

54. Ibid.

55. Forsmo, S., H. M. Hvam, et al. 2007. Height Loss, Forearm Bone Density and Bone Loss in Menopausal Women: A 15-Year Prospective Study. The Nord-Trøndelag Health Study, Norway. *Osteoporosis International* 18:1261–1269.

56. National Institutes of Health. 2015 *Osteoporosis Overview.* Available at www.niams.nih.gov/Health_Info/Bone/Osteoporosis/overview.asp. Accessed March 2017.

57. Ibid.

58. Modalsli, E. H., B. O. Åsvold, et al. 2016. Psoriasis, Fracture Risk and Bone Mineral Density: The HUNT Study, Norway. *British Journal of Dermatology.* doi: 10.1111/bjd.15123.

59. Frisco, D. 2017. What Is Osteoporosis? Available at www.spine-health.com. Accessed March 2017.

60. Ibid.

61. National Osteoporosis Foundation. 2013 *Osteoporosis Report.* Available from www.nof.org. Accessed March 2017.

62. Ibid.

63. Sacco. 2013. Phytonutrients for Bone Health during Ageing.

64. Hamidi, M. S., O. Gajic-Veljanoski, et al. 2013. Vitamin K and Bone Health. *Journal of Clinical Densitometry* 16(4): 409–413.

65. Mangano, K., J. Kerstetter, et al. 2014. An Investigation of the Association between Omega-3 FA and Bone Mineral Density among Older Adults: Results from the National Health and Nutrition Examination Survey Years 2005–2008. *Osteoporosis International* 25(3):1033–1041.

66. Langsetmo, L., S. I. Barr, et al. 2016. Dietary Patterns in Men and Women Are Simultaneously Determinants of Altered Glucose Metabolism and Bone Metabolism. *Nutrition Research* 36(4):328–336. doi: 10.1016/j.nutres.2015.12.010.

67. Movassagh, E. Z., and H. Vatanparast. 2017. Current Evidence on the Association of Dietary Patterns and Bone Health: A Scoping Review. *Advanced Nutrition* 8(1):1–16. doi: 10.3945/an.116.013326.

68. Ibid.

69. Lind, T., A. Sundqvist, et al. 2013. Vitamin A Is a Negative Regulator of Osteoblast Mineralization. *PLoS One* 8(12):e82388.

70. Kim, M. H., and H. J. Lee. 2016. Osteoporosis, Vitamin C Intake, and Physical Activity in Korean Adults Aged 50 Years and Over. *Journal of Physical Therapy Science* 28(3):725–730. doi: 10.1589/jpts.28.725

71. Berz, K., and T. McCambridge. 2016 Amenorrhea in the Female Athlete: What to Do and When to Worry. *Pediatrci Annals* 45(3):e97–e102. doi: 10.3928/00904481-20160210-03.

72. Gabel, L., H. M. Macdonald, et al. 2017. Physical Activity, Sedentary Time, and Bone Strength From Childhood to Early Adulthood: A Mixed Longitudinal HR-pQCT Study. *Journal of Bone Mineral Research*. doi: 10.1002/jbmr.3115.

73. Bilek, L. D., N. L. Waltman, et al. 2016. Protocol for a Randomized Controlled Trial to Compare Bone-loading Exercises with Risedronate for Preventing Bone Loss in Osteopenic Postmenopausal Women. *BMC Women's Health*. 16(1):59. doi:10.1186/s12905-016-0339-x.

74. McCrory, J. L., A. J. Salacinski, et al. 2013. Competitive Athletic Participation, Thigh Muscle Strength, and Bone Density in Elite Senior Athletes and Controls. *Journal of Strength and Conditioning Research*

27(11):3132–3141. doi: 10.1519/JSC.0b013e31828bf29d.

75. Gómez-Bruton, A., A. Gónzalez-Agüero, et al. 2013. Is Bone Tissue Really Affected by Swimming? A Systematic Review. *PLoS* doi: 10.1371/journal.pone.0070119.

76. Gombos Császár, G., V. Bajsz, et al. 2014. The Direct Effect of Specific Training and Walking on Bone Metabolic Markers in Young Adults with Peak Bone Mass. *Acta Physiologica Hungarica* 6:1–11.

77. Boudreaux, R. D., J. M. Swift, et al. 2014. Increased Resistance During Jump Exercise Does Not Enhance Cortical Bone Formation. *Medicine and Science in Sports and Exercise* 46(5):982–989. doi:10.1249/MSS.0000000000000195.

78. Hamilton, K. C., G. Fisher, et al. 2013. The Effects of Weight Loss on Relative Bone Mineral Density in Premenopausal Women. *Obesity* 21(3):441–448.

79. Misra, M., N. H. Golden, et al. 2016. State of the Art Systematic Review of Bone Disease in Anorexia Nervosa. *International Journal of Eating Disorders* 49(3):276–292. doi:10.1002/eat.22451.

80. Emaus, N., T. Wilsgaard, et al. 2014. Impacts of Body Mass Index, Physical Activity,

and Smoking on Femoral Bone Loss: The Tromso Study. *Journal of Bone Mineral Research*. doi:10.1002/jbmr.2232.

81. Weaver, C. M., C. M. Gordon, et al. 2016. The National Osteoporosis Foundation's Position Statement on Peak Bone Mass Development and Lifestyle Factors: A Systematic Review and Implementation Recommendations. *Osteoporosis International* 27:1281–1386. doi:10.1007/s00198-015-3440-3.

82. Ibid.

83. Emaus, N., T. Wilsgaard, et al. 2014. Impacts of Body Mass Index, Physical Activity, and Smoking on Femoral Bone Loss: The Tromso Study.

84. Ibid.

85. Gaddini, G. W., R. T. Turner, et al. 2016. Alcohol: A Simple Nutrient with Complex Actions on Bone in the Adult Skeleton. *Alcoholism. Clinical and Experimental Research* 40(4):657–671. doi: 10.111/acer.13000.

86. Ibid.

87. Mafi Golchin, M., L. Heidari, et al. 2015. Osteoporosis: A Silent Disease with Complex Genetic Contribution. *Journal of Genetics and Genomics* 43(2):49–61. doi: 10.1016/j.jgg.2015.12.001.

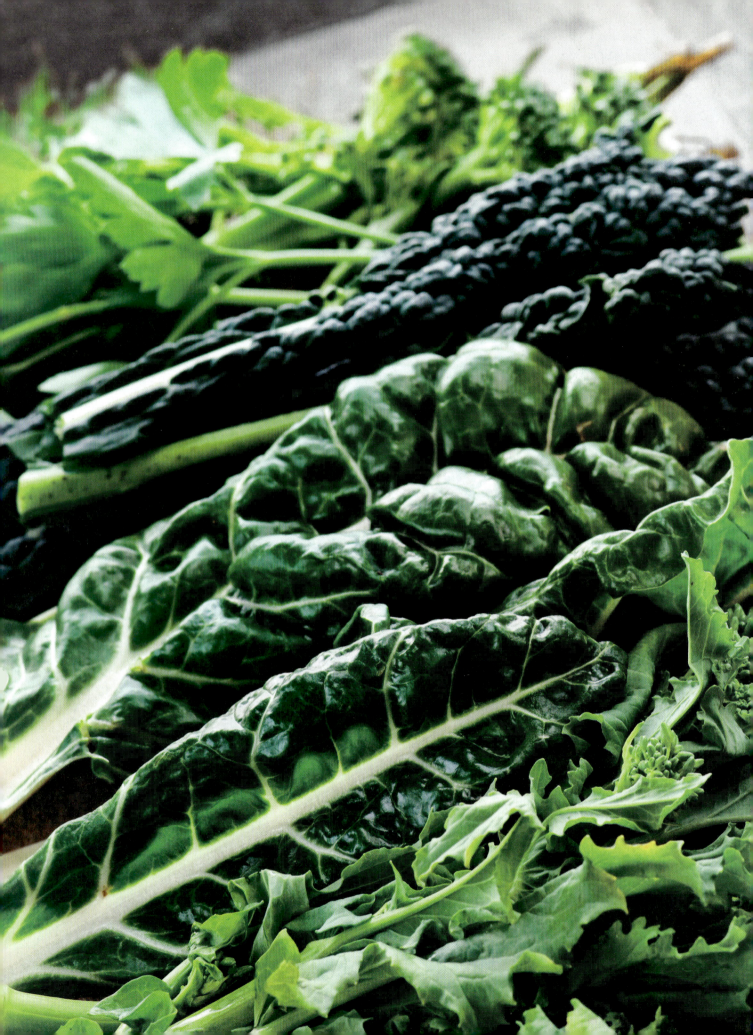

Trace Minerals

Learning Outcomes

After reading this chapter, you will be able to:

13.1 Discuss the characteristics and functions of trace minerals in the body.

13.2 Describe the mechanisms of iron absorption and transport, functions, recommended intakes, food sources, and toxicity and deficiency effects of iron.

13.3 Describe the functions, recommended intakes, food sources, and toxicity and deficiency effects of copper.

13.4 Describe the functions, recommended intakes, food sources, and toxicity and deficiency effects of zinc.

13.5 Describe the functions, recommended intakes, food sources, and toxicity and deficiency effects of selenium.

13.6 Describe the functions, recommended intakes, food sources, and toxicity and deficiency effects of fluoride.

13.7 Describe the functions, recommended intakes, food sources, and toxicity and deficiency effects of chromium.

13.8 Describe the functions, recommended intakes, food sources, and toxicity and deficiency effects of iodine.

13.9 Describe the functions, recommended intakes, food sources, and toxicity and deficiency effects of molybdenum.

13.10 Describe the functions, recommended intakes, food sources, and toxicity and deficiency effects of manganese.

13.11 Identify several minerals that may contribute to body functions but are not considered essential nutrients.

13.12 Explain the causes and treatments for the various nutrient-deficiency anemias.

True or False?

1. Trace minerals are called "trace" because food contains such small amounts. **T**/**F**

2. Meat is the primary source of iron in the American diet. **T**/**F**

3. Taking iron supplements can cause a copper deficiency. **T**/**F**

4. Zinc can cure the common cold. **T**/**F**

5. Consuming too much selenium can cause vomiting and diarrhea. **T**/**F**

6. Most bottled waters contain fluoride. **T**/**F**

7. Chromium can help weightlifters build bigger muscles. **T**/**F**

8. Iodized salt is the only reliable source of iodine. **T**/**F**

9. Cinnamon is a good source of manganese. **T**/**F**

10. Consuming leafy green vegetables ensures a diet rich in molybdenum. **T**/**F**

See page 503 for the answers.

There has been an eruption of new evidence in trace mineral research in the past decade. Science is now able to track the biochemical movement of these trace elements and is finding new links that connect a lack of these intriguing nutrients to disease. In this chapter, we examine the important functions and unique qualities of the trace minerals. We also discuss the amounts needed in the diet, the absorption and transport of each, and the best foods from which to obtain them.

What Are Trace Minerals and Why Do You Need Them?

LO 13.1 Discuss the characteristics and functions of trace minerals in the body.

Iron, zinc, selenium, fluoride, chromium, copper, iodine, manganese, and molybdenum are known as the **trace minerals** (or microminerals). The human body needs them in much smaller amounts than it needs the major minerals. Collectively, less than 5 grams of trace minerals are found in the body,[1] and even though the daily dietary need for each is less than 20 milligrams, they are just as necessary for health as other nutrients. **Table 13.1** identifies the trace minerals, their functions, food sources, and nutrient interactions that we cover in this chapter.

Similar to the major minerals, trace minerals are found in both plant and animal foods, but the best food sources are whole grains, legumes, dairy, meat, and seafood. The trace mineral amount found in a given plant food depends partly on the mineral content in the soil in which the food was grown. In addition, processing removes trace minerals found in the bran and germ of grains. For this reason, whole grains contain more trace minerals than do refined grains. Trace minerals found in all foods are stable in cooking.

Bioavailability of Trace Minerals Can Vary

As with the major minerals, the bioavailability of trace minerals can vary according to an individual's nutritional status, other foods that are eaten, and the form of the mineral.

Trace minerals often compete with each other for absorption in the GI tract. Some trace minerals, such as iron, copper, and zinc, are absorbed in their ionic state, have the same ionic charge $\left(^{+2}\right)$, and use the same protein carriers during absorption. Too much of one of these minerals, such as iron, Fe^{+2}, can cause a decrease in the absorption and metabolism of another, for example, copper, Cu^{+2}, leading to an imbalance.[2] Thus, bioavailability of each mineral depends on the amount of both minerals in the GI tract at the time of absorption. This is one reason why most people should avoid taking single-mineral supplements. Some trace minerals, such as iron, are recycled in the body and can be used repeatedly.

Most Trace Minerals Function as Cofactors

Several trace minerals function as cofactors within an enzyme complex. The enzymes that trace minerals attach to and activate are referred to as **metalloenzymes**. For example, iron, copper, and selenium are important cofactors within antioxidant enzyme systems.

Other essential roles of trace minerals include helping hormones function; for example, iodine is a component of the thyroid hormone thyroxine. Iron, copper, and zinc

trace minerals Minerals required in amounts smaller than 100 milligrams per day that are essential to health; also called *microminerals*.

metalloenzymes Active enzymes that contain one or more metal ions that are essential for their biological activity.

TABLE 13.1

TABLE 13.1 Metabolic Function, Daily Needs, Food Sources, and Symptoms of Toxicity and Deficiency of the Trace Minerals

Trace Mineral	Metabolic Function	Daily Needs (19 years +)	Food Sources	Toxicity Symptoms/ UL	Deficiency Symptoms	Interaction with Other Nutrients
Iron (Fe)	• Major component of hemoglobin and myoglobin; carries oxygen and carbon dioxide • Part of cytochromes • Enhances immune system	Women: 18 mg/day Men: 8 mg/day	Meat, fish, poultry, enriched and fortified breads and cereals	• Nausea and vomiting, diarrhea, constipation • Organ damage, including the kidney and liver UL: 45 mg	• Fatigue • Microcytic anemia • Poor immune function • Growth retardation in infants	• Zinc • Calcium • Ascorbic acid
Copper (Cu)	• A component of several metalloenzymes • Enzymes involved in iron metabolism • Connective tissue enzymes • Antioxidant enzymes	900 μg/day	Cocoa, whole grains, legumes, and shellfish	• Nausea and vomiting, abdominal pain, diarrhea • Liver damage UL: 10,000 μg	• Anemia • Impaired immune function • Impaired growth and development	• Zinc • Iron
Zinc (Zn)	• Cofactor for several metalloenzymes • DNA and RNA synthesis • Part of the enzyme superoxide dismutase	Women: 8 mg/day Men: 11 mg/day	Seafood, meat, whole grains	• Nausea and vomiting, cramps, diarrhea • Loss of appetite • Headaches • Impaired immune function UL: 40 mg	• Skin rash and hair loss • Diarrhea • Loss of taste and smell • Depressed growth and development	• Iron • Calcium and phosphorus • Copper • Folate • Protein • Phytates
Selenium (Se)	• A component of antioxidant enzymes	55 μg/day	Meat, seafood, fish, eggs, whole grains	• Brittle hair and nails • Skin rash • Garlic breath odor • Fatigue • Irritability UL: 400 μg	• Muscle weakness and pain • May trigger Keshan disease	Unknown
Fluoride (F)	• Part of fluoroapatite, which makes teeth stronger • Enhances bone formation	Women: 3 mg/day Men: 4 mg/day	Fluoridated water, tea, seaweed	• Fluorosis in teeth and skeletal fluorosis UL: 10 mg	• Increased susceptibility to dental caries	• Calcium
Chromium (Cr)	• Improves insulin response	Women: 20–25 μg/day Men: 30–35 μg/day	Pork, egg yolks, whole grains, nuts	• Unconfirmed toxicity effects Data insufficient to establish a UL	• Elevated postmeal blood glucose	• Vitamin C • Phytates • Simple sugars
Iodine (I)	• Component of the thyroid hormone thyroxine	150 μg/day	Iodized salt, seafood, dairy products	• Thyroiditis • Goiter • Hypothyroidism and hyperthyroidism UL: 1,100 μg	• Goiter • Cretinism	Unknown
Molybdenum (Mo)	• Cofactor for a variety of metalloenzymes	45 μg/day	Legumes, nuts, leafy vegetables, dairy, cereals	Unknown in humans UL: 2,000 μg	Unknown in humans	Unknown
Manganese (Mn)	• Cofactor for metalloenyzmes involved in carbohydrate metabolism	Women: 1.8 mg/day Men: 2.3 mg/day	Beans, oats, nuts, tea	• Abnormal central nervous system effects UL: 11 mg	Unknown in humans	• Calcium • Iron • Phytates

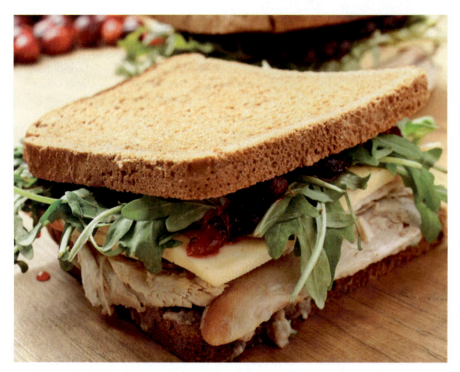

The ingredients of this sandwich are good sources of trace minerals: The whole-wheat bread contributes zinc, copper, chromium, iodine, and manganese to your diet, while a few slices of low-fat turkey add iron, zinc, and selenium. Top off your sandwich with manganese-rich leafy greens and cranberries packed with selenium to make this a meal brimming with a variety of essential trace minerals.

support the health of red blood cells. Some trace minerals, such as fluoride, are part of the structure of bones and teeth.

Trace Mineral Deficiencies and Toxicities Are Hard to Identify

Because trace minerals are found in short supply in the body, symptoms of deficiency are hard to identify, and deficiencies are often overlooked. This fact also makes it difficult to establish recommended intakes, including Tolerable Upper Intake Limits (ULs) to prevent toxicity.

In this chapter we cover each individual trace mineral in detail, beginning with iron.

LO 13.1: THE TAKE-HOME MESSAGE Trace minerals are inorganic nutrients that the human body needs in small amounts. Their bioavailability is affected by the amount in the body and whether the mineral competes with other substances for absorption. Trace minerals act as cofactors within enzyme systems, contribute to hormones, maintain red blood cells, and are part of the structure of bones and teeth.

EXPLORING Iron

LO 13.2 Describe the mechanisms of iron absorption and transport, functions, recommended intakes, food sources, and toxicity and deficiency effects of iron.

heme iron Iron that is part of a heme group found in hemoglobin in the blood, myoglobin in muscles, and in the mitochondria as part of the cytochromes.

nonheme iron Iron that is not attached to heme.

hemoglobin Oxygen-carrying, heme-containing protein found in red blood cells.

myoglobin Oxygen-carrying, heme-containing protein found in muscle cells.

What Is Iron?

Iron (Fe) is the most abundant mineral on Earth, and the most abundant trace mineral in the body. A 130-pound female has over 2,300 milligrams (2.3 grams) of iron—about the weight of a dime—in her body, whereas a 165-pound male has 4,000 milligrams (4.0 grams)—slightly less than the weight of two dimes.[3] Iron deficiency is the most common nutrient deficiency around the world, and iron-deficiency anemia is common in women of childbearing age and children, particularly in the developing world, but also in the United States.

Two forms of iron are found in foods: **heme iron** and **nonheme iron**. Heme iron is part of the proteins **hemoglobin** (in red blood cells) and **myoglobin** (in muscle cells) and part of cytochromes in the electron transport chain. It is therefore found in animal foods such as meat, poultry, and fish. Plant foods don't contain heme iron but do contain nonheme iron, as do animal foods. Nonheme iron comprises more than 80 percent of the iron consumed in foods (100 percent for vegans). Nonheme iron is the form of iron used to enrich breads and fortify cereals.

Iron Bioavailability

The bioavailability of iron is influenced by several factors, including the molecular form of the iron, the iron status of the individual, and the types of food eaten at the same time. Iron is found in foods either as an oxidized form $\left(Fe^{+3}\right)$ called **ferric iron** or nonheme iron, or the reduced form $\left(Fe^{+2}\right)$ called **ferrous iron**, which is the heme form of iron.

Heme iron is two to three times more bioavailable than nonheme iron. Nonheme iron is often bound to acids, such as oxalates in leafy vegetables or polyphenols in tea and coffee, which makes it more difficult to absorb. A serving of cooked spinach, for example, contains approximately 6 milligrams of nonheme iron, but less than 1 percent is absorbed because of the oxalates in the spinach. The polyphenols in tea or coffee can reduce the absorption of nonheme iron in a meal by as much as 70 percent.[4]

There are ways in which nonheme iron bioavailability can be improved (see **Table 13.2**). For example, adding vitamin C to a meal that contains nonheme iron can enhance its rate of absorption. In the GI tract, vitamin C donates an electron to the ferric form, which reduces it to the more bioavailable ferrous form. As little as 25 milligrams of vitamin C—the amount in about one-quarter cup of orange juice—can double the amount of nonheme iron absorbed from a meal and 50 milligrams of vitamin C can increase the amount absorbed by about sixfold.

Another way to enhance nonheme iron absorption from foods is to eat meat, fish, or poultry at the same meal as the nonheme iron source; this is referred to as the MFP (*meat, fish, and poultry*) factor. The peptides in these animal-derived foods are thought to be the enhancing factors. The meat in a turkey sandwich helps enhance the absorption of the nonheme iron in whole-wheat bread.

Let's look more closely at the mechanisms that affect iron absorption.

Iron Absorption and Transport

The absorption–transport mechanism of iron (**Figure 13.1**) is tightly controlled, thereby regulating the amount of iron absorbed into the body and preventing iron toxicity. Once the iron is absorbed into the blood, only 1–2 grams is lost daily from the body (except during blood loss).

Iron must cross two cell membranes in the small intestine, the brush border and the basolateral membrane, before it is absorbed into the portal vein. Heme iron crosses the brush border of the enterocyte attached to a protein carrier. Once inside the enterocyte, the enzyme *heme oxygenase* releases the ferrous iron $\left(Fe^{+2}\right)$ from hemoglobin.[5] If the body does not need the iron immediately, ferrous iron is oxidized to the ferric form and binds to the protein **ferritin**, which acts as a temporary storage form of iron in the intestine.

Once ferritin becomes saturated with iron, additional iron can be attached to another protein called **hemosiderin** for storage. If not needed by the body, this iron remains stored until the intestinal cells are sloughed off and excreted through the feces.

Nonheme iron is absorbed less efficiently than heme iron. Nonheme iron must first be released during digestion and reduced to ferrous iron $\left(Fe^{+2}\right)$ by stomach acids and pepsin to improve its absorption rate across the brush border. Both the ferrous $\left(Fe^{+2}\right)$ and ferric $\left(Fe^{+3}\right)$ forms of iron from nonheme sources are absorbed across the brush border attached to a transport protein. The alkaline environment of the small intestine renders nonheme iron less soluble and thus less bioavailable. Like heme iron, once inside the enterocyte, nonheme iron is stored attached to ferritin until needed or excreted as intestinal cells are sloughed off. Any nonheme iron that remains bound to food or other compounds in the GI tract remains unabsorbed and is excreted in the feces.

When the body needs iron, the ferritin stored within the enterocyte releases the ferric $\left(Fe^{+3}\right)$ iron, which is again reduced to the ferrous $\left(Fe^{+2}\right)$ form. Ferrous iron attaches to **ferroportin**, a protein that transports the iron across the basolateral membrane into the portal vein. Once ferroportin crosses the basolateral membrane, it releases the ferrous iron $\left(Fe^{+2}\right)$. Ferrous iron is once again oxidized to ferric iron $\left(Fe^{+3}\right)$ by a copper-containing enzyme called **hephaestin** and attaches to a protein carrier in the blood called **transferrin**, which transports the iron throughout the body.[6]

TABLE 13.2	Factors That Influence Iron Absorption
Enhance Iron Absorption	**Decrease Iron Absorption**
• Sufficient hydrochloric acid in the stomach • The form of iron in the food; heme iron is more easily absorbed than nonheme iron • Increased need for iron (blood loss, pregnancy, growth) • Vitamin C in the small intestine at the same time • Presence of MFP factor (meat, fish, poultry)	• Phytates in cereal grains (dietary fiber) • Oxalates • Polyphenols (tea or coffee) • Reduced hydrochloric acid in stomach • Excess use of antacids • Excess minerals such as calcium, zinc, and magnesium

ferric iron Oxidized form of iron $\left(Fe^{+3}\right)$.

ferrous iron Reduced form of iron $\left(Fe^{+2}\right)$.

ferritin Protein that stores iron in the intestine.

hemosiderin Protein that stores iron in the body.

ferroportin Protein found on the basolateral surface of the enterocyte that transports iron out of the enterocyte into the portal vein.

hephaestin Copper-containing enzyme that catalyzes the conversion of ferrous to ferric iron before attaching to transferrin for transport.

transferrin Iron-transporting protein.

(continued)

Iron (continued)

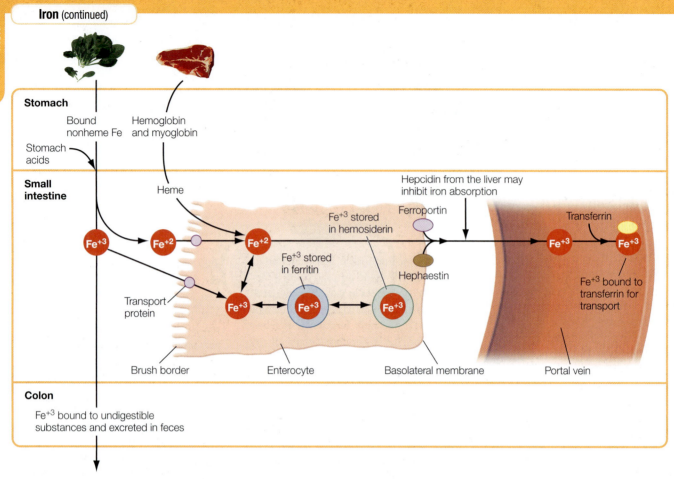

Stomach

Bound nonheme Fe

Hemoglobin and myoglobin

Stomach acids

Small intestine

Heme

Hepcidin from the liver may inhibit iron absorption

Ferroportin

Transferrin

Fe^{+3} stored in hemosiderin

Fe^{+3}

Fe^{+2}

Fe^{+2}

Fe^{+3} stored in ferritin

Hephaestin

Fe^{+3}

Fe^{+3}

Fe^{+3} bound to transferrin for transport

Transport protein

Fe^{+3}

Fe^{+3}

Fe^{+3}

Brush border

Enterocyte

Basolateral membrane

Portal vein

Colon

Fe^{+3} bound to undigestible substances and excreted in feces

▲ **Figure 13.1 The Absorption and Transport of Iron**
Iron is absorbed into the enterocyte and attached to ferritin in the enterocyte. When the body requires iron, it is released from ferritin, attached to ferroportin, oxidized to ferric iron by hephaestin, and transported through the blood attached to transferrin. The liver hormone hepcidin controls the process. Additional iron can be attached to the protein hemosiderin for storage.

Hormonal Regulation of Iron Absorption

A hormone produced by the liver called **hepcidin** controls iron absorption.[7] When iron stores are high, the liver produces more hepcidin, which inhibits ferroportin from transporting iron across the basolateral membrane—in a sense, trapping the iron in the enterocyte. When iron stores are low, hepcidin levels are decreased, which allows ferroportin to actively transport iron out of the enterocyte into the portal blood.

Stored Iron Affects Iron Absorption

Iron status influences the amount of ferritin produced in the GI tract. Thus, if the iron stores in the body are low, less

ferritin is produced, to allow more iron to be absorbed directly into the bloodstream. In other words, the lower the stores, the greater the percentage of iron absorbed. If the body contains adequate iron stores, it absorbs an average of 14–18 percent of the iron consumed in the average mixed diet. When iron stores are high, the amount of iron absorbed can be as low as 5 percent of the iron consumed because more ferritin and hepcidin are produced to block iron from absorption and to store the iron in the enterocytes.

Iron Recycling

As a key component of blood, iron is highly valuable to the body and is treated accordingly. The amount of iron absorbed is not sufficient to meet the body's daily iron needs; therefore, approximately 95 percent of the iron in the body is recycled and reused.[8] In blood, the iron found in the heme portion of hemoglobin is broken down in the liver and spleen, with 20–25

milligrams of iron salvaged per day. This iron is then used for synthesizing new red blood cells in the bone marrow, incorporated into iron-containing enzymes, or stored as ferritin for use later. Very little iron is excreted or shed in hair, skin, and sloughed-off intestinal cells. In fact, most iron loss is due to bleeding.

Metabolic Functions of Iron

Iron plays a major role in a variety of key functions. It participates in oxidation-reduction reactions because of its ability to be changed from its ferrous $\left(Fe^{+2}\right)$ to ferric $\left(Fe^{+3}\right)$ forms and back again. This is illustrated in the nearby Chemistry Boost.

Hemoglobin and Myoglobin Transport Oxygen

Approximately two-thirds of the iron in the body is in hemoglobin and myoglobin

hepcidin Hormone produced in the liver that regulates the absorption and transport of iron.

Chemistry Boost

The Oxidation and Reduction of Iron

Iron can exist in two valence states: ferrous (Fe^{+2}) and ferric (Fe^{+3}). Ferric (Fe^{+3}) iron is *reduced* to ferrous (Fe^{+2}) iron, meaning it has gained electrons and has a more negative oxidation number $(^{+2}$ vs. $^{+3})$. The opposite is true when ferrous iron is oxidized to ferric iron; it loses an electron and the oxidation number increases.

$$Fe^{+2} \leftrightarrow Fe^{+3} + e^-$$

Recall that:

When a substance is oxidized, it . . .	When a substance is reduced, it . . .
Loses electrons	Gains electrons
Has a more positive oxidation number	Attains a more negative oxidation number
Is the reducing agent	Is the oxidizing agent

(**Figure 13.2**). The heme in hemoglobin binds with oxygen from the lungs and transports it to the tissues for their use. Hemoglobin also picks up a small amount of carbon dioxide waste products from the cells and transports them back to the lungs to be exhaled.

Similarly, iron is part of the protein myoglobin that transports and stores oxygen in the muscles. Heme in myoglobin accepts oxygen from hemoglobin and transports it to the muscle cells, including those of the heart. Myoglobin also transports the carbon dioxide produced in the muscle cells to hemoglobin in the blood for excretion. In other words, myoglobin in the muscle works with hemoglobin in the blood in the exchange of oxygen and carbon dioxide.

Iron Participates in Energy Metabolism

Iron performs as a cofactor in enzymes involved in energy metabolism. Recall from Chapter 8 that electrons produced during glycolysis and in the TCA cycle are delivered to the electron transport chain by nicotinamide adenine dinucleotide plus hydrogen and flavin adenine dinucleotide $(NADH^+ + H^+$ and $FADH_2)$. Along with flavoproteins, iron-containing cytochromes in the inner mitochondrial membrane transfer the electrons down the chain to eventually produce ATP, carbon dioxide, and water. Iron also participates in the conversion of citrate to isocitrate in the TCA cycle. In iron-deficiency anemia, both of these functions are diminished, which leads to fatigue.

Iron Is Important for Immune Function

Iron is necessary for the production of the lymphocytes and macrophages that help fight infection, and macrophages may store iron to prevent pathogens from using the mineral to multiply.[9] Iron is also a cofactor for several antioxidant enzyme systems involved in protecting cell membranes from free radical damage.

Iron Is Needed for Brain Function

In the brain, iron helps enzymes that are involved in the synthesis of neurotransmitters, including dopamine, epinephrine, norepinephrine, and serotonin, which send messages to the rest of the body.[10] A deficiency of iron in children can impact cognitive development and their ability to learn and retain information. Studies have shown that children with iron-deficiency anemia in their early years can have persistent, decreased cognitive ability during their later school years.[11]

Daily Needs for Iron

The current RDA for iron needed by adult females, age 19–50, is 18 milligrams a day to cover the iron lost during menstruation. After menopause, usually around age 50, a woman's daily iron needs drop to 8 milligrams because she is no longer losing blood monthly. Adult males need 8 milligrams of dietary iron daily. The recommendations for women and men take into account a typical American diet, which

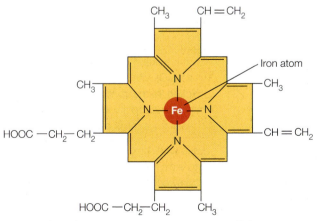
Heme portion containing iron (Fe)

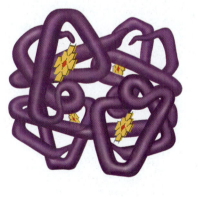
Hemoglobin

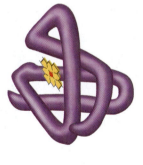
Myoglobin

▲ **Figure 13.2 Iron-Containing Hemoglobin and Myoglobin**
Iron is part of the heme in hemoglobin and myoglobin.

(continued)

Iron (continued)

includes both heme and nonheme iron sources. Vegetarians may need to eat as much as 1.8 times the amount of iron as nonvegetarians. This is due to the lower bioavailability of iron from plant foods.[12]

Adult men consume more than twice their recommended iron needs—over 16 milligrams, on average, daily. Adult premenopausal women consume only about 70 percent of their daily need, or approximately 13 milligrams, on average. Postmenopausal women consume slightly over 12 milligrams of iron daily, so, like men, they are more than meeting their needs.

Food Sources of Iron

About half of Americans' dietary iron intake comes from iron-enriched bread and other grain foods such as cereals (see **Figure 13.3**).[13] Meat, fish, poultry, and egg yolks are rich sources of efficiently absorbed heme iron, which contributes 12 percent of the dietary needs of males and females.[14] Cooking foods in iron pans and skillets can also increase their nonheme iron content, as foods absorb iron from cookware.[15] For more information on boosting your iron intake, see the Table Tips.

Iron Toxicity

Hepcidin, the liver hormone that circulates in the blood, controls iron balance and prevents iron toxicity. Hepcidin binds to ferroportin, the protein that exports iron out of the enterocyte and prevents excess iron from entering the blood. The iron is stored in the enterocyte until the intestinal cells slough off and the iron is lost in the feces. In

◄ **Figure 13.3 Food Sources of Iron**
Source: Data from *USDA What's In The Food You Eat?* 2016. Available at https://www.ars.usda.gov. Accessed March 2017.

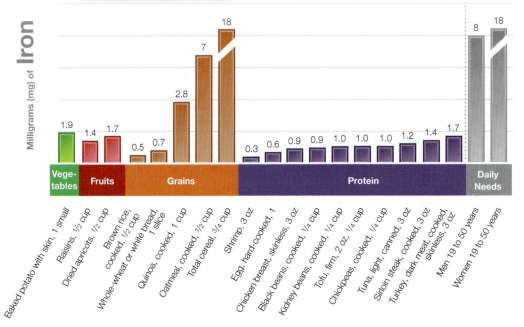

Cooking foods in a cast-iron skillet can increase the nonheme iron content of the food.

TABLE TIPS

Increase Your Iron Intake

Enjoy an iron-enriched whole-grain cereal along with a glass of vitamin C–rich orange juice to boost the nonheme iron absorption in cereal.

Add plenty of salsa (vitamin C) to bean burritos to enhance the absorption of the nonheme iron in both the beans and the flour tortilla.

Stuff a baked potato (nonheme iron, vitamin C) with shredded cooked chicken (heme iron) and broccoli (vitamin C) and top it with melted low-fat cheese for a quick and iron-rich dinner.

Eat a small box of raisins (nonheme iron) and a clementine or tangerine (vitamin C) as a sweet snack that's abundant in iron.

Add chickpeas (nonheme iron) to salad greens (vitamin C). Don't forget the tomato wedges for another source of iron-enhancing vitamin C.

healthy people, hepcidin increases when the storage of iron is high and decreases when iron storage is low.[16] When iron is overconsumed in supplements, this *mucosal block* is overwhelmed and too much iron is absorbed, causing iron toxicity. Consuming too much iron from supplements can cause constipation, nausea and vomiting, and diarrhea. The UL for iron for adults is set at 45 milligrams daily, as this level is slightly less than the amount known to cause these intestinal symptoms. This upper level doesn't apply to, and is too high for, individuals with liver disease or certain genetic disorders that can affect iron stores in the body.

Iron Poisoning in Children

In the United States the accidental consumption of supplements containing iron is the leading cause of poisoning deaths in children under age 6. Ingestion of as little as 200 milligrams has been shown to be fatal. Children who swallow iron supplements can experience symptoms such as nausea and vomiting and diarrhea within minutes. Intestinal bleeding can also occur, which can lead to shock, coma, and even death. The FDA has mandated that a warning statement about the risk of iron poisoning in small children be put on every iron supplement label and that pills that contain 30 milligrams or more of iron must be individually wrapped.[17]

Iron Overload

Undetected excessive storing of iron in the body over several years is called *iron overload*

hemochromatosis Genetic disorder that causes the body to store excessive amounts of iron.

and can damage tissues and organs, including the heart, kidneys, liver, and nerves. **Hemochromatosis**, a genetic disorder in which individuals absorb too much dietary iron, can cause iron overload. Though this condition is congenital, its symptoms often don't manifest until adulthood. If not diagnosed and treated early enough, organ damage can occur. Individuals with hemochromatosis need to avoid iron supplements throughout their lives, as well as large amounts of vitamin C supplements, which enhance iron absorption.

Other Effects of Iron Toxicity

Some studies suggest that excessive iron can stimulate free radical production in the body, which can damage the coronary arteries and contribute to heart disease. It has also been suggested that iron's role in free radical production may increase the risk of cancer. Though this association is not definite, unless you are medically diagnosed with iron deficiency, it doesn't make any sense to consume excessive amounts of iron.

Iron Deficiency

If the diet is deficient in iron, body stores will be slowly depleted so as to keep blood hemoglobin in a normal range. Iron-deficiency anemia occurs when body stores are so depleted that blood hemoglobin levels decrease. Red blood cells contain less heme and become small and pale. This diminishes the delivery of oxygen through the body, causing fatigue and weakness. Individuals with iron-deficiency anemia are also more susceptible to and have a reduced ability to fight infections.[18] Health Connection: What Are

Nutrient-Deficiency Anemias? provides more information on this deficiency.

Because of their increased iron needs, pregnant women, menstruating women, and teenage girls, especially those with heavy blood losses, and preterm or low-birthweight infants, as well as older infants and toddlers, often don't meet their iron needs and are at risk of becoming deficient.[19]

The best way to prevent iron deficiency is through an iron-rich diet as described in Nutrition in Practice: Evelyn on page 478.

LO 13.2: THE TAKE-HOME MESSAGE

The absorption of iron is controlled by iron status, the molecular form of the iron, and types of foods eaten together. Iron is stored as ferritin or hemosiderin and transported attached to transferrin. Iron functions in energy metabolism and is needed for a healthy immune system and brain function. The RDA for iron is 18 milligrams per day for menstruating women and 8 milligrams per day for men and postmenopausal women. There are two different forms of iron in the foods we eat: heme iron, which is found only in animal-based foods, and nonheme iron, which is found in both animal and plant foods. Adults with normal GI tract functioning have little risk of developing iron toxicity from food. Iron toxicity can develop from taking supplements. Hemochromatosis caused by a genetic mutation is associated with iron buildup in the body and possibly death. Iron deficiency results in iron-deficiency anemia. A deficiency of iron in children can impact their ability to learn and retain information.

(continued)

NUTRITION *in* PRACTICE:
Nurse Practitioner

Evelyn is a college freshman majoring in hospitality. In addition to a full-time class credit load, she is waitressing on weekends at a local Italian restaurant. Evelyn is trying to gain some restaurant experience during the school year so that she can secure a hospitality internship at a large restaurant chain during the summer. While she always seems to be tired because of her school work and job commitments, this semester she is extremely lethargic and her appetite has decreased. She has lost weight over the last three months. Evelyn has complained to her roommate that she is sometimes light-headed, especially during her menstruation, which has become more intense and lasts longer than usual. Her roommate mentioned to her that she looked very pale and volunteered to walk with her to the college Student Health Center.

As soon as she reached the receptionist at the Health Center, her knees started to buckle, and she felt as though she was going to faint. The nurse practitioner (NP) attended to her immediately. After obtaining a medical history, the NP ordered a complete blood count (CBC) from the lab. The blood test revealed that she had iron-deficiency anemia. While the NP recommended that Evelyn take an iron supplement, he also wanted her to meet with a Registered Dietitian Nutritionist (RDN) to make sure that her diet contained adequate kilocalories and iron-rich foods.

Evelyn's Stats

- ❑ Age: 17
- ❑ Height: 5 feet 7 inches
- ❑ Weight: 120 pounds
- ❑ BMI: 18.8

Critical Thinking Questions

1. What factors might have contributed to Evelyn's diagnosis of iron deficiency anemia?
2. Based on her food log, which iron-rich food group is Evelyn likely falling short of in her diet?

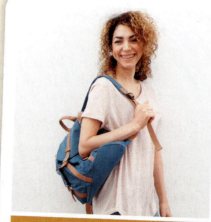

Evelyn

EVELYN'S FOOD LOG

Food/Beverage	Time Consumed	Hunger Rating*	Location
Muffin	7:00 A.M.	3	Dining Hall
Coffee with milk	11:30 A.M.	3	Coffee shop
Peanut butter jelly sandwich, water	1:30 P.M.	5	Dining Hall
Pasta and tomato sauce	6:30 P.M.	5	Dining Hall
Iced tea	10:00 P.M.	3	Bedroom, Watching Netflix

*Hunger Rating (1–5): 1 = not hungry; 5 = super hungry.

3. What foods can be added to her meatless meals that would improve her body's absorption of nonheme iron?

RDN's Observation and Plan for Evelyn

- ❑ Support the NP's recommendation to take an iron supplement.
- ❑ Discuss the difference between heme and nonheme iron in the diet and the role of vitamin C and MFP Factor in increasing the absorption of nonheme iron.
- ❑ Add a source of vitamin C, such as orange or grapefruit juice, with her morning muffin.
- ❑ Suggest adding an iron-fortified whole grain cereal on some mornings with the vitamin C-rich juice.
- ❑ Add a tossed salad with vitamin C-rich foods, such as tomatoes and broccoli, with her meatless lunches.

- ❑ Alternate her meatless lunches with sandwiches containing meat, fish or poultry, such as roast beef, tuna, or turkey breast.
- ❑ Snack on raisins along with a vitamin C-rich fruit, such as kiwis or strawberries, in the evening.

Two weeks later, Evelyn returns for a follow-up visit with the RDN. She is feeling less tired and enjoys eating roast beef and turkey breast sandwiches at lunch. She is eating more vitamin C-rich fruit, but doesn't like the raisins as an evening snack. The RDN suggested Evelyn continue to take the iron supplement and eat sandwiches at lunch as well as snacking on nuts more frequently to increase her iron intake. She also suggested that Evelyn try dried apricots, which are a good source of iron and can be purchased at the campus convenience store.

EXPLORING **Copper**

LO 13.3 Describe the functions, recommended intakes, food sources, and toxicity and deficiency effects of copper.

What Is Copper?

Copper (Cu) may bring to mind ancient tools, great sculptures, or American pennies (although pennies are no longer made of solid copper), but it is also associated with several key body functions. Copper is found in two forms in the body: the oxidized **cupric** $\left(Cu^{+2}\right)$ form and the reduced **cuprous** $\left(Cu^{+}\right)$ form.

Copper Absorption and Transport

Copper is absorbed mostly in the small intestine. As with iron, the absorption of copper is based on the body's need for the mineral and the ability to free copper from food complexes during digestion with the aid of hydrochloric acid and pepsin in the stomach.

The absorption mechanisms for copper are not clear. However, the current understanding is that once copper is free, it is reduced to the cupric $\left(Cu^{+2}\right)$ state by enzymes on the surface of the enterocytes and then absorbed across the brush

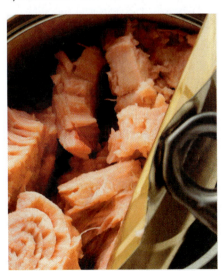

border, mostly by active transport. After crossing the brush border, copper is either used by the enterocyte, stored attached to a zinc-containing protein called metallothionein, or transported across the basolateral membrane into the blood.

The bioavailability of copper can be enhanced by amino acids, especially those that contain sulfur. However, phytates in legumes and cereals bind copper and can reduce its bioavailability, as with iron. Excess zinc can also reduce the bioavailability of copper because zinc stimulates more metallothionein, which binds copper in the enterocyte. Because of their electron configuration, iron, calcium, molybdenum, and phosphorus compete with copper for absorption. Vitamin C supplements reduce the absorption of copper, at least in animals, and can contribute to a copper deficiency.[20]

Absorbed copper crosses the basolateral membrane and attaches to the protein albumin to be transported through the portal vein to the liver. In the liver, copper is incorporated into another protein called **ceruloplasmin**. Very little copper, about 100 milligrams, is stored in the body. Most excess copper is excreted through the feces as part of bile.

Metabolic Functions of Copper

Copper is part of several metalloenzymes and proteins. Many of these proteins are essential for oxidation reactions and in reducing damage by free radicals. Copper-containing ceruloplasmin is the enzyme mentioned earlier that oxidizes iron from the ferrous form $\left(Fe^{+2}\right)$ to the ferric form $\left(Fe^{+3}\right)$ (**Figure 13.4**). If the diet is deficient in copper, the amount of copper-containing enzymes hephaestin and ceruloplasmin are reduced and iron accumulates in the enterocyte rather than being attached to and transported by transferrin. A copper deficiency can thus result in iron-deficiency anemia.[21]

As part of the cytochromes, copper assists in energy production in the electron transport chain. And as part of the enzyme lysyl oxidase, copper links the proteins collagen and elastin together in connective tissue. Superoxide dismutase is a copper-containing enzyme that protects cells from free-radical damage.

In addition, copper also helps synthesize melanin (the dark pigment found in skin) and plays an important role as a cofactor in blood clotting and immune response.[22]

cupric copper Oxidized form of copper $\left(Cu^{+2}\right)$.

cuprous copper Reduced form of copper $\left(Cu^{+}\right)$.

ceruloplasmin Protein found in the blood that transports copper.

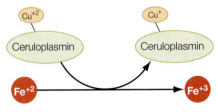

▲ **Figure 13.4 Ceruloplasmin Oxidizes Iron**
The copper-containing protein ceruloplasmin oxidizes ferrous iron $\left(Fe^{+2}\right)$ to ferric iron $\left(Fe^{+3}\right)$ before iron can bind to transferrin for transport in the blood.

(continued)

Copper (continued)

Daily Needs for Copper

The Adequate Intake (AI) for copper for adult women and men is set at 900 micrograms daily. U.S. women consume 1,000–1,100 micrograms, whereas men consume 1,300–1,500 micrograms daily, on average.

Food Sources of Copper

Organ meats (such as liver), seafood, nuts, and seeds are abundant in copper. Bran cereals, whole-grain products, and cocoa are also good sources (see **Figure 13.5**). Although potatoes, milk, and chicken are low in copper, they are consumed in such abundant amounts that they contribute a fair amount of copper to Americans' diets. For more information on increasing your copper intake, see the Table Tips.

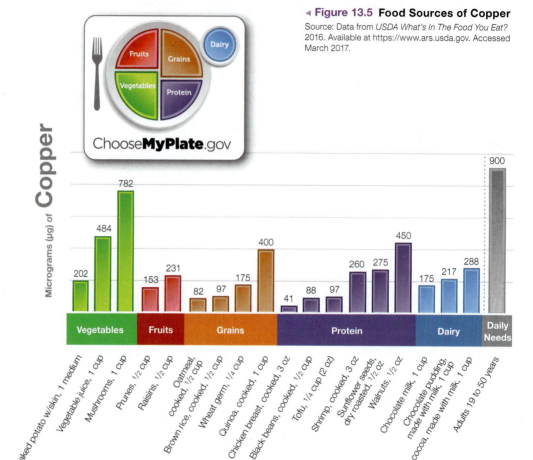

◄ **Figure 13.5** **Food Sources of Copper**
Source: Data from *USDA What's In The Food You Eat?* 2016. Available at https://www.ars.usda.gov. Accessed March 2017.

TABLE TIPS

Counting Copper

Make hot cocoa with milk, rather than water, for two sources (cocoa and milk) of copper.

Mix raisins with brown rice at dinner.

Top chocolate pudding with a sprinkling of crushed walnuts for a dessert that is both sweet and crunchy.

Choose sunflower seeds for an afternoon snack.

Ladle black beans and salsa into a whole-wheat pita. Top with reduced-fat cheddar cheese. Zap it in the microwave for a Mexican lunch with a copper kick.

Menkes' disease Genetic disorder that interferes with copper absorption.

Wilson's disease Rare genetic disorder that results in accumulation of copper in the body.

Copper Toxicity and Deficiency

Excessive intakes of copper supplements can cause stomach pain and cramps, nausea and vomiting, diarrhea, and even liver damage. The upper level for copper for adults is set at 10,000 micrograms daily.

Copper deficiency is rare in the United States. Its symptoms resemble those of iron deficiency: fatigue and weakness. It has occurred in premature babies fed milk formulas, in malnourished infants fed cow's milk, and in individuals given intravenous feedings that lacked adequate amounts of copper.

Two genetic diseases affect copper metabolism. **Menkes' disease** is a copper transport disorder. Copper accumulates in the kidney, brain, and liver and can cause developmental problems, osteoporosis, cardiovascular disease, and death. **Wilson's disease** prevents the body from excreting copper through the bile.

An accumulation of copper in the brain and liver results in severe liver and brain damage if left untreated.

LO 13.3: THE TAKE-HOME MESSAGE
Copper is absorbed in the small intestine and transported attached to albumin. The bioavailability of copper is reduced by iron, zinc, molybdenum, calcium, phosphorus, and vitamin C supplements. Copper is part of ceruloplasmin, the cytochromes, and other metalloenzymes and proteins involved in energy production and the synthesis of connective tissue. It is also part of the superoxide dismutase enzyme. The AI for copper is 900 micrograms for adults. Copper is found in seafood, nuts, and seeds. Copper toxicity is caused by some genetic diseases but deficiencies are rare.

EXPLORING Zinc

LO 13.4 Describe the functions, recommended intakes, food sources, and toxicity and deficiency effects of zinc.

What Is Zinc?

Zinc (Zn^{+2}) is found in very small amounts in almost every cell of the body, but mostly in bone and muscle. It is involved in the function of more than 100 metalloenzymes, including those used for protein synthesis.

Zinc Absorption, Transport, and Recycling

Like iron and copper, the absorption of zinc is controlled at the small intestine (**Figure 13.6**). Once it has been absorbed into the enterocyte, zinc is bound to a protein called **metallothionine**, which stores it and temporarily prevents it from being absorbed into the portal vein. The body produces more metallothionine when zinc stores are high, to prevent toxicity,

and less when zinc is deficient. If the zinc isn't needed, it diffuses into the lumen of the small intestine and is excreted through the feces. When it is needed, zinc stored in enterocytes is released from metallothionine and attaches to a transport protein for absorption across the basolateral membrane. The zinc is then released to attach to albumin for transport through the portal vein to the liver.

Zinc absorption can be reduced when high levels of nonheme iron are present in the GI tract. The use of iron supplements may be a factor in zinc status, and diets high in fiber and phytates also reduce zinc absorption. Consuming animal protein improves zinc absorption.

Zinc is found in the intestine as part of the pancreatic digestive juices. Because these juices are repeatedly excreted into and reabsorbed by the small intestine, zinc is recycled back to the pancreas to be reused. The zinc that is not recycled is excreted in the feces. Zinc can also be excreted in small amounts in the urine, sweat, and sloughed-off skin and hair.

Metabolic Functions of Zinc

Zinc plays a role in growth and development, in the immune system, and in the healing of wounds. It also influences taste and can help fight macular degeneration.

Zinc Is Needed for DNA Synthesis

Zinc is necessary for DNA and RNA synthesis. Zinc helps regulate gene expression by turning genes on and off, thus controlling transcription.[23] Delayed growth and maturation in children is a characteristic of zinc deficiency.

Zinc Supports the Immune System

Zinc affects a variety of key factors involved in maintaining a healthy immune system. For example, zinc is a component

metallothionine Metal-binding protein rich in sulfur-containing amino acids that transports ions.

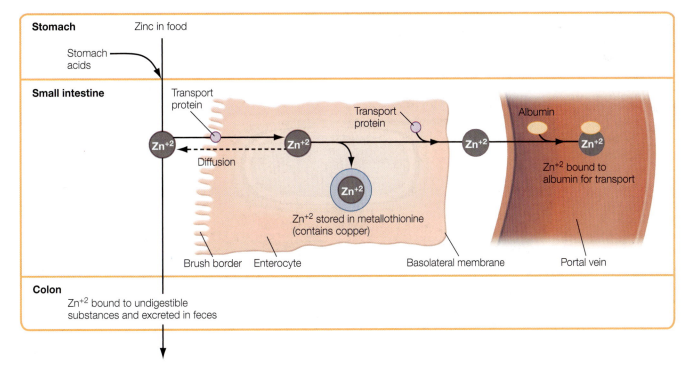

▲ **Figure 13.6 Zinc Absorption**
Zinc is absorbed into the enterocyte and attached to metallothionine for storage. When the body needs more zinc, it is released from metallothionine, transported across the basolateral membrane, and attached to albumin for transport through the body.

(continued)

Zinc (continued)

of thymic hormone, which controls and facilitates the maturation of lymphocytes and killer macrophages. Zinc also acts as an antioxidant and stabilizes cell membranes to provide a barrier to infection.[24] Without sufficient zinc, cell membranes become more susceptible to damage by free radicals and oxidation. Zinc helps reduce the inflammation that can accompany skin wounds and helps wounds heal by being part of enzymes and proteins that repair skin cells and enhance their proliferation.[25]

Zinc lozenges are sometimes advertised to help reduce the severity and duration of the common cold. Whereas early research found little benefit to using them,[26] more recent research from Finland suggests zinc lozenges or syrup, if taken within 24 hours of the first sign of the sniffles, reduce a cold's severity and duration.[27] Zinc gluconate used as a nasal gel may also show promise, as it has lessened the duration[28] and the severity of cold symptoms in some cases.[29] Though the mechanism is still unclear, researchers suggest that zinc gels may reduce the duration of colds by blocking the viral infection at the site where cold viruses enter the body— the nasal passage. But not everyone is convinced. Possible side effects of the use of zinc nasal gels or lozenges include loss of smell, bad taste in the mouth, and nausea. More research is needed to understand the dosage and possible side effects before any recommendations can be made.

Zinc Improves Taste Perception

Zinc activates areas of the brain that perceive taste

and smell. Its importance to appetite was first demonstrated in 1972 when researchers showed that taste disorders responded to zinc supplementation. Zinc has also been reported to influence taste preferences especially for salty foods.[30] This may be related to zinc's role in taste and smell.

Zinc May Help Prevent Age-Related Macular Degeneration

Research studies show that zinc may play a role in reducing the risk of age-related macular degeneration (AMD), a condition that hampers central vision. Zinc may work with an enzyme in the eyes that is needed to properly use vitamin A for vision. Zinc may also help mobilize vitamin A from the liver to ensure adequate blood levels of this vitamin. Supplements that contain antioxidants along with zinc have been shown to reduce the risk of AMD. (For more information about the causes and treatment of AMD, see Chapter 9.)

Daily Needs for Zinc

The current RDA for adult men is 11 milligrams of zinc daily, whereas women need 8 milligrams daily. American adults, on average, are meeting their zinc needs. Men are consuming from 11 milligrams to over 14 milligrams daily and women are consuming 8–9 milligrams of zinc daily, on average.

Vegetarians, especially strict vegetarians, may need to consume 50 percent more zinc compared to nonvegetarians. The bioavailability of zinc is lower in a vegetarian meal plan because it excludes meat. The foods that vegetarians consume, such as grains and legumes that are high in phytates, can bind with zinc, reducing its absorption in the GI tract and stores of zinc in the body.[31]

Food Sources of Zinc

Red meat, some seafood, and whole grains are excellent sources of zinc (**Figure 13.7**). The dark meat in chicken and turkey is higher in zinc than the white meat.

▼ **Figure 13.7** **Food Sources of Zinc**
Source: Data from *USDA What's In The Food You Eat?* 2016. Available at https://www.ars.usda.gov. Accessed March 2017.

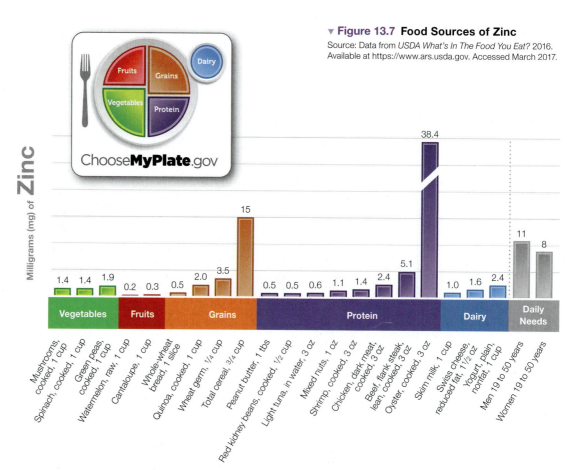

Because zinc is found in the germ and bran portion of grains, refined grains have as much as 80 percent less zinc than whole grains. This is yet another reason to favor whole-grain products over those made with refined grains. For more ways to boost your zinc intake, see the Table Tips.

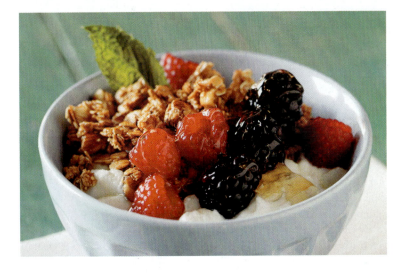

TABLE TIPS
Rethink Your Zinc

Enjoy a tuna fish sandwich on whole-wheat bread at lunch for a double serving (fish and bread) of zinc.

Add kidney beans to a soup or salad.

Pack a small handful of mixed nuts and raisins in a zip-closed bag for a snack on the run.

Make oatmeal with milk for two servings of zinc in one bowl.

Add cooked green peas to casseroles, stews, soups, and salads.

Zinc Toxicity and Deficiency

The upper level for zinc in food and/or supplements for adults is set at 40 milligrams daily. Consuming too much zinc, as little as 50 milligrams, can cause stomach pains, nausea and vomiting, and diarrhea. Approximately 60 milligrams of zinc daily has been shown to lower body levels of copper by competing for absorption in the GI tract. This is an excellent example of how the overconsumption of one mineral can compromise the benefits of another. Excessive amounts, such as 300 milligrams of zinc

daily, have been shown to suppress the immune system and lower HDL ("good") cholesterol.

A zinc deficiency can result from too much iron, which can interfere with zinc transport. The transport protein transferrin transports both zinc and iron. In an iron overload, transferrin becomes saturated with iron. This saturation reduces the sites available for zinc transport. Iron transport is also impaired if transferrin is saturated with zinc.

A deficiency of zinc can cause hair loss, loss of appetite, impaired taste of foods, diarrhea, and delayed sexual maturation, as well as impotence and skin rashes.

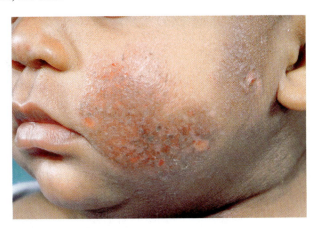

Skin rash is one of the symptoms of zinc deficiency.

A chronic deficiency of zinc during childhood can slow and impair growth. Classic studies of groups of people in the Middle East showed that people who consumed a diet mainly of unleavened bread, which is high in zinc-binding phytates, experienced impaired growth and dwarfism.[32] Impaired growth may be partially reversed if zinc is restored in the diet.

LO 13.4: THE TAKE-HOME MESSAGE
Zinc is part of the RNA and DNA structure, functions in taste acuity, and helps prevent age-related macular degeneration. Zinc isn't effective in preventing the common cold but may reduce the duration of a cold. The RDA for zinc is 11 mg for adult males and 8 mg for adult females. Zinc is found in meat, fish, and whole grains. Zinc toxicity causes vomiting and diarrhea, suppresses the immune system, and lowers HDL cholesterol, whereas a zinc deficiency impairs growth, causes loss of hair and appetite, and delays sexual maturation.

EXPLORING Selenium

LO 13.5 Describe the functions, recommended intakes, food sources, and toxicity and deficiency effects of selenium.

What Is Selenium?

The mineral selenium (Se) is a component of a class of proteins called **selenoproteins**, many of which are enzymes. Most dietary selenium is in the form of **selenomethionine**. Unlike iron and zinc, selenium absorption is based on the individual's needs. In fact, more than 85 percent of dietary selenium is absorbed mostly in the duodenum by passive diffusion.[33] Once absorbed, selenium is stored as selenomethionine or selenoprotein in a variety of tissues, including the liver, muscles, kidneys, and bone (**Figure 13.8**).

selenoproteins Proteins that contain selenomethionine.

selenomethionine Amino acid that contains selenium rather than sulfur.

Homeostasis of selenium is maintained by the kidneys, which excrete excess amounts through the urine.

Metabolic Functions of Selenium

Three selenium-containing enzymes help regulate thyroid hormones in the body. These enzymes activate and deactivate thyroid hormone to maintain balance and promote normal development and growth by regulating the thyroid gland.

Selenoproteins, such as glutathione peroxidase, function as antioxidants that protect the cells from free-radical damage. Research studies have suggested that deaths from cancers, such as lung, colon, and prostate cancers, are lower in groups of people who consume more selenium.[34] Selenium's antioxidant capabilities, and its ability to potentially slow the growth of tumors, are thought to be the mechanism behind its anticancer effects.[35]

The FDA allows a Qualified Health Claim on food labels and dietary supplements that states, "Selenium may reduce the risk of certain cancers but the evidence is limited and not conclusive to date."[36]

Daily Needs for Selenium

The RDA for both adult females and males is set at 55 micrograms of selenium daily. American adults are more than meeting their needs—they consume about 80–160 micrograms daily, on average. The RDA is set to maintain optimal activity of the enzyme glutathione peroxidase. Most manufacturers do not include selenium on food labels unless the food has been fortified with the mineral. In this case, the label uses 70 micrograms as the standard for the percent Daily Value.

Food Sources of Selenium

Nuts, meat, seafood, cereal, grains, dairy foods, and fruits and vegetables can all contribute to dietary selenium (see **Figure 13.9**). However, the amount of selenium in foods depends on the soil where the plants were grown and the animals grazed. For example, wheat grown

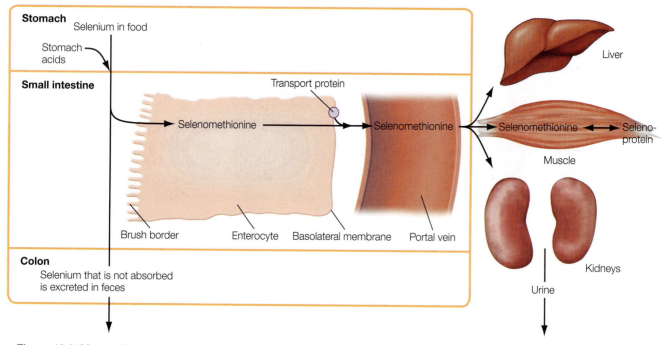

▲ **Figure 13.8 Metabolism of Selenium**
Selenium is easily absorbed, transported, and stored in the body, mostly as selenomethionine.

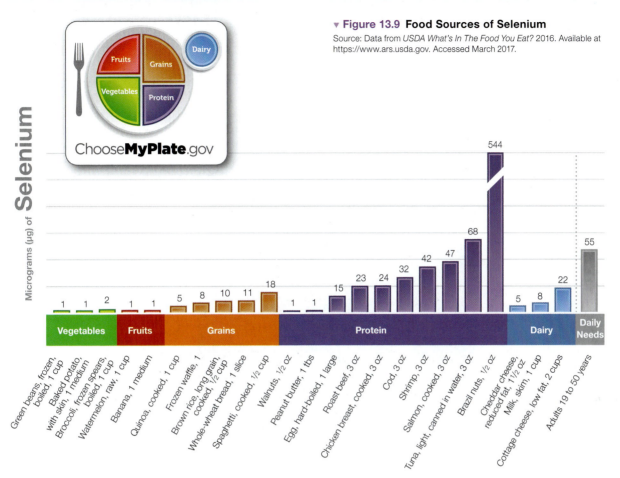

▼ **Figure 13.9** **Food Sources of Selenium**
Source: Data from *USDA What's In The Food You Eat?* 2016. Available at https://www.ars.usda.gov. Accessed March 2017.

in selenium-rich soil can have more than a tenfold higher amount of the mineral than wheat grown in selenium-poor soil. See the Table Tips for suggestions on boosting your selenium intake.

TABLE TIPS

Seek Selenium

Top a toasted whole-wheat bagel with a slice of reduced-fat cheddar cheese for a hot way to start the day.

Spread peanut butter on whole-wheat crackers. Top each cracker with a slice of banana.

Top dinner pasta with broccoli for a selenium-smart meal.

Zap sliced apples, sprinkled with a little apple juice and cinnamon, in the microwave and top with vanilla yogurt for a tasty snack.

Spoon a serving of low-fat cottage cheese into a bowl and top with canned sliced peaches and almonds for a fabulous dessert.

Selenium Toxicity and Deficiency

Too much selenium can cause toxicity and a condition called **selenosis**. A person with selenosis will have brittle nails and hair, both of which may fall out. Other symptoms include stomach and intestinal discomfort, a skin rash, garlicky breath, fatigue, and damage to the nervous system. A chronic intake of as little as 1–3 milligrams per day can result in toxicity. Thus, the upper level for selenium for adults is set at 400 micrograms daily to prevent the loss and brittleness of nails and hair.

Though rare in the United States, a selenium deficiency can cause **Keshan disease**, which damages the heart. This disease typically only occurs in children who live in rural areas that have selenium-poor soil. However, some researchers speculate that selenium deficiency alone may not cause Keshan disease, but the selenium-deficient individual may also be exposed to a virus, which, together with the selenium deficiency, causes the damaged heart.[37]

Some reports suggest that selenium deficiencies may result in changes in thyroid hormone.[38] For example, there is a higher incidence of thyroiditis, such as the autoimmune thyroid disease called Hashimoto's, in individuals with lower levels of selenium.[39] This may be due to a decrease in activity of enzymes that require selenium as a cofactor within thyroid cells.

> **LO 13.5: THE TAKE-HOME MESSAGE**
> Selenium is part of selenoproteins, which act as antioxidants. Selenium also regulates thyroid function. Adults need 55 micrograms of selenium per day. All food groups contribute selenium, including nuts, meat, and seafood. Selenium toxicity causes brittle teeth and fingernails, garlic odor in the breath, gastrointestinal problems, and damage to the nervous system. A selenium deficiency can lead to Keshan disease and changes in thyroid hormone production.

selenosis Presence of toxic levels of selenium.

Keshan disease Disease related to a deficiency of selenium.

(continued)

EXPLORING Fluoride

LO 13.6 Describe the functions, recommended intakes, food sources, and toxicity and deficiency effects of fluoride.

What Is Fluoride?

Fluoride (F^-) is the safe ionic form of fluorine, a poisonous gas. Fluoride is not classified as essential because the body does not require it for normal growth and development. However, it plays a critical role in developing strong teeth that are resistant to decay.

Fluoride is found naturally in plants and animals and is often added to the water supply. Almost all the fluoride consumed in the diet is absorbed in the small intestine and taken up by the bones and developing teeth.

Metabolic Functions of Fluoride

While no tissue or cellular process requires fluoride to function, fluoride has been shown to help maintain healthy teeth. Fluoride forms **fluoroapatite** by replacing the OH in hydroxyapatite crystals with fluoride. Fluoroapatite helps harden the outer layer of the tooth (the *enamel*) and makes the tooth more resistant to damage (see **Figure 13.10**). Over time, acids produced by bacteria in the mouth, and from acidic foods and beverages, erode tooth enamel. Continual exposure of the teeth to these acids, especially during tooth formation, or if fluoride is lacking, can result in dental caries.

Fluoride from food, beverages, and dental products, such as toothpaste, can repair enamel that has already started to erode. Fluoride also interferes with the ability of the bacteria to metabolize carbohydrates, thus reducing the amount of acid they produce, and provides a protective barrier between the tooth and the destructive acids. Fluoride in the saliva continually

fluoroapatite Crystalline structure that results when hydroxyapatite has been changed by exposure of the tooth to fluoride.

bathes the teeth's surface, which helps remineralize the hydroxyapatite structure of the tooth and reduce the effect of the

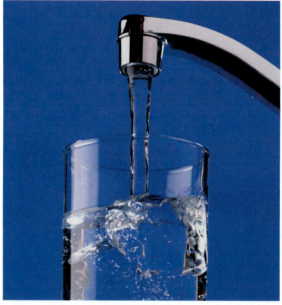

Tap water can be a good source of fluoride in communities that have fluoridated water.

bacteria.[40] Consuming adequate amounts of fluoride is extremely important during infancy and childhood, when teeth are developing, and for maintenance of healthy teeth throughout life.

In the 1930s, scientists noticed lower rates of dental caries among individuals

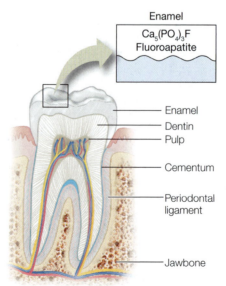

▲ **Figure 13.10 Structure of Fluoroapatite in Teeth**

whose community water systems contained significant amounts of fluoride. Studies confirmed that the fluoride was the protective factor in the water. Since 1945, most communities have fluoridated their water, and today 67 percent of Americans live in communities that have a fluoridated water supply.[41] The increase in access to fluoridated water is the major reason there has been a decline in dental caries in the United States, and fluoridation of water is considered one of the 10 greatest public health advances of the twentieth century.[42]

Fluoride also helps maintain strong bones by stimulating the osteoblasts. Fluoride in combination with calcium and vitamin D may increase bone mineral density and reduce the incidence of osteoporosis.

Daily Needs for Fluoride

The AI for fluoride for adult men has been set at 3.8 milligrams and 3.1 milligrams for adult women. The Department of Health and Human Services estimates the optimal level of fluoridated tap water to prevent tooth decay is 0.7 milligrams per liter.[43] At this level, an individual would have to consume at least 15 cups of water daily, through either beverages or cooking, to meet fluoride needs $(1 \text{ liter} = 4.2 \text{ cups})$.

Currently, adults consume 1.4–3.4 milligrams of fluoride daily if they are living in communities with fluoridated water. The number drops to only 0.3–1.0 milligram consumed daily if the water isn't fluoridated.[44] In 2012 more than 74.6 percent of people were drinking fluoridated water.[45] This is close to the *Healthy People 2020* goal that 79.6 percent of people consume water that has the optimum level of fluoride recommended for preventing tooth decay.[46]

Food Sources of Fluoride

Foods in general are not a good source of fluoride. The best sources are fluoridated water and beverages and foods made with this water, such as coffee, tea, and soups. Another source of fluoride can be juices made from concentrate using fluoridated tap water (remember, not all tap water contains fluoride). Water and processed beverages such as soft drinks account for up to 75 percent of Americans' fluoride intake.[47] Tea is also a good source of fluoride, as tea leaves accumulate fluoride. Because the decaffeination process involves the use of mineral water, which is naturally high in fluoride, decaffeinated tea has twice the amount of fluoride as the caffeinated variety.[48] Want more ideas on increasing your fluoride intake? See the Table Tips.

Most bottled waters sold in the United States have less than the optimal amount of fluoride. It is difficult to determine the fluoride content of many bottled waters because currently fluoride amounts only have to be listed on the label if fluoride has been specifically added. Consumers need to check the label to see if the bottled water they purchase contains added fluoride.

Fluoride Toxicity and Deficiency

Having some fluoride is important for healthy teeth, but too much can cause **fluorosis**, a condition whereby the teeth

TABLE TIPS
Find More Fluoride

Pour orange juice into ice cube trays and pop a couple of frozen cubes into a glass of tap water for a refreshing and flavorful beverage.

Use tap water when making coffee, tea, or juice from concentrate and for food preparation.

Brew a mug of flavored decaffeinated tea, such as French vanilla or gingerbread, to keep you warm while you're hitting the books.

become mottled (pitted) and develop white patches or stains on the surface (**Figure 13.11**). Fluorosis creates teeth that are extremely resistant to caries but cosmetically unappealing.

Fluorosis occurs when teeth are forming, so only infants and children up to 8 years of age are at risk. Once teeth break through the gums, fluorosis can't occur. Fluorosis results from overfluoridation of water, swallowing toothpaste, or excessive use of dental products that contain fluoride. Some research suggests that fluorosis may be reversible, but more studies are needed to determine this.

Skeletal fluorosis can occur in bones when a person consumes at least 10 milligrams of fluoride daily for 10 or more years. This is a rare situation that may

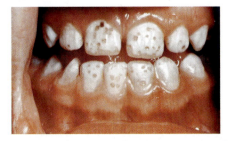

▲ **Figure 13.11 Fluorosis**
Teeth pitted by fluorosis.

happen when water is mistakenly overfluoridated. Skeletal fluorosis can cause bone concentrations of fluoride that are up to five times higher than normal and result in stiffness or pain in joints, osteoporosis, and calcification of the ligaments.

The UL for adults has been set at 10 milligrams to reduce the risk of fluorosis in the bones. Note, however, that the UL for infants and children is much lower to prevent fluorosis in teeth. Infants in their first 6 months of age should ingest no more than 0.7 milligrams per day or 0.9 milligrams per day for infants 7–12 months old. Children from 1 to 3 years of age should not ingest more than 1.3 milligrams per day or 2.2 milligrams per day for children age 4–8.

Because of fluoride's protective qualities, too little exposure to or consumption of fluoride increases the risk of dental caries.

LO 13.6: THE TAKE-HOME MESSAGE
Fluoride helps maintain the structure of bones and teeth and helps prevent dental caries. Adult males should consume 3.8 milligrams and women 3.1 milligrams of fluoride daily. The primary dietary source of fluoride is a fluoridated water supply and the consumption of foods and beverages prepared using fluoridated water. In children too much fluoride can result in fluorosis; in adults it can cause skeletal fluorosis. Too little fluoride increases the risk of dental caries.

fluorosis Condition caused by excess amounts of fluoride, resulting in mottling of the teeth.

EXPLORING **Chromium**

LO 13.7 Describe the functions, recommended intakes, food sources, and toxicity and deficiency effects of chromium.

What Is Chromium?

Chromium (Cr) is the most recent mineral to be found necessary in humans.[49] **Trivalent chromium** $\left(Cr^{+3} \right)$ is the active form of chromium found in foods.

Very little chromium is absorbed (less than 2.5 percent).[50] Once absorbed, the mineral is stored in a variety of tissues, including the liver, muscle, and spleen. Chromium can be excreted in the urine, especially when the diet is high in simple sugars.[51]

Metabolic Functions of Chromium

Chromium plays an essential role in how the body makes use of insulin. It also has an impact on prediabetes, metabolic syndrome, and weight.

Chromium Helps Insulin in the Body

The main function of chromium is to increase insulin's effectiveness in cells. The role of chromium in this mechanism is not clearly understood, but recent studies suggest that once insulin binds to the insulin receptor on the surface of the cells, chromium moves inside the cell and stimulates the transport of glucose across the cell membrane.[52] Chromium may also improve insulin's effects on the metabolism and storage of carbohydrates, fats, and protein.

Because it works with insulin, some researchers believe that chromium may help individuals who have diabetes or prediabetes improve their blood glucose control. One small study suggests that a chromium

trivalent chromium Oxidized form of chromium $\left(Cr^{+3} \right)$ found in food.

supplement may reduce the risk of insulin resistance and, therefore, favorably affect the handling of glucose in the body.[53] Improving the body's sensitivity to insulin and maintaining a normal blood glucose level can possibly lower the incidence of

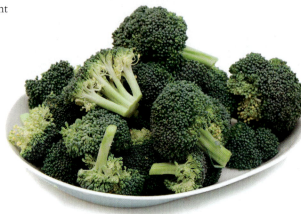

type 2 diabetes in individuals at risk.[54] However, a large research study has yet to be reported that might confirm this theory.

Chromium May Prevent or Improve Metabolic Syndrome

Individuals with insulin resistance may not develop diabetes but could develop other health-related problems including metabolic syndrome, which comprises a cluster of risk factors including obesity, high lipid levels in the blood, hypertension, and hyperglycemia. Additionally, insulin resistance has been associated with cardiovascular disease.[55] Because chromium reduces insulin resistance, some researchers suggest that chromium supplements, particularly those that contain niacin, might reduce the symptoms of metabolic syndrome as well as lower blood glucose. Nutrigenomics could shed some light on these mechanisms and lead to new dietary strategies to prevent these insulin-resistance disorders.[56]

Based on this research, the FDA has allowed a Qualified Health Claim on chromium supplements. However, the supplement label must state that the evidence regarding the relationship between chromium supplements and either insulin

resistance or type 2 diabetes is not certain at this time.[57]

Chromium Does Not Improve Body Composition

Although advertisements have sometimes touted chromium supplements as an aid to losing weight and building lean muscle, research doesn't support the claim.

A review of over 20 research studies found no benefits from taking up to 1,000 micrograms of chromium daily.[58]

Daily Needs for Chromium

The AI for adult men age 19–50 is 30–35 micrograms of chromium daily, whereas women need 20–25 micrograms daily, on average, depending on their age. American men consume an estimated 33 micrograms of chromium from foods, and women consume 25 micrograms, on average, daily.[59]

Food Sources of Chromium

Many foods contain chromium, but the amount varies and is influenced by the amount of chromium in the soil. Whole grains are good sources of chromium, while refined grains contain much less. Meat, fish, and poultry and some fruits and vegetables can also provide chromium, whereas dairy foods are low in the mineral (**Figure 13.12**). More ways to increase your chromium intake are in the nearby Table Tips.

Chromium Toxicity and Deficiency

Excess chromium, such as from supplements, may reduce the absorption, transport, and utilization of iron by binding to transferrin.[60] However, there are no known risks in humans from consuming excessive amounts of chromium from food or supplements, so no UL has been set.

Chromium deficiency is very rare in the United States. Individuals who have a chromium deficiency show signs similar

TABLE TIPS
Cram in the Chromium

Toast a whole-wheat English muffin and top it with a slice of lean ham for a chromium-laden breakfast.

Add broccoli florets to salad for a chromium-packed lunch.

Try an afternoon glass of cold grape juice for a refreshing break. Add an apple for a double dose of chromium.

Combine mashed potatoes and peas for a sweet and starchy addition to dinner.

Split a firm banana in half, lengthwise, and spread a small amount of peanut butter on each side.

to those observed in diabetics, such as elevated blood glucose, and in people with cardiovascular disease, such as elevated fatty acids in the blood.[61] When a chromium deficiency has been shown to exist in individuals with type 2 diabetes, they experienced lower blood glucose levels and less insulin resistance when they were given chromium supplements. However, it is not clear if individuals with diabetes who do not have a chromium deficiency would benefit by taking a supplement.

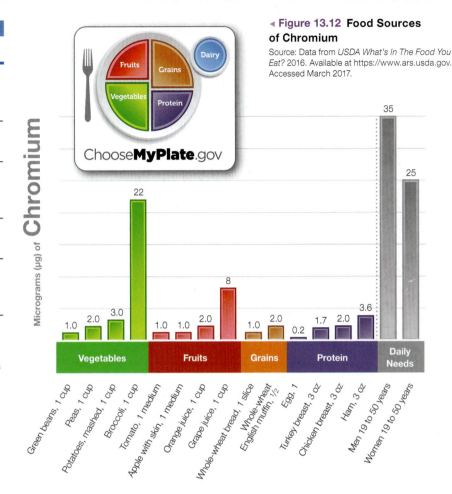

◄ **Figure 13.12 Food Sources of Chromium**
Source: Data from *USDA What's In The Food You Eat?* 2016. Available at https://www.ars.usda.gov. Accessed March 2017.

LO 13.7: THE TAKE-HOME MESSAGE Chromium may improve insulin function, the metabolism and storage of carbohydrates and fats, and metabolic syndrome and prediabetes. The AI for adult men is 30–35 micrograms of chromium daily and women need 20–25 micrograms daily. Many plant foods contain chromium, depending on the soil levels. Chromium toxicity interferes with iron metabolism. Deficiencies of chromium are very rare.

EXPLORING Iodine

LO 13.8 Describe the functions, recommended intakes, food sources, and toxicity and deficiency effects of iodine.

What Is Iodine?

Iodine (I) in the ionic form **iodide** (I^-) is an essential mineral. Like the fluoridation of community drinking water,

the iodization of salt was a significant advance for public health in the United States. Prior to the 1920s, many Americans suffered from the iodine-deficiency disease **goiter** (**Figure 13.13**). A goiter epidemic in the midwestern United States prompted the campaign for mandatory iodization of salt. Once salt manufacturers began adding iodine to their product, incidence of the disease dropped. Today,

rates of the disease are very low in the United States, though not in other parts of the world.

iodide Ionized form of iodine in the body (I^-).

goiter Enlargement of the thyroid gland, mostly due to iodine deficiency.

(continued)

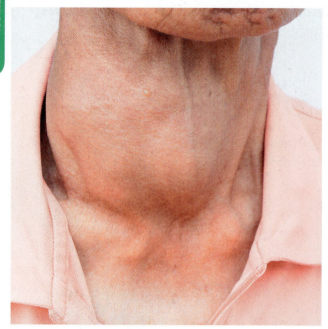

▲ **Figure 13.13 Goiter**
Goiter refers to the enlarged thyroid gland caused by an iodine deficiency.

Metabolic Functions of Iodine

Iodine is essential for the thyroid, a butterfly-shaped gland that wraps around the trachea. The thyroid gland has evolved to trap iodine from the blood to make thyroid hormones and to store these thyroid hormones during times of iodine deficiency. Approximately 60 percent of thyroid hormones are comprised of iodine. The thyroid gland converts iodide to *tetraiodothyronine*, also referred to as T_4, or **thyroxine**. One of the iodide ions is removed from T_4 to form *triiodothyronine*, or T_3. The amount of T_4 produced by the thyroid is much greater than the amount of T_3, but T_3 is more potent. Both of these active thyroid hormones are released from the thyroid gland into the blood.

The powerful thyroid hormones affect the majority of cells. They help regulate

thyroxine Less active form of thyroid hormone; also known as *tetraiodothyronine* (T_4).

thyroxine-releasing hormone (TRH)
Hormone secreted by the hypothalamus that stimulates the pituitary gland to release thyroxine-stimulating hormone (TSH).

thyroxine-stimulating hormone (TSH)
Hormone released by the pituitary that stimulates the thyroid gland to trap more iodine to produce more thyroid hormone (T_4 and T_3).

metabolic rate, reproduction, and nerve, muscle, and heart function. Thyroid hormones also control the rate of ATP production in the TCA cycle. Children need thyroid hormones for normal growth of bones and brain development.[62]

The metabolism of the thyroid gland and the production of thyroxine are controlled by the hypothalamus. When the blood level of T_4 (thyroxine) is reduced, the hypothalamus responds by releasing **thyroxine-releasing hormone (TRH)**, which stimulates the pituitary gland to produce **thyroxine-stimulating hormone (TSH)**. TSH stimulates the thyroid to trap more iodide ions from the blood to produce more T_4. When the blood levels of T_4 rise, the hypothalamus shuts off the production of TRH and TSH to maintain thyroid hormone homeostasis. When the diet is low in iodine, the blood levels of iodide ions become low and T_4 synthesis decreases, stimulating the process all over again (**Figure 13.14**).

Daily Needs for Iodine

The RDA for both adult men and women is 150 micrograms of iodine daily, an amount easily met by consuming seafood and iodized salt. In fact, Americans currently consume 230–410 micrograms of iodine daily, on average, depending on their age and gender.

Food Sources of Iodine

The amount of iodine that occurs naturally in foods is typically low, approximately 3–75 micrograms in a serving, and is influenced by the amount of iodine in the soil, water, and fertilizers used to grow foods. Fish can provide higher amounts of iodine, as they concentrate it from seawater (**Figure 13.15**). Seaweed is also a highly concentrated source of iodine, with an average of 4,500 micrograms of iodine in one-quarter ounce of seaweed, or 30 times the percent Daily Value. Iodized salt provides 400 micrograms of iodine per teaspoon. Note that not all salt has added iodine. Kosher salt, for example, has no additives, including iodine. Processed foods that use iodized salt or iodine-containing preservatives are also a source. For more ideas on increasing your iodine intake, see the Table Tips.

TABLE TIPS

Increase Your Iodine

Add a hard-cooked egg to your breakfast.

Add beans to your lunchtime soup.

Sprinkle tuna fish flakes on your dinner salad.

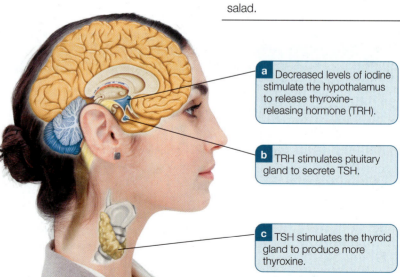

a Decreased levels of iodine stimulate the hypothalamus to release thyroxine-releasing hormone (TRH).

b TRH stimulates pituitary gland to secrete TSH.

c TSH stimulates the thyroid gland to produce more thyroxine.

▲ **Figure 13.14 The Thyroid Gland Produces the Hormone Thyroxine**

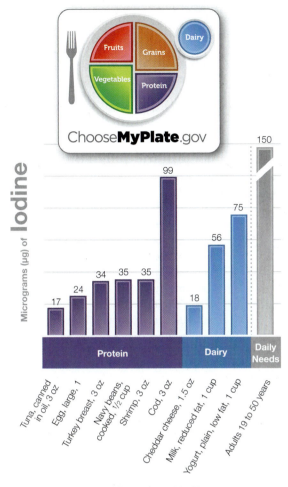

Figure 13.15 Food Sources of Iodine

Source: Data from *USDA What's In The Food You Eat?* 2016. Available at https://www.ars.usda.gov. Accessed March 2017.

Iodine Toxicity and Deficiency

It is rare in the United States to consume too much iodine through the intake of whole foods. Diets that contain large amounts of seaweed may provide iodine intakes of 50,000–80,000 micrograms of iodine per day,[63] which is at least 45 times greater than the UL set at 1,100 micrograms per day. Consuming too much iodine can challenge the thyroid, impairing its function and reducing the synthesis and release of thyroxine. The result is similar to an iodine deficiency and hypothyroidism.

An early sign of iodine deficiency is the enlarged thyroid gland known as *simple goiter*.[64] Consuming naturally occurring substances called **goitrogens**, found in foods such as rutabagas, cabbage, soybeans, and peanuts, can also result in a secondary deficiency and goiter if a person is iodine deficient. These antithyroid compounds reduce the absorption of iodide ions by the thyroid gland and decrease the amount of thyroid hormone released into the blood.

A deficiency of iodine during the early stages of fetal development can damage the fetal brain, causing mental retardation. If the iodine deficiency is severe, **cretinism**, also known as *congenital hypothyroidism* (*congenital* = born with, *hypo* = under, *ism* = condition), can occur. Individuals with cretinism can experience abnormal sexual development, mental retardation, and dwarfism. Early detection of an iodine deficiency and treatment in women of childbearing age is critical to avoid irreversible damage in their offspring. Worldwide, programs encouraging iodization of salt protect children from brain damage.

LO 13.8: THE TAKE-HOME MESSAGE

Iodine is essential to make the thyroid hormones T_3 and T_4, which help regulate metabolic rate and stimulate growth and development. The RDA for both adult men and women is 150 micrograms of iodine daily. Iodine is found mostly in iodized salt, seafood including shellfish, and dairy products. Iodine toxicity impairs thyroid function. Iodine deficiency during pregnancy causes mental retardation and cretinism in the offspring and during childhood and adulthood causes goiter.

goitrogens Substances in food that reduce the utilization of iodine by the thyroid gland, resulting in goiter.

cretinism Condition caused by a deficiency of thyroid hormone during prenatal development, resulting in abnormal mental and physical development in children.

EXPLORING Molybdenum

LO 13.9 Describe the functions, recommended intakes, food sources, and toxicity and deficiency effects of molybdenum.

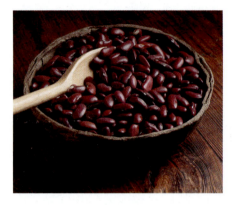

What Is Molybdenum?

Molybdenum (Mo) is part of several metalloenzymes involved in the metabolism of certain amino acids and oxidation-reduction reactions. For example, molybdenum is a cofactor for sulfate oxidase, the mitochondrial enzyme that converts sulfite (SO_3^{2-}) to sulfate (SO_4^{2-}) in the metabolism of methionine and cysteine.

Daily Needs for Molybdenum

The RDA for adult men and women is set at 45 micrograms of molybdenum daily. American women currently consume 76 micrograms and men consume 109 micrograms of molybdenum daily, on average.

Food Sources of Molybdenum

Legumes are excellent sources of molybdenum. Other molybdenum-rich foods include grains, nuts, dairy products, and leafy green vegetables.[65]

Molybdenum Toxicity and Deficiency

There is limited research on the adverse effects of too much dietary molybdenum in humans. In animal studies, too much molybdenum can cause reproductive problems and kidney disorders.[66] Because of this finding in animals, the UL for molybdenum in humans has been set at 2 milligrams for adults.

A dietary deficiency of molybdenum has not been seen in healthy individuals.[67]

LO 13.9: THE TAKE-HOME MESSAGE
Molybdenum functions as a cofactor for protein synthesis, including DNA and RNA. The RDA for adult men and women is 45 micrograms daily. Molybdenum is found in legumes, whole grains, and nuts. Molybdenum is not toxic and a dietary deficiency has not been reported in humans.

EXPLORING Manganese

LO 13.10 Describe the functions, recommended intakes, food sources, and toxicity and deficiency effects of manganese.

What Is Manganese?

Manganese (Mn) is a trace mineral that is either part of, or activates, many enzymes in the body. Much of the manganese in the body is found in bones and the accessory organs of digestion, including the liver and pancreas.

Metabolic Functions of Manganese

Manganese acts as a cofactor for a variety of metalloenzymes involved in the metabolism of carbohydrates, fats, and amino acids. For example, in glycolysis, the conversion of pyruvate to oxaloacetate in the TCA cycle requires manganese. Manganese participates in the formation of the bone matrix and helps build cartilage that supports the joints.

Daily Needs for Manganese

The AI for manganese for adult women has been set at 1.8 milligrams and at 2.3 milligrams for men. Americans are easily meeting their manganese needs. Adult women consume over 2 milligrams of manganese daily, and adult men consume over 2.8 milligrams daily, on average, in their diet.[68]

Food Sources of Manganese

Manganese is prevalent in plant foods. Whole grains, nuts, legumes, tea, vegetables, and fruits such as pineapples, strawberries, and bananas are all robust sources of manganese (**Figure 13.16**). A teaspoon of ground cinnamon provides just under 0.5 milligram of manganese. See the Table Tips for ways to include more manganese in your diet.

Manganese Toxicity and Deficiency

Manganese toxicity generally only occurs upon exposure to environmental pollutants, such as in manganese mining, battery manufacturing, and steel production.[69] For example, welders in the United States have inhaled manganese in welding fumes because of lack of ventilation.[70] Toxicity can damage the nervous system and result in symptoms that resemble Parkinson's

◀ **Figure 13.16** **Food Sources of Manganese**
Source: Data from *USDA What's In The Food You Eat?* 2016. Available at https://www.ars.usda.gov. Accessed March 2017.

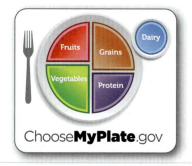

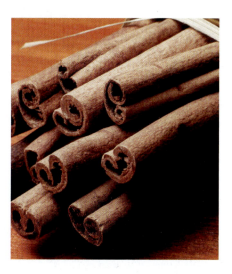

TABLE TIPS
Managing Manganese

Sprinkle whole-wheat toast with a dusting of cinnamon.

Combine cooked brown rice, canned and rinsed lentils, and chickpeas for dinner in a snap.

Spoon vanilla yogurt over canned crushed pineapples and sliced bananas for a tropical snack.

disease, including tremors, facial spasms, and difficulty walking.[71]

While toxicity is usually due to environmental pollutants, there have been reports of toxicity resulting from dietary intake. Manganese is found naturally in soil and under certain circumstances naturally high levels can be found in groundwater. A study of children in Canada who drank tap water with high levels of manganese showed lower IQ scores.[72] Most sources of water contain low levels (less than 10 μg/liter) of manganese. The Environmental Protection Agency (EPA) recommends that drinking water have no more than 50 μg/liter.[73] In addition, to protect against this toxicity, the UL for dietary intake of manganese has been set at 11 milligrams daily.

A deficiency of manganese is rare in healthy individuals who consume a balanced diet. However, as with some other minerals, phytates can reduce the absorption of manganese. Excessive intake of

(continued)

Milligrams (mg) of Manganese

Chart data:

Food	Milligrams
Peas, green, frozen, boiled without salt, 1 cup	0.5
Spinach, boiled, 1 cup	1.7
Banana, raw, 1 medium	0.3
Strawberries, raw, 1 cup	0.6
Blackberries, raw, 1 cup	0.9
Pineapple, fresh, 1 cup	1.8
Whole-wheat bread, 1 slice	0.7
Quinoa, cooked, 1 cup	1.2
Brown rice, long grain, cooked, 1/2 cup	1.8
Lentils, boiled, 1/4 cup	0.3
Pecans, 1/2 oz	0.6
Clams, canned, drained, 3 oz	0.9
Yogurt, fruit flavor, low fat, 1 cup	0.2
Milk, chocolate, low fat, 1 cup	0.2
Men 19 to 50 years	2.3
Women 19 to 50 years	1.8

Categories: Vegetables, Fruits, Grains, Protein, Dairy, Daily Needs

other minerals from dietary supplements, including iron and calcium, may also reduce manganese absorption. Consuming a diet deficient in manganese can cause low serum cholesterol, a rash and scaly skin, and impaired growth in children.[74]

LO 13.10: THE TAKE-HOME MESSAGE

Manganese assists enzymes involved in energy metabolism and functions as an antioxidant and in the synthesis of bone. The AI for men is 2.3 milligrams and women 1.8 milligrams daily. Legumes, nuts, and whole grains are good sources of manganese. Manganese is generally not toxic and deficiencies are rare.

Are Any Other Minerals Important to Health?

LO 13.11 Identify several minerals that may contribute to body functions but are not considered essential nutrients.

A few other minerals exist in the body, but their nutritional importance in humans has not yet been established. These minerals include arsenic, boron, nickel, silicon, and vanadium. Whereas limited research suggests that these may have a function in animals, there isn't enough data to confirm an essential role in humans.[75]

Arsenic may be needed in the metabolism of a specific amino acid in rats. A deficiency may impair growth and reproduction in other animals. The best food sources of arsenic are dairy products, meat, poultry, fish, grains, and cereal products. There are no adverse toxicity effects in humans from the organic arsenic compounds found in foods. The inorganic element is poisonous for humans.

A deficiency of boron may be associated with reproductive abnormalities in certain fish and frogs, which suggests a possible role in normal development in other animals. Grape juice, legumes, potatoes, pecans, peanut butter, apples, and milk are all good food sources of boron. No known adverse effect from boron has been reported from foods. Some research suggests that high amounts of boron may cause reproductive and developmental problems in animals.[76] Because of this, the upper limit for human adults has been set at 20 mg daily, which is more than 10 times the amount American adults consume daily, on average.

Specific enzymes in the human body may need nickel. It is considered an essential mineral in animals. Grains and grain products, vegetables, legumes, nuts, and chocolate are good sources of nickel. No known toxicity of nickel has been shown in humans when consuming a normal diet. In rats, high exposure to nickel salts can cause toxicity, with symptoms such as lethargy, irregular breathing, and a lower than normal weight gain.[77] Because of this, the upper limit for adults is set at 1 mg daily for nickel salts.

Silicon may be needed for bone formation in animals. Grains, grain products, and vegetables are good sources of silicon. There is no known risk of silicon toxicity to animals from food sources.

Vanadium has insulin-like actions in animals. A deficiency of vanadium increases the risk of miscarriage. Vanadium can be purchased in supplement form, but mushrooms, shellfish, parsley, and black pepper are good food sources. There is no known risk of vanadium toxicity in humans by consuming foods. Too much vanadium has been shown to cause kidney damage in animals.[78] Because of the known toxicity in animals, the UL for adults is set at 1.8 mg daily.

LO 13.11: THE TAKE-HOME MESSAGE Other minerals, including arsenic, boron, nickel, silicon, and vanadium, may play a role in maintaining health, at least in animals. More research is needed in humans.

What Are Nutrient-Deficiency Anemias?

LO 13.12 Explain the causes and treatments for the various nutrient-deficiency anemias.

Do you donate blood more than two to four times a year? Are you a female of childbearing age, a vegetarian, or just don't eat right? If you answered *yes* to any one of these questions, you may be at risk of developing a nutrient-deficiency anemia. Unfortunately, you are not alone.

Anemia is a condition in which the blood lacks enough healthy, normal-sized red blood cells to deliver oxygen to the tissues. According to the National Heart, Lung, and Blood Institute, more than 3.5 million people have anemia.[79] Most of the more than 400 known anemias are caused by non-nutritional factors, including losing too much blood, insufficient red blood cell production, or red blood cells being destroyed.

Lack of nutrient intake, malabsorption, or abnormal metabolism of certain nutrients can also cause anemia. The most common nutrient deficiencies that result in anemias are deficiencies of iron, folate, vitamin B_{12}, and vitamin B_6.

Anemias can be classified by the size of red blood cells. A complete blood count (CBC) can provide a mean cell volume measurement identifying the red blood cells as *microcytic* (small), *normocytic* (normal), or *macrocytic* (large). Nutrient-deficiency anemias are usually either microcytic or macrocytic (**Figure 13.17**).

In Microcytic Anemia, Red Blood Cells Are Smaller than Normal

Microcytic anemia is a blood condition in which the mean cell volume of red blood cells is smaller than normal (*microcytosis*) and often *hypochromic* (pale) due to a lack of sufficient hemoglobin. The most common reason for microcytic anemia is having low iron stores in the body.

Iron-Deficiency Anemia

As the name suggests, **iron-deficiency anemia**, which is the most common form of anemia, results from insufficient iron stores in the body. An estimated 20 percent of women, 3 percent of men, and 50 percent of all pregnant women are iron deficient but may not have iron-deficiency anemia.[80] Anemia develops slowly when the levels of stored iron have been depleted and the number of red blood cells falls below normal. As

the iron stores are decreasing, the bone marrow gradually produces fewer red blood cells. When the reserves of iron are depleted, there are fewer and abnormally smaller red blood cells.

Women, who have smaller stores of iron and who lose more blood (due to menstruation) than men, are at a higher risk. In men and postmenopausal women, iron deficiency is often the result of blood loss due to ulcers, increased use of aspirin, and specific cancers such as colon, esophagus, and stomach cancer.

Signs and Symptoms

Mild iron-deficiency anemia may go unnoticed. The most common symptom is fatigue, especially during physical exertion, due to the lack of red blood cells and, thus, the inability to carry sufficient oxygen to the muscle cells. Other possible signs may include pale skin color, irritability, shortness of breath, sore tongue, brittle nails, headache, a blue tinge to the whites of the eyes, and decreased appetite (especially in children).[81] In young children, a mild iron-deficiency anemia can result in intellectual impairment that is irreversible even after adding iron

---

iron-deficiency anemia Type of anemia due to a lack of dietary iron or excessive loss of blood.

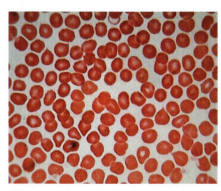

a Normal healthy red blood cells

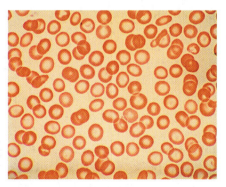

b Microcytic red blood cells affected by anemia

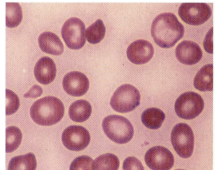

c Macrocytic red blood cells affected by anemia

▲ **Figure 13.17 Normal, Microcytic, and Macrocytic Red Blood Cells**
Microcytic red blood cells affected by anemia (b) are small and pale in color compared with normal red blood cells (a) due to lower heme concentration. Macrocytic red blood cells affected by anemia (c) are large, pale, and fewer in number compared with normal red blood cells due to the inability to normally divide.

supplements to the diet.[82] Mild iron-deficiency anemia during pregnancy may cause premature births, low birth weight, and even maternal mortality.

Individuals who have been diagnosed with iron-deficiency anemia may also practice *pica*, a condition characterized by eating clay and other nonfood items, including burnt matches and rubber bands.[83] Pica may exacerbate iron-deficiency anemia because the nonfood substances reduce the bioavailability of iron.

Testing

In an individual with iron-deficiency anemia, a CBC will show a low hemoglobin level and an abnormal number, shape, or size of red blood cells. A normal range for hemoglobin is 11.1–15.0 grams per deciliter. Anemia is diagnosed if the test reveals a hemoglobin level below 11.1. A CBC also determines the hematocrit, or the ratio of red blood cells to fluid in the blood. A normal hematocrit is between 32 and 43 percent red blood cells. If the tests reveal lower than normal hemoglobin, hematocrit, or both, the individual is diagnosed with anemia. The CBC also provides a mean cell volume measurement that can establish whether red blood cells are microcytic or macrocytic.

Another test can be conducted to measure serum iron. This test directly measures the amount of iron in the blood, but it doesn't accurately reflect the stores of iron. To estimate iron stores, the **total iron-binding capacity (TIBC)**, or transferrin levels, are measured. If iron-deficiency anemia exists, the total iron-binding capacity and the ability to transport more iron will be high.

Treatment

Iron supplements, along with an optimum intake of dietary iron, are usually

total iron-binding capacity (TIBC) Blood test that measures the amount of iron that transferrin can bind; a higher TIBC indicates iron-deficiency anemia.

macrocytic anemia Condition that results in abnormally large, pale, and fewer than normal red blood cells.

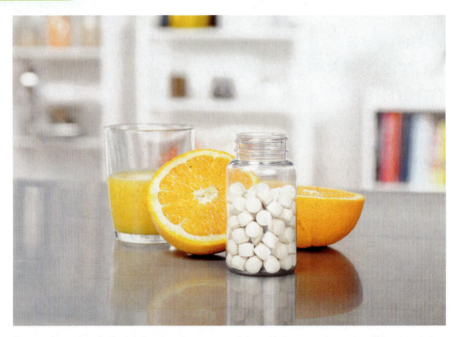

Consuming a vitamin C–rich food such as orange juice with iron supplements will improve iron absorption.

necessary to correct iron-deficiency anemia and restore the iron reserves. Oral iron supplements in the ferrous, or Fe^{+2}, form, sold as ferrous sulfate, ferrous gluconate, or ferrous fumarate, are the most easily absorbed.[84] These supplements, taken for several weeks or even months, are best taken with orange juice or another vitamin C–rich substance to improve iron absorption. Recall that vitamin C makes iron more bioavailable. Avoid taking iron supplements with milk or antacids, which may interfere with the absorption of iron.

Vitamin B₆ Microcytic Anemia

A deficiency of vitamin B_6 (pyridoxine) may also result in microcytic anemia, although this is not as common as iron-deficiency anemia.[85] Recall from Chapter 10 that the active form of vitamin B_6, pyridoxal phosphate or PLP, acts as a coenzyme for more than 100 enzymes, most of which are involved in protein metabolism. PLP is required as a coenzyme in the synthesis of heme, the part of hemoglobin that is used to transport oxygen in the blood. If the diet is deficient in vitamin B_6, insufficient heme production results in hypochromic, microcytic anemia. The symptoms are undistinguishable from those of iron-deficiency anemia.

In Macrocytic Anemia, Red Blood Cells Are Larger than Normal

Macrocytic anemia is characterized by fewer, but abnormally large red blood cells (*macrocytosis*) that lack sufficient hemoglobin (see Figure 13.17). Macrocytic anemia is also referred to as *megaloblastic anemia* because the larger than normal immature (blast) cells cannot produce DNA quickly enough to divide and mature properly and become too large. The most common cause of nutritional macrocytic anemia is a deficiency of either folate or vitamin B_{12}.

Folate and Vitamin B₁₂ Deficiencies

The mechanisms that result in macrocytic anemia are the same whether the diet is deficient in folate or vitamin B_{12}. The difference between a folate and a vitamin B_{12} deficiency is that the liver has abundant stores of vitamin B_{12} but the body doesn't store folate; thus, it takes longer to manifest macrocytic anemia due to vitamin B_{12} deficiency.

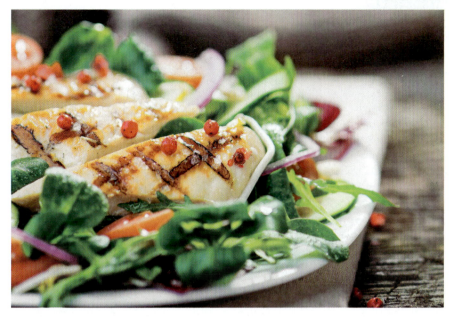

A leafy green salad topped with grilled chicken is a good source of both folate and vitamin B_{12}.

Remember that in Chapter 10 you learned that a key function of folate is to transfer a single-carbon compound in the first step that converts homocysteine to methionine in DNA metabolism. If this step is impaired due to a lack of folate, the synthesis of DNA is disrupted and the red blood cells don't divide and increase in adequate numbers, causing macrocytic anemia.

In addition to activating folate, vitamin B_{12} also activates coenzyme methylcobalamin, which is used in the conversion of homocysteine to the amino acid methionine, and in turn provides the methyl group used in DNA and RNA synthesis. Without adequate vitamin B_{12}, homocysteine levels accumulate and DNA synthesis is slowed, which results in macrocytic anemia.

Signs and Symptoms

Mild macrocytic anemia may be asymptomatic, especially in younger individuals. The most common symptoms include loss of appetite, sore mouth and tongue, shortness of breath, fatigue, heart palpitations, and pale lips and eyelids.

Testing

As with other forms of anemia, a CBC can be used to measure the mean cell volume or size of the red blood cells and the mean cell hemoglobin. In a normal CBC, the hemoglobin concentration will increase in proportion to the size of the cell, but in macrocytic anemia the hemoglobin concentration is less than expected. A mean cell volume greater than 100 fL (called *femtoliters*) indicates macrocytosis, or the presence of abnormally large cells (see Figure 13.18). Once macrocytosis has been confirmed, tests of serum levels of folate and vitamin B_{12} are conducted to determine whether the cause is a folate or a vitamin B_{12} deficiency.

Treatment

Individuals deficient in folate or vitamin B_{12} are prescribed supplements to overcome the anemia. If the macrocytic anemia is caused by a folate deficiency, 1 milligram per day of folate is usually the first line of treatment.[86] In macrocytic anemia due to a vitamin B_{12} deficiency, the individual is treated with vitamin B_{12} intramuscular injections.[87] A diet rich in folate, including green leafy vegetables and citrus, and animal products or vitamin B_{12}–fortified vegetarian alternatives, is essential to support supplementation and prevent a recurrence.

Pernicious Anemia

Pernicious anemia is a form of macrocytic anemia caused by the inability to absorb vitamin B_{12}. The cause is most often a lack of sufficient intrinsic factor secreted from the parietal cells in the stomach. This lack of intrinsic factor can be due to either gastritis or an autoimmune reaction in which the body's immune system attacks the parietal cells.[88] The symptoms include diarrhea or constipation, fatigue or light-headedness, loss of appetite, pale skin, shortness of breath, and difficulty concentrating. Serum vitamin B_{12} and the presence of antibodies against intrinsic factor or parietal cells are blood tests used to diagnose pernicious anemia. The treatment for pernicious anemia involves intramuscular shots of vitamin B_{12} given once per month to circumvent the malabsorption.[89]

LO 13.2: THE TAKE-HOME MESSAGE
Microcytic and macrocytic anemias can be caused by nutrient deficiencies. A deficiency of iron and vitamin B_{6} can cause microcytic anemia. Folate and vitamin B_{12} deficiencies or malabsorption can cause macrocytic anemia, and malabsorption of vitamin B_{12} can result in pernicious anemia. A complete blood count is used to determine the form and cause of anemia, followed by treatment with supplements and an optimal diet to supply the lacking nutrient.

---

pernicious anemia Form of macrocytic anemia caused by a lack of intrinsic factor due to either gastritis or an autoimmune disorder.

Visual Chapter Summary

LO 13.1 Trace Minerals Are Essential Inorganic Nutrients

Trace minerals are inorganic elements the body needs in small amounts. The bioavailability and absorption of trace minerals are affected by soil content, nutrient status, and the composition of the diet. The bioavailability of trace minerals depends on the individual's nutrient status, other foods eaten at the same time, and the form of the mineral. Once absorbed, several trace minerals, including iron and zinc, are recycled repeatedly for use in the body. For this reason, toxicity can be a concern.

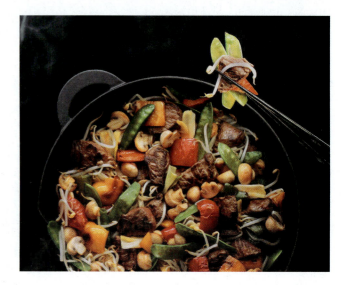

LO 13.2 Iron

Iron absorption is tightly controlled and depends on the iron status of the individual, the form of iron in the food, and the types of foods eaten together. Iron is stored as ferritin or hemosiderin and transported attached to transferrin. Iron functions as part of the oxygen-carrying transport proteins—hemoglobin in the red blood cells and myoglobin in the muscles. As part of cytochromes in the electron transport chain, iron is involved in energy production. It is also a component of antioxidant enzyme systems.

The RDA for iron is 18 milligrams per day for menstruating women and 8 milligrams per day for men and postmenopausal women. Heme iron, as well as nonheme iron, is found in meat, poultry, and fish. Nonheme iron is also found in plant foods, such as grains and vegetables. Nonheme iron is the predominant source of iron in the diet but isn't absorbed as readily as is heme iron.

Adults with normal GI tract functioning have little risk of developing iron toxicity from food. Iron toxicity from supplements greater than 20 mg/kg can develop and cause gastrointestinal distress. Hemochromatosis caused by a genetic mutation is associated with iron buildup in the body and possibly death. Iron deficiency is the most common nutrient deficiency in the world. A deficiency of iron in children can impact their ability to learn and retain information. Iron-deficiency anemia can cause fatigue and weakness.

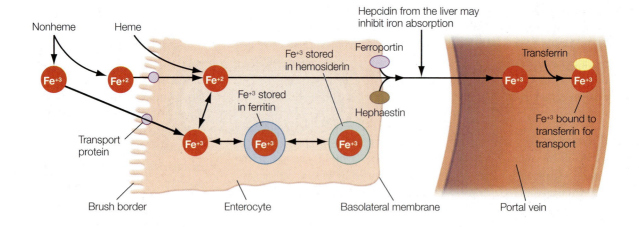

LO 13.3 Copper

Copper status is regulated by absorption in the small intestine. Copper is absorbed attached to albumin. Very little copper is stored and the excess is excreted through the bile into the feces. Copper is part of the protein ceruloplasmin, which converts ferrous iron to ferric iron. Copper is thus necessary for the synthesis of hemoglobin and red blood cells. Copper is a cofactor for metalloenzymes involved in energy production, is a component of cytochromes, and supports the synthesis of connective tissue. Copper is part of the superoxide dismutase enzyme, which reduces free-radical damage in cells.

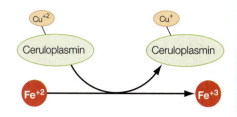

The AI for copper is 900 micrograms for adults. Copper is found in a variety of foods, especially seafood, nuts, and seeds. Some genetic diseases result in the accumulation of copper and cause tissue damage and even death if left untreated.

A deficiency of copper results in anemia and weakened bones and connective tissue.

LO 13.4 Zinc

Zinc plays a role in the structure of RNA and DNA, in taste acuity, and in helping prevent age-related macular degeneration. Zinc does not cure the common cold, but zinc lozenges or gels used in nasal passages may reduce the duration of a cold.

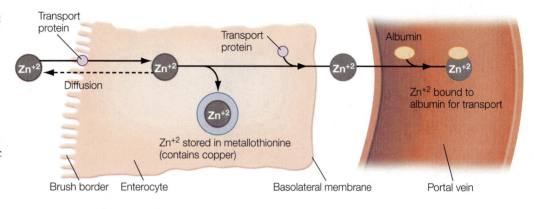

The RDA for zinc is 11 milligrams per day for adult males and 8 milligrams per day for adult females. Meat, fish, and whole grains are good sources of zinc.

Consuming too much zinc can cause vomiting and diarrhea, suppress the immune system, and lower HDL cholesterol. Eating too little can impair growth, cause loss of hair and loss of appetite, and delay sexual maturation.

LO 13.5 Selenium

Selenium is a component of a group of proteins called selenoproteins, which act as antioxidants in the body and may help fight cancer. Selenium also regulates thyroid function.

The AI for adults is set at 55 micrograms of selenium per day. All food groups contribute selenium, including nuts, meat, and seafood.

Toxicity of selenium results in brittle teeth and fingernails, garlic odor in the breath, gastrointestinal problems, and damage to the nervous system. A deficiency of selenium can lead to Keshan disease, which damages the heart. Selenium deficiency may also result in changes in thyroid hormone production.

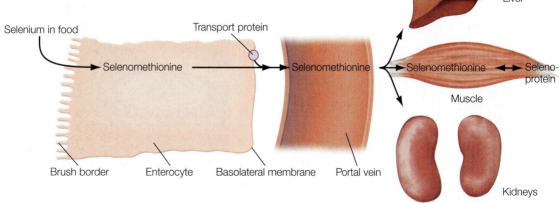

LO 13.6 Fluoride

Fluoride is not an essential nutrient, but it helps maintain the structure of bones and teeth and helps prevent dental caries.

The AI is 3.8 milligrams for men and 3.1 milligrams for women. The primary dietary source of fluoride is a fluoridated water supply and the consumption of foods and beverages prepared using fluoridated water.

In children, consumption of too much fluoride during tooth development can result in fluorosis. In adults, too much fluoride can cause skeletal fluorosis, which results in joint stiffness or pain, osteoporosis, and calcification of the ligaments.

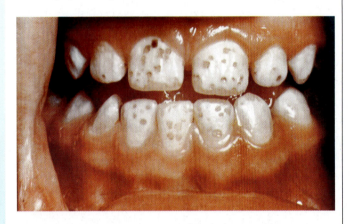

LO 13.8 Iodine

Iodine is essential to make the thyroid hormones T_3 and T_4, which help regulate metabolic rate and stimulate growth and development. The RDA for adult men and women is 150 micrograms of iodine daily. Iodine is found mostly in iodized salt, seafood including shellfish, and dairy products. A deficiency of iodine during pregnancy causes mental retardation and cretinism in the offspring. A deficiency of iodine during childhood or adulthood causes simple goiter, which is characterized by an enlarged thyroid gland.

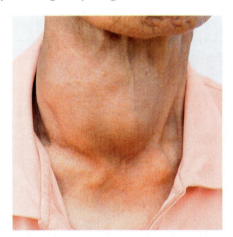

LO 13.7 Chromium

Chromium helps insulin function, may improve the metabolism and storage of carbohydrates, fats, and protein, may reduce prediabetes, and may improve metabolic syndrome. It has not been proven to enhance weight loss or build muscle mass during exercise. Adult men need 30–35 micrograms of chromium daily and women need 20–25 micrograms daily. Many plant foods contain chromium, depending on the soil levels. Chromium toxicity from taking supplements interferes with iron metabolism. Deficiencies of chromium are very rare in the United States.

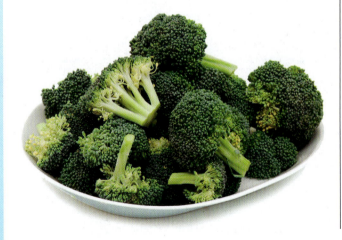

LO 13.9 Molybdenum

Molybdenum is a cofactor for enzymes that synthesize proteins, including DNA and RNA. The RDA for adult men and women is 45 micrograms daily. Molybdenum is found in legumes, whole grains, and nuts. A dietary deficiency of molybdenum is rare and molybdenum does not appear to be toxic in humans.

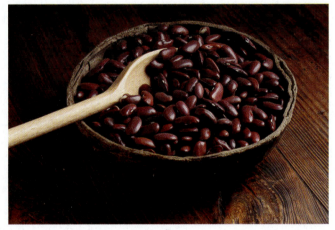

LO 13.10 Manganese

Manganese assists enzymes involved in energy metabolism and functions in synthesis of bone and as an antioxidant. The AI for manganese is 2.3 milligrams for men and 1.8 milligrams for women daily. Manganese is found in legumes, nuts, and whole grains. A deficiency of manganese is rare in healthy individuals who consume a balanced diet. Some food components, such as phytates, or excessive use of supplements that contain iron and calcium can reduce the absorption of manganese and cause a rash and dry, scaly skin, low serum cholesterol levels, and impaired growth in children. Toxicity can damage the nervous system and result in symptoms that resemble Parkinson's disease, including tremors, facial spasms, and difficulty walking.

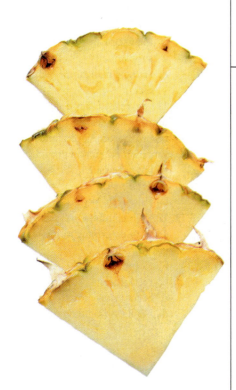

LO 13.11 Other Minerals Might Be Important to Body Functioning

Other minerals, including arsenic, boron, nickel, silicon, and vanadium, may play a role in maintaining health. Arsenic in its organic form may be used for growth and both arsenic and boron may function in reproduction. Nickel may activate enzymes, silicon may be needed for bone formation, and vanadium may have insulin-like properties. More research is needed to understand the role each of these trace minerals plays in the human body.

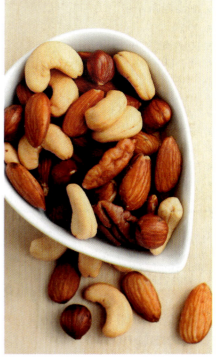

LO 13.12 Microcytic and Macrocytic Anemias Can Be Caused by Micronutrient Deficiencies

Microcytic and macrocytic anemias can be caused by mineral and vitamin deficiencies. Symptoms are often similar for both forms of anemia. A deficiency of iron and vitamin B_6 can cause microcytic anemia, characterized by pale and smaller than normal red blood cells. A lack of dietary folate or vitamin B_{12} can cause pale and abnormally large red blood cells, a condition called macrocytic anemia. Both microcytic and macrocytic red blood cells lack sufficient hemoglobin. Insufficient release of intrinsic factor either due to gastritis or an autoimmune disorder can cause a malabsorption of vitamin B_{12} and result in pernicious anemia. A complete blood count is used to determine the form and cause of anemia, followed by treatment with supplements and an optimal diet to supply the lacking nutrient.

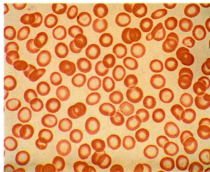

Microcytic red blood cells

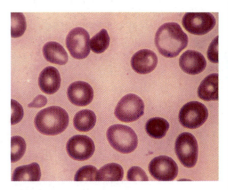

Macrocytic red blood cells

Terms to Know

- trace minerals
- metalloenzymes
- heme iron
- nonheme iron
- hemoglobin
- myoglobin
- ferric iron
- ferrous iron
- ferritin
- hemosiderin
- ferroportin
- hephaestin

- transferrin
- hepcidin
- hemochromatosis
- cupric
- cuprous
- ceruloplasmin
- Menkes' disease
- Wilson's disease
- metallothionine
- selenoproteins
- selenomethionine
- selenosis
- Keshan disease
- fluoroapatite

- fluorosis
- trivalent chromium
- iodide
- goiter
- thyroxine
- thyroxine-releasing hormone (TRH)
- thyroxine-stimulating hormone (TSH)
- goitrogens
- cretinism
- iron-deficiency anemia
- total iron-binding capacity (TIBC)
- macrocytic anemia
- pernicious anemia

Mastering Nutrition

Visit the Study Area in Mastering Nutrition to hear an MP3 chapter summary.

Check Your Understanding

LO 13.1 1. The bioavailability of trace minerals is affected by
- a. the time of day you consume foods containing trace minerals.
- b. the form of the trace mineral.
- c. the protein content of your diet.
- d. the fat content of your diet.

LO 13.2 2. The iron-containing protein that carries oxygen from the lungs to the tissues is called
- a. hemosiderin.
- b. myoglobin.
- c. hemoglobin.
- d. transferrin.

LO 13.3 3. Copper is transported through the circulation by the blood protein called
- a. transferrin.
- b. albumin.
- c. hemoglobin.
- d. myoglobin.

LO 13.4 4. A zinc deficiency may result in which of the following conditions?
- a. Cretinism
- b. Dental caries
- c. Stunted growth
- d. Inability to reduce ferrous iron to ferric iron

LO 13.5 5. Selenium may help prevent cancer through its role as a(an)
- a. toxin.
- b. enzyme.
- c. antioxidant.
- d. supplement.

LO 13.6 6. Which of the following statements regarding fluoride is true?
- a. Fluoride is considered an essential nutrient.
- b. Fluoride is found mostly in animal products such as meat and dairy products.
- c. Fluoride is part of the fluoroapatite crystal that makes your teeth stronger and resistant to decay.
- d. Ingesting more than the recommended amount of fluoride increases your susceptibility to tooth decay.

LO 13.7 7. Chromium increases the effectiveness of which hormone?
- a. Thyroid-stimulating hormone
- b. Insulin
- c. Antidiuretic hormone (ADH)
- d. Glucagon

LO 13.8 8. Goitrogens may be found in
- a. poultry.
- b. cabbage.
- c. seafood.
- d. bananas.

LO 13.9 9. There have been no reported risks of deficiency associated with molybdenum.
- a. True
- b. False

LO 13.10 10. The amount of manganese absorbed in the body is increased by
- a. a good source of phytates in the meal.
- b. the use of calcium supplements.
- c. the use of iron supplements.
- d. eating a manganese-rich diet.

LO 13.11 11. Several studies done on humans have established the role of boron, silicon, and vanadium in human growth and metabolism.
- a. True
- b. False

LO 13.12 12. Which of the following is a test to determine iron stores in the body?
- a. Complete blood count
- b. Hematocrit
- c. Serum iron
- d. Total iron-binding capacity

Answers

1. (b) The bioavailability of trace minerals in the food you consume can vary depending on the form of the mineral, your nutrient status, and the foods you choose to eat. The protein and fat content of the food does not influence trace mineral bioavailability, nor does the time of day the food is eaten.

2. (c) Hemoglobin is the iron-containing protein in red blood cells that carries oxygen. Hemoglobin exchanges oxygen with myoglobin, another protein found in muscle.

Hemosiderin is the stored form of iron and transferrin is the protein that transports iron throughout the body.

3. (b) Albumin is the blood protein that transports copper. Transferrin transports iron, and hemoglobin and myoglobin are iron-containing proteins that participate in oxygen and carbon dioxide exchange.

4. (c) Zinc plays a significant role in growth and cell division. A deficiency of this trace mineral results in stunted growth. A deficiency of iodine during pregnancy results in cretinism. Fluoride makes the tooth enamel resistant to dental caries and copper functions as a cofactor to reduce ferrous iron to ferric iron.

5. (c) As part of selenoproteins, selenium functions as an antioxidant that protects cells from free radical damage.

6. (c) Fluoride, which is not considered an essential nutrient because the body doesn't require it for normal growth and development, makes up part of the fluoroapatite crystal that strengthens tooth structure and helps the tooth resist decay. It is found mostly in fluoridated water, tea, and seaweed. Consuming too much fluoride can cause fluorosis, a discoloration of the teeth.

7. (b) Chromium increases insulin's effectiveness in promoting glucose uptake by the cells. Iodine is needed to make thyroid hormones; ADH is the hormone that directs kidneys to minimize water loss and concentrate urine; and glucagon is the hormone that has the opposite effect to insulin, stimulating the release of glucose into the blood.

8. (b) Goitrogens are found in certain whole foods including cabbage, rutabagas, soybeans, and peanuts and can result in secondary deficiency of iodine if too much is consumed.

9. (a) A dietary deficiency of molybdenum has not been reported in healthy individuals.

10. (d) Tissue levels of manganese are related to the amount present in your diet; thus, eating a manganese-rich diet improves the amount of

manganese absorbed. Phytates in food bind or inhibit the absorption of manganese, and other minerals in supplement form, such as iron and calcium supplements, decrease the absorption of manganese.

11. (b) Only animal studies have been conducted to research the effects of boron, silicon, and vanadium.

12. (d) Total iron-binding capacity is the best test to determine iron storage. If iron-deficiency anemia exists, the total iron-binding capacity will be high indicating a greater ability to transport iron. A complete blood count measures hemoglobin levels in the blood, hematocrit is the ratio of the volume of red blood cells to the total volume of blood, and serum iron reflects the amount of iron in the blood.

Answers to True or False?

1. **False.** Trace minerals are called *trace* because they are needed in small dietary amounts (less than 100 milligrams per day) and are found in small amounts in the body (less than 5 grams).

2. **False.** Although meat and seafood are rich sources of iron in the American diet, they are not the primary sources. Enrichment and fortification processes make many bread products and cereals the primary sources of iron in the American diet.

3. **False.** Even though iron competes with other minerals, including zinc and copper, for binding to a transport protein in the small intestine, iron supplements do not appear to affect copper absorption or cause copper deficiency. Iron supplements do significantly reduce zinc absorption and could result in a zinc deficiency.

4. **False.** Zinc lozenges and gels do not prevent or cure the common cold. Some studies have reported that zinc lozenges or nasal gels may reduce the severity and duration of cold symptoms.

5. **True.** Excess selenium intake from dietary supplements is toxic.

The symptoms include vomiting, diarrhea, fatigue, and hair loss.

6. **False.** Most bottled water sold in the United States does not contain fluoride. However, most tap water in the United States has been fluoridated.

7. **False.** Chromium supplementation does not appear to increase protein synthesis or have a beneficial effect on body composition or muscle mass.

8. **True.** While iodine is found in saltwater fish and in small amounts in dairy products, the only reliable source of iodine is iodized salt. Plants can be a good source of iodine, but only if they are grown in iodine-rich soil.

9. **True.** Two teaspoons of cinnamon contain 0.76 milligrams of manganese, or about 38 percent of the AI.

10. **False.** Vegetables are generally low in molybdenum. Other plant-based foods such as legumes, nuts, and grains are considered good sources of this trace mineral.

Web Resources

- To find out if your community water is fluoridated and how much fluoride is added, visit the Centers for Disease Control and Prevention website, My Water's Fluoride, at http://apps.nccd.cdc.gov/MWF/Index.asp

- For more information on trace minerals, visit the U.S. Department of Health and Human Services website at www.healthfinder.org

- For more information on iron and the symptoms associated with iron deficiency and iron overload, visit the Iron Overload Diseases Association at www.ironoverload.org

- Visit the American Cancer Society website for more information on selenium's role in cancer prevention at www.cancer.org

- For more information on thyroid health, visit the American Thyroid Association at www.thyroid.org

- For more information on the importance of minerals and mineral supplements, visit MedlinePlus, a service of the U.S. National Library of Medicine and the National Institutes of Health, at www.nlm.nih.gov/medlineplus

References

1. Institute of Medicine. 2001. *Dietary Reference Intakes: Vitamin A, Vitamin K, Arsenic, Boron, Chromium, Copper, Iodine, Iron, Manganese, Molybdenum, Nickel, Silicon, Vanadium, and Zinc.* Washington, DC: National Academies Press.

2. Olivares, M. 2012. Acute Inhibition of Iron Bioavailability by Zinc: Studies in Humans. *BioMetals* 25(4):657–664.

3. Ibid.

4. Olivares, M., C. Castro, et al. 2013. Effect of Increasing Levels of Zinc Fortificant on the Iron Absorption of Bread Co-Fortified with Iron and Zinc Consumed with a Black Tea. *Biological Trace Element Research* 154(3):321–325.

5. Wallace, D. F. The Regulation of Iron Absorption and Homeostasis. 2016. *Clinical Biochemist Reviews* 37(2):51–62.

6. Ibid.

7. Gropper, S. S., and J. L. Smith. 2013. *Advanced Nutrition and Human Metabolism.* 7th ed. Belmont, CA: Wadsworth—Cengage Learning.

8. Ibid.

9. Wessling-Resnick, M. 2014. Iron. In *Modern Nutrition in Health and Disease.* A. C. Ross, B. Caballero, R. J. Cousins, K. L. Tucker, and T. R. Ziegler, eds. Philadelphia: Lippincott Williams & Wilkins.

10. Lam, L. F., and T. R. Lawlis. 2016. Feeding the Brain—The Effects of Micronutrient Interventions on Cognitive Performance Among School-aged Children: A systematic Review of Randomized Controlled Trials. *Clinical Nutrition* pii: S0261-5614(16)30146-7. doi: 10.1016/j.clnu.2016.06.013.

11. Jáuregui-Lobera, I. 2014. Iron Deficiency and Cognitive Functions. *Neuropsychiatric Disease and Treatment* 10:2087–2095. doi: 10.2147/NDT.S72491.

12. Institute of Medicine. 2006. *Dietary Reference Intakes: The Essential Guide to Nutrient Requirements.* J. J. Otten, J. P. Helwig, and L. D. Meyers, eds. Washington, DC: National Academies Press.

13. Office of Disease Prevention and Health Promotion. Dietary Guidelines for Americans 2015-2020, 8th ed. Available at https://health.gov/dietaryguidelines/2015/guidelines. Accessed March 2017.

14. Ibid.

15. Britton, H. C., and C. E. Nossamn. 1986. Iron Content of Food Cooked in Iron Utensils. *Journal of the American Dietetic Association* 86:897–901.

16. Galy, B., D. Ferring-Appel, et al. 2013. Iron Regulatory Proteins Control a Mucosal Block to Intestinal Iron Absorption. *Cell Reports* 3(3):844–857.

17. FDA. 2015. Dietary Supplement Labeling Guide: Chapter VIII. Other Labeling Information. Available at https://www.fda.gov. Accessed March 2017.

18. Dao, M. C., and S. N. Meydani. 2013. Iron Biology, Immunology, Aging, and Obesity: Four Fields Connected by the Small Peptide Hormone Hepcidin. *Advanced Nutrition* 4(6):602–617.

19. Centers for Disease Control and Prevention. 2013. *Hemochromatosis (Iron Storage Disease).* Available at www.cdc.gov. Accessed March 2017.

20. Collins, J. F. 2018. Copper. In *Modern Nutrition in Health and Disease.* A. C. Ross, B. Caballero, R. J. Cousins, K. L. Tucker, and T. R. Ziegler, eds. Philadelphia: Lippincott Williams & Wilkins.

21. Chen, H., G. Huang, et al. 2006. Decreased Hephaestin Activity in the Intestine of Copper-Deficient Mice Causes Iron Deficiency. *Journal of Nutrition* 136:1236–1241.

22. Collins. 2018. Copper. In *Modern Nutrition in Health and Disease.*

23. Institute of Medicine. 2006. *Dietary Reference Intakes : The Essential Guide to Nutrient Requirements.*

24. Hojyo, S., and T. Fukada. 2016. Roles of Zinc Signaling in the Immune System. *Journal of Immunological Research* 2016:6762343.

25. Haase, H., and L. Rink. 2014. Multiple Impacts of Zinc on Immune Function. *Metallomics* doi: 10.1039/C3MT00353A.

26. Hiroyuki, Y., T. Kawashima, et al. 2016. Validity of the Copper/Zinc Ratio as a Diagnostic Marker for Taste Disorders Associated with Zinc Deficiency. *Journal of Trace Elements in Medicine and Biology* 36:80–83.

27. Hemilä, H, E. J. Petrus, et al. Zinc Acetate Lozenges for Treating the Common Cold: An Individual Patient Data Meta-analysis. *British Journal of Clinical Pharmacology* 82(5):1393–1398. doi: 10.1111/bcp.13057

28. Hemilä, H. 2015. Common Cold Treatment Using Zinc. *JAMA* 314(7):730. doi: 10.1001/jama.2015.8174

29. Ibid.

30. Baltaci, A. K., and R. Mogulkoc. 2017. Leptin, NPY, Melatonin and Zinc Levels in Experimental Hypothyroidism and Hyperthyroidism: The Relation to Zinc. *Biochemistry and Genetics* doi: 10.1007/s10528-017-9791-z.

31. Institute of Medicine. 2001. *Dietary Reference Intakes: Vitamin A, Vitamin K, Arsenic, Boron, Chromium, Copper, Iodine, Iron, Manganese, Molybdenum, Nickel, Silicon, Vanadium, and Zinc.*

32. King, J. C., and R. J. Cousins. 2018. Zinc. In *Modern Nutrition in Health and Disease.* A. C. Ross, B. Caballero, R. J. Cousins, K. L. Tucker, and T. R. Ziegler, eds. Philadelphia: Lippincott Williams & Wilkins.

33. Sunde, R. A. 2018. Selenium. In *Modern Nutrition in Health and Disease.* A. C. Ross, B. Caballero, R. J. Cousins, K. L. Tucker, and T. R. Ziegler, eds. Philadelphia: Lippincott Williams & Wilkins.

34. Vinceti, M., G. Dennert, et al. 2014. Selenium for Preventing Cancer. *Cochrane Database of Systematic Reviews* doi: 10.1002/14651858.CD005195.pub3.

35. Cui, Z., D. Liu, et al. 2017. Serum Selenium Levels And Prostate Cancer Risk: A MOOSE-Compliant Meta-Analysis. Alves. MG, ed. *Medicine* 96(5):e5944. doi:10.1097/MD.0000000000005944.

36. FDA. 2014. *Summary of Qualified Health Claims Subject to Enforcement Discretion.* Available at www.fda.gov. Accessed March 2017.

37. Sunde. 2018. Selenium.

38. Liontiris, M. I., and E. E. Mazokopakis. 2017. A Concise Review of Hashimoto Thyroiditis (HT) and the Importance of Iodine, Selenium, Vitamin D and Gluten on the Autoimmunity and Dietary Management of HT Patients. *Hellenic Journal of Nuclear Medicine* pii:s002449910507. doi: 10.1967/s002449910507.

39. Ibid.

40. American Dental Association. *2013. Fluoride and Fluoridation.* Available at www.ada.org. Accessed March 2017.

41. Brissette, S. 2011. Water Fluoridation: Has It Outlived Its Usefulness? Available at http://www.healthworldnet.com. Accessed March 2017.

42. Centers for Disease Control and Prevention. 2016. *Dental Fluorosis.* Available at www.cdc.gov. Accessed March 2017.

43. Federal Register. 2015. Public Health Service Recommendation for Fluoride Concentration in Drinking Water for the Prevention of Dental Caries. Available at https://www.federalregister.gov. Accessed March 2017.

44. Institute of Medicine. 2006. *Dietary Reference Intakes: The Essential Guide to Nutrient Requirements.*

45. Centers for Disease Control and Prevention. 2016. *Community Water Fluoridation. General Fact Sheet Overview.* Available at www.cdc.gov. Accessed March 2017.

46. Centers for Disease Control and Prevention. 2016. *Water Fluoridation Basics.* Available at www.cdc.gov. Accessed March 2017.

47. American Dental Hygienists' Association. 2015. ADHA Supports New Water Fluoridation. Available at www.adha.org. Accessed March 2017.

48. Centers for Disease Control and Prevention. 2016. *Community Water Fluoridation.*

49. Chan, S., X. Jin, et al. 2017. Inverse Association of Plasma Chromium Levels with Newly Diagnosed Type 2 Diabetes: A Case-Control Study. *Nutrients* 9(3). pii: E294. doi: 10.3390/nu9030294.

50. Institute of Medicine. 2006. *Dietary Reference Intakes: The Essential Guide to Nutrient Requirements.*

51. Ibid.

52. Hoffman, N. J., B. A. Penque, et al. 2014. Chromium Enhances Insulin Responsiveness via AMPK. *Journal of Nutritional Biochemistry* 25(5):565–572.

53. Chan, S., X. Jin, et al. 2017.

54. Ibid.

55. Ganguly, R., A. M. Wen, et al. 2016. Anti-atherogenic Effect of Trivalent Chromium-loaded CPMV Nanoparticles in Human Aortic Smooth Muscle Cells under

Hyperglycemic Conditions *in vitro*. *Nanoscale* 8(12), 6542–6554. http://doi.org/10.1039/c6nr00398b

56. Liu, Y., A. Cotillard, et al. 2015. A Dietary Supplement Containing Cinnamon, Chromium and Carnosine Decreases Fasting Plasma Glucose and Increases Lean Mass in Overweight or Obese Pre-Diabetic Subjects: A Randomized, Placebo-Controlled Trial. *PLoS ONE* 10(9), e0138646. doi: 10.1371/journal.pone.0138646

57. Suksomboon, N., N. Poolsup, et al. 2014. Systematic Review and Meta-Analysis of the Efficacy and Safety of Chromium Supplementation in Diabetes. *Journal of Clinical Pharmacy and Therapeutics* 39(3):292–306.

58. Tian, H., X. Guo, et al. 2013. Chromium Picolinate Supplementation for Overweight or Obese Adults. *Cochrane Database of Systematic Reviews* doi: 10.1002/14651858. CD010063.pub2.

59. Institute of Medicine. 2006. *Dietary Reference Intakes: The Essential Guide to Nutrient Requirements.*

60. Tian. 2013. Chromium Picolinate Supplementation for Overweight or Obese Adults.

61. Roussel, A. M., A. Andriollo Sanchez, et al. 2007. Food Chromium Content, Dietary Chromium Intake and Related Biological Variables in French Free-Living Elderly. *British Journal of Nutrition* 98:326–331.

62. Laurberg, P. Iodine. 2018. In *Modern Nutrition in Health and Disease.* A. C. Ross, B. Caballero, R. J. Cousins, K. L. Tucker, and T. R. Ziegler, eds. Philadelphia: Lippincott Williams & Wilkins.

63. Ibid.

64. Institute of Medicine. 2006. *Dietary Reference Intakes: The Essential Guide to Nutrient Requirements.*

65. Ibid.

66. Institute of Medicine. 2001. *Dietary Reference Intakes: Vitamin A, Vitamin K, Arsenic, Boron,*

Chromium, Copper, Iodine, Iron, Manganese, Molybdenum, Nickel, Silicon, Vanadium, and Zinc.

67. Ibid.

68. Ibid.

69. Long, Z., Y. M. Jiang, et al. 2014. Vulnerability of Welders to Manganese Exposure—A Neuroimaging Study. *Neurotoxicology.* doi: 10.1016/j.neuro.2014.03.007.

70. Ibid.

71. Barceloux, D. G. 1999. Manganese. *Clinical Toxicology* 37:293–307.

72. Vollet, K., E. N. Haynes, et al. 2016. Manganese Exposure and Cognition Across the Lifespan: Contemporary Review and Arguments for Biphasic Dose Respnse Health Effects. *Current Environment Health Reports* 13(4):392–404.

73. Environmental Protection Agency. 2013. *Drinking Water Contaminants.* Available at http://water.epa.gov. Accessed March 2017.

74. Vollet, K., E. N. Haynes, et al. 2016. Manganese Exposure and Cognition Across the Lifespan: Contemporary Review and Arguments for Biphasic Dose Response Health Effects.

75. Institute of Medicine. 2006. *Dietary Reference Intakes: The Essential Guide to Nutrient Requirements.*

76. Bhasker, T. V., N. K. Gowda, et al. 2016. Boron Influences Immune and Antioxidant Responses by Modulating Hepatic Superoxide Dismutase Activity Under Calcium Deficit Abiotic Stress in Wister Rats. *Journal of Trace Elements in Medical Biology* 36:73–79. doi: 10.1016/j.jtemb.2016.04.007.

77. Institute of Medicine. 2001. *Dietary Reference Intakes: Vitamin A, Vitamin K, Arsenic, Boron, Chromium, Copper, Iodine, Iron, Manganese, Molybdenum, Nickel, Silicon, Vanadium, and Zinc.*

78. Ibid.

79. National Heart, Lung, and Blood Institute. 2013. *What Is Anemia?* Available at www.nhlbi.nih.gov. Accessed March 2017.

80. Centers for Disease Control and Prevention. 2016. *Anemia or Iron Deficiency.* Available at www.cdc.gov. Accessed March 2017.

81. National Institutes of Health. 2014. *Iron-Deficiency Anemia.* Available at www.nlm.nih.gov. Accessed March 2017.

82. Low, M., A. Farrell, et al. 2013. Effects of Daily Iron Supplementation in Primary-School-Aged Children: Systematic Review and Meta-Analysis of Randomized Controlled Trials. *Canadian Medical Association Journal* 185(17):E791–E802.

83. Bay, A., M. Dogan, et al. 2013. A Study on the Effects of Pica and Iron-Deficiency Anemia on Oxidative Stress, Antioxidant Capacity and Trace Elements. *Human and Experimental Toxicology* 32(9):895–903.

84. Dara, R. C., N. Marwaha, et al. 2016. A Randomized Control Study to Evaluate Effects of Short-term Oral Iron Supplementation in Regular Voluntary Blood Donors. *Indian Journal of Hematologic Blood Transfusions* 32(3):299–306. doi: 10.1007/s12288-015-0561-y.

85. Da Silva, V. R., A. D. Mackey, et al. 2018. Vitamin B_6. In *Modern Nutrition in Health and Disease.* A. C. Ross, B. Caballero, R. J. Cousins, K. L. Tucker, and T. R. Ziegler, eds. Philadelphia: Lippincott Williams & Wilkins.

86. Maakaron, J. E., and E. C. Basa. 2014. Macrocytosis Treatment and Management. Available at http://emedicine.medscape.com. Accessed March 2017.

87. Ibid.

88. Yousaf, F., B. Spinowitz, et al. 2017. Pernicious Anemia Associated Cobalamin Deficiency and Thrombotic Microangiopathy: Case Report and Review of the Literature. *Case Reports in Medicine* 2017:9410727. doi: 10.1155/2017/9410727.

89. Green, R., and A. Datta Mitra. 2017. Megaloblastic Anemias: Nutritional and Other Causes. *Medical Clinics of North American Medicine* 101(2):297–317. doi: 1016/j.mcna.2016.09.013.

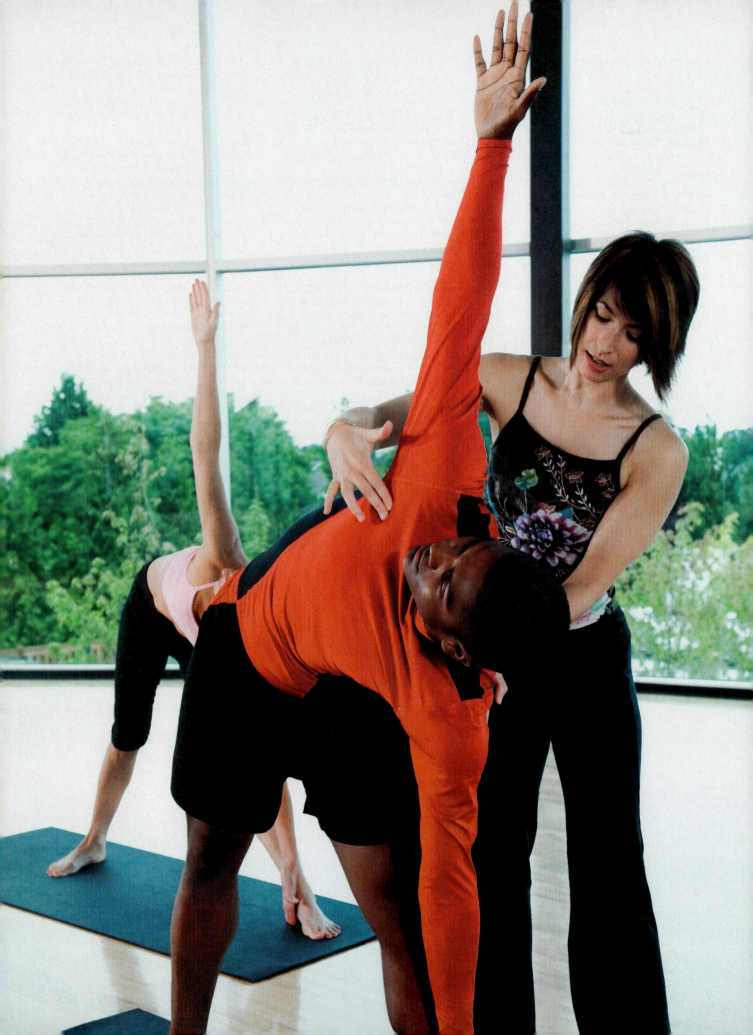

Energy Balance and Body Composition

14

Learning Outcomes

After reading this chapter, you will be able to:

14.1 Define the terms *energy balance*, *positive energy balance*, and *negative energy balance* as they relate to body weight.

14.2 Discuss the factors that contribute to total daily energy expenditure, including basal metabolism, the thermic effect of food, and the thermic effect of exercise.

14.3 Explain how energy expenditure is measured and calculate basal metabolic rate and estimated energy requirement using equations and physical activity factors.

14.4 Define the term *body composition*, and explain the methods used to assess lean body mass and body fat.

14.5 Explain the methods used to estimate a healthy body weight, and the link between body weight and mortality.

14.6 List the criteria used to diagnose eating disorders and discuss the shared traits and options for treatment.

True or False?

1. Exercise isn't necessary to lose weight. **T/F**

2. Being underweight is always healthier than being overweight. **T/F**

3. Men burn more kilocalories than women. **T/F**

4. Body mass index (BMI) can be used to determine if you are at a healthy weight, overweight, or obese. **T/F**

5. Storing fat around the hips is as unhealthy as storing it around the waist. **T/F**

6. Body composition is the same thing as body weight. **T/F**

7. Eating an excess 100 kilocalories per day will result in a weight gain of a pound a week. **T/F**

8. Skinfold calipers are used to measure body composition. **T/F**

9. Disordered eating and eating disorders are the same thing. **T/F**

10. Eating disorders can be fatal. **T/F**

See page 535 for the answers.

Flip through a magazine, watch a little television, or spend some time online, and before long you'll find someone talking about how to lose or gain weight. Maintaining a healthy body weight is all about balance—that is, balancing the food and drinks you consume with the amount of kilocalories your body burns over time. While this equation seems simple enough, food intake is not the sole cause of an unbalanced equation. Genetics, the environment, and other factors also play a strong role.

In this chapter, we discuss the concept of energy balance, the methods used to assess energy intake and energy expenditure, and the factors that influence a healthy body weight and body composition.

What Is Energy Balance and Why Is It Important?

LO 14.1 Define the terms *energy balance*, *positive energy balance*, and *negative energy balance* as they relate to body weight.

The concept of **energy balance** can be boiled down to five simple words: energy in versus energy out. When the amount of energy (in the form of kilocalories) consumed equals the amount expended, the body does not store excess kilocalories as fat or break down stored fat for energy.

An Energy Imbalance Results in Weight Gain or Loss

Body weight remains constant when the energy equation is balanced. If energy intake is greater than the amount of energy expended, the body is in a state of **positive energy balance** (**Focus Figure 14.1**). In this situation, weight gain can occur from an increase in muscle mass, an increase in adipose tissue, or both. Positive energy balance is essential during growth periods such as pregnancy, infancy, childhood, and adolescence. Strength training requires a positive energy balance to increase muscle mass, and when the body is in a state of repair following surgery or an illness. However, nonpregnant, healthy adults will experience weight gain if they are in a regular state of positive energy balance. Even a small but chronic positive energy balance can result in weight gain over time. For every 3,500 excess kilocalories consumed, about a pound of body weight is gained. So if an individual takes in 100 excess kilocalories per day, he or she will gain a little less than one pound after a month, and about 10 pounds after a year. Most likely this weight gain will be stored as fat in the adipose tissue.

A **negative energy balance** occurs when the amount of energy consumed doesn't meet the amount of energy expended. When inadequate energy is consumed, energy needs are met by mobilizing energy reserves such as stored fat. The result of a negative energy balance is usually weight loss, mostly from adipose tissue. However, some of the weight loss may reflect a decrease in muscle mass, stored glycogen, and water.

The energy balance equation appears to be quite simple. If we would simply consume the same number of kilocalories as we expend, we could maintain a healthful body weight. However, energy balance is more complex than it seems.

Food and Beverages Provide Energy In

As you learned in earlier chapters, the kilocalories that make up energy intake come from the carbohydrates, proteins, fats, and alcohol found in foods and beverages. The number of kilocalories found in a given food or beverage can be determined in one of two ways: either in a lab using a **bomb calorimeter** or by calculating the grams of carbohydrate, fat, protein, and alcohol in the food.

energy balance State at which energy (kilocalorie) intake from food and beverages is equal to energy (kilocalorie) output for basal metabolism, the thermic effect of exercise, and the thermic effect of food.

positive energy balance State in which energy intake is greater than energy expenditure; over time, this results in weight gain.

negative energy balance State in which energy intake is less than energy expenditure; over time, this results in weight loss.

bomb calorimeter Instrument used to measure the amount of heat released from food during combustion; the amount of heat produced is directly related to the number of kilocalories in a given food.

Head to Mastering Nutrition and watch a narrated video tour of this figure by author Joan Salge Blake.

A chronic state of positive or negative energy balance will result in a change in body weight.

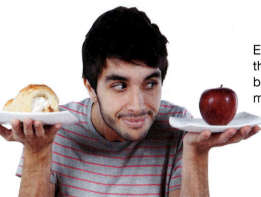

Energy balance is the relationship between the food we eat and the energy we expend each day. Finding the proper balance between energy intake and energy expenditure allows us to maintain a healthy body weight.

ENERGY BALANCE

When the kilocalories you consume meet your needs, you are in energy balance. Your weight will be stable.

ENERGY INTAKE = ENERGY EXPENDITURE = WEIGHT MAINTENANCE

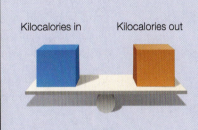

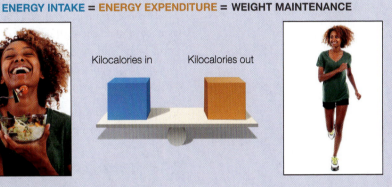

Kilocalories in   Kilocalories out

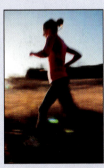

NEGATIVE ENERGY BALANCE

When you consume fewer kilocalories than you expend, your body will draw upon your stored energy to meet its needs. You will lose weight.

ENERGY INTAKE < ENERGY EXPENDITURE = WEIGHT LOSS

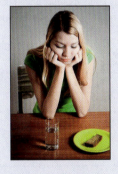

Kilocalories in   Kilocalories out

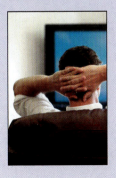

POSITIVE ENERGY BALANCE

When you take in more kilocalories than you need, the surplus calories will be stored as fat. You will gain weight.

ENERGY INTAKE > ENERGY EXPENDITURE = WEIGHT GAIN

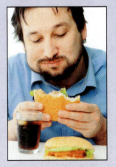

Kilocalories in   Kilocalories out

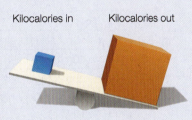

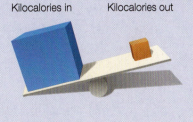

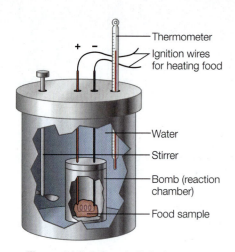

Thermometer

Ignition wires for heating food

Water

Stirrer

Bomb (reaction chamber)

Food sample

▲ **Figure 14.2 A Bomb Calorimeter Measures Energy in Foods**
A bomb calorimeter directly measures the kilocalorie content of food by measuring the heat released during combustion.

A bomb calorimeter (**Figure 14.2**) measures the amount of heat produced when a given food is burned. The energy released when the chemical bonds in the food are broken raises the temperature of the water in the calorimeter. Because one kilocalorie is the heat required to raise the temperature of one kilogram of water one degree Celsius, the rise in water temperature indicates the number of kilocalories in the food.

The burning of food also releases carbon and hydrogen, which combine with oxygen to form carbon dioxide and water. Hence, measuring the amount of oxygen consumed during combustion in the calorimeter provides an indirect measurement of the energy content of a food.

The body is not as efficient as a bomb calorimeter and does not completely digest or metabolize the fuels it consumes. The fuels that are not metabolized to energy are stored as either glycogen or body fat. The kilocalorie values obtained from a bomb calorimeter must be adapted to reflect the inefficiency of the body. For example, the heat of combustion of protein in meat is approximately 5.65 kilocalories per gram. However, because protein is only 97 percent digested and absorbed, the net kilocalories are actually 4.27 kilocalories per gram.[1] These corrected energy values are called **physiological fuel values** and reflect the kilocalories actually transformed into energy in the body. These are the energy values presented in food composition tables and databases.

Because bomb calorimeters are available only in laboratories, most individuals who want to estimate energy intake use nutrition analysis software or food composition tables to track and add up the kilocalories contained in meals. These resources provide the kilocalorie content of a given food as calculated by multiplying the grams of each energy nutrient in the food by the kilocalories per gram (see the Calculation Corner).

 Calculation Corner

Calculating the Energy Content of a Meal

Calculate the total energy content of this breakfast meal using the fuel values of 4 kilocalories per gram for carbohydrates and protein and 9 kilocalories per gram for fat.

Food	Carbohydrate (g)	Protein (g)	Fat (g)		Kilocalories
½ cup cooked oatmeal	12	3	0	=	_____
½ cup nonfat milk	6	4	0	=	_____
½ cup orange juice	12	0	0	=	_____
2 slices whole-wheat toast	30	6	2	=	_____
1 Tbsp margarine	0	0	10	=	_____
8 fl oz coffee	0	0	0	=	_____
Total kilocalories				=	_____

(a) Complete the table by calculating the total kilocalories for each food. Multiply the fuel value of each macronutrient by the number of grams found in each food. For example, ½ cup of cooked oatmeal would be calculated as follows:

Total kcal = (12 g carbohydrate × 4 kcal/g) + (3 g protein × 4 kcal/g) + (0 g fat × 9 kcal/g)

Total kcal = 60 kcal

(b) After you have calculated the total kilocalories for each food, add the kilocalories for each food together to determine the total kilocalories for the meal.

physiological fuel values Real energy value of foods that are digested and absorbed; adjusted from the results of bomb calorimetry because of the inefficiency of the body.

Body Processes and Physical Activity Result in Energy Out

The other side of the energy equation is the expenditure of energy. Body processes, from digestion to respiration to circulation, expend energy, as does physical activity, from texting a friend to running up a flight of stairs. Obviously, then, each individual varies in the energy he or she expends throughout the day. Knowing your average daily energy expenditure is essential if you want to either stay in energy balance to maintain your body weight or create an energy imbalance to gain or lose weight. We explain how to estimate your total daily energy expenditure next.

> **LO 14.1: THE TAKE-HOME MESSAGE** Energy balance is the relationship between energy intake and energy expenditure. In positive energy balance, more kilocalories are consumed than are expended, resulting in weight gain. In negative energy balance, more kilocalories are expended than are consumed, resulting in weight loss. The kilocalories in foods and beverages provide energy in, whereas basic body processes and physical activity account for energy out.

How Is Total Daily Energy Expenditure Calculated?

LO 14.2 Discuss the factors that contribute to total daily energy expenditure, including basal metabolism, the thermic effect of food, and the thermic effect of exercise.

Several components contribute to our **total daily energy expenditure (TDEE)**; that is, the total kilocalories needed to keep the body functioning and fuel physical activity (**Figure 14.3**).

Basal Metabolism Contributes to TDEE

The energy needed to fuel the body's vital functions, such as pumping blood, expanding the lungs, and brain function, is known as its **basal metabolism** and is expressed as a **basal metabolic rate (BMR)**. This is the amount of energy spent to meet the body's basic physiological needs when it's at physical, emotional, and digestive rest, but not asleep—in other words, the minimum amount of energy needed to keep your awake, resting body alive. If you sit on the couch to watch television, you aren't engaged in any physical activity but your cells are still active and require energy for basic functions.

The BMR determines approximately 50–70 percent of your total daily energy use (see Figure 14.3). Your **lean body mass (LBM)** is the factor that most affects your BMR. Lean body mass is defined as the muscle, bone, and other nonfat tissue that makes up your body weight. Because lean body mass is more active tissue than body fat, it burns kilocalories at a higher rate than stored fat, even at rest. Thus, the more lean body mass you have, the greater your BMR—about 70 percent of your BMR is attributable to the metabolic activity of your LBM. Additional factors such as age, gender, body size, genes, ethnicity, emotional and physical stress, thyroid hormone levels, nutritional state, and environmental temperature, as well as caffeine and nicotine intake, affect BMR. **Table 14.1** explains each of these factors.

BMR, which is determined by an indirect measurement of the amount of oxygen consumed, is measured when a person is awake and cellular activity is the lowest. To get an accurate BMR measurement, your sympathetic nervous system cannot be stimulated. This is the reason a person's BMR is usually measured in a laboratory setting in the morning while the person lies motionless in a controlled (no shivering or sweating) environment

total daily energy expenditure (TDEE) Total kilocalories needed to meet daily energy requirements.

basal metabolism Amount of energy expended by the body to meet its basic physiological needs, including muscle tone and heart and brain function.

basal metabolic rate (BMR) Measure of basal metabolism taken when the body is at rest in a warm, quiet environment after a 12-hour fast; expressed as kilocalories per kilogram of body weight per hour.

lean body mass (LBM) Total body weight minus the fat mass; consists of water, bones, vital organs, and muscle; metabolically active tissue in the body.

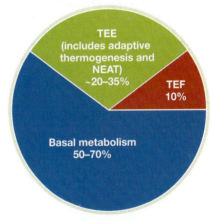

▲ **Figure 14.3 Requirements for the Total Daily Energy Expenditure** The amount of total energy expended during a 24-hour period is composed of an individual's basal metabolism, the thermic effect of exercise or physical activity, which includes adaptive thermogenesis and nonexercise activity thermogenesis, and the thermic effect of foods. A sedentary individual will expend a larger percentage of energy from basal metabolism compared with an active person who would have a greater need for energy to fuel physical activity.

TABLE 14.1 Factors That Affect Basal Metabolism

Factor	Explanation
Lean body mass	Lean body mass, which is mostly muscle mass, is more metabolically active than fat tissue, so more kilocalories are needed to maintain it. Athletes who have a large percentage of lean body mass due to their increased muscle mass have a higher BMR than individuals who aren't athletic.
Age	For adults, BMR declines about 1–2 percent per decade after the early adult years but it increases by 15 percent during pregnancy. For children, BMR increases during times of rapid growth such as infancy and adolescence.
Gender	Women have less lean body mass, and typically have a higher percentage of body fat than men. This results in women having a BMR up to 10 percent lower than men's. Women also tend to have a smaller body size.
Body size	Taller individuals have a higher BMR due to increased surface area compared with shorter individuals. More surface area means more heat lost from the body, which causes the metabolism rate to increase to maintain the body's temperature.
Genes	Research suggests that genes may affect BMR, as individuals within families have similar metabolic rates.
Race	African Americans have BMRs that are about 10 percent lower than those of Caucasians.
Stress	Hormones such as epinephrine, which are released during emotional stress, increase BMR. Physiological stress on the body caused by injury, fever, burns, and infections also causes the release of hormones that raise BMR. Heat loss from the body through wounds, as well as the response of the immune system during infection, increase BMR.
Hormones	An increase in thyroid hormone increases BMR, whereas too little of this hormone lowers BMR. Hormone fluctuations during a woman's menstrual cycle lower BMR during the phase before ovulation.
Starvation	Starvation and fasting for more than about 48 hours lower BMR.
Environmental temperature	Being very cold or very hot can increase BMR. The change is minimal if clothing or air temperature are adjusted.
Caffeine	Caffeine can raise BMR, but only slightly when consumed regularly in moderate amounts.
Drugs	Nicotine may increase BMR.* Stimulant drugs such as amphetamine and ephedrine increase BMR.

*Note: Smoking is not a weight-management strategy. Some people may think that replacing snacks with cigarettes helps them stay slim, but the health risks associated with smoking, such as lung cancer, heart disease, and stroke, make it a foolish habit. Anyone concerned about weight gain when quitting smoking can minimize the chances of this with exercise.

Source: Data from Food and Nutrition Board, National Institute of Medicine, *Dietary Reference Intakes: The Essential Guide to Nutrient Requirements* (Washington, DC: National Academies Press, 2006).

after a 12-hour overnight fast. Neither the digestion of food nor physical activity (which both require energy) is factored into the BMR.

Because such precise circumstances are needed to measure BMR, it is a challenge to obtain. For this reason, the **resting metabolic rate (RMR)** is often used instead. The RMR is the amount of energy used by the body, measured when the person is lying calmly after only a 3- to 4-hour fasting period. The RMR is about 6 percent higher than the BMR, as it reflects increases in energy expenditure related to any recent food intake or physical activity.

The Thermic Effect of Food Contributes to TDEE

The digestive system requires kilocalories to digest and absorb the foods you eat, and the amount of energy required for this is called the **thermic effect of food (TEF)**. The body uses energy to process the fuels and extract kilocalories during catabolism. Immediately after eating and for several hours after a meal, energy expenditure increases to provide ATP for chewing, peristalsis, digestion, absorption, and transport of nutrients. Approximately 10 percent of the kilocalories in food consumed is used for TEF. In other words, about 10 kilocalories in a 100-kilocalorie cookie are used to process the cookie. Likewise

resting metabolic rate (RMR) Measure of the amount of energy expended by the body at rest and after approximately a 3- to 4-hour fasting period; about 6 percent higher than BMR.

thermic effect of food (TEF) Amount of energy expended by the body to digest, absorb, transport, metabolize, and store energy-yielding nutrients from foods.

due to TEF, the gross kilocalories found in a food are slightly more than the net amount available for energy expenditures.

The type of nutrients consumed influences the TEF. For instance, a meal high in protein has the highest thermic effect (approximately 20–30 percent), probably because of the synthesis of body proteins after a protein meal. Carbohydrates have a greater TEF (5–10 percent) than fat (0–3 percent), most likely due to the energy cost to convert glucose into glycogen. The energy cost of converting fat into stored triglycerides is minimal. Other factors that influence the TEF, such as composition of a meal, alcohol intake, age, and athletic training status, are presented in **Table 14.2**. A trained athlete appears to be able to digest and absorb food using fewer kilocalories than the untrained.[2] An obese individual may also have a reduced TEF. The reason for the decrease in TEF in obesity may be due to insulin insensitivity.[3] Note that the number of kilocalories used for TEF is small compared with the number expended by BMR and physical activity.

The Thermic Effect of Exercise Contributes to TDEE

Energy can also be expended by producing heat (**thermogenesis**). *Adaptive thermogenesis* is the term used for the processes by which the body regulates heat production. It is influenced by environmental changes such as stress, temperature, or diet, which result in a change in metabolism. Shivering when the temperature drops is an example of adaptive thermogenesis.

Experts are still not sure how adaptive thermogenesis relates to total daily energy expenditure. A reduced ability to produce heat from food energy rather than store the kilocalories in fat tissue may be partly responsible for greater weight gain in overweight individuals versus their lighter peers.[4] Some researchers believe adaptive thermogenesis explains why two people can have the same diet and exercise patterns but have completely different body compositions.[5]

Researchers do know, however, that physical activity is thermogenic. In fact, the heat produced by contracting muscle during physical activity or exercise can contribute significantly to the amount of energy expended each day. Walking across campus, vacuuming your home, or pulling weeds in the garden are all activities that require energy above the minimum needed for BMR. This expenditure of kilocalories is referred to as the **thermic effect of exercise (TEE)**. The number of kilocalories you need each day for TEE

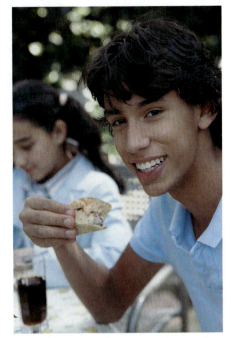

The process of digesting and absorbing foods requires energy called the thermic effect of food.

TABLE 14.2	Factors That Influence the Thermic Effect of Food
Factor	**Effects on the Thermic Effect of Food**
Type of fuel	Fat has the least effect on TEF; protein has the greatest effect.
Meal composition	Consuming all three macronutrients together produces a lower TEF than would be produced by protein or carbohydrates separately.
Fiber content	A high-fiber meal produces a lower TEF.
Age	TEF declines as we age.
Environmental temperature	Consuming a meal in a cold environment increases TEF.
Alcohol	Alcohol consumption increases TEF but reduces TEF if alcohol is consumed in a cold environment.
Intense exercise	TEF is higher following intense exercise.
Training status	Individuals who are trained athletes have a lower TEF than untrained individuals.
Obesity	Obese individuals have a lower TEF than normal-weight individuals.

Source: Data from J. Kang, *Bioenergetics Primer for Exercise Science* (Champaign, IL: Human Kinetics, 2008).

thermogenesis Generation of heat from the basal metabolism, digestion of food, and all forms of physical activity.

thermic effect of exercise (TEE) Increase in muscle contraction that occurs during physical activity, which produces heat and contributes to the total daily energy expenditure.

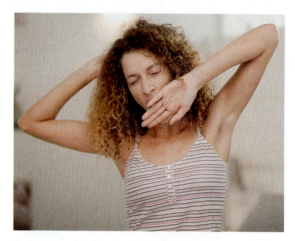

Once you crawl out of bed in the morning, the kilocalories you expend to stretch, take a shower, and get dressed are classified as TEE.

depends on the activity itself, the amount of time you perform the activity, and how much you weigh. For instance, if two males run together at the same pace for an hour, but one male weighs 10 kilograms more than the other, the heavier male will burn 496 kilocalories compared with 400 kilocalories for his lighter running partner.

The kilocalories expended for TEE for sedentary people is less than half of their BMR. For very physically active individuals who have a greater muscle mass, TEE can be as much as double their BMR. In short, the more physical activity people incorporate into their daily routine, the more kilocalories they need to consume to maintain energy balance. For example, two females who weigh the same and are similar in age both have a BMR of 1,200 kilocalories. One female is sedentary and her TEE is only 600 kilocalories, while the second female has a much higher TEE of 2,000 kilocalories because of her physically active lifestyle. Based on her TEE, the sedentary female can only consume 1,800 kilocalories per day (BMR + TEE) to maintain energy balance and not gain weight. In contrast, because of her higher TEE, the physically active female must eat 3,200 kilocalories per day to meet her energy requirements and not lose weight.

The amount of energy expended during physical activity goes beyond the activity itself. Exercise causes a small increase in energy expenditure for some time after the activity has stopped because of the recovery and adaptation the body undergoes following the exercise.[6]

In addition to the energy required to walk, jog, or lift weights, TEE also includes the cost of energy to maintain posture and body position, and for fidgeting and other activities we don't normally consider exercise. This form of energy expenditure is called **nonexercise activity thermogenesis (NEAT)**. NEAT may play a key role in energy balance. Adults who fidget or are hyperactive tend to burn more kilocalories than people who do not. While sitting in front of a computer all day does expend kilocalories, the amount is minimal.[7] Read the nearby Examining the Evidence box to learn more on the influence of NEAT on energy expenditure.

Figure 14.4 summarizes the factors on both sides of the energy balance equation that contribute to your total daily energy expenditure.

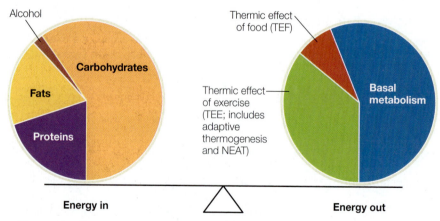

▲ **Figure 14.4 The Factors Involved in Energy Balance**
Basal metabolism, the thermic effect of food, and the thermic effect of exercise account for the energy-out side of the energy balance equation. The protein, carbohydrate, fat, and alcohol found in foods and beverages contribute to energy intake.

nonexercise activity thermogenesis (NEAT) Energy expended for all activities not related to sleeping, eating, or exercise, including fidgeting, performing work-related activities, and playing.

What Is NEAT About Fidgeting?

Fidgeting is one aspect of the energy expenditure referred to as NEAT, or nonexercise activity thermogenesis.[1] The term *NEAT*, coined by cardiologist Dr. James A. Levine, is a component of TEE that refers to the energy we expend for everything we do while awake except eating or participating in structured exercise such as jogging, aerobics, or power walking. NEAT includes walking to work, dancing, gardening, and, yes, even fidgeting.

As a nation, the less often we move, the more obese we become.[2] Research has reported a strong correlation between a drop in NEAT and an increase in weight gain, specifically body fat.[3] Studies report that lean people who are sedentary stand and move 152 minutes longer per day than obese individuals do. And obese subjects sit 164 minutes per day (over 2.5 hours) more than lean subjects. In other words, people who are classified as obese have low NEAT.[4] Sitting, it would seem, increases your risk of obesity and all of the health risks associated with excess weight.

The number of kilocalories burned by NEAT activities can vary substantially between individuals. Levine and colleagues report that NEAT can vary by almost 2,000 kilocalories per day.[5] What accounts for these large differences in daily energy expenditure? Let's examine the evidence.

Your Occupation Impacts NEAT

The advancement of technology has reduced NEAT by limiting the physical activity of jobs in the workplace. According to current research, working in a sedentary occupation is the main factor contributing to lower NEAT.[6] Among workers, men with sedentary jobs (secretaries, motor vehicle operators) were 22 percent less active and women were 30 percent less active than those with more active professions, such as farm or construction workers.[7] If you compare this to steps taken per day, a desk-bound man or woman takes only 5,000–6,000 steps a day. That compares with about 18,000 steps a day for the average man and 14,000 for the average woman in an Amish farming community.[8]

In controlled studies of sedentary adults, changes in the work environment that encourage NEAT, such as fidgeting and standing, have been shown to reduce weight gain. For example, standing rather than sitting is an example of passive work that burns more kilocalories. **Figure 1** illustrates the differences of energy expenditure in standing versus sitting during work. For those who find it difficult to stand during the workday, sitting on a therapy ball, which requires the individual to contract core muscles, may be another passive means to increase energy expenditure.[9] In fact, standing still for hours is not recommended. The important concept is to mix both sitting and standing to avoid injury and burn more kilocalories.[10]

Research is currently being conducted in a variety of office settings on the feasibility of using walking stations in the workplace and the impact these stations may have on body composition, cognitive

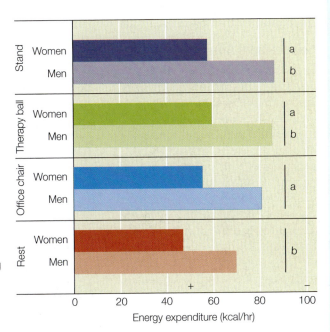

▲ **Figure 1**
Energy expenditure in males and females expressed as kilocalories per hour during rest, office chair, therapy ball, and standing postures. Data are mean $\pm$ S.E.; $p < 0.05$ for means with the same letter.

Based on: E. A. Beers, J. N. Roemmich, L. H. Epstein, and P. J. Horvath. 2008. Increasing Passive Energy Expenditure during Clerical Work. *European Journal of Applied Physiology* 103:353–360. Copyright © by Springer. Reprinted with permission of Springer Science + Business Media.

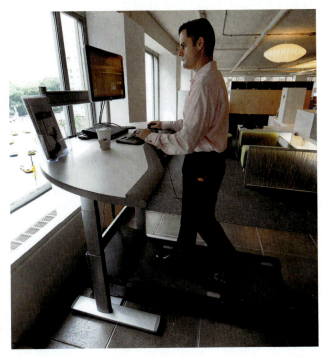

Walking slowly at the rate of about 1 mile per hour while working at your desk increases energy expenditure by about 200 kilocalories per hour compared with sitting at your desk.

function, and job productivity. The use of walking desks should increase NEAT energy expenditure and may improve overall health in the workplace.

Leisure Time Affects NEAT

Labor-saving devices and technology make it possible to squelch much leisure-time NEAT through the use of riding lawnmowers, electronically programmed vacuum cleaners, bread machines, microwave ovens, electric hammers, and handheld video games.[11] Consider your leisure-time hours after work or school and on the weekends. Do you surf the Internet or watch television for hours until bedtime, just moving the mouse or using the remote control? If this were your routine after work, the average energy expenditure for that sedentary activity would be about 70 kilocalories per hour.[12] What if you cleaned the house, walked your dog after dinner, or worked in the garden as an alternative? Instead of 70 kilocalories per hour, you could burn 200–400 kilocalories per hour. This change in NEAT could potentially increase the amount of energy you burn by more than 800 kilocalories per day.

NEAT Changes with Food Intake

Research suggests that when you eat too much, NEAT increases, and when you eat too little, NEAT decreases. This was illustrated in a study that overfed nonobese subjects 1,000 kilocalories per day for 8 weeks. As expected, the subjects gained between 1.4 kilograms and 7.2 kilograms of weight. What was unexpected was that there was also an increase in NEAT, including changes in posture, fidgeting, and daily activities. The increase in NEAT seemed to be a factor in those who gained less weight than the others. The researchers concluded that the increase in NEAT helped resist additional weight gain even when subjects overate.[13]

Move and Walk More to Prevent Obesity

Even if you engage in regular structured exercise, your overall daily energy expenditure may be relatively low if you spend the rest of your time sitting. The

FITNESS TIPS
Increase Your NEAT

Find a friend at work to walk with at lunch.

Stand or pace while talking on the telephone.

Put on your headset and listen to your favorite music while you walk during your morning break.

When you watch television, stretch your shoulders, back, and legs.

Fold laundry while watching your favorite TV show.

Take the stairs instead of riding the elevator or escalator.

If you drive to work or school, park farther from the building.

Buy a pedometer to measure your steps; aim for 10,000 per day.

secret to increasing your NEAT and burning more kilocalories during the day, especially during work hours, is to get up out of the chair and move more. Find ways to work simple movements into your day—tap your feet, pace while you talk on the phone, stand while you read, get up and walk to a coworker's desk instead of emailing. Any additional NEAT activities will help minimize the potential health risks of a chair-sitting lifestyle. See the Fitness Tips for helpful suggestions.

References

1. Villablanca, P. A., J. R. Alegria, et al. 2015. Nonexercise Activity Thermogenesis in Obesity Management. *Mayo Clinic Proceedings* 90(4):509–519. doi: 10.1016/j.mayocp.2015.02.001.
2. Lear, S. A., et al. 2014. The Association between Ownership of Common Household Devices and Obesity and Diabetes in High, Middle, and Low Income Countries. *Canadian Medical Association Journal*. doi: 10.1503/cmaj.131090.
3. Müller, M. J., and A. Bosy-Westphal. 2013. Adaptive Thermogenesis with Weight Loss in Humans. *Obesity* 21(2):218–228. doi: 10.1002/oby.22027.
4. Gupta, N., D. M. Hallman, et al. 2016. Are Temporal Patterns of Sitting Associated with Obesity Among Blue-Collar Workers?: A Cross Sectional Study Using Accelerometers. *BMC Public Health* 16:148. doi: 10.1186/s12889-016-2803-9.
5. Levine, J. A., W. M. W. Vander, et al. 2006. Non-Exercise Activity Thermogenesis: The Crouching Tiger Hidden Dragon of Societal Weight Gain. *Arteriosclerosis, Thrombosis, and Vascular Biology* 26:729–736.
6. Villablanca, P. A., J. R. Alegria, et al. 2015. Nonexercise Activity Thermogenesis in Obesity Management. *Mayo Clinic Proceedings* 90:509–519.
7. Aittasalo, M., M. Livson, et al. 2017. Moving to Business – Changes in Physical Activity and Sedentary Behavior after Multilevel Intervention in Small and Medium-Size Workplaces. *BMC Public Health* 17:319. doi: 10.1186/s12889-017-4229-4.
8. Hairston, K. G., J. L. Ducharme, et al. 2013. Comparison of BMI and Physical Activity Between Old Order Amish Children and Non-Amish Children. *Diabetes Care* 36(4):873–878. doi: 10.2337/dc12-0934.
9. Pederson, S. J., et al. 2013. An E-Health Intervention Designed to Increase Workday Energy Expenditure by Reducing Prolonged Occupational Sitting Habits. *Work*. doi: 10.3233/WOR-131644.
10. Van Nassau, F., J. Y. Chau, et al. 2015. Validity and Responsiveness of Four Measures of Occupational Sitting and Standing. *International Journal of Behavioral Nutrition and Physical Activity* 12:144. doi: 10.1186/s12966-015-0306-1
11. Lear. 2014. The Association between Ownership of Common Household Devices and Obesity and Diabetes in High, Middle, and Low Income Countries.
12. ChooseMyPlate. 2015. *How Many Calories Does Physical Activity Use?* Available at www.choosemyplate.gov. Accessed March 2017.
13. Villablanca, P. A., J. R. Alegria, et al. 2015. Nonexercise Activity Thermogenesis in Obesity Management.

LO 14.2: THE TAKE-HOME MESSAGE About 50–70 percent of total daily energy expenditure (TDEE) is attributable to basal metabolic rate (BMR), the amount of energy spent to meet the body's basic physiological needs when it is at rest. Lean body mass accounts for about 70 percent of BMR. In addition to BMR, TDEE includes the thermic effect of food (TEF), or the energy spent to digest and absorb nutrients from food; adaptive thermogenesis, the processes by which the body regulates heat production; and the thermic effect of exercise (TEE), which includes the energy spent on physical activities and nonexercise activity thermogenesis (NEAT).

How Do We Measure Energy Expenditure?

LO 14.3 Explain how energy expenditure is measured and calculate basal metabolic rate and estimated energy requirement using equations and physical activity factors.

Have you ever wondered how many kilocalories you burn walking to class or washing your car? Or how resting metabolic rate is calculated? Several methods have been developed to measure energy expenditure. Some of these methods require the skills of a trained technician using expensive equipment. Other methods involve simple equations and a calculator.

Direct and Indirect Calorimetry Measure Energy Expenditure

An individual's energy expenditure can be measured by *direct* or *indirect calorimetry*. Both methods quantify the amount of energy produced during rest and physical activity.

Direct calorimetry measures the amount of heat the body generates and can be determined using a metabolic chamber in a specialized laboratory. Briefly, a metabolic chamber is an airtight room designed with the comforts an individual would need for normal daily living such as a bed, chair, TV, telephone, treadmill for exercise, and bathroom. The temperature and relative humidity in the room are controlled and the oxygen and carbon dioxide concentrations of the air supply and exhaust are measured for 24 hours. The concept is similar to the bomb calorimeter, but rather than measuring the amount of heat generated by burning food, this method measures the change in water temperature caused by heat that dissipates from the body of a person in the chamber. Although this method provides a precise answer to the question of how many kilocalories an individual expends, for most people its use is too expensive and impractical.

The more practical and less expensive approach is to use **indirect calorimetry** to estimate the amount of energy expended. Indirect measurements sample the amount of oxygen consumed and carbon dioxide produced during exercise and for a specific amount of time. Metabolic calculations can then be done to determine energy expenditure. **Figure 14.5** illustrates two examples of indirect calorimetry—at rest and during physical activity. Figure 14.5a illustrates the use of a metabolic cart, which measures the uptake of oxygen and the output of carbon dioxide to determine resting energy expenditure while sitting in a metabolic chamber. Figure 14.5b illustrates the use of a collection bag, which collects expired carbon dioxide, allowing researchers to calculate oxygen consumption and thereby energy expenditure during exercise.

direct calorimetry Direct measurement of the energy expended by the body; obtained by assessing heat loss.

indirect calorimetry Indirect measurement of energy expenditure obtained by measuring the amount of oxygen consumed and carbon dioxide produced.

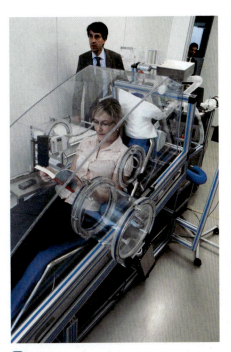

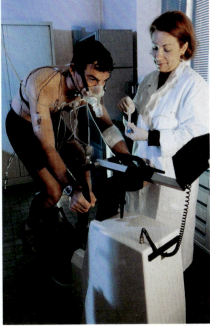

(a) Measuring metabolic rate at rest

(b) Measuring metabolic rate during exercise

▲ **Figure 14.5 Medical Tools Can Indirectly Measure Energy Expenditure**
Researchers can use (a) a metabolic cart to measure the amount of oxygen consumed and carbon dioxide produced at rest or (b) a collection bag to calculate oxygen consumed and carbon dioxide produced during exercise. This information can then be used to indirectly calculate an individual's energy expenditure.

Simple Calculations Are Used to Estimate Energy Expenditure

Recall from Chapter 2 that the DRIs include the **estimated energy requirement (EER)**, which is the average kilocalorie intake that is estimated to maintain energy balance. An individual's EER is based on gender, age, height, body weight, and level of physical activity. The physical activity levels are assigned numerical values from sedentary (1.00) to very active (1.45–1.48), as shown in **Table 14.3**. The calculation used by the DRI committee to estimate EER is presented in the Calculation Corner.[8] You can obtain an even more precise EER by assessing every minute of movement and physical activity that you do throughout the day and, based on this, calculating the energy that you expend.

Calculation Corner

What's Your Estimated Energy Requirement (EER)?
You can estimate your energy requirement for kilocalories using this two-step calculation:

(1) First, complete the information below.
  (a) My age is _____.
  (b) My physical activity during the day based on Table 14.3 is _____.
  (c) My weight in pounds is _____ divided by 2.2 = _____ kilograms.
  (d) My height in inches is _____ divided by 39.4 = _____ meters.

(2) Using your answers from each part of step 1, complete the following calculation based on your gender and age.

Males, 19+ years old, use this calculation:

$$\text{EER} = [662 - (9.53 \times \underline{})] + \underline{} \times [(15.91 \times \underline{}) + (539.6 \times \underline{})]$$
$$\qquad\qquad\quad (a)\qquad\qquad (b)\qquad\qquad\quad (c)\qquad\qquad\qquad (d)$$

Females, 19+ years old, use this calculation:

$$\text{EER} = [354 - (6.91 \times \underline{})] + \underline{} \times [(9.36 \times \underline{}) + (726 \times \underline{})]$$
$$\qquad\qquad\quad (a)\qquad\qquad (b)\qquad\qquad\quad (c)\qquad\qquad\qquad (d)$$

(3) Now calculate Will's EER. Will is 21 years old, weighs 180 pounds, and stands at 5 feet 11 inches tall. He describes his physical activity level as active. What is Will's estimated energy requirement?

> Go to Mastering Nutrition and complete a Math Video activity similar to the problem in this Calculation Corner.

TABLE 14.3 Physical Activity Factors for Men and Women

Physical Activity Level	Physical Activity Factor for Men	Physical Activity Factor for Women
Sedentary	1.00	1.00
Low level of activity (walking approximately 2 miles per day at 3 to 4 miles per hour)	1.11	1.12
Active (walking approximately 7 miles per day at 3–4 miles per hour)	1.25	1.27
Very active (walking approximately 17 miles per day at 3–4 miles per hour)	1.45	1.48

Source: Data from Food and Nutrition Board, National Institute of Medicine, *Dietary Reference Intakes: The Essential Guide to Nutrient Requirements* (Washington, DC: National Academies Press, 2006).

estimated energy requirement (EER)
Average kilocalorie intake that is estimated to maintain energy balance based on a person's gender, age, height, body weight, and level of physical activity.

Another calculation often used is the Harris-Benedict equation, which also calculates RMR based on gender, age, height, and weight and applies an activity factor to determine total daily energy expenditure. The drawback to this equation is that it does not include lean body mass, so it may not be accurate for individuals who are very muscular (for whom it underestimates kilocalorie needs) or who are very fat (for whom it overestimates kilocalorie needs). In those circumstances, other calculations may be used in clinical settings.

Want to increase your energy expenditure? Check out the nearby Fitness Tips.

LO 14.3: THE TAKE-HOME MESSAGE Energy expenditure can be measured by direct calorimetry using a metabolic chamber or by indirect calorimetry using a metabolic cart or collection bag. Simple calculations can also be used to estimate energy expenditure using age, height, weight, and level of physical activity.

What Is Body Composition and How Is It Assessed?

LO 14.4 Define the term *body composition*, and explain the methods used to assess lean body mass and body fat.

Body tissues include bone, skin, muscle, fat, organs, and blood, which are made up of the same basic nutrients: water, protein, minerals, and fat. The ratio of fat tissue to lean body mass is called **body composition**. This ratio, stated as *percent body fat*, is particularly important for the sake of measuring health risks associated with too much body fat.

Most Body Fat Is Stored in Adipose Tissue

Two types of fat make up total body fat: **essential fat**, which includes the fat found in the bone marrow, heart, lungs, liver, spleen, kidneys, intestines, muscles, and central nervous system, and *stored fat*, found in adipocytes. Essential fat is just that—essential for the body to function. Women have four times (12 percent) more essential fat than men (3 percent) because of the fat deposits in breast tissue and surrounding the uterus.

Every cell contains some fat, but most body fat is the stored fat found in adipocytes, either as **subcutaneous fat** under the skin or as **visceral fat** around the internal organs. Subcutaneous and visceral fat insulate the body from cold temperatures and help protect and cushion the internal organs (**Figure 14.6**). Men and women store subcutaneous fat slightly differently, with men more likely to accumulate it in the belly, hips, and thighs, and women more apt to store it in the breasts, neck, and upper arms, as well as in the hips and thighs.

Adipocytes release fat to be used as fuel when the body is in negative energy balance. An adipocyte shrinks as more fat is hydrolyzed from storage and overall body weight is lost. When the body is in positive energy balance, fat accumulates in the adipocytes, which expand in size, and weight gain occurs.

Adipose tissue is described as *white fat* because of its creamy white appearance. Another type of adipose tissue, called **brown adipose tissue (BAT)**, is made up of specialized fat cells that contain more mitochondria and are rich in blood (**Figure 14.7**). While white adipose tissue is used as a storage depot for excess kilocalories, the function of BAT is to generate heat. Found primarily in infants, BAT protects infants from heat loss and cold. Recent research suggests that adults, especially older adults, have more BAT than once thought. Studies have shown that the more BAT an adult has, the lower their body mass index, suggesting that this active tissue plays an important role in adult metabolism.[9] This may be due to the fact that brown adipose tissue converts kilocalories into heat rather than storing them.

body composition Ratio of fat to lean tissue (muscle, bone, and organs) in the body; usually expressed as percent body fat.

essential fat Component of body fat that is necessary for health and normal body functions; includes the fat stored in the bone marrow, heart, lungs, liver, spleen, kidneys, intestines, muscles, and the lipid-rich tissues of the central nervous system.

subcutaneous fat Fat located under the skin and between the muscles.

visceral fat Body fat associated with the internal organs and stored in the abdominal area.

brown adipose tissue (BAT) Type of adipose tissue, found primarily in infants, that produces body heat; gets its name from the large number of mitochondria and capillaries responsible for the brown color.

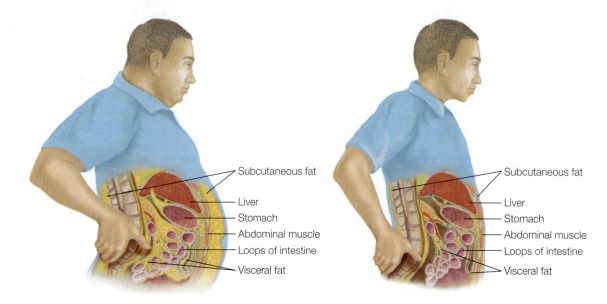

▲ **Figure 14.6 Visceral and Subcutaneous Fat Storage in the Body**
Visceral fat stored around the abdominal organs is more likely to lead to health problems than is subcutaneous fat sandwiched between the muscle and skin.

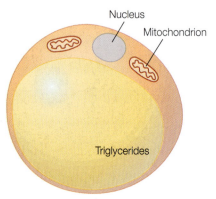

White adipocyte

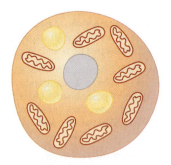

Brown adipocyte

▲ **Figure 14.7 White Adipocyte and Brown Adipocyte**
Brown adipose tissue has significantly more mitochondria and less stored triglyceride than white adipose tissue.

Body Fat Level and Distribution Affect Health

Carrying either too much or too little body fat can affect body functions and impair health. Everyone needs to have a certain amount of body fat to meet basic needs, but excess amounts of body fat can impair overall health. For this reason, specific body composition standards have been developed over the years from a variety of research studies to help individuals avoid health risks (**Table 14.4**). These body fat ranges, which can be measured using a variety of indirect methods (discussed shortly), are based on epidemiological studies of the general population of Americans.

How *much* fat you carry isn't the only determinant of health risk—*where* you carry it also matters. Storing excess fat around the waist versus carrying it around the hips and thighs has been shown to increase the risk of heart disease, diabetes, and hypertension.[10] **Central** (or android) **obesity** occurs when excess visceral and subcutaneous fat is stored in the abdomen (**Figure 14.8**). This is sometimes referred to as an "apple-shaped" fat distribution pattern and is more common in men than in women. **Gynoid obesity** is due to excess fat stored in the lower part of the body around the thighs and buttocks. This "pear-shaped" fat distribution pattern is more frequently found in women than in men.

TABLE 14.4	Body Composition Reference Standards for Adult Men and Women	
	Men	**Women**
Essential fat	3 percent of total body fat	12 percent of total body fat
Desirable fatness for good health	10–20 percent body fat	16–26 percent body fat
Overfat	More than 25 percent body fat	More than 30 percent body fat

Source: Data from W. D. McArdle, F. I. Katch, and V. L. Katch, *Sports and Exercise Nutrition*, 4th ed. (Baltimore: Lippincott Williams & Wilkins, 2012).

Fatty acids released from visceral fat located near the liver are believed to travel to the liver and contribute to hyperlipidemia. Visceral fat also contributes to insulin resistance, high levels of blood triglyceride, low levels of the good HDL cholesterol, and high levels of LDL cholesterol in the blood, which all increase the risk of heart disease and diabetes. Insulin resistance also increases the risk for hypertension. Men, postmenopausal women, and obese people tend to have more visceral fat than young adults and lean individuals.

Body Composition Is Assessed Indirectly

There are several indirect measurements used to estimate the percentage of body fat and lean body mass in the body. The most popular indirect techniques are found in laboratory settings and include hydrostatic weighing, air displacement, dual-energy X-ray absorptiometry (DEXA), bioelectrical impedance, and skinfold measurement (Table 14.5).

Percent Body Fat

Because fat mass has a lower density than either muscles or bones, it is possible to estimate body fat percentage from body volume. **Hydrostatic weighing** and **air-displacement plethysmography** are two methods that use body volume to measure percent body fat. Hydrostatic weighing is based on the principle that an object immersed in water is buoyed up by a force equal to the weight of the fluid displaced by the object. In other words, if the density of an object is greater than the density of water, the object sinks. If the density of the object is less than water, the object floats. We can use this principle to determine body composition by measuring the difference in body weight in air compared with under water. With a 2–3 percent margin of error, hydrostatic weighing is considered one of the most accurate assessment tools. The BodPod, an air displacement plethysmography device that measures air rather than water displacement, is similarly accurate within 3 percent. Both hydrostatic weighing and the BodPod have pros and cons. While both are accurate, hydrostatic weighing takes longer; some people find it difficult to be submersed under water; and the equipment is usually only found in research facilities. The BodPod, on the other hand, is faster and it only requires you to sit quietly in a chamber. See the Calculation Corner for the equation used to determine body composition from either of these body volume methods.

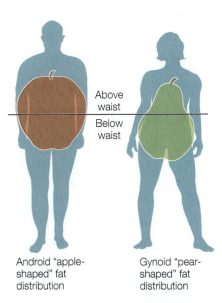

▲ **Figure 14.8 Android and Gynoid Fat Distribution Patterns**
Men and women store fat differently. Men tend to store it in the upper body including the abdomen, chest, neck, and back—often referred to as "apple-shaped" fat distribution—whereas women tend to store it below the waist including the buttocks, hips, and thighs for more of a "pear-shaped" appearance.

Android "apple-shaped" fat distribution

Gynoid "pear-shaped" fat distribution

 Calculation Corner

Body Volume and Density

The body volume determined by either hydrostatic weighing or air displacement is mathematically converted to density and then to percentage of body fat using this equation:

Body density = body weight (kg)/body volume (L)

Percentage of body fat = (495/body density) − 450

Example: The body volume of an 83-kilogram male (182.6 pounds) was determined from hydrostatic weighing to be 79.4 L. Dividing body weight by body volume yields a body density of 1.0453. Body density can then be used to determine percent body fat as follows:

(495/1.0453) − 450 = 23.5 percent body fat

central or android obesity Excess storage of visceral fat in the abdominal area, indicated by a waist circumference greater than 40 inches in males and 35 inches in females; central obesity increases the risk of heart disease, diabetes, and hypertension.

gynoid obesity Excessive storage of body fat in the thighs and hips of the lower body.

hydrostatic weighing Method used to assess body volume by underwater weighing.

air-displacement plethysmography Procedure used to estimate body volume based on the amount of air displaced.

TABLE 14.5 Ways to Measure Percentage of Body Fat

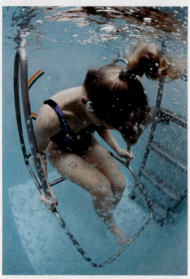

▲ Hydrostatic Weighing

How It Is Done: To determine the density of the body, a person is weighed both on land and suspended in a water tank. Fat is less dense and weighs less than muscle mass and this is reflected in the person's weight in the water. The difference of a person's weight in water and on land is then used to calculate the percentage of body fat.

Cost: $$

Accuracy: 2–3% margin of error

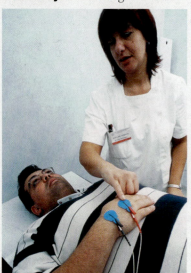

▲ Bioelectrical Impedance (BIA)

How It Is Done: An electric current flows through the body and its resistance is measured. Lean tissue is highly conductive and less resistant than fat mass. Based on the current flow, the volume of lean tissue can be estimated. From this information, the percentage of body fat can be determined.

Cost: $

Accuracy: 3–4% margin of error

▶ Air Displacement Plethysmography Using a BodPod

How It Is Done: A person's body volume is determined by measuring air displacement. The person sits in a special chamber (called the BodPod) and the air displacement in the chamber is measured. From this measurement, the percentage of body fat can be estimated.

Cost: $$$

Accuracy: 2–3% margin of error

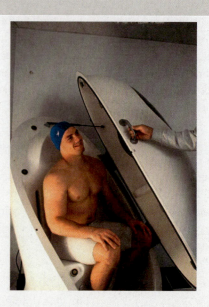

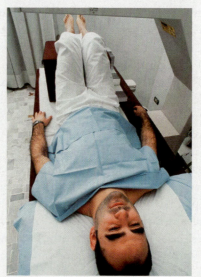

◀ Dual-Energy X-Ray Absorptiometry (DEXA)

How It Is Done: Beams of X-ray energy from two different sources are used to measure bone, fat, and lean tissue. The different types of tissue that the beams pass through absorb different amounts of energy. The percentage of body fat can be determined from the difference in the readings.

Cost: $$$

Accuracy: 1–4% margin of error

▶ Skinfold Thickness Measurements

How It Is Done: Calipers are used to measure the thickness of fat that is located just under the skin in the arm, in the back, on the upper thigh, and in the waist area. From these measurements, percent body fat can be determined.

Cost: $

Accuracy: 3–4% margin of error

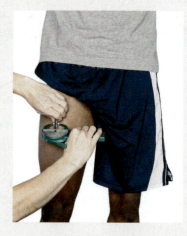

$, very affordable;
$$, less affordable;
$$$, expensive

Dual-energy X-ray absorptiometry (DEXA) is the most accurate method of determining body composition; its margin of error is only 1–4 percent. DEXA is a noninvasive method that can estimate three body compartments: fat mass, lean body mass, and bone mass. This noninvasive method uses two low-energy X-ray beams: one detects all tissues including fat mass and bone mass and the other detects only lean body mass. The computer then calculates the difference between lean body mass and fat mass to determine the percentage of body fat.

Bioelectrical impedance analysis (BIA) measures the resistance to a low-energy current as it travels through muscle and body fat. The current travels more quickly through lean tissue, which is high in body water and electrolytes, than through fat tissue. The resistance of the fat tissue is used to calculate body composition. BIA is not as accurate as body density tests and can be affected by age, hydration status, and consuming food and alcohol prior to the test.

Anthropometric (relating to body measurement) techniques are the simplest methods available and involve using a **skinfold caliper** to measure fat in various body locations. The metal calipers are used to pinch the subcutaneous fat at selected sites on the body. A trained technician grasps the skin and fat between the thumb and forefinger and pulls it gently away from the muscle. The caliper exerts a constant pressure while measuring the skinfold thickness in millimeters. These values are then used to calculate percent body fat. When conducted by a trained technician, skinfold caliper tests are fairly accurate.

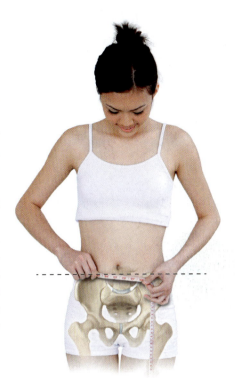

Waist Circumference

Because abdominal fat can be particularly detrimental to health, measuring a person's **waist circumference** can quickly reveal whether he or she is at increased risk (**Figure 14.9**). A woman with a waist measurement of more than 35 inches or a man with a measurement of more than 40 inches is at a higher risk for disease than people with slimmer middles. Carrying extra fat around the waist can increase health risks even if you are not overweight. In other words, a person who may be at a healthy weight based on their height, but who has excess fat around the middle, is at a higher risk for disease.

▲ **Figure 14.9 Measuring Waist Circumference**
The waist circumference measurement is taken at the top of the iliac crest (top of the hip bone), as shown by the dashed line.

LO 14.4: THE TAKE-HOME MESSAGE The body is composed of lean and fat tissue. Adipose tissue is classified as essential fat or fat that is stored as either subcutaneous or visceral fat. How much fat a person has and the placement of that fat can increase the risk of heart disease, diabetes, and hypertension, especially if the fat is distributed in the abdomen. Hydrostatic weighing, air displacement plethysmography, dual-energy X-ray absorptiometry (DEXA), bioelectrical impedance analysis (BIA), and skinfold measurements are all techniques used to determine body composition. Measuring waist circumference can determine whether an individual has excess abdominal (central) fat, which can increase the risk of several chronic diseases.

How Do We Estimate a Healthy Body Weight?

LO 14.5 Explain the methods used to estimate a healthy body weight, and the link between body weight and mortality.

The terms *body weight* and *body composition* are not synonymous. Body weight is defined as total mass expressed in either pounds (lb) or kilograms (kg). As you just learned, body composition is the percentage of body weight that is composed of fat and lean body mass. Even though the terms *body weight* and *body composition* do not measure the same component, they are often used interchangeably in the popular media.

dual-energy X-ray absorptiometry (DEXA) Method that uses two low-energy X-rays to measure body density and bone mass.

bioelectrical impedance analysis (BIA) Method used to assess the percentage of body fat by using a low-level electrical current; body fat resists or impedes the current, whereas water and muscle mass conduct electricity.

skinfold caliper Tool used to measure the thickness of subcutaneous fat.

waist circumference Measurement taken at the top of the iliac crest or hip bone; used to determine the pattern of obesity.

Two common methods used to help individuals estimate whether their own percent body fat falls within a healthy range are height–weight tables and body mass index (BMI). These reference standards are indirect estimates of body composition, and therefore somewhat imprecise, but they can be used as a rough guide for most people.

Height and Weight Tables Are Problematic

Height–weight tables have been used since the 1940s in large-scale studies that were designed to investigate the relationship between body weight and disease. The Metropolitan Life Insurance Company developed the most commonly used height–weight table. The company published the Desirable Weights for Men and Women table in 1959 based on data collected from millions of policyholders. The most recent version of the table was published in 1999 and provides a recommended desirable weight range for a given height based on gender and body frame size.

Several factors make the data used in these tables problematic. For example, the data does not represent the American population as a whole. The tables were originally designed with data from 25- to 59-year-olds, which means they may underrepresent older adults and individuals younger than 25 years of age. The researchers did not standardize the original data. For instance, subjects self-reported their height and weight; the weights were measured at different times of the year; and there was no standard procedure regarding wearing shoes or clothing when taking the height and weight measurements. Lastly, the tables were constructed with the assumption that weight is associated with body fat. Today, mostly insurance companies use height–weight tables to determine mortality rates. Most health experts use body mass index rather than height–weight tables to determine healthy weight.

Body Mass Index Is a Useful Indicator of Healthy Weight for Most People

Body mass index (BMI) (**Figure 14.10**) is a convenient method of calculating body weight in relationship to height, and is a useful screening tool to determine an individual's risk of disease. It is calculated using either of the following formulas:

$$\text{BMI} = \frac{\text{body weight (in kilograms)}}{\text{height}^2 \text{ (in meters)}}$$

$$\text{BMI} = \frac{\text{body weight (in pounds)} \times 703}{\text{height}^2 \text{ (in inches)}}$$

body mass index (BMI) Calculation of body weight in relationship to height.

healthy weight Body weight in relationship to height that doesn't increase the risk of developing any weight-related health problems or diseases. A BMI between 18.5 and 24.9 is considered healthy.

underweight Weighing too little for your height; defined as a BMI less than 18.5.

overweight Body weight that increases risk of developing weight-related health problems; defined as having a BMI between 25 and 29.9.

obese Condition of excess body weight due to an abnormal accumulation of stored body fat; a BMI of 30 or more is considered obese.

severe obesity Defined as a BMI greater than 40 or more than 100 pounds over ideal body weight.

A BMI of 18.5–24.9 kg/m^2 is considered a **healthy weight** based on height. A BMI below 18.5 kg/m^2 is considered **underweight** or having a body weight that is below normal, average, or considered healthy. A BMI between 25 and 29.9 kg/m^2 is considered **overweight**, and a BMI between 30 and 39.9 kg/m^2 is considered **obese**. **Severe obesity** is a BMI at or above 40. **Table 14.6** summarizes the BMI criteria for defining these terms in adults, and **Table 14.7** compares three ways to classify obesity specifically.

As the BMI decreases below 18.5, or increases above 25, the risk of premature death increases. That risk is modest for those with a BMI between 25 and 29.9;[11] however, obese individuals have a 50–100 percent higher risk of dying prematurely than those at a healthy weight. Again, underweight is also risky. Adults with a BMI below 18.5 have a greater risk of premature death than those with a BMI of 18.5–24.9.[12] BMI has been shown to correlate with health risks associated with excess body fat, and an equation can be used to estimate body fat percentage from BMI (see the Calculation Corner).

While BMI can be useful in determining disease risks, it is important to note that BMI is not a *direct* measure of the percentage of body fat, and it doesn't specify if body weight is predominantly muscle or fat.[13] Therefore, athletes and people with a high

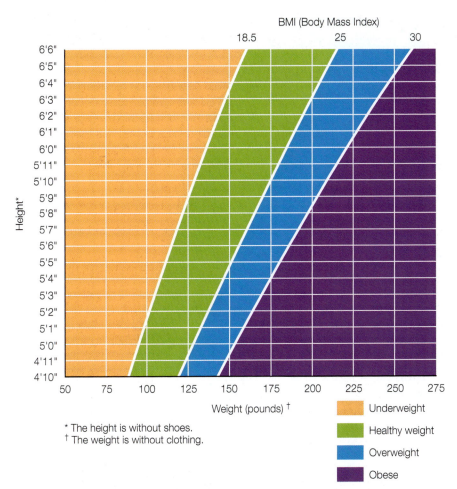

A BMI between 18.5 and 24.9 is considered healthy. A BMI over 25 is considered overweight, and a BMI over 30 is obese. A BMI under 18.5 is considered underweight, and can also be unhealthy.

* The height is without shoes.
† The weight is without clothing.

- Underweight
- Healthy weight
- Overweight
- Obese

TABLE 14.6	Definitions of Underweight, Overweight, and Obesity in Adults
Classification	**BMI (kg/m^2)**
Underweight	< 18.5
Normal weight	18.5–24.9
Overweight	25–29.9 (also defined as being 10–15 pounds above a healthy weight)
Obesity	30–39.9
Severe obesity	> 40

TABLE 14.7	Ways to Classify Obesity in Adults
Obesity Is Classified by . . .	
Percent of body fat	Women: > 32% Men: > 25%
Distribution of body fat	Excess subcutaneous and visceral fat stored in the upper body (abdomen and waist); referred to as central or android obesity • Waist circumference > 35 inches in women • Waist circumference > 40 inches in men Excess subcutaneous fat stored in the lower body (hips, buttocks, thighs); referred to as gynoid obesity • Waist-to-hip ratio < 0.8 in women • Waist-to-hip ratio < 0.95 in men
Body mass index (BMI)	Women: > 30 kg/m^2 Men: > 25 kg/m^2

Source: Adapted from A. G. Kazaks and J. Stern, *Nutrition and Obesity. Assessment, Management, and Prevention* (Burlington, MA: Jones & Bartlett Publishing, 2013).

Converting BMI to Percent Body Fat

Now that you have learned how to calculate body mass index (BMI), how does this number correlate to the amount of stored body fat? Researchers have developed equations that show a correlation between BMI and percent body fat in adults.[1] The formulas, which are age and gender specific, can yield valid estimates of body fat comparable to those obtained from skinfold thickness measurements or BIA. The prediction equations do, however, overestimate percent body fat in obese individuals. Follow these steps to practice using these prediction equations.

(1) If you are a female, use this formula: 1.2 (BMI) + 0.23 (age(y)) − 5.4

For example, a 21-year-old female with a BMI of 25 would calculate percent body fat as follows:

$$1.2 (25) + 0.23 (21) − 5.4 = 30 + 4.83 − 5.4 = 29.43 \text{ percent body fat}$$

(2) A male would use this formula: 1.2 (BMI) + 0.23 (age(y)) − 16.2

For example, a 31-year-old male with a BMI of 21 would calculate percent body fat as follows:

$$1.2 (21) + 0.23 (31) − 16.2 = 25.2 + 7.13 − 16.2 = 16.13 \text{ percent body fat}$$

Now, using your own BMI, complete the calculation for percent body fat.

Note that these calculations do not consider race/ethnicity. The BMI–body fat relationship varies between different racial/ethnic groups[2] and should be used in conjunction with other measurements such as waist circumference and percent body fat to provide a true picture of a healthy body weight.

References

1. P. Deurenbert, J. A. Weststrate, and J. C. Seidell. 1991. Body–Mass Index as a Measure of Body Fatness: Age- and Sex-Specific Prediction Formulas. *British Journal of Nutrition* 65:105–114.
2. Balasubramanian, B. A., M. P. Garcia, D. A. Corley, et al. 2017. Racial/Ethnic Differences in Obesity and Comorbidities Between Safety-Net and Non Safety-Net Integrated Health Systems. *Medicine* 96(11):e6326. doi: 10.1097/MD.0000000000006326.

Go to **Mastering** Nutrition and complete a Math Video activity similar to the problem in this Calculation Corner.

Extremely High Risk
BMI 40+ and high waist circumference

Very High Risk
BMI 30–39.9 and high waist circumference

High Risk
BMI 25–29.9 and high waist circumference
or
BMI 30–34.9 and low waist circumference

Increased Risk
BMI 25–29.9 and low waist circumference

Low Risk
BMI under 25

▲ **Figure 14.11 Using BMI and Waist Circumference to Determine Health Risk**
Considering both BMI and waist circumference can give you a good idea of total risk levels for several chronic diseases.

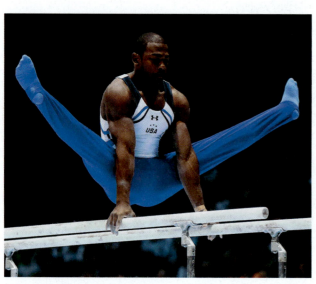

This male gymnast stands 5 feet 5 inches tall and weighs 160 pounds. His BMI of 26.6 would place him in the overweight category without considering his low percentage of body fat.

percentage of muscle mass may have a BMI over 25 kg/m², yet have a low percentage of body fat. Although these individuals are overweight based on their BMI, they are not "overfat" and unhealthy, and their muscular weight doesn't increase their health risk. In contrast, an older adult may be in a healthy weight range, but steadily lose weight due to an unbalanced diet or poor health. This chronic weight loss is a sign of loss of muscle mass and the depletion of nutrient stores in the body, which increases health risks even though the BMI seems healthy. Also, because height is factored into the BMI, individuals who are very short—less than 5 feet—may have a high BMI but, similar to athletes, may not be unhealthy.[14]

Combining indirect measurements is one way to get a better estimate of body composition. For example, a person who has both a BMI greater than 25 and a large waist circumference is considered at a higher risk for health problems than if he or she only had a high BMI but a low waist circumference (**Figure 14.11**).

Again, a healthy body weight does not increase the risk of premature death or any weight-related health problems or diseases. In contrast, being underweight or overweight increases the risk for premature death and for numerous diseases. The health risks associated with both underweight and overweight are discussed in detail in Chapter 15.

Height and weight tables and BMI are used to screen for overweight and obesity. Height–weight tables do not necessarily indicate a healthy weight for everyone. The body mass index (BMI) is a calculation of the ratio of weight to height and can be used to assess health risks. A BMI less than 18.5 kg/m² is considered underweight. A BMI of 18.5–24.9 kg/m² is normal weight. A BMI of 25–29.9 kg/m² is overweight. A BMI of 30–39.9 kg/m² is considered obesity, and 40 kg/m² or above is considered severe obesity. Both underweight and overweight, especially obesity, are associated with an increased risk of premature death and numerous health problems.

HEALTHCONNECTION

What Is Disordered Eating?

LO 14.6 List the criteria used to diagnose eating disorders and discuss the shared traits and options for treatment.

Attaining a healthy weight, whether it means gaining or losing a few pounds, is a worthwhile goal that can result in lowered risk of disease and a more productive life. However, patterns of eating that involve severe kilocalorie restriction, binge eating, purging, or other abnormal behaviors can be severely damaging to health. Whereas disordered eating and eating disorders are sometimes thought of as psychological rather than nutrition-related topics, it's important to be aware of them and recognize their symptoms.

The term *disordered eating* is used to describe a variety of eating patterns considered abnormal and potentially harmful. Refusing to eat, compulsive eating, binge eating, restrictive eating, vomiting after eating, and abusing diet pills, laxatives, or diuretics are all examples of disordered eating behaviors. **Eating disorders**, in contrast, are psychiatric disorders diagnosed when a person meets specific criteria that include disordered eating behaviors as well as other factors. It is possible for someone to have disordered eating without having an actual eating disorder.

Eating Disorders Occur in Both Women and Men

In the United States, an estimated 30 million people of various genders and ages struggle with eating disorders.[15] Adolescent and young adult females in predominantly white upper-middle- and middle-class families are the population

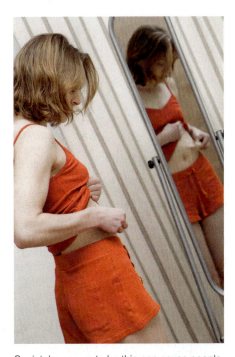

Societal pressure to be thin can cause people to feel fat when they look in the mirror regardless of their body weight. Dissatisfaction with one's body can lead to disordered eating behaviors.

with highest prevalence. However, eating disorders and disordered eating among males, racial and ethnic minorities, and other age groups are increasing.[16,17] Anyone can develop an eating disorder.

Societal pressure to be thin and have a "perfect" figure is one factor that likely contributes to disordered eating among girls and women. Images of models and celebrities with abnormally low body weights are portrayed as ideal; therefore, many normal-weight females believe that they cannot be beautiful, successful, or happy unless they are thin. Many females will try to achieve a perfect figure at any cost, including plastic surgery, liposuction, and engaging in disordered eating behaviors.

The prevalence of eating disorders in males is difficult to assess because many men, as well as women, feel ashamed or embarrassed and may hide their problem. In fact, the prevalence of eating disorders among both males and females is probably higher than reported. Researchers have found that men diagnosed with eating disorders have higher rates of other psychiatric illness such as depression and anxiety disorders compared with men who do not have eating disorders.[18]

disordered eating Abnormal and potentially harmful eating behaviors that do not meet specific criteria for a clinical eating disorder.

eating disorders Psychiatric illnesses that involve specific abnormal eating behaviors.

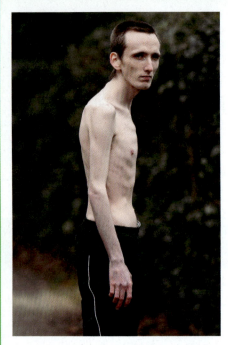

Although the highest rates of disordered eating patterns occur among females, males are not immune. Adolescents in particular can feel pressure to achieve a certain body image.

The three clinically recognized eating disorders are anorexia nervosa, bulimia nervosa, and binge eating disorder. The diagnostic criteria for each are listed in **Table 14.8**.

Anorexia Nervosa Involves Severe Kilocalorie Restriction

Anorexia nervosa is a serious, potentially life-threatening eating disorder that is characterized by self-starvation and excessive weight loss. People who suffer from anorexia nervosa have an intense fear of gaining weight or being "fat." This fear causes them to control their food intake by restricting the amount of food they consume, resulting in significant weight loss.

Many people with anorexia nervosa have a fear of eating certain foods, such as those that contain fat and sugar. They believe that these foods will make them "fat," regardless of how little of them they eat. A distorted

anorexia nervosa Eating disorder in which people intentionally starve themselves, causing extreme weight loss.

TABLE 14.8	Diagnostic Criteria for Eating Disorders
Eating Disorder	**Diagnostic Criteria**
Anorexia nervosa	• Restriction of energy intake relative to requirements leading to a significantly low body weight in the context of age, sex, developmental trajectory, and physical health • Intense fear of gaining weight or becoming fat, even though underweight • Disturbance in the way one's body weight or shape is experienced, excessive influence of body weight or shape on self-esteem or denial of the seriousness of the current low body weight

Bulimia nervosa	• Recurrent episodes of binge eating. An episode of binge eating is characterized by *both* of the following:
	  • Eating in a discrete amount of time (within a 2-hour period) large amounts of food
	  • Sense of lack of control over eating during an episode
	• Recurrent inappropriate compensatory behavior in order to prevent weight gain (purging)
	• The binge eating and compensatory behaviors both occur, on average, at least twice a week for 3 months
	• Self-evaluation is unduly influenced by body shape and weight
	• The disturbance does not occur exclusively during episodes of anorexia nervosa

Binge eating disorder (BED)	• Recurrent and persistent episodes of binge eating. An episode of binge eating is characterized by *both* of the following:
	  • Eating, in a discrete period of time, an amount of food that is definitely larger than most people would eat in a similar period of time under similar circumstances
	  • A sense of lack of control over eating during the episode (for example, a feeling that one cannot stop eating or control what or how much one is eating)
	• Binge eating episodes are associated with three (or more) of the following:
	  • Eating much more rapidly than normal
	  • Eating until feeling uncomfortably full
	  • Eating large amounts of food when not feeling physically hungry
	  • Eating alone because of being embarrassed by how much one is eating
	  • Feeling disgusted with oneself, depressed, or very guilty after overeating
	• Marked distress regarding binge eating is present
	• The binge eating occurs, on average, at least once a week for three months
	• The binge eating is not associated with the recurrent use of inappropriate compensatory behavior (for example, purging) and does not occur exclusively during the course of anorexia nervosa, bulimia nervosa, or avoidant/restrictive food intake disorder

Other specified feeding or eating disorder (OSFED)	• A pattern of disordered eating that does not meet the criteria for anorexia nervosa, bulimia nervosa, or binge eating disorder; includes orthorexia and night eating syndrome

Source: American Psychiatric Association, *Diagnostic and Statistical Manual of Mental Disorders (DSM-5®)*, 5th ed. (Arlington, VA: American Psychiatric Association, 2013).

body image is also present. Typically, sufferers see themselves as fat even though they are underweight. They therefore continue to restrict their food intake in order to lose more weight. For instance, someone with anorexia nervosa might eat only a piece of fruit and a small container of yogurt during an entire day. Some may also exercise excessively as a means of controlling their weight.

Numerous health consequences can occur with anorexia nervosa and some can be fatal. One of the most serious is an electrolyte imbalance, specifically low blood potassium, which can lead to an irregular heart rhythm and cardiac arrest. Additionally, because of their extreme lack of body fat, their internal body temperature drops and they feel cold even when it is hot outside. In an effort to regulate body temperature, their body may begin to grow **lanugo** (downy hair), particularly on the face and arms. Loss of body fat also disrupts levels of reproductive hormones, resulting in amenorrhea (cessation of menstruation) in women.

Because the body of a person with anorexia nervosa is not getting enough nutrients, nonessential body functions begin to slow or shut down in an effort to conserve energy for the most vital functions. The person may begin to experience a decrease in heart rate and blood pressure, overall weakness and fatigue, hair loss, and a slowing of digestive process, which often results in constipation, bloating, and delayed gastric emptying. Dehydration, iron deficiency, and osteoporosis can also result from inadequate nutrient intake.

Bulimia Nervosa Involves Cycles of Binge Eating and Purging

Bulimia nervosa is another clinical eating disorder that can be life-threatening. During times of binge eating, the person lacks control over eating and consumes larger than normal amounts of food in a short period of time. Following the binge, the person counters the excess food consumption with some type of purging. Many

people assume that bulimics always purge by vomiting, but purging can be described as any behavior that assists in "getting rid" of food to prevent weight gain or to promote weight loss. This can include vigorous exercise, abuse of diet pills, laxatives, or diuretics, and strict dieting or fasting.

As with anorexia nervosa, people with bulimia nervosa often suffer from depression and have low self-esteem. They may feel shame and guilt about their eating behaviors and may try to hide their eating problems from others. Those who have bulimia nervosa are overly concerned with body shape and weight, but usually do not have the same distorted body image as someone with anorexia nervosa.

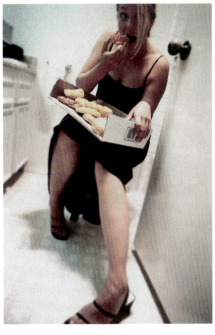

People with bulimia nervosa often eat in secret.

Most of the health consequences that occur with bulimia nervosa are associated with self-induced vomiting, such as tearing of the esophagus, swollen parotid glands (the salivary glands located on each side of the face in front of the ears), tooth decay and gum disease (due to stomach acid), and broken blood vessels in the eyes (due to pressure from vomiting). One sign of bulimia nervosa is often scar tissue on the knuckles of a person's fingers, which forms from their being frequently used to induce

vomiting. Electrolyte imbalance can occur with bulimia nervosa and can be fatal. People with bulimia nervosa may experience dehydration and constipation due to frequent episodes of binge eating and purging.

Laxative abuse can cause serious medical complications. The repeated use of laxatives can cause constipation, dehydration due to fluid loss in the intestines, electrolyte imbalances, fluid retention, bloody stools, and impaired bowel function.

Binge Eating Disorder Involves Compulsive Overeating

Binge eating disorder is characterized by recurrent episodes of binge eating without purging. People who have binge eating disorder eat without regard to physiological cues. They may eat for emotional reasons, which results in an out-of-control feeling while eating and physical and psychological discomfort after eating. Many people who struggle with this type of eating disorder will eat in secret and feel ashamed about their behaviors.

Because people who struggle with binge eating disorder do not typically purge, they are typically overweight or obese. Health effects therefore may include hypertension, high cholesterol levels, heart disease, type 2 diabetes, and gallbladder disease.

Other Disordered Eating Behaviors Can Be Harmful

In addition to anorexia nervosa, bulimia nervosa, and binge eating disorder, there are other abnormal eating behaviors that

---

body image How you perceive your physical appearance.

lanugo Very fine, soft hair typically found on a newborn or a person who is malnourished.

bulimia nervosa Eating disorder characterized by binging (consuming large quantities of food in a short period of time) and then purging through vomiting or other means.

binge eating disorder Eating disorder characterized by recurrent episodes of binge eating without purging.

can be harmful and require treatment. These include orthorexia, night eating syndrome, and pica.

Orthorexia is defined as an obsession with "healthy or righteous eating" and often begins with someone's simple desire to live a healthy lifestyle. Someone with orthorexia fixates on defining the "right" foods, and will spend just as much time and energy thinking about food as someone with anorexia nervosa or bulimia nervosa. While this person may not obsess about calories, they think about the overall health benefits and how the food was processed, prepared, etc. Various factors can contribute to this obsession for healthy foods, including hearing something negative about a food or food group, which then leads to completely eliminating the food or foods from their diet. The restrictive nature of orthorexia has the potential to develop into anorexia nervosa.

Night eating syndrome is a unique combination of disordered eating, a sleep disorder, and a mood disorder.[19] Someone with this syndrome consumes the majority of daily kilocalories after the evening meal, as well as wakes up during the night, possibly even several times, to eat. In addition, the person typically does not have an appetite during the morning hours and consumes very little throughout the day. One study found that people with night eating syndrome consume 56 percent of their 24-hour kilocalorie intake between the hours of 8:00 P.M. and 6:00 A.M. This study also found that people with night eating syndrome generally do not binge eat with each awakening; rather, they eat smaller portions of food on several occasions throughout the night.[20]

Pica refers to a strong, persistent desire to eat, lick, or chew non-nutritive substances, such as clay, dirt, or chalk. Consuming nonfood substances can cause serious medical complications such as intestinal obstruction, intestinal perforation, infections, or lead poisoning.

Because orthorexia and night eating syndrome do not meet the diagnostic criteria for anorexia nervosa, bulimia nervosa, or binge eating disorder, but still require treatment, they fall into the diagnostic category of "other specified feeding and eating

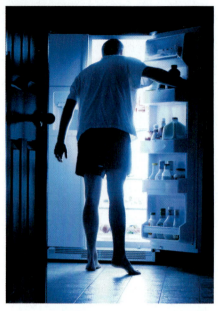

People with night eating syndrome may consume more than half their day's kilocalories between 8:00 P.M. and 6:00 A.M.

disorders" (OSFED).[21] Other behaviors in this category include purging without binging, restrictive eating by people who are in a normal weight range despite having significant weight loss, binging and purging but not frequently enough to meet criteria for

bulimia, and chewing and spitting out food instead of swallowing it.

Different Eating Disorders Share Some Common Traits

A common trait of people with eating disorders is obsession with food and eating.[22] Unrealistic standards can produce a sense of self-loathing, guilt, and low self-esteem. Many people who struggle with eating disorders are trying to gain some control in their lives. When external factors feel out of control, they get a sense of security from being able to control food consumption and body weight. They may withdraw from social interactions where food is present and where they might have to eat around others. Also, depression is more common among people who have eating disorders as compared to the general population.[23]

You might know someone with an eating disorder, but may not know how to help the person. First, learn the warning signs (**Table 14.9**). If you're concerned about your own eating behaviors, take the

TABLE 14.9	Warning Signs for Eating Disorders
Warning Sign	**Explanation/Example**
Weight is below 85% of ideal body weight	Even if underweight, refusal to accept and maintain current body weight
Excessive exercise	Often exercises daily for long periods of time to burn kilocalories and prevent weight gain. May skip work or class to exercise.
Preoccupation with food and weight	Constantly worries about amount and type of food eaten and potential weight gain. May check body weight daily or several times per day.
Refusal to eat appropriate variety and/or quantity of food	Will avoid food in order to lose weight or prevent weight gain. May avoid only certain foods, such as those with fat or sugar.
Avoidance of social eating	Wants to eat alone. Makes excuses to avoid eating with others.
Diet pill use or laxative use	Evidence of pill bottles, boxes, or packaging
Distorted body image	Does not see himself/herself as he or she truly is. May comment on being fat even if underweight.
Changes in mood	May become more withdrawn, depressed, or anxious, especially around food
Loss of menstrual period	Periods become irregular or completely absent
Hair loss	Hair becomes thinner and falls out in large quantities

Are You at Risk for an Eating Disorder?

Mark the following statements True or False to help you find out.

1. I constantly think about eating, weight, and body size.

   True ☐ **False** ☐

2. I'm terrified about being overweight.

   True ☐ **False** ☐

3. I binge eat and can't stop until I feel sick.

   True ☐ **False** ☐

4. I weigh myself several times each day.

   True ☐ **False** ☐

5. I exercise too much or get very rigid about my exercise plan.

   True ☐ **False** ☐

6. I have taken laxatives or forced myself to vomit after eating.

   True ☐ **False** ☐

7. I believe food controls my life.

   True ☐ **False** ☐

8. I feel extremely guilty after eating.

   True ☐ **False** ☐

9. I eat when I am nervous, anxious, lonely, or depressed.

   True ☐ **False** ☐

10. I believe my weight controls what I do.

    True ☐ **False** ☐

Analysis

These statements are designed to help you identify potentially problematic eating behavior. These statements do *not* tell you if you have an eating disorder. Look carefully at any statement you marked as true and decide if this behavior prevents you from enjoying life or makes you unhealthy. Changing these behaviors should be done gradually, making small changes one at a time. Contact your student health services center or your health care provider if you suspect you need help.

Adapted from National Eating Disorders Association. 2016. Available at https://www.nationaleatingdisorders .org/learn/help/educators/school-setting. Accessed April 2017.

Self-Assessment "Are You at Risk for an Eating Disorder?" to find out.

If you are concerned about a friend's eating behaviors, find a good time and place to gently express your concerns without criticism or judgment. Realize that you may be rejected or your friend may deny the problem. Be supportive and let the person know that you are available if they want to talk to you at another time. You should also realize that there are many things that you cannot do to help a loved one or friend get better. You cannot force an anorexic to eat, keep a bulimic from purging, or make a binge eater stop overeating. It is up to the individual to decide when he or she is ready to deal with the issues in life that led to the eating disorder.

Eating Disorders Can Be Treated

The most effective treatment for eating disorders is a multidisciplinary team approach including psychological, medical, and nutrition professionals. All members of the team should be knowledgeable and experienced with eating disorders treatment. A physician or other medical professional should closely monitor the person. In severe cases, a physician may require the patient to be hospitalized as part of the treatment. A psychologist can help the person deal with emotional and other psychological issues that may be contributing to the eating disorder.

A registered dietitian nutritionist can help someone with an eating disorder establish normal eating behaviors. Some nutritional approaches to eating disorders include identifying binge triggers, safe and unsafe foods, and hunger and fullness cues. Food journals are often helpful to identify eating patterns, food choices, moods, disordered eating triggers, eating cues, and timing of meals and snacks. Meal plans are also used in some instances to ensure adequate kilocalorie and nutrient intake among those with anorexia nervosa and to help avoid overeating among those with bulimia nervosa or binge eating disorder.

Most people recover from eating disorders. When treatment is sought in the early stages, there is a better chance that the person will recover fully and have a shorter recovery process than someone who begins treatment after many years. In some people, the recovery process takes years. Some continue throughout life to have the desire to engage in disordered eating behaviors; however, they are able to refrain from actually engaging in these behaviors. Unfortunately, some individuals never fully recover.

LO 14.6: THE TAKE-HOME MESSAGE
Disordered eating is characterized by an abnormal eating pattern. Eating disorders are psychiatric disorders diagnosed in people who meet specific diagnostic criteria. The three clinical eating disorders are anorexia nervosa, bulimia nervosa, and binge eating disorder. Eating disorders are most effectively treated with a multidisciplinary approach including psychological, medical, and nutrition professionals. A full recovery takes time but is possible, especially if the disorder is treated in the early stages.

Visual Chapter Summary

LO 14.1 Energy Balance Is Achieved When Energy In Equals Energy Out

Energy balance is the relationship between energy consumed and energy expended. Body weight remains constant when energy intake equals energy expenditure. When more energy is consumed than expended, the body is in positive energy balance and weight gain occurs. When the intake of kilocalories falls short of energy needs or you expend more energy than you consume, the body is in negative energy balance and weight loss occurs.

ENERGY INTAKE = ENERGY EXPENDITURE

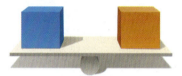

WEIGHT MAINTENANCE

LO 14.2 Three Factors Contribute to TDEE

Total daily energy expenditure (TDEE) is the sum of energy expended on basal metabolism, the thermic effect of food (TEF), and the thermic effect of exercise (TEE). An individual's basal metabolic rate (BMR) is influenced mainly by lean body mass. The thermic effect of food is the energy used to process recently eaten foods. The thermic effect of exercise (TEE) includes the energy required to exercise, maintain posture while standing and sitting, and engage in nonexercise activity thermogenesis, or NEAT, which is all activity that is not structured exercise, including unconscious muscle activity.

Total Daily Energy Expenditure (TDEE)

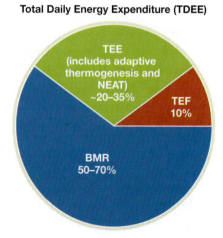

- TEE (includes adaptive thermogenesis and NEAT) ~20–35%
- TEF 10%
- BMR 50–70%

LO 14.3 Energy Expenditure Can Be Measured Directly or Indirectly

Energy expenditure can be measured directly with a metabolic chamber or indirectly based on oxygen consumed and carbon dioxide produced during activity. The estimated energy requirement (EER) can be calculated using an individual's age, weight, height, and physical activity level.

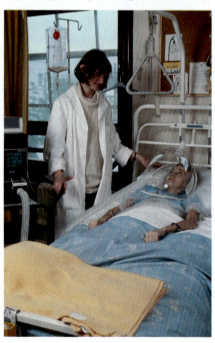

LO 14.4 Body Composition Is a Ratio of Fat to Lean Body Mass

Body composition refers to the ratio of fat to lean body mass and is measured as a percent body fat. Total body fat comprises essential fat, found in bone marrow, organs, muscles, and the central nervous system, and storage fat, found in adipose tissue. Stored fat can be visceral, located around the organs, or subcutaneous, located just beneath the skin. White adipose tissue is primarily a storage tissue; brown adipose tissue contains more mitochondria, is rich in blood, and generates heat.

The placement of body fat also affects overall health. Storing excess fat around the waist has been shown to increase the risk of heart disease, diabetes, and hypertension. The more visceral fat stored near the liver, the greater the risk of insulin resistance, hyperlipidemia, and low levels of HDL cholesterol, all of which increase the risk of heart disease and diabetes.

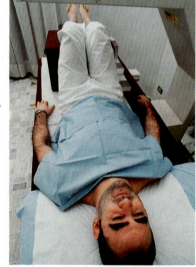

The most accurate instrument to measure body composition is dual-energy X-ray absorptiometry (DEXA). Body composition is also estimated from body volume using hydrostatic weighing and air displacement plethysmography. Bioelectrical impedance analysis measures resistance by body fat; skinfold calipers estimate subcutaneous fat; and waist circumference measures android obesity.

LO 14.5 BMI Is Used to Determine Body Weight and Health Risks

Reference standards have been developed as indirect measurements of a healthy body weight. Body mass index (BMI) is a calculation of body weight related to height and is correlated with health risks. A BMI of 18.5–24.9 kg/m² is considered healthy. A BMI from 25 to 29.9 kg/m² is considered overweight and a BMI of 30 kg/m² or greater is considered obese. A BMI lower than 18.5 kg/m² is considered underweight.

A healthy body weight doesn't increase the risk of any weight-related health problems. Overweight and obesity increase the individual's risk of chronic disease and premature death. Underweight is also associated with a variety of health risks, including an increased risk of premature death.

Extremely High Risk
BMI 40+ and high waist circumference

Very High Risk
BMI 30–39.9 and high waist circumference

High Risk
BMI 25–29.9 and high waist circumference
or
BMI 30–34.9 and low waist circumference

Increased Risk
BMI 25–29.9 and low waist circumference

Low Risk
BMI under 25

LO 14.6 Eating Disorders Are Psychiatric Disorders

Disordered eating describes a variety of abnormal eating patterns, such as restrictive eating, binge eating, vomiting after eating, and abusing laxatives or diet pills. Eating disorders are psychiatric disorders diagnosed according to specific criteria that include disordered eating behaviors and other factors.

Anorexia nervosa is characterized by self-starvation and excessive weight loss. Bulimia nervosa involves repeated cycles of binge eating and purging. Binge eating disorders are characterized by binge eating without purging. Night eating syndrome is described as excessive kilocalorie intake in the evening and waking up during the night to eat.

The most effective treatment for eating disorders involves a multidisciplinary team approach including psychological, nutrition, and medical professionals.

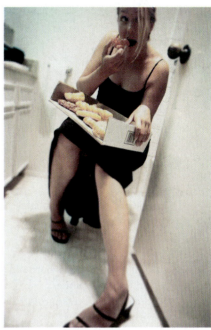

Terms to Know

- energy balance
- positive energy balance
- negative energy balance
- bomb calorimeter
- physiological fuel values
- total daily energy expenditure (TDEE)
- basal metabolism
- basal metabolic rate (BMR)
- lean body mass (LBM)
- resting metabolic rate (RMR)
- thermic effect of food (TEF)
- thermogenesis
- thermic effect of exercise (TEE)
- nonexercise activity thermogenesis (NEAT)
- direct calorimetry
- indirect calorimetry
- estimated energy requirement (EER)
- body composition
- essential fat
- subcutaneous fat
- visceral fat
- brown adipose tissue (BAT)
- central (android) obesity
- gynoid obesity
- hydrostatic weighing
- air-displacement plethysmography
- dual-energy X-ray absorptiometry (DEXA)
- bioelectrical impedance analysis (BIA)
- skinfold caliper
- waist circumference
- body mass index (BMI)
- healthy weight
- underweight
- overweight
- obese
- severe obesity
- disordered eating
- eating disorders
- anorexia nervosa
- body image
- lanugo
- bulimia nervosa
- binge eating disorder

Mastering Nutrition
Visit the Study Area in
Mastering Nutrition to hear
an MP3 chapter summary.

Check Your Understanding

LO 14.1 1. An individual who is regularly in negative energy balance will most likely
  a. lose weight.
  b. gain weight.
  c. maintain current body weight.
  d. burn more muscle weight than fat weight.

LO 14.1 2. A negative energy balance means that you
  a. eat more than you burn off in total kilocalories.
  b. eat less than you burn off in total kilocalories.
  c. are gaining weight.
  d. are maintaining weight.

LO 14.2 3. The basal metabolic rate (BMR) is a measure of
  a. the amount of energy expended during physical activity.
  b. the amount of energy expended during digestion.
  c. the amount of energy consumed daily.
  d. the amount of energy expended to meet basic physiological needs.

LO 14.2 4. Will's breakfast contains 525 kilocalories. How many kilocalories will he expend (TEF) to process this meal?
  a. 5–10 kilocalories
  b. 50–100 kilocalories
  c. 125–140 kilocalories
  d. 150–175 kilocalories

LO 14.3 5. An individual's estimated energy requirement is based on all of the following *except*:
  a. body posture.
  b. age.
  c. activity level.
  d. gender.

LO 14.4 6. The method that uses the fact that lean tissue is denser than water to measure body composition is called
  a. air-displacement plethysmography.
  b. bioelectrical impedance analysis.
  c. dual-energy X-ray absorptiometry.
  d. hydrostatic weighing.

LO 14.4 7. Approximately what percentage of the body is made up of essential fat?
  a. 9 percent for women, 5 percent for men
  b. 15 percent for women, 18 percent for men
  c. 12 percent for women, 3 percent for men
  d. 18 percent for women, 20 percent for men

LO 14.5 8. Being underweight increases the risk of which of the following?
  a. Premature death
  b. Cancer
  c. Heart disease
  d. Diabetes

LO 14.6 9. Which of the following is a clinical eating disorder?
  a. Orthorexia
  b. Night eating syndrome
  c. Pica
  d. Binge eating disorder

LO 14.6 10. What causes those who suffer from anorexia nervosa to control their food intake?
  a. Intense distaste for healthy foods
  b. Loss of appetite
  c. Busy lifestyle
  d. Intense fear of becoming overweight

Answers

1. (a) Negative energy balance means the amount of energy intake is less than the energy output. If maintained over time, negative energy balance most likely results in weight loss.

2. (b) If you are in negative energy balance, you are consuming fewer kilocalories than you expend. You are in energy balance when your weight is stable—you are consuming and expending the same number of kilocalories. You are in positive energy balance when you are consuming more energy than you expend.

3. (d) BMR is a measure of the amount of energy needed to meet basic physiological needs; for example, to maintain cellular functions and keep blood circulating and lungs breathing. The amount of energy expended during physical activity is not factored into the BMR. The energy cost of digesting, absorbing, and processing food is called the thermic effect of food (TEF) and is also not part of BMR. The amount of energy consumed doesn't factor into the BMR.

4. (b) The thermic effect of food costs approximately 10 percent of the total kilocalories to process a normal mixed meal. Ten percent of 525 kilocalories equals 52 kilocalories.

5. (a) Estimated energy requirement is based on gender, age, and activity level. Body posture is not a factor.

6. (d) Hydrostatic weighing is the method used to measure body composition based on the fact that lean tissue is denser than water. Air-displacement plethysmography is based on the amount of air the body displaces. Bioelectrical impedance measures the resistance of a current by body fat, and dual-energy X-ray absorptiometry measures body fat by passing X-rays through fat-free mass and fat mass.

7. (c) Essential body fat makes up approximately 12 percent of total body fat for women and 3 percent for men.

8. (a) Being underweight increases the risk of premature death. Being overweight increases the risk of developing diabetes, cancer, or heart disease.

9. (d) Binge eating disorder is a clinical eating disorder. Night eating syndrome, orthorexia, and pica are patterns of behavior involving disordered eating but are not classified as psychiatric disorders.

10. (d) An intense fear of becoming overweight generally causes those who suffer from anorexia nervosa to control their food intake.

Answers to True or False?

1. **True.** Technically, exercise isn't necessary to produce a negative energy balance. People who are ill, for example, commonly lose weight, as do breastfeeding mothers. Exercise is, however, an important component of healthy weight loss programs, because in addition to burning kilocalories directly, it speeds up your metabolism and has multiple health benefits.

2. **False.** Being underweight increases the risk of serious health consequences, including anemia, heart irregularities, osteoporosis, amenorrhea, depression, and anxiety. It can therefore be more harmful to health than moderate overweight.

3. **True.** Males have a higher basal metabolic rate than females mostly because they have more muscle mass and lower levels of body fat. This means that men, on average, burn more kilocalories than women.

4. **True.** The *Dietary Guidelines for Americans* recommend using weight for height or body mass index calculations to estimate whether you are at a healthy weight.

5. **False.** Android obesity, or storing excess fat around the abdomen, puts an individual at higher risk for cardiovascular disease and diabetes than does gynoid obesity, which is the storage of excess fat around the hips.

6. **False.** Body weight is a sum of an individual's body fat plus lean body mass, whereas body composition indicates the ratios of body fat to total body weight and lean body mass to total body weight.

7. **False.** If you eat an extra 100 kilocalories per day for a week, that is equal to 700 additional kilocalories, not the 3,500 kilocalories needed to gain a pound.

8. **True.** Skinfold calipers are an inexpensive and practical method for measuring body composition in a gym or recreation center. Fitness labs use more expensive and more precise tools.

9. **False.** Disordered eating describes a variety of eating patterns considered abnormal and potentially harmful. Eating disorders are diagnosed by clinicians according to specific criteria that include disordered eating behaviors as well as other factors. It is possible for someone to engage in disordered eating without having an actual eating disorder.

10. **True.** The long-term starvation of anorexia nervosa and consistent purging of bulimia nervosa (which can lead to electrolyte imbalance) can be fatal.

Web Resources

- For more on overweight and obesity, visit the Centers for Disease Control and Prevention at www.cdc.gov
- For more information on assessing body composition and health risks, visit the National Heart, Lung, and Blood Institute at www.nhlbi.nih.gov
- Additional information on eating disorders and their prevention and treatment can be found at the National Eating Disorders Association at www.nationaleatingdisorders.org

References

1. Merrill, A. L., and B. K. Watt. 1973. *Energy Values of Foods: Basis and Derivation.* Agricultural Handbook no. 74. Washington, DC: USDA.

2. Apolzan, J. W., H. J. Leidy, R. D. Mattes, and W. W. Campbell. 2011. Effects of Food Form on Food Intake and Postprandial Appetite Sensations, Glucose and Endocrine Responses, and Energy Expenditure in Resistance Trained v. Sedentary Older Adults. *British Journal of Nutrition* 106(7):1107–1116.

3. Petzke, K. J., A. Freudenberg, and S. Klaus. 2014. Beyond the Role of Dietary Protein and Amino Acids in the Prevention of Diet-Induced Obesity. *International Journal of Molecular Sciences* 15(1):1374–1391. doi: 10.3390/ijms15011374.

4. Wu, C. S., O. Y. N. Bongmba, J. Yue, J. H. Lee, L. Lin, K. Saito, et al. 2017. Suppression of GHS-R in AgRP Neurons Mitigates Diet-Induced Obesity by Activating Thermogenesis. *International Journal of Molecular Science* 18:832.

5. Ibid.

6. Pedersen, S. J., P. D. Cooley, and C. Mainsbridge. 2013. An E-Health Intervention Designed to Increase Workday Energy Expenditure by Reducing Prolonged Occupational Sitting Habits. *Work.* doi: 10.3233/WOR-131644.

7. Food and Nutrition Board. 2005. *Dietary Reference Intakes for Energy, Carbohydrate, Fiber, Fat, Fatty Acids, Cholesterol, Protein, and Amino Acids (Macronutrients).* Washington, DC: National Academies Press.

8. Ibid.

9. Orava, J., L. Nummenmaa, T. Noponen, T. Viljanen, R. Parkkola, P. Nuutila, and K. A. Virtanen. 2014. Brown Adipose Tissue Function Is Accompanied by Cerebral Activation in Lean But Not in Obese Humans. *Journal of Cerebral Blood Flow and Metabolism.* doi: 10.1038/jcbfm.2014.50.

10. National Institutes of Health. 2000. *Clinical Guidelines on the Identification, Evaluation, and Treatment of Overweight and Obesity in Adults.* Available at www.nhlbi.nih.gov. Accessed April 2017.

11. Tanisawa, K., H. Taniguchi, X. Sun, T. Ito, R. Kawakami, S. Sakamoto, and M. Higuchi. 2017. Visceral Fat Area is a Strong Predictor of Leukocyte Cell-Derived Chemotaxin 2, a Potential Biomarker of Dyslipidemia. *PLoS ONE* 12(3):e0173310. doi: 10.1371/journal.pone.0173310.

12. Centers for Disease Control and Prevention. 2013. *Body Mass Index: Considerations for Practioners.* Available at www.cdc.gov. Accessed April 2017.

13. National Institutes of Health. 2000. *Clinical Guidelines on the Identification, Evaluation, and Treatment of Overweight and Obesity in Adults.*

14. Diemer, E. W., J. D. Grant, M. A. Munn-Chernoff, D. Patterson, and A. E. Duncan. (2015). Gender Identity, Sexual Orientation, and Eating-Related Pathology in a National Sample of College Students. *Journal of Adolescent Health* 57(2):144–149.

15. Schoenefeld, S. J., and J. B. Webb. 2013. Self-Compassion and Intuitive Eating in College Women: Examining the Contributions of Distress Tolerance and Body Image Acceptance and Action. *Eating Behaviors* 14(4):493–496.

16. Räisänen, U., and K. Hunt. 2014. The Role of Gendered Constructions of Eating Disorders in Delayed Help-Seeking in Men: A Qualitative Interview Study. *British Medical Journal Open* 4(4):e004342.

17. Chao, A. M., C. M. Grilo, and R. Sinha. 2016. Food Cravings, Binge Eating, and Eating Disorder Psychopathology: Exploring the Moderating Roles of Gender and Race. *Eating Behaviors* 21:41–47. doi: 10.1016/j.eatbeh.2015.12.007.

18. Ibid.

19. Kucukgoncu, S., M. Midura, and C. Tek. 2015. Optimal Management of Night Eating Syndrome: Challenges and Solutions. *Neuropsychiatric Disease and Treatment* 11:751–760. doi: 10.2147/NDT.S70312.

20. Ibid.

21. *Diagnostic and Statistical Manual of Mental Disorders (DSM-5®), Fifth Edition.* 2015. Washington, DC: American Psychiatric Association.

22. National Eating Disorders Collaboration. 2016. What Is an Eating Disorder? Available at http://nedc.com.au/eating-disorders-explained. Accessed April 2017.

23. Eating Disorders: A Professional Resource for General Practitioners. 2014. Available at http://www.nedc.com.au/files/Resources//GPs%20Resource.pdf. Accessed April 2017.

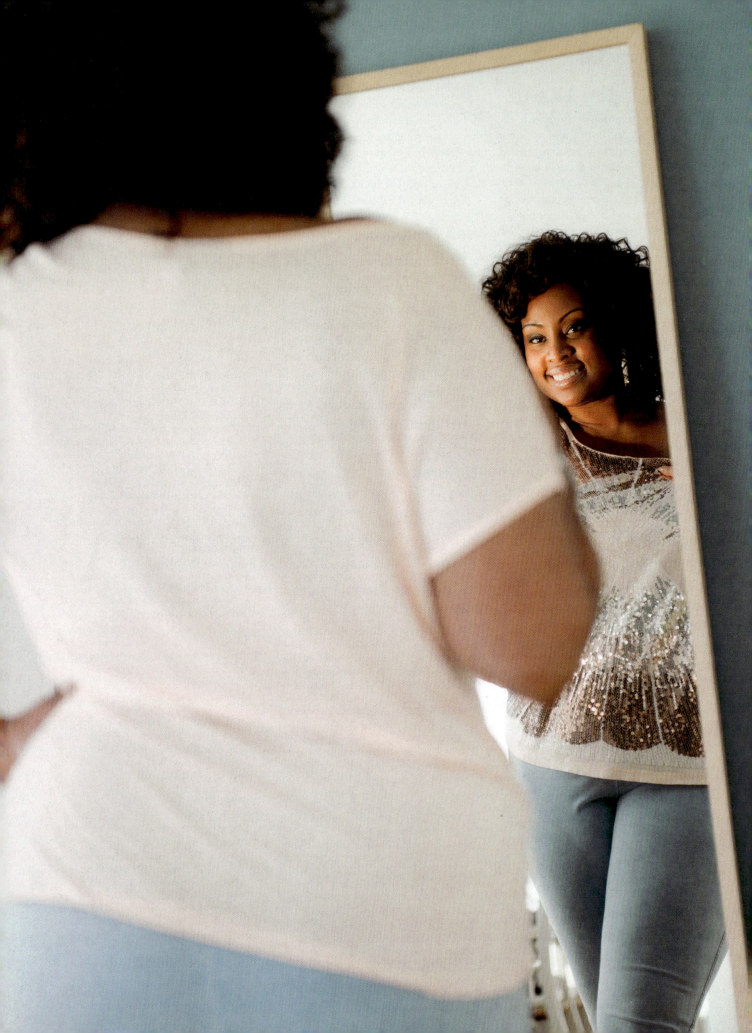

Weight Management

15

Learning Outcomes

After reading this chapter, you will be able to:

15.1 Explain why weight management is important to health and well-being.

15.2 Define the terms *appetite*, *hunger*, and *satiety*, and describe the physiological factors involved in regulating food intake.

15.3 Describe the role of hyperplasia and hypertrophy of adipocytes in the development of obesity.

15.4 Discuss the role of genetics and the environment in the development of underweight, overweight, and obesity.

15.5 Describe the role of diet and exercise in achieving a reasonable rate of weight loss.

15.6 Design a food and exercise plan to maintain a healthy weight.

15.7 Describe the role of diet and exercise in achieving a healthy weight gain.

15.8 Describe the role of weight-loss drugs and surgery for reducing obesity.

True or False?

1. Healthy weight loss occurs only with at least 2 hours of daily exercise. **T**/**F**

2. The body stops synthesizing fat cells after adolescence. **T**/**F**

3. Grazing throughout the day helps curb appetite and control body weight. **T**/**F**

4. Losing even 10 pounds can improve health. **T**/**F**

5. Genetics and the environment both affect body weight. **T**/**F**

6. Eating more vegetables and fruits can help an individual lose weight. **T**/**F**

7. Obesity is the result of consuming more energy than is expended. **T**/**F**

8. The nutrient that has the most effect on satiety is fat. **T**/**F**

9. You don't need to diet and exercise if you are taking a weight-loss drug. **T**/**F**

10. Bariatric surgery results in weight loss without restricting food intake. **T**/**F**

See page 572–573 for the answers.

In the last two decades, rates of overweight and obesity have exploded in the United States. In the early 1960s, fewer than 32 percent of Americans were overweight.[1] Today, that number has risen to an alarming 67 percent of Americans classified as overweight, and more than 33 percent of adults (about 72 million people) and 17 percent of children are obese.[2] Not surprisingly, as more and more individuals cross the threshold from a healthy body weight to being overweight, the topic has garnered much interest in popular culture. In fact, people often turn to social media sites such as Facebook, Pinterest, and Twitter to talk about weight management and locate helpful tools to help manage their body weight.[3]

Despite its prevalence, people do not enjoy being overweight, and regularly spend large amounts of money in search of a "cure." In fact, Americans annually spend over $60 billion[4] on everything from over-the-counter diet pills to books, magazines, online support groups, and commercial dieting centers to help shed their excess weight. It has been estimated that 21 percent of the total U.S. health care budget is spent to treat the medical complications associated with being overweight.[5]

If you are currently struggling with your weight or know someone who is, don't despair. Weight loss takes work, but it is achievable. This chapter emphasizes the key components of how to achieve and sustain a healthy body weight.

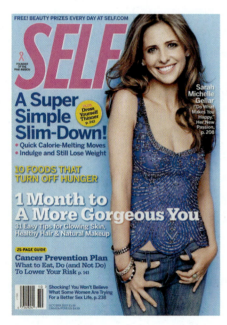

Weight management is such a hot topic in the United States that the mainstream media frequently covers it.

weight management Maintaining a healthy body weight; defined as having a BMI of 18.5–24.9.

Why Is Weight Management Important?

LO 15.1 Explain why weight management is important to health and well-being.

The term *weight management* means maintaining body weight within a healthy range. Achieving a healthy body weight is essential for physical and emotional well-being. It helps you feel good about yourself, provides the energy you need to enjoy life, and lowers the risk of chronic disease. In addition, weight management reduces costs to society. The costs for treating obese individuals are several thousand dollars higher than for their lean counterparts. It has been estimated that each additional pound of extra body weight above healthy body weight could add up to $13 a year per pound in added medical costs for men and up to $45 for women.[6]

Being Overweight or Obese Increases Health Risks

As you learned in Chapter 14, a healthy weight is a body weight that doesn't increase the risk of developing any weight-related health problems or diseases.[7] In contrast, overweight—and especially obesity—is associated with numerous health problems. In fact, in 2013, the American Medical Association declared obesity a disease in itself—specifically a *multi-metabolic and hormonal disease state*.[8] This new classification of obesity as a disease helps focus attention and resources on the problem, opening the door for the 90 million obese Americans to receive treatment for their obesity. It may also be changing the way physicians approach obesity management, increasing the use of drug therapies and surgery. Alternatively, the obesity-as-a-disease message suggests that body weight is uncontrollable, and—if it discourages patients—might hinder weight management efforts that focus on healthy eating and exercise.

People who are overweight or obese have an increased risk for cardiovascular disease—including hypertension, heart disease, and stroke—and the risk increases as BMI increases.[9] This increased risk may be due in part to the fact that overweight people tend to have high blood levels of both triglycerides and LDL cholesterol and low levels of HDL cholesterol.[10]

Overweight and obesity are also strongly linked to type 2 diabetes. Excessive adipose tissue contributes to insulin resistance, which forces the pancreas to work harder to produce more insulin. Eventually, the pancreas can stop producing insulin altogether, causing diabetes. Nearly 85 percent of people with type 2 diabetes are overweight or obese.[11]

A higher BMI can also increase the risk of gallbladder disease, joint stress, sleep apnea, reproductive problems, and some cancers, including endometrial, breast, and colon cancer. Central obesity is especially harmful: It is one of the five risk factors that comprise metabolic syndrome, a condition that in turn increases the risk for cardiovascular disease and type 2 diabetes. Obesity also increases the risk for osteoarthritis, a condition in which the tissue that protects the joints of the knees, hips, and lower back wears away.

Carrying extra body weight is so detrimental to health that for overweight individuals, losing as little as five to ten percent of body weight can be lifesaving.[12] For example, if you currently weigh 200 pounds, a weight loss of 10–20 pounds can reduce your risk of type 2 diabetes and other chronic diseases.

Being Underweight Also Increases Health Risks

As with being overweight, being underweight can lead to numerous diseases and conditions. These include anemia, heart irregularities, and amenorrhea (loss of menstruation in women). Underweight older adults are at risk for low body protein and fat stores and a depressed immune system, which makes it more difficult to fight infections. Injuries, wounds, and illnesses that would normally improve in healthy individuals can result in serious complications in individuals with a depressed immune system.

Individuals who are underweight are more likely to lack vital nutrients, such as calcium, which is important to maintain strong, dense bones. Being underweight increases the risk for osteoporosis and bone fractures later in life.[13] Sustaining a normal, healthy body weight can reduce this risk.

Certain diseases, such as cancer, inflammatory bowel disease, and celiac disease, can cause malabsorption and result in significant weight loss. Other inadvertent causes of underweight include certain medications—such as some antidepressant, osteoporosis, and blood pressure drugs—all of which can decrease appetite. Smoking and substance abuse can also lead to unhealthy weight loss.

Overweight and Underweight Have Social and Psychological Risks

Beyond the physical effects of carrying too much body weight, obese and overweight individuals are often at a social, educational, and economic disadvantage. Overweight people suffer more discrimination and are more likely to be denied job promotions and raises than normal-weight individuals.[14] Obese females are less likely to be accepted into college, especially higher-ranked schools.[15] Social situations, such as attending movies or sporting events, and travel on buses and airplanes may be limited for obese individuals due to restrictive seat sizes.[16] These prejudices and limitations can result in lower self-esteem.[17]

Popular perceptions of overweight individuals as being lazy or weak-willed can further affect their feelings of self-confidence and self-worth.[18] Images of slender models as the ideal in advertising and other media help perpetuate the notion that overweight individuals are less desirable. Living in an antagonistic environment may compromise

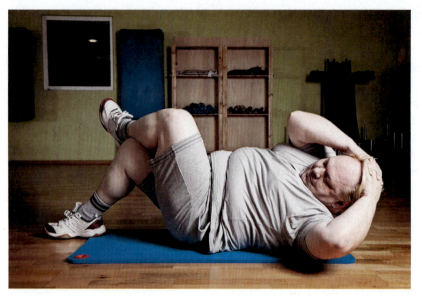
Overweight and obese people are often embarrassed to exercise in a gym or change clothes in a locker room because of their body weight.

attempts at achieving a healthy body weight. For example, obese and overweight people are less likely to exercise because they are embarrassed to change in the locker room or work out at a gym.[19] Obese people have higher rates of suicide than healthy-weight people[20] and are more likely to use alcohol and drugs when compared with their normal-weight peers.[21]

The psychological consequences of being underweight can be just as debilitating. Research has suggested that people who are underweight are at greater risk for irritability, anger, and depression.[22] For example, underweight males are reported to have a 12 percent increased risk of committing suicide compared with healthy-weight males.[23] People who are underweight can be more socially withdrawn compared with those with a healthy body weight.[24]

LO 15.1: THE TAKE-HOME MESSAGE Weight management means maintaining a healthy weight to reduce the risk of specific health problems. Classifying obesity as a disease may improve treatment options but may also raise health care costs, increase drug and surgical procedures, and hamper lifestyle changes to lose weight. The physical risks of overweight and obesity include an increased risk for cardiovascular disease, type 2 diabetes, certain cancers, and other disorders, whereas underweight increases the risk for anemia, heart irregularities, amenorrhea, and osteoporosis. The social and psychological effects of obesity and underweight include discrimination, low self-esteem, depression, suicide, and alcohol and drug problems.

How Is Food Intake Regulated?

LO 15.2 Define the terms *appetite*, *hunger*, and *satiety*, and describe the physiological factors involved in regulating food intake.

Why do you feel hungry or full? A variety of factors influence not only how much we eat, but also the type of food we choose to eat. These factors include strong physiological and psychological influences that go beyond the need for energy.

Appetite Often Triggers Eating for Unnecessary Reasons

Distinguishing between true hunger and **appetite**, or the desire to eat based on signals other than hunger, can be difficult. Have you ever groaned after a huge meal, "I'm so full!" only to turn around and eat a thick slice of apple pie with ice cream? Appetite is often stimulated even when we are satiated. This desire to eat the apple pie may be triggered by the smell, taste, texture, or color of the food, or by external cues such as time of day, social occasions, or other people. Appetite can also be triggered by learned behavior and by emotions such as stress, fear, and depression. Identifying the triggers that affect your desire to eat is one of the key strategies in maintaining a healthy body weight.

appetite Desire to eat food whether or not there is hunger; a taste for particular foods and cravings in reaction to cues such as the sight, smell, or thought of food.

Hunger and Satiation Affect the Desire to Eat and Stop Eating

Two strong physiological factors, hunger and satiety, affect the amounts of food individuals consume. **Hunger** is the physical sensation associated with the need or intense desire for food. Physiological signals such as low blood sugar or an empty stomach trigger hunger and searching for food. Once eating begins, hunger subsides as the feeling of fullness, or **satiation**, sets in and you stop eating. **Satiety** describes how you feel after a meal and before hunger is triggered again.

Satiety and hunger are both controlled by hormones produced in the brain and the gastrointestinal tract. In the brain, two regions of the hypothalamus control the trigger mechanisms that stimulate hunger and satiety: the *ventromedial nucleus* and the *lateral hypothalamus*. These regions receive signals from both inside and outside the brain. **Focus Figure 15.1** explains the signals that control hunger and satiation.

Regulation of Satiety

Satiety is triggered in the ventromedial nucleus in response to a variety of physiological cues. After a meal, the stomach becomes distended, sending signals from stretch receptors in the lining of the stomach to the brain to suppress hunger. As protein, fatty acids, and monosaccharides reach the small intestine, two hormones, cholecystokinin (CCK) and peptide YY (PYY), are released, sending feedback to the hypothalamus to increase satiety and decrease hunger.[25] Once these nutrients are absorbed, the hormone insulin is released, which also results in a decrease in hunger.[26]

Other hormones, including leptin, produced in adipose tissue, influence satiety. The production of leptin is controlled by the obese gene (*ob*) and increases in amount as the fat stores increase. Leptin is a satiety signal. It acts on receptors found in the hypothalamus to decrease hunger and food intake, probably by inhibiting neuropeptide Y, a hormone that stimulates hunger. At the same time, leptin creates a negative energy balance by raising the body temperature, which in turn increases energy expenditure and stimulates the oxidation of fatty acids in the liver and muscles. Thus, leptin regulates the amount of fat stored in the adipose tissue.[27]

In addition to the influence of hormones, certain macronutrients, especially protein, influence satiety and reduce the intake of food. Researchers have reported that protein intake ranging from 15 to 30 percent of total kilocalorie intake significantly reduces food intake.[28]

Regulation of Hunger

Whereas the ventromedial nucleus affects satiety, the lateral hypothalamus controls hunger. The hormone ghrelin, produced in the gastric cells of the stomach, stimulates the lateral hypothalamus. Thus ghrelin has the opposite effect of leptin—it stimulates hunger. Ghrelin concentrations rise in the blood before a meal. Ghrelin travels through the blood to the hypothalamus, where it activates neuropeptide Y to stimulate hunger.

The production of ghrelin changes throughout the day. More ghrelin is produced between meals, during sleep, or when you fast. This increase in ghrelin production signals the hypothalamus that the body needs energy. Ghrelin levels drop following a meal, especially one that contains high amounts of carbohydrate and/or kilocalories. This drop in ghrelin levels signals satiety and decreases the urge to eat.

Lean individuals tend to have higher levels of ghrelin than individuals with more body fat, especially in the morning hours. Ghrelin levels increase when an individual is on a low-kilocalorie diet, a fact that might help explain why people on weight-reduction diets continually feel hungry and find it difficult to lose weight.[29]

Leptin may also be partly responsible for hunger. When adipocytes shrink during weight loss, leptin levels drop. This reduction in leptin stimulates hunger and may drive the body to eat more to reestablish fat stores.

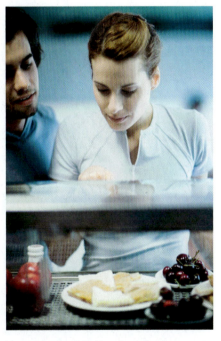

Hunger is stimulated by circulating hormones and signals from your intestinal tract.

hunger Strong sensation indicating a physiological need for food.

satiation State of being satisfactorily full during a meal, which inhibits the ability to eat more food.

satiety Feeling of satiation or "fullness" after a meal before hunger sets in again.

Head to Mastering Nutrition and watch a narrated video tour of this figure by author Joan Salge Blake.

Two regions of the brain—the ventromedial nucleus and the lateral hypothalamus—control eating behaviors in response to hormones released from the stomach, pancreas, small intestine, adipocytes, and the hypothalamus. The ventromedial nucleus responds to hormones to stimulate satiety. Hunger is triggered by hormones that stimulate the lateral hypothalamus.

HORMONES THAT STIMULATE SATIETY

HORMONES THAT STIMULATE HUNGER

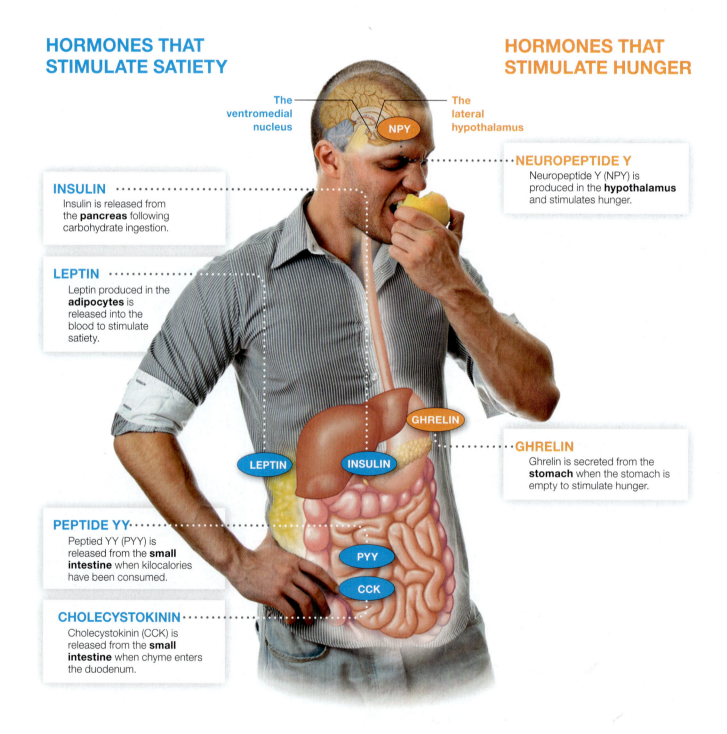

The ventromedial nucleus

The lateral hypothalamus

NPY

NEUROPEPTIDE Y
Neuropeptide Y (NPY) is produced in the **hypothalamus** and stimulates hunger.

INSULIN
Insulin is released from the **pancreas** following carbohydrate ingestion.

LEPTIN
Leptin produced in the **adipocytes** is released into the blood to stimulate satiety.

GHRELIN

LEPTIN INSULIN

GHRELIN
Ghrelin is secreted from the **stomach** when the stomach is empty to stimulate hunger.

PEPTIDE YY
Peptied YY (PYY) is released from the **small intestine** when kilocalories have been consumed.

PYY

CCK

CHOLECYSTOKININ
Cholecystokinin (CCK) is released from the **small intestine** when chyme enters the duodenum.

Certain vitamins and minerals have been shown to lower leptin concentrations and affect hunger levels. For example, zinc supplements have been reported to lower leptin in obese individuals and may be responsible for overeating.[30] On the other hand, ingesting too little vitamin A and C also appears to inhibit leptin secretion.[31] The mechanism of how vitamin and mineral intake affects the hormone leptin and hunger is still unclear.

LO 15.2: THE TAKE-HOME MESSAGE Food intake is controlled by hunger, satiation and satiety, and appetite. Appetite is a desire for food prompted by factors other than hunger. Hunger is a strong physiological need for food. Satiety is the physiological response to food intake, resulting in satisfaction. Hunger, satiation, and satiety are controlled by the hypothalamus and regulated by neuropeptides, hormones, and neural signals from the gastrointestinal tract and adipocytes. The hormones leptin and ghrelin play key roles in triggering hunger and satiety, with ghrelin triggering hunger and leptin triggering satiation.

How Do Fat Cells Form and Expand?

LO 15.3 Describe the role of hyperplasia and hypertrophy of adipocytes in the development of obesity.

The increase in the stores of body fat occurs in two ways: (1) Adipocytes, like muscle cells and many other body cells, can grow in size. This process is known as **hypertrophy**. In adipocytes, hypertrophy is caused by increased storage of fat. (2) Once an adipocyte fills to capacity, the production of more adipocytes is stimulated. The stimulation of excessive cell division—which occurs in tumor formation and other physiological processes, is known as **hyperplasia**. Adipocyte hyperplasia causes a buildup of excess fat tissue, which is stored throughout the body (**Figure 15.2**).

The Number of Fat Cells in the Body Never Decreases

The average nonobese adult's body contains approximately 30 billion to 50 billion adipocytes, each of which holds between 0.4 and 0.5 micrograms of fat. Overweight or obese adults most likely have the same number of adipocytes as healthy-weight adults but their fat cells are much larger, holding between 0.6 and 1.2 micrograms of fat. Thus, when a healthy-weight adult gains weight, it is likely due to hypertrophy.

When an overweight or obese adult loses weight, the size of the fat cell shrinks, but the number of cells does not. After weight loss, the smaller fat cells remain and can easily be filled up again when energy intake is greater than energy output.

hypertrophy Increase in size; in adipocytes, hypertrophy refers to the increase in size of the cells.

hyperplasia Increase in the number of cells due to cell division.

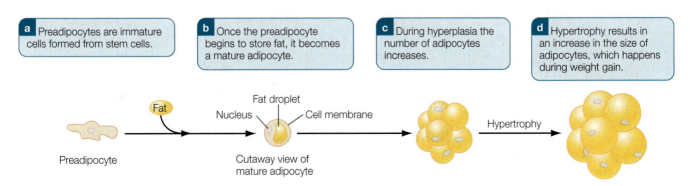

a Preadipocytes are immature cells formed from stem cells.

b Once the preadipocyte begins to store fat, it becomes a mature adipocyte.

c During hyperplasia the number of adipocytes increases.

d Hypertrophy results in an increase in the size of adipocytes, which happens during weight gain.

Fat

Fat droplet

Nucleus — Cell membrane

Hypertrophy

Preadipocyte

Cutaway view of mature adipocyte

▲ Figure 15.2 **The Formation of Adipocytes**

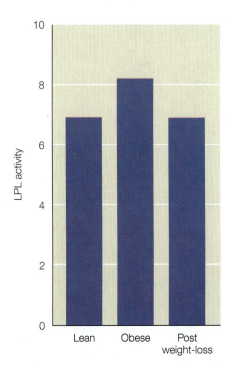

▲ **Figure 15.3 Lipoprotein Lipase Activity in Lean, Obese, and Post-Weight-Loss Adults**
LPL increases lipogenesis, or the accumulation of fat in the adipocyte.

Source: J. English. 2013. *Reversing Altered Metabolic Functions to Enhance Long-Term Weight Control.* Available at http://nutritionreview.org/2013/04/reversing-altered-metabolic-functions-enhance-longterm-weight-control/. Accessed April 2017.

gene–environment interaction Interaction of genetics and environmental factors that increases the risk of obesity in susceptible individuals.

Although hyperplasia appears to slow with age,[32] the growth and production of fat cells may continue throughout life, especially in obese individuals. Every year about 10 percent of fat cells die and are replaced by new ones. The number of fat cells you create as a child remains with you for life.[33]

Fat Cells Can Grow and Shrink

The size of fat cells is regulated by the enzyme lipoprotein lipase (LPL), which is made in the adipose tissue and lies on the surface of the adipocyte. As you learned in Chapter 5, LPL increases lipogenesis, or the accumulation of fat in the adipocyte. Another enzyme, called *hormone-sensitive lipase (HSL)*, plays the opposite role in fat metabolism. HSL stimulates lipolysis, or the hydrolysis of triglycerides inside the adipocyte, and frees the fatty acids, which are then released into the bloodstream. The balance between lipogenesis and lipolysis affects the size of the adipocyte. This is similar to a savings account—as you save money, the balance grows until you take it out and the balance shrinks.

The activity of LPL and HSL differs in overweight and lean individuals.[34] Heavier people have much more LPL activity, especially after eating (**Figure 15.3**). This makes it much easier to store energy from the meal. The activity of LPL increases following weight loss, which makes it much easier to regain lost weight.

Differences in LPL activity are also noted between genders.[35] In men, LPL is more active in the visceral, abdominal fat cells than in females, but females have higher LPL activity rates in the hips and thighs than do males. This is probably the reason women deposit more fat in the lower body and why adipose tissue in these areas is more stable and takes longer to lose. Overall, women oxidize more fat for fuel during exercise than men do and a male's LPL activity is higher following exercise than a female's. The reason for this remains unclear.

LO 15.3: THE TAKE-HOME MESSAGE The average adult body contains 30 billion to 50 billion adipocytes. Once adipocytes are formed, they can increase or decrease in size as fat storage needs change, but they can never decrease in number. Every year 10 percent of fat cells die and are replaced. The enzymes lipoprotein lipase and hormone-sensitive lipase influence the balance between lipolysis and lipogenesis, and thus the growing or shrinking of fat cells.

How Do Genetics and Environment Influence Obesity and Weight Management?

LO 15.4 Discuss the role of genetics and the environment in the development of underweight, overweight, and obesity.

The relationship of genes to obesity was first demonstrated in studies on separated identical twins raised in different home environments who have similar weight gain and body fat distribution.[36] On the other hand, our genetic code has not changed since the obesity epidemic began. Therefore the environment in which we work and live must also influence body weight. Indeed, most health professionals now agree that obesity arises from a **gene–environment interaction**.[37] The question is, which is stronger, nature or nurture?

Nutrigenomics and Epigenetics May Influence Weight Control

Two new areas of study introduced in Chapter 1, nutritional genomics and epigenetics, may help answer this question. The science of nutrigenomics has identified specific genes that are involved in the body's response to certain nutrients, such as how we absorb, store, or break down dietary fat, and can pinpoint the variation in the gene that may be responsible for the body's response. However, even with identical twins that have the same genetic makeup, the response to overeating or restricting kilocalories varies.

Researchers are still unclear what mechanism causes genes and nutrients to interact. This is where epigenetics comes into play. Recall that epigenetics studies changes in gene activity and gene expression that occur without changing the DNA sequence itself. The DNA in the body is wrapped around proteins called *histones*, much as thread is wrapped around a spool. Both the DNA and the histones are covered with chemical tags that can react to signals within the body, such as diet, stress, toxins, and physical activity. These chemical tags are collectively called the *epigenome* (**Figure 15.4**). The epigenome can cause the DNA-histone structure to tightly wrap, hiding genes. These genes are not accessible to the cell and therefore are not translated into proteins. However, the epigenome can also cause the DNA-histones to partially unwind, exposing the genes that were hidden and allowing them to be used to assemble proteins.

Food is one epigenetic factor that can cause the DNA-histones to partially unwind and expose inactive genes. For example, the B vitamins thiamin, riboflavin, and vitamin B_{12} donate methyl groups during metabolic reactions. These methyl groups tag the DNA-histones and thereby influence the expression of certain genes. These genes may, for example, trigger or inhibit fat synthesis, although how the mechanism might work is still unknown.[38] In other words, while we can't alter the genetic makeup we are born with, we may eventually be able to control the factors that turn obesity genes on or off.

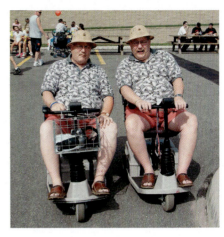

People who share genes often have similar body weights.

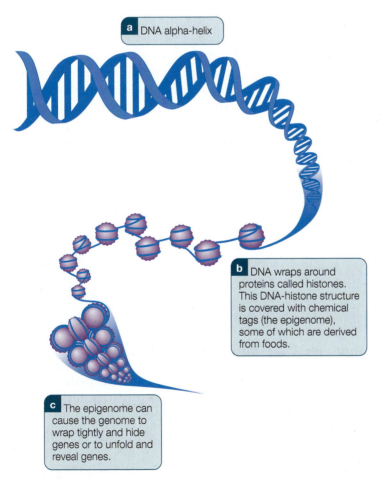

a DNA alpha-helix

b DNA wraps around proteins called histones. This DNA-histone structure is covered with chemical tags (the epigenome), some of which are derived from foods.

c The epigenome can cause the genome to wrap tightly and hide genes or to unfold and reveal genes.

▲ **Figure 15.4 The Epigenome**
The epigenome consists of chemical tags that influence the use of genes to assemble proteins. The epigenome can cause the genome to wind more tightly, thereby hiding genes, or unwind, making genes accessible for expression as proteins.

Genetic Variants Can Influence Body Weight

Scientists currently associate more than 40 genetic variants with obesity.[39] Some of these gene variants influence your levels of hunger-satiety hormones. Others affect eating behavior, insulin response, thermogenesis, and other factors.[40] But how do these gene variants occur?

Recall that even small changes in a gene can affect its ability to code for protein assembly. Among the most common of these small changes are *single-nucleotide polymorphisms*, referred to as SNPs, or "snips." Unlike epigenetic factors, which don't change the structure of the DNA itself, SNPs are copy errors that occur during DNA replication and do change the building blocks—the nucleotide bases—of DNA. For example, in a gene with an SNP, a length of DNA might have the nucleotide thymine (T) in place of the nucleotide cytosine (C). This shift in a single nucleotide changes the way the gene behaves. This is similar to dialing a telephone number with one wrong digit. Most SNPs have no direct effect whatsoever on body weight, but some play an important role in how individuals respond to food intake.

SNPs of certain genes can influence the level or the functioning of some hormones that influence hunger, satiety, and appetite.[41] Earlier in the chapter, you learned that the hypothalamus regulates hunger and satiety by responding to signals from the adipocytes, the pancreas, the stomach, and the small intestine. These signals are conveyed to the brain by the hormones leptin, insulin, CCK, peptide YY, and ghrelin. The hypothalamus then instructs you to eat more or eat less. Multiple gene variants can influence the way the body receives and responds to these signals. For example, an SNP of the ghrelin gene may cause high levels of ghrelin secretion, which could cause some people to overeat and become obese.[42] Individuals who are genetically prone to a leptin deficiency (remember, leptin suppresses hunger) become massively obese, yet when they are given leptin, their hunger decreases and their weight falls to within a healthy range.[43] Ironically, many obese people have adequate amounts of leptin, but the brain has developed a resistance to it, rendering its hunger control ineffective.[44] For these individuals, other mechanisms prevent leptin from functioning as a regulator of hunger.

The adipocytes also secrete another hormone called **adiponectin**, which improves the body's response to insulin, reduces fat accumulation in the liver and muscle, and enhances energy expenditure.[45] The levels of this hormone are higher in lean people but are low in people who are obese and those with type 2 diabetes. This difference may be explained by SNPs involving the adiponectin gene and may explain why obesity increases the risk for diabetes.

Genetics may also affect thermogenesis, which in turn affects energy expenditure. Gene variants may cause different rates of thermogenesis in brown adipose tissue and in nonexercise activity thermogenesis (NEAT). When some individuals overeat, they burn rather than store excess kilocalories and are thus better able to manage their energy balance.[46] Many overweight individuals don't appear to have this compensatory mechanism.

Gene Theories May Help Explain Weight Variations

Some researchers have described a genetic "**set point**" that determines body weight. This theory holds that the body fights to remain at a specific body weight and opposes attempts at either weight loss or weight gain. In other words, a person's weight remains fairly constant because the body "has a mind of its own." Given that the average weight of Americans has increased dramatically over the last few decades relative to previous decades, this theory either isn't true or the set point can be overridden.[47]

Other researchers have observed that, when excessive amounts of food are available, some people store more fat than others, and in environments where food is scarce, they lose less fat than others.[48] Research comparing the Pima Indians in Arizona with their

adiponectin Hormone produced in the adipocytes that controls the body's response to insulin and may be involved in reducing the risk of obesity and type 2 diabetes.

set point Weight-control theory proposing that each individual has a genetically established body weight and that significant deviation from this point stimulates changes in body metabolism to reestablish the normal weight.

ancestors in Mexico reveals that the environment can encourage weight gain in genetically susceptible populations; that is, populations with so-called thrifty genes.[49] The Arizona Pima Indians are descended from the Pima Indians of northwestern Mexico. The original population of Mexican Pima Indians passed their genetic heritage on to their Arizona descendants, but not their lifestyle. This genetic inheritance is theorized to have included genes that have helped the Pimas expend less energy during times of famine and store more energy in times of plenty. However, as compared to the Arizona Pimas, the traditional Mexican Pimas engage in more physical activity and consume a diet higher in complex carbohydrates and lower in animal fats. Mexican Pimas have, on average, a BMI of about 25, compared with Arizona Pimas who have, on average, a BMI of over 33.[50] Because they have a healthier lifestyle, the traditional Pimas have lower rates of obesity than the Arizona Pimas. This suggests that even if you have a genetic predisposition to being overweight, it's not a done deal. If you are determined to make healthy dietary choices and engage in regular physical activity, you can overcome your genetic predisposition.

Environmental Factors Can Increase Appetite and Decrease Physical Activity

As we saw with the Mexican and Arizona Pimas, the environment around us has changed in ways that have made it easier for people to gain weight. To explain how genetics and environment interact to produce obesity, researchers have used the analogy that genes load the gun but an obesity-promoting environment pulls the trigger.[51] Environmental factors that seem particularly important include lack of time, an abundant food supply coupled with portion distortion, and lack of physical activity. Take the Self-Assessment: Does Your Environment Affect Your Energy Balance? to consider how your environment influences the lifestyle decisions you make throughout the day.

Self-Assessment

How Much Does Your Environment Affect Your Energy Balance?

1. Do you eat out at least once a day?

   Yes ☐ **No** ☐

2. Do you often buy snacks at convenience stores or vending machines?

   Yes ☐ **No** ☐

3. Do you buy the supersized portions of fast foods or snacks?

   Yes ☐ **No** ☐

4. When you order pizza, do you have it delivered?

   Yes ☐ **No** ☐

5. Do you drive around the parking lot to get the closest parking space to the entrance?

   Yes ☐ **No** ☐

6. Do you get off at the subway or bus stop that is nearest to your destination?

   Yes ☐ **No** ☐

7. Do you take the elevator when stairs are available in a building?

   Yes ☐ **No** ☐

Answer

All of the above habits contribute to an obesity-promoting environment. If you answered "yes" to three or more, you should think about how you can improve your lifestyle habits.

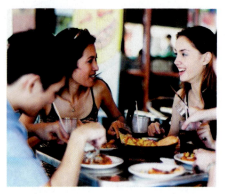

Research has shown that women who dine out five or more times weekly consume close to 300 kilocalories more on dining-out days than do women who eat at home.

Lack of Time

Research shows that adults spend more time traveling to work and devote more of their daily hours to work than in previous decades.[52] This longer workday means there is less time to devote to everyday activities, such as food preparation. Today, almost a third of Americans' daily kilocalories come from ready-to-eat foods that are not prepared at home.[53] Between 1972 and 1995, the prevalence of eating out in the United States increased by almost 90 percent, a trend that is expected to increase steadily to the year 2020.[54] To accommodate this demand, the number of food service establishments in the United States has almost doubled—to nearly 900,000—during the last three decades.[55]

Dining out frequently is associated with a higher BMI.[56] An Economic Research Service study found an average increase in kilocalorie intake for adults of 134 kilocalories for every meal eaten away from home.[57] Eating out also reduces fruit and vegetable intake and adds more fat, sugar, and alcohol.[58] The top foods selected when eating out, especially among college-age diners, are energy-dense French fries and hamburgers.[59] Dining out also tends to displace nutrient-dense vegetables and fruits.

An Abundant Food Supply and Portion Distortion

In the United States food is plentiful, there's a lot to choose from, and portion sizes are generous. All of these factors are associated with consuming too many kilocalories.[60]

Years ago, people went to a bookstore for the sole purpose of buying a book. Now they go to a bookstore to sip a vanilla latte and nibble on biscotti while they ponder which book to buy. Americans can grab breakfast at a fast-food drive-through, lunch at a museum, a sub sandwich at many gas stations, and a three-course meal of nachos, pizza, and ice cream at a movie theater.

This access to a variety of foods is problematic for weight-conscious individuals. The appeal of a food diminishes as it continues to be eaten (that is, the first bite tastes the best and each subsequent bite loses some of that initial pleasure), but having a variety of foods available allows the eater to move on to another food once boredom sets in.[61] The more good-tasting foods that are available, the more a person eats. For example, during that three-course meal at the movie theater, once you're tired of the nachos, you can move on to the pizza, and when that loses its appeal, you can dig into the ice cream. If the pizza and ice cream weren't available, you would have stopped after the nachos and consumed fewer kilocalories.

As you learned from Chapter 2, the portion sizes of many foods, such as French fries and sodas, have doubled, if not tripled, compared with the portions listed on food labels. Consumers perceive "supersized" portions as bargains because they often cost only slightly more than the regular size. Research shows that people tend to eat more of a food, and thus more kilocalories, when larger portions are served.[62] In other words, when served a supersized soft drink, a person consumes more, if not all, of it even though a smaller drink would have provided the same level of satisfaction.

At home, the size of the serving bowl or package of food influences the amount that ends up on the plate. Serving from a large bowl or package has been shown to increase the serving size by more than 20 percent.[63] This means that you are more likely to scoop out (and eat) a bigger serving of ice cream from a half-gallon container than from a pint container. To make matters worse, most people don't compensate for these extra kilocalories by reducing the portions at the next meal.[64]

You have probably heard competing claims about the superiority of diets high in either protein or carbohydrate for promoting weight loss. Does the macronutrient composition of the diet really influence body weight? To find out, see Examining the Evidence: Do Diets Rich in Carbohydrates Make Us Fat?

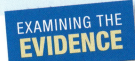
Do Diets Rich in Carbohydrates Make Us Fat?

In recent years, there has been a renewed interest in altering the nutrient composition of diets to achieve weight loss. The recommended AMDR (Acceptable Macronutrient Distribution Range) is for 45–65 percent of daily kilocalories to come from carbohydrates, 20–35 percent of daily kilocalories to come from fat, and 10–35 percent of daily kilocalories to come from proteins. Some nutrition experts believe that people who wish to lose weight should increase their protein consumption to as much as 45 percent of total kilocalories, at the same time reducing carbohydrates to 25 percent.[1] They cite studies reporting that high-protein diets produce greater weight loss when compared with high-carbohydrate diets of the same kilocalorie content.[2] A diet lower in carbohydrate and higher in protein also was reported to prevent weight regain after weight loss had been achieved.[3] Epidemiological evidence also suggests that carbohydrates may be contributing to America's weight gain: According to a 2013 meta-analysis, our increased intake in carbohydrate-rich, sugar-sweetened beverages correlates with the weight gain observed in both children and adults in recent decades.[4] This would suggest that as dietary intake of carbohydrates increases, so do our waistlines.

One big challenge is pinpointing the mechanism that might be responsible for weight gain with a higher carbohydrate intake. Some researchers argue that the culprit is insulin, while others suggest high-glycemic foods and beverages, such as sugary drinks, are the cause. A third theory is that carbohydrates alter appetite-suppressing hormones, causing hunger after a carbohydrate meal. Let's take a closer look at the evidence.

The Insulin Connection

As you learned in Chapter 4, the body requires insulin to facilitate the transport of glucose into body cells. But that's not the only function of insulin. This pancreatic hormone also promotes the synthesis of fatty acids, or lipogenesis, in the liver. Excess glucose

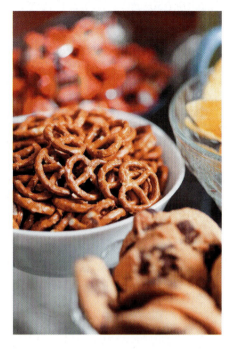

not converted to glycogen in the liver, or used for energy, is converted to fatty acids and stored as fat. In theory, the more carbohydrate ingested, the more insulin the pancreas releases, the greater the potential for glucose to be stored as fatty acids in the adipocytes.

Insulin also prevents beta-oxidation of fatty acids by inhibiting lipolysis of stored fat in the adipose tissue, trapping fatty acids in the adipocytes.[5] Thus, the effects of insulin on lipid metabolism tend toward conservation of fat. To avoid elevated insulin levels, a diet lower in carbohydrates would be a logical strategy.

Hunger Control and Carbohydrate Intake

The composition of the diet may influence the release of hunger-suppressing hormones. Recall that hunger is stimulated when ghrelin levels increase or is reduced when leptin levels increase. In one study, total ghrelin levels were shown to decrease significantly when protein was consumed, compared with carbohydrates or lipids.[6] The researchers also noted that after 3 hours, ghrelin levels rebounded following carbohydrate intake but not following

protein intake, supporting the theory that protein suppresses hunger for longer than does carbohydrate.

Ghrelin levels may be regulated by insulin, at least initially. In one study, a higher carbohydrate intake, which increased the amount of insulin released, led in turn to a reduction in the amount of ghrelin in the blood.[7] Researchers suggest that this may be due to the impact of insulin on circulating ghrelin levels. Or insulin may be affected by whether the carbohydrates ingested were simple or complex carbohydrates.[8] The theory is that the release of insulin following a meal regulates the reduction of ghrelin, thus influencing satiety.

Carbohydrate and protein may also affect the satiety hormone peptide YY. PYY levels have been shown to increase gradually without declining after consumption of a high-protein meal, whereas PYY levels peak and then begin to decline after consumption of a high-carbohydrate meal.[9] Researchers suggest that the increase in PYY following a high-protein/low-carbohydrate meal leads to more sustained feelings of satiety and may play a role in promoting a reduction in overall food intake and weight loss.

Glycemic Index and Weight Loss

The typical Western diet, based on high-glycemic-index staples such as potatoes, bread, and rice, may affect hunger and ultimately body weight. Foods with a high glycemic index are digested quickly, and in turn quickly raise blood glucose, thereby increasing insulin secretion to a greater extent compared with lower-glycemic foods. Consumption of high-glycemic foods has also been shown to be followed by hunger earlier than consumption of low-glycemic foods.[10] The increase in satiety with low-glycemic, high-fiber foods also results in lower kilocalorie intakes and potential weight loss.

Consuming a low-glycemic-index diet may also be effective in reducing total body fat. As noted above, increased levels of insulin may increase lipogenesis and decrease lipolysis, thereby preserving body fat. A 2013 study measured the impact of a low-glycemic diet (average 49 on the glycemic index) compared with a high-glycemic diet (average 60 on the glycemic index) for 16 weeks. Results showed that at the end of the 16-week study, the low-glycemic group had dropped 4.4 percent more intra-abdominal fat compared with the high-glycemic group (**Figure 1**).[11] Another study reported that a low-glycemic diet is associated

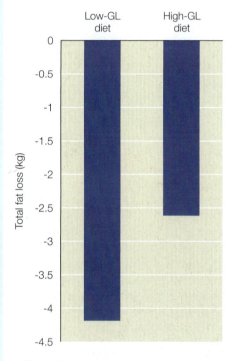

▲ **Figure1**

The Effects of a High versus Low Glycemic Diet on Fat Loss A low-glycemic diet resulted in a greater loss of abdominal fat compared to a high-glycemic diet.

Source: A. M. Goss, L. L. Goree, A. C. Ellis, P. C. Chandler-Laney, K. Casazza, M. E. Lockart, and B. A. Gower. 2013. Effects of Diet Macronutrient Composition and Fat Distribution during Weight Maintenance and Weight Loss. *Obesity* 21(6):1139–1142.

with a smaller waist circumference.[12] The results of these studies suggest that consuming low-glycemic foods reduces the impact of insulin on lipid metabolism and may enhance fat loss.

The evidence supporting the premise that a high-carbohydrate diet may promote weight gain is promising; however, when researchers compare the effects of isocaloric diets that are low in carbohydrate (less than 45 percent carbohydrate) versus moderate in carbohydrate (45–65 percent carbohydrate), the weight loss is similar.[13] Until more conclusive evidence is presented, a healthy weight-loss diet should include lean meats, low-fat dairy, whole grains, legumes and other vegetables, and fresh fruits and limit high-glycemic refined carbohydrates.[14]

References

1. Astrup, A., A. Raben, and N. Geiker. 2015. The Role of Higher Protein Diets in Weight Control and Obesity-Related Comorbidities. *International Journal of Obesity* 39(5):721–726. doi: 10.1038/ijo.2014.216.

2. Bray, G. A., D. H. Ryan, W. Johnson, et al. 2017. Markers of Dietary Protein Intake Are Associated with Successful Weight Loss in the POUNDS Lost Trial. *Clinical Obesity.* doi: 10.1111/cob.12188.

3. M. P. Lejeune, E. M. Kovacs, and M. S. Westerterp-Plantenga. 2005. Additional Protein Intake Limits Weight Regain After Weight Loss in Humans. *British Journal of Nutrition* 93:281–289.

4. V. S. Malik, A. Pan, W. C. Willett, and F. B. Hu. 2013. Sugar-Sweetened Beverages and Weight Gain in Children and Adults: A Systematic Review and Meta-Analysis. *American Journal of Clinical Nutrition* 98(4):1084–1102.

5. DiPilato, L. M., F. Ahmad, M. Harms, P. Seale, V. Manganiello, and M. J. Birnbaum. 2015. The Role of PDE3B Phosphorylation in the Inhibition of Lipolysis by Insulin. *Molecular and Cellular Biology* 35(16):2752–2760. doi: 10.1128/MCB.00422-15

6. Vancleef, L., T. Van Den Broeck, T. Thijs, S. Steensels, L. Briand, J. Tack, and I. Depoortere. 2015. Chemosensory signalling pathways involved in sensing of amino acids by the ghrelin cell. *Scientific Reports* 5:15725. doi: 10.1038/srep15725.

7. Steensels, S., L. Vancleef, and I. Depoortere. 2016. The Sweetener-Sensing Mechanisms of the Ghrelin Cell. *Nutrients* 8(12):795. doi: 10.3390/nu8120795.

8. Penaforte, F. R., C. C. Japur, L. P. Pigatto, P. G. Chiarello, and R. W. Diez-Garcia. 2013. Short-Term Impact of Sugar Consumption on Hunger and Ad Libitum Food Intake in Young Women. *Nutrition Research and Practice* 7(2):77–81.

9. Sedlackova, D., J. Kopeckova, H. Papezova, V. Hainer, H. Kvasnickova, M. Hill, and J. Nedvidkova. 2012. Comparison of a High-Carbohydrate and High-Protein Breakfast Effect on Plasma Ghrelin, Obestatin, NPY and PYY Levels in Women with Anorexia and Bulimia Nervosa. *Nutrition and Metabolism* 9:52. doi: 10.1186/1743-7075-9-52.

10. S. Wang, L. Yang, J. Lu, and Y. Mu. 2014. High Protein Breakfast Promotes Weight Loss by Suppressing Subsequent Food Intake and Regulating Appetite Hormones in Obese Chinese Adolescents. *Hormonal Research in Paediatrics.* doi: 10.1159/000362168.

11. A. M. Goss, L. L. Goree, A. C. Ellis, P. C. Chandler-Laney, K. Casazza, M. E. Lockart, and B. A. Gower. 2013. Effects of Diet Macronutrient Composition and Fat Distribution During Weight Maintenance and Weight Loss. *Obesity* 21(6):1139–1142.

12. J. Halkjaer, T. I. Sorensen, A. Tjonneland, et al. 2004. Food and Drinking Patterns as Predictors of 6-year BMI-Adjusted Changes in Waist Circumference. *British Journal of Nutrition* 92:735–748.

13. Naude, C. E., A. Schoonees, M. Senekal, T. Young, P. Garner, and J. Volmink. 2014. Low Carbohydrate versus Isoenergetic Balanced Diets for Reducing Weight and Cardiovascular Risk: A Systematic Review and Meta-Analysis. *PLoS ONE* 9(7):e100652. doi: 10.1371/journal.pone.0100652.

14. Astrup, A., and J. Brand-Miller. 2014. Obesity: Have New Guidelines Overlooked the Role of Diet Composition? *Natural Review of Endocrinology* 10(3):132–133.

Lack of Physical Activity

Since 1985, Americans have been consuming about 300 more kilocalories daily while also expending less energy during their entire day.[65] The increase in "kilocalories in" and decrease in "kilocalories out" is a recipe for a positive energy imbalance and weight gain. Compared with years past, Americans expend less energy both at work and in the little leisure time that they have.

When your great-grandparents went to work in the morning in the 1940s, chances are good they headed out to the fields or into factories. Your parents, though, are more likely to head to an office and sit in front of a computer, and you will probably sit at a desk for much of your workday. This shift in work from jobs that required manual labor to jobs that are sedentary has contributed to the rising rates of overweight and obesity in

America.[66] One study found that men who sit for more than 6 hours during their workday are at higher risk of being overweight than those who sit for less than an hour daily.[67]

Technology in the workplace now allows us to communicate with everyone without having to leave our desks. This means that people no longer have to get up and walk to see the colleague down the hall or the client down the street. Researchers estimate that a 145-pound person expends 3.9 kilocalories for each minute of walking, compared with 1.8 kilocalories per minute sitting. Thus, walking 10 minutes during each workday to communicate in person with coworkers would expend 10,000 kilocalories annually, yet only about 5,000 kilocalories would be expended if the person sat in the office sending e-mails or calling colleagues on the phone. Over the course of a year, these extra 5,000 kilocalories not expended could add up to over a pound of body weight. After 5 years in the workforce, there would be around seven extra pounds of body weight sitting in the chair.

Another form of technology, mechanized transportation, may negatively affect your weight-management goals. Research on urban sprawl has shown that the greater the distance between home and school or work, the more people drive or use public transportation and the less they engage in biking or walking. In addition, the more you drive, the more you weigh.[68] For each hour you spend driving to work or school, the likelihood of obesity increases 6 percent, whereas for each half-mile walked per day, the likelihood of obesity is reduced by almost 5 percent.[69] This may be one of the factors in the increase in obesity rates among children. In a recent study in Canada, only 25–30 percent of children and youth reported walking or bicycling to school.[70] Changing these behaviors while providing a safe way for children to arrive at school requires creative solutions. One such solution is the "walking school bus." A walking school bus is similar to a car pool except students walk to school with one or more adults. Children arrive at school safely and increase their daily physical activity.[71]

As technology continues to advance and allows for less energy expenditure during the day, *planned* physical activity at another time of day must make up the difference. Unfortunately, more than 20 percent of Americans report no daily leisure-time physical activity.[72] Research shows that those age 2–18 years old spend over 5 hours daily, on average, on a combination of "screen-time" activities. These include watching TV, playing video games, and non-work/school-related computer time—even though experts have suggested limiting screen time to 2 hours daily.[73]

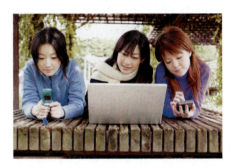

Students who walk to school accompanied by their parents demonstrate the concept of a "walking school bus."

Increased amounts of "screen time" are contributing to decreased amounts of physical activity.

LO 15.4: THE TAKE-HOME MESSAGE Many genetic influences play a role in obesity and weight management. Nutrigenomics has identified specific genes that are involved in how we absorb, store, or break down dietary fat. Epigenetics—changes in gene expression rather than DNA—may help to explain the effects on body weight when certain foods are eaten. Gene variants, such as single-nucleotide polymorphisms that affect hormone levels, can influence body weight, as can so-called thrifty genes. Several environmental factors—which include lack of time, easy access to a variety of energy-dense foods and large portions, and lack of physical activity—also encourage obesity.

How Can You Lose Weight Healthfully?

LO 15.5 Describe the role of diet and exercise in achieving a reasonable rate of weight loss.

The easiest way to avoid having to lose weight is to not gain weight in the first place. But for people who do need to shed pounds, following the principles discussed here can help.

Avoid Fad Diets

The low-carbohydrate, high-protein, and high-fat diets of the 1970s (Dr. Atkins' Diet Revolution) were replaced by the very high-carbohydrate and very low-fat diets of the 1980s and early 1990s (Pritikin and Dr. Ornish's diets), which were in turn replaced by the carbohydrate-restricted, moderate-protein and -fat diets of the late 1990s (the Zone diet), only to flip back to the low-carbohydrate, high-protein and high-fat diets in the early 2000s (Dr. Atkins' New Diet Revolution, South Beach). Fifteen years later, we're back to lower-carbohydrate and higher-protein diets (Paleo and New Atkins diets).

Fad diets promise quick weight loss by means that are typically unproven and unhealthy. For example, the latest fad diets claim that consumption of pasta, breads, rice, and many fruits and vegetables should be limited, whereas fatty meats, butter, and cheeses should be on the menu often. A diet high in saturated fat and low in fiber and phytochemicals is a recipe for heart disease, cancer, constipation, and deficiencies in many vitamins and minerals, such as vitamins A, E, C and folate, calcium, iron, zinc, and potassium.

Whereas each of the fad diets just mentioned provides a different percentage of carbohydrates, protein, and fat, they all had one important thing in common: They all reduced energy intake. A very interesting point emerged from a recent study comparing several of these diets: People who were most diligent about adhering to the diet—no matter which one—experienced the most weight loss.[74] However, more than 20 percent of the dieters quit just two months into the study, and more than 40 percent of them dropped out after 1 year. The highest dropout rates occurred among followers of the Atkins or Ornish diets. The researchers speculate that the rigidity of these extreme diets may have caused the higher dropout rates. Thus, the problem with many fad diets is that people give up on them long before they meet their weight-loss goals. A fad diet doesn't fix anything in the long term. If it did, new (or recycled) fad diets wouldn't continually be appearing on the market.

Strive for a Reasonable Rate of Weight Loss

The National Institutes of Health advises that overweight individuals aim to lose about 10 percent of their body weight over a 6-month period.[75] This means that the goal for an overweight, 180-pound person would be to shed 18 pounds in half a year, which would be about 3 pounds a month or $^3/_4$ pound weekly. Because a person must have an energy deficit of approximately 3,500 kilocalories to lose a pound of fat, a deficit of 250–500 kilocalories daily will result in a reasonable weight loss of about $^1/_2$ to 1 pound weekly. Any diet that promises quicker weight-loss results is likely to restrict kilocalories to the point of falling short of nutrient needs. Practice calculating the amount of reasonable weight loss you can expect in the Calculation Corner.

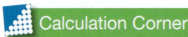

Calculation Corner

Calculating Percentage of Weight Loss
If an overweight individual weighs 237 pounds at the beginning of a weight-loss program, what would he or she weigh after 6 months if the recommendations for healthy weight loss were followed?

Answer:
The individual's initial weight minus 10 percent

$$237 \text{ lbs} - (237 \times 0.10) = 213.3 \text{ lbs}$$

> Go to **Mastering** Nutrition and complete a Math Video activity similar to the problem in this Calculation Corner.

fad diet Diet that promises rapid weight loss via a method that is typically unproven and unhealthy.

Though there is no single diet approach that has been universally embraced, many health experts agree that a person needs to modify three areas of life for successful, long-term weight loss. These three areas are diet, physical activity, and behavior. Let's begin with the diet.

Remember That Kilocalories Count

When it comes to losing weight, two important words need to be remembered: *kilocalories count*—no matter where they come from. An energy imbalance of too many kilocalories in and too few kilocalories out causes weight gain, and reversing the imbalance causes the opposite: Taking in fewer kilocalories and burning off more results in weight loss. The dietary goal, then, is to reduce the number of kilocalories consumed in foods. This can be done in several ways: by choosing lower-kilocalorie foods, by eating less food overall, or by doing both.

However, cutting back too drastically on kilocalories is the culprit behind many failed weight-loss attempts. If a person skips meals or isn't satiated at each meal because of skimpy portions, the person will experience hunger between meals and be more inclined to snack on energy-dense foods. Thus a key factor for success during the weight-loss process is for the person to eat a healthy, balanced diet that provides fewer kilocalories but is also *satisfying*. One strategy that many find helpful is to eat three small, nutritious meals throughout the day combined with a midmorning and a midafternoon snack. Eating more frequently keeps a person from getting too hungry and overeating at one sitting, while keeping meals small and nutrient dense ensures adequate nutrient intake without an over-consumption of kilocalories. Note that eating three small meals plus snacks is not the same thing as *grazing*. Grazing involves constant eating or nibbling throughout the day without allowing for feelings of hunger or satiation. This mindless eating behavior results in overconsumption of kilocalories and is considered a high-risk behavior for weight gain.[76]

Reducing the intake of kilocalories a little at a time can add up to healthy weight loss. A 180-pound, overweight person who consumes 2,800 kilocalories daily can reduce his or her intake to 2,400–2,600 kilocalories, incurring a kilocalorie deficit of 200–400 kilocalories daily. He or she will then lose 10 pounds in about 3 months. Small changes, like switching from full-fat to nonfat dairy products or replacing an afternoon soda with a glass of water, can contribute to this kilocalorie reduction.

Eat More Vegetables, Fruits, and Fiber

Research suggests that the volume (or bulk) of food consumed at a meal is very important. High-volume (high-bulk) meals and snacks have a high water and/or fiber content and are filling. Thus, consuming high-volume, low-energy-density vegetables and fruits at meals and snacks is associated with increased satiety and reduced feelings of hunger and kilocalorie intake—all helpful in weight management.[77] In contrast, people tend to eat the same amount of food regardless of its energy density—that is, the number of kilocalories in the meal.[78] In other words, energy-dense, low-volume foods can easily fill you *out* before they fill you *up*. Try calculating the energy density of foods in the Calculation Corner.

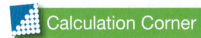

Calculation Corner

Calculating Energy Density

Energy density of foods can be calculated and compared using the method described by Barbara Rolls, PhD.[1] Divide the kilocalories in a serving of food by the weight in grams of a serving of the food. Try calculating the energy density of the following foods to determine which one is more energy dense.

(1) Chocolate ice cream: $^1/_2$-cup serving (111 grams); 340 kilocalories

(2) Frozen broccoli florets: 1-cup serving (85 grams); 25 kilocalories

To calculate the energy density of each food, divide the kilocalories by the weight in grams.

Answer:

Ice cream: 340 kcals/111 g = 3.1

Frozen broccoli florets: 25 kcals/85 g = 0.3

Reference

1. Vernarelli, J., D. C. Mitchell, B. J. Rolls, and T. J. Hartman. 2013. Methods for Calculating Dietary Energy Density in a Nationally Representative Sample. *Procedia Food Science* 2:68–74.

> Go to Mastering Nutrition and complete a Math Video activity similar to the problem in this Calculation Corner.

In fact, consuming a large, high-volume, low-energy-density salad at the beginning of a meal can reduce the kilocalories eaten at that meal by over 10 percent.[79] Adding vegetables to sandwiches and soups increases both the volume of food consumed and meal satisfaction and helps displace higher-kilocalorie items (**Figure 15.5**). Feeling full after eating a sandwich loaded with vegetables reduces the consumption of energy-dense potato chips. This is important because you don't need to eliminate chips from your diet if you enjoy them. Any food—from chocolate to chips—can be modest in kilocalories if eaten in modest amounts. Again, to lose weight, limit your intake of energy-dense, low-bulk foods and choose more nutrient-dense, high-bulk foods. **Table 15.1** provides examples of foods low, moderate, and high in energy density.

High-energy-dense foods

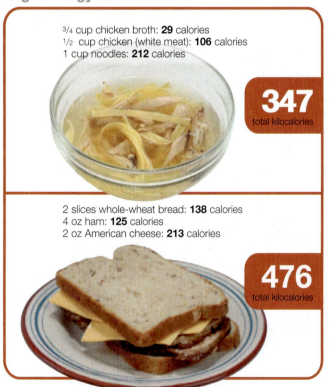

³/₄ cup chicken broth: **29** calories
¹/₂ cup chicken (white meat): **106** calories
1 cup noodles: **212** calories

347 total kilocalories

2 slices whole-wheat bread: **138** calories
4 oz ham: **125** calories
2 oz American cheese: **213** calories

476 total kilocalories

Low-energy-dense foods

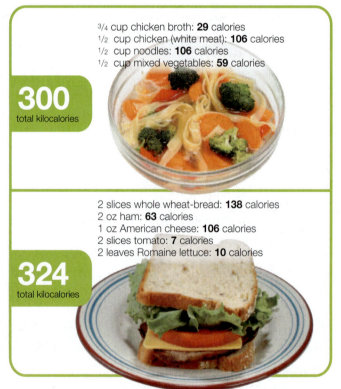

³/₄ cup chicken broth: **29** calories
¹/₂ cup chicken (white meat): **106** calories
¹/₂ cup noodles: **106** calories
¹/₂ cup mixed vegetables: **59** calories

300 total kilocalories

2 slices whole wheat-bread: **138** calories
2 oz ham: **63** calories
1 oz American cheese: **106** calories
2 slices tomato: **7** calories
2 leaves Romaine lettuce: **10** calories

324 total kilocalories

▲ **Figure 15.5 Adding Volume to Meals**
Adding high-volume, low-energy-dense foods like fruits and vegetables to sandwiches, soups, and meals can add to satiety and displace foods higher in kilocalories, two factors that can improve weight management.

TABLE 15.1 The Energy Density of Foods

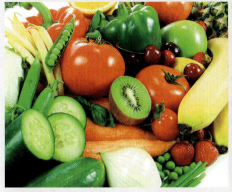

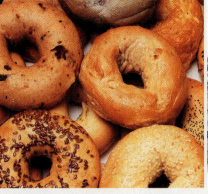

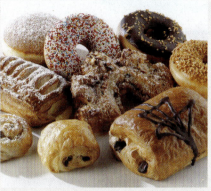

▲ Low

These foods provide 0.7–1.5 kilocalories per gram and are high in water and fiber. Examples include most vegetables and fruits—tomatoes, cantaloupe, strawberries, broccoli, cauliflower, broth-based soups, fat-free yogurt, and cottage cheese.

▲ Medium

These foods have 1.5–4 kilocalories per gram and contain less water. They include bagels, hard-cooked eggs, dried fruits, lean sirloin steak, hummus, whole-wheat bread, and part-skim mozzarella cheese.

▲ Hight

These foods provide 4–9 kilocalories per gram, are low in moisture, and include chips, cookies, crackers, cakes, pastries, butter, oil, and bacon.

Source: Adapted from B. J. Rolls and R. A. Barnett, *The Volumetrics Weight-Control Plan* (New York: HarperCollins, 2000) and Centers for Disease Control and Prevention, *How to Use Fruits and Vegetables to Manage Your Weight,* 2012. Available at www.cdc.gov/healthyweight/healthy_eating/fruits_vegetables.html. Accessed May 2014.

We just noted that dietary fiber contributes to the bulk of vegetables and fruits and their ability to prolong satiety.[80] Intriguingly, overweight individuals have been shown to consume less dietary fiber than normal-weight people.[81] The Table Tips provide easy ways to add these foods to your diet.

The composition of the diet alters the composition of the GI flora. This in turn may influence body weight. Read Examining the Evidence: The Microbiome: Is There a Link to Obesity? on page 556 to find out more.

Add Some Protein and Fat to Meals

Protein has the most dramatic effect on satiety; therefore, high-protein diets tend to reduce hunger and support weight loss.[82] Because fat slows the movement of food out of the stomach into the intestines, it can also prolong satiety. Therefore, adding some lean protein and healthy fat at all meals and even with snacks can help reduce hunger. This is not to say that carbohydrates should be severely restricted or eliminated; rather, all macronutrients are necessary in the correct proportions.

Keep in mind, however, that a diet high in saturated fat increases the risk for cardiovascular disease. To boost protein, choose lean meat, skinless chicken, fish, legumes, and nuts and seeds, which are kinder to the waist and heart.

Meals that contain fruits, vegetables, and whole grains, as well as some lean protein and a modest amount of fat, are sensible for weight loss. These meals are also balanced, meeting daily nutrient needs.

Increase Physical Activity

Regular physical activity can not only add to the daily energy deficit needed for weight loss, but can also displace sedentary activity such as watching television, which often leads to mindless snacking on energy-dense foods.[83] Going for a walk and expending kilocalories rather than watching a movie while snacking on a bag of tortilla chips provides kilocalorie benefits beyond the exercise alone.

TABLE TIPS
Eat More to Weigh Less

Eat more whole fruit and drink less juice at breakfast. The orange has more fiber and bulk than the OJ.

Make the vegetable portions on your dinner plate twice the size of the meat portion.

Have a side salad with low-fat dressing with a lunchtime sandwich instead of a snack bag of chips.

Order your next pizza with less pepperoni and more peppers, onions, and tomatoes. A veggie pizza can have 25 percent fewer kilocalories and about 50 percent less fat and saturated fat than a meat pizza.

Cook up a whole-wheat-blend pasta for your next Italian dinner. Ladle on plenty of tomato sauce and don't forget the big tossed salad as the appetizer.

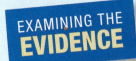

EXAMINING THE EVIDENCE

The Microbiome: Is There a Link to Obesity?

The term *microbiome* refers to the billions of microscopic organisms that live within an individual's body, including in the GI tract, on the skin, and in the lungs. The majority of these microbes are the GI flora living in the large intestine. Recall from Chapter 3 that GI flora participate in digestion and metabolism. For instance, they extract energy from undigested foods; synthesize vitamins, including vitamin K; regulate fatty acid tissue composition; and control peptides secreted from the GI tract.

More than 1,000 different types of bacteria live in the GI tract, but the precise species and the size of their populations vary.[1] Recently, scientists have suggested that when specific intestinal microbes are significantly high in the gut, obesity may result.[2] If this is true, could we alter the composition of our GI flora and eliminate the obesity epidemic?

Effect of Diet on Intestinal Bacteria

Different diets, whether followed briefly or persistently, influence the types of intestinal bacteria that live in the GI tract and the types of genes expressed by those bacteria.[3] In fact, differences in diet may explain up to 57 percent of the differences in the type of intestinal bacteria.[6] The changes are thought to occur because diet influences the bacteria's metabolism and your body's immune functions.

For example, breast-fed infants have more *Bifidobacterium* and *Ruminococcus*, with significantly less *Escherichia coli*, *Clostridium difficile*, *Bacteroides fragilis*, and *Lactobacillus* than infants fed formula.[4] As soon as infants begin to eat solid food, the composition of the GI flora changes again, resembling that of an adult, with *Firmicutes* and *Bacteroidetes* becoming dominant.[5] In addition, a change from a low-fat, high-fiber diet to a high-fat, high-sugar diet increases the bacteria *Firmicutes* and decreases *Bacteroidetes*.[7] These changes can occur within just 24 hours.[8,9] In other studies, people eating a vegetarian or vegan diet had significantly lower levels of *Bacteroidetes*, *Bifidobacterium*, *E. coli*, *Enterobacteriaceae*, and *Clostridium*

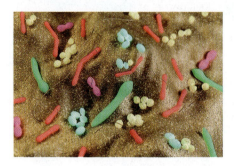

bacteria than people eating a normal mixed diet.[10,11] What effect, if any, do these variations in microbiome have on obesity?

Intestinal Bacteria and Obesity

The first clue that intestinal bacteria could influence obesity was the discovery that obese mice have a higher proportion of *Firmicutes* and significantly fewer *Bacteroidetes* than lean mice.[12] Similarly, 12 obese human subjects were found to have a larger proportion of *Firmicutes* and very few *Bacteroidetes* compared with two lean subjects.[13] Other studies report slightly different patterns,[14,15,16] but the question remains: Do these differences in the type of intestinal bacteria cause or contribute to obesity?

Just as the diet affects the different forms of bacteria that live in the GI tract, the presence of certain strains of intestinal bacteria can also influence human metabolism. Several theories have been proposed for the role of the microbiome in physiological mechanisms contributing to obesity. Different species of intestinal bacteria may control the amount of energy produced from nondigested food in the intestinal tract. For instance, an increase in *Firmicutes* and a drop in *Bacteroidetes* could increase the amount of energy produced. The *Firmicutes* bacteria are genetically prone to increase the digestion of polysaccharides, producing monosaccharides and short-chain fatty acids. These short-chain fatty acids attach to the enterocytes on the surface of the intestinal villi, slowing intestinal motility and transit. These short-chain fatty acids attach to the epithelial cells that cover the villi lining the intestinal cells, slowing intestinal motility and transit. Not only does the intestinal tract have receptor sites for

ghrelin to stimulate hunger, but there are also receptor sites on the intestinal cells to which short-chain fatty acids attach that may also stimulate hunger. Certain bacteria may also cause inflammation and alter human genes that stimulate fat synthesis in the adipocyte.[17]

If we altered the diet of obese people in order to change the composition of intestinal bacteria, would they lose weight? Perhaps. One case study involved a morbidly obese male whose intestinal bacteria were 35 percent *Enterobacter*. This form of intestinal bacteria produces lipopolysaccharide endotoxins that, if they leak through the intestinal tract into the blood, can cause inflammation and contribute to obesity, at least in animal models. The subject in this case study was placed on a 9-week dietary regimen composed of whole grains, prebiotics, and foods promoted in traditional Chinese medicine. After 9 weeks, the subject lost 66 pounds and reduced the *Enterobacter* population to 1.8 percent.[18] As the level of *Enterobacter* decreased, the inflammation and levels of lipopolysaccharide endotoxins also dropped.

The majority of the research reported thus far, however, has been in animal models. Well-designed research in humans is needed to unravel the complex relationship between microbiome composition and obesity. At this point, manipulating the GI flora is not a realistic weight-management tool.

References

1. Komaroff, A. L. 2017. The Microbiome and Risk for Obesity and Diabetes. *Journal of the American Medical Association* 317(4):355–356. doi: 10.1001/jama.2016.20099.
2. Gérard, P. 2016. Gut Microbiota and Obesity. *Cellular and Molecular Life Sciences* 73(1):147–162. doi: 10.1007/s00018-015-2061-5.
3. Ibid.
4. Stearns, J. C., M. A. Zulyniak, R. J. de Souza, N. C. Campbell, M. Fontes, and M. Shaikh. 2017. Ethnic and Diet-Related Differences in the Healthy Infant Microbiome. *Genome Medicine* 9:32. doi: 10.1186/s13073-017-0421-5
5. F. Turroni, C. Peano, D. A. Pass, E. Foroni, M. Severgnini, M. J. Claesson, et al. 2012. Diversity of *Bifidobacteria* within the Infant Gut Microbiota. *PLoS ONE* 7:e36957. doi: 10.1371/journal.pone.0036957.

6. Cong, X., W. Xu, R. Romisher, S. Poveda, S. Forte, A. Starkweather, and W. A. Henderson. 2016. Gut Microbiome and Infant Health: Brain-Gut-Microbiota Axis and Host Genetic Factors. *Yale Journal of Biology and Medicine* 89(3):299–308.

7. Murphy, E. A., K. T. Velazquez, and K. M. Herbert. 2015. Influence of High-Fat-Diet on Gut Microbiota: A Driving Force for Chronic Disease Risk. *Current Opinion in Clinical Nutrition and Metabolic Care* 18(5):515–520. doi: 10.1097/MCO.0000000000000209

8. Wu, G. D., J. Chen, C. Hoffmann, K. Bittinger, Y. Y. Chen, S. A. Keilbaugh, et al. 2011. Linking Long-Term Dietary Patterns with Gut Microbial Enterotypes. *Science* 334:105–108.

9. De Filippo, C., D. Cavalieri, M. Di Paola, M. Ramazzotti, J. B. Poullet, S. Massart, et al. 2010. Impact of Diet in Shaping Gut Microbiota Revealed by a Comparative Study in Children from Europe and Rural Africa. *Proceedings of the National Academy of Science U.S.A.* 107:14691–14696.

10. Glick-Bauer, M., M. C. Yeh. 2014. The Health Advantage of a Vegan Diet: Exploring the Gut Microbiota Connection. *Nutrients* 6(11), 4822–4838. doi: 10.3390/nu6114822.

11. Zimmer, J., B. Lange, J. Frick, H. Sauer, K. Zimmermann, A. Schwiertz, et al. 2011. A Vegan or Vegetarian Diet Substantially Alters the Human Colonic Faecal Microbiota. *European Journal of Clinical Nutrition* 66:53–60.

12. Brahe, L. K., A. Astrup, and L. H. Larsen. 2016. Can We Prevent Obesity-Related Metabolic Diseases by Dietary Modulation of the Gut Microbiota? *Advances in Nutrition* 7(1):90–101. doi: 10.3945/an.115.010587.

13. Ibid.

14. John, G. K., and G. E. Mullin. 2016. The Gut Microbiome and Obesity. *Current Oncology Report* 18(7):45. doi: 10.1007/s11912-016-0528-7.

15. Ibid.

16. Blaut, M. 2015. Gut Microbiota and Energy Balance: Role in Obesity. *The Proceedings of the Nutrition Society* 74(3):227-234. doi: 10.1017/S0029665114001700.

17. Moreno-Indias, I., F. Cardona, and M. I. Queipo-Ortuño. 2014. Impact of the Gut Microbiota on the Development of Obesity and Type 2 Diabetes Mellitus. *Frontiers in Microbiology* 5:190–200.

18. Cani, P. D., J. Amar, M. A. Iglesias, M. Poggi, C. Knauf, D. Bastelica, et al. 2007. Metabolic Endotoxemia Initiates Obesity and Insulin Resistance. *Diabetes* 56:1761–1772.

Individuals are advised to devote 60–90 minutes daily to moderate-intensity activities to aid in weight loss and prevent weight gain.[84] Moderately intense physical activity would be the equivalent of walking 3.5 miles per hour (**Table 15.2**). The longer your exercise session, the more oxygen is consumed after the exercise ends, which contributes to a higher sustained metabolic rate and more kilocalories burned throughout the day, even at rest.[85] Establishing an exercise program that incorporates cardiorespiratory and strength-training activities has even greater benefits, one of which is the increased metabolic rate that occurs with an increase in muscle mass. For more information on the influence of exercise on losing weight, see Examining the Evidence: Which Exercise Is Most Effective for Weight Loss? on page 558.

Research suggests that accumulating 10,000 steps daily, which generally is the equivalent of walking 5 miles, can help reduce the risk of becoming overweight.[86] Americans, on average, accumulate only 900–3,000 steps daily.[87] To reach 10,000 steps, most people need to make a conscious effort to keep moving. Using a pedometer can help you track the number of steps you take and let you know if you are hitting this target, or if you need to get up and move much more often. The Fitness Tips provide more suggestions on how to expend more energy during the day.

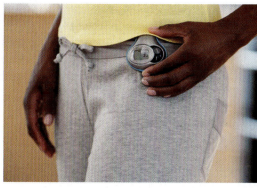

Wearing a pedometer, like the one shown here, can help you track your steps. Remember to aim for 10,000 steps per day.

FITNESS TIPS
Get UP and MOVE

Skip the text messages and walk to visit your friends on campus.

Don't go to the closest coffee shop for your morning latte; walk to the java joint that is a few blocks farther away.

Take a 5-minute walk at least twice a day. A little jolt of exercise can help break the monotony of studying and work off some stress.

Accomplish two goals at once by cleaning your dorm room or apartment. A 150-pound person burns about 4 kilocalories for every minute spent cleaning. Scrub, sweep, or vacuum for 30 minutes and you could work off about 120 kilocalories.

Offer to walk your neighbor's dog daily.

TABLE 15.2 Kilocalories Used during Activities

Moderate Physical Activity	Approximate Kilocalories/Hour for a 154-lb Person*	Vigorous Physical Activity	Approximate Kilocalories/Hour for a 154-lb Person*
Hiking	370	Running/jogging (5 mph)	590
Light gardening/yard work	330	Bicycling (> 10 mph)	590
Dancing	330	Swimming (slow freestyle laps)	510
Golf (walking and carrying clubs)	330	Aerobics	480
Bicycling (< 10 mph)	290	Walking (4.5 mph)	460
Walking (3.5 mph)	280	Heavy yard work (chopping wood)	440
Weight lifting (general light workout)	220	Weightlifting (vigorous effort)	440
Stretching	180	Basketball (vigorous)	440

Note:* Calories burned per hour will be higher for persons who weigh more than 154 lbs (70 kg) and lower for persons who weigh less.

Source: Adapted from 2015–2020 *Dietary Guidelines for Americans.* 2017. Available at https://health.gov/dietaryguidelines/2015/. Accessed April 2017.

Which Exercise Is the Most Effective for Weight Loss?

Weight loss occurs when the amount of energy you expend is greater than the amount of energy you consume, creating an energy deficit. Adding exercise to your daily routine can help create this energy deficit. Exercise mobilizes energy stores, including fat stored in adipocytes, to fuel the exercise, ultimately reducing the size of adipocytes, increasing the ratio of lean body mass to fat mass, and reducing risk factors correlated with obesity.[1]

The American College of Sports Medicine recommends that most adults engage in moderate-intensity cardiorespiratory exercise for at least 225–300 minutes per week to maintain a healthy body weight and prevent weight gain.[2] For weight loss, however, some researchers advocate more intense exercise regimens. What are the potential weight-loss benefits of different types and intensities of exercise?

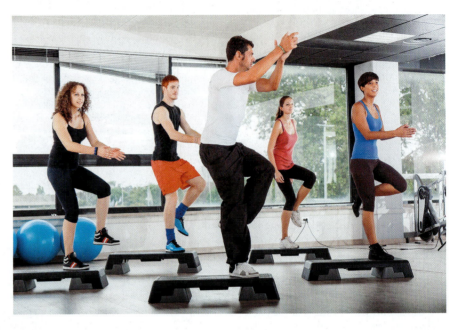

Aerobic Exercise and Weight Loss

Even though aerobic exercise provides numerous health benefits, including blood glucose control, reduced blood pressure, and an increase in high-density lipoproteins for overweight or obese subjects, clinical trials report only modest weight-loss effects related to the exercise itself.[3] Aerobic exercise is classified as exercise of low to moderate intensity that utilizes the aerobic reactions that produce ATP. Carbohydrates, fats, and protein all provide energy to perform aerobic-type exercise, which includes brisk walking, jogging, hiking, and cross-country skiing.

Recall from Chapter 8 that lipolysis, or the breakdown of stored fatty acids for energy production, occurs during aerobic metabolism. However, in the first few minutes of any moderate exercise, carbohydrates, creatine phosphate, and the 3–5 seconds' worth of stored ATP—not fat—provide most of the fuel. As aerobic metabolism begins to fully power up, lipolysis of stored fat and beta-oxidation of fatty acids increases, eventually exceeding carbohydrate as the main fuel source. Does this mean

that moderate aerobic exercise is the key to successful weight loss?

A classic 3-month study reported the influence of diet and exercise on body composition in obese women. Ninety-one obese women were randomly assigned to diet only, exercise only, diet plus exercise, or control group. Those in the exercise groups were asked to complete 45 minutes of moderate-intensity cardiorespiratory exercise per day, 5 days a week. The results were surprising: those in the diet-plus-exercise group lost the same amount of weight as those who only dieted.[4] The aerobic exercise–only group did not differ in weight loss from the control group at the end of the study. A more recent study found similar results. Subjects who increased the cardiorespiratory exercise to 50 minutes, 5 days a week without dieting lost a similar amount of weight to those who restricted kilocalories without exercise.[5] In another study involving obese women, moderate-intensity aerobic exercise without dieting had the same effect as dieting without exercise. Both groups lost an average of 8 kilograms (about 17.5 pounds) over the course of 12 weeks.[6]

Over the course of a 1-year study, subjects who performed aerobic

exercise without dieting for 60 minutes a day, 6 days a week, lost only an average of 3.5 pounds over the year.[7] Unless the overall volume of accumulated time devoted to aerobic exercise is high, according to the experts, significant weight loss is unlikely from aerobic exercise alone.[8] Moreover, as you already learned in this chapter, finding—or making—the time to exercise is a barrier for most adults. Perhaps the answer lies in short, intense bouts of anaerobic exercise?

Anaerobic Exercise and Weight Loss

Anaerobic exercise is more intense than aerobic, but it is also by necessity shorter in duration because the body's glucose and glycogen stores are rapidly depleted. For instance, heavy weightlifting, sprinting, jumping rope, and climbing stairs are all examples of anaerobic, high-intensity exercise. The higher the intensity of anaerobic exercise, the less fat is oxidized and the more glycogen and blood glucose are used to produce energy.

Performing intermittent cycles of high-intensity exercise, also known as high-intensity intermittent exercise (HIIE) or high-intensity interval training (HIIT), has been shown to result in greater fat loss than aerobic exercise in some studies.[9] For example, one 15-week study involved women performing either three 20-minute HIIE exercise sessions per week or a steady-state exercise (SSE) at 60 percent of their maximum heart rate for 40 minutes three times per week. The HIIE group's exercise sessions consisted of 8 seconds of sprint cycling followed by 12 seconds of slow cycling repeated for 20 minutes. The HIIE subjects lost 2.5 kilograms, or 5.5 pounds, of subcutaneous body fat over the 15-week study, whereas women who performed SSE aerobic exercise for the 15 weeks experienced no change in body fat (**Figure 1**).[10] Notice that fat loss was achieved with 50 percent less time exercising and a similar energy expenditure. Researchers suggested that the significant loss of body fat in the HIIE group might be due to the impact of high-intensity exercise on reducing hunger hormones and overall kilocalorie intake. Another explanation may be that high-intensity exercise enhances lipolysis and fatty-acid oxidation. And

finally, while the changes in lean muscle mass were not significantly different between groups, the high-intensity exercise group gained lean muscle, while the steady-state group lost lean muscle. This is important for weight loss, as loss of lean muscle reduces basal metabolic rate, whereas an increase in active muscle tissue continues to burn more fatty acids even at rest.

One of the advantages of anaerobic exercise is that it burns more total kilocalories per minute than moderate aerobic exercise. For instance, a 150-pound female who jogged at a pace of 12 minutes per mile would burn approximately 220 kilocalories in 30 minutes compared with running a 7-minute-mile pace, which would burn approximately 390 kilocalories in 30 minutes. Even though less fat is burned during anaerobic exercise, anaerobic exercise increases resting metabolic rate and lean muscle mass that continues to burn kilocalories (mostly fat kilocalories) after the exercise is complete, for up to 14 hours.

Whether you enjoy anaerobic or aerobic exercise, the key is to exercise every day. Gradually increase the duration and intensity of the exercises, and if you are overweight or obese, slow down or stop if you experience chest pains, joint pain, or nausea or become dehydrated.[11]

Aerobic Exercise Combined with Resistance Training

If aerobic exercise utilizes fatty acids for energy but anaerobic exercise increases lean muscle mass and resting metabolic rate, why not combine the two in one exercise bout? In a recent study at Duke University, researchers followed 234 overweight and obese adults who were randomly assigned to an aerobic-exercise

group, a resistance-training group, or a group that performed both aerobic exercise and resistance training. The aerobic-exercise group exercised the equivalent of 12 miles per week either on a treadmill or elliptical trainer. The resistance-training group lifted weights 3 days per week, three sets per day, with 8–12 repetitions per set. The aerobic-exercise plus resistance-training group completed both protocols. After 10 weeks, the aerobic-exercise group and the aerobic-plus-resistance-training group lost more total body weight and fat loss than the resistance-training group.[12] Interesting to note, however, is that the subjects in the combined group significantly reduced their waist circumference compared with the aerobic-only group or the resistance-training group.

Another study tested the hypothesis that short-term aerobic activity combined with anaerobic exercise might improve weight loss compared with aerobic activity alone. Sixteen obese subjects performed one of two exercise protocols for 4 weeks. Group one performed an aerobic cycle workout for 30 minutes while group two completed a 25-minute aerobic workout followed by 5 minutes of anaerobic exercise. Shifting 5 minutes to anaerobic exercise achieved a significantly greater reduction in body fat compared with aerobic exercise alone.[13] Total body fat, visceral fat, and abdominal fat also appear to be significantly reduced with the addition of anaerobic resistance training. The addition of anaerobic resistance training may have produced greater lipolysis of stored body fat.

Choosing the Right Exercise for You

Not all individuals respond to the same type of exercise. Most research compares the group mean response of weight loss to exercise, not the individual variation. Just because one study failed to show results for the group of subjects doesn't mean it may not work for you. In other words, if you enjoy a specific type of exercise and you find it effective in weight loss or maintaining a healthy weight—don't stop! Any exercise is better than not exercising at all.

▲ **Figure 1** **The Effects of High-Intensity Intermittent Exercise on Fat Loss**

Source: E. G. Trapp, D. J. Chisholm, J. Freud, and S. H. Boutcher. 2008. The Effects of High-Intensity Intermittent Exercise Training on Fat Loss and Fasting Insulin Levels of Young Women. *International Journal of Obesity* 32:684–691.

In addition, research is clear that achieving healthy weight loss requires not just exercise but dieting as well.[14] In an 18-month study of 288 obese men and women, the results reported a significant drop in body fat and an increase in lean muscle mass when subjects participated in both exercise and a weight-loss diet compared with those who just exercised without dieting.[15] The bottom line? If you want to lose weight, eat a healthy, lower-energy diet and engage in a combination of aerobic and anaerobic exercise.

References

1. Swift, D. L., N. M. Johannsen, C. J. Lavie, C. P. Earnest, and T. S. Church. 2014. The Role of Exercise and Physical Activity in Weight Loss and Maintenance. *Progress in Cardiovascular Diseases* 56(4):441–447.

2. Garber, C. E., B. Blissmer, M. R. Deschenes, B. A. Franklin, M. J. Lamonte, et al. 2011. American College of Sports Medicine Position Stand. Quantity and Quality of Exercise for Developing and Maintaining Cardiorespiratory, Musculoskeletal, and Neuromotor Fitness in Apparently Healthy Adults: Guidance for Prescribing Exercise. *Medicine and Science in Sports and Exercise* 43(7):1334–1359.

3. Kemmler, W., M. Scharf, M. Lee, C. Petrasek, and S. von Stengel. 2014. High versus Moderate Intensity Running Exercise to Impact Cardiometabolic Risk Factors: The Randomized Controlled RUSH-Study. *BioMed Research International* doi: 10.1155/2014/843095.

4. Utter, A. C., D. C. Nieman, E. M. Shannonhouse, et al. 1998. Influence of Diet and/or Exercise on Body Composition and Cardiorespiratory Fitness in Obese Women. *International Journal of Sport Nutrition* 8(3):213–222.

5. Redman, L. M., L. K. Helbronn, C. K. Martin, A. Alfonso, S. R. Smith, and E. Ravussin. 2007. Effect of Calorie Restriction With or Without Exercise on Body Composition and Fat Distribution. *Journal of Clinical Endocrinology and Metabolism* 92(3):865–872.

6. Hoppes, E., and G. Caimi. 2011. Exercise in Obesity Management. *Journal of Sports Medicine and Physical Fitness* 51(2):275–282.

7. McTiernan, A., B. Sorensen, M. L. Irwin, A. Morgan, Y. Yasui, R. E. Rudolph, et al. 2007. Exercise Effect on Weight and Body Fat in Men and Women. *Obesity* 15(6):1496–1512.

8. Swift, D. L., N. M. Johannsen, C. J. Lavie, C. P. Earnest, and T. S. Church. 2014. The Role of Exercise and Physical Activity in Weight Loss and Maintenance. *Progress in Cardiovascular Diseases* 56(4):441–447.

9. Heydari, M., J. Freund, and S. H. Boutcher. 2012. The Effect of High-Intensity Intermittent Exercise on Body Composition of Overweight Young Males. *Journal of Obesity* doi: 10.1155/2012/4804.

10. Trapp, E. G., D. J. Chisholm, J. Freud, and S. H. Boutcher. 2008. The Effects of High-Intensity Intermittent Exercise Training on Fat Loss and Fasting Insulin Levels of Young Women. *International Journal of Obesity* 32:684–691.

11. Willis, L. H., C. A. Slentz, L. A. Bateman, A. T. Shields, L. W. Piner, C. W. Bales, J. A. Houmard, W. E. Kraus. Effects of Aerobic and/or Resistance Training on Body Mass and Fat Mass in Overweight or Obese Adults. *Journal of Applied Physiology* 113(12):1831. doi: 10.1152/japplphysiol.01370.2011.

12. Ibid.

13. Salvadori, A., P. Fanari, P. Marzullo, F. Codecase, I. Tovaglieri, M. Cornacchia, et al. 2014. Short Bouts of Anaerobic Exercise Increase Non-Esterified Fatty Acids Release in Obesity. *European Journal of Nutrition* 53(1):243–249.

14. Fletcher, G., F. F. Eves, E. I. Glover, et al. 2017. Dietary Intake is Independently Associated with the Maximal Capacity for Fat Oxidation During Exercise. *American Journal of Clinical Nutrition* 105(4):864–872. doi: 10.3945/ajcn.116.133520.

15. Beavers, K. M., D. P. Beavers, B. A. Nesbit, W. T. Ambrosium, A. P. Marsh, B. J. Niclas, and W. J. Rejeski. 2014. Effect of an 18-Month Physical Activity and Weight-Loss Intervention on Body Composition in Overweight and Obese Older Adults. *Obesity* 22(2):325–331.

Modify Your Eating Behaviors

Many incoming college freshmen worry more about gaining weight—the "freshman 15"—than about how they'll manage their course load. The term *freshman 15* was coined to describe a gain in weight that some college students experience during their first year away from home. However, little data supports the theory. As with adults, freshman weight gain can be prevented by establishing healthy eating and exercise behaviors that lead to a healthy weight.

Behavior modification focuses on changing the eating behaviors that contribute to weight gain or impede weight loss. Several behavior modification techniques can be used to identify and improve eating behaviors. These techniques include self-monitoring by keeping a food log, controlling environmental cues that trigger eating when not hungry, and learning how to better manage stress.[88] Understanding the habits and emotions that drive your eating and exercise patterns is a key element of behavior modification. Once you have identified the less-than-healthy behaviors, you can replace them with new behaviors that promote weight loss and weight management.

A food log allows individuals to track the kinds of foods they eat during the day, when and where they eat them, their moods, and their hunger ratings. Based on this information, people can restructure their environment, how they respond to their environment, or both to improve the eating behaviors and manage their weight. A typical day's log may be similar to the one in **Figure 15.6**.

You might have habits that work against your desire to maintain a healthy weight. These include skipping breakfast, which causes people to be very hungry in the late morning and increases impulsive snacking on energy-dense, low-nutrition foods from vending machines. A study of overweight women who typically skipped breakfast showed that once

behavior modification Changing behaviors to improve health outcomes. In the case of weight management, it involves identifying and altering eating patterns that contribute to weight gain or impede weight loss.

Food Log

For: Hannah

Date: Monday, September 6

Food and drink	Time eaten	What I ate/ Where I ate it	Hunger level*	Mood †
Breakfast		Skipped it	3	G
Snack	11 a.m.	Oreo cookies, PowerAde from vending machine during morning class.	5	E
Lunch	1:30 p.m.	Ham and cheese sandwich, 2 large M&M cookies in student union cafeteria.	4	B
Snack				
Dinner	6:30 p.m.	Hamburger, french fries, salad at kitchen table	4	F
Snack	7 p.m. to 10 p.m.	Large bag of tortilla chips and entire bag of Pepperidge Farm Milano cookies while studying at kitchen table	1	I

*Hunger levels (1–5): 1 = not hungry; 5 = super hungry

† **Moods:**
A = Happy; B = Content; C = Bored; D = Depressed; E = Rushed; F = Stressed; G = Tired; H = Lonely; I = Anxious; J = Angry

◄ **Figure 15.6 Food Log**
Keeping track of when, where, and what you eat, as well as why you ate it, can yield some surprising information. Do you think you sometimes eat out of boredom or stress, rather than because you're hungry?

they started consuming cereal for breakfast, they indulged in less impulsive snacking.[89] Eating a bowl of high-fiber, whole-grain cereal with skim milk (approximately 200 kilocalories) can help you bypass an 11:00 A.M. vending machine snack of 270-kilocalorie cookies. This one behavior change would not only save you 70 kilocalories, but also reduce your intake of added sugars and boost your intake of essential nutrients and fiber. Additionally, adding a high-volume, low-energy salad to your sandwich at lunch could help increase your satiety and displace at least one of the energy-dense cookies that people often grab with a sandwich.

Stress-induced eating associated with studying can be modified by a change in environment—for example, by going to the campus library, where eating is prohibited. In fact, removing access to snacks altogether is an excellent environmental change—once snacks are "out of sight" they are more likely to be "out of mind." Exercising before or after studying would be a healthier way to relieve stress than eating a bag of chips. The nearby Table Tips list some additional healthy behaviors that can easily be incorporated into your life.

Based on the information presented in the Nutrition in Practice on page 562, what recommendations would you have for Adam in his quest to lose weight?

LO 15.5: THE TAKE-HOME MESSAGE For successful, long-term weight loss, people can reduce their daily kilocalorie intake, increase their physical activity, and improve their eating behaviors. Choosing low-energy-density, high-volume vegetables and fruits, along with lean-protein foods, can help increase satiety and reduce unplanned snacking. Incorporating approximately 60–90 minutes of physical activity daily can facilitate weight loss. Establishing healthy eating and exercise habits by restructuring the environment to minimize or eliminate unhealthy eating behaviors can also help shed extra pounds.

TABLE TIPS

Adopt Some Healthy Habits

Don't eat out of boredom or stress; go for a jog instead.

Food-shop with a full stomach and a grocery list. Walking around aimlessly while hungry means you are more likely to grab items on a whim.

The next time you pass a difficult course or get that long-awaited raise, celebrate without a plate. Replace the traditional restaurant dinner with a no-kilocalorie reward such as a new music download or a weekend hike.

Declare a vending machine–free day at least once a week, save money, and stop the impulsive snacking. On that day, pack two pieces of fruit as satisfying snacks.

NUTRITION *in* PRACTICE:
Sports Medicine Specialist and PT

Adam is a 40-year-old Fine Arts professor who has gained 20 pounds over the last year. He blames his weight gain on the nagging pain in his shoulder, which has caused him to drop out of the faculty tennis league. Adam used to play league tennis games three to four times a week and practice drills on the weekend. Unhappy with his excess weight, Adam decided to visit the campus health center. While he was at the center, he saw a flyer advertising the new Sports Medicine Clinic on campus, adjacent to the Health Center. Adam made an appointment with the sports medicine specialist, a physician who specializes in sports medicine, for the next day. The doctor diagnosed his shoulder soreness as impingement syndrome, which is pain sometimes experienced by tennis players when they lift and rotate their arm. The doctor referred Adam to the physical therapist (PT) at the clinic for guidance for an exercise program that would strengthen his shoulder muscles to ease the pain. To help him lose his excess weight, the doctor recommended that Adam visit with the registered dietitian nutritionist (RDN) at the clinic.

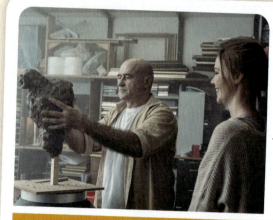

Adam

ADAM'S FOOD LOG

Food/Beverage	Time Consumed	Hunger Rating*	Location
Granola with whole milk, orange juice, coffee with cream	7:00 A.M.	3	Kitchen
Coffee with cream, donut	10:30 A.M.	2	Campus coffee shop
Ham and cheese sub	1:30 P.M.	5	Sub shop on campus
Cookies	4:00 P.M.	1	Vending machine in faculty lounge
Steak, rice, and corn	6:30 P.M.	3	Kitchen
Peanuts	9:00 P.M.	1	Watching TV

*Hunger Rating (1–5): 1 = not hungry; 5 = super hungry.

Adam's Stats
- Age: 40
- Height: 6 feet
- Weight: 210 pounds
- BMI: 28.5

Critical Thinking Questions
1. Based on Adam's food log, which waist-friendly food groups are missing from his diet?
2. Why do you think Adam is snacking between meals, even when he isn't very hungry?
3. What beverage recommendations would you make based on Adam's food log?

PT's Observation and Plan for Adam
- Explain that impingement syndrome occurs when the tissues in the shoulder are pitched or compressed due to poor mechanics.

- Provide Adam with a strengthening program for shoulder stabilizing muscles.

RDN's Observation and Plan for Adam
- Discuss the lack of adequate amounts of whole fruits and vegetables in his diet and the role these high-fiber, high-volume, lower-energy-dense foods play in weight reduction. Explain the concept that these foods displace other higher-kilocalorie foods in the diet and "fill you up before they fill you out."
- Discuss the issue of routinely snacking when not hungry. Consider alternatives to eating when bored.
- Replace the bowl of energy-dense granola cereal with lower-kilocalorie shredded wheat cereal with a sprinkling of granola as a topping.
- Substitute skim milk for whole milk on his cereal and the cream in his coffee.

- Decrease the size of the sandwich at lunch. Instead of a large sub, order a small sub and a side salad with light dressing.

Two weeks later, Adam returns for a follow-up visit with the RDN and PT. While he has only lost a pound, he is feeling better about this diet and the strengthening program that the PT designed for him, although his overhead tennis serve is still somewhat painful. He has added more fruits and vegetables to his diet and, surprisingly, doesn't feel hungry. The RDN works with Adam to choose leaner sources of protein at lunch and dinner. Adam agrees to try a smaller turkey sandwich at lunch and grilled salmon or chicken for dinner more often. He made another appointment to see the RDN in a month. The PT tweaks Adam's strengthening program and continues to work with him through the month.

How Can Weight Loss Be Maintained?

LO 15.6 Design a food and exercise plan to maintain a healthy weight.

Losing weight can be difficult, but not regaining the lost weight over time can be just as challenging. You or someone you know may be familiar with the typical weight-loss experience: the triumphant rush associated with dropping 10 pounds of weight, the disappointment that sets in when 15 pounds are regained, then a new round of hope when 10 of them are re-shed.

But don't be discouraged! Weight loss can be maintained when the right strategies are used. The National Weight Control Registry (NWCR) was developed to follow those individuals who have not only succeeded at weight loss but kept it off. In a recent study of 3,000 individuals who had lost at least 30 pounds, researchers reported that 87 percent of the subjects who lost at least 10 percent of their body weight had maintained the weight loss when measured at 5 and 10 years.[90] The researchers reported that low-fat diets, avoiding overeating, being physically active, and daily self-weighing were successful strategies in maintaining the subjects' weight loss.

Diet and Exercise Can Aid in Maintaining Weight Loss

Consuming a healthy diet is as essential to weight-loss maintenance as it was to the weight loss. Individuals who lose weight often experience an **energy gap**. After weight loss, a person will have lower overall energy needs, as there is less body weight to maintain. The energy gap is the difference in daily kilocalories that are needed for weight maintenance before and after weight loss.[91] Researchers have estimated that the energy gap is about 8 kilocalories per pound of lost weight.[92] For example, someone who lost 30 pounds would need approximately 240 fewer kilocalories a day to maintain the new, lower body weight.

One problem with maintaining weight loss is that once the weight has been lost, individuals revert to the unhealthy eating habits that caused the excess weight in the first place. To adapt your eating patterns to the new body weight, limit the intake of fatty foods, monitor your kilocalorie intake, and follow a pattern of eating three small meals and two snacks a day. For many people, eating more frequent, smaller meals allows them to avoid becoming ravenous and overeating at the next meal. If weight loss continues even though you've reached your goal weight, gradually add about 200 kilocalories of healthy, low-fat, high-fiber foods to your daily intake until weight balance is achieved.

Another way to close the energy gap and help the body adjust to its new lower weight is to increase exercise. Because the environment we live in seems to encourage eating more than discourage it, researchers believe that increasing daily physical activity is likely the easier way to close the energy gap.[93] *Adding* something (physical activity) to one's lifestyle is often easier than *removing* something (kilocalories). Thus, the recommendation is to engage in 60–90 minutes of moderate physical activity daily in order to maintain weight loss.[94]

energy gap Difference between the numbers of kilocalories needed to maintain weight before and after weight loss.

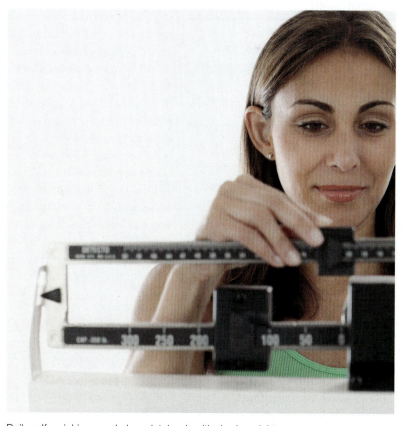

Daily self-weighing may help maintain a healthy body weight.

Self-Weighing Is a Positive Strategy to Maintain Weight Loss

Daily or weekly self-weighing has often been discouraged to prevent increasing the risk of disordered eating, negative body image, mood disorders, or binge eating. Recent research refutes these claims and reports that daily self-weighing improved body satisfaction[95] and helped maintain weight loss.[96]

> **LO 15.6: THE TAKE-HOME MESSAGE** People who lose weight are most likely to keep it off if they maintain the positive diet and lifestyle habits that helped them lose the weight. Exercise improves muscle mass, prevents a decline in basal metabolism, and helps overcome plateaus often associated with weight loss. Eating less and/or exercising more helps close the energy gap that occurs after weight loss.

What Is the Healthiest Way to Gain Weight?

LO 15.7 Describe the role of diet and exercise in achieving a healthy weight gain.

For people who are underweight, trying to gain weight can be as challenging and frustrating as trying to lose weight is for an overweight individual. The major difference is that the thin person rarely gets sympathy from others.

Like overweight individuals, those who are underweight experience an energy imbalance. In their case, however, they consume fewer kilocalories than they expend each day. Because those who wish to gain weight generally want to add muscle mass, rather than large amounts of fat, the challenge is to eat sufficient energy to meet their basal metabolic needs plus provide fuel for the exercise needed to stimulate muscle synthesis.

People who want to gain weight need to do the opposite of those who are trying to lose weight—they need to make each bite more energy dense. Adding at least 500 kilocalories to their daily energy intake will enable them to add about a pound of extra body weight weekly.

Of course, someone who wants to gain weight should not just load up on high-fat, high-kilocalorie foods. The quality of the extra kilocalories is very important. Snacking on an extra 500 kilocalories of jellybeans adds 500 kilocalories of sugar and little nutrient value. Instead, these individuals should make energy-dense, nutritious choices from a variety of foods within each food group. For example, instead of eating a slice of toast in the morning, they should choose a whole-grain waffle. In a salad bar lunch, adding coleslaw provides 10 times the kilocalories of plain cabbage. **Figure 15.7** contrasts more- and less-energy-dense foods within each food group. Eating larger portion sizes at meals and energy-dense snacks during the day also adds kilocalories. The Table Tips provide easy and portable snack ideas.

Regular exercise and resistance training stimulate muscle growth and help avoid excess fat storage. Remember that it takes time to gain weight and build sufficient muscle mass. Be patient and continue to choose healthy foods until you reach your goal weight.

> **LO 15.7: THE TAKE-HOME MESSAGE** People who want to gain weight need to consume additional kilocalories through energy-dense foods so that they take in more energy than they expend. Adding nutrient-dense snacks between meals and increasing portion sizes during meals are easy ways to increase the number of kilocalories consumed. Add resistance exercise to build muscle mass and avoid excess fat storage.

TABLE TIPS

Healthy Snacks for Healthy Weight Gain

Stash an 8-ounce container of 100 percent fruit juice (about 100 kilocalories) in your bag, plus one of the 150-kilocalorie snacks listed below for a quick 250-kilocalorie snack (food and juice combined) between meals.

Graham crackers, 5 crackers ($2\frac{1}{2}$″ square)

Mixed nuts, 1 oz

Fig bars, 2-oz package

Pudding, individual serving sizes, 4 oz

Peanut butter on whole-wheat crackers (1 Tbsp peanut butter on six crackers)

Kilocalories

Value	Food
161	Potato, 1 medium baked
237	Potatoes, mashed, 1 cup
55	Apple, 1 small
194	Applesauce, 1 cup
128	Whole-wheat flakes, 1 cup
464	Granola, 1 cup
138	Chicken breast, cooked, 1 oz
313	Chicken salad, homemade, 3/4 cup
102	Low-fat milk, 1 cup
158	Low-fat chocolate milk, 1 cup
154	Yogurt, low fat, plain, 1 cup
238	Yogurt, low fat, strawberry, 1 cup
49	Mayonnaise, light, 1 tbs
100	Mayonnaise, 1 tbs

Food groups: Vegetables, Fruits, Grains, Protein, Dairy, Oils

HEALTHCONNECTION

What Are the Medical Interventions for Severe Obesity?

LO 15.8 Describe the role of weight-loss drugs and surgery for reducing obesity.

For most people, the best path to a healthy body weight is to commit to improving their diet and exercising more. However, those who are severely obese are at such a high risk for conditions such as heart disease and stroke, and even of dying, that medications and/or surgery may be necessary.

Weight-Loss Medications May Improve Weight Loss but Have Side Effects

Some prescription medications can help a person lose weight by either suppressing hunger or inhibiting the absorption of fat in the GI tract. These drugs typically have potentially dangerous side effects; because of this, they are almost always available only by prescription and must be taken under the care of a health care provider.

One hunger suppressant is the drug sibutramine (trade name Meridia), which also increases thermogenesis and thereby increases energy expenditure. However, the drug can also increase a person's heart rate and blood pressure, and therefore may not be appropriate for those who have hypertension, which is common in obese individuals.

The fat-absorption-inhibitor orlistat (trade name Xenical) is a prescription medication that inhibits an intestinal enzyme needed to break down fat. If fat isn't broken down, the body doesn't absorb the fat (and kilocalories). In patients using orlistat, up to about a third of the dietary fat in a meal is blocked and expelled in the stool. Orlistat needs to be taken at each meal and should be used with a diet that provides no more than about 30 percent of its kilocalories from fat. Because fat is lost in the stool, the drug can cause oily and more frequent stools, flatulence, and oily discharge.[97] Ironically, these side effects may help an individual adhere to a low-fat diet, as these effects are more pronounced if a high-fat meal is consumed.

A reduced-strength version of orlistat (brand named Alli) is approved as an over-the-counter medication for overweight adults 18 years and older. Alli, combined with a low-kilocalorie, low-fat diet and regular exercise, aids in modest weight loss. Because of the recent reports of rare, but serious, cases of liver damage in individuals

using Xenical and Alli, both of these drugs must now carry warnings on their labels.[98]

The latest weight loss drug to be approved by the FDA is called liraglutide (trade name Saxenda). This injectable drug stimulates the release from the GI tract of GLP-1, a hormone that stimulates satiety and may therefore contribute to weight loss.[99] A 2017 study showed benefits of liraglutide using a randomized, double-blind study of 2,254 adults with prediabetes and a body mass index of at least 30 kg/m^2. Either liraglutide or a placebo was given over 3 years. The results showed that after 3 years, subjects receiving liraglutide lost more weight and improved glucose control compared to the placebo group.[100] Unfortunately, this drug may cause serious side effects, including severely low blood glucose leading to extreme weakness, confusion, tremors, fast heart rate, trouble speaking, nausea and vomiting, rapid breathing, fainting, and seizures.[101]

The side effects of certain weight-loss supplements are so serious that the FDA has required the supplement be withdrawn from the market. For instance, the FDA has prohibited the sale of supplements that contain ephedra (also called *Ma huang*), the plant source for ephedrine. Ephedrine has

been shown to cause chest pains, palpitations, hypertension, and an accelerated heart rate and has been linked to numerous deaths.[102]

Bariatric Surgery Restricts Food Intake

Bariatric surgery has been shown to be an effective means of weight loss for moderately to severely obese people compared with low-kilocalorie diets and medication.[103] A variety of bariatric surgery procedures either reduce the absorption of food or restrict food intake.

The most common form of bariatric surgery is **gastric bypass surgery**. This surgical technique was developed in the middle of the twentieth century and quickly grew in popularity. The first gastric bypass surgery was performed in 1967 by Dr. Edward Mason, a surgeon at the University of Iowa.[104] By 1998, approximately 13,000 obese patients each year underwent gastric bypass. Ten years later that number had increased to over 190,000.[105] During gastric bypass surgery, the stomach is reduced in size by making a small pouch at the top of the stomach with surgical staples (**Figure 15.8**). The pouch is

Alli promotes weight loss by reducing the digestion and absorption of fat.

bariatric surgery Surgical procedure that promotes weight loss by limiting the amount of food that can be eaten or absorbed.

gastric bypass surgery Type of bariatric surgery that reduces the functional volume of the stomach to minimize the amount of food eaten. Such surgeries are sometimes used to treat extreme obesity.

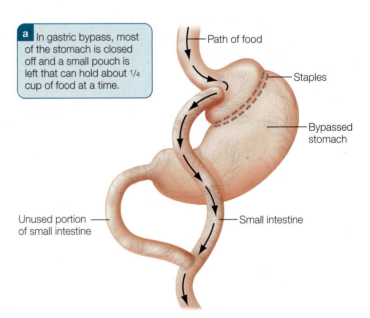

a In gastric bypass, most of the stomach is closed off and a small pouch is left that can hold about 1/4 cup of food at a time.

Path of food — Staples — Bypassed stomach — Small intestine — Unused portion of small intestine

▲ **Figure 15.8 Gastric Bypass Surgery**
In gastric bypass surgery, much of the stomach is closed off and a small pouch is left that can hold about $1/4$ cup of food at a time. The pouch is reattached to the jejunum, bypassing the duodenum.

then connected to the jejunum, bypassing the rest of the stomach and the duodenum (the upper small intestine). This reduces the size of the stomach so that it holds less than $\frac{1}{4}$ cup of food and also reduces the small intestine's ability to absorb food. After the surgery, individuals need to consume frequent, small meals because the stomach pouch can only expand to a maximum of about 5 ounces, the size of a woman's fist. Bypass patients not only eat less because of their smaller stomachs, but also have higher levels of satiety and lower levels of hunger after the surgery. This loss of appetite is thought to be due to lower levels of ghrelin associated with the loss of stomach area.[106]

Because food is rerouted past the majority of the stomach and the duodenum, individuals can experience deficiencies of vitamin B_{12}, iron, and calcium. Recall from Chapter 10 that vitamin B_{12} needs to be separated from the protein in food before it can be absorbed. Also, intrinsic factor (IF) secreted from the gastric cells is needed for vitamin B_{12} to be absorbed. Levels of IF are significantly reduced after surgery. To be absorbed, iron must be converted from ferric iron to ferrous iron by hydrochloric acid secreted in the stomach. Bariatric surgery reduces the amount of hydrochloric acid

released, which results in less iron available for absorption. Iron and calcium are also typically absorbed in the upper part of the small intestine, which is now bypassed.

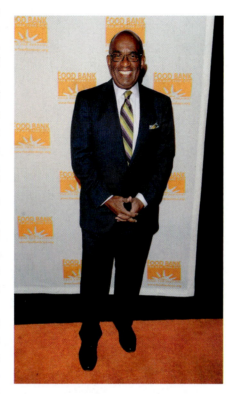

Al Roker, a weatherman on NBC's *Today Show*, lost approximately 140 pounds after gastric bypass surgery.

Vitamin B_{12} injections or supplements as well as calcium and iron supplements, plus vitamin C, are prescribed to help maintain a healthy balance.

Although weight loss varies from one individual to the next, the average weight loss with gastric bypass surgery is approximately 5–15 pounds per week for the first 2 or 3 months.[107] The weight loss gradually tapers off to about 1–2 pounds per week after the first 6 months. Other benefits of gastric bypass include a reduction in diabetes in 76.8 percent of patients, improved lipid profiles in more than 70 percent of patients, and the elimination of hypertension (in 61.7 percent) and sleep apnea (in 85.7 percent).[108]

Although dramatic amounts of weight loss can occur with gastric bypass, there are also risks involved. About 10 percent of those undergoing gastric bypass surgery experience complications such as gallstones, ulcers, and bleeding in the stomach and intestines. Approximately 1–2 percent die from complications relating to the surgery.[109] After surgery, individuals need to be monitored long term by their physician and nutrition professionals to ensure that they remain healthy and meet their nutritional needs.

LO 15.8: THE TAKE-HOME MESSAGE

Pharmacological or surgical weight loss approaches may be necessary for obese individuals. The current weight-loss drugs suppress appetite, reduce fat absorption, or increase satiety; however, they have serious side effects. Gastric bypass surgery is the most common form of bariatric (weight-loss) surgery. It reduces the size of the stomach and bypasses the duodenum, thereby restricting both food intake and absorption of food. Patients typically experience not only weight loss, but reduction in chronic disease risks.

Visual Chapter Summary

LO 15.1 Weight Management Is Important for Physical and Emotional Well-Being

Weight management means maintaining a healthy weight to reduce the risk of specific health problems. Classifying obesity as a disease may improve treatment options but may also raise health care costs, increase drug and surgical procedures, and reduce emphasis on lifestyle changes to lose weight. Physical problems associated with obesity include an increased risk for cardiovascular disease, type 2 diabetes, certain cancers, and many other disorders. Both obesity and underweight significantly increase the risk of premature death. Social and psychological misperceptions and prejudices toward people who are obese or underweight may contribute to discrimination, low self-esteem, depression, suicide, and alcohol and drug problems.

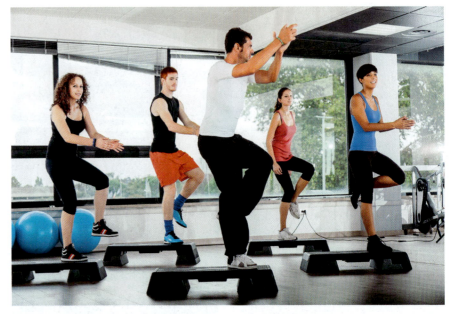

LO 15.2 Food Intake Is Regulated by the Hypothalamus

Food intake is regulated by the physiological responses known as hunger and satiety. Hunger prompts the body to eat and subsides soon after eating begins. Satiety determines the length of time between meals or snacks. Appetite is psychological, not physiological, and can be affected by the sight, smell, taste, and thought of food, as well as emotions, environment, and social settings.

Hunger is controlled by the lateral hypothalamus and satiety is controlled by the ventromedial nucleus of the hypothalamus. Both areas of the brain respond to hormonal and neural signals from the GI tract. Certain hormones, including neuropeptide Y from the hypothalamus and ghrelin from the stomach, stimulate hunger. Other hormones, including cholecystokinin and peptide YY from the small intestine, insulin from the pancreas, and leptin from adipose tissue, increase satiety.

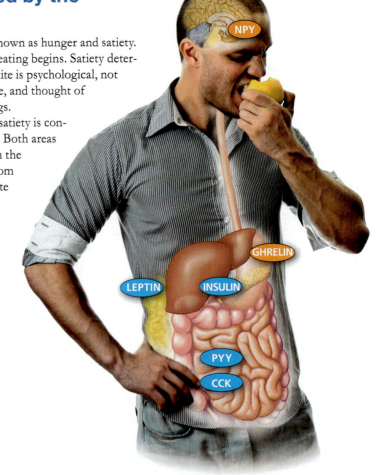

LO 15.3 Fat Cells Form, Expand, and Shrink

Fat cells can increase in size to store additional fat (hypertrophy) and new fat cells can be produced (hyperplasia) to replace old cells and to create additional cells once existing ones fill to capacity. During weight loss, fat cells shrink but are not destroyed.

The enzyme lipoprotein lipase (LPL) stimulates lipogenesis and the enzyme hormone-sensitive lipase stimulates lipolysis. LPL activity is greater in obese individuals; in males, LPL is more active in the abdominal fat cells than in females, but females have higher LPL activity rates in the hips and thighs.

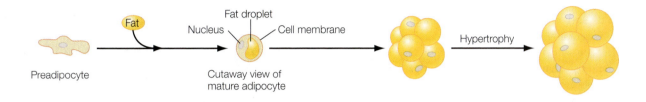

Preadipocyte → Fat → Nucleus / Fat droplet / Cell membrane — Cutaway view of mature adipocyte → Hypertrophy

LO 15.4 Genetics and Environment Both Influence Body Weight

Obesity is explained as a gene–environment interaction in which genetically prone individuals have easy access to a variety of large portions of food and an environment that encourages a sedentary lifestyle. Nutrigenomics has identified specific genes that influence how we absorb, store, or break down foods. Epigenetic factors, including components of the foods we eat, can turn gene expression on or off, thereby influencing many physiological factors that affect body weight. Single-nucleotide polymorphisms result in variant genes, some of which influence the secretion of hormones such as ghrelin and leptin that affect hunger and satiety. Populations with "thrifty genes" may experience increased fat storage and reduced energy expenditure as compared to other populations. Environmental factors such as lack of time, an abundant food supply and portion distortion, and lack of physical activity due to the advances in technology increase the risk of obesity.

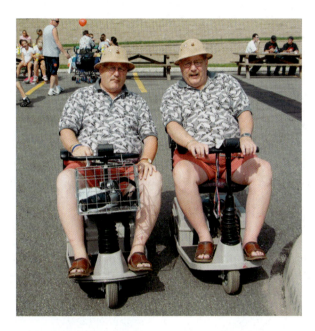

LO 15.5 Losing Weight Healthfully Involves Eating Less and Exercising More

A healthy, reasonable rate of weight loss is losing 10 percent of body weight over a 6-month period. Losing weight rapidly can cause a person to fall short of meeting nutrient needs. Many fad diets promise quick results but can be unhealthy for the long term.

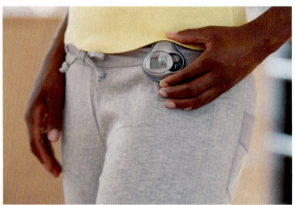

Expending more kilocalories than consumed is the key to weight loss. Eating more low-energy-density, high-volume (high in water and fiber) foods, such as vegetables and fruits, improves satiation, which results in fewer kilocalories consumed. Protein has the most dramatic effect on satiety. Eating high-protein foods such as lean meats, chicken, and fish at meals can help reduce hunger between meals. Because fat slows the movement of food out of the stomach into the intestines, it can also prolong satiety.

Routine physical activity and exercise can add to the daily energy deficit needed for weight loss. To support weight loss, overweight individuals should engage in 60–90 minutes of moderate-intensity exercise daily.

Individuals who wish to lose weight must change the eating behaviors that contributed to weight gain or impeded weight loss. Keeping a food record, controlling environmental cues that trigger eating when not hungry, and learning how to better manage stress are all behavior modification techniques that can be used by individuals who eat "out of habit" and in response to their environment.

LO 15.6 Behavior Modification Helps Maintain a Healthy Weight

To maintain weight loss, individuals must modify their food intake to reflect their smaller body's reduced energy requirements. After weight loss, there is an energy gap between the original body weight and the new healthy weight, which may be as high as 8 kilocalories per pound of lost body weight. The energy gap can also be reduced with an increase in exercise of about 60–90 minutes per day. Self-weighing each day can improve body satisfaction and help maintain weight loss.

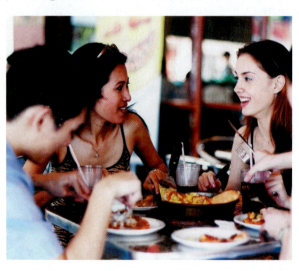

LO 15.7 Increase Kilocalories and Exercise to Gain Weight Healthfully

Individuals who wish to gain weight must increase kilocalorie intake and engage in strength training to build muscle mass. Consuming larger portions of nutrient-dense foods at mealtimes and snacking on nutritious foods between meals can help with weight gain.

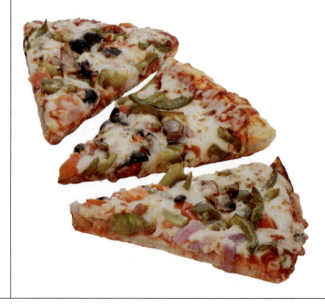

LO 15.8 Medications or Surgery May Be Necessary to Treat Severe Obesity

For severely obese individuals who have tried diet and exercise and failed to achieve a healthy body weight, pharmacological or surgical treatments may be necessary. The current weight-loss drugs approved by the FDA suppress appetite, reduce fat absorption, or increase satiety. However, they have serious side effects and their use must be monitored by the patient's physician. Bariatric (weight-loss) surgery reduces the consumption and absorption of food. Gastric bypass surgery, the most common procedure, involves reducing the size of the stomach to a small pouch and connecting it to the jejunum, in order to bypass the duodenum. Gastric bypass is effective in helping patients lose significant body weight and reduce their risk for chronic disease.

Gastric bypass

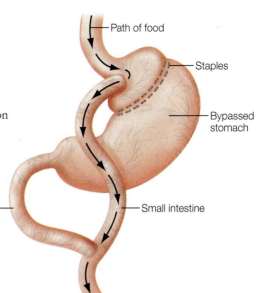

- Path of food
- Staples
- Bypassed stomach
- Unused portion of small intestine
- Small intestine

Terms to Know

- weight management
- appetite
- hunger
- satiation
- satiety
- hypertrophy
- hyperplasia
- gene–environment interaction
- adiponectin
- set point
- fad diet
- behavior modification
- energy gap
- bariatric surgery
- gastric bypass surgery

 Mastering Nutrition
Visit the Study Area in Mastering Nutrition to hear an MP3 chapter summary.

Check Your Understanding

LO 15.1 1. A healthy body weight can be defined as a body weight that
   a. does not increase the risk of developing weight-related health problems or diseases
   b. enhances an individual's physical attributes
   c. is generally acceptable in society
   d. is the easiest to maintain by all individuals of a given height and age

LO 15.2 2. Which region of the brain responds to hormones by stimulating satiety?
   a. Lateral hypothalamus
   b. Ventromedial nucleus
   c. Hippocampus
   d. Pineal gland

LO 15.3 3. When an individual loses body fat
   a. there is a decrease in the number of adipocytes due to hyperplasia.
   b. there is a decrease in the size of the fat cells due to hypertrophy.
   c. subcutaneous fat, not visceral fat, is lost.
   d. the adipocytes shrink but their number stays the same.

LO 15.4 4. Which of the following is a factor that increases the risk of obesity?
   a. Increased time
   b. Increased physical activity
   c. Low consumption of fruits and vegetables.
   d. Small portion sizes

LO 15.5 5. Which of the following can increase the risk of becoming obese?
   a. Having a parent who is obese
   b. Consuming more meals at home than dining out
   c. Reducing the amounts of "screen time" during the day
   d. Decreasing the size of your food portions at meals

LO 15.5 6. What is the best dietary approach to losing weight?
a. Eliminate all sweets from the diet
b. Reduce kilocalorie intake by reducing portion sizes
c. Consume foods high in carbohydrate to stimulate satiety
d. Limit fat intake to less than 5 grams per day

LO 15.6 7. Mary Ellen was obese and lost 30 pounds during the last year by eating a well-balanced, kilocalorie-reduced diet and being physically active daily. To maintain her weight loss, she should continue to eat a healthy diet, monitor her eating behaviors, and
a. accumulate 30 minutes of physical activity three times a week.
b. accumulate 45 minutes of physical activity three times a week.
c. accumulate at least 60 minutes of physical activity daily.
d. accumulate more than 2 hours of physical activity daily.

LO 15.7 8. After recovering from a lengthy illness, Simon has been trying to regain the weight he lost while he was sick. It seems easy enough to load up on doughnuts and French fries, but Simon would prefer to return to his normal weight in a healthy way. Which of the following strategies would help Simon reach his goal?
a. Decreasing his portions at meals
b. Eliminating all exercise
c. Eating salads without salad dressing
d. Drinking 100% fruit juice with a nutrient-dense snack between meals

LO 15.8 9. Which of the following weight-loss medications may stimulate thermogenesis?
a. Meridia
b. Xenical
c. Alli
d. Saxenda

LO 15.8 10. Which of the following occurs in the majority of patients who undergo gastric bypass surgery?
a. Iron toxicity
b. Gallstones
c. Elimination of hypertension
d. All of these are correct.

Answers

1. (a) A healthy body weight can be defined as a body weight that does not increase the risk of developing weight-related health problems or diseases.

2. (b) The ventromedial nucleus responds to certain hormonal signals by inducing satiety. The lateral hypothalamus controls hunger, the hippocampus is a structure involved in memory consolidation, and the pituitary gland, located beneath the hypothalamus, secretes many hormones important to homeostasis; it is not technically part of the brain.

3. (d) When the body loses fat, adipocytes shrink in size, but their number remains constant. Adipocytes are the specialized cells that make up all adipose tissue, including both subcutaneous and visceral fat. Hyperplasia is an increase, not a decrease, in number of cells, and hypertrophy is an increase, not a decrease, in cell size.

4. (a) Low consumption of fruits and vegetables increases the risk of becoming obese. Having more time, increasing physical activity, and eating smaller portions will all decrease your risk of obesity.

5. (a) Having a parent who is obese increases the probability that you have a genetic predisposition to obesity. Increasing your regular physical activity by reducing screen time, eating more meals at home, and reducing food portions are methods that reduce your risk.

6. (b) The best healthy dietary approach to losing weight is to reduce kilocalorie intake by eating smaller portion sizes. Eliminating all sweets would be unnecessarily restrictive, as would reducing fat intake to less than 5 grams per day, which would also be unhealthful. Foods high in

carbohydrate are less satiating than foods high in protein and fat.

7. (c) If Mary Ellen wants to continue to maintain the weight she has lost, she should try to accumulate 60–90 minutes of exercise daily.

8. (d) To gain weight, Simon should drink 100% fruit juice with a nutrient-dense snack, such as nuts, between meals. Decreasing his portions at meals and eating salads without salad dressing would cause him to lose more weight rather than gain weight. Eliminating all exercise is unhealthful.

9. (a) Meridia (or sibutramine) increases thermogenesis and energy expenditure. Xenical, also known as orlistat, and Alli, the less potent over-the-counter weight-loss medication, inhibit fat absorption. Liraglutide, sold as Saxenda, increases satiety.

10. (c) The majority of people who undergo gastric bypass surgery experience an elimination of hypertension. A minority of patients experience gallstones. Iron deficiency, not toxicity, is a concern following gastric bypass surgery.

Answers to True or False?

1. **False.** While the recommendation for weight loss is to accumulate at least 60–90 minutes of daily physical activity, the bottom line is that for weight loss to occur, more energy must be expended than is consumed. This can be accomplished by consuming less, exercising more, or a combination of both.

2. **False.** While the overall number of fat cells generally doesn't increase in adulthood, fat cell synthesis continues to replace old cells. Ten percent of fat cells are replaced with new cells every 10 years.

3. **False.** Grazing is considered a high-risk behavior for weight management because the foods that are typically chosen are low in protein and not satiating. Individuals may also consume higher amounts of kilocalories by eating mindlessly rather than consuming planned, smaller meals.

4. **True.** Weight loss of as little as 10 pounds can improve health if an individual is overweight.

5. **True.** Nature and nurture both play a role in regulating body weight. Nature (genes) often sets the stage, while nurture (environment and personal behavior) directly affects weight management.

6. **True.** Increasing the volume of food and the fiber content of meals by eating more vegetables and fruits can improve appetite control, reducing kilocalorie intake and thus helping attain weight loss.

7. **True.** At its most basic, weight gain occurs because of a positive energy balance. However, genetics and the environment play strong roles.

8. **False.** Of all the nutrients, protein has the most powerful effect on satiety.

9. **False.** Most weight-loss supplement labels indicate that you need to eat a healthy diet and exercise regularly if you want to shed the pounds.

10. **False.** Bariatric surgery alters the gastrointestinal tract and requires permanent changes to eating habits.

Web Resources

- For more on overweight and obesity, visit the Centers for Disease Control and Prevention at www.cdc.gov/nccd-php/dnpa/obesity/index.htm
- For more information on weight control and physical activity, visit the Weight-control Information Network (WIN) at http://win.niddk.nih.gov/index.htm
- For more weight-loss shopping tips, recipes, and menu makeovers, visit the USDA's Nutrition and Weight Management website at www.nutrition.gov
- For more information on gastric bypass surgery, visit the American Society for Metabolic and Bariatric Surgery at www.asbs.org

References

1. Weight Control and Information Network. 2014. *Overweight and Obesity Statistics*. Available at http://win.niddk.nih.gov/statistics/. Accessed April 2017.
2. Ibid.
3. Li, J. S., T. A. Barnett, E. Goodman, R. C. Wasserman, and A. R. Kemper. 2012. Approaches to the Prevention and Management of Childhood Obesity: The Role of Social Networks and the Use of Social Media and Related Electronic Technologies: A Scientific Statement from the American Heart Association. *Circulation.* doi: 10.1161/CIR.0b013e3182756d8e.
4. Williams, J. 2013. *The Heavy Price of Losing Weight.* Available at www.money.usnews.com. Accessed April 2017.
5. Center for Disease Control and Prevention. 2016. Community-Based Interventions to Decrease Obesity and Tobacco Exposure and Reduce Health Care Costs: Outcome Estimates From Communities Putting Prevention to Work for 2010–2020. Available at https://www.cdc.gov. Accessed April 2017.
6. Conover, Chris. 2013. *Declaring Obesity a Disease: The Good, the Bad, the Ugly.* Available at www.forbes.com/sites/theapothecary/2013/06/28/declaring-obesity-a-disease-the-good-the-bad-the-ugly. Accessed April 2017.
7. Weight-Control Information Network. 2013. *Do You Know the Health Risks of Being Overweight?* Available at http://win.niddk.nih.gov/publications/health_risks.htm. Accessed April 2017.
8. The Global Burden of Metabolic Risk Factors for Chronic Diseases Collaboration (BMI Mediated Effects). 2014. Metabolic Mediators of the Effects of Body-Mass Index, Overweight, and Obesity on Coronary Heart Disease and Stroke: A Pooled Analysis of 97 Prospective Cohorts with 1·8 Million Participants. *Lancet* 383(9921):970–983. doi: 10.1016/S0140-6736(13)61836-X.
9. Ibid.
10. Ibid.
11. Chao, A.M., et al. 2017. Binge Eating and Weight Loss Outcomes in Individuals with Type 2 Diabetes: 4-Year Results from the Look AHEAD Study. 25(11):1830-1837. doi: 10.1002/oby.21975.
12. Paniagua, J. A. 2016. Nutrition, insulin resistance and dysfunctional adipose tissue determine the different components of metabolic syndrome. *World Journal of Diabetes* 7(19):483–514. doi: 10.4239/wjd.v7.i19.483.
13. Bialo, S. R., and C. M. Gordon. 2014. Underweight, Overweight, and Pediatric Bone Fragility: Impact and Management. *Current Osteoporosis Reports.* doi: 10.1007/s11914-014-0226-z.
14. Jackson, S. E., et al. 2015. Obesity, Perceived Weight Discrimination, and Psychological Well-Being in Older Adults in England. *Journal of Obesity* 23(5):1105–11.
15. Richards, E. 2013. College Admissions Bias Reflects Cultural Sterotypes. Available at www.examiner.com/article/college-admissionsbias-reflects-cultural-stereotypes. Accessed April 2017.
16. U. S. News Report and Travel. 2014. Who Is Too Fat to Fly? Airlines Are Working It Out. Available at www.huffingtonpost.com/usnews-travel/too-fat-to-fly_b_2101347.html. Accessed April 2017..
17. Khan, S. S., M. Tarrant, D. Weston, P. Shah, and C. Farrow. 2017. Can Raising Awareness about the Psychological Causes of Obesity Reduce Obesity Stigma? *Health Communications* 19:1–8. doi: 10.1080/10410236.2017.1283566.
18. Adachi-Mejia, A. M., C. Lee, H. A. Carlos, B. E. Saelens, E. M. Berke, and M. P. Doescher. 2017. Geographic Variation in the Relationship Between Body Mass Index and the Built Environment. pii: S0091-7435(17)30116-0. doi:10.1016/j.ypmed.2017.03.018.
19. Hemmingsson, E. 2014. A New Model of the Role of Psychological and Emotional Distress in Promoting Obesity: Conceptual Review with Implications for Treatment and Prevention. *Obesity Review.* doi: 10.1111/obr.12197.
20. Henriksen, C. A., A. A. Mather, C. S. Mackenzie, O. J. Bienvenu, and J. Sareen. 2014. Longitudinal Associations of Obesity with Affective Disorders and Suicidality in the Baltimore Epidemiologic Catchment Area Follow-Up Study. *Journal of Nervous and Mental Disease* 202(5):379–385..
21. Field, A. E., K. R. Sonneville, R. D. Crosby, et al. 2014. Prospective Associations of Concerns about Physique and the Development of Obesity, Binge Drinking, and Drug Use among Adolescent Boys and Young Adult Men. *JAMA Pediatrics* 168(1):34–39.
22. Calugi, S., M. El Ghoch, M. Conti, and R. Dalle Grave. 2014. Depression and Treatment Outcome in Anorexia Nervosa. *Psychiatry Research* 218(1–2):195–200.
23. Gao, S., J. Juhaeri, S. Reshef, and W. S. Dai. 2013. Association between Body Mass Index and Suicide, and Suicide Attempt among British Adults: The Health Improvement Network Database. *Obesity* 21(3):E334–E342.
24. Ibid.
25. Crespo, C. S., A. P. Cachero, L. P. Jiménez, V. Barrios, and E. A. Ferreiro. 2014. Peptides and Food Intake. *Frontiers in Endocrinology.* doi: 10.3389/fendo.2014.00058.
26. Wauman, J., L. Zabeau, and J. Tavernier. 2017. The Leptin Receptor Complex: Heavier Than Expected? *Frontiers in Endocrinology* 8:30. doi: 10.3389/fendo.2017.00030
27. Leidy, H. J. 2014. Increased Dietary Protein as a Dietary Strategy to Prevent and/or Treat Obesity. *Missouri Medicine* 111(1):54–58.
28. Pradhan, G., S. L. Samson, and Y. Sun. 2013. Ghrelin: Much More Than a Hunger Hormone. *Current Opinion in Clinical Nutrition and Metabolic Care* 16(6):619–624.
29. Ibid.
30. Garcia, O. P., D. Ronquillo, M. del Carmen, M. Camacho, K. Z. Long, and J. L. Rosado. 2012. Zinc, Vitamin A, and Vitamin C Status Are Associated with Leptin Concentrations and Obesity in Mexican Women: Results from a Cross-Sectional Study. *Nutrition and Metabolism* 9:59–79.
31. Ibid.
32. Arner, P., S. Bernard, M. Salehpour, et al. 2011. Dynamics of human adipose lipid turnover in health and metabolic disease. *Nature* 478(7367):110–113. doi: 10.1038/nature10426.

33. Ibid.
34. English, J. 2013. *Reversing Altered Metabolic Functions to Enhance Long-Term Weight Control.* Available at http://nutritionreview.org/2013/04/reversing-altered-metabolic-functions-enhance-longterm-weight-control. Accessed April 2017.
35. Lundsgaard, A. M., & B. Kiens. 2014. Gender Differences in Skeletal Muscle Substrate Metabolism – Molecular Mechanisms and Insulin Sensitivity. *Frontiers in Endocrinology* 5:195. doi: 10.3389/fendo.2014.00195.
36. Nead, K. T., A. Li, M. R. Wehner, et al. 2015. Contribution of Common Non-Synonymous Variants in *PCSK1* to Body Mass Index Variation and Risk of Obesity: A Systematic Review and Meta-Analysis with Evidence from up to 331,175 Individuals. *Human Molecular Genetics* 24(12):3582–3594. doi: 10.1093/hmg/ddv097.
37. Youngson, N. A., and M. J. Morris. 2013. What Obesity Research Tells Us about Epigenetic Mechanisms. *Philosophical Transactions of the Royal Society B.* Available at http://dx.doi.org/10.1098/rstb.2011.0337.
38. Kaur, Y., R. J. de Souza, W. T. Gibson, and D. Meyre. 2017. A Systematic Review of Genetic Syndromes with Obesity. *Obesity Review.* doi: 10.1111/obr.12531.
39. Corella, D., and J. M. Ordovás. 2013. Can Genotype Be Used to Tailor Treatment for Obesity? State of the Art and Guidelines for Future Studies and Applications. *Minerva Endocrinologica* 38(3):219–235.
40. Centers for Disease Control and Prevention. 2013. *Public Health Genomics: Genes and Obesity.* Available at www.cdc.gov/genomics/resources/diseases/obesity/obesedit.htm. Accessed April 2017.
41. Polsky, S., V. A. Catenacci, H. R. Wyatt, and J. O. Hill. 2014. Obesity: Epidemiology, Etiology, and Prevention. In Ross, C. A., et al., eds. *Modern Nutrition in Health and Disease.* 11th ed. Philadelphia: Lippincott Williams & Wilkins.
42. Fallah-Fini, S., H. Rahmandad, T. Huang, R. M. Bures, and T. A. Glass. 2014. Modeling US Adult Obesity Trends: A System Dynamics Model for Estimating Energy Imbalance Gap. *American Journal of Public Health* 104(7):1230–1239. doi: 10.2105/AJPH.2014.301882
43. Brodsky, I. 2014. Hormones and Growth Factors. In Ross, C. A., et al., eds. *Modern Nutrition in Health and Disease.* 11th ed. Philadelphia: Lippincott Williams & Wilkins.
44. Yu, N., Ruan, Y., Gao, X., and Sun, J. 2017. Systematic Review and Meta-Analysis of Randomized, Controlled Trials on the Effect of Exercise on Serum Leptin and Adiponectin in Overweight and Obese Individuals. *Hormone and Metabolism Research* 49(3):164–173. doi: 10.1055/s-0042-121605.
45. Polsky, et al. 2014. Obesity: Epidemiology, Etiology, and Prevention.
46. Ibid.
47. Sifferlin, A. 2013. *New Genes ID'd in Obesity: How Much of Weight Is Genetic?* Available at http://healthland.time.com/2013/07/19/news-genes-idd-in-obesity-how-much-of-weight-is-genetic/. Accessed April 2017.
48. Urquidez-Romero, R., J. Esparaza-Romero, L. S. Chaudhari, et al. 2014. Study Design of the Maycoba Project: Obesity and Diabetes in Mexican Pimas. *American Journal of Health Behaviors* 38(3):370–378.
49. Esparza-Romero, J., Valencia, M. E., Urquidez-Romero, R., Chaudhari, L. S., Hanson, R. L., Knowler, W. C., . . . Schulz, L. O. 2015. Environmentally Driven Increases in Type 2 Diabetes and Obesity in Pima Indians and Non-Pimas in Mexico Over a 15-Year Period: The Maycoba Project. *Diabetes Care* 38(11):2075–2082. doi: 10.2337/dc15-0089.
50. Carr, K. A., H. Lin, K. D. Fletcher, et al. 2013. Two Functional Serotonin Polymorphisms Moderate the Effect of Food Reinforcement on BMI. *Behavioral Neuroscience* 127(3):387–399.
51. Fuglestad, P. T., R. W. Jeffery, and N. E. Sherwood. 2012. Lifestyle Patterns Associated with Diet, Physical Activity, Body Mass Index and Amount of Recent Weight Loss in a Sample of Successful Weight Losers. *International Journal of Behavioral Nutrition and Physical Activity.* doi: 10.1186/1479-5868-9-79.
52. Ibid.
53. Saguy, et al. 2014. Reporting Risk, Producing Prejudice.
54. Fuglestad, et al. 2012. Lifestyle Patterns Associated with Diet, Physical Activity, Body Mass Index and Amount of Recent Weight Loss.
55. Wenwen, D., S. Chang, W. Huijun, W. Zhihong, W. Youfa, and Z. Bing. 2014. Is Density of Neighborhood Restaurants Associated with BMI in Rural Chinese Adults? A Longitudinal Study from the China Health and Nutrition Survey. *BMJ Open.* doi: 10.1136/bmjopen-2013.
56. Todd, J., and R. M. Morrison. 2014. *Less Eating Out, Improved Diets, and More Family Meals in the Wake of the Great Recession.* Available at www.ers.usda.gov. Accessed April 2017.
57. Ibid.
58. Larson, N., D. Neumark-Sztainer, M. N. Laska, and M. Story. 2011. Young Adults and Eating Away from Home: Associations with Dietary Intake Patterns and Weight Status Differ by Choice of Restaurant. *Journal of the American Dietetic Association* 111: 1696–1703.
59. DeCosta, P., Møller, P., Frøst, M. B., and Olsen, A. 2017. Changing Children's Eating Behaviour-A Review of Experimental Research. *Appetite* 113:327–357. doi: 10.1016/j.appet.2017.03.004.
60. Spence, C., Okajima, K., Cheok, A.D., Petit, O., and Michel, C. 2016. Eating with Our Eyes: From Visual Hunger to Digital Satiation. *Brain Cognition* 110:53–63. doi: 10.1016/j.bandc.2015.08.006.
61. Rolls, B. 2003. The Supersizing of America. *Nutrition Today* 38:42–53.
62. Wansink, B. 1996. Can Package Size Accelerate Usage Volume? *Journal of Marketing* 60:1–14.
63. Zuraikat, F. M., Roe, L. S., Privitera, G. J., & Rolls, B. J. 2016. Increasing the Size of Portion Options Affects Intake But Not Portion Selection at a Meal. *Appetite, 98,* 95–100. doi: 10.1016/j.appet.2015.12.023.
64. Ashton, L. M., Hutchesson, M. J., Rollo, M. E., Morgan, P. J., Thompson, D. I., & Collins, C. E. 2015. Young Adult Males' Motivators and Perceived Barriers Towards Eating Healthily and Being Active: A Qualitative Study. *International Journal of Behavioral Nutrition and Physical Activity, 12,* 93. doi: 10.1186/s12966-015-0257-6.
65. Ibid.
66. Gupta, N., Hallman, D. M., Mathiassen, S. E., Aadahl, M., Jørgensen, M. B., & Holtermann, A. 2016. Are Temporal Patterns of Sitting Associated with Obesity among Blue-Collar Workers?: A Cross Sectional Study Using Accelerometers. *BMC Public Health* 16:148. doi: 10.1186/s12889-016-2803-9.
67. Mackenbach, J. D., Rutter, H., Compernolle, S., Glonti, K., Oppert, J.-M., Charreire, H., . . . Lakerveld, J. 2014. Obesogenic Environments: A Systematic Review of the Association between the Physical Environment and Adult Weight Status, the SPOTLIGHT Project. *BMC Public Health* 14:233. doi: 10.1186/1471-2458-14-233.
68. Berrigan, D., Tatalovich, Z., Pickle, L. W., Ewing, R., & Ballard-Barbash, R. 2014. Urban Sprawl, Obesity, and Cancer Mortality in the United States: Cross-Sectional Analysis and Methodological Challenges. *International Journal of Health Geographics* 13:3. doi: 10.1186/1476-072X-13-3.
69. Larouche, R., J. Barnes, and M. S. Tremblay. 2013. Too Far to Walk or Bike? *Canadian Journal of Public Health* 104(7):e487–e489.
70. Berrigan, D., Tatalovich, Z., Pickle, L. W., Ewing, R., & Ballard-Barbash, R. 2014. Urban Sprawl, Obesity, and Cancer Mortality in the United States.
71. Chang, P.-J., Wray, L., & Lin, Y. 2014. Social Relationships, Leisure Activity, and Health in Older Adults. *Health Psychology: Official Journal of the Division of Health Psychology, American Psychological Association* 33(6), 516–523. doi: 10.1037/hea0000051.
72. Colley, R. C., D. Garriguet, K. B. Adamo, V. Carson, I. Janssen, B. W. Timons, and M. S. Tremblay. 2013. *Physical Activity and Sedentary Behavior during the Early Years in Canada: A Cross-Sectional Study.* Available at www.ijbnpa.org/content/pdf/1479-5868-10-54.pdf. Accessed July 2014.
73. National Institutes of Health. 2014. *Clinical Guidelines on the Identification, Evaluation, and Treatment of Overweight and Obesity in Adults.* Available at http://www.medstarfamily-choice.com/documents/guidelines/obesity.pdf. Accessed April 2017.
74. Salley, J. N., Hoover, A. W., Wilson, M. L., and Muth, E. R. 2016. Comparison between Human and Bite-Based Methods of Estimating Calorie Intake. *Journal of the Academy of Nutrition and Dietetics* 116(10):1568–1577. doi: 10.1016/j.jand.2016.03.007.

75. National Institutes of Health. 2014. *Clinical Guidelines on the Identification, Evaluation, and Treatment of Overweight and Obesity in Adults*.

76. Nicolau, J., Ayala, L., Rivera, R. et al. 2015. Postoperative Grazing as a Risk Factor for Negative Outcomes After Bariatric Surgery. *Eating Behavior* 18:147–150. doi: 10.1016/j.eatbeh.2015.05.008.

77. Stookey, J. J. D. 2016. Negative, Null and Beneficial Effects of Drinking Water on Energy Intake, Energy Expenditure, Fat Oxidation and Weight Change in Randomized Trials: A Qualitative Review. *Nutrients* 8(1):19. doi: 10.3390/nu8010019.

78. Karl, J. P., & Roberts, S. B. 2014. Energy Density, Energy Intake, and Body Weight Regulation in Adults. *Advances in Nutrition* 5(6):835–850. doi: 10.3945/an.114.007112.

79. Schwingshackl, L., Hoffmann, G., Kalle-Uhlmann, T., Arregui, M., Buijsse, B., & Boeing, H. 2015. Fruit and Vegetable Consumption and Changes in Anthropometric Variables in Adult Populations: A Systematic Review and Meta-Analysis of Prospective Cohort Studies. *PLoS ONE* 10(10):e0140846. doi: 10.1371/journal.pone.0140846.

80. Harrington, D. M., Martin, C. K., Ravussin, E., & Katzmarzyk, P. T. 2013. Activity Related Energy Expenditure, Appetite and Energy Intake: Potential Implications for Weight Management. *Appetite* 67:1–7. doi: 10.1016/j.appet.2013.03.005.

81. Ibid.

82. Morales, F. E., Tinsley, G. M., and Gordon, P. M. 2017. Actue and Long-Term Impact of High Protein Diets on Endocrine and Metabolic Function, Body Composition, and Exercise-Induced Adaptations. *Journal of American College of Nutrition* 1–11. doi: 10.1080/07315724.2016.1274691.

83. Swift, D. L., Johannsen, N. M., Lavie, C. J., Earnest, C. P., & Church, T. S. 2014. The Role of Exercise and Physical Activity in Weight Loss and Maintenance. *Progress in Cardiovascular Diseases* 56(4):441–447. doi: 10.1016/j.pcad.2013.09.012.

84. Jakicic, J. and A. Otto. 2005. Physical Activity Consideration for the Treatment and Prevention of Obesity. *American Journal of Clinical Nutrition* 82:226S–229S.

85. U. S. News and World Report. 2014. Why 10,000 Steps a Day Won't Make You Thin. Available at http://health.usnews.com. Accessed April 2017.

86. Alamuddin, N., Bakizada, Z., and Wadden, T. A. 2016. Management of Obesity. *Journal of Clinical Oncology* 34(35):4295–4305.

87. Ibid.

88. Thomas, J. G., D. S. Bond, S. Phelan, J. O. Hill, and R. R. Wing. 2014. Weight-Loss Maintenance for 10 Years in the National Weight Control Registry. *American Journal of Preventive Medicine* 46(1):17–21.

89. Camps, S., S. Verhoef, and K. Westerterp. 2013. Weight Loss, Weight Maintenance, and Adaptive Thermogenesis. *American Journal of Clinical Nutrition* 97:990–994.

90. Alamuddin, N., bakizada, Z., and Wadden, T. A. 2016. Management of Obesity.

91. Ibid.

92. U.S. Department of Health and Human Services. 2015. *2015–2020 Dietary Guidelines for Americans*. Available at https://www.cnpp.usda.gov. Accessed April 2017.

93. Steinberg, D. M., D. F. Tate, G. G. Bennett, S. Ennett, C. Samuel-Hodge, D. and S. Ward. 2014. Daily Self-Weighing and Adverse Psychological Outcomes: A Randomized Controlled Trial. *American Journal of Preventive Medicine* 46(1):24–29.

94. Thomas, et al. 2014. Weight-Loss Maintenance for 10 Years.

95. Ibid.

96. Ibid.

97. Food and Drug Administration. 2017. *Medications Target Long Term Weight Management Control*. Available at www.fda.gov. Accessed April 2017.

98. Ibid.

99. Astrup, A., Fujioka, K., leRoux, C. W., Greenway, F., et al. 2017. 3 Years of Liraglutide versus Placebo for Type 2 Diabetes Risk Reduction and Weight Management in Individuals with Prediabetes: A Randomized, Double-blind Trial. *The Lancet*. doi: http://dx.doi.org/10.1016/S0140-6736(17)30069-7.

100. Armstrong, M. J., Gaunt, P., Guruprasal, P., et al. 2015. Liraglutide Safety and Efficacy in Patients with Non-alcoholic Steatohepatitis (LEAN): A Multicentre, Double-blind, Randomized, Placebo-controlled Phase 2 Study. *The Lancet* 387(10019):679–690.

101. Yen, M., and M. B. Ewald. 2012. Toxicity of Weight-Loss Agents. *Journal of Medicinal Toxicology* 8(2):145–152.

102. Ibid.

103. Colquitt, J. L., Pickett, K., Loveman,, E. and Frampton, G. K. 2014. Surgery for Weight Loss in Adults. *Cochrane Database for Systematic Review* (8):CD003641. doi: 10.1002/14651858.CD003641.pub4.

104. Puzziferri, N., Roshek, T. B., Mayo, H. G. et al. 2014. Long-term Follow-up After Bariatric Surgery: A Systematic Review. *Journal of the American Medical Association* 312(9):934–942. doi: 10.1001/jama.2014.10706.

105. Padwal, R., S. Klarenbach, N. Wiebe, D. Birch, S. Karmali, B. Manns, et al. 2011. Bariatric Surgery: A Systematic Review and Network Meta-Analysis of Randomized Trials. *Obesity Reviews* 12(8):602–621.

106. Buchwald, H., Y. Avidor, E. Braunwald, M. D. Jensen, W. Pories, K. Fahrbach, and K. Schoelles. 2004. Bariatric Surgery: A Systematic Review and Meta-Analysis. *Journal of the American Medical Association* 292:1724–1737.

107. Crookes, P. 2006. Surgical Treatment of Morbid Obesity. *Annual Reviews of Medicine* 57:243–264.

108. Ibid.

109. Ibid.

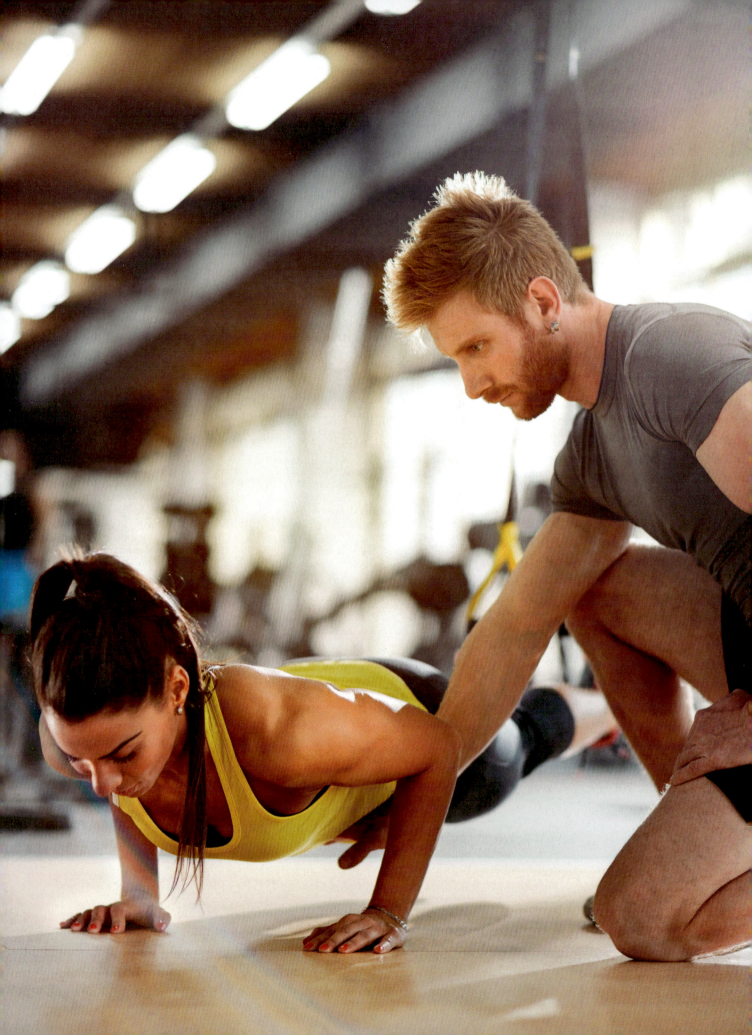

Nutrition and Fitness

16

Learning Outcomes

After reading this chapter, you will be able to:

16.1 List and describe the five basic components of fitness.

16.2 Explain the main features of a successful fitness program.

16.3 Describe the role of carbohydrate, fat, and protein in exercise.

16.4 Discuss the timing and types of foods to consume before, during, and after exercise.

16.5 Describe the importance of vitamins and minerals for physical fitness.

16.6 Explain the relationship between exercise and fluid intake.

16.7 Identify the most common ergogenic aids and summarize the current research on their benefits and side effects.

True or False?

1. Most people in the United States are physically fit. **T**/**F**

2. As little as 60 minutes of physical activity per week provides health benefits. **T**/**F**

3. Carbohydrate, fat, and protein provide energy during exercise. **T**/**F**

4. Low- to moderate-intensity exercise uses more fat than carbohydrate for fuel. **T**/**F**

5. Athletes should eat immediately after training. **T**/**F**

6. Vitamin and mineral supplements always improve athletic performance. **T**/**F**

7. Many athletes are at risk for iron deficiency. **T**/**F**

8. Everyone who exercises should consume sports drinks. **T**/**F**

9. You can never drink too much water. **T**/**F**

10. The NCAA classifies caffeine as a banned substance when consumed in high amounts. **T**/**F**

See page 615 for the answers.

Whether you are a weekend warrior, walking for fitness, or a triathlete, eating the right foods is just as important to your fitness and athletic performance as the exercise itself. Food preserves lean body mass, repairs cells, maximizes oxygen utilization, maintains strong bones, regulates all metabolic reactions, and provides the energy to contract muscles. The more you move, the more energy is required.

Imagine you are participating in a 5k race. To fuel your competition, your body will initially derive energy from the limited amount of ATP in your cells. As exercise progresses, the size of your carbohydrate stores and the rate at which your cells are able to break down fat and produce ATP will determine the outcome of the race. Once the race ends, nutrients consumed at the right time and in the right amounts will help your body recover and restore energy reserves. Fueling your body with the proper balance of nutrients is necessary to achieve optimal fitness levels and optimal athletic performance.

In this chapter, we explore the components and health benefits of physical fitness, the role the various nutrients play in physical activity, and how nutrition relates to physical fitness and athletic performance. You do not have to be an athlete to find the information in this chapter beneficial. It is intended for anyone seeking to understand the relationship between nutrition and physical fitness and apply that knowledge to her or his life.

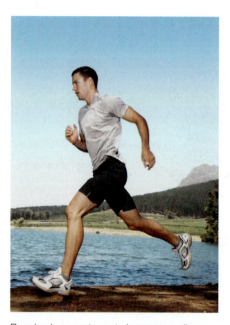

Running is a great way to improve cardiorespiratory fitness.

physical fitness Ability to perform physical activities requiring cardiorespiratory endurance, muscle endurance, strength, and/or flexibility, typically acquired through exercise and adequate nutrition.

physical activity Voluntary movement that results in energy expenditure.

exercise Any type of structured or planned physical activity.

cardiorespiratory endurance Body's ability to sustain cardiorespiratory exercise for a prolonged period of time.

muscular strength Greatest amount of force that can be exerted by the muscle at one time.

muscular endurance Ability of the muscle to produce prolonged effort.

What Is Physical Fitness and Why Is It Important?

LO 16.1 List and describe the five basic components of fitness.

What does it mean to be physically fit? Can you carry a heavy bag of groceries up a flight of steps without becoming winded, lift a heavy box from a shelf without straining a muscle, or feel invigorated after a long bike ride on the weekend? And are you at a healthy body weight? If the answer to these questions is yes, you are probably fit. **Physical fitness** can be defined as good health or physical condition, primarily as the result of exercise and proper nutrition.

The terms *physical activity* and *exercise* are often used interchangeably, but technically they are not the same thing. **Physical activity** refers to body movement that expends energy (kilocalories). Activities such as gardening, walking the dog, and playing with children can all be regarded as physical activity. **Exercise** is formalized training or structured physical activity, like step aerobics, running, or weightlifting. However, for our purposes in this chapter, the terms are used interchangeably.

Physical Fitness Has Five Components

Cardiorespiratory endurance, muscular strength, muscular endurance, flexibility, and body composition are the five basic components that contribute to physical fitness.

Cardiorespiratory endurance is the ability to sustain cardiorespiratory exercise, such as running and biking, for an extended length of time. This requires that the heart, blood, and lungs provide enough oxygen and nutrients to the working muscles to avoid fatigue. Someone who can run a mile without being too out of breath to talk has good cardiorespiratory endurance. Someone who is out of breath after climbing one flight of stairs, on the other hand, does not.

Muscular strength is the ability to produce force for a brief period of time, whereas **muscular endurance** is the ability to exert force over a long period of time without fatigue. Together muscular strength and endurance produce muscular fitness. Increasing muscle strength and endurance is best achieved with **resistance training**. You probably associate muscle strength with bodybuilders or weightlifters, and it is true that these people train to be particularly strong. However, other athletes, such as cheerleaders and ballet dancers, also work hard to strengthen their muscles. A dancer who holds another dancer over his head for several minutes shows exceptional muscular endurance.

Flexibility is the range of motion around a joint. Improved flexibility is achieved with stretching. Athletic performance, joint function, and muscular function are all enhanced with improved flexibility. In addition, improved flexibility reduces the likelihood of injury. A gymnast exhibits high flexibility when performing stunts and dance routines. In contrast, people with low flexibility may not be able to bend over and touch their toes from a standing or sitting position. Although a person does not need to be as flexible as a gymnast, lack of flexibility can lead to a reduction in activities of daily living. Thus, it is important that people continue to maintain flexibility over their lifetime.

Finally, recall from Chapter 14 that body composition is the proportion of lean tissue (primarily muscle and water) and fat tissue in the body. Body composition can change without total body weight changing because muscle takes up less space per pound than body fat. This is why an individual can lose inches without noticing a drop in body weight. Contrary to popular belief, body fat does not "turn into" muscle nor does muscle "turn into" body fat. Both muscle and fat can be lost with weight loss or increased with weight gain, but neither directly converts into the other.

Physical Fitness Provides Numerous Health Benefits

It is common knowledge that eating a balanced diet and exercising regularly helps maintain good health. It is also clear that even modest amounts of exercise provide health benefits, and the more you exercise, the more fit you'll be. However, despite the fact that the benefits of exercise are well known and well documented, only one in five adults living in the United States meets the *2008 Physical Activity Guidelines* recommendations for regular physical activity.[1]

The U.S. Department of Health and Human Services developed the *2008 Physical Activity Guidelines for Americans* to improve the health of American adults and children through regular physical activity. This publication gives information and guidance on the types and amounts of physical activity that provide substantial health benefits for Americans age 6 years and older. The recommendations are based on a review of scientific research on the benefits of physical activity and conclude with the main idea that regular physical activity over time can produce long-term health benefits.[2]

How does physical activity maintain good health? It reduces the risk of developing chronic diseases like type 2 diabetes mellitus, some forms of cancer, and cardiovascular disease. Physical activity improves body composition, bone health, and immune function. Being physically active also enhances mental well-being, increases the likelihood of restful sleep, and helps reduce stress.[3] **Table 16.1** lists some of the numerous health benefits that result from being physically active on a regular basis. Individuals have to be cautious, however, not to **overexercise** and increase the risk of injury.

LO 16.1: THE TAKE-HOME MESSAGE Physical fitness is the state of being in good physical condition attained through proper nutrition and regular physical activity. The five components of physical fitness are cardiorespiratory endurance, muscular strength, muscular endurance, flexibility, and body composition. To achieve optimal fitness, all five components must be considered. The numerous health benefits of physical activity include reduced risk of several chronic diseases, including type 2 diabetes and cardiovascular disease; improved body composition, bone health, and immune function; more restful sleep; enhanced mental well-being; and reduced stress.

resistance training Exercising with weights to build, strengthen, and tone muscle to improve or maintain overall fitness; also called *strength training*.

flexibility Ability to move joints freely through a full and normal range of motion.

overexercise To perform excessive physical activity without adequate rest periods for proper recovery.

TABLE 16.1 The Benefits of Physical Fitness

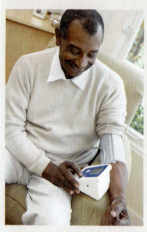

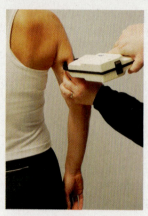

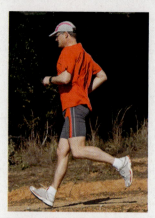

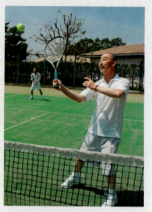

▲ **Reduced Risk of Cardio-vascular Disease**

How It Works: Research has shown that moderate physical activity lowers blood pressure.[1] In addition, exercise is positively associated with high-density lipoprotein (HDL) cholesterol.[2]

▲ **Improved Body Composition**

How It Works: Individuals with moderate cardiorespiratory fitness have less total fat and abdominal fat compared with people with low cardiorespiratory fitness.[3]

▲ **Reduced Risk of Type 2 Diabetes**

How It Works: Exercise helps control blood glucose levels by increasing insulin sensitivity.[4] This not only reduces risk for type 2 diabetes, but also improves blood glucose control for those who have been diagnosed with type 2 diabetes.

▲ **Reduced Risk of Some Forms of Cancer**

How It Works: Increased physical activity has been associated with a reduced risk of colon, breast, endometrial, and lung cancers. This reduced risk is likely the result of a reduction in overall body weight and other hormonal and metabolic mechanisms.[5]

Sources:
1. B. Bushman. 2014. Promoting Exercise as Medicine for Prediabetes and Prehypertension. *Current Sports Medicine Report* 13(4):233–239.
2. N. Sousa, R. Mendes, C. Abrantes, J. Sampaio, and J. Oliveira. 2014. A Randomized Study on Lipids Response to Different Exercise Programs in Overweight Older Men. *International Journal of Sports Medicine*. doi: 10.1055/s-0034-1374639.
3. I. Janssen, P. T. Katzmarzyk, R. Ross, A. S. Leon, J. S. Skinner, D. C. Rao, J. H. Wilmore, et al. 2004. Fitness Alters the Associations of BMI and Waist Circumference with Total and Abdominal Fat. *Obesity* 12:525–537.
4. J. W. Van Dijk, M. Venema, W. van Mechelen, C. D. Stehouwer, F. Hartgens, and L. L. van Loon. 2013. Effect of Moderate-Intensity Exercise versus Activities of Daily Living on 24-Hour Blood Glucose Homeostasis in Male Patients with Type 2 Diabetes. *Diabetes Care* 36(11):3448–3453.
5. U.S. Department of Health and Human Services. 2008. *Physical Activity Guidelines Advisory Committee Report*. Washington, DC: ODPHP Publication No. U0049. Available from www.health.gov/paguidelines/Report/pdf/CommitteeReport.pdf. Accessed July 2014.

What Does a Successful Physical Fitness Program Look Like?

LO 16.2 Explain the main features of a successful fitness program.

Physical fitness programs generally incorporate activities that are based on the five components of fitness, including aerobic exercise, resistance training, and stretching. A successful fitness program should be tailored to meet the needs of the individual and performed consistently so that any gains in physical fitness are not lost. It is also important to incorporate activities that are enjoyable so that they are more likely to become a regular part of one's lifestyle. Someone who hates to jog, for example, is not likely to be consistent about jogging daily.

Cardiorespiratory Exercise Improves Cardiorespiratory Endurance and Body Composition

Cardiorespiratory exercise, such as high-impact aerobics, stair climbing, and brisk walking, often involves continuous activities that use large muscle groups (abdomen, legs, and buttocks). This type of exercise is predominantly aerobic because it uses oxygen. During cardiorespiratory exercise, the heart beats faster and more oxygen-carrying blood is delivered to tissues.

TABLE 16.1 The Benefits of Physical Fitness

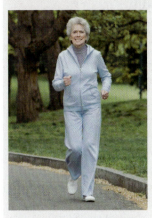

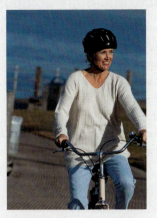

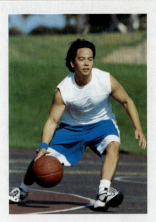

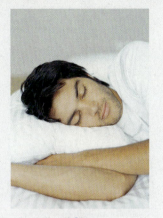

▲ **Improved Bone Health**

How It Works: Bone density has been shown to improve with weight-bearing exercise and resistance training, thereby reducing the risk for osteoporosis.[6,7]

▲ **Improved Immune System**

How It Works: Regular exercise can enhance the immune system, which may result in fewer colds and other infectious diseases.[8]

▲ **Improved Mental Well-Being**

How It Works: Regular exercise protects against the onset of depression and anxiety disorders, reduces symptoms in people diagnosed with depression and anxiety, delays the incidence of dementia, and overall enhances mental well-being.[9]

▲ **Improved Sleep**

How It Works: People who engage in regular exercise often have better quality of sleep. This is especially true for older adults.[10]

Sources:
6. L. A. Tucker, J. E. Strong, J. D. Lecheminant, and B. W. Bailey. 2014. Effect of Two Jumping Programs on Hip Bone Mineral Density in Premenopausal Women: A Randomized Controlled Trial. *American Journal of Health Promotion*. doi: 10.4278/ajhp.
7. F. D. Saraví and F. Sayegh. 2013. Bone Mineral Density and Body Composition of Adult Premenopausal Women with Three Levels of Physical Activity. *Journal of Osteoporosis*. doi: 10.1155/2013/953271.
8. D. Menicucci, A. Piarulli, F. Mastorci, L. Sebastiani, et al. 2013. Interactions between Immune, Stress-Related Hormonal and Cardiovascular Systems Following Strenuous Physical Exercise. *Archives Italiennes de Biologie* 151(3):126–136.
9. U.S. Department of Health and Human Services. 2008. *Physical Activity Guidelines Advisory Committee Report*.
10. A. A. Akbari Kamrani, D. Shamsipour Dehkordi, and R. Mohajeri. 2014. The Effect of Low and Moderate Intensity Aerobic Exercises on Sleep Quality in Men Older Adults. *Pakistan Journal of Medical Sciences* 30(2):417–421.

How does this work? As exercise begins, the body requires more oxygen to break down nutrients for energy, so it increases blood flow (volume) to the working muscles. It accomplishes this by increasing heart rate and **stroke volume**. The body also redistributes blood from internal organs to maximize the volume of blood that is delivered to the muscles.

An individual's level of cardiorespiratory fitness can be measured by the maximum amount of oxygen the muscles can consume during exercise, or **VO_2max**. A person who is more physically fit has a higher VO_2max and can exercise at a higher intensity without fatigue than someone who is not as fit. A trained athlete, for example, might have a VO_2max of 50–80 milliliters per kilogram per minute (ml/kg/min), whereas a sedentary, unfit individual might have a VO_2max of 25–30 ml/kg/min.[4] Two of the highest VO_2max ever recorded were for two cross-country skiers, a male and a female, who measured 94 and 77 ml/kg/min, respectively.[5]

Cardiorespiratory conditioning, which includes making gradual increases in exercise intensity, helps increase VO_2max, and therefore improves cardiorespiratory endurance and overall physical fitness. In addition, cardiorespiratory exercise can help individuals maintain a healthy body weight and improve body composition by reducing body fat. Cardiorespiratory exercise also reduces stress and lowers the risk of heart disease by maintaining normal cholesterol levels and lowering heart rate and blood pressure. As the heart becomes a more efficient pump, it does not have to work as hard with each beat.

stroke volume Amount of blood pumped by the heart with each heartbeat.

VO_2max Maximum amount of oxygen (ml) a person uses in 1 minute per kilogram of body weight.

cardiorespiratory conditioning
Improvements in the delivery of oxygen to working muscles as a result of aerobic activity.

Strength Training Improves Muscle Strength, Muscle Endurance, and Body Composition

Strength (or resistance) training is designed to increase muscle mass, strength, and endurance. Maintaining adequate muscle mass and strength is important for everyone. Contrary to common belief, resistance training does not necessarily lead to large, bulky muscles. Many females, as well as males, use resistance training to define their muscles and improve their physical appearance and body composition.

In general, individuals should perform a low number of repetitions using heavy weights to increase muscle strength. To increase muscular endurance, perform a high number of repetitions using lighter weights. Heavier weights can also be used to improve muscular endurance by allowing short rest intervals between repetition sets.

Rest periods between sets of an exercise and between workouts are important to avoid overworking muscles and increasing risk of injury. Muscle that is not adequately rested may break down and not recover, leading to a loss of muscle mass. The amount of rest recommended during a workout depends on a person's fitness goals and level of **conditioning**. If increasing strength is the goal, long rest periods of 2–3 minutes between sets are best. If the goal is to increase muscular endurance, shorter rest periods of 30 seconds or less are recommended.

The general guideline for rest periods between workouts is 2 days, or a total of 48 hours, between workouts that use the same muscle groups. However, strength training can be performed daily as long as different muscles are used on consecutive days. For example, you can perform upper body strength training on one day—working your biceps, triceps, and pectoral muscles—and on the following day do leg lifts, squats, and lunges to work your lower body muscles.

Stretching Improves Flexibility

Most people associate flexibility with gymnasts or dancers, but everyone can benefit from being more flexible. Improving flexibility can reduce muscle soreness and the risk of injury, as well as improve balance, posture, and circulation of blood and nutrients throughout the body. Stretching, such as through yoga, is the most common exercise used to improve flexibility.

The FITT Principle Can Be Used to Design a Fitness Program

FITT is an acronym for *frequency, intensity, time, and type*. The FITT principle provides an easy way to design a successful physical fitness regimen or conditioning program.

Frequency is how often an individual performs the activity, such as the number of times per week. **Intensity** refers to the degree of difficulty at which the activity is performed. *Time*, or *duration*, is how long the activity is performed, such as a 30-minute run. And lastly, *type* means the specific activity performed.

Frequency, time, and type are easy to assess. But what about intensity? Common terms used to describe intensity are *low*, *moderate*, and *vigorous (high)*. One measure of intensity for cardiorespiratory exercise is **rating of perceived exertion (RPE)**, in which the person performing the activity self-assesses the level of intensity. The RPE is based on your current level of fitness and your perception of how hard you are working. The scale ranges from 1 (rest) to 10 (maximal exertion). A range of 5–7 on the RPE scale (somewhat hard to hard) is recommended for most adults to achieve fitness. A more precise method of measuring intensity is using your **target heart rate**. Your target heart rate is the range (given in percentages of maximal heart rate) that your heart rate should fall within to ensure that you are training at your desired level of intensity. For example, a target heart

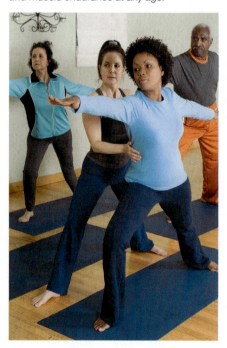

Resistance training improves muscle strength and muscle endurance at any age.

Improving flexibility can help reduce muscle soreness and lower the risk of injury.

conditioning Process of improving physical fitness through repeated activity.

intensity Level of difficulty of an activity.

rating of perceived exertion (RPE) Subjective measure of the intensity level of an activity using a numerical scale.

target heart rate Heart rate in beats per minute (expressed as a percentage of maximum heart rate) achieved during exercise that indicates the level of intensity at which fitness levels can increase.

rate of 60 percent would be considered low intensity compared with a target heart rate of 80 percent, which is considered high intensity. The Calculation Corner illustrates how to calculate your target heart rate. For weight training, intensity is referred to as **repetition maximum (RM)**. For example, 1 RM is the maximum amount of weight that can be lifted once.

Calculation Corner

Target Heart Rate

Target heart rate can be useful in determining the intensity level of cardiorespiratory exercise. One method used to calculate your target heart rate (THR) begins with calculating an estimate of your maximal heart rate (HRmax). Use the following formula to calculate an estimated HRmax.

$$206.9 - (\text{age in years} \times 0.67) = \text{estimated HRmax}$$

Before you can calculate your THR, you must first decide the intensity level at which you wish to exercise. Use the following as a guideline:

- Light/low intensity – 55–64% of HRmax
- Moderate intensity – 65–84% of HRmax
- High intensity – 85–95% of HRmax

Now, multiply your estimated HRmax by the desired intensity level to determine your target heart rate.

$$THR = HRmax \times \text{intensity level}$$

Example: John, a 45-year-old office manager, wants to know what his target heart rate should be as he begins his new training program at moderate intensity.

(1) Calculate John's estimated HRmax:

$$206.9 - (45 \times 0.67) = 177 \text{ estimated HRmax}$$

(2) Multiply John's estimated HRmax × intensity at 65% and 84% to determine his THR.

$$177 \times 0.65 = 115 \text{ THR}$$
$$177 \times 0.84 = 149 \text{ THR}$$

John's THR for moderate intensity is between 115 and 149 bpm. John can adjust his THR based on his RPE.

Source: Data from B. Bushman, ed. 2011. *ACSM's Complete Guide to Fitness & Health.* Chicago: IL: Human Kinetics.

Go to **Mastering** Nutrition and complete a Math Video activity similar to the problem in this Calculation Corner.

The frequency, intensity, time (duration), and types of exercise that are right for a person depend partly on what goal the individual is trying to achieve. For individuals seeking health benefits, the *2008 Physical Activity Guidelines* state that as little as 60 minutes a week of moderate-intensity activity offers some health benefits.[6] However, a total amount of 150 minutes (2 hours and 30 minutes) a week of moderate-intensity aerobic activity provides substantial health benefits for adults by reducing the risk of many chronic diseases. To gain additional health benefits, such as a lower risk of colon and breast cancer, up to 300 minutes (5 hours) per week of moderate-intensity physical activity is recommended. Additionally, resistance training at a moderate or high intensity and that involves all major muscle groups should be performed 2 or more days a week.

Do you feel like you don't have the time to exercise? This is a common barrier that keeps many people from engaging in regular physical activity. The good news is that aerobic activity can be performed in sessions as short as 10 minutes to get some health benefits.

repetition maximum (RM) Maximum amount of weight that can be lifted for a specified number of repetitions.

Get Moving!

Schedule physical activity into your day, just as you would schedule a meeting, class, or work.

Find activities that you enjoy. Make exercise something you look forward to, so that you're more likely to keep it up.

Ask a friend or coworker to exercise with you. Many people are more likely to exercise if they have a partner to motivate them.

Track your exercise in a log or journal so you see how much you are getting and note improvement over time.

Take advantage of activities that are offered at your college or university, including club sports, intramurals, group fitness classes, and personal training sessions.

Be adventurous and try new activities. If you're used to jogging or going to the gym, try hiking or racquetball. Mixing up your routine will help prevent boredom.

Of course, the more activity performed, the greater the benefits. Taking advantage of short periods of time during the day for a brisk 10-minute (or longer) walk will help you meet the recommendations for physical activity. For more suggestions, see the Fitness Tips.

Engaging in more vigorous-intensity activities, such as jogging or fast-paced swimming, for longer duration results in even greater health benefits. Individuals striving to maintain body weight and prevent gradual weight gain should participate in approximately 60 minutes of moderate- to vigorous-intensity activity on most days of the week and avoid consuming excess kilocalories. Those striving to lose weight should participate in at least 60–90 minutes of daily moderate-intensity physical activity and adjust kilocalorie intake so that more kilocalories are expended than are consumed.

The Physical Activity Pyramid is another tool that can be used as a guide to meeting physical activity needs. It is designed to show examples of activities and how often they should be performed for optimal health and physical fitness (**Figure 16.1**). People with diabetes mellitus, hypertension, heart disease, and other chronic diseases should consult with a health care provider before participating in any exercise program, especially one to be performed at a vigorous intensity.

Individuals seeking improved physical fitness in addition to health benefits can follow the general recommendations outlined by the American College of Sports Medicine. These guidelines for cardiorespiratory endurance, muscular fitness, and flexibility for healthy adults are summarized in **Table 16.2** using the FITT principle.

High-Intensity Interval Training Is More Time-Efficient

If you are strapped for time, but want to increase your physical activity levels, high-intensity interval training may be the answer. **High-intensity interval training (HIIT)** is defined as any exercise or physical activity that switches between intense bursts of

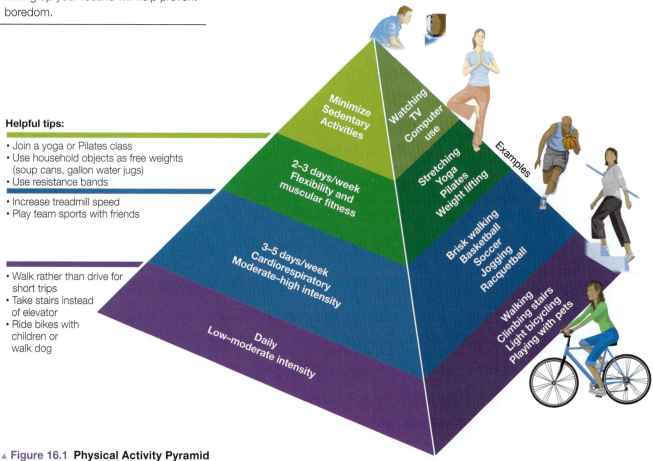

Helpful tips:

- Join a yoga or Pilates class
- Use household objects as free weights (soup cans, gallon water jugs)
- Use resistance bands

- Increase treadmill speed
- Play team sports with friends

- Walk rather than drive for short trips
- Take stairs instead of elevator
- Ride bikes with children or walk dog

▲ **Figure 16.1 Physical Activity Pyramid**

TABLE 16.2 Using FITT to Improve Fitness

	Cardiorespiratory Fitness	Muscular Fitness	Flexibility
Frequency	3–5 days per week	2–3 days per week	2–3 days per week
Intensity	64–95% of maximum heart rate	60–80% of 1 RM	To the point of feeling tightness or slight discomfort
Time	20–60 minutes per day (150 minutes per week), continuous or intermittent (minimum of 10-minute bouts)	8–10 different exercises performed in 2–4 sets, 8–12 repetitions	2–4 repetitions for each muscle group; hold static stretch for 10–30 seconds
Type	Brisk walking, jogging, biking, step aerobics	Free weights, machines with stacked weights, resistance bands	Stretching, yoga

Source: Data from the American College of Sports Medicine. 2011. Position Stand: Quantity and Quality of Exercise for Developing and Maintaining Cardiorespiratory, Musculoskeletal, and Neuromotor Fitness in Apparently Healthy Adults: Guidance for Prescribing Exercise. *Medicine and Science in Sports and Exercise* 43(7):1334–1359.

activity and fixed periods of rest. For example, a HIIT workout might include running, biking, jump roping, and rowing for short, high-intensity workouts for 1 minute followed by walking for 2 minutes. This 3-minute interval might then be repeated five times for a total of 15 minutes.

Research has shown that HIIT can be more effective than moderate-intensity training, especially in overweight or obese individuals.[7] One study suggested that just 2 weeks of high-intensity intervals improves aerobic capacity as much as 6–8 weeks of endurance training.[8] HIIT is more time-efficient, improves cardiorespiratory fitness and fasting blood glucose, and improves body composition.[9] Another study found that participants who performed HIIT had a better aerobic and anaerobic capacity. This was compared to the group who trained at a moderately intense level and only improved their aerobic capacity.[10]

Progressive Overload Can Help Improve Fitness over Time

During conditioning, the body gradually adapts to the activities that are being performed. Over time, if the activity is kept exactly the same, the body doesn't have to work as hard and fitness levels plateau. To continue to improve fitness, the body must be challenged by performing different workout regimens on a regular basis. This can be done using the **progressive overload principle**. Modifying one or more elements of the FITT principle challenges the body in different ways so that the level of fitness improves. For example, someone trying to improve cardiorespiratory endurance might gradually increase both the pace and the duration of a run. To increase muscle strength, an individual might gradually increase the amount of weight being lifted.

As the body responds to the work it is being asked to do, it becomes more physically fit. The muscle cells increase in size (hypertrophy), endurance, and strength, and cardiorespiratory endurance and flexibility improve. However, if conditioning is executed improperly or nutrient intake is inadequate for physical activity, muscles can lose mass (**atrophy**), endurance, and strength, and cardiorespiratory fitness levels will decline.

LO 16.2: THE TAKE-HOME MESSAGE Cardiorespiratory exercise improves cardiorespiratory endurance and body composition. Strength training can improve muscle strength and endurance as well as body composition. Stretching can enhance flexibility. An effective conditioning program can be designed using the FITT principle, which stands for frequency, intensity, time, and type of activity. The *2008 Physical Activity Guidelines* state that most people should aim for at least 60 minutes of moderate activity per week for some health benefits. Greater amounts of exercise are needed for substantial health benefits, weight loss, and to improve physical fitness. Applying the progressive overload principle to workouts helps individuals achieve optimal fitness.

high-intensity interval training (HIIT) Interval training that includes short periods of intense anaerobic exercise alternating with less intense recovery periods.

progressive overload principle Gradual increase in exercise demands resulting from modifications to the frequency, intensity, time, or type of activity.

atrophy To shrink in size.

How Are Carbohydrate, Fat, and Protein Used During Exercise?

LO 16.3 Describe the role of carbohydrate, fat, and protein in exercise.

Food meets our nutrient needs for physical activity in two ways. Food supplies the energy, particularly from carbohydrate and fat, which the body needs to perform an activity. And food provides nutrients, predominantly from carbohydrate and protein, which help the body recover properly so that it can repeat the activity. The type of food used to supply energy depends on whether the physical activity is anaerobic or aerobic, reactions you learned about in Chapter 8. Let's review these energy-producing reactions.

Anaerobic Energy Production Fuels Quick, Intense Exercise

Recall that all body actions require energy in the form of adenosine troposphere (ATP), produced either aerobically (requiring oxygen) or anaerobically (without oxygen) from macronutrients in foods. Much of the energy production during cardiorespiratory exercise is aerobic. By contrast, anaerobic energy production is typically used for quick, intense activities that require strength, such as lifting weights; agility and speed, such as sprinting; or a sudden burst of power, such as jumping for a slam dunk during a basketball game.

During the first few seconds of physical activity the body relies heavily on anaerobic energy production from ATP and creatine phosphate (PCr) found in muscle cells (see the Chemistry Boost). Most anaerobic activities are fueled by ATP and rely on creatine phosphate to resynthesize ATP—a total of about 10 seconds. Thus, the ATP-CP stored in the muscle can provide enough energy to fuel all-out exercise for about 10 seconds. If maximal exercise continues beyond 10 seconds, ATP will be recharged during anaerobic glycolysis.

Energy is released from ATP when the bond connecting the end phosphate is hydrolyzed from the ATP molecule, leaving adenosine diphosphate (ADP) (**Figure 16.2**). ADP

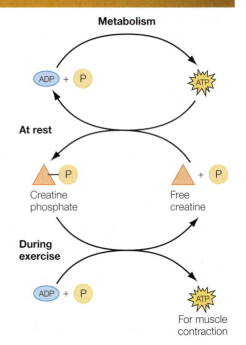

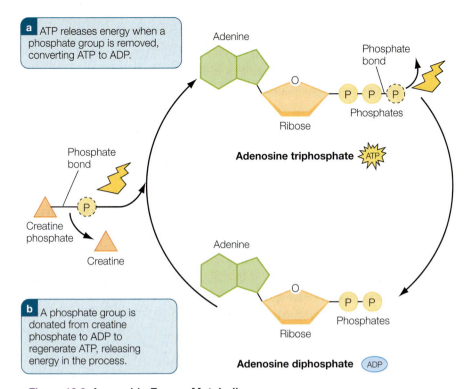

a ATP releases energy when a phosphate group is removed, converting ATP to ADP.

Adenine

Ribose

O

Phosphate bond

P — P — P

Phosphates

Adenosine triphosphate ATP

Phosphate bond

P

Creatine phosphate

Creatine

b A phosphate group is donated from creatine phosphate to ADP to regenerate ATP, releasing energy in the process.

Adenine

Ribose

O

P — P

Phosphates

Adenosine diphosphate ADP

▲ **Figure 16.2 Anaerobic Energy Metabolism**
During anaerobic metabolism, energy is released during the breakdown of ATP and the breakdown of creatine phosphate.

is regenerated to ATP in the mitochondria of the cell when creatine phosphate donates a phosphate molecule. Creatine phosphate is a quick source of phosphate with a dual role in energy production. Energy is directly produced when the phosphate group is removed from the creatine phosphate molecule. This is an example of a catabolic reaction releasing energy. Energy is indirectly produced because the released phosphate group is donated to ADP, which regenerates ATP, and sets up another round of energy production.

The body produces a small amount of creatine from foods, including meat and fish, or creatine can be supplied to the body directly from dietary supplements. With the help of the liver and kidneys, creatine is converted to creatine phosphate and stored in skeletal muscle and other tissues, including the cardiac muscle and brain. The amount of creatine phosphate stored in the muscles is limited and becomes depleted after up to 10 seconds of maximum-intensity activity. Creatine phosphate is regenerated when the muscle cell is at rest, such as between sprints or in between sets during weight training, to prepare for the next exercise effort.

Aerobic Energy Production Fuels Sustained Exercise

Just like creatine phosphate, the amount of ATP in cells is limited and can support only a few seconds of intense exercise, such as is needed to perform a 100-meter sprint. When the ATP and creatine phosphate stores are unable to meet sustained energy demands, breathing becomes heavier and oxygen intake increases. At this point the pace of exercise slows down and the body begins to rely more on aerobic production of ATP because the amount needed to support the quick bursts or sprints cannot be generated fast enough by anaerobic energy production. With oxygen in the cell, pyruvate formed from glucose during glycolysis is converted into acetyl CoA and is metabolized through aerobic metabolism to produce ATP.

The body relies on a mixture of carbohydrate, fat, and protein for energy during exercise, but the type and amount of these nutrients that are used depends on the intensity and duration of the exercise, the body's nutritional status, and the level of physical fitness. Remember that carbohydrate contributes to both anaerobic and aerobic energy production and fat contributes to the aerobic generation of ATP. Protein can be used for energy production when kilocalorie needs haven't been met; however, the body prefers to use protein to promote muscle growth and recovery.

Carbohydrate Is the Primary Energy Source During High-Intensity Exercise

Carbohydrate is the predominant fuel used during high-intensity, short-duration, anaerobic exercise. Carbohydrate provides energy to the working muscle either through blood glucose, stored glycogen in the muscles and the liver, or the consumption of dietary carbohydrates (**Figure 16.3**). In adults, the amount of glycogen stored in the muscles ranges from about 200 to 500 grams. In addition, the liver stores around 60–120 grams of glycogen, which can be converted into glucose through glycogenolysis and released into the blood. The amount of glycogen that each person stores depends on many factors, including the person's nutritional intake and fitness levels.

The average adult body stores about 2,600 kilocalories of energy as glycogen, of which 2,000 kilocalories can be used. The rate at which glycogen stores are used depends on the intensity and duration of the exercise. If the exercise is of high intensity and short

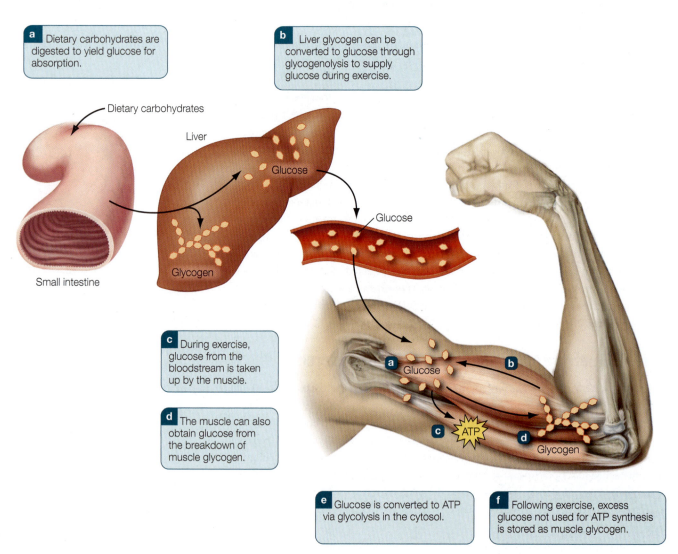

a Dietary carbohydrates are digested to yield glucose for absorption.

b Liver glycogen can be converted to glucose through glycogenolysis to supply glucose during exercise.

Dietary carbohydrates

Liver

Glucose

Glucose

Small intestine

Glycogen

c During exercise, glucose from the bloodstream is taken up by the muscle.

a Glucose

b

d The muscle can also obtain glucose from the breakdown of muscle glycogen.

c ATP

d Glycogen

e Glucose is converted to ATP via glycolysis in the cytosol.

f Following exercise, excess glucose not used for ATP synthesis is stored as muscle glycogen.

▲ **Figure 16.3 Glucose Utilization During Exercise**

duration, glycogen stores are depleted in about 20 minutes, compared with low-intensity, long-duration exercise, during which glycogen stores can last up to 90 minutes.

Glucose derived from stored muscle glycogen is the preferred source for energy during exercise; however, liver glycogen stores are just as important. Glycogen stored in the liver is converted into glucose and delivered to the bloodstream to maintain normal blood glucose levels, both during periods of activity and at rest. Muscle cells first rely on glycogen stored in the muscles for energy during activity, but also blood glucose formed from the breakdown of liver glycogen. Liver glycogen is depleted faster when a person's muscle glycogen stores are suboptimal at the start of exercise.

Whereas muscle and liver glycogen provide glucose for the muscle cells during activity, blood glucose is also the energy source for the brain. If the brain does not receive the glucose to meet its energy needs, individuals may feel a lack of coordination or lack of concentration—two things no one wants to experience, especially during exercise or a sport competition.

Recall that during glycolysis, the pyruvate formed is reduced to lactate when the mitochondria lack sufficient oxygen to transform pyruvate into acetyl CoA. When lactate is produced at a low rate, as during aerobic metabolism, muscles can effectively clear it from the blood and use it as an energy source. For example, during low-intensity exercise, the body is able to oxidize the lactate that is produced by the muscle during glycolysis and therefore it does not accumulate in the working muscle tissue. The body also shuttles excess lactate to other tissues, such as the brain, heart, and liver, to prevent excessive accumulation in the muscle. Lactate from the muscle diffuses into the blood, is picked up by the liver, and enters the Cori cycle. In the Cori cycle (see Figure 8.8 in Chapter 8), lactate undergoes gluconeogenesis, is converted back to glucose, and is returned to the bloodstream to be used for energy again.

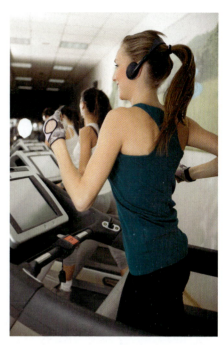
Less glycogen is used as fuel compared to fat during low-intensity, long-duration exercise.

As exercise intensity increases, the energy demands are greater than the amount of ATP the cell can produce aerobically using available oxygen. As a result, more hydrogen ions are rapidly generated as glucose is anaerobically metabolized to pyruvate. These excess hydrogen ions combine with pyruvate to form lactate, which diffuses quickly into the blood. As exercise intensity continues, the levels of lactate and hydrogen ions increase as the body attempts to produce enough ATP to meet energy demands. The increase in hydrogen ions may negatively affect exercise performance as pH in the muscle cell drops. The good news is that the ability of the muscles to effectively use and shuttle lactate to other tissues improves with training. Lactate in the muscle will rise before it diffuses out of the cell into the blood where it is transferred to the liver to undergo transformation to glucose.

For many years, lactate in muscles was thought to be a cause of muscle fatigue, but now scientists report that lactate produced during anaerobic glycolysis can also be an important fuel during exercise. In several types of exercise, muscle is the major site of lactate production and removal. Some researchers believe that as exercise continues, there is a shift from lactate diffusing out of the muscle into the blood, to the muscle itself oxidizing lactate for energy in the mitochondria.[11] The rate at which muscles consume lactate for energy depends on the metabolic rate, the pH in the muscle, blood flow, and the fitness level of the individual.[12]

Intensity Affects the Use of Glucose and Glycogen

Muscles use glucose for energy no matter how intense the exercise. However, research shows that as the intensity of exercise increases, the percentage of energy derived from glucose and glycogen also increases.[13] Carbohydrates are the preferred energy source at high intensity levels because, unlike fat and protein, carbohydrate is efficiently oxidized for energy as the intensity of activity increases. At very high intensities, carbohydrates supply most of the energy in the form of muscle glycogen. Although carbohydrates are not the main energy source during prolonged low- to moderate-intensity exercise, they still provide some energy for the working muscles.

Duration Affects the Use of Glucose and Glycogen

In addition to intensity, the duration of exercise also affects the source and amount of carbohydrate used to fuel physical activity. At the start of low- to moderate-intensity exercise, stored muscle glycogen is the main source of energy. As muscle glycogen stores diminish, the liver also contributes its glycogen to be converted to glucose for energy and to prevent hypoglycemia. During prolonged exercise, the body relies more on blood glucose (generated from stored liver glycogen) and less on muscle glycogen as its carbohydrate source of energy.

In addition to affecting the source of carbohydrate, duration also affects how much carbohydrate is used. After about 20 minutes, as low- to moderate-intensity exercise continues, muscles rely less on glycogen and glucose and more on fat for fuel (more on this in a later discussion). Even when fat is being used for some energy production during exercise, the body always uses glycogen for energy as well, and if the intensity and duration of the exercise last long enough, muscle and liver glycogen stores become depleted and the activity can no longer be sustained at the same intensity. Many endurance runners refer to this as "hitting the wall."

Conditioning Affects the Use of Glucose and Glycogen

Research has shown that the amount of glycogen that the muscles can hold can be affected by training.[14,15] Well-trained muscles have the ability to store 20–50 percent more glycogen than untrained muscles. More stored glycogen means more fuel for working muscles to use, which means individuals can exercise for a longer period of time and increase endurance. Just eating a high-carbohydrate meal before competition will not improve performance; individuals need to train their muscles *and* eat a high-carbohydrate diet regularly to maximize the effect.

Carbohydrate Requirement Depends on Exercise Duration

Recall that most adults should get 45–65 percent of their daily energy intake from carbohydrates. As we've already learned, the amount of carbohydrate needed to fuel physical activity depends greatly on the duration of the activity. Glycogen stores are continuously being depleted and replenished. For those who exercise often, eating carbohydrate-rich foods on a regular basis is important to provide the muscles with adequate glycogen. When glycogen stores are inadequate, the muscles have only a limited amount of energy available to support activity, which has been shown to reduce athletic performance and promote fatigue.[16,17] Keep in mind that the glycogen storage capacity of both the muscles and the liver is limited. Once the muscles and liver have stored all of the glycogen possible, the body converts any excess glucose into fatty acids and stores it in the form of body fat.

Carbohydrate loading is one training strategy that athletes use to build up muscle glycogen stores before a competition. See Spotlight: Carbohydrate Loading for an explanation of this beneficial strategy for endurance athletes.

The best types of carbohydrates to eat during and immediately after exercise are simple carbohydrates, such as sports drinks, bars and gels, bananas, bagels, or corn flakes, because they are absorbed and enter the bloodstream quickly, and therefore can be used immediately for energy (glucose) or to replenish glycogen stores. Complex carbohydrates like whole-grain rice and pasta, oatmeal, and whole wheat are ideal to eat a couple of hours before exercise because they take longer to digest than simple carbohydrates and enter the bloodstream much more slowly, thereby providing a sustained source of energy. Remember, however, that complex carbohydrates are generally high in fiber, and too much fiber before a workout can cause bloating, gas, and diarrhea.

carbohydrate loading Diet and training strategy that maximizes glycogen stores in the body before an endurance event.

Carbohydrate Loading

The goal of carbohydrate loading is to maximize the storage capacity of muscle glycogen before an endurance event. Increasing the amount of stored muscle glycogen can improve an athlete's endurance performance by providing the energy to fuel activity at an optimal pace for a longer period of time.

Not all athletes or physically active people will have improved performance with carbohydrate loading, however. The people who are likely to benefit the most from this strategy are those who participate in endurance events or exercise that lasts more than 90 minutes. Examples of endurance events include marathons, triathlons, cross-country skiing, and long-distance cycling and swimming. Individuals who exercise or train for less than 90 minutes should follow the standard recommendations for carbohydrate intake for athletes to ensure adequate muscle glycogen stores. Research has also shown that women are less likely than men to have improved performance with carbohydrate loading because women oxidize significantly more fat and less carbohydrate and protein during endurance exercise compared with men.[1]

So how do athletes start carbohydrate loading? When this concept was first developed, athletes began by training very hard for 3–4 days in addition to eating a low-carbohydrate diet (less than 5–10 percent of total kilocalories). This period was called the *depletion phase* and was thought to be necessary to increase glycogen stores during the next phase, called the *loading phase*. The loading phase involved three to four days of minimal or no training while eating a diet high in carbohydrates. This resulted in higher muscle glycogen stores and better endurance performance.

Many people found the depletion phase hard to endure and would often experience irritability, hypoglycemia, and fatigue. Today, many endurance athletes exclude the depletion phase. Research

has shown that depleting muscle glycogen stores is not necessary to increase the amount of stored muscle glycogen. However, there will be greater increases in muscle glycogen by initially depleting muscle glycogen stores.[2]

To begin a modified carbohydrate-loading regimen, athletes taper exercise about 7 days prior to the event by doing a little less activity each day (**Figure 1**). This is often the hardest recommendation to follow because many athletes feel that they will be out of shape if they stop training before competition. But tapering exercise is necessary to increase muscle glycogen; otherwise, the body continues to burn glycogen for fuel rather than storing it to be used for energy during the upcoming event. One study showed that athletes can decrease training by 70 percent about 1 week prior to an endurance event without negatively affecting performance.[3]

In addition to tapering exercise, carbohydrate loading involves eating

a high-carbohydrate diet that provides about 4–5 grams of carbohydrate per kilogram of body weight for the first 3–4 days. During the last 3 days of tapering exercise, carbohydrate intake is increased to 10 grams per kilogram of body weight. Lastly, a meal that is high in carbohydrate (providing about 250–300 grams), moderate in protein, and low in fat should be consumed about 3–4 hours prior to the start of the event to further maximize glycogen stores.

Despite the emphasis on carbohydrate, athletes need to be sure not to compromise intake of protein and fat. They still need to include at least 0.8 grams of protein per kilogram of body weight (some athletes may require more protein) in their training diet, as well as about 20–25 percent of kilocalories coming from fat, preferably unsaturated fats.

Table 1 is a sample 1-day menu that might be used the day before an event. This menu is high in carbohydrate, adequate in protein, and low in fat.

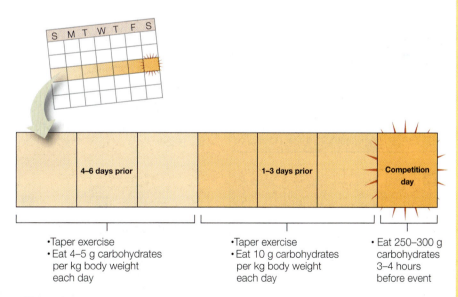

▲ **Figure 1**
Carbohydrate loading involves tapering exercise and gradually increasing carbohydrate intake the week before a competitive event. On the day of the competition, a high-carb meal is eaten 3–4 hours before the event begins.

References

1. Cermak, N. M., and L. J. van Loon. 2013. The Use of Carbohydrates During Exercise as an Erogenic Aid. *Sports Medicine* 43(11):1139–1155. doi: 10.1007/s40279-013-0079-0.

2. Goforth, W. H., D. Laurent, W. K. Prusaczyk, K. E. Schneider, K. F. Peterson, and G. I. Shulman. 2003. Effects of Depletion Exercise and Light Training on Muscle Glycogen Super-Compensation in Men. *American Journal of Physiology—Endocrinology and Metabolism* 285:E1304–E1311.

3. Gilgen-Ammann, R., T. Wyss, S. Troesch, L. Heyer, and W. Taube. 2017. Postive Effects of Augmented Feedback to Reduce Time on Ground in Well-Trained Runners. *International Journal of Sports and Physiological Performance* 122. doi: 10.1123/ijspp.2016-0746.

TABLE 1 Sample Carbohydrate-Loading Menu

Breakfast	Lunch	Dinner	Snack
1 cup orange juice $1/2$ cup Grape-Nuts cereal 1 medium banana 1 cup 2% milk 1 English muffin 1 tbsp jelly	2 slices oatmeal bread 3 oz turkey breast with lettuce, tomato 8 oz apple juice 1 cup frozen yogurt	3 cups spaghetti (6 oz uncooked) 1 cup tomato sauce 2 oz ground turkey $1/4$ loaf multigrain bread (4 oz)	1 cup vanilla yogurt 6 fig bars
750 kilocalories	*750 kilocalories*	*1,300 kilocalories*	*500 kilocalories*
85% carbohydrates	*65% carbohydrates*	*70% carbohydrates*	*80% carbohydrates*

Total: 3,300 kilocalories: 75% carbohydrates (610 g), 15% protein (125 g), 10% fat (40 g)

Reprinted, with permission, from N. Clark, *Nancy Clark's Nutrition Guidebook*, 5th ed. (Champaign, IL: Human Kinetics, 2013), p. 148.

Fat Is the Primary Energy Source during Low- to Moderate-Intensity Exercise

Fat is supplied to muscles as an energy source in two forms: fatty acids stored in muscle tissue and free fatty acids in the blood derived from those stored in adipose tissue. Fatty acids in the muscle directly supply energy to the muscles, so they are used for energy during exercise before the fatty acids in adipose tissue. Recall from Chapter 8 that when the body breaks down stored body fat for energy (lypolysis), triglycerides in adipose tissue are first hydrolyzed into fatty acids and glycerol and then released into the bloodstream. Circulating free fatty acids are taken up by the muscles and go through beta-oxidation inside the mitochondria to produce energy. The liver takes up glycerol, where it is converted into glucose through gluconeogenesis to help maintain blood glucose levels and provide energy (see **Figure 16.4**).

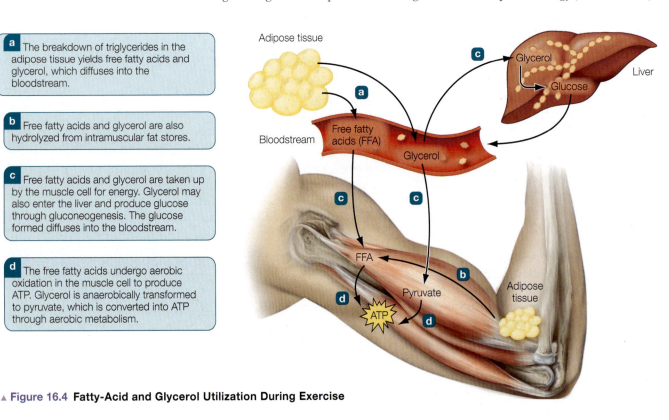

a The breakdown of triglycerides in the adipose tissue yields free fatty acids and glycerol, which diffuses into the bloodstream.

b Free fatty acids and glycerol are also hydrolyzed from intramuscular fat stores.

c Free fatty acids and glycerol are taken up by the muscle cell for energy. Glycerol may also enter the liver and produce glucose through gluconeogenesis. The glucose formed diffuses into the bloodstream.

d The free fatty acids undergo aerobic oxidation in the muscle cell to produce ATP. Glycerol is anaerobically transformed to pyruvate, which is converted into ATP through aerobic metabolism.

▲ **Figure 16.4** **Fatty-Acid and Glycerol Utilization During Exercise**

There are advantages to storing excess energy as fat rather than carbohydrate and protein. Fat is a more concentrated source of energy because it provides more than twice the kilocalories of carbohydrate or protein; this is because, unlike glycogen and protein, stored fat does not contain water. In addition, greater amounts of energy can be stored as fat because, while glycogen stores are limited, the capacity of fat cells is unlimited.

Intensity Affects the Use of Fat

Just as with carbohydrates, fat is used for energy during rest and aerobic exercise. The exercise intensity affects the source and amount of fat used. Recall that fatty acids require oxygen to be converted into energy (beta-oxidation). Therefore, the availability of oxygen is one of the most important factors for determining what nutrient the muscles use the most for energy.

During low- to moderate-intensity exercise, sufficient oxygen is available to oxidize fat efficiently enough to keep up with the demand for energy. Fat supplies nearly all of the energy required during low- to moderate-intensity activity, relative to the amount of carbohydrate and protein that is used. At low-intensity exercise, the body uses mostly free fatty acids in the blood (released from adipose tissue), rather than fatty acids stored in muscle, for energy. During moderate-intensity exercise, the body begins to use more fatty acids from muscle triglycerides and less fatty acids released from adipose tissue. At the same time, more muscle glycogen is used and contributes to about half of total energy.

As exercise intensity increases and greater demands are placed on the cardiorespiratory system, the availability of oxygen declines. With less oxygen, fatty acids cannot be converted into energy fast enough to meet the demand. Because glucose oxidation is more efficient than fat oxidation at higher intensities, muscles begin to rely less on fat and more on glucose for fuel.

Duration Affects the Use of Fat

In general, the use of fat for energy increases throughout the duration of low- to moderate-intensity exercise. During the first 15–20 minutes of exercise, fat utilization by the muscles increases at a slow rate because of the time required to oxidize fat for energy. During this time, free fatty acids in the bloodstream are taken up by the muscles and used for energy, which causes blood levels to drop. This in turn stimulates an increase in lypolysis, by way of the hormone epinephrine, and more fatty acids are hydrolyzed from adipose tissue and released into the bloodstream to provide (more) energy for the working muscles.

Once the duration of moderate-intensity activity exceeds 20 minutes, the level of fatty acids in the bloodstream becomes greater than normal as the body continues to use and release stored fat for energy. Because of this increase in blood levels, the body increases its use of fatty acids for energy.

The body relies mostly on the energy produced from carbohydrate and fat during exercise. **Focus Figure 16.5** summarizes the preferred sources used to fuel muscular work based on the duration and intensity of the exercise.

Conditioning Affects the Use of Fat

An individual's level of conditioning can affect how much fat the body uses for energy. Endurance training results in an increase in the amount of fatty acids stored in the muscles. This can increase the total amount of fat used for energy because these fatty acids supply fuel directly to the muscles. Training also causes muscle cells to produce new and larger mitochondria, which oxidize fatty acids to produce ATP. Lastly, training is thought to increase enzymes that aid in fatty-acid oxidation. For these reasons, muscles that are well trained use more fat for energy than muscles that are not as well trained. Because they use more fat and less glycogen, conditioned individuals have the potential to increase endurance by "sparing" glycogen stores for later use.

Head to Mastering Nutrition and watch a narrated video tour of this figure by author Joan Salge Blake.

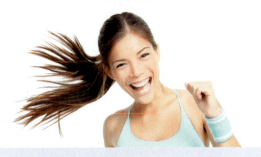

Depending on the duration and intensity of the activity, our bodies may use ATP-CP, carbohydrate, or fat in various combinations to fuel muscular work. Keep in mind that the amounts and sources shown below can vary based on the person's fitness level and health, how well fed the person is before the activity, and environmental temperatures and conditions.

SPRINT START (0–3 seconds)
A short, intense burst of activity like sprinting is fueled by ATP and creatine phosphate (CP) under anaerobic conditions.

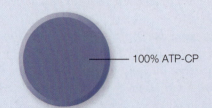

— 100% ATP-CP

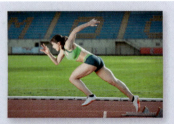

100-M DASH (10–12 seconds)
ATP and CP provide energy for about 10 seconds of quick, intense activity, after which energy is provided as ATP from the breakdown of carbohydrates.

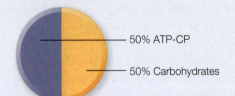

— 50% ATP-CP

— 50% Carbohydrates

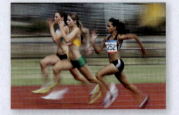

1500-M RACE (4–6 minutes)
Energy derived from ATP and CP is small and would be exhausted after about 10 seconds of the race. At this point, most of the energy is derived from aerobic metabolism of primarily carbohydrates.

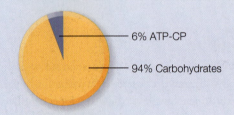

— 6% ATP-CP

— 94% Carbohydrates

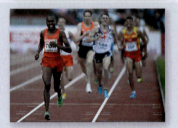

10-KM RACE (30–40 minutes)
During moderately intense activities such as a 10-kilometer race, ATP is provided by fat and carbohydrate metabolism. As the intensity increases, so does the utilization of carbohydrates for energy.

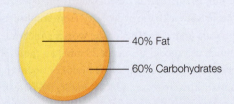

— 40% Fat

— 60% Carbohydrates

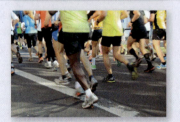

MARATHON (2.5–3 hours)
During endurance events such as marathons, ATP is primarily derived from carbohydrates, and to a lesser extent fat. A very small amount of energy is provided by the breakdown of amino acids to form glucose.

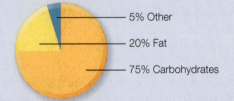

— 5% Other

— 20% Fat

— 75% Carbohydrates

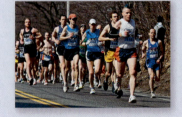

DAY-LONG HIKE (5.5–7 hours)
The primary energy source for events lasting several hours at low intensity is fat (free fatty acids in the bloodstream, which derive from triglycerides stored in fat cells). Carbohydrates contribute a small percentage of energy needs.

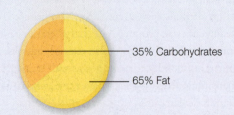

— 35% Carbohydrates

— 65% Fat

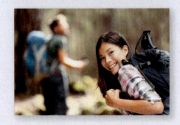

Recall that the body requires oxygen to convert fatty acids into energy. This demand for oxygen appropriately stresses the cardiovascular system. Conditioning the body through regular exercise results in the ability of the heart and lungs to deliver oxygen to working muscles more efficiently at higher intensity; thus, the oxidation of fatty acids for energy is greater.

Athletes Should Meet the AMDR for Fat

Dietary recommendations for fat intake are generally the same for active people as for the average adult population, with 25–30 percent of kilocalories coming from fat.[18] Remember from Chapter 5 that high intakes of saturated and *trans* fats have been linked to high cholesterol levels and heart disease. Physically active people sometimes assume that because they're in shape, they don't have to worry about these conditions. Although it is true that physical activity greatly benefits the cardiovascular system, athletes and other fit people can have high cholesterol and experience heart attacks and strokes. Everyone, regardless of activity level, should consume primarily unsaturated fats to meet the body's need for dietary fat.[19]

Some athletes, such as endurance runners and those in sports where low body weight is important, such as gymnasts and figure skaters, may feel they can benefit from a very low-fat diet (less than 20 percent). Though consuming too much dietary fat is a concern, limiting fat intake too much is also undesirable. Consuming less than adequate amounts of fat is more likely to result in inadequate consumption of kilocalories, essential fatty acids, and fat-soluble vitamins, which can negatively affect exercise performance.[20,21]

Protein Is Primarily Used to Build and Repair Muscle

Protein is the nutrient most commonly associated with muscle and its relationship to physical activity, especially strength training. Recall from Chapter 6 that, in the process of protein turnover, dietary and body proteins are broken down into amino acids and then reassembled into the various proteins that the cells need. When protein synthesis occurs more often than breakdown, conditions are favorable for increases in muscle protein, which can translate to more muscle mass, strength, and endurance.

Exercise is a form of physiological stress and prompts the release of cortisol, a stress hormone. Cortisol affects protein turnover by triggering muscle protein breakdown. This protein breakdown can be counterbalanced nutritionally by consuming adequate dietary protein, in addition to carbohydrate and fat, for protein synthesis. The amino acids and other nutrients consumed in foods are especially critical in promoting muscle growth (hypertrophy) and recovery after exercise. This postworkout protein synthesis is necessary to maintain or improve performance.

The Body Can Use Protein for Energy

Just as during rest, the body prefers to use carbohydrate and fat as its main energy sources during exercise. All active people use small amounts of protein for energy, but greater amounts are used when kilocalorie intake and carbohydrate stores are insufficient.

When dietary and body proteins are used for energy, they are broken down into amino acids that are then released into the bloodstream. The amino acids are carried to the liver, where they get converted through gluconeogenesis into glucose, which supplies the working muscles with energy. Remember that once amino acids are transformed to glucose, they cannot be changed back into amino acids. If the glucose is not used for energy, it is converted into fatty acids and stored as body fat.

If the body has to use a significant amount of protein for energy, that protein is not available to perform its vital functions and the rate of protein breakdown exceeds protein synthesis. Muscle atrophy is a likely consequence of protein breakdown when dietary intakes are inadequate to support physical activity. This commonly occurs in athletes who are trying to lose weight, those who need to "make weight" for a specific sport like wrestling, or in individuals who unintentionally do not eat enough to compensate for nutrients expended during physical activity.

Protein Needs Depend on the Level of Training

Many athletes and people who exercise assume that they need substantially more protein than people who do not exercise. Although it is true that those who are fit and physically active need more protein than those who are sedentary, their need is not significantly higher. For this reason, the RDA for protein for most healthy adults, including recreational exercisers, is 0.8 grams per kilogram of body weight per day. Most people, including athletes, exceed this amount, with intake ranging from 0.9 to 2.3 grams per kilogram of body weight.

Competitive and elite athletes, as well as bodybuilders, do have a higher RDA for protein. Endurance athletes are advised to consume 1.2–1.4 grams of protein per kilogram of body weight daily. People who primarily participate in resistance and strength activities may need to consume as much as 1.6–1.7 grams per kilogram of body weight daily.[22]

> **LO 16.3: THE TAKE-HOME MESSAGE** Energy is provided by ATP-CP, carbohydrate, or fat, depending on the intensity and duration of exercise. Carbohydrate, in the form of blood glucose and muscle and liver glycogen, is the primary source of ATP during anaerobic, high-intensity, short-duration exercise. Fat is the main energy source during rest and aerobic, low-intensity, long-duration exercise. Protein provides the amino acids that are necessary to promote muscle growth and repair muscle breakdown caused by exercise.

How Do the Timing and Composition of Meals Affect Physical Activity?

LO 16.4 Discuss the timing and types of foods to consume before, during, and after exercise.

The timing and composition of meals and snacks before, during, and after exercise or athletic performance has a significant impact on energy stores, fatigue, and recovery time. For competitive athletes, modifying food intake to ensure optimal stores of liver and muscle glycogen before an athletic event is essential. In addition, the breakdown of muscle protein that can result from inadequate total energy and/or carbohydrate intake can lead to loss of muscle mass and strength and lack of energy, which can negatively affect exercise performance.

Food Intake Should Be Timed Appropriately

The wisdom of consuming a precompetition meal depends on timing: The body needs time to digest the food so that it doesn't negatively affect performance by causing cramps, bloating, or other discomforts. In general, larger meals (those that make you feel quite full) may take 3–4 hours to digest, whereas smaller meals (those that make you feel satisfied but not overly full) may take only 2–3 hours to digest. A liquid supplement or small snack may be digested within about 30 minutes to 1 hour. For athletes competing in the early morning, a high-carbohydrate, low-fat dinner the night before will maintain glycogen stores during sleep, and a small snack in the morning will provide the energy needed for performance. If an athlete competes in the afternoon, the morning meal becomes the critical feeding to pack muscle and liver glycogen stores. For a late-afternoon or evening event, lunch should provide the carbohydrate necessary to top off the glycogen stores.

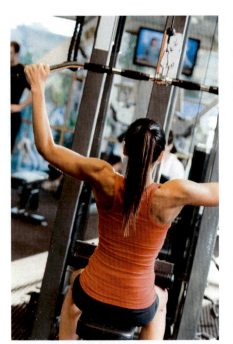

Consuming protein immediately after weight training enhances muscle recovery.

Endurance athletes or those who engage in high-intensity intermittent exercise, such as soccer, ice hockey, or basketball, are at risk of depleting glycogen stores during the event. Ingesting carbohydrate during the competition supports blood glucose levels and delays the depletion of glycogen stores.

Consuming the appropriate foods after exercise is important to support muscle recovery. During exercise, especially strength training, muscles are under a great deal of stress, which can result in overstretching and tearing of proteins and potential inflammation. After exercise, the body is in a catabolic (breaking-down) state: Muscle and liver glycogen stores are low or depleted, muscle protein is broken down, and the immune system is suppressed.

Foods eaten after exercise affect how fast the body recovers, which in turn may affect how soon it is ready for the next workout or training session. This is especially important for competitive athletes who may train more than once per day.

These are general guidelines and may not apply to everyone. Individuals should experiment with their own eating and exercise schedule to learn how long to wait before starting an activity.

Carbohydrate and Protein Are Optimal Before Exercise

A pre-exercise meal should contain adequate amounts of carbohydrate to maximize muscle and liver glycogen stores and maintain normal blood glucose levels. In general, the pre-exercise meal should contain 150–300 grams of carbohydrate (3–4.5 grams of carbohydrate per kilogram of body weight) and be consumed 3–4 hours prior to exercise (see **Table 16.3**). High-fiber carbohydrates and carbonated drinks should be avoided to prevent intestinal cramping and distress.

Consuming simple carbohydrates (1 gram per kilogram of body weight) immediately before exercise (about 15–30 minutes prior to the start), especially if the carbohydrate is in liquid form, may be beneficial. The extra glucose gives muscles an immediate source of energy and spares glycogen stores, which allows for exercise for a longer duration or at a higher intensity without the body becoming tired as quickly.[23,24]

Protein intake has a significant impact on muscle preservation, growth, and recovery. Combining both protein *and* carbohydrate before exercise increases the muscle glycogen content in both the liver and the muscle more than eating carbohydrate alone.[25] With more glycogen in the liver and muscles and proper training, endurance increases. Another benefit of consuming both protein and carbohydrate before exercise is that it results in greater protein synthesis after the exercise is over, compared with either protein or carbohydrate alone.[26] The making of new body proteins, including muscles, is necessary for optimal fitness and muscle preservation, repair, and growth.

Foods with a higher fat content take longer to digest than foods that are higher in carbohydrate and protein, and can lead to feelings of sluggishness or discomfort, which can impair performance. For this reason, high-fat foods should generally be avoided several hours before exercise. Of course this is a general guideline, and not all active people who consume higher fat foods before exercise experience difficulty.

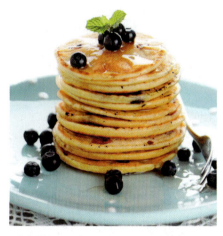

A pre-exercise meal must contain adequate amounts of carbohydrate.

TABLE 16.3	Timing and Amount of Macronutrients for Performance			
		During Exercise		
Nutrient	**Pre-Exercise**	**Endurance**	**Ultra-Endurance**	**Postexercise Recovery**
Carbohydrate	150–300 g (3–4.5 per kg body weight)	30–60 g per hour	Up to 90 g per hour	Immediately after exercise 0.3–0.6 g per pound of body weight
Protein	Low protein	0	0	20 g of high-quality protein
Fat	Limit intake	0	0	Limit intake

Simple Carbohydrates Are Beneficial During Exercise

For exercise lasting longer than 1 hour, food intake during exercise should begin shortly after the start of exercise to maintain a blood supply of glucose, delay glycogen depletion, and reduce the perception of fatigue.[27] For long-lasting endurance activities, a total of 30–60 grams of carbohydrate should be consumed per hour.[28] Ultra-endurance athletes such as ultra-marathon runners or long-distance cyclists may need as much as 90 grams of carbohydrate per hour.[29]

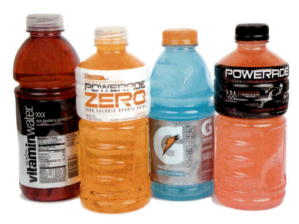

Sports drinks including VitaminWater, Powerade, and Gatorade can be a good source of carbohydrate during exercise.

Sports drinks and gels are one way to take in carbohydrate immediately before or during activity, but foods such as crackers and sports bars are also commonly eaten. Recent research has reported improved performance with a 6 percent carbohydrate mouth rinse for 5–10 seconds four times during a race.[30]

Glucose, sucrose, and maltodextrin are the best forms of carbohydrate to consume during exercise because the body absorbs them more quickly than other forms. Fructose, the sugar found in fruits and fruit juice, should generally be avoided during exercise because it may cause gastrointestinal problems or stomach discomfort in some individuals.[31]

Many sports drinks and gels contain only carbohydrate and electrolytes, while some also contain protein. For endurance athletes, consuming both carbohydrate and protein during exercise has been shown to improve net protein balance at rest as well as during exercise and postexercise recovery.[32] This net balance has, in turn, a positive effect on muscle maintenance and growth.

Consume Carbohydrate and Protein Shortly After Exercise

Consuming carbohydrate after exercise helps replenish muscle and liver glycogen stores and stimulate muscle protein synthesis. The muscles are most receptive to storing new glycogen within the first 30–45 minutes after the end of exercise. Consuming 0.3–0.6 grams per pound of body weight of simple carbohydrates within that time frame will promote maximum glycogen storage.[33] Waiting longer than 1 hour results in less glycogen stored. Research shows that eating carbohydrate immediately after exercise also results in a more positive body protein balance.[34]

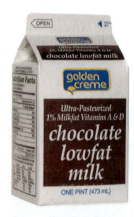

Low-cost options like this Golden Creme lowfat chocolate milk provide the whey protein and carbohydrate that help with muscle and glycogen synthesis after exercise. For vegan athletes, rice protein can be used effectively.

Consuming both protein and carbohydrate after exercise results in increased muscle protein synthesis. In addition, protein intake immediately after exercise rather than several hours later results in greater muscle protein synthesis. Research studies have shown that the addition of protein to carbohydrate intake causes an even greater increase in glycogen synthesis than either carbohydrate or protein alone, and therefore both nutrients should be consumed both before and after exercise.[35,36] Postexercise consumption of carbohydrate and protein in a ratio of approximately 4:1 (in grams) is ideal to stimulate muscle glycogen synthesis, repair muscle cells, stimulate protein synthesis, and promote faster recovery time.[37]

What is the best way to get these two nutrients? Most athletes and regular exercisers prefer to consume a liquid supplement that contains carbohydrate and protein rather than solid foods immediately after exercising. Whey protein (found in milk) is the preferred protein source because it is rapidly absorbed and contains all of the essential amino acids that the body needs. Commercial shakes and drinks containing whey protein are one option, but they can be expensive. A cheaper alternative is low-fat chocolate milk, which provides adequate amounts of carbohydrate and protein to assist in recovery.[38] For vegan athletes, rice protein supplements mixed with water have been shown to be effective following a resistance-training workout.[39] A liquid supplement or small snack consumed after exercise should be followed by a high-carbohydrate, moderate-protein, low-fat meal within the next 2 hours for optimal recovery.

The importance of carbohydrate and protein for recovery is clear. What about fat? Some people who load up on high-fat foods after a workout or competition experience fatigue that can reduce performance during the next workout.[40] Again, competitive athletes should experiment with timing and composition of food intake during training and not on the day of competition. An hour prior to a competition is not the time to find out that a particular food doesn't agree with you. Apply these timing concepts to the athlete described in Nutrition in Practice on page 600.

LO 16.4: THE TAKE-HOME MESSAGE Consuming the right balance of nutrients at the right time can improve exercise performance and recovery time. Pre-exercise meals should contain 150–300 grams of carbohydrate, be low in protein and fat to promote faster digestion, and be low in fiber to prevent intestinal problems. Fructose and higher-fat foods should generally be avoided before exercise. During prolonged exercise, 30–60 grams of carbohydrates should be consumed per hour to delay glycogen depletion and support blood glucose. Immediately after exercise, simple carbohydrates plus protein should be consumed to replenish depleted glycogen and begin protein repair.

What Vitamins and Minerals Are Important for Fitness?

LO 16.5 Describe the importance of vitamins and minerals for physical fitness.

Recall that vitamins and minerals play a major role in the metabolism of carbohydrate, fat, and protein for energy during exercise. Some also act as antioxidants and help protect cells from the oxidative stress that can occur with exercise.

Some Vitamins and Minerals Contribute to the Processes of Energy Metabolism

The B vitamins thiamin, riboflavin, niacin, pantothenic acid, biotin, and vitamin B_6 activate the enzymes that transform carbohydrates, proteins, and fats to ATP. Folate and vitamin B_{12} act together to maintain healthy red blood cells, which carry oxygen to the muscle used during aerobic metabolism. A deficiency in either of these two vitamins will result in fatigue and, potentially, anemia.

In addition to their important roles in normal body functioning, minerals are essential to physical fitness and athletic performance. The major mineral phosphorus is part of the energy currency adenosine triphosphate (ATP). A lack of phosphorus can lead to fatigue and weakness. Iron (discussed further below) is an integral part of hemoglobin in red blood cells to carry and exchange oxygen with myoglobin in the muscle. And finally, the trace mineral iodine is necessary to produce thyroid hormone that controls metabolic rate and the rate at which the body produces energy.

Antioxidants Can Help Protect Cells from Damage Caused by Exercise

Muscles use more oxygen during exercise than at rest. As a result, the body increases production of free radicals that damage cells, especially during intense, prolonged exercise.

NUTRITION *in* PRACTICE:
Athletic Trainer

Dalton was recruited with a full scholarship to be a guard on the college basketball team. He was the star basketball player in high school and played with a travelling team. While he was used to heavy schedule of games and practices in high school, his college routine of games, practices, and weight training six days a week is taking a toll on this energy level. He finds he is getting tired before the end of practices and doesn't have the stamina to play all four quarters of the game. Dalton understands how important his performance is to retaining his athletic scholarship, so he met with the team Athletic Trainer (AT) to see if he should change his training routine. The AT asked Dalton if he is getting adequate sleep and how he is doing in school. Dalton told the AT that he sleeps soundly at night and that his school work was manageable. The AT then asked about his diet. When Dalton told him what he typically eats daily, the AT recommended that Dalton make an appointment with the team's Registered Dietitian Nutritionist (RDN), who has a specialty in sports nutrition.

Dalton's Stats
- ❏ Age: 18
- ❏ Height: 6 feet 4 inches
- ❏ Weight: 205 pounds
- ❏ BMI: 25
- ❏ Percent Body Fat: 9%

Critical Thinking Questions
1. What nutrient is missing from Dalton's diet, possibly contributing to his fatigue?
2. Is Dalton's food timing appropriate for his exercise performance? What recommendations would you make to improve the timing of his meals and snacks?
3. What changes should Dalton make in his diet in the evening and why?

RDN's Observation and Plan for Dalton:
- ❏ Discuss the importance of consuming adequate amounts of carbohydrates at his meals to achieve optimal energy storage as liver and muscle glycogen. If there is not adequate carbohydrate intake before a practice and game,

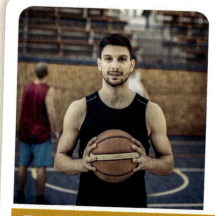

Dalton

DALTON'S FOOD LOG			
Food/Beverage	**Time Consumed**	**Hunger Rating***	**Location**
3-egg omelet with ham and cheese, hash browns, and sports drink	8 AM	5	Dining hall
3 oz. cheeseburger, fries, sports drink	1:00 PM	4	Dining hall
16 ounces sports drink; 3 protein bars	3:00 PM (before and during his 3 hour practice)	3	Basketball court
10 oz. fried chicken, mashed potatoes, corn	7 PM (after practice)	5	Fast-food eatery with teammates

* Hunger Rating (1–5): 1 = not hungry; 5 = super hungry.

the body's fuel storage will be quickly depleted.

- ❏ Recommend Dalton add vegetables to his omelet and add a salad, fresh fruit, or vegetables to his lunch. The RDN also recommends Dalton change his dinner choices to include grilled or sautéed chicken, rice, and more vegetables to increase his carbohydrates. The increased fat content of fried chicken may slow the absorption of carbohydrate and protein.
- ❏ Discuss the need for Dalton to have more snacks during the day to allow increased accessibility to kilocalories and to better balance intake and output of energy. The large gap between breakfast and lunch should be reduced to help sustain his energy over the course of the day. The RDN recommends that Dalton eat cereal and milk as a midmorning snack.

- ❏ Recommend Dalton continue drinking a carbohydrate-containing sports drink during games to maintain blood glucose levels, slow glycogen depletion, and provide fluid for hydration. Also recommend he eat a protein bar before and after the event, rather than during, to help with protein sparing and muscle recovery.

Two weeks later, Dalton returns for a follow-up visit with the RDN. He is feeling less fatigued and the increased food opportunities during the day are enabling him to have more stamina during his games and practices. However, he is getting bored with the evening snacking and wants more food choices. The RDN recommends that he try baked beans on toast, beef jerky and crackers, potatoes and eggs, granola and cottage cheese, or chicken and rice as an evening snack.

Antioxidants, such as vitamins E and C and selenium, are known to protect cells from the damage of free radicals. Vitamin C also assists in the production of collagen, which provides most of the structure of connective tissues like bone, tendons, and ligaments. This, in turn, can reduce the likelihood of developing strains, sprains, and fractures that may occur as a result of exercise.

Adequate intake of vitamins E and C through nutrient-rich foods has been linked to good health, which in turn can positively affect exercise and training. Research has not shown, however, that the use of antioxidants in levels above the RDA improves athletic performance, nor that it decreases oxidative stress in highly trained athletes.[41]

Highly Active People Are at Increased Risk for Iron and Calcium Deficiencies

In general, active people do not need more minerals than less active individuals. However, some active people are at increased risk for deficiencies of iron and calcium.

Iron

Iron is important to exercise because it is necessary for energy metabolism and transporting oxygen within muscle cells and throughout the body. Iron is a structural component of hemoglobin and myoglobin, two proteins that carry and store oxygen in the blood and muscle, respectively. If iron levels are low, hemoglobin and myoglobin levels can also fall, diminishing the blood's ability to carry oxygen to the cells. Individuals with low iron levels will therefore feel tired during physical activity, even when they are not vigorously exercising. Iron supplementation can improve aerobic performance for people with depleted iron stores.[42]

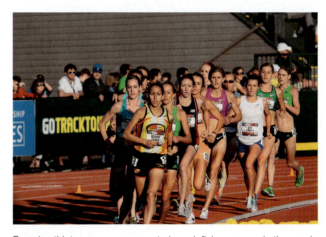

Female athletes are more prone to iron-deficiency anemia than male athletes.

When iron levels are severely diminished, anemia can occur. Athletes and physically fit people are prone to iron-deficiency anemia for many reasons, including poor dietary intake or increased iron losses. Women can lose a lot of iron during menstruation, depending on their iron status and menstrual blood flow. This is one reason why female athletes are at a greater risk for iron-deficiency anemia than male athletes. Long-distance runners and athletes in sports where they must "make weight" have been noted to be at higher risk for iron-deficiency anemia. Athletes in other sports such as basketball, tennis, softball, and swimming also have a greater risk of suboptimal iron status.[43,44] Some vegetarian athletes are especially susceptible to iron deficiency and need to plan their diets appropriately so they consume adequate amounts of foods plentiful in iron.

Some people experience decreased levels of hemoglobin because of training, especially when the training is quite strenuous. During exercise, blood volume increases and concentrations of hemoglobin in the blood decrease. This is often referred to as **sports anemia**, or *pseudoanemia*, and is not the same as iron-deficiency anemia. Iron-deficiency anemia typically has to be treated with iron supplementation. Sports anemia can be corrected on its own because a body with sufficient iron stores can adapt to training and produce more red blood cells, which restores normal hemoglobin levels.

Another effect of exercise on iron is intravascular hemolysis (*hemo* = blood, *lysis* = breaking down), the bursting of red blood cells. Also called "foot strike hemolysis," this condition occurs when feet repeatedly hit a hard surface (the ground) during running, causing red blood cells to burst and release iron. The iron is recycled by the body and not lost, and therefore does not typically contribute to iron deficiency.

sports anemia Low concentrations of hemoglobin in the blood; results from an increase in blood volume during strenuous exercise.

Calcium

Most people know about the importance of calcium to maintain bone health. Some people, including athletes, are particularly susceptible to broken bones and fractures. Having adequate calcium in the diet can reduce one's risk for these types of injuries. In addition, calcium affects both skeletal and heart muscle contraction and hormone and neurotransmitter activity during exercise. It also assists in blood clotting in response to a cut or other minor hemorrhage, which may occur during exercise or competition.

Many athletes do not consume enough iron or calcium to meet their needs. This is especially true for athletes who exhibit disordered eating patterns. For more information, see the Spotlight on page 603.

Calcium is lost in sweat; the more individuals sweat, the more calcium they lose. One study concluded that exercise could increase bone mineral content (the mass of all minerals in bone) sufficiently to compensate for the calcium lost through sweating.[45]

While adequate calcium intake is essential, calcium supplements are not recommended unless intake from food and beverages does not meet the RDA. Choosing foods and beverages that are high in calcium, including fortified foods, can ensure that all individuals, including athletes, meet their needs for calcium.

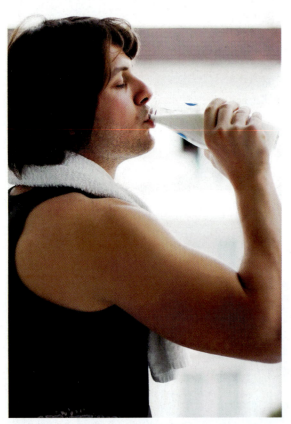

Milk is an effective postexercise beverage that adds calcium, protein, and fluid to an athlete's diet.

Vitamin and Mineral Supplements Are Generally Not Necessary

Many athletes mistakenly believe that vitamins and minerals themselves supply energy, or that consuming extra vitamins and minerals can enhance performance. Previous studies have shown that multivitamin and mineral supplements are the supplements most commonly used by college athletes.[46] Can these supplements really improve athletic performance? The answer is: not unless the body is already deficient in the nutrient. Vitamins and minerals can be used repeatedly in metabolic reactions; thus, for people who consume enough vitamins and minerals in their diet, taking more than the RDA will not result in improved performance.[47]

Everyone, not just athletes, should obtain vitamins and minerals by consuming adequate amounts of a wide variety of nutrient-dense foods. For most people, taking vitamin and mineral supplements is a waste of money. In addition, excess intakes of some vitamins and minerals, especially from supplements, can be harmful (see Chapters 9, 10, 12, and 13). Anyone, including athletes, should consult with a physician or a registered dietitian nutritionist before taking dietary supplements.

LO 16.5: THE TAKE-HOME MESSAGE Vitamins and minerals play important roles in metabolism, and vitamins E and C can act as antioxidants. Some athletes need to pay special attention to their intakes of iron and calcium. Iron is important because of its role in transporting oxygen in blood and muscle. Iron deficiency is prevalent among athletes, especially females and vegetarians. Calcium intake is important for bone health and muscle contraction. Adequate amounts of all nutrients can be consumed in foods, so supplements are not usually necessary.

Relative Energy Deficiency in Sport (RED-S)

Christy Henrich joined the U.S. gymnastics team in 1986 weighing 95 pounds at 4 feet, 11 inches tall. Shortly after joining the team, Christy succeeded as a gymnast, but after a judge told her she needed to lose weight, she developed anorexia nervosa. Sadly, her weight plummeted to 47 pounds, and she died from multiple organ failure at the age of 22.

The anorexia that Christy battled was part of a syndrome that used to be known as the *female athlete triad*. The problem with this nomenclature, however, is that it referred only to women, whereas male athletes can also be afflicted. The term was therefore changed in 2014 to **relative energy deficiency in sport (RED-S)**.

RED-S is a combination of interrelated health conditions existing on a continuum of severity in athletes. These interrelated conditions include low energy availability and a variety of physiological impairments affecting metabolic rate, menstrual function, bone health, immunity, protein synthesis, and cardiovascular function, along with reduced psychological health (**Figure 1**). Thus, this disorder not only reduces the performance of the athlete but may have serious medical and psychological consequences.[1]

Low Energy Availability or Disordered Eating

RED-S occurs when female or male athletes in certain sports are pressured to reach or maintain an unrealistically low body weight and/or level of body fat. This pressure contributes to the development of disordered eating, which helps to initiate the syndrome. At one extreme are athletes who fulfill the diagnostic criteria for anorexia nervosa or bulimia nervosa. However, disordered eating occurs on a continuum and is not always so pronounced. At the other end are those who unintentionally take in fewer kilocalories than they need. They may appear to be eating a healthy diet—one that would be adequate for a sedentary individual—but their kilocalorie needs are higher because of their level of physical activity.

Disordered eating can occur in both male and female athletes in all types of sports, but is most common in sports where appearance is important, such as figure skating, gymnastics, and ballet, and sports in which individuals strive to maintain a low body weight, such as wrestling, rowing, and horse racing.

Menstrual Dysfunction or Amenorrhea

In a female athlete, the failure to consume enough energy to compensate for the "energy cost" of the exercise can lead to disruption of the menstrual cycle.[2] **Amenorrhea**, the absence of at least three consecutive menstrual cycles, is the most extreme and recognizable form of disruption. Unfortunately, many females welcome the convenience of not menstruating and do not report it; however, this may put them at risk for reduced bone mass and increased rate of bone loss caused by decreased levels of estrogen in the body.[3]

Low Bone Mineral Density or Osteoporosis

Energy deficiency and—in females—decreased estrogen levels due to

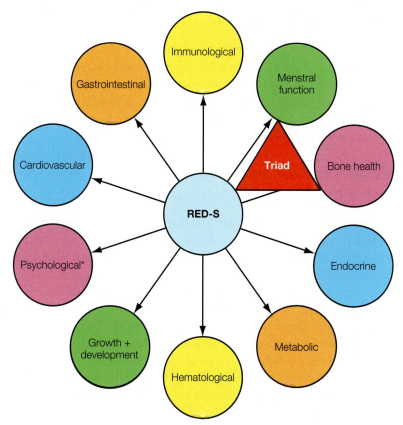

Source: doi:10.1136/bjsports-2014-093502

▲ **Figure 1** The health consequences of relative energy deficit in sport (RED-S), which has a much broader range of outcomes and application to male athletes than the female athlete triad.

Source: Mountjoy, M., Sundgot-Borgen, J., Burke, L., et al. 2014. The IOC Consensus Statement: Beyond the Female Athlete Triad—Relative Energy Deficiency in Sport (RED-S). *British Journal of Sports Medicine* 48:491–497. doi: 10.1136/bjsports-2014-093502.

relative energy deficiency in sport (RED-S) Syndrome of low energy availability based on the balance between energy intake through food and energy expenditure for daily activities, growth, and training and competition.

amenorrhea Absence of menstruation for at least three consecutive cycles.

menstrual dysfunction contribute to bone loss and low bone mineral density. At its most extreme this causes premature osteoporosis, which puts the athlete at risk for stress fractures and hip and vertebral fractures, as well as the loss of bone mass that may be irreplaceable.[4]

Signs and Treatment

All individuals, including friends, teachers, health care providers, and coaches, involved with at-risk athletes should be aware of the warning signs of RED-S. These include weight changes, disordered eating patterns, cardiac arrhythmia, depression, or stress fractures.

Those working with at-risk athletes should provide a training environment in which athletes are not pressured to lose weight and should be able to recommend appropriate nutritional, medical, and/or psychological resources if needed. Treatment of an athlete with this disorder is multidisciplinary, and needs to involve cooperation among the athlete's physician, psychologist, sports nutritionist, coach or trainer, family, and friends.

References

1. Slater, J., McLay-Cooke, R., Brown, R., and Black, K. 2016. Female Recreational Exercisers at Risk for Low Energy Availability. *International Journal of Sport Nutrition and Exercise Metabolism* 26(5):421–427.

2. Melin, A., Torstveit, M. K., Burke, L., Marks, S., and Sundgot-Borgen, J. 2014. Disordered Eating and Eating Disorders in Aquatic Sports. *International Journal of Sport Nutrition and Exercise Metabolism* 24(4): 450–459.

3. Eberman, L. E., Myrick, K., Feinn, R., and Harkins, M. 2014. The Prevalence of and Attitudes Toward Oligomenorrhea and Amenorrhea in Division I Female Athletes *International Journal of Athletic Therapy and Training* 19(6):41–47.

4. M. T. Barrack, J. C. Gibbs, M. J. De Souza, N. I. Williams, J. F. Nichols, M. J. Rauh, and A. Nattiv. 2014. Higher Incidence of Bone Stress Injuries with Increasing Female Athlete Triad–Related Risk Factors: A Prospective Multisite Study of Exercising Girls and Women. *American Journal of Sports Medicine* 42(4):949–958.

How Does Exercise Influence Fluid Needs?

LO 16.6 Explain the relationship between exercise and fluid intake.

As basic as it sounds, water is one of the most important nutrients during physical activity. Drinking too little fluid to replace fluid and electrolyte losses through sweating can cause physiological changes that can negatively affect exercise performance and even endanger health. Consuming adequate fluids before and during physical activity is key to maintaining optimal performance and preventing dehydration (also called *hypohydration*) and electrolyte imbalance.

Exercise Affects Fluid and Electrolyte Balance and Regulation of Body Temperature

Exercise causes the body to lose more water and electrolytes via sweat. The amount of water lost through sweating varies from person to person. Regardless of how much you sweat, it is important that you replace the fluid lost. Sweat contains not only water, but also sodium and chloride and, to a lesser extent, potassium. An imbalance in any of these electrolytes can cause heat cramps, as well as nausea, lowered blood pressure, and edema in the hands and feet, all of which can hinder performance. When electrolyte losses are within the range of normal daily dietary intake, they can easily be replaced by consuming foods rich in sodium, chloride, and potassium within 24 hours after exercise. If you prefer, you can replace electrolytes by drinking beverages that contain them, such as sports drinks.

As you learned in Chapter 11, the body loses fluid in breathing, via the exhalation of water vapor. Moderate to vigorous exercise increases these losses. This in turn increases the body's need for fluids.

Exercise also affects regulation of body temperature. Sweat releases the heat generated by muscular activity and the breakdown of nutrients to keep body temperature normal. However, if the air is very humid (i.e., it contains a lot of water), sweat may not evaporate off the skin and the body can't cool down. This can cause **hyperthermia**, and increase the risk of heat exhaustion or heat stroke. Heat exhaustion occurs when the body overheats. Symptoms of heat exhaustion include heavy sweating and rapid pulse rate.

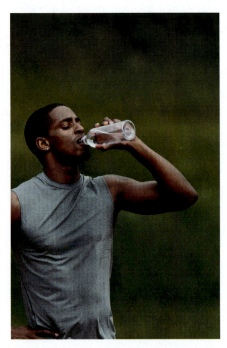

Staying hydrated during physical activity is important to maintain electrolyte balance and help regulate body temperature.

hyperthermia Rise in body temperature above normal.

TABLE 16.4 Warning Signs of Heat Exhaustion and Heat Stroke

Heat Exhaustion	Heat Stroke
Profuse sweating	Red, hot, and dry skin (no sweating)
Fatigue	Rapid, strong pulse
Thirst	Rapid, shallow breathing
Muscle cramps	Throbbing headache
Headache	Dizziness
Dizziness or lightheadedness	Nausea
Weakness	Extreme confusion
Nausea and vomiting	Unconsciousness
Cool, moist skin	Extremely high body temperature (above 103°F [39.4°C], orally)

If heat exhaustion is allowed to continue, it can progress to heat stroke, which is a life-threatening condition. One significant warning sign of heat stroke is a complete lack of sweating. This happens when an individual is extremely dehydrated and cannot produce sweat. This failure of evaporative cooling allows body temperature to soar to lethal levels. Other warning signs of heat exhaustion and heat stroke are shown in **Table 16.4**.

Many athletes and other active people may not realize that they can be at risk for **hypothermia**, which is just as serious as hyperthermia. Cold weather, especially if wet, can contribute to hypothermia when a person is exercising for a long period of time. Someone who is running at a slow pace in cold weather may produce very little heat, and the body temperature may gradually fall. Keep in mind that the body still sweats when exercising in cold weather, so meeting fluid needs is still important. Wearing adequate clothing and drinking fluids at least at room temperature or warmer helps prevent hypothermia.

Fluids Are Needed Before, During, and After Exercise

Being hydrated prior to exercise is essential to performance. The timing and amount of fluid depends on the individual's current hydration status. Too much fluid can cause bloating and result in excess urine produced during exercise. Too little fluid intake prior to exercise can result in dehydration during the exercise and impaired performance. Most healthy adult women need 9 cups of water daily, while most healthy adult men need about 13 cups. This amount does not, however, include the additional needs associated with exercising.

Proper hydration during and after exercise is essential to replace sweat losses. As you learned in Chapter 11, you can determine fluid needs during exercise by weighing yourself both before and after an activity. After exercise, you should consume 20–24 fluid ounces (about 2–3 cups) of fluid for every pound of body weight lost (weight loss is mainly due to water loss).[48] The American College of Sports Medicine has specific recommendations for how much fluid to drink before, during, and after exercise. See **Table 16.5** for these recommendations.

Some Beverages Are Better than Others

Beverages like tea, coffee, soft drinks, fruit juice, and, of course, water contribute to daily fluid needs. But what is the best type of fluid for preventing dehydration prior to and during activity? What about for rehydrating your body after activity? For these purposes, not all beverages are equal.

hypothermia Drop in body temperature to below normal.

TABLE 16.5	ACSM Hydration Recommendations	
When?	**How Much Fluid?**
4 hours before exercise	16–20 fl oz (2–2 1/2 cups)
10–15 minutes before exercise	8–12 fl oz (1–1 1/2 cups)
At 15- to 20-minute intervals when exercising less than 60 minutes	3–8 fl oz (3/8–1 cup)
At 15- to 20-minute intervals when exercising more than 60 minutes	3–8 fl oz (3/8–1 cup) sports beverage (5–8 percent carbohydrate with electrolytes)
After exercise for every pound of body weight lost	20–24 fl oz (2 1/2–3 cups)

Source: Simpson, Michael R., and Tom Howard. 2011. *Selecting and Effectively Using Hydration for Fitness.* Copyright © 2011 by the American College of Sports Medicine. Reprinted with permission.

Sports drinks are popular in the fitness world and are often marketed to all people, not just athletes. They replace fluid and electrolytes that are lost through sweating, which is vital to prevent or treat muscle cramps associated with exercise. Sports drinks have been shown to be superior to water for rehydration, mostly because their flavor causes people to drink more than they would of just plain water.[49]

Sports drinks typically contain sodium and potassium, two electrolytes that are critical in muscle contraction and maintaining fluid balance. The concentration of electrolytes found in sports drinks will differ depending on the manufacturer.

Sports drinks also provide carbohydrate to prevent glycogen depletion. This is beneficial during long endurance events or exercise when glycogen stores may be running low. Consuming sports drinks during exercise provides glucose, which can be used as an immediate energy source and prevent further decline in muscle glycogen stores. The amount of carbohydrate in sports drinks (6–8 percent) is formulated for optimal absorption, which makes them preferred over other beverages, such as soft drinks and fruit juice, which have higher concentrations and different types of carbohydrate.

However, not everyone needs sports drinks to stay adequately hydrated. For exercise that lasts less than 60 minutes, water can sufficiently replace fluids lost through sweating and food consumption following exercise can adequately replace electrolytes. Generally, a sports drink is most beneficial when physical activity lasts longer than 60 minutes because fluids, electrolytes, and/or glucose are inevitably lost in greater amounts and need to be replenished to avoid fatigue and other negative effects on performance.[50] Sports beverages provide approximately 60 kilocalories for each 8-ounce cup, so remember that they can be a source of extra kilocalories.

Other beverages may be suboptimal for hydration during physical activity. Fruit juice and juice drinks contain a larger concentration of carbohydrate and do not hydrate the body as quickly during exercise as beverages with a lower concentration of carbohydrate (like sports drinks). However, fruit and vegetable juices can be a good choice to add simple carbohydrates and fluid after exercise. Carbonated drinks contain a large amount of water; however, the air bubbles from the carbonation can cause stomach bloating and may limit the amount of fluid consumed. In addition, fructose (the type of carbohydrate provided by carbonated soft drinks) is not as well absorbed as the glucose or sucrose that is found in sports drinks.

Though alcohol may seem like an unlikely choice for rehydration, some people drink alcoholic beverages, such as beer, in order to quench their postexercise thirst. But because alcohol is a diuretic, it can actually contribute to dehydration. Alcohol is also absorbed more quickly on an empty stomach, and therefore can impair judgment and reasoning more when consumed after exercise.

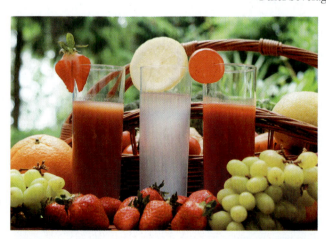

Fluids such as milk and fruit and vegetable juices can help meet daily water needs and make good postexercise beverage choices. Whole fruits and many other foods are also good sources of water.

Caffeinated beverages, such as coffee, energy drinks, and some soft drinks, contribute to the DRI for water but are not optimal sources for meeting fluid needs for physical activity. Caffeine, a diuretic, should only be consumed in moderate amounts (less than about 300 milligrams, or the amount found in three 8-ounce cups of coffee, per day) because excessive intake can cause increased heart rate, nausea and vomiting, excessive urination, restlessness, anxiety, and difficulty sleeping.[51] However, recall from Chapter 11 that caffeine does not contribute to dehydration in individuals who regularly consume it. A discussion of caffeine use during exercise is presented in the Health Connection section on page 609.

Consuming Too Little or Too Much Fluid Can Be Harmful

As the body loses fluid during physical activity, it sends signals of thirst to stimulate fluid consumption. However, by the time an individual feels thirsty, he or she may already be dehydrated. **Figure 16.6** shows the effect of dehydration on exercise performance. Athletes need to know the warning signs of dehydration so they can respond by drinking adequate fluids and prevent health consequences and impaired exercise performance.

Becoming dehydrated over a short period of time, such as during a single exercise session or sports competition, can result in **acute dehydration**. Acute dehydration most commonly occurs if an individual is not adequately hydrated before beginning a hard exercise session, especially if that person has been sick, if it is extremely hot and humid, or if the temperature is significantly different from what the person is used to. To prevent acute dehydration, follow a regimented hydration schedule using water or sports drinks to hydrate before, during, and after exercise sessions or competition.

Chronic dehydration refers to being inadequately hydrated over an extended period of time, such as during several sports practices or games. The most common warning signs of chronic dehydration include fatigue, muscle soreness, poor recovery from a workout, headaches, and nausea. Very dark urine and infrequent bathroom trips (less than every

acute dehydration Dehydration that sets in after a short period of time.

chronic dehydration Dehydration over a long period of time.

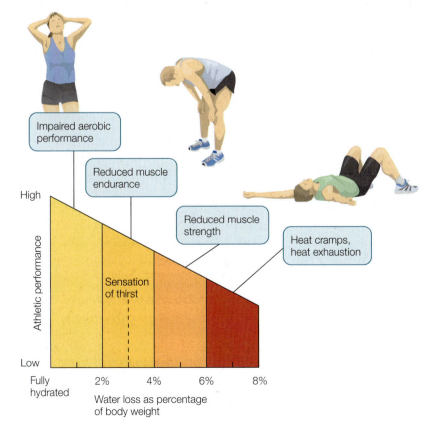

◄ **Figure 16.6 Effects of Dehydration on Exercise Performance**
Failing to stay hydrated during exercise or competition can result in fatigue and cramps and, in extreme cases, heat exhaustion. Because the thirst mechanism doesn't kick in until after dehydration has begun, replacing fluids throughout physical activity is important.
Source: Adapted from L. Burke. 2007. *Practical Sports Nutrition.* Champaign, IL: Human Kinetics.

Are You Meeting Your Fitness Recommendations and Eating for Exercise?

Now that you know how to plan an effective fitness strategy and eat for optimal fitness and performance, think about your current dietary and exercise habits. Take this brief assessment to find out if your daily habits are as healthful as they could be:

1. Do you participate in at least 60 minutes of moderately intense physical activity during the week?

   Yes ☐ **No** ☐

2. Do you participate in strength training two to three times per week?

   Yes ☐ **No** ☐

3. Do you drink 6–12 ounces of fluid every 15–20 minutes during exercise?

   Yes ☐ **No** ☐

4. Do you drink a sports beverage after moderate- or high-intensity exercise lasting longer than 1 hour?

   Yes ☐ **No** ☐

5. Do you consume carbohydrate and protein within 30–45 minutes after stopping exercise?

   Yes ☐ **No** ☐

Answer

If you answered "yes" to all of the questions, you are well on your way to optimal fitness. Participating in regular exercise, including aerobic exercise and strength training, helps you maintain optimal health and improves your level of fitness. Eating and drinking adequate nutrients also improves fitness. If you answered "no" to any of the questions, review this chapter to learn more on fitness and eating for exercise.

3 or 4 hours) can be signs of chronic dehydration. As with acute dehydration, following a regimented hydration schedule throughout the day helps prevent chronic dehydration.

When speaking of hydration and physical activity, we are usually concerned about consuming *enough* fluids so that we do not become dehydrated. However, consuming *too much* fluid without sufficient electrolytes can also be harmful. Symptoms of severe hyponatremia (review Chapter 11) occur more often in those who participate in endurance sports or prolonged exercise periods (greater than 4 hours), in which fluid and sodium loss is more likely.

If you are a distance runner, see the Calculation Corner for a hydration test to determine your fluid needs during long-distance races.[52] Keep in mind that you should perform this hydration test well before a competition or event, and perform the test again if your level of fitness improves or if the climate changes from when you initially determined fluid needs.

Take the nearby Self-Assessment to determine if you are meeting exercise and dietary recommendations.

> **LO 16.6: THE TAKE-HOME MESSAGE** Being adequately hydrated before, during, and after exercise is important to sustain fluid and electrolyte balance and a normal body temperature. Inadequate hydration can impair performance. Water is the preferred beverage for hydration, but sports drinks can be beneficial during moderate- or vigorous-intensity exercise lasting more than 60 minutes. Overhydration can be just as important to avoid as dehydration, but is more likely to occur among people engaging in endurance sports or prolonged exercise.

Calculation Corner

Fluid Needs for Distance Runners

The next time you take a 1-hour training run, use the following process to determine your fluid needs.

(1) Make sure that you are properly hydrated before the workout. Your urine should be colorless.

(2) Do a warm-up run to the point where you start to sweat, then stop. Urinate if necessary.

(3) Weigh yourself on an accurate scale.

(4) Run for 1 hour at an intensity similar to your targeted race.

(5) Drink a measured amount of a beverage of your choice during the run to quench your thirst. Be sure to keep track of how much you drink.

(6) Do not urinate during the run.

(7) After you have finished the run, weigh yourself again on the same scale you used in step 3.

(8) Calculate your fluid needs using the following formula:

   a. Enter your body weight from step 3 in pounds _____

   b. Enter your body weight from step 7 in pounds _____

   c. Subtract b. from a. _____

   d. Convert the pounds of weight in c. to fluid ounces by multiplying by 15.3 _____

   e. Enter the amount of fluid you consumed during the run in ounces _____

   f. Add e. to d. _____

The final figure is the number of ounces of fluid that you must consume per hour to remain well hydrated.

Source: D. Casa. 2007. *USATF Self-Testing Program for Optimal Hydration,* from the USA Track and Field website. Copyright © 2007 by Douglas Casa. Reprinted with permission of the author.

HEALTH**CONNECTION**

Can Ergogenic Aids Contribute to Exercise Performance and Fitness?

LO 16.7 Identify the most common ergogenic aids and summarize the current research on their benefits and side effects.

Competitive athletes are always looking for an edge, and many turn to supplements in the hope of improving their performance. Supplement manufacturers may claim that their products enhance immunity, boost metabolism, improve memory, or provide some other physical enhancement. Because the Food and Drug Administration does not strictly regulate dietary supplements, however, manufacturers do not have to prove the validity of these claims or the safety or quality of their products. As a result, many athletes risk their health and, in some cases, eligibility for competition by taking supplements that can be ineffective or even dangerous.

The term **ergogenic aid** describes any substance used to improve athletic performance, including dietary supplements. Research studying the effects of several supplements on athletic performance have indicated that some have a positive effect on performance, whereas others do not. Furthermore, some ergogenic aids cause serious side effects.

Creatine Monohydrate Improves Muscle Strength, Muscle Mass, and Anaerobic Metabolism during Some Activities

Creatine monohydrate is one of the most well-known dietary supplements in the fitness industry today. In the early 1990s, some research found that creatine

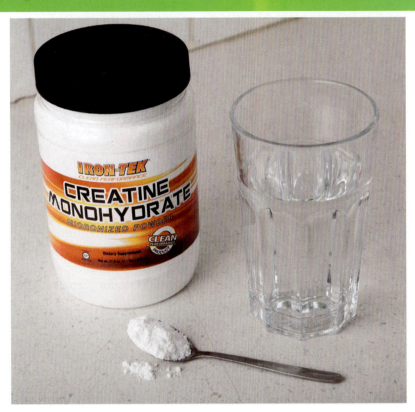

Athletes sometimes take creatine monohydrate, such as Iron-Tek, or caffeine supplements, to enhance their athletic performance. Supplements are not regulated by the FDA, so their quality and effectiveness can vary widely.

monohydrate supplementation increased creatine stores in the muscles (in the form of creatine phosphate), which increased the amount of ATP generated and improved performance during high-intensity, short-duration exercise.[53]

However, the results of later studies on whether creatine monohydrate supplements enhance performance have been mixed. Studies have supported the hypothesis that creatine monohydrate supplementation improves athletic performance in high-intensity, short-duration activities such as weight training, when the body relies on anaerobic energy metabolism and increased muscle strength and muscle mass.[54] But research has shown mixed results in creatine monohydrate supplementation improving sprint-running performance, with some studies showing improvement and others showing no benefit.[55,56]

The most common side effect of creatine monohydrate supplementation is water retention. However, when taken at higher than recommended doses for several months, creatine monohydrate

supplementation has been linked to liver and kidney problems.[57] Anyone considering taking creatine monohyrate supplements should check with a health care provider first.

Caffeine Improves Perception and Aerobic Metabolism

Caffeine has become popular as an ergogenic aid among athletes, trainers, and coaches. Caffeine may decrease perception of effort by stimulating the central nervous system, directly affect the breakdown of muscle glycogen, and increase the availability of fatty acids during exercise, therefore sparing glycogen stores.

Studies on the effects of drinking caffeine prior to exercise have shown that caffeine enhances athletic performance, mostly during endurance events.[58] However,

ergogenic aid Substance, such as a dietary supplement, used to enhance athletic performance.

research has not shown that caffeine provides any benefit during short-duration activities, such as sprinting.[59]

Some athletic associations consider caffeine a banned substance when consumed in high amounts. For example, the National Collegiate Athletic Association (NCAA) classifies caffeine as a banned substance only when urine concentrations exceed 15 micrograms per milliliter. Because individuals weigh different amounts and metabolize caffeine at different rates, it is difficult to determine how many cups of coffee or another caffeinated beverage it would take to test positive for caffeine.

Bicarbonate Loading May Improve Anaerobic Metabolism during Exercise

Athletes who participate in anaerobic, high-intensity sports, including sprint cycling, 400- or 800-meter sprints, and swimming, strive to find ways to buffer lactate buildup during their event. Recall from Chapter 8 that anaerobic metabolism involves the conversion of glucose to pyruvate. When there is insufficient oxygen, pyruvate is reduced to lactate and results in hydrogen ion buildup in the muscle cell and a drop in pH. The more acidic pH inhibits muscle contraction and the phosphorylation of ADP to form ATP, leading to muscle fatigue.

Sodium bicarbonate, or baking soda, has been reported to buffer or neutralize the acid in the blood and improve performance.[60] Some research presented positive results when sodium bicarbonate was ingested pre-exercise. For example, ingestion of sodium bicarbonate significantly reduced fatigue in intermittent repeated sprint performance,[61] improved maximal sprint swimming performance,[62] and improved the number of accumulated repetitions in weightlifters.[63]

Unfortunately, there are side effects with ingesting sodium bicarbonate. Some subjects have reported nausea, bloating, and gastric reflux within an hour of consumption.

Diarrhea, flatulence, and intestinal discomfort have also been reported.[64]

Amino Acid Supplementation Shows Some Benefit

Amino acid supplements have become popular as ergogenic aids. For resistance-trained athletes, amino acid powders and pills have been proposed to enhance muscle synthesis and accelerate recovery following exercise. Endurance athletes take amino acid supplements to improve their physiological response during endurance exercise and training. Do these supplements work?

Numerous research studies have tested the benefits of ingesting branched-chain amino acid (BCAA) supplements (leucine, isoleucine, and valine) to enhance exercise performance. These studies have failed to demonstrate any benefit of BCAAs during exercise. However, some evidence suggests that these amino acids may improve muscle recovery after exercise and support the immune system.[65]

A few other amino acid supplements show promise. Beta-alanine has been shown to buffer hydrogen ions produced during high-intensity intermittent exercise

and to improve endurance performance and lean body mass.[66] Carnitine reduces free-radical formation during exercise, reduces muscle damage, and improves muscle recovery after exercise.[67] The amino acid leucine taken as a supplement after endurance exercise may improve protein synthesis and muscle recovery.[68] Glutamine supplementation may help maintain the immune system,[69] improve glucose utilization, and stimulate muscle glycogen synthesis postexercise.[70] Glutamine has not been shown, however, to reduce muscle soreness or improve muscle repair.[71]

It is important to avoid single amino acid supplementation because high doses of individual amino acids can compete for one another in the body and impair protein synthesis. If athletes want to try amino acid supplements, they should look for a multi–amino acid formula that is balanced.

Sports Bars and Shakes May Provide Some Nutritional Benefits

Sports bars and shakes are not defined as dietary supplements by the FDA because they are more like food and contain one

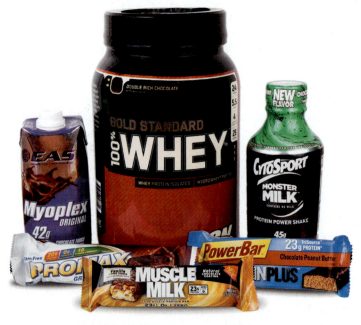

Sports bars and shakes, such as PowerBar, Gold Standard, CyroSport, Myoplex, Muscle Milk, and Promax, should supplement—not replace—whole, nutritious foods.

or more macronutrients. However, people often refer to these items as supplements because they are typically eaten in addition to whole-food meals and snacks.

The main energy source in most commercial sports bars and shakes is carbohydrate, with protein and fat contributing smaller amounts of energy. The ratio of the macronutrients in these foods varies depending on the purpose. Bars and shakes that are intended to provide energy for and recovery from exercise have a greater proportion of carbohydrates.

Those that are promoted for muscle protein synthesis typically contain more protein. Vegetarians and some athletes who need additional sources of protein in their diet often use bars and shakes that are high in protein. Most bars and shakes also contain a variety of vitamins and minerals. These vitamins and minerals may not be necessary for individuals who consume regular, balanced meals or take a daily multivitamin.

Sports bars and shakes can be convenient, but they are often expensive.

An energy bar may be trendy and easy to stash in a gym bag, but an old-fashioned peanut butter sandwich on whole-grain bread would cost less, fit a vegan athlete's diet, and be just as easy to carry. In addition, when athletes consume dietary protein within the recommended guidelines, there is little scientific evidence that adding more protein through sports bars and shakes enhances exercise performance. Overall, it is best to limit intakes of commercial sports bars and shakes so that they don't become a substitute for whole, nutritious foods.

LO 16.7: THE TAKE-HOME MESSAGE Dietary supplements and ergogenic aids may enhance performance, but can have side effects. Creatine improves performance during high-intensity, short-duration exercise and increases muscle strength and muscle mass, but causes water retention and at high doses may negatively affect liver and kidney function. Caffeine may decrease perception of effort by stimulating the central nervous system and improve endurance performance by sparing glycogen stores and increasing fatty-acid utilization during exercise. The NCAA bans caffeine in high amounts. Sodium bicarbonate buffers the blood and improves anaerobic performance in some sports, but can cause unpleasant gastrointestinal side effects. Some amino acid supplements, including branched-chain amino acids, alanine, carnitine, leucine, and glutamine, may show some benefit in improving muscle recovery but should not be taken as individual amino acids. Sports bars and shakes are convenient sources of energy, but are often more expensive than whole foods and are not necessary in a healthy diet.

Visual Chapter Summary

LO 16.1 Physical Fitness Includes Five Components for Health

Physical fitness, defined as good health or physical condition, includes five basic components: cardiorespiratory endurance, muscular strength, muscular endurance, flexibility, and body composition. Physical activity reduces the risk of developing type 2 diabetes, some forms of cancer, and cardiovascular disease. It improves body composition, bone health, immune function, mental well-being, and sleep and reduces stress.

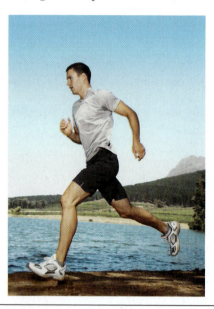

LO 16.2 A Successful Physical Fitness Program Uses FITT Principles

Fitness programs generally incorporate activities that are based on the five components of fitness, including aerobic exercise, resistance training, and stretching. FITT is an acronym for frequency (how often), intensity (degree of difficulty or effort), time (how long), and type (specific activity). Rating of perceived exertion (RPE) and target heart rate are used to measure intensity for cardiorespiratory exercise, while repetition maximum (RM) measures intensity for weight training.

A successful fitness program should be tailored to meet the needs of the individual and performed consistently so that any gains in fitness are maintained. The progressive overload principle of gradually increasing the exercise demands placed on the body will improve fitness levels over time.

Minimize Sedentary Activities

2–3 days/week Flexibility and muscular fitness

3–5 days/week Cardiorespiratory Moderate–high intensity

Daily Low–moderate intensity

LO 16.3 Carbohydrate, Fat, and Protein Fuel Exercise

The body uses carbohydrate, fat, and protein during exercise. The source of energy used depends on the intensity and duration of the activity and an individual's current fitness level.

The body relies heavily on anaerobic energy from ATP and creatine phosphate (PCr) during the first few seconds of exercise. As exercise continues, the body relies on aerobic production of ATP mainly from carbohydrate obtained from blood glucose and stored glycogen, fatty acids stored in muscle tissue, and free fatty acids in the blood derived from lipolysis. Fat supplies nearly all of the energy required during rest and low- to moderate-intensity activity.

Protein primarily functions to maintain, build, and repair tissues, including muscle tissue. As long as the diet is adequate in total kilocalories, carbohydrate, and fat, only small amounts of protein are used for energy during exercise.

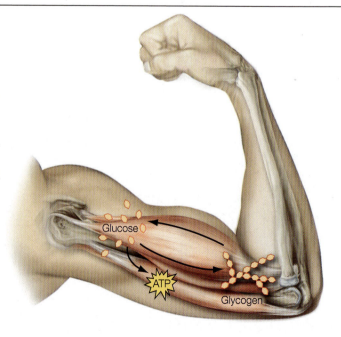

Glucose

ATP

Glycogen

LO 16.4 Timing and Composition of Meals Affects Fitness Performance

The timing of meals before, during, and after exercise influences energy levels, performance, and recovery time. Consuming both carbohydrate (about 150–300 grams) and small amounts of protein up to 4 hours before exercise produces a greater increase in muscle glycogen synthesis, promotes greater endurance, and results in greater protein synthesis after exercise is over. Ingesting 1 gram of carbohydrate per kilogram of body weight 15–30 minutes prior to the start of exercise gives muscles an immediate source of energy, spares glycogen stores, and protects muscles from damage. For longer events, 30–60 grams of carbohydrate should be consumed per hour of activity. As much as 90 grams of carbohydrate per hour may be necessary for ultra-endurance events.

Consumed within the first 30–45 minutes postexercise, 0.3–0.6 grams of carbohydrate per pound of body weight helps replenish glycogen stores and stimulates muscle protein synthesis. Carbohydrate and protein in a ratio of 4:1 (in grams) after exercise results in increased muscle protein synthesis, with protein intake immediately following exercise resulting in greater muscle protein synthesis.

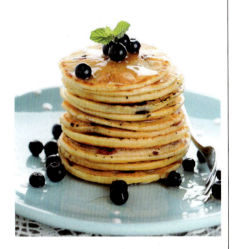

LO 16.5 Some Vitamins and Minerals May Improve Athletic Performance

Thiamin, riboflavin, niacin, pantothenic acid, and vitamin B_6 assist as coenzymes in energy metabolism. Folate, vitamin B_{12}, and iron contribute to healthy red blood cells that deliver oxygen to the cells for aerobic metabolism.

Antioxidants, such as vitamins E and C and selenium, can protect cells from damage by free radicals; however, consuming high levels of these in supplement form has not been shown to improve athletic performance or decrease oxidative stress. Athletes are at greater risk of developing iron deficiency and should consume iron-rich foods regularly. Athletes also need to be sure their calcium intake is adequate to help reduce their risk of bone fractures during physical activity.

Athletes do not have greater needs for vitamins and minerals than do nonathletes, and intakes above the RDA do not improve athletic performance. Supplements containing vitamins and minerals are not necessary when adequate amounts are obtained through a varied diet.

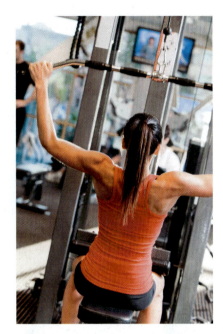

LO 16.6 Fluid Intake Affects Fitness and Performance

Being adequately hydrated before, during, and after exercise helps maintain fluid and electrolyte balance and normal body temperature. Sports drinks that contain a 6–8 percent concentration of carbohydrates, as well as electrolytes, are beneficial for moderate- to vigorous-intensity exercise lasting 60 minutes or more to replace fluid and electrolytes and provide carbohydrates for fuel. For exercise that lasts less than 60 minutes, water can sufficiently replace fluids lost through sweating, and food consumption following exercise can adequately replace electrolytes. Dehydration and overhydration should both be avoided because they can be harmful to health.

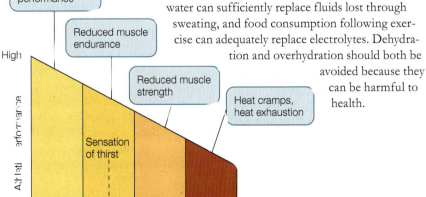

LO 16.7 Some Ergogenic Aids Can Contribute to Fitness

Dietary supplements, including ergogenic aids, are not regulated for their safety and efficacy; individuals who choose to use them may be placing their health, and possibly their eligibility for competition, at risk. Creatine improves performance during high-intensity, short-duration exercise and increases muscle strength and muscle mass, but causes water retention and may impair liver and kidney function when taken at high doses. Caffeine has been shown to improve endurance performance by sparing glycogen stores and increasing fatty-acid utilization, and may decrease perception of effort, but has not shown any benefit in activities of short duration. The NCAA restricts caffeine during competition. Sodium bicarbonate buffers the blood and improves anaerobic performance in some sports, but causes unpleasant gastrointestinal side effects. Amino acid supplements including branched-chain amino acids, alanine, carnitine, leucine, and glutamine have demonstrated some benefit in improving muscle recovery, but amino acids should be taken in a balanced formula rather than as single amino acids. Sports bars and shakes are convenient but expensive sources of energy, carbohydrate, and protein.

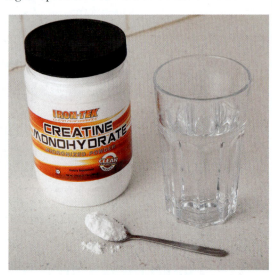

Terms to Know

- physical fitness
- physical activity
- exercise
- cardiorespiratory endurance
- muscular strength
- muscular endurance
- resistance training
- flexibility
- overexercise
- stroke volume
- VO_2max
- cardiorespiratory conditioning
- conditioning
- intensity
- rating of perceived exertion (RPE)
- target heart rate
- repetition maximum (RM)
- high-intensity interval training (HIIT)
- progressive overload principle
- atrophy
- carbohydrate loading
- sports anemia
- relative energy deficiency in sport (RED-S)
- amenorrhea
- hyperthermia
- hypothermia
- acute dehydration
- chronic dehydration
- ergogenic aid

Mastering Nutrition
Visit the Study Area in Mastering Nutrition to hear an MP3 chapter summary.

Check Your Understanding

LO16.1 1. Which of the following is one of the five components of physical fitness?
   a. Hydration
   b. Cardiorespiratory endurance
   c. Stress
   d. Body mass index

LO16.2 2. Gradually increasing the exercise demands on the body is called
   a. cardiorespiratory endurance.
   b. VO_2max.
   c. progressive overload.
   d. hypertrophy.

LO16.3 3. Well-trained muscles have the ability to store
   a. an unlimited amount of glycogen.
   b. up to 100 grams of glycogen.
   c. up to 300 grams of glycogen.
   d. up to 500 grams of glycogen.

LO16.3 4. During the first few minutes of physical activity the body relies on anaerobic energy production from ATP and what other high-energy molecule?
   a. Adenosine phosphate
   b. GTP
   c. Creatine phosphate
   d. GMP

LO16.3 5. Under what conditions does the body use significant amounts of protein for energy during exercise?
   a. Inadequate kilocalorie and fluid intake
   b. Inadequate carbohydrate and protein stores
   c. Inadequate protein stores and fluid intake
   d. Inadequate kilocalorie intake and carbohydrate stores

LO16.4 6. A pregame meal should be
   a. high in carbohydrate, low in fat.
   b. high in carbohydrate and high in fat.
   c. low in carbohydrate, high in fat.
   d. low in protein, high in fat.

LO16.4 7. How much carbohydrate should you consume 15–30 minutes before an activity to give muscles an immediate source of energy?
   a. 1 gram of carbohydrate per kilogram of body weight
   b. 2 grams of carbohydrate per kilogram of body weight
   c. 5 grams of carbohydrate per kilogram of body weight
   d. 7 grams of carbohydrate per kilogram of body weight

LO16.5 8. Athletes should take a daily vitamin and mineral supplement to improve their overall exercise performance.
   a. True
   b. False

LO16.6 9. An appropriate exercise recovery beverage would be
   a. a soft drink.
   b. coffee.
   c. low-fat chocolate milk.
   d. orange juice.

LO16.7 10. Which ergogenic aid can cause water retention and potentially kidney and liver problems if taken in high doses over an extended period of time?
   a. Creatine monohydrate
   b. Sodium bicarbonate
   c. Caffeine
   d. Amino acid supplements

Answers

1. (b) Cardiorespiratory endurance, muscular strength, muscular endurance, body composition, and flexibility are the five basic components of physical fitness. Hydration, stress, and body mass index are not components of physical fitness.

2. (c) The progressive overload principle allows an individual to improve his or her performance as the body adapts to increasingly difficult physical activity. Cardiorespiratory endurance is one aspect of physical fitness. VO_2max is the maximum amount of oxygen a person uses in 1 minute, and hypertrophy is the building of new muscle mass.

3. (d) Muscles that are well trained are able to store about 20–50 percent more glycogen than normal, or up to 500 grams; however, the storage capacity is limited.

4. (c) Creatine phosphate is another source of phosphate to regenerate ATP from ADP during high-intensity exercise.

5. (d) The body uses larger amounts of protein for energy if overall kilocalorie intake is inadequate and if carbohydrate stores are low. Fluid intake does not affect the use of protein for energy during exercise.

6. (a) A meal before a game or workout should be high in carbohydrate to maximize glycogen stores and low in fat to prevent feelings of fatigue or discomfort.

7. (a) One gram of carbohydrate per kilogram of body weight is the recommended amount to provide an immediate source of energy for the muscles.

8. (b) Ingesting vitamin or mineral supplements does not improve athletic performance. Athletes should focus on obtaining sufficient vitamins and minerals by consuming a variety of foods.

9. (c) Low-fat chocolate milk is a good exercise recovery beverage because it contains an appropriate ratio of carbohydrate and protein that is necessary for optimal recovery. Soft drinks, coffee, and orange juice provide the body with fluids, but lack sufficient protein that is ideal for recovery after exercise.

10. (a) Creatine monohydrate improves short, high-intensity anaerobic exercise but also increases water retention and may result in liver and kidney problems.

Answers to True or False?

1. **False.** Fewer than half of all Americans meet recommendations for physical activity.

2. **True.** According to the *2008 Physical Activity Guidelines*, as little as 60 minutes of physical activity per week bestows health benefits, including improved bone health and lowered risk of certain diseases.

3. **True.** The body does use carbohydrate, fat, and protein for energy during exercise, but the amount of each that is used partly depends on the intensity of the exercise.

4. **True.** The body prefers to use fat as its primary fuel source during low- to moderate-intensity exercise.

5. **True.** Consumption of nutrients immediately after stopping exercise will improve recovery.

6. **False.** Taking vitamin and/or mineral supplements is only beneficial if an individual is deficient in vitamins or minerals.

7. **True.** Female and vegetarian athletes in particular are at higher risk for iron deficiency.

8. **False.** Sports drinks are generally beneficial only when exercise lasts for longer than 1 hour.

9. **False.** Overhydration can dilute the blood and alter the body's delicate fluid and electrolyte balance.

10. **True.** Caffeine is a banned substance at urine concentrations of more than 15 micrograms per milliliter.

Web Resources

- For more information on The President's Council on Fitness, Sports, and Nutrition, visit www.fitness.gov
- For more information on exercise, presented by the American Council on Exercise, visit www.acefitness.org
- For more information from the American College of Sports Medicine, go to www.acsm.org
- For more information on nutrition and fitness, visit the Academy of Nutrition and Dietetics at www.eatright.org
- For more information from Sports, Cardiovascular, and Wellness Nutrition, a dietetic practice group of the Academy of Nutrition and Dietetics, visit www.scandpg.org
- For more information on the National Collegiate Athletic Association, go to www.ncaa.org

References

1. Centers for Disease Control and Prevention. 2014. *Facts About Physical Activity.* Available at www.cdc.gov. Accessed April 2017.
2. U.S. Department of Health and Human Services. 2008. *Physical Activity Guidelines for Americans.* Available at www.health.gov/paguidelines. Accessed April 2017.

3. Sagatun, Å., Heyerdahl, S., Wentzel-Larsen, T., and Lien, L. (2015). Medical Benefits in Young Adulthood: A Population-Based Longitudinal Study of Health Behaviour and Mental Health in Adolescence and Later Receipt of Medical Benefits. *BMJ Open* 5(5):e007139. doi: 10.1136/bmjopen-2014-007139.

4. Kenney, W. L., J. H. Wilmore, and D. L. Costill. 2015. *Physiology of Sport and Exercise.* 6th ed. Champaign, IL: Human Kinetics.

5. Astrand, P., K. Rodahl, H. A. Dahl, and S. B. Stromme. 2003. *The Textbook of Work Physiology: Physiological Bases of Exercise.* 4th ed. Champaign, IL: Human Kinetics.

6. U.S. Department of Health and Human Services. 2008. *Physical Activity Guidelines for Americans.*

7. Kong, Z., Sun, S., Liu, M., and Shi, Q. 2016. Short-Term High-Intensity Interval Training on Body Composition and Blood Glucose in Overweight and Obese Young Women. *Journal of Diabetes Research* 2016:4073618. doi: 10.1155/2016/4073618.

8. Cruz, R. S., R. A. de Aguiar, T. Turnes, R. Penteado Dos Santos, M. F. de Oliveira, and F. Caputo. 2012. Intracellular Shuttle: The Lactate Aerobic Metabolism. *Scientific World Journal.* doi: 10.1100/2012/420984.

9. Thum, Jacob S. et al. 2017. High-Intensity Interval Training Elicits Higher Enjoyment than Moderate Intensity Continuous Exercise. *PLoS ONE* 12(1):e0166299.

10. Osawa Y, Azuma K, Tabata S, et al. 2014. Effects of 16-Week High-Intensity Interval Training Using Upper and Lower Body Ergometers on Aerobic Fitness and Morphological Changes in Healthy Men: A Preliminary Study. *Open Access Journal of Sports Medicine* 5:257–265. doi: 10.2147/OAJSM.S68932.

11. Cruz, R. S., R. A. de Aguiar, T. Turnes, R. Penteado Dos Santos, M. F. de Oliveira, and F. Caputo. 2012. Intracellular Shuttle: The Lactate Aerobic Metabolism.

12. Eskelinen, J. J., Heinonen, I., Löyttyniemi, E., et al. 2016. Left Ventricular Vascular and Metabolic Adaptations to High-intensity Interval and Moderate Intensity Continuous Training: A Randomized Trial in Healthy Middle-aged Men. *Journal of Physiology* 594(23):7127–7140. doi: 10.1113/JP273089.

13. Katz, A. 2016. Role of Reactive Oxygen Species in Regulation of Glucose Transport in Skeletal Muscle During Exercise. *Journal of Physiology* 594(11):2787–2794. doi: 10.1113/JP271665.

14. Knuiman, P., Hopman, M. T., and Mensink, M. 2015. Glycogen Availability and Skeletal Muscle Adaptations with Endurance and Resistance Exercise. *Nutrition and Metabolism* 12:59. doi: 10.1186/s12986-015-0055-9.

15. Marquet, L. A., Brisswalter, J., Louis, J., et al. 2016. Enhanced Endurance Performance by Periodization of Carbohydrate Intake: "Sleep Low" Strategy. *Medicine and Science in Sports and Exercise* 48(4):663–672. doi: 10.1249/MSS.0000000000000823.

16. Alghannam, A. F., Jedrzejewski, D., Bilzon, J., et al. 2016. Influence of Post-Exercise Carbohydrate-Protein Ingestion on Muscle Glycogen Metabolism in Recovery and Subsequent Running Exercise. *International Journal of Sport Nutrition and Exercise Metabolism* 26(6):572–580. doi: 10.1123/ijsnem.2016-0021.

17. Jensen, et al. 2012. Regulation of Glucose and Glycogen Metabolism.

18. American College of Sports Medicine, American Dietetic Association, and Dietitians of Canada. 2016. Nutrition and Athletic Performance Joint Position Statement. Available at http://www.dietitians.ca. Accessed April 2017.

19. Ibid.

20. da Silva Santos, J. F., Takito, M. Y., Artioli, G. G., and Franchini, E. 2016. Weight Loss Practices in Taekwondo Athletes of Different Competititve Levels. *Journal of Exercise Rehabilitation* 12(3):202–208. doi: 10.12965/jer.1632610.305.

21. Horvath, P. J., C. K. Eagen, S. D. Ryer-Calvin, and D. R. Pendergast. 2000. The Effects of Varying Dietary Fat on the Nutrient Intake in Male and Female Runners. *Journal of the American College of Nutrition* 19:42–51.

22. American College of Sports Medicine, et al. 2016. Nutrition and Athletic Performance Joint Position Statement.

23. Cermak, N. M., and van Loon, L. J. 2013. The Use of Carbohydrates During Exercise as an Ergogenic Aid. *Sports Medicine* 43(11):1139–1155. doi: 10.1007/s40279-013-0079-0.

24. Alghannam, A. F., Jedrzejewski, D., Tweddle, M. G., et al. 2016. Impact of Muscle Glycogen Availability on the Capacity for Repeated Exercise in Man. *Medicine and Science in Sports and Exercise* 48(1):123–131. doi: 10.1249/MSS.0000000000000737.

25. Cermak, N. M., and L. J. van Loon. 2013. The Use of Carbohydrates during Exercise as an Ergogenic Aid. *Sports Medicine* 43(11):1139–1155.

26. Miller, S. L., K. D. Tipton, D. L. Chinkes, S. E. Wolf, and R. R. Wolfe. 2003. Independent and Combined Effects of Amino Acids and Glucose after Resistance Exercise. *Medicine and Science in Sports and Exercise* 35:449–455.

27. Temesi, J., N. A. Johnson, J. Raymond, C. A. Burdon, and H. T. O'Connor. 2011. Carbohydrate Ingestion during Endurance Exercise Improves Performance in Adults. *Journal of Nutrition* 141(5):890–897.

28. Ibid.

29. Heung-Sang Wong, S., Sun, F. H., Chen, Y. J., et al. 2017. Effect of Pre-Exercise Carbohydrate Diets with High vs Low Glycemic Index on Exercise Performance: A Meta-analysis. *Nutrition Reviews.* doi: 10.1093/nutrit/nux003.

30. Hawkins, K. H., Krishnan, S., Ringos, L., Garcia, V., and Cooper, J. A. 2017. Running Performance with Nutritive and Non-Nutritive Sweetened Mouth Rinses. *International Journal of Sports Physiology and Performance* 1–23. doi: 10.1123/ijspp.2016-0577.

31. Stellingwerff, T., and G. R. Cox. 2014. Systematic Review: Carbohydrate Supplementation on Exercise Performance or Capacity of Varying Durations. *Applied Physiology, Nutrition, and Metabolism* 25:1–14.

32. Williamson, E. 2016. Nutritional Implications for Ultra-Endurance Walking and Running Events. *Extreme Physiology and Medicine* 5:13.

33. Alghannam, A. F., Jedrzejewski, D., Bilzon, J., et al. 2016. Influence of Post-Exercise Carbohydrate-Protein Ingestion on Muscle Glycogen Metabolism in Recovery and Subsequent Running Exercise. *International Journal of Sport Nutrition and Exercise Metabolism* 26(6):572–580. doi: 10.1123/ijsnem.2016-0021.

34. Phillips, S. M. 2016. The Impact of Protein Quality on the Promotion of Resistance Exercise-Induced Changes in Muscle Mass. *Nutrition and Metabolism* 13:64.

35. Witard, O. C., Cocke, T. L., Fernando, A. A., Wolfe R. R., and Tipton, K. D. 2014. Increased Net Muscle Protein Balance in Response to Simulataneous and Separate Ingestion of Carbohydrate and Essential Amino Acids Following Resistance Exercise. *Applied Physiology, Nutrition and Metabolism* 39(3):329–339. doi: 10.1139/apnm-2013-0264.

36. Rustad, P. I., Sailer, M., Cumming, K, T,, et al. 2016. Intake of Protein Plus Carbohydrate during the First Two Hours after Exhaustive Cycling Improves Performance the Following Day. *PLoS ONE* 11(4):e0153229. doi: 10.1371/journal.pone.0153229.

37. Beck, K. L., Thomson, J. S., Swift, R. J., and von Hurst, P. R. (2015). Role of nutrition in performance enhancement and postexercise recovery. *Open Access Journal of Sports Medicine* 6:259–267. doi: 10.2147/OAJSM.S33605.

38. Pritchett, K., and R. Pritchett. 2012. Chocolate Milk: A Post-Exercise Recovery Beverage for Endurance Sports. *Medicine and Sport Science* 59:127–134.

39. Joy, J. M., R. P. Lowery, J. M. Wilson, M. Purpura, E. O. De Souza, S. M. C. Wilson, D. S. Kalman, et al. 2013. The Effects of 8 Weeks of Whey or Rice Protein Supplementation on Body Composition and Exercise Performance. *Nutrition Journal.* doi:10.1186/1475-2891-12-86.

40. Temesi, et al. 2011. Carbohydrate Ingestion during Endurance Exercise Improves Performance in Adults.

41. Mariacher, C., H. Gatterer, J. Greilberger, R. Djukic, M. Greilberger, M. Philippe, and M. Burtscher. 2014. Effects of Antioxidant Supplementation on Exercise Performance in Acute Normobaric Hypoxia. *International Journal of Sport Nutrition and Exercise Metabolism* 24:227–235.

42. Alaunyte, I., Stojceska, V., and Plunkett, A. (2015). Iron and the Female Athlete: A Review of Dietary Treatment Methods for Improving Iron Status and Exercise Performance. *Journal of the International Society*

of Sports Nutrition 12:38. doi: 10.1186/s12970-015-0099-2.

43. Łagowska, K., Kapczuk, K., Friebe, Z., and Bajerska, J. (2014). Effects of Dietary Intervention in Young Female Athletes with Menstrual Disorders. *Journal of the International Society of Sports Nutrition* 11:21. doi: 10.1186/1550-2783-11-21.

44. Alaunyte, I., Stojceska, V., and Plunkett, A. (2015). Iron and the Female Athlete.

45. Nasri, R., S. Hassen Zrour, H. Rebai, F. Neffeti, M. F. Najjar, N. Bergaoui, H. Mejdoub, and Z. Tabka. 2013. Combat Sports Practice Favors Bone Mineral Density among Adolescent Male Athletes. *Journal of Clinical Densitometry.* doi: 10.1016/j.jocd.2013.09.012.

46. Darvishi, L., G. Askari, M. Hariri, M. Bahreynian, R. Ghiasvand, S. Ehsani, N. S. Mashhadi, et al. 2013. The Use of Nutritional Supplements among Male Collegiate Athletes. *International Journal of Preventive Medicine* 4(Suppl. 1):S68–S72.

47. Fry, A. C., R. J. Bloomer, M. J. Falvo, C. A. Moore, B. K. Schilling, and L. W. Weiss. 2006. Effect of a Liquid Multivitamin/Mineral Supplement on Anaerobic Exercise Performance. *Research in Sports Medicine* 14(1):53–64.

48. Rosenbloom, C., and E. J. Coleman, eds. 2012. *Sports Nutrition: A Practice Manual for Professionals.* Chicago: IL: Academy of Nutrition and Dietetics.

49. Driller M. W., Gregory J. R., Williams A. D., and Fell J. W. 2013. The Effects of Chronic Sodium Bicarbonate Ingestion and Interval Training in Highly Trained Rowers. *International Journal of Sport Nutrition and Exercise Metabolism* 23(1):40–47.

50. American College of Sports Medicine. 2007. Exercise and Fluid Replacement. *Medicine and Science in Sports and Exercise* 39(2):377–390.

51. National Institutes of Health. 2013. *Caffeine in the Diet.* National Institutes of Health Medline Plus Medical Encyclopedia. Available at www.nlm.nih.gov/medlineplus/ency/article/002445.htm. Accessed April 2017.

52. USA Track & Field. Press Release, April 19, 2003. *USATF Announces Major Change in Hydration Guidelines.* Available at www.usatf.org/news/showRelease.asp?article=/news/releases/2003-04-19-2.xml. Accessed April 2017.

53. Kalhan, S. C., Gruca, L., Marczewski, S., Bennett, C., and Kummitha, C. (2016). Whole Body Creatine and Protein Kinetics in Healthy Men and Women: Effects of creatine and amino acid supplementation. *Amino Acids* 48(3):677–687. doi: 10.1007/s00726-015-2111-1.

54. Antonio, J., and V. Ciccone. 2013. The Effects of Pre Versus Post Workout Supplementation of Creatine Monohydrate on Body Composition and Strength. *Journal of the International Society of Sports Nutrition.* doi: 10.1186/1550-2783-10-36.

55. Williams, J., G. Abt, and A. E. Kilding. 2014. Effects of Creatine Monohydrate Supplementation on Simulated Soccer Performance. *International Journal of Sports Physiology and Performance* 9(3):503–510.

56. Antonio, J., and Ciccone, V. (2013). The effects of pre versus post workout supplementation of creatine monohydrate on body composition and strength. *Journal of the International Society of Sports Nutrition* 10:36. doi: 10.1186/1550-2783-10-36.

57. Hall, M., and T. H. Trojian. 2013. Creatine Supplementation. *Current Sports Medicine Reports* 12(4):240–244.

58. Spriet, L. L. (2014). Exercise and Sport Performance with Low Doses of Caffeine. *Sports Medicine (Auckland, New Zealand)* 44(Suppl. 2):175–184. doi: 10.1007/s40279-014-0257-8.

59. Brown, S. J., J. Brown, and A. Foskett. 2013. The Effects of Caffeine on Repeated Sprint Performance in Team Sport Athletes—A Meta-Analysis. *Sport Science Review* 22:25–32.

60. Saunders, B., C. Sale, R. C. Harris, and C. Sunderland. 2014. Effect of Sodium Bicarbonate and Beta-Alanine on Repeated Sprints during Intermittent Exercise Performed in Hypoxia. *International Journal of Sport Nutrition and Exercise Metabolism* 24:196–205.

61. Afman, G., R. M. Garside, N. Dinan, N. Gant, J. A. Betts, and C. Williams. 2014. Effect of Carbohydrate or Sodium Bicarbonate Ingestion on Performance during a Validated Basketball Simulation Test. *International Journal of Sport Nutrition and Exercise Metabolism.* doi: 10.1123/ijsnem.2013-0168.

62. Mero, A. A., P. Hirvonen, J. Saarela, J. J. Hulmi, J. R. Hoffman, and J. R. Stout. 2013. Effect of Sodium Bicarbonate and Beta-Alanine Supplementation on Maximal Sprint Swimming. *Journal of the International Society of Sports Nutrition.* doi: 10.1186/1550-2783-10-52.

63. Carr, B. M., M. J. Webster, J. C. Boyd, G. M. Hudson, and T. P. Scheet. 2013. Sodium Bicarbonate Supplementation Improves Hypertrophy-Type Resistance Exercise Performance. *European Journal of Applied Physiology* 113(3):743–752.

64. Afman, et al. 2014. Effect of Carbohydrate or Sodium Bicarbonate Ingestion on Performance.

65. Waldron, M., Whelan, K., Jeffries, O., Burt, D., Howe, L., and Patterson, S. D. 2017. The Effects of Acute Branched-chain Amino Acid Supplementation on Recovery From a Single Bout of Hypertrophy Exercise in Resistance-trained Athletes. *Applied Physiology, Nutrition, and Metabolism* 1–7. doi: 10.1139/apnm-2016-0569.

66. Brisola, G. M., Milioni, F., Papoti, M., and Zagatto, A. M. 2016. Effects of 4 Weeks of β-Alanine Supplementary L-Carnitine in Exercise and Exercise Recovery. *International Journal of Sports Physiology Performance* 1–25.

67. Huang, A., and K. Owen. 2012. Role of Supplementary L-Carnitine in Exercise and Exercise Recovery. *Medicine in Sport Science* 59:135–142.

68. Rowlands, D. S., A. R. Nelson, S. M. Phillips, J. A. Faulkner, J. Clarke, N. A. Burd, D. Moore, and T. Stellingwerff. 2014. Protein-Leucine Fed Dose Effects on Muscle Protein Synthesis after Endurance Exercise. *Medicine and Science in Sports and Exercise.* doi: 10.1249/MSS.0000000000000447.

69. Kreider, R. B., C. D. Wilborn, L. Taylor, et al. 2010. ISSN Exercise and Sport Nutrition Review: Research and Recommendations. *Journal of the International Society of Sports Nutrition.* doi: 10.1186/1550-2783-7-7.

70. Mason, B. C., and M. E. Lavallee. 2012. Emerging Supplements in Sports. *Sports Health* 4(2):142–147.

71. Ibid.

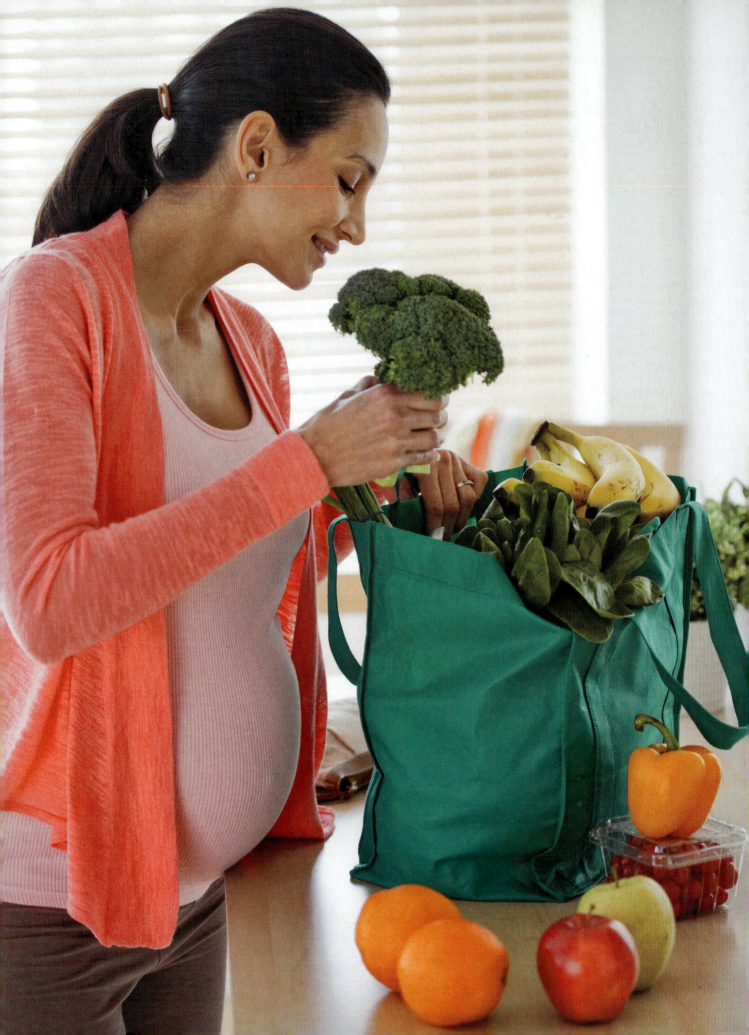

Life Cycle Nutrition

Pregnancy through Infancy

17

Learning Outcomes

After reading this chapter, you will be able to:

17.1 Identify the stages of pregnancy and the critical periods of prenatal development.

17.2 Discuss the key diet and lifestyle factors associated with a successful pregnancy.

17.3 Identify key nutrient needs, health behaviors, and nutrition-related concerns during the first trimester of pregnancy.

17.4 Identify key nutrient needs, health behaviors, discomforts, and potential complications during the second and third trimesters of pregnancy.

17.5 Discuss nutrition-related challenges of younger, older, and low-income mothers-to-be.

17.6 Describe the benefits and dietary requirements of breastfeeding.

17.7 Explain why infant formula is a healthy alternative to breast milk.

17.8 Discuss the nutritional needs of infants.

17.9 Explain when and how solid foods should be introduced to infants.

17.10 Explain how a food allergen causes a potentially life-threatening reaction.

True or False?

1. A man's health habits have little impact on his fertility. **T**/**F**

2. Drinking red wine is healthy during pregnancy. **T**/**F**

3. Morning sickness only happens between 8:00 A.M. and noon during the first trimester. **T**/**F**

4. Pregnant women shouldn't exercise. **T**/**F**

5. Commercially prepared infant formula is better for babies than breast milk. **T**/**F**

6. Breast milk helps boost a baby's immune system. **T**/**F**

7. Chubby babies should be put on diets. **T**/**F**

8. Infants never need dietary supplements. **T**/**F**

9. Commercially prepared baby food is always less nutritious than homemade. **T**/**F**

10. Infants should never eat highly allergenic foods, such as products made with peanuts or wheat. **T**/**F**

See page 659 for the answers.

When a woman is pregnant, her body facilitates the division, growth, and specialization of millions of new cells in her developing child. Nearly all of the raw materials for this rapid growth are provided by the nutrients found in food. A pregnant woman's diet, then, must be sufficient to maintain her health while fostering the proper growth and development of her baby.

The lifestyle choices a woman makes before conception help to give her baby a better chance for good health at birth and beyond. The father's preconception habits, including what he eats and drinks, also play a role in the pregnancy.

This chapter highlights the specific nutrient requirements of pregnancy. We also explore the diet and lifestyle factors in both the mother and father that can help ensure successful conception and healthy prenatal development, as well as the nutritional needs and concerns of infants in their first year of life.

What Are the Key Events of Prenatal Development?

LO 17.1 Identify the stages of pregnancy and the critical periods of prenatal development.

A full-term pregnancy is defined as 39 weeks, 0 days to 40 weeks, 6 days from **conception** to birth and is divided into three roughly equal 13-week trimesters (*tri* = three, *mester* = month).[1]

The initial 2 weeks after conception, called the *preembryonic period*, begin as the fertilized egg, or **zygote**, travels down the fallopian tube. Along the way, it divides rapidly, forming a mass (a preembryo) that becomes embedded in the lining of the uterus (**Figure 17.1**). Once attached, the preembryo begins receiving nutrients from the mother.

conception Moment when a sperm fertilizes an egg.

zygote Fertilized egg prior to the first cleavage (which occurs at approximately 72 hours)

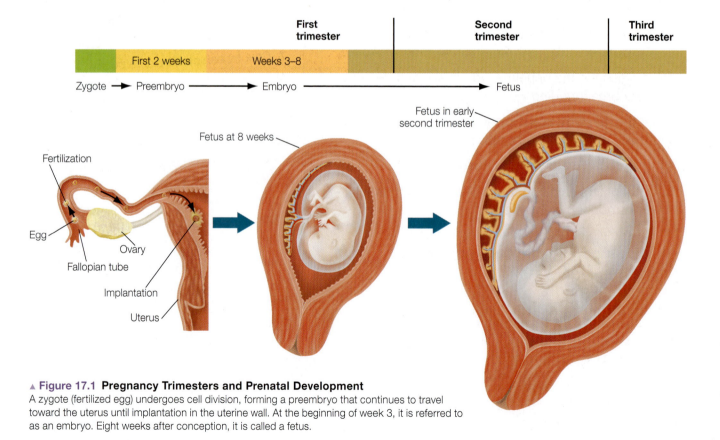

▲ Figure 17.1 **Pregnancy Trimesters and Prenatal Development**
A zygote (fertilized egg) undergoes cell division, forming a preembryo that continues to travel toward the uterus until implantation in the uterine wall. At the beginning of week 3, it is referred to as an embryo. Eight weeks after conception, it is called a fetus.

Many important physiological changes occur during this preembryonic period, even before a woman may be aware that she is pregnant.

During week 3, the cell mass (now called an **embryo**) develops three distinct layers from which all tissues and organs will eventually develop. Also at this time, the placenta begins to develop. The **placenta** is the site of common tissue between the mother and the embryo (later to be called a **fetus**) where nutrients, oxygen, and waste products are exchanged through the **umbilical cord** (**Figure 17.2**). It allows the mother's mature organ systems to perform physiological functions for the embryo/fetus while its own organs develop.

Notice that, because the placenta has distinct maternal and fetal tissue layers, maternal and fetal blood do not mix; instead, substances diffuse between the two circulatory systems. Although this dual lining prevents the passage of red blood cells, bacteria, and many large proteins from mother to fetus, potentially harmful substances, such as alcohol, illicit drugs, and common prescription and over-the-counter medications, can cross the placenta into fetal blood vessels. The placenta also releases hormones required to support the physiological changes of pregnancy, including the hormones that trigger labor and birth.

During the remainder of the first trimester of pregnancy, cells multiply, differentiate, and establish functional tissues and organs. Because of this rapid cellular activity, the embryo/fetus is most vulnerable to nutritional deficiencies, toxins, and other potentially harmful factors (also called *insults*) during this time. **Figure 17.3** identifies the **critical periods** of prenatal development during which such insults can cause irreversible damage.

The second and third trimesters are characterized by further differentiation of cells and tissues, rapid growth, and maturation of organ systems. A premature birth—one that occurs prior to the beginning of the 37th week of pregnancy—increases the risk for medical complications. The fetal lungs, for example, fully mature only by about week 36. Birth before that time can cause moderate to severe respiratory distress. Prematurity also increases the risk for brain hemorrhage, heart disorders, gastrointestinal problems, and many other disorders.

embryo Fertilized egg during the third through the eighth week of pregnancy.

placenta Organ that allows nutrients, oxygen, and waste products to be exchanged between a mother and fetus.

fetus Developing offspring that is at least 8 weeks old.

umbilical cord Cord of blood vessels connecting the fetus to the placenta.

critical periods Developmental stages during which cells and tissues rapidly grow and differentiate to form body structures.

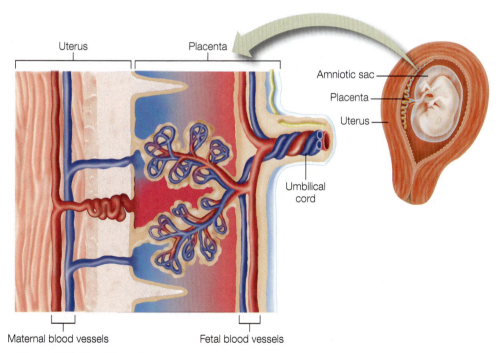

Uterus Placenta

Amniotic sac
Placenta
Uterus

Umbilical cord

Maternal blood vessels   Fetal blood vessels

▲ **Figure 17.2 The Placenta**
The placenta is the site of common tissue between the mother and the embryo where nutrients, oxygen, and waste products are exchanged through the umbilical cord. The maternal blood vessels exchange nutrients and oxygen with the fetal vessels, and the fetal vessels deliver waste products for the maternal blood to carry away for excretion. Note that while substances diffuse between the two circulatory systems, no mixing of maternal and fetal blood occurs.

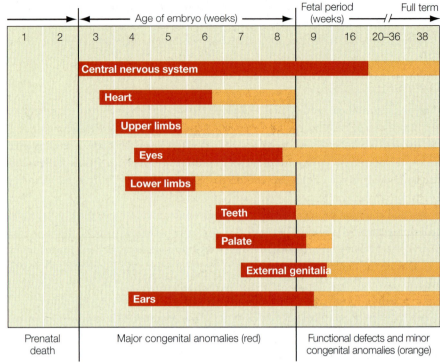

▶ **Figure 17.3 Prenatal Development**
The damage caused by toxins or lack of nutrients during pregnancy can vary according to the stage of prenatal development. Damage done during critical periods may be irreversible.

*Red indicates highly sensitive periods when teratogens may induce major anomalies.

In addition to affecting the growth and development of the embryo/fetus, maternal nutrition can influence the health of the offspring throughout the life course. Through a natural, yet tragic, human experiment, researchers studying birth records from the Dutch Famine (1944–1945) found a strong link between the timing of maternal famine exposure (i.e., lack of macronutrients and micronutrients in the first, second, or third trimesters) and birth outcomes. Babies exposed to famine during the first trimester of development had normal birthweights, whereas those who were exposed during the third trimester had low birthweights.[2] Through subsequent follow-up of this cohort, however, it became clear that suboptimal maternal nutrition early in gestation had long-term metabolic consequences; specifically, as a region's food supply increased and stabilized, the affected children and adults were found to have an increased risk for obesity, diabetes, and cardiovascular disease.[3]

These findings and others have led to the Developmental Origins of Health and Disease paradigm, which posits that altered maternal nutrition as well as exposure to environmental toxins, drugs, and/or stress during specific times of development can alter gene expression, lead to functional tissue changes, and ultimately predispose an individual to disease later in life.[4] Thus, **metabolic programming** (also known as *fetal programming*) is not influenced solely by maternal energy intake. Even when the food supply is abundant, inadequate intake of the minerals iron or iodine, for example, may impair cognitive development.[5] Moreover, research suggests that maternal obesity at the time of conception increases the risk for birth defects, increased birthweight, childhood overweight and obesity, and early mortality in adulthood.[6,7,8]

LO 17.1: THE TAKE-HOME MESSAGE A healthy pregnancy lasts 39–40 weeks and is divided into three trimesters. The placenta is an organ through which oxygen, nutrients, and waste products are exchanged; however, the maternal and fetal blood supplies do not mix. Toxins and insufficient nutrient intake during critical periods may cause irreversible damage to the embryo or fetus. Proper nutrition positively influences the metabolic programming during pregnancy and may help limit future chronic disease in the child and adult.

metabolic programming Process by which the prenatal environment interacts with genetic and other factors to produce permanent change; also called *fetal programming*.

What Health Behaviors Are Most Important for a Successful Pregnancy?

LO 17.2 Discuss the key diet and lifestyle factors associated with a successful pregnancy.

You're probably aware of some of the suggested lifestyle changes pregnant women should make, including avoiding cigarettes and alcohol. Healthy preconception habits in future moms—and dads—are also important to support fertility and the healthiest pregnancy possible. Are you ready for a healthy pregnancy? Take the Self-Assessment below to find out.

Are You Ready for a Healthy Pregnancy?

Both men and women should practice healthy habits before becoming parents. Take the following self-assessment to see if you need some diet and lifestyle fine-tuning before trying to get pregnant.

For Both Men and Women

1. Are you overweight?

   Yes ☐ **No** ☐

2. Do you smoke?

   Yes ☐ **No** ☐

3. Do you have more than two alcoholic drinks per day (men) or one drink per day (women) on a regular basis and do you consume four drinks or more within a 2-hour span (women) or five or more drinks within the same time span (men)?

   Yes ☐ **No** ☐

4. Do you use any illicit drugs such as marijuana, cocaine, and/or Ecstasy?

   Yes ☐ **No** ☐

Additional Questions for Women Only

1. Do you drink alcohol?

   Yes ☐ **No** ☐

2. Do you take herbal supplements or drink herbal teas other than what's available on supermarket shelves?

   Yes ☐ **No** ☐

3. Do you drink more than 12 ounces of caffeinated coffee or energy drinks or four cans of caffeinated soft drinks daily?

   Yes ☐ **No** ☐

4. Do you eat albacore (white canned) tuna, swordfish, mackerel, tilefish, and/or shark?

   Yes ☐ **No** ☐

5. Do you consume less than 400 micrograms of folic acid daily from dietary supplements, fortified grains, or a combination?

   Yes ☐ **No** ☐

Answers

If you answered yes to any of these questions, study this section to find out how these diet and lifestyle habits can impact a pregnancy.

Prospective Fathers Should Practice Healthy Habits

A healthy baby is the product of two healthy parents, so fathers-to-be who make appropriate diet and lifestyle choices prior to conception help ensure the health of their offspring. A man's lifestyle choices may affect his fertility. Smoking, alcohol abuse, drug abuse, the use of certain prescription medications, and obesity have been linked to decreased production and function of sperm.[9] Adequate intake of zinc and folate are linked to the production of healthy sperm, and antioxidants—such as vitamins E and C and carotenoids—may help protect sperm from damage by free radicals.[10] Moreover, evidence now suggests that a man's health-related lifestyle choices can affect embryonic development and influence the risk for disease in his adult offspring.[11]

Men should consume a balanced diet that contains adequate kilocalories to achieve and maintain a healthy weight and that provides a variety of fruits, legumes and other vegetables, whole grains, lean proteins, nuts, and dairy. Men should not smoke and should drink alcohol only in moderation (no more than two drinks daily), if at all. A future father who eats healthfully and practices other positive health habits supports his partner's efforts to do the same.

Women Should Practice Healthy Habits Before and During Pregnancy

Anyone who has run a marathon, or knows someone who has, is aware of the tremendous amount of effort and diligence it takes to train for the event. Ask any woman who has had a baby and she will tell you that planning for, carrying, and giving birth to a healthy child was the marathon of her life. Achieving a healthy body weight, eating a nutritious diet, and practicing other healthy lifestyle habits are important for preconception health and fertility as well as for pregnancy.

Achieve and Maintain a Healthy Weight

Women who are capable of becoming pregnant should strive for a healthy weight before conception. Women who begin pregnancy at a healthy weight are likely to conceive more easily, have an uncomplicated pregnancy, and have an easier time nursing the baby.[12] Overweight or obese women may have a harder time getting pregnant, possibly due to irregular menstrual cycles. When they do become pregnant, they are at increased risk of complications, including hypertension and gestational diabetes.[13] Research indicates that women who begin pregnancy obese are also less likely to initiate breastfeeding and more likely to have shorter duration of any breastfeeding.[14]

Overweight and obese women also have a greater chance of requiring an induced labor or a cesarean section.[15] Being overweight can increase a woman's risk of hypertension, which increases the risk of several pregnancy complications.[16] Children born to overweight or obese women are at greater risk of certain birth defects, preterm birth, and difficult deliveries because they tend to be larger.[17] These babies are also at a higher risk of developing childhood obesity[18] and, later in life, cardiovascular disease and diabetes.[19] Overweight or obese women should consider losing excess weight prior to conception to improve the chances of a healthier pregnancy and baby. Once an overweight or obese woman becomes pregnant, she should follow guidelines for the recommended weight gain based on her pre-pregnancy weight and should not try to lose weight.

Underweight women should also strive for a healthy weight before getting pregnant. A low pre-pregnancy BMI may indicate chronic nutritional insufficiency, and women with a low BMI may have a harder time conceiving. A woman who is underweight has an increased risk of delivering preterm and having a **low-birthweight** baby, or a baby weighing less than 5 pounds, 8 ounces.[20] As compared to a normal-weight baby, a

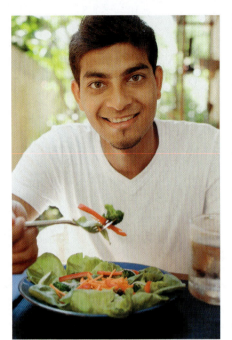

Prospective fathers should practice healthy habits prior to conception.

low birthweight Describes a baby weighing less than $5\frac{1}{2}$ pounds at birth.

low-birthweight baby is usually born too early and is at a higher risk of health problems, including developmental and intellectual disabilities, vision and hearing loss, and dying within the first year of life, than an infant born at a healthy weight.[21]

Underweight mothers are also at higher risk for delivering **small for gestational age (SGA)** babies, who may be born full term but weigh less than the 10th percentile of weight for gestational age. Although some babies are smaller because of genetics (their parents are small), most SGA babies are small because of growth problems that occur during pregnancy. The fetus may not have received the nutrients and oxygen needed for proper growth and development of organs and tissues.

Consume Adequate Folic Acid

Folic acid, the synthetic form of folate or vitamin B$_9$, is needed to create new cells and help a fetus grow and develop properly in utero. Consuming the DRI of folic acid (400 μg per day) beginning at least 1 month prior to conception, and preferably earlier, helps reduce the risk of giving birth to a newborn with a neural tube defect (NTD) such as anencephaly or spina bifida. NTDs occur when the embryonic neural tube fails to fold properly (**Figure 17.4**).[22] This improper folding results in incomplete brain and skull development (anencephaly) or a herniation and exposure of the spinal cord (spina bifida) (see Figure 10.22 on page 380). While both conditions are irreversible, anencephaly is incompatible with survival after birth.

The neural tube closes within 1 month of conception—a time when a woman may not be aware that she's pregnant. Recent estimates from a nationally representative sample suggest that 75 percent of women of childbearing age do not consume adequate folic acid.[23] Accordingly, in the United States 6.5 out of every 10,000 births results in an NTD.[24] For this reason, women who are capable of becoming pregnant should consume 400 micrograms of folic acid daily through supplements, fortified foods, or a combination (see Chapter 10). Women who have had a pregnancy affected by a NTD should consult with their health care provider, as higher daily doses of folic acid may help to prevent neural tube defects in future pregnancies.

Eat Safe Fish

Although the Food and Drug Administration (FDA) recommends that all women of childbearing age, including pregnant women, eat two to three servings of fish a week, they are advised to avoid certain fish with higher amounts of methylmercury. This form of mercury can harm the developing nervous system of the fetus and young child. All fish contain some methylmercury, but some are much safer than others; **Table 17.1** summarizes the fish consumption guidelines for women of childbearing age based on methylmercury content.

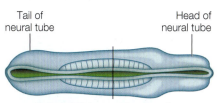

Neural plate (future brain and spinal cord)

Embryo 20 days post-conception

Tail of neural tube — Head of neural tube

Embryo 26 days post-conception

▲ **Figure 17.4 Folding of the Neural Tube**
During normal prenatal development, the embryonic neural plate folds inward to form a tube within which the brain and spinal cord develop properly. Inadequate maternal folate (folic acid) can lead to incomplete brain and skull development (anencephaly) or a herniation and exposure of spinal cord (spina bifida). However, not all neural tube defects are linked to inadequate folate.

TABLE 17.1	Fish Intake for Women of Childbearing Age

Women of childbearing age, especially those who are pregnant or breastfeeding, should eat two to three 4-ounce servings of fish each week (two 4-ounce servings from the *Best Fish* list and one 4-ounce serving from the *Good Fish* list)

Fish to Avoid	Good Fish	Best Fish
Shark, swordfish, king mackerel, tilefish, orange roughy, bigeye tuna	Albacore (white) tuna, bluefish, carp, grouper, halibut, mahi mahi, snapper, striped bass	Canned light tuna, cod, haddock, catfish, pollack, salmon, scallops, shrimp, crab, clams, sardines, anchovies

Source: Adapted from The Food and Drug Administration. 2017. Eating Fish: What Pregnant Women and Parents Should Know. Available at https://www.fda.gov/Food/FoodborneIllnessContaminants/Metals/ucm393070.htm. Accessed March 2017.

small for gestational age (SGA) Term for babies who weigh less than the 10th percentile of weight for gestational age.

TABLE 17.2	Common Sources of Caffeine
Beverage	**Caffeine (mg)**
Coffee (8 oz)	
Brewed, drip	85
Brewed, decaffeinated	3
Espresso (1 oz)	40
Tea (8 oz)	
Brewed	40
Iced	25
Soft drinks (8 oz)	24
Energy drinks (8 oz)	80
Hot cocoa (8 oz)	6
Chocolate milk (8 oz)	5

Source: Data from National Toxicology Program, Department of Health and Human Services. 2014. Caffeine. http://ntp.niehs.nih.gov; International Food Information Council (IFIC), www.foodinsight.org.

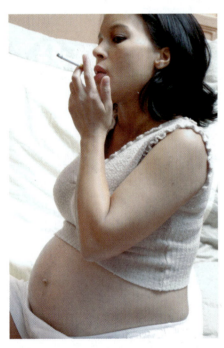

Smoking during pregnancy is harmful to the mother and to the fetus.

sudden infant death syndrome (SIDS) Unexplained death of an infant at less than 1 year of age.

Keep Caffeine Intake Moderate

During pregnancy, the caffeine a mother consumes from coffee, soft drinks, and energy drinks is passed on to her baby. Because the fetus cannot metabolize caffeine, it may linger in his or her body longer than in the mother's. Research on the effects of caffeine on female fertility and fetal health are conflicting, but experts suggest limiting caffeine intake before and during pregnancy to 200 milligrams a day or less.[25] The average cup of coffee has 85 mg of caffeine, so this means that if a woman does not want to avoid caffeine altogether, she should limit her intake to a cup or two per day. See **Table 17.2** for the caffeine content in several common beverages.

Avoid Cigarettes

Cigarette smoking increases the risk of infertility in women, possibly making conception more difficult.[26] Prenatal exposure to cigarette smoke may stunt the fetus' growth and development, affect a child's future intellect and behavior, and increase the risk of birth defects, stillbirth, premature birth, and **sudden infant death syndrome (SIDS)**.[27] Though there are thousands of harmful substances in tobacco and cigarette smoke, nicotine and carbon monoxide are particularly dangerous because they reduce the amount of oxygen that reaches the baby, thus intensifying adverse effects. In addition, pregnant smokers may weigh less and gain less weight during pregnancy than nonsmokers, which can contribute to a low-birthweight baby.

Even secondhand smoke can affect the health of a mom-to-be and her infant. Exposure to passive smoke in utero is associated with stillbirth, preterm birth, low birthweight, congenital anomalies, neonatal and infant mortality, asthma, and respiratory infections.[28] In part, these research findings are behind the World Health Organization's call for smoke-free legislation globally.[29] Accordingly, pregnant women, new mothers, and their children should avoid work, home, or social environments where they are exposed to secondhand smoke.

Don't Drink Alcohol

Because alcohol can affect embryonic development before a woman is even aware that she is pregnant, the U.S. Surgeon General recommends that all women who may become pregnant abstain from alcohol.[30] As you read in Chapter 7, drinking alcohol during pregnancy can lead to fetal alcohol spectrum disorders (FASDs) in the baby. Children exposed to even low levels of alcohol during pregnancy can be born with learning and behavioral disabilities that last a lifetime. Because there is no known safe level of alcohol consumption, pregnant women should abstain completely to eliminate the chance of having a baby with these disorders.

Avoid Illicit Drugs

Marijuana, cocaine, and other illegal drugs can cross the placenta from the mother to the fetus. Illicit drug use during pregnancy may be linked to miscarriage, preterm birth, hypertension, cognitive and behavioral problems, and other health issues. Babies born to cocaine-using mothers are more likely to have low birthweight and may have an increased risk of stillbirth and SIDS.[31] Newborns whose mothers used illicit drugs during pregnancy may experience drug withdrawal symptoms, such as excessive crying, trembling, and seizures, as well as long-term health problems such as heart defects and behavioral and learning problems.

Women who use illicit substances, even occasionally, should speak with their health care provider about how to stop, preferably before pregnancy. They can also visit the National Drug and Alcohol Treatment Referral Routing Service at *www.niaaa.nih.gov* or phone 1-800-662-HELP (4357).

Beware of Botanicals

Whereas many women trying to conceive wouldn't even consider taking over-the-counter drugs without clearance from their health care provider, they often don't have the same level of caution when it comes to taking dietary supplements, including **botanicals**—roots, leaves, or other plant parts that are believed to have medicinal effects. Perceiving botanicals as "natural," people often assume they can take them without risk. This isn't always true: some botanicals can be harmful or even dangerous, especially during pregnancy. Pregnant women—and women hoping to become pregnant—should always check with their health care provider before consuming any dietary supplement, including botanicals.

Blue cohosh, for example, is a botanical that is sometimes used to induce labor, but it has been associated with seizures, strokes, and heart attacks in newborns.[32] Juniper, pennyroyal, goldenseal, and thuja, as well as teas such as raspberry tea, may also cause contractions of the uterus, which can lead to a miscarriage or premature labor.[33]

Although most teas sold on supermarket shelves are safe during pregnancy in moderate amounts, such as a cup or two daily, green tea contains a compound that inhibits folic acid uptake. While it's unclear how strong the link between green tea intake and folic acid deficiency is, women of childbearing age should avoid excessive amounts of green tea to ensure that there is sufficient folic acid for the embryo and fetus.[34]

Effective Management of Chronic Disease Is Essential Before a Woman Conceives

Chronic diseases, including diabetes, hypertension, and phenylketonuria, can have a negative effect on the outcome of a pregnancy and therefore must be successfully managed before a woman conceives.

Diabetes mellitus increases the risk for maternal and fetal complications. An estimated 13.4 million (11.2 percent of) women in the United States age 20 and older have diabetes, and many are unaware of their condition.[35] Women with poorly controlled type 1 or type 2 diabetes are more likely to deliver an infant with a birth defect than are women without diabetes or those who enter pregnancy with normal glucose levels.[36] Optimal blood glucose control can help ensure a successful pregnancy. Medications used by women with diabetes should be evaluated before conception, as drugs commonly used to treat diabetes and its complications may be contraindicated or not recommended during pregnancy.

Women with preexisting, or chronic, hypertension are more likely to have certain complications during pregnancy than those with normal blood pressure. Hypertension can harm the mother's kidneys and other organs and it can cause low birthweight and premature birth.[37]

Women with the genetic disorder phenylketonuria (PKU) can have healthy children as long as they are aware of and maintain strict adherence to their low-phenylalanine diet throughout their pregnancy. As discussed in Chapter 4, PKU is an inability to metabolize phenylalanine, one of the amino acids. Phenylalanine is present in most foods high in protein, including meat, poultry, fish, eggs, dairy products, and soy. It is also found in the artificial sweetener aspartame. Women with poorly controlled PKU during a pregnancy put their baby at risk for delayed development, mental retardation, poor growth, heart defects, and other structural birth defects.

Women—especially those with one or more chronic diseases—benefit from pre-pregnancy nutritional counseling. In fact, nutritional counseling is also important throughout pregnancy and the postpartum period (the first 6 weeks after birth).

botanicals Part of a plant, such as its root, that is believed to have medicinal or therapeutic attributes.

What Nutrients and Health Behaviors Are Important in the First Trimester?

LO 17.3 Identify key nutrient needs, health behaviors, and nutrition-related concerns during the first trimester of pregnancy.

Several developmental milestones mark the first trimester. Organs begin to develop and function. The liver starts forming red blood cells, the heart begins beating, the limbs take shape, and the brain grows rapidly. During the first trimester, the head is actually much larger than the body to accommodate the developing brain. In spite of all the activity, the fetus weighs just a half ounce and measures only about 3 inches long by the end of the first 3 months; it still has a long way to go before birth.

Adequate Weight Gain Reduces the Risk of Complications

In a singleton (one-baby) pregnancy, the fetus typically comprises about a third of the total weight gained. Maternal tissues and fluids account for the remainder (**Figure 17.5**). The amount of overall weight a woman should gain during her pregnancy depends on her pre-pregnancy weight and health. Starting pregnancy at a healthy weight and gaining appropriately during pregnancy translates into a lower risk of complications for mother and child. Expert recommendations for pregnancy weight gain are based on a woman's pre-pregnancy BMI.[38] For example, women having a single baby who conceive at a healthy

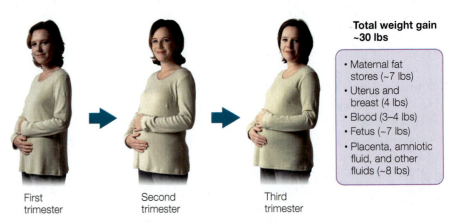

Total weight gain ~30 lbs

- Maternal fat stores (~7 lbs)
- Uterus and breast (4 lbs)
- Blood (3–4 lbs)
- Fetus (~7 lbs)
- Placenta, amniotic fluid, and other fluids (~8 lbs)

First trimester   Second trimester   Third trimester

▲ **Figure 17.5 Components of Weight Gain during Pregnancy for Healthy-Weight Women**
Healthy-weight women should gain 25–35 pounds during pregnancy.

weight (with a BMI between 18.5 and 24.9) should gain 25–35 pounds, whereas under-weight or overweight women have different weight gain goals (see **Table 17.3**).

The pattern of weight gain—that is, the rate of weight gained per week of pregnancy after the first trimester—as well as total weight gain influence the outcome of the pregnancy, especially for twin and triplet pregnancies, which tend to be shorter than single-ton pregnancies. Weight gain guidelines for pregnancy are designed to strike a balance between the baby's development and the mother's health. Appropriate weight gain during pregnancy provides for adequate growth so that the baby reaches a healthy weight of about 6.5–8.5 pounds, and it does not increase the risk of complications during birth. Gaining excess weight increases the odds that the mother will be overweight or obese for decades post pregnancy.[39] **Figure 17.6** shows healthy patterns of weight gain during a singleton pregnancy. The recommended pattern serves as a goal and helps providers identify women who are at risk for insufficient or excessive gain.

Notice in Figure 17.6 that most pregnancy weight gain occurs in the second and third trimesters. During the first trimester, because the embryo/fetus is so small, most pregnant women need to gain just $1-4\frac{1}{2}$ pounds.[40] However, it has been suggested that women having more than one baby need about 500 additional kilocalories a day starting in the first trimester to help maximize fetal growth, as their pregnancies may not go to full term.[41]

Adequate Micronutrient Intake Is a Concern throughout Pregnancy

Starting in the first trimester, a pregnant woman needs up to 50 percent more of certain vitamins and minerals than prior to pregnancy (**Figure 17.7**). A mother-to-be can increase her intake of these micronutrients by including nutrient-dense foods and taking a daily prenatal vitamin supplement.

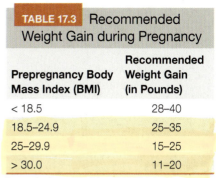

TABLE 17.3	Recommended Weight Gain during Pregnancy
Prepregnancy Body Mass Index (BMI)	Recommended Weight Gain (in Pounds)
< 18.5	28–40
18.5–24.9	25–35
25–29.9	15–25
> 30.0	11–20

Source: Institute of Medicine. 2009. Weight Gain during Pregnancy: Reexamining the Guidelines. Copyright 2009 by the National Academy of Sciences, Courtesy of the National Academies Press, Washington, DC. Reprinted with permission.

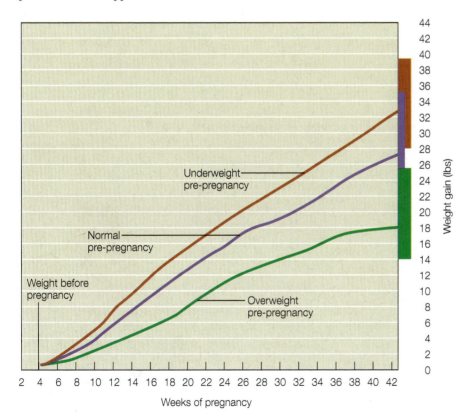

▲ **Figure 17.6 Patterns of Weight Gain**
A chart such as this is often used to monitor the rate of weight gain during pregnancy. Pregnant women should chart their weight gain every 2–4 weeks.
Source: Parent Link Centre, Alberta Children's Services. www.parentlinkalberta.ca/publish/474.htm. Accessed June 2012.

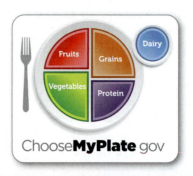

Vegetables	Fruits	Grains	Protein	Dairy	Oils
2.5 cups	2 cups	6 oz eq	5.5 oz eq	3 cups	6 tsp

Nutrient	Recommended DRI for Nonpregnant Women Aged 19–50 Years	Recommended Nutrient Intake during Pregnancy
Protein	46 g	71 g
Carbohydrates	130 g	175 g (minimum)
Linoleic acid	12 g	13 g
Alpha-linolenic acid	1.1 g	1.4 g
Dietary folate equivalents	400 µg	600 µg*
Thiamin	1.1 mg	1.4 mg
Riboflavin	1.1 mg	1.4 mg
Niacin equivalents	14 mg	18 mg
Vitamin B$_6$	1.3–1.5 mg	1.9 mg
Vitamin B$_{12}$	2.4 µg	2.6 µg
Vitamin C	75 mg	85 mg
Vitamin E	15 mg	15 mg
Vitamin A	700 µg	770 µg
Vitamin D	15 µg	15 µg
Calcium	1,000 mg	1,000 mg
Magnesium	310–320 mg	350–360 mg
Copper	900 µg	1,000 µg
Iron	18 mg	27 mg†
Phosphorus	700 mg	700 mg
Zinc	8 mg	11 mg
Calories	**2,000–2,200‡**	**§**

* Supplemented and/or fortified foods are recommended.
† A supplement is recommended.
‡ Varies depending upon activity level and weight.
§ Doesn't increase until second and third trimester.

▲ **Figure 17.7 Nutrient Needs during Pregnancy**
A balanced 2,000-calorie diet can meet most pregnant women's nutrient needs during the first trimester. Additional healthy foods in the second and third trimesters help to satisfy increased requirements.

Folate or Folic Acid

The DRI for folate is 400 micrograms daily; it increases to 600 micrograms daily throughout pregnancy. If a woman takes a dietary supplement with 400 micrograms of folic acid prior to conception and continues to take it while also consuming folic acid–fortified grains, it's reasonable to assume that she will satisfy her pregnancy folic acid needs. Foods rich in the naturally occurring form of this B vitamin—folate—are also helpful for meeting the DRI. These include lentils, beets, broccoli, and most leafy green vegetables.

Iron

A woman's daily iron needs increase from 18 milligrams to 27 milligrams during pregnancy. Even though a woman loses less iron during pregnancy because she's not menstruating, and she absorbs up to three times more iron from foods than before she was pregnant, she must increase her iron intake for several reasons. She needs more iron to make additional red blood cells, which increase her oxygen-carrying capacity and help replace possible significant iron losses from bleeding during birth. Iron is essential for fetal growth and development and for the growth of the placenta. A woman also needs extra iron to prevent iron-deficiency anemia, a condition associated with premature birth and an increased risk of death for both mother and baby.[42]

A pregnant woman's increased iron needs are not easy to meet with food alone. Although meat, fish, poultry, and enriched grains supply iron, nearly all women need a dietary supplement to satisfy the suggested intake during pregnancy.[43] Women should not take iron supplements with foods that have components that inhibit its absorption, including milk products (calcium), high-fiber foods (phytate), and coffee and tea (polyphenolic compounds).

Zinc and Copper

Because iron can interfere with the absorption of other minerals, a woman taking more than 30 milligrams of iron daily should also take 15 milligrams of zinc and 2 milligrams of copper to prevent a deficiency of these minerals.[44] Zinc is needed in protein metabolism and in the synthesis of DNA so that cells can replicate and differentiate. Copper, as part of enzymes, is needed in the production of energy, the synthesis of connective tissues, and the transport and use of iron.

Calcium

Calcium needs do not increase during pregnancy. A pregnant woman absorbs more calcium during pregnancy, which offsets the additional calcium needed by the growing fetus. However, many women fail to get adequate calcium before pregnancy to help build and preserve their own bone mass and to prevent osteoporosis later in life. More than half of women of childbearing age in the United States do not eat the suggested number of servings from the dairy and vegetable groups as suggested by MyPlate, putting them at risk of inadequate intake for several nutrients, including calcium.[45]

Drinking milk or calcium-fortified soymilk can ensure adequate calcium intake during pregnancy. Both beverages are also rich in protein, and most are fortified with vitamin D (see below). Sugary drinks, such as regular soda, on the other hand, contain kilocalories, sugar, and not much else and are not a good beverage choice for anyone, including mothers-to-be.

Vitamin D

Vitamin D is another important nutrient that women of childbearing age frequently underconsume. Suggested intakes for vitamin D don't increase during pregnancy; however, there is a high prevalence of low levels of serum vitamin D among women of childbearing age in the United States. Insufficient vitamin D during pregnancy can lead to poor absorption and use of calcium, which in turn impairs fetal bone formation. Maternal vitamin D deficiency during pregnancy has also been linked to hypertension, preterm birth, low birthweight, and gestational diabetes.[46] To avoid vitamin D deficiency, experts suggest consumption of adequate vitamin D from vitamin D–rich foods and dietary supplements, if necessary.

Other Nutrients of Concern during Pregnancy

Other nutrients are also of concern throughout pregnancy, especially if the mother is vegan or doesn't eat the recommended daily servings from each food group. Choline, found in high amounts in animal foods, is important during pregnancy and breastfeeding. Choline is needed for healthy cells to divide and grow, especially in the brain.[47] Vegans who don't consume any animal products need to make sure that they are getting adequate amounts of vitamin B_{12} from reliable sources, such as dietary supplements and fortified foods.

All pregnant women should be mindful about meeting their needs for alpha-linolenic acid (ALA), an omega-3 essential fatty acid found in flaxseeds, walnuts, soybeans, and canola oil. ALA and its derivatives EPA and DHA are needed in the development of cell membranes and are important in the formation of new tissues, particularly those of the central nervous system.[48]

Avoid Overconsumption of Vitamin A

While it's important that pregnant women meet their nutrient needs, it is equally important that they not consume too much of certain nutrients. Excessive amounts of preformed vitamin A (retinol) can increase the risk of birth defects, especially when taken during the first trimester (see Chapter 9). Women who take dietary supplements should consume no more than 5,000 IU (1,500 micrograms RAE) of preformed vitamin A daily and should avoid other vitamin and mineral supplements with more than 100 percent of the DRI.

Morning Sickness and Cravings Are Common

The mother's body is changing rapidly during the first trimester. Her breasts may be tender, and she may start to experience other effects of pregnancy, such as a newly heightened sense of taste or smell. She may also experience "morning sickness" as well as food aversions and food cravings.

Morning Sickness

"Morning sickness," or nausea related to pregnancy, is so common that some health care professionals consider it an initial sign of pregnancy.[49] In spite of its name, "morning" sickness can occur at any time of the day. It usually begins during the first trimester and often ends by the 20th week of pregnancy, although about 10 percent of women experience it longer.[50] The causes of morning sickness are unknown, but lower blood glucose during early pregnancy or fluctuating hormone levels, particularly increased estrogen, may play a role.[51]

Though there are no known dietary deficiencies that cause morning sickness or dietary changes that can prevent it, some women find relief in eating frequent, small meals that are high in carbohydrates such as pasta, rice, and crackers and avoiding an empty stomach. Salty foods such as potato chips combined with sour and tart beverages such as lemonade have been shown to help. Vitamin B_6 (100 milligrams or less daily) may

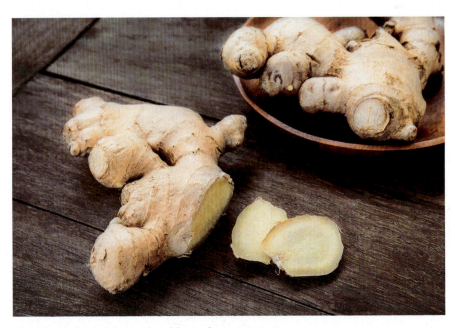

Ginger can help alleviate morning sickness for some women.

also reduce the nausea and vomiting.[52] Because there is an upper limit for safe vitamin B_6 intake, pregnant women should consult their health care provider before increasing it.

Ginger consumption has also been shown to help ease morning sickness. However, ginger root may inhibit a specific enzyme in the body, causing potentially adverse effects, including interfering with blood clotting.[53] As with vitamin B_6, pregnant women should not consume ginger supplements or extracts without first consulting their health care provider.

Though morning sickness is uncomfortable, it usually does not harm the health of the woman or her fetus. However, in rare cases (less than 1 percent of pregnancies) some women experience a more severe form of morning sickness called **hyperemesis gravidarum** (*hyper* = overstimulated, *emesis* = vomiting, *gravida* = pregnant), which can cause serious complications including dehydration, electrolyte imbalances, and weight loss. Women with hyperemesis gravidarum often have to be hospitalized for treatment.

The loss of appetite that often accompanies nausea can be harmful if it causes the mother to reduce her intake of nutritious foods. Whereas avoiding coffee, tea, and fried or spicy foods (common aversions for pregnant women) is fine, limiting consumption of fruits, vegetables, and whole grains, along with an inability to tolerate prenatal supplements, may result in certain nutrient deficiencies. When the fetus does not receive adequate amounts of an array of nutrients during pregnancy, fetal development may be irreversibly harmed.

Although morning sickness is not usually severe, it can cause the pregnant woman significant discomfort. The nearby Nutrition in Practice explains how a registered dietitian nutritionist (RDN) helps a client manage it.

Cravings

Pregnant women can have aversions to certain foods while craving others. Chocolate, citrus fruits, pickles, snack chips, and ice cream are foods that women commonly report craving when they are pregnant. There's no scientific basis for pregnancy food cravings and there's no research that substantiates the common belief that women crave foods because their body needs certain nutrients, such as snack chips for the sodium or ice cream for calcium.

Whereas there may be no harm in occasionally indulging food cravings as part of a balanced diet, there is potential harm when women crave and consume nonfood substances. **Pica** is the abnormal, compulsive intake of nonedible items such as laundry starch, burnt matches, cornstarch, clay, dirt, paint chips, or baking soda. Pica has been associated with low blood levels of iron, which has led to the theory that pregnant women seeking out nonfood substances have an iron deficiency.[54] However, other research suggests that pica causes the iron deficiency in these women.[55] Consuming nonfood substances can lead to the ingestion of toxic compounds, such as lead, that could lead to lead poisoning and other ill effects in both the mother and the baby.[56]

Food Safety Is a Concern

During pregnancy, a woman's immune system is weakened and the fetus' immune system is undeveloped, which makes pregnancy a time of heightened susceptibility to foodborne pathogens. The bacterium *Listeria monocytogenes*, for example, can cause miscarriage, premature labor, low birthweight, developmental problems, and even infant death.

Raw and undercooked animal products are more likely to carry pathogens and should be avoided during pregnancy. Pregnant women should also avoid unpasteurized milk, cheese, and juices and raw sprouts. You learn more about foodborne pathogens and how to safeguard your food in Chapter 20.

Sugar substitutes such as aspartame (Equal), sucralose (Splenda), acesulfame-K (Sunett), and saccharin (Sweet 'N Low) have been deemed safe to consume within the FDA's level of acceptable daily intake.[57] Whereas consumption of sugar substitutes in pregnancy may not pose a direct health risk, it is recommended that women use them sparingly so as not to displace the nutrients that are essential to a healthy pregnancy.[58] Women with PKU, however, should avoid using aspartame.

hyperemesis gravidarum Excessive vomiting during pregnancy that can lead to dehydration and loss of electrolytes.

pica Eating nonfood substances such as dirt and clay.

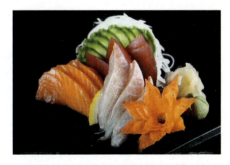

Food that may carry pathogens, including raw animal foods such as sashimi, should be avoided by pregnant women for their own safety and the safety of their fetus.

NUTRITION *in* PRACTICE:
WIC Nutritionist

Kayla was anxious when her doctor confirmed that she was pregnant at her last appointment, 2 weeks ago. This pregnancy—she and her husband already have a 1-year-old boy—was unexpected. Kayla had been planning to take night classes to finish her degree and become a paralegal.

During her last pregnancy, Kayla worked with a registered dietitian nutritionist (RDN) at her local WIC center. WIC is the federal Special Supplemental Nutrition Program for Women, Infants and Children, which assists low-income families. Kayla still has the diet that the WIC RDN prescribed her, but her nausea during most of the day has been preventing her from following it. Kayla decides to make another appointment with a WIC nutritionist to discuss her diet. When she explains her situation to the nutritionist, she begins to cry. Her husband was just laid off from his construction job. Kayla is scared her monthly income will not be enough to pay her bills and provide herself and her family with a healthy diet. After listening to Kayla's concerns, the WIC nutritionist recommends she speak with a WIC community coordinator. The community coordinator is employed by the WIC to help people in similar situations obtain food and other resources for themselves and their families.

Kayla's Stats
- Age: 22
- Height: 5 feet 6 inches
- Weight 132 pounds
- BMI: 21.3

Critical Thinking Questions
1. What should the WIC nutritionist's first priority be in Kayla's situation?
2. What changes can the WIC nutritionist suggest to help Kayla with her nausea and improve her diet?
3. Which nutrients are missing from Kayla's current diet? What foods could be added to her diet to ensure she's consuming enough of these vital nutrients?

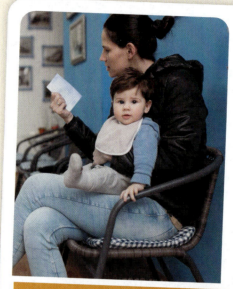

Kayla

KAYLA'S FOOD LOG

Food/Beverage	Time Consumed	Hunger Rating*	Location
Toast, OJ	7:00 A.M.	2	In kitchen at home
Crackers	9:30 A.M.	4	Kitchen at home
Chicken soup, crackers	12:30 P.M.	5	Staff break room
Cheese stick and crackers	3:00 P.M.	2	Playground with daughter
Chicken soup, crackers	6:30 P.M.	3	In the dining room at home
Crackers	9 P.M.	2	In front of the TV at home

* Hunger Rating (1–5); 1 = not hungry; 5 = super hungry.

WIC Nutritionist's Observation and Plan for Kayla
- Remind Kayla that she is eligible for food subsidies from WIC in the form of vouchers. These vouchers can be used at the supermarket to buy bread, milk, cheese, whole-grain cereals, fruits, vegetables, beans, and tuna.
- Recommend that Kayla "eat around her nausea." In other words, if she feels less nausea in the afternoon and evening, she should try to add more solid foods, such as yogurt and whole-grain cereals, to her meals later in the day. Sipping on ginger ale when she is nauseated may also help. Suggest that Kayla take her prenatal supplement at night, which may help with the nausea. Iron supplements can sometimes contribute to nausea during pregnancy.
- Also recommend Kayla add beans to her soup to add more protein to her meals.
- Review Kayla's previous pregnancy diet. Since Kayla's nausea during her last pregnancy ended in the first trimester, the WIC nutritionist creates a new diet plan, anticipating that she will be able to consume a more varied and balanced diet soon.

During their meeting, the community coordinator noted Kayla's anxiety and provided her with a referral to the Supplemental Nutrition Assistance Program (SNAP). This program provides her and her family with additional food vouchers to buy healthy foods at the supermarket. The coordinator gave Kayla vouchers to use at the local farmers' market and the names of local food pantries to supplement the vouchers during the month. Additionally, Kayla received the contact information for the unemployment office so that her husband could apply for benefits.

A few weeks later, Kayla set up another appointment with the WIC nutritionist and community coordinator. The WIC nutritionist helped Kayla develop a diet plan to combine the foods Kayla buys using the vouchers provided by the WIC. The coordinator gave Kayla the contact information for a service that can assist her with housing costs until her husband finds another job. Kayla left the meetings feeling much more optimistic.

LO 17.3: THE TAKE-HOME MESSAGE Women who begin their pregnancy at a healthy weight should gain from 25 to 35 pounds during pregnancy; underweight and overweight women will be advised to gain different amounts. The need for many micronutrients increases during the first trimester, but, with the exception of iron, most can be met with a balanced diet. For pregnant women to obtain the iron they need, a supplement is often prescribed. Pregnant women must avoid excessive intake of preformed vitamin A, as it can cause birth defects. Morning sickness and cravings are common during the first trimester and are usually not dangerous; however, hyperemesis gravidarum and pica can seriously threaten the health of the mother and the embryo/fetus. Pregnant women should avoid raw or undercooked animal foods and unpasteurized milk, cheese, and juice to reduce their chances of foodborne illness. Sugar substitutes are safe to consume in moderation during pregnancy.

What Nutrients and Health Behaviors Are Important in the Second and Third Trimesters?

LO 17.4 Identify key nutrient needs, health behaviors, discomforts, and potential complications during the second and third trimesters of pregnancy.

For many pregnant women, the nausea and fatigue of the first trimester resolve during the second and third trimesters, and appetite begins to increase. The baby is growing rapidly: blood cells are forming in the baby's bone marrow, the body grows bigger than the head, the ears become prominent, the eyes blink, and the lips are capable of a sucking motion. The fetus weighs just under 2 pounds by the end of the second trimester, and at the time of birth, the average newborn weighs 7 pounds, 7 ounces.[59]

The mother's body is also changing as her amniotic fluid and blood volume increase, her breasts get larger, and she stores more fat. She is likely to have a harder time getting around because of her expanding body. By the end of the third trimester, climbing stairs may take her breath away and finding a comfortable sleeping position could take some maneuvering. During this period of growth, the mother should get adequate kilocalories, protein, and other nutrients; exercise on a regular basis if her pregnancy is healthy; and become more aware of potential pregnancy complications.

Adequate Kilocalories, Carbohydrate, and Protein Are Critical

The mother's kilocalorie needs increase at the beginning of the second trimester. Women who begin pregnancy at a healthy weight need to eat an additional 340 kilocalories to gain between one-half and 1 pound weekly from this point until birth.[60] Underweight women may need more kilocalories and overweight women, fewer. A whole-wheat English muffin topped with peanut butter and some baby carrots (**Figure 17.8**) has about 340 kilocalories. See the Table Tips for more suggestions.

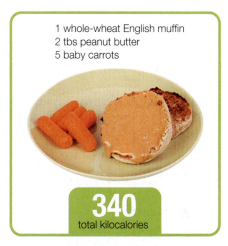

1 whole-wheat English muffin
2 tbs peanut butter
5 baby carrots

340 total kilocalories

▲ **Figure 17.8 Adding Kilocalories and Nutrients**
The extra kilocalorie and nutrient needs of the second and third trimesters can be met with additional nutrient-dense foods.

TABLE TIPS

340 Snacks

Create a "340 snack" to meet the extra energy needs of the second trimester. Start with a whole- or enriched-grain English muffin and top it with a serving of protein, low-fat dairy, and/or fruit/vegetable (like $\frac{1}{4}$ cup low-fat shredded mozzarella and $\frac{1}{4}$ cup tomato sauce).

Spread 3 tablespoons of low-fat ricotta cheese on two brown rice cakes topped with a small sliced banana for a 340-kilocalorie pick-me-up.

Layer $\frac{1}{4}$ cup low-fat granola cereal and $\frac{3}{4}$ cup berries with 1 cup low-fat vanilla yogurt for a 340-kilocalorie refreshing yogurt parfait.

Layer one whole-wheat tortilla with $\frac{1}{2}$ cup low-fat refried beans, 2 tablespoons salsa, $\frac{1}{4}$ cup shredded cheddar cheese, and $\frac{1}{4}$ cup shredded lettuce. Roll up and enjoy.

TABLE TIPS

Going from 340 to 450

Add an apple or banana to your 340 snack.
A small handful of chopped nuts can top a yogurt parfait.
Melt a slice of cheese on a burger.
Garnish a green salad with an ounce of whole-grain croutons.
Sip a fruit smoothie made with 1 cup low-fat vanilla yogurt, 1 cup low-fat milk, a small banana, $\frac{1}{2}$ cup berries, and 2 tablespoons wheat germ.

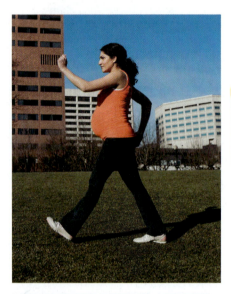

Walking is one form of exercise that is safe for both mother and baby and helps reduce the risk of diabetes.

TABLE 17.4 Safe and Unsafe Exercises during Pregnancy

Safe Activities	Unsafe Activities (Contact Sports and High-Impact Activities)
Walking	Hockey (field and ice)
Stationary cycling	Basketball
	Football
Low-impact aerobics	Soccer
	Gymnastics
Swimming	Horseback riding
Dancing	Skating
Jogging	Skiing (snow and water)
	Vigorous racquet sports
	Weightlifting

Source: Adapted from American College of Obstetrics and Gynecology. 2016. Exercise during Pregnancy. Available at http://www.acog.org/Patients/FAQs/Exercise-During-Pregnancy#exercises. Accessed May 2017.

During the third trimester, a woman who started pregnancy at a healthy weight should be eating 450 kilocalories more every day than before she became pregnant, and she should continue to gain between one-half and 1 pound weekly. Adding a banana to the English muffin with peanut butter and carrots shown in Figure 17.8 will provide about 450 kilocalories. Check out the Table Tips for more suggestions.

Pregnant women need a minimum of 175 grams of carbohydrates per day (versus 130 grams for nonpregnant women) to supply the amount of glucose required for both the developing brain and the energy needs of the fetus and to prevent ketosis in the mother. A balanced diet easily provides 175 grams of carbohydrate.

A pregnant woman's protein needs also increase by about 35 percent, to about 71 grams daily, during the second and third trimesters. Three servings of dairy foods and about 8 ounces of meat, poultry, or seafood provide the protein most pregnant women need for the day.

Experts Recommend Exercise

Daily exercise during pregnancy can help improve sleep, lower the risk of hypertension and diabetes, prevent backaches, help relieve constipation, shorten labor, and allow women to return more quickly to their prepregnancy weight after birth. Exercise may also provide an emotional boost by reducing stress, depression, and anxiety. Experts recommend healthy pregnant women get at least 150 minutes (2 hours, 30 minutes) each week of moderate-intensity aerobic activity, such as brisk walking, during and after their pregnancy. It is best to spread this activity throughout the week.[61] Pregnant women should check with their health care provider before exercising to see if it is appropriate.

Low-impact activities such as walking, swimming, and stationary cycling are best because they pose less risk of injury for both mother and baby. In contrast, high-impact activities, such as tennis and basketball, could injure the baby and cause joint injuries for the mother (Table 17.4). As long as there are no health complications, pregnant women who already do vigorous-intensity aerobic activity, such as running, can continue doing so during and after their pregnancy provided they stay healthy and discuss with their health care provider how and when activity should be adjusted over time.[62] Exercising moms-to-be should take special care to avoid a significant increase in their core body temperature and to drink plenty of fluids to avoid dehydration.[63] Check out the Fitness Tips for more suggestions for exercising during pregnancy.

Heartburn and Constipation Are Common Discomforts

As the growing baby exerts pressure on the mother's intestines and stomach, she may experience heartburn due to reflux of gastric juices into the lower esophagus (see Chapter 3). Hormonal changes may also slow the movement of food through the GI tract and increase the likelihood of heartburn. To minimize discomfort, pregnant women should eat frequent, small meals rather than fewer, larger meals and avoid foods that may irritate the esophagus, such as spicy or highly seasoned foods. They also shouldn't lie down immediately after meals, and they should elevate their head and shoulders during sleep to minimize reflux.[64]

Constipation is common near the end of pregnancy. The slower movement of food through the GI tract, the iron in prenatal supplements, and a tendency for less physical activity are contributing factors. Regular physical activity and a fiber-rich diet that features whole grains, fruits, and legumes and other vegetables, along with plenty of fluids, can help prevent or alleviate constipation.

Gestational Diabetes and Hypertension Are Potential Complications

Women may develop complications during pregnancy that can endanger their health and the health of their child. Two potential problems, gestational diabetes and hypertension, often first make their appearance in the second trimester.

Gestational Diabetes

Gestational diabetes (*gestation* = pregnancy), or having high blood glucose levels during pregnancy, affects an estimated 4–9 percent of pregnancies in the United States after about the 20th week.[65] A pregnant woman should be tested for gestational diabetes during her second trimester. Though the cause of gestational diabetes is still unknown, the hormones from the placenta may cause insulin resistance in the mother, which in turn causes hyperglycemia. Extra blood glucose crosses the placenta, stimulating the baby's pancreas to make more insulin, which leads to the storage of excess glucose as fat and can result in **macrosomia** (*macro* = large, *somia* = body), or a large baby.[66] A larger than normal baby may be at risk of injury to its shoulders during vaginal birth or may require cesarean birth.[67] Because the fetus is producing extra insulin during its gestation, the newborn may have elevated insulin levels, causing a rapid drop in blood glucose levels, which can cause hypoglycemia.[68] Gestational diabetes also increases the risk of **jaundice** and breathing problems in newborns and birth defects.[69]

Gestational diabetes typically goes away with birth. However, immediately after pregnancy, 5–10 percent of women with gestational diabetes are found to have diabetes, usually type 2.[70] In addition, women with gestational diabetes and the babies they carry are at higher risk of developing type 2 diabetes, as well as hypertension and being overweight, later on in life.[71] Certain factors can increase a woman's risk for gestational diabetes:

- Being overweight or obese
- Being over 25 years old
- Having a history of higher-than-normal blood glucose levels
- Having a family history of diabetes
- Being of Hispanic, African American, Native American, or Pacific Islander descent
- Having previously given birth to a very large baby (> 9 pounds) or a stillborn baby
- Having had gestational diabetes in a prior pregnancy

A woman with two or more of these risk factors is at high risk for developing gestational diabetes and should be tested during the first trimester of her pregnancy.[72] Having one risk factor indicates average risk, while having no risk factors indicates low risk.[73] Eating healthfully, maintaining a healthy weight, and exercising regularly can help reduce the risk of developing gestational diabetes.

To achieve normal maternal blood glucose levels, women with gestational diabetes should receive nutritional counseling by a registered dietitian nutritionist. Because gestational diabetes is a major risk factor for future maternal diabetes, it presents a "teachable moment" during which women can be alerted to take action to decrease risk.

Hypertension

Hypertension during pregnancy can damage the woman's kidneys and other organs and increase the risk of low birthweight and premature birth.[74] Though some women have hypertension prior to conceiving, others develop it during their pregnancy.

FITNESS TIPS
Exercising while Pregnant

According to the Physical Activity Guidelines for Americans:
Healthy women should get at least 150 minutes (2 hours and 30 minutes) per week of moderate-intensity aerobic activity, such as brisk walking, during and after their pregnancy. It is best to spread this activity throughout the week.

Women who already exercise longer or at a higher intensity can continue doing so during and after their pregnancy provided they stay healthy and discuss with their health care provider how and when activity should be adjusted over time.

Consult your health care provider before beginning or continuing an exercise program.

Drink plenty of fluids to stay hydrated.

Report any problems or unusual symptoms such as chest pains, contractions, dizziness, headaches, calf swelling, blurred vision, vaginal discharge or bleeding, and/or abdominal pain immediately to your health care provider.

Source: Centers for Disease Control and Prevention. 2017. Healthy Pregnant and Postpartum Women. Available from https://www.cdc.gov/physicalactivity/basics/pregnancy/. Accessed April 2017.

---

gestational diabetes Diabetes that occurs in women during pregnancy.

macrosomia Term for a large newborn, weighing more than 8 pounds, 13 ounces.

jaundice Yellowish coloring of the skin due to the presence of bile pigments in the blood.

Pregnancy-induced hypertension (PIH) includes gestational hypertension, preeclampsia, and eclampsia, each a progressively greater medical threat to mother and baby.

Gestational hypertension is a form of PIH that develops in a pregnant woman with no history of high blood pressure. It is more likely to develop about halfway through pregnancy. Because gestational hypertension increases the risk for future chronic hypertension, women who develop it should continue to have their blood pressure monitored after the birth.[75]

Gestational hypertension is often a precursor to **preeclampsia**, the most common form of PIH, which is characterized by both hypertension and protein in the urine, which signals kidney damage.[76] Women with preeclampsia may therefore experience mild to severe edema. Though some edema in a woman's feet and ankles is normal during pregnancy, the dramatic edema seen in preeclampsia is visible in her face and hands and can cause rapid weight gain. Preeclampsia can also prevent oxygen- and nutrient-rich blood from reaching the placenta.[77] The cause is unknown, but women at higher risk of developing preeclampsia include those who have hypertension prior to pregnancy or develop it during pregnancy, are overweight, under the age of 20 or over the age of 40, are carrying more than one baby, or have diabetes.[78] If left untreated, preeclampsia can lead to **eclampsia**, which can cause seizures in the mother and is a major cause of death of women during pregnancy.[79]

The only cure for preeclampsia and eclampsia is childbirth. Because birth before 32 weeks is unsafe for the baby, bedrest, medications, and hospitalization are used to treat preeclampsia until the baby can be born safely.[80] Some research suggests that antioxidants, specifically vitamins C and E, may reduce the risk, but more research is needed to confirm a connection.[81]

LO 17.4: THE TAKE-HOME MESSAGE Pregnant women who conceive at a healthy weight should consume an additional 340 kilocalories daily during the second trimester. During the third trimester, a woman who began her pregnancy at a healthy weight needs an additional 450 kilocalories daily and should continue gaining about a pound per week. A varied selection of nutrient-dense foods helps to satisfy increased kilocalorie needs. Exercise can provide numerous benefits during pregnancy. Heartburn and constipation commonly occur during the third trimester. Regular exercise, increasing fiber in the diet, and consuming plenty of fluids can help reduce constipation. Some women develop gestational diabetes and pregnancy-induced hypertension and need to be closely monitored by a health care provider.

pregnancy-induced hypertension High blood pressure resulting from pregnancy; includes gestational hypertension, preeclampsia, and eclampsia.

gestational hypertension Hypertension occurring during pregnancy in a woman without prior history of high blood pressure.

preeclampsia Serious medical condition developed late in pregnancy in which hypertension, severe edema, and protein loss occur.

eclampsia Seizures or coma in a woman with preeclampsia.

What Special Situations Do Younger, Older, or Low-Income Mothers-to-Be Face?

LO 17.5 Discuss nutrition-related challenges of younger, older, and low-income mothers-to-be.

Pregnancy and childbirth stress the body of a mother-to-be no matter what her age, but teenage moms and those over the age of 35 may encounter certain age-related challenges.

Adolescent Mothers Face Nutritional Challenges

For several years, the birthrate for women under the age of 20 has been on the decline in the United States.[82] This is good news because teenagers face some unique nutritional and health challenges.

An adolescent's body is still growing; thus, pregnant teens have higher nutrient needs than pregnant adults. At the same time, adolescents are more likely to eat on the run, skip meals, eat nutrient-poor snacks, and consume inadequate amounts of whole grains, fruits, vegetables, and dairy products. A pregnant teen's inadequate diet can mean not only a low-birthweight or SGA baby, but her own diminished health status.[83]

Teenage mothers are also more likely to develop pregnancy-induced hypertension and iron-deficiency anemia and to give birth prematurely, putting both baby and mother at risk for health problems.[84] In addition, adolescents are less likely to receive adequate prenatal care than their older counterparts.[85] If she receives prenatal care, pays close attention to her nutrition, and avoids unhealthy habits, a teenage mother can experience a normal, healthy pregnancy.

Older Mothers May Have Special Concerns

More women are having babies during their later childbearing years. The number of women who fall into this category has increased significantly in the last two decades: Since 1990, the number of births to women over age 35 has risen 40 percent. Today, births to mothers over age 35 represent over 35 percent of overall births in the United States. Fertility typically begins to decline in women starting in their early 30s, so getting pregnant may take longer, but when they do conceive, older women have a higher rate of multiple births. The more advanced age of women at childbirth accounts for about one-third of the rise in twin pregnancies over the previous 30 years.[86]

Though women in their late 30s and 40s often experience normal, healthy pregnancies, they are at higher risk for certain complications, including gestational diabetes and PIH; moreover, an older woman's fetus is more likely to be affected by Down syndrome or other birth defects.[87] Like all women, older women should try to achieve a healthy body weight prior to conception, avoid smoking, eat a balanced diet before and during pregnancy, consume adequate amounts of folic acid before and throughout pregnancy, limit their caffeine intake, and avoid alcohol and illicit drugs. If they regularly take prescription or over-the-counter medications, they should check with their doctor to see if these are safe during pregnancy. See **Table 17.5** for a summary of factors that relate to high-risk pregnancy.

Low-Income Mothers May Need Food Assistance

Adequate nutrition during pregnancy is critical for the health of both the mother and the child. The government program Special Supplemental Nutrition Program for Women, Infants, and Children (WIC) is designed to ensure that pregnant women and mothers with young children have access to nutrition information and nutritious foods during the most critical years of growth and development. WIC provides supplemental foods, health care referrals, and nutrition education for low-income pregnant and postpartum women and children up to age 5 who are at nutritional risk and who meet the program's eligibility requirements.[88] Supplemental foods include iron-fortified infant formula and infant cereal, iron-fortified breakfast cereal, fruits, legumes and other vegetables, whole-grain bread, eggs, milk, cheese, peanut butter, and canned fish.[89]

Evaluation studies have shown that the WIC program has been playing an important role in improving birth outcomes and containing health care costs. The program improved the nutritional status of nearly 9 million WIC participants in 2012.[90] For example, the WIC program reduced the incidence of iron-deficiency anemia in pregnant and postpartum women, improved babies' birthweights, reduced premature births and infant

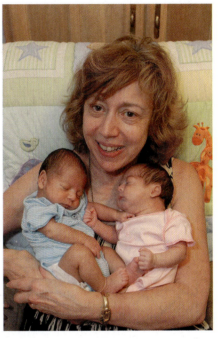

Older mothers often deliver multiples—twins, triplets, or quads.

TABLE 17.5	Factors That May Negatively Affect a Pregnancy
Factor	**Conditions Associated with Increased Risk**
Lifestyle	Smoking, alcohol, and abuse of illicit drugs Use of over-the-counter medications or dietary supplements without consulting with a health care provider Use of certain prescription medications Sedentary lifestyle
Age	Under age 20 Over age 35
Weight	Pre-pregnancy: underweight, obese During pregnancy: insufficient or excessive weight gain
Health history	Chronic diseases, including diabetes and hypertension Past history of a pregnancy affected by a birth defect, such as a neural tube defect Gestational diabetes, pregnancy-induced hypertension
Diet	Environmental contaminants (methylmercury, pica) Insufficient or excessive kilocalorie intake Nutrient deficiencies (folic acid, iron, calcium, vitamins D and B_{12}) Excessive caffeine intake Foodborne illness
Socioeconomic status	Poverty Limited food supply Low educational level

mortality, and increased prenatal care.[91] Every $1.00 spent on prenatal WIC participation for low-income women saves between $1.77 and $3.13 in health care costs within the first 60 days after birth.[92]

LO 17.5: THE TAKE-HOME MESSAGE Teens who become pregnant are at higher risk of hypertension, anemia, and premature birth and having a low-birthweight baby. Because a teen is still growing, she may have difficulty meeting both her own nutrient needs and her baby's, unless she is diligent about eating a well-balanced diet. Women over age 35 may have a harder time conceiving, are at higher risk for hypertension and diabetes during pregnancy, and have higher rates of babies born with developmental disabilities. The Special Supplemental Nutrition Program for Women, Infants, and Children (WIC) is a government-funded program that provides food assistance for nutritionally at-risk mothers during pregnancy and for at-risk children through the first 5 years of life.

What Are the Benefits and Dietary Requirements of Breastfeeding?

LO 17.6 Describe the benefits and dietary requirements of breastfeeding.

A woman who has just given birth begins a period of **lactation**, that is, her body produces milk to nourish her new infant. The infant's suckling at the mother's nipple stimulates milk production (**Figure 17.9**). Nerve signals sent from the nipple to the hypothalamus in the mother's brain prompt the pituitary gland to release two hormones: prolactin and oxytocin. Prolactin causes milk to be produced in the breast, while oxytocin triggers a **letdown response**, which releases milk so the infant can receive it through the nipple.[93]

lactation Production of milk in a woman's body after childbirth and the period during which it occurs.

letdown response Release of milk from the mother's breast to feed a nursing baby.

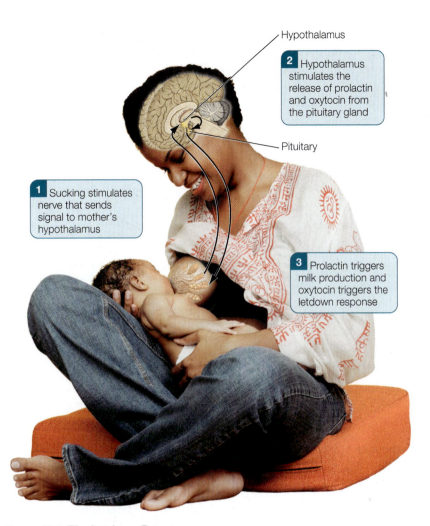

Labels on figure:

Hypothalamus

2 Hypothalamus stimulates the release of prolactin and oxytocin from the pituitary gland

Pituitary

1 Sucking stimulates nerve that sends signal to mother's hypothalamus

3 Prolactin triggers milk production and oxytocin triggers the letdown response

▲ **Figure 17.9 The Letdown Response**

The adage "breast is best" when nourishing an infant is true. Through **breastfeeding**, or nursing, mothers provide food that is uniquely tailored to meet their infant's nutritional needs in an easily digestible form. Breastfeeding also provides many other advantages for both the mother and the baby.

Breastfeeding Provides Nutritional and Health Benefits for Infants

The more than 200 compounds in breast milk, both nutritive and non-nutritive, work in concert to benefit an infant's health. For example, breast milk is rich in maternal immune factors, which provide direct immunity, as well as oligosaccharides, which are thought to provide indirect immunity by supporting the development of the infant's microbiome.[94] Numerous research studies indicate that breastfeeding provides nutritional and health advantages that can last years beyond infancy, ranging from reduced risk for childhood overweight and obesity to improved cognitive outcomes.[95] Breastfeeding is one of the most important strategies for improving an infant's long-term health prospects.

Best for an Infant's Unique Nutrition Needs

The nutritional composition of breast milk changes as an infant grows, varies within feeds, throughout the day, and between women. Right after birth, a new mother produces a carotenoid-rich, yellowish fluid called **colostrum** that has little fat and lactose but a lot of protein, vitamin A, and minerals. Colostrum also contains maternal immune factors that help protect the infant from infections, particularly in the GI tract.

breastfeeding Act of feeding an infant milk from a woman's breast.

colostrum Fluid that is expressed from the mother's breast after birth and before the development of breast milk.

Four to 7 days later, mature breast milk begins to flow. While its content varies, research supports that its macronutrient consumption is relatively stable to meet the infant's nutrient needs and developmental stage. Specifically, mature milk contains approximately 0.9–1.2 g/dL protein, 3.2–3.6 g/dL fat, and 6.7–7.8 g/dL lactose. Energy estimates, which vary according to fat content, range from 65 to 70 kcals/dL in mature milk.[96] Breast milk is high in B vitamins and relatively low in fat-soluble vitamins, sodium, and other minerals. These nutrients are proportionally balanced to enhance their absorption. Breast milk contains the right amount of protein so as not to stress an infant's immature kidneys with excessive amounts of nitrogen waste products. The protein is also mostly in the form of alpha-lactalbumin, which is highly digestible.[97] The nutrient composition of breast milk continues to change as the baby grows and his or her needs change.[98] To determine the precise kilocalorie and fat content of breast milk, visit the nearby Calculation Corner.

Calculation Corner

Determining Kilocalorie and Fat Content of Breast Milk

The daily energy needs of infants 0–6 months are typically met with a liter of breast milk. One liter of breast milk provides about 60 grams of carbohydrate, 9.1 grams of protein, and 31 grams of fat. Approximately how many kilocalories are found in a liter of breast milk?

$$60 \text{ g of carbohydrate} \times 4 \text{ kcal/g} = 240 \text{ kcal}$$
$$9.1 \text{ g of protein} \times 4 \text{ kcal/g} = 36.4 \text{ kcal}$$
$$31 \text{ g of fat} \times 9 \text{ kcal/g} = 279 \text{ kcal}$$

Answer: A liter of breast milk provides approximately 555 kilocalories.

The fat in breast milk contributes what proportion of the kilocalories?
Answer: From the above calculations, 279 kilocalories come from fat.

$$279 \text{ kcal from fat} \div 555 \text{ total kcal} = 50.3 \times 100 = 50\%$$

Answer: Fat represents 50 percent of the total kilocalories found in breast milk.

Go to Mastering Nutrition and complete a Math Video activity similar to the problem in this Calculation Corner.

Breast milk alone does not provide infants with an adequate intake of vitamin D because the vitamin D concentration is typically 25 IU per liter or less.[99] Therefore, the American Academy of Pediatrics (AAP) recommends that all breastfed infants consume 400 IU of vitamin D per day. Vitamin D supplementation should be continued unless the infant begins drinking at least one quart of vitamin D–fortified formula or vitamin D–fortified whole milk daily (after 12 months of age).[100]

Protection against Infections and Other Health Problems

Breast milk provides the infant with a disease-fighting boost until the baby's own immune system matures. Research supports that breastfeeding decreases the risk and severity of diarrhea and other intestinal disorders, respiratory infections, meningitis, ear infections, and urinary tract infections.[101]

One particular protein in breast milk, lactoferrin, protects the infant against bacteria, viruses, fungi, and inflammation by binding with iron and making it unavailable to bacteria that need it to flourish.[102] Lactoferrin also inhibits the ability of bacteria to stick to the walls of the intestines, which impedes their growth.

Breast milk provides other beneficial compounds, such as antioxidants, hormones, enzymes, and growth factors, that support infant development and offer protection from pathogens, inflammation, diseases, and allergies.[103] Some research suggests that breast milk may also protect against SIDS, asthma, leukemia, heart disease, and diabetes mellitus.[104]

Reduced Childhood Obesity Risk

Breastfeeding, especially if continued beyond 6 months, may help reduce the risk of childhood obesity. The reason for this isn't clear, but could be associated with the tendency of breast-fed infants to gain less weight during the first year of life than formula-fed infants. The lower weight gain may be due to breast-fed infants having more control over when they start and stop eating as compared to infants who are bottle-fed.[105]

Brain Development

Breast milk may enhance an infant's cognitive development. When a lactating mother eats properly, her breast milk is rich in the unsaturated fatty acids arachidonic acid (AA) and docosahexaenoic acid (DHA), which are important for the development of vision and the central nervous system, particularly the brain (see Chapter 5). Many commercial infant formulas also supply AA and DHA, but their effect on cognitive development is not clear.[106]

Breastfeeding Provides Physical, Emotional, and Financial Benefits for Mothers

Breastfeeding not only provides optimal nutrition and immunological benefits for the baby, it helps improve the health of the mother and can be less expensive, safer, and more convenient than bottle-feeding. The health and emotional benefits of breastfeeding may last for years after it ends.

Pregnancy Recovery and the Risk of Some Chronic Diseases

In addition to stimulating the release of breast milk, the hormone oxytocin stimulates contractions in the uterus, which helps the organ return to its pre-pregnancy size and shape. Breastfeeding also reduces blood loss in the mother after delivery.[107] It may help some women better manage their weight after delivery. Breastfeeding women have a lower risk for type 2 diabetes, cancer of the breasts and ovaries, and postpartum depression.[108]

Expense and Convenience

Moms who breastfeed can save between $1,200–1,500 in expenditures on infant formula in the first year alone.[109] These savings do not include the costs of clean water, energy, or time that goes into sterilizing, preparing, heating, and cleaning bottles. Furthermore, they do not include the health care savings. One study concluded that the national health care cost of not breastfeeding infants in their first year of life is as much as $13 billion.[110]

In addition, considerable natural resources are used to produce, package, and ship formula throughout the United States. The wastes generated include 550 million formula cans and 800,000 pounds of paper and plastic packaging that are disposed of in landfills each year.[111]

Feeding from the breast is also more convenient than bottle-feeding because the milk is always sterile and at the right temperature, and there is no need to prepare bottles or mix infant formula. In addition, there is less cleanup associated with breastfeeding.

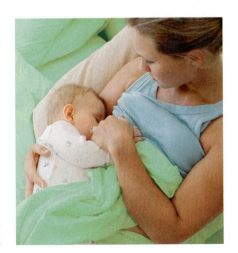

The intimacy of breastfeeding promotes bonding between mother and child.

Stress Reduction and Bonding

Recent research suggests that exclusive breastfeeding is associated with a mother's reduced reactivity to psychological stress.[112] In addition, the close interaction between mother and child during nursing promotes a unique bonding experience. The physical contact helps the baby feel safe, secure, and emotionally attached to the mother.[113]

Breastfeeding Is Recommended by Experts

Because of all of the benefits breastfeeding provides for mother and child, the AAP and the Academy of Nutrition and Dietetics recommend that women exclusively breastfeed for the first 6 months and then use a combination of appropriate foods and breastfeeding during the remainder of the first year of life, and breastfeed for longer, if desired. Currently, 79 percent of American women initiate breastfeeding when their infants are born, which is below the goal of 81.9 percent set for the nation in *Healthy People 2020*.[114,115] However, only 49 percent still breastfeed their infants at 6 months and only 27 percent continue until the baby is 1 year of age. These rates are well below the national goals of 60.6 percent at 6 months and 34.1 percent at 1 year.[116]

The breast-fed infant doesn't always have to consume breast milk directly from the breast. Milk can be expressed with a breast pump, refrigerated, and fed to the baby in a bottle by another caregiver at another time. This allows the mother to work outside the home or enjoy a few hours "off duty" and it allows others to feed the child. Expressed breast milk needs to be used within 24 hours or it can be stored in the freezer for 3–6 months. The Spotlight: Breastfeeding at Work Can Work addresses the dilemma of moms who want to breastfeed but who also want or need to return to work.

Breastfeeding Mothers Have Special Dietary Needs

During the first 6 months of breastfeeding, the mother produces about three-fourths of a liter of breast milk daily. In the second 6 months, she produces a little over half a liter daily. To support this production, a mother needs to consume about 13 cups of fluid daily, and most of it should be plain water. Recall from Chapter 11 that most healthy nonpregnant women need 9 cups of water daily.

A breast-feeding woman's body requires 500 kilocalories daily during the first 6 months of lactating to make enough milk to feed her child. However, not all of these kilocalories have to come from the food she eats. Approximately 170 kilocalories are mobilized daily from fat that was stored during pregnancy, so she needs to eat about an extra 330 kilocalories to make up the difference.[117] This use of stored fat allows for a potential weight loss of about 2 pounds a month during the first 6 months of breastfeeding, assuming the mother's diet aligns with her energy needs.

After the first 6 months of breastfeeding, less energy is available from stored body fat, so a lactating woman needs to consume about 400 extra kilocalories daily to meet her needs.[118] A well-balanced diet similar to the one she consumed during pregnancy will meet her breastfeeding nutrient needs. Lactating women who are vegans should make sure that they consume adequate amounts of vitamin B_{12} from dietary supplements and fortified foods.

Breastfeeding Mothers Should Limit or Entirely Avoid Certain Substances

Anything that goes into a breastfeeding mother's body can potentially pass into her breast milk and ultimately to her baby. Both illicit drugs and medications, for example, can be transferred to a breast-fed infant and cause harm. Methylmercury, which a mother can overconsume if she eats certain fish, can also be harmful, so nursing mothers should adhere to the FDA's guidelines about fish to minimize the infant's exposure (refer to Table 17.1 on page 625).

Nursing women should limit their consumption of coffee, energy drinks, and other caffeinated beverages, as caffeine can interfere with a baby's sleep and cause crankiness. They should also avoid alcohol because it can inhibit the mother's milk production and enter what breast milk is made. Whereas long-term effects of infant alcohol exposure

Breastfeeding at Work Can Work

Many women feel uncomfortable about breastfeeding or pumping breast milk outside the home, especially at their place of employment. Consider that 54 percent of mothers with babies 1 year of age or younger are employed and you can see that this reluctance is a big issue.[1] And the hesitation isn't just one-sided: Despite the requirement in the Patient Protection and Affordable Care Act of 2010 that companies must provide reasonable break time and a private, non-bathroom place for an employee to express breast milk for her nursing child for 1 year after the child's birth, many women still have to fight for their legal right to breastfeed at work in a safe, private space.[2] The reality is that many women must choose between breastfeeding and a paycheck, and work usually wins out.

This may be slowly changing. In 1998, the state of Minnesota mandated that its companies aid and support breastfeeding moms. From 1998 to 2002, the percentage of women still breastfeeding at 6 months more than doubled within that state.[3] Currently, 28 U.S. states, Puerto Rico, and the District of Columbia have laws to support breastfeeding in the workplace.[4] The requirement of the Patient Protection and Affordable Care Act that employers accommodate breastfeeding mothers does not preempt state laws that provide greater protections to employees.[5]

Worksite support is not only healthy for the infant and mother but, in many ways, healthy for the corporate bottom line. Because breast-fed infants are sick less often than formula-fed

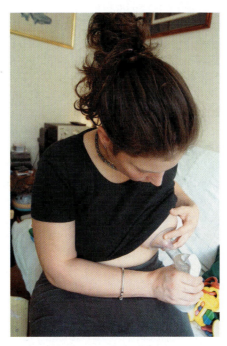

Women can express breast milk using a breast pump and store the milk in the refrigerator or freezer for later use.

babies, the United States could save $13 billion annually if 90 percent of mothers exclusively breastfeed their infants for 6 months as is recommended.[5] Employees who are able to breastfeed are also happier, miss fewer workdays (whether for their own illness or to tend to a sick infant), are more productive, and show greater loyalty to the employer. In fact, Cigna Health Insurance reports that they save $240,000 in health care expenses for women who breast-fed their infants.[6] Moreover, providing breastfeeding accommodations to women has been shown to improve retention post childbirth from 59 to 94 percent, on average.[7]

Women who return to work while lactating need only minimal worksite resources to accommodate their breastfeeding. First, they need adequate break times throughout the day and access to a private, comfortable room with an electrical outlet in order to pump their breast milk. They also need a sink in which to wash their hands and the pumping equipment and a refrigerator for storing the milk.[8] It's a small investment with a big pay-off for American families and American companies.

References

1. U.S. Department of Labor, Bureau of Labor Statistics. Table 6. Employment status of mothers with own children under 3 years old by single year of age of youngest child and marital status, 2014–2015 annual averages; 2016. Available at www.bls.gov/news.release/famee.t06.htm. Accessed April 2017.
2. US Department of Labor. Break Time for Nursing Mothers. Available from www.dol.gov/whd/nursingmothers/. Accessed April 2017.
3. M. Johnson. 2008. Letter to the Editor: Twentieth Anniversary Issue. *Journal of Human Lactation* 22:14–15.
4. National Conference of State Legislatures. 2017. *Breastfeeding State Laws.* Available at www.ncsl.org/research/health/breast feeding-state-laws.aspx. Accessed March 2017.
5. Office on Women's Health. *The Business Case for Breastfeeding Support* Available at https://www.womenshealth.gov/breastfeeding/employer-solutions/business-case.html. Accessed April 2017.
6. Ibid.
7. Ibid.
8. U.S. Breast-Feeding Committee. 2010. *Workplace Accommodations to Support and Protect Breast-Feeding.*

remain unknown, research supports that alcohol exposure through breast milk can affect infant sleep and mood.[119]

Neither breastfeeding women nor their partners or other caregivers should smoke. Maternal smoking is associated with a decrease in milk production and causes nicotine to enter the breast milk. Evidence suggests that this may have neurobehavioral effects on the infant in the short term, while affecting infant weight gain and growth in the longer term.[120] Secondhand smoke is associated with more frequent and severe asthma attacks, respiratory infections, ear infections, and SIDS.[121]

Breast milk can reflect the foods a mother eats and cause problems for the baby. For example, babies can become fussy if the mother has consumed certain spicy foods. The mother can abstain from that food, wait a few days, and then try it again. If the infant reacts the same way, it's best to stop eating that food while nursing.

In the past, medical experts and organizations such as the AAP advised mothers to avoid consuming highly allergenic foods, such as peanuts, while breastfeeding. However, there is a lack of evidence that avoiding allergens plays a significant role in the prevention of food allergy in infants. For infants at high risk of developing a food allergy (because a parent or sibling has food or other allergies), there is evidence that exclusive breastfeeding for at least 4 months compared with feeding cow's milk–based infant formula decreases the risk early in life.[122] For more on infant food allergies, see the Health Connection later in this chapter.

> **LO 17.6: THE TAKE-HOME MESSAGE** Breastfeeding helps reduce the risk for type 2 diabetes, certain cancers, and postpartum depression and may help mothers return to their pre-pregnancy weight. Breastfeeding is the least expensive and most convenient way to nourish an infant and helps the mother and baby bond. Human milk is rich in nutrients, antibodies, and other compounds that protect the infant against infections, allergies, and chronic diseases and may enhance the child's cognitive development. Women are advised to breastfeed exclusively for the first 6 months of their baby's life, and then breastfeed to supplement solid food for the remainder of the first year, or longer if desired. A mother must increase her fluid and nutrient intake to help her body produce breast milk. Nursing mothers should limit caffeine consumption and avoid illicit drugs, alcohol, smoking, and overly spicy foods.

Why Is Formula a Healthy Alternative to Breast Milk?

LO 17.7 Explain why infant formula is a healthy alternative to breast milk.

Commercial infant formula is the only healthy alternative to breast milk. Formula is designed to match the energy-nutrient composition of breast milk; but thus far, no formulas have been able to mimic the immune-related compounds in breast milk. For some women, formula-feeding is a personal preference. For others, it is necessary, as breastfeeding may not be possible because of illness or other circumstances.

Some Women Are Not Able to Breastfeed

Some health conditions or lifestyle choices make breastfeeding unsafe for an infant. Women taking prescription or over-the-counter medications should check with their health care provider to ensure that the medications are safe to consume while breastfeeding. Women who have untreated, active tuberculosis, who are infected with human

T-lymphotrophic virus type I or type II, or who have untreated brucellosis are among those who should not breastfeed.[123] An infant born with a genetic disorder of metabolism such as galactosemia can't metabolize breast milk and needs specialized infant formula.[124] In developed countries, women who are infected with HIV (human immunodeficiency virus), the virus that causes AIDS, should not breastfeed, as the virus can be transmitted to the child through breast milk. However, for HIV-infected women living in under-developed regions of the world where there is inadequate food, an unsafe food and water supply, and/or frequent incidences of nutritional deficiencies and infectious diseases, the benefits of breast milk often outweigh the risks of HIV infection for the baby.

Infant Formula Is Patterned After Breast Milk

Commercial infant formula is developed to be as similar as possible to breast milk, and formula-fed infants grow and develop normally. The FDA regulates all infant formulas sold in the United States and has established specific requirements for the nutrients that the formula must contain.

Formula is typically made from cow's milk that has been altered to improve its nutrient content and digestibility. Soy protein–based formulas are free of cow's milk protein and lactose and can be used for infants who can't tolerate cow's milk protein–based formula or who are in vegan families. Hypoallergenic infant formulas are also available for infants who are unable to tolerate cow's milk or soy formulas. The AAP recommends that all formula-fed infants consume iron-fortified formulas to reduce the risk of iron deficiency during infancy.[125] Regular cow's milk should not be fed to infants, as it lacks sufficient vitamin E, essential fatty acids, and iron and provides more protein, sodium, and potassium than an infant's body can process.[126]

Commercially made infant formulas can be purchased as powder, as a concentrated liquid, or in ready-to-use forms. Care must be taken to mix the powder or concentrated liquid with the correct amount of water so the formula is not too diluted or too concentrated.

If the infant doesn't finish the bottle, the formula must be discarded rather than saved for another feeding. The bacteria in the infant's mouth can contaminate the formula and multiply to levels that could be harmful even if the formula is reheated. Constant reheating of the formula also destroys some of the heat-sensitive nutrients.[127] Formula should not be left out at room temperature for more than 2 hours, as bacteria can multiply to unhealthy levels.

Infants of any age should not be allowed to sleep with a bottle containing liquids (milk, formula, fruit juice, soda, or other sweetened drinks), as this practice can lead to **early-childhood caries**, sometimes called *nursing bottle tooth decay* (see **Figure 17.10**). Liquids from bottles tend to pool in the mouth during sleep. The normal bacteria in the mouth change the sugar to an acid, which gradually dissolves the immature enamel and allows tooth decay to occur.[128] In addition, drinking from the bottle while lying down allows liquid to pool in the eustachian tubes, increasing the risk of ear infection. The American Academy of Pediatric Dentistry recommends against putting infants to sleep with bottles or sweetened pacifiers.[129] To prevent tooth decay, parents can massage and cleanse infant gums with a soft cloth after each feeding.

Early-childhood caries Tooth decay from prolonged tooth contact with formula, milk, fruit juice, or other sugar-rich liquid offered to an infant in a bottle.

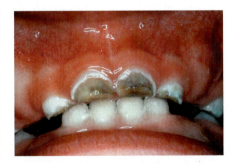

▲ **Figure 17.10 Early-Childhood Caries** When infants are allowed to fall asleep with a bottle, the sugar in the beverage can pool in the mouth. Bacteria act upon the sugar, creating an acid that can dissolve immature tooth enamel.

LO 17.7: THE TAKE-HOME MESSAGE Commercially prepared infant formula is the only healthy alternative to breastfeeding. Commercially made formulas are modified from soy or cow's milk and patterned after human breast milk. Cow's milk should not be given before age 1, as it is too high in protein and some minerals and too low in fat. Powdered and concentrated formulas need to be mixed carefully so they are not too diluted or concentrated for the baby's digestive system. Avoid putting infants to sleep with baby bottles to help prevent early childhood tooth decay and ear infections.

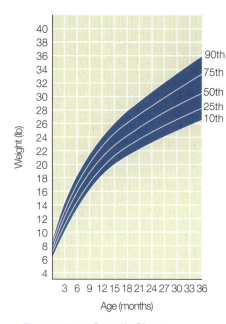

▲ **Figure 17.11 Growth Chart**
Growth charts can help determine if a child is growing at a healthy rate for her age.

What Are an Infant's Nutrient Needs and Why Are They So High?

LO 17.8 Discuss the nutritional needs of infants.

Parents and caregivers can be confident that adequate amounts of breast milk and commercial formulas will meet their infants' nutritional needs. Nevertheless, they benefit from knowing exactly what those nutrient needs are and why they are so high.

Infants Grow at an Accelerated Rate

During **infancy**, or the first year of life, a child experiences tremendous growth. Typically, an infant doubles his or her birthweight by about 6 months of age and triples it by the age of 12 months. Length doubles around the end of the first year as well.

Health care providers use **growth charts** to track physical development. Typically, measures of head circumference, length, weight, and weight for length are used to assess growth. These measures are taken at each pediatric wellness check, about once a month for the first year. The information obtained from the measurements is plotted on a growth chart, placing the child into a **percentile**. Percentiles rank the infant with regard to other infants of the same age in a reference group (**Figure 17.11**). For example, a 4-month-old who is in the 25th percentile for weight for that age has a body weight lower than that of 75 percent of 4-month-olds.[130] Regular checkups enable health care providers to identify and address any inconsistencies in patterns of growth.

Infants are doing much more than getting heavier and longer. Cognitive and social developments are also under way. As time goes by, infant communication skills go beyond crying, and by about 3 months of age a baby starts to smile. As infant brain development continues, their preferences become clearer, too: for particular people (such as the mom), for specific activities (such as getting kisses or being held), and for certain foods (such as mashed bananas).[131]

An infant who does not receive adequate nutrition may have difficulty reaching developmental **milestones** (**Figure 17.12**), which can be thought of as checkpoints of physical, social, and cognitive development. A child who doesn't reach the appropriate milestones

infancy Age range from birth to 12 months.

growth charts Series of percentile curves that illustrate the distribution of selected body measurements in U.S. children.

percentile Most commonly used clinical indicator to assess the size and growth patterns of children in the United States. An individual child is ranked according to the percentage of the reference population he or she equals or exceeds.

milestones Objectives or significant events that occur during development.

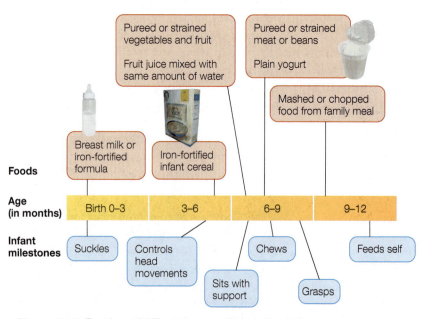

▲ **Figure 17.12 Foods and Milestones for Baby's First Year**
During the first year after birth, an infant's diet will progress from breast milk or formula to age-appropriate versions of family meals.

may develop a condition called *failure to thrive (FTT)*. A child with FTT is delayed in physical growth or size or does not gain enough weight. Poor appetite, poor diet, or a medical problem that has not yet been diagnosed can all cause FTT.[132] Sometimes, FTT results from inappropriate care or neglect. Caregivers and health care providers need to be aware of the signs of this condition and watch for those signs in their children and patients.

Optimal infant nutrition is sometimes hindered by circumstance. In less-developed countries where poverty is the norm and food is scarce, problems such as protein-energy malnutrition (see Chapter 6) are common. Even in developed countries, problems with poor infant nutrition may affect growth. For example, infants fed juice, water, or cow's milk instead of adequate amounts of breast milk or iron-fortified formula may develop iron-deficiency anemia (see Chapter 13). Depletion of iron stores in breast-fed infants who do not begin consuming iron in solid foods by 4–6 months of age may also pave the way for anemia.

Infants Have Specific Energy, Iron, and Other Nutrient Needs

Though every child is different, there are certain guidelines to follow to meet an infant's nutrient needs. For examples, infants under the age of 6 months require, on average, 108 kilocalories per kilogram of body weight every day.[133] Imagine a similar proportion of kilocalories at the scale of an adult who weighs 150 pounds (68 kilograms)—it would work out to 7,344 (68 kg $\times$ 108) kilocalories per day, more than twice the kilocalories required by some elite Olympic athletes!

Carbohydrate, protein, and fat needs change within the first year of life. Infants up to 6 months of age should consume 60 grams of carbohydrate per day and 95 grams per day at 7–12 months. Infants need about 9 grams of protein per day during the first 6 months of life and 11 grams daily in the second 6 months. (The DRIs for infants are listed on the inside front cover of this textbook.) There's no need to limit fat in the first year of life, and doing so could negatively impact physical and mental growth and development. Babies should never be put on weight-loss diets.

Three nutrients should be added to an infant's diet: vitamin K, vitamin D, and iron. All newborns should receive an injection of vitamin K, which participates in the synthesis of clotting proteins. This is necessary because infants are born with a sterile gut and lack the intestinal bacteria that produce vitamin K.[134] It is recommended that an infant receive this bolus of vitamin K after initiation of breastfeeding.

The amount of vitamin D in breast milk is inadequate to prevent rickets, so infants should also receive 400 IU of vitamin D drops daily beginning during the first 2 months of life. Emerging evidence suggests that maternal supplementation may improve the vitamin D content of breast milk; however, given a limited amount of research, infant supplementation is still required.[135] Infants exclusively fed adequate amounts of vitamin D–fortified formula do not require additional vitamin D. Once they reach age 1, children can drink vitamin D–fortified milk instead of infant formula or breast milk; however, if they don't get enough vitamin D through foods, including fortified milk, they may still need supplementation. Exposure of the infant's skin to sunlight to obtain vitamin D is not recommended because it can cause sunburns and increases the risk of skin cancer.[136]

Iron-rich foods, such as enriched cereals, should be introduced at around 6 months, as the infant's stores of iron are depleted by this time. Premature infants, who have lower iron stores because they were born early, may need iron supplementation before age 6 months.[137]

Because vitamin B_{12} is naturally found only in animal foods, supplementation may be recommended if the infant is being breast-fed by a strictly vegan mother. If the child's water supply is nonfluoridated, or if bottled water is used for mixing formula, a fluoride supplement may also be necessary.[138]

An infant's fluid needs are nearly always met with adequate consumption of breast milk or formula. Extra fluid is only necessary in hot climates or to rehydrate following episodes of diarrhea, fever, or vomiting, when the body loses fluid and electrolytes. Extra fluid should still be limited even in these circumstances, to ensure the baby remains hungry for nutrient-rich breast milk or formula.[139]

Beverages such as apple juice are a popular component of infant diets; however, the AAP suggests avoiding the introduction of juice until the child is a toddler. Juice should not be given to an infant until at least 6–9 months of age and should be limited to 4–6 ounces per day.[140] Though juice provides nutrients, it often displaces more nutrient-dense foods. Only 100 percent juice, not juice drinks, should be used.

LO 17.8: THE TAKE-HOME MESSAGE Infants grow at a dramatic rate during the first year of life. Caregivers and health care providers can monitor infant growth by making sure the child achieves appropriate developmental milestones and by using CDC growth charts. Nutrient needs during the first year of life are substantial, and supplementation of vitamin K, vitamin D, and iron may be required.

When Are Solid Foods Safe to Introduce to Infants?

LO 17.9 Explain when and how solid foods should be introduced to infants.

Often, proud parents can hardly wait to show off how their baby is eating "real food." It is an exciting time because eating **solid foods** represents infant maturity. Solid foods should be introduced at around 4–6 months of age.[141] However, the infant must be nutritionally, physiologically, and physically ready.

Solid Foods May Be Introduced Once Certain Milestones Are Met

Common sense tells us that as babies get bigger in size, they need more nutrients. Thus, an older, larger infant has higher nutrient needs than a younger, smaller one. Though breast milk can technically still provide most nutrients until age 4–6 months, introducing solid foods helps infants to meet their nutritional needs and develop feeding skills. Emerging obesity research suggests that very early introduction of solid foods may increase risk for childhood overweight, particularly among those who are formula fed.[142]

Before solid foods are introduced, the infant needs to be physiologically ready; that is, body systems must be able to process solid foods. At birth, and in early infancy, the GI tract and organs such as the kidneys cannot process solid foods.

An infant who is nutritionally and physiologically ready for solid foods may or may not be physically ready. Physical readiness is specific to the individual child and depends on whether he or she has met the necessary developmental milestones. To determine physical readiness, the following questions must be answered:

- Has the **tongue-thrust reflex** faded? The tongue-thrust reflex protects infants against choking. The tongue automatically pushes outward when a substance is placed on it. The reflex fades at around 4–6 months of age.
- Does the infant have head and neck control? Without such control, the infant is at greater risk for choking on solids.
- Does the infant swallow with ease?
- Is the infant able to sit with support?
- Does the infant have the ability to turn his or her head away when full?

solid foods Foods other than breast milk or formula given to an infant, usually around 4–6 months of age.

tongue-thrust reflex Forceful protrusion of the tongue in response to an oral stimulus, such as a spoon.

When the answer to all of these questions is "yes," it is safe and realistic to begin offering solid foods. If the answer to any question is "no," parents and caregivers should wait until the infant does develop the appropriate skills.[143] Parents who have any doubts about their child's readiness for solid foods should consult their pediatrician.

Solid Foods Should Be Introduced Gradually

Once an infant is ready for solids, foods should be introduced gradually to make sure the child isn't allergic or intolerant and to increase acceptance as children learn to take food from a spoon. The best practice is to introduce only one new food per week.[144] Infant cereal heavily diluted with breast milk or infant formula is often offered to infants as a first food, so there is a familiar taste mixed in with the new taste. There is no scientific evidence regarding the best progression of foods for infants, although parents are often advised to leave fruits for last, so that babies become accustomed to foods that are less sweet. As long as foods are introduced one at a time, the order of introduction of cereal, meat, fruits, and vegetables doesn't much matter in the long run.[145] Research supports that parents and caregivers should introduce a varied diet so as to expand their child's food repertoire.[146] Additionally, infants may need several exposures to a new food before they accept it. Children should not have cow's milk of any type until after 1 year of age.

After introducing a new food, parents should wait at least 2–3 days to monitor the baby for an allergic reaction.[147] Iron-fortified infant cereal, pureed meats, and pureed vegetables are the least likely to cause an allergic reaction. (The Health Connection ahead explains the mechanism of allergic reactions.) Parents may introduce highly allergenic foods such as egg, soy, or wheat once a few other foods are well tolerated first. To be safe, highly allergenic foods are best first introduced at home, rather than at a daycare center or restaurant.[148]

Solid foods should be phased in over a period of several months. Infants should eat pureed foods at first. As the infant's chewing and swallowing skills improve with practice, pureed foods can be replaced with soft, cooked foods. Refer again to Figure 17.12, which shows the progression in the infant's diet from breast milk or formula to age-appropriate versions of family meals.

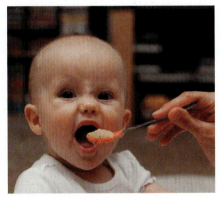

Solid foods such as iron-fortified rice cereal, oatmeal, and pureed meats can be introduced to infants between 4 and 6 months of age.

Many parents wonder if they should make homemade baby food. This is an admirable idea and gives the child exposure to fresh, unprocessed meals. However, many store-bought baby foods are of high quality and comparable to homemade. While some companies opt to add sugar, salt, or other less-desirable ingredients, others use organic produce or no preservatives or additives. One benefit of homemade food that everyone might agree upon is the financial savings—there are no added costs for fancy packaging and labels. The choice to use homemade or commercial baby food is up to the parent or caregiver.

Some Foods Are Not Appropriate for Infants

Not surprisingly, many foods are not appropriate for a baby. Some foods, like hot dog rounds or raw carrot slices, present a choking hazard and need to be cut into very small pieces or avoided altogether. Because infants have few teeth, foods should have a soft texture so they do not require excessive chewing; ideally, foods with texture should easily melt in the mouth, like a cracker. No matter what the food, infants should always be supervised by a responsible adult when eating.

Though some cultures and families have used honey-dipped pacifiers to calm infants for generations, this is a dangerous practice. Honey has been known to carry spores of *Clostridium botulinum*, which can develop in an infant's GI tract and secrete a toxin that causes infant **botulism**. Untreated infant botulism may cause paralysis of the arms, legs, trunk, and respiratory muscles, causing a potentially fatal respiratory failure. Older children (1 year and older) and adults can consume honey without these concerns because the mature GI tract can destroy the spores.[149]

botulism A rare but serious paralytic illness caused by a toxin secreted by the bacterium *Clostridium botulinum*.

The high salt, sugar, and fat content of restaurant and processed foods along with our own habits in the kitchen and at the table have conditioned us to think that food only tastes good if it is salty, sweet, or buttery. Some of the earliest work done on childhood food preferences suggests that in 3- to 4-year-old children, 50–60 percent of variance in food preference comes from our desire for sweetness, while the other 40–50 percent comes from familiarity.[150] Since familiarity is modifiable, parents and caregivers should avoid adding butter, salt, or sugar to their infant's foods. Doing so will help their child develop preferences for more healthy foods.

Whereas fiber is needed for GI health in adults, too much can actually be harmful to an infant. Because fiber is not digested in the GI tract, it can cause nutrients to leave the GI tract before they have a chance to be absorbed. At this time, no recommendations have been established for fiber during the first year of life.

> **LO 17.9: THE TAKE-HOME MESSAGE** An infant must be physically and physiologically ready before being introduced to solid foods. Solid foods should be introduced gradually and cautiously. Choking hazards and honey should be avoided, and infants should always be supervised while eating. Avoid excessive amounts of seasonings such as salt, sugar, and butter in the infant's diet, as well as too much fiber.

HEALTH CONNECTION

What Causes Food Allergies?

LO 17.10 Explain how a food allergen causes a potentially life-threatening reaction.

One-year-old Adam was playing in the sandbox at the neighborhood playground when his babysitter pulled a peanut butter cookie from her backpack. She broke off a small bite of the cookie and handed it to Adam, assuming that he must be hungry for his afternoon snack.

After a minute of chewing, Adam started to wheeze and have difficulty

food allergy Abnormal reaction by the immune system that occurs reproducibly in response to consumption of a particular food.

food allergens Proteins that are not broken down by cooking or digestion and enter the body intact, causing an adverse reaction by the immune system of a susceptible individual.

mast cells Cells in connective tissue to which antibodies attach, setting the stage for potential future allergic reactions.

breathing. Then he vomited. The sitter quickly used her cell phone to call for emergency help. She gave the rest of the cookie to one of the paramedics who rushed Adam to the hospital. Unbeknownst to the sitter, Adam had developed a food allergy to peanuts.

A **food allergy** is an abnormal reaction of the immune system that occurs reproducibly in response to the consumption of a particular food. The offending food component, called a **food allergen**, is usually a large protein that is not broken down during cooking or digestion. Because they are not degraded, food allergens are absorbed intact and trigger an adverse reaction by the immune system, which responds to the allergen as a foreign invader.

Food Allergies Are Immune System Reactions

Allergic reactions to foods occur in two stages: the "sensitization stage" followed by the actual response, or "allergic

reaction stage." In the first stage, a food allergen doesn't produce a reaction (**Figure 17.13**, steps 1–3). Instead, it sensitizes, or introduces, itself to the immune system. In response, the immune system creates an army of antibodies that enter the blood. The antibodies attach to **mast cells** found in connective tissues, setting the stage for a potential future allergic reaction.

The "allergic reaction stage" occurs when a person consumes the food allergen again. The food allergen comes in contact with the mast cells carrying the antibody for the particular allergen. The mast cells release chemicals such as heparin and histamine that trigger a chain of reactions in the body. The areas in the body that manifest a food allergy reaction are those where mast cells are most prevalent, such as under the skin and in the mucosa. In very sensitive individuals, even a small amount of a food allergen—just one peanut, for example—can trigger an allergic reaction.[151] Reactions appear quickly after eating the food. In fact, itchiness in the mouth may occur

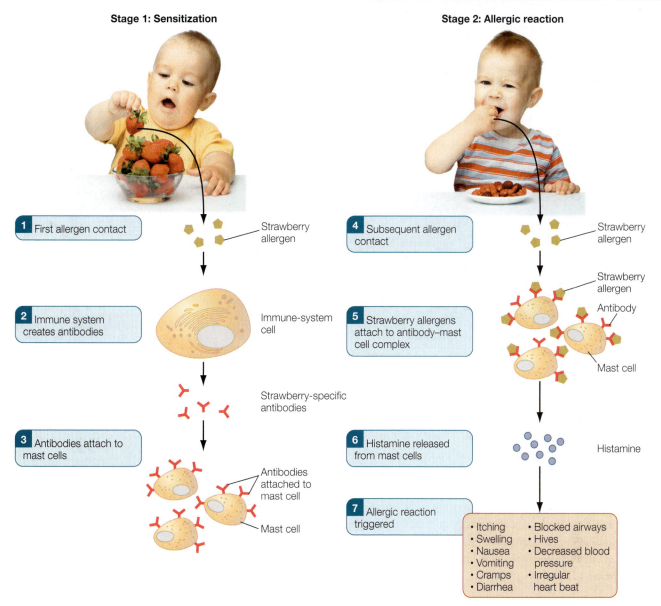

Stage 1: Sensitization

1 First allergen contact

Strawberry allergen

2 Immune system creates antibodies

Immune-system cell

Strawberry-specific antibodies

3 Antibodies attach to mast cells

Antibodies attached to mast cell

Mast cell

Stage 2: Allergic reaction

4 Subsequent allergen contact

Strawberry allergen

Strawberry allergen

5 Strawberry allergens attach to antibody–mast cell complex

Antibody

Mast cell

6 Histamine released from mast cells

Histamine

7 Allergic reaction triggered

- Itching
- Swelling
- Nausea
- Vomiting
- Cramps
- Diarrhea
- Blocked airways
- Hives
- Decreased blood pressure
- Irregular heart beat

▲ **Figure 17.13 Reactions to Allergens**
The reaction stage occurs when a person eats the food allergens for the second and subsequent times.

as soon as the food touches the tongue, and skin reactions and difficulty breathing may develop within minutes. After the food reaches the stomach and begins to be digested, vomiting and/or diarrhea may result. Once they enter the bloodstream, food allergens can cause blood pressure to plummet. A severe allergic reaction can lead to **anaphylaxis**, a potentially life-threatening condition. Individuals with allergies or their caretakers often carry a syringe injector of epinephrine (adrenaline) to help treat a reaction. Epinephrine constricts blood vessels, relaxes the muscles in the lungs to help with breathing, and decreases swelling and hives.

Eight Foods Are Highly Allergenic

Any food can cause an allergy, but 90 percent of food allergies are caused by eggs, cow's milk, peanuts, soy, wheat, tree nuts (such as walnuts), fish, and shellfish. The FDA requires that the food label state whether the product contains protein from any of these eight foods. The FDA is continually working with food manufacturers and consumer groups to improve public education about food allergies and the seriousness of anaphylactic reactions, in particular for the most common sources of food allergies.[152]

The proportion of children in the United States age 0–17 with a reported food allergy rose from 3.4 percent in 1997–1999

anaphylaxis Severe, life-threatening allergic reaction involving a sudden drop in blood pressure and constriction of the airways in the lungs, which inhibits the ability to breathe.

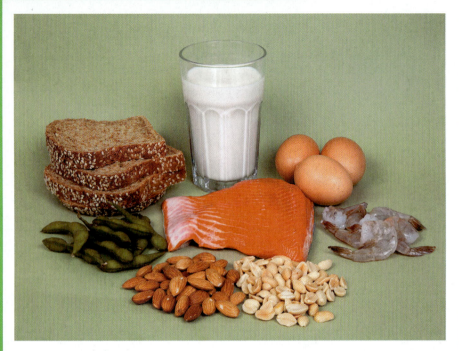

The eight most common food allergens are milk, eggs, fish, shellfish, tree nuts, peanuts, soy, and wheat.

children with a peanut allergy will eventually outgrow it.[157] Food allergies that are not outgrown cannot be cured; only strict avoidance of food allergens and early recognition and management of allergic reactions to food help to prevent serious health consequences.

A food allergy is different from a **food intolerance**. The symptoms of a food intolerance may mimic a food allergy, but a food intolerance does not involve the immune system. An example is lactose intolerance, the inability to digest lactose, which occurs when the small intestine fails to synthesize adequate levels of the enzyme lactase.

LO 17.10: THE TAKE-HOME MESSAGE

Food allergies are caused by proteins called allergens, which are interpreted by the body as foreign and trigger an immune response that ranges in severity from uncomfortable to life-threatening. They are on the rise in children. The reason for the increased prevalence is not known, but may be due to delayed introduction of allergenic foods. Most food allergies are caused by eggs, cow's milk, peanuts, soy, wheat, tree nuts, fish, and shellfish. Children may outgrow food allergies, but the only way to safely manage them is to avoid the offending allergen.

---

to 5.1 percent in 2009–2011, according to the Centers for Disease Control and Prevention.[153] Whereas it is unclear what has caused the increase in food allergies among American children, research supports that it may be due to delayed introduction. It was previously recommended that parents hold off in introducing specific allergens, including peanuts and tree nuts, until 1 year of age, particularly among high-risk children (those with eczema or a family history of food allergies). However, findings from a randomized clinical trial showed that high-risk children who were exposed to peanuts during infancy had lower rates of peanut allergies as compared to those who were not exposed until 5 years of age. Based on these findings, the AAP has revised their guidelines.[154] Specifically, they now recommend that parents or caregivers not delay the introduction of peanuts and tree nuts, even in infants at high risk of allergy.[155] An estimated 80–90 percent of egg, milk, wheat, and soy allergies disappear by age 5 years,[156] and up to 20 percent of

food intolerance Adverse reaction to a food that does not involve an immune response.

Visual Chapter Summary

LO 17.1 There Are Three 13-Week Trimesters of Prenatal Development

An average healthy pregnancy lasts about 39–40 weeks and is divided into three 13-week trimesters. In the initial 2 weeks after conception, the preembryo implants into the uterine wall. The preembryo gradually develops into an embryo during weeks 3–8. This is a critical developmental period when major congenital anomalies can occur if the embryo is exposed to insults. After 8 weeks, the embryo is called a fetus. Nutrients, oxygen, and waste products begin to be exchanged between the mother and fetus through the placenta. During the second and third trimesters, the fetus grows and organ systems mature. Proper nutrition and avoidance of known toxins, such as alcohol, are important to support the proper development of the embryo and the fetus throughout pregnancy.

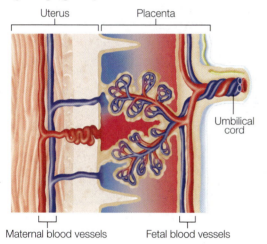

Uterus Placenta

Umbilical cord

Maternal blood vessels   Fetal blood vessels

LO 17.2 Nutrient Intake and Healthy Behaviors Are Important Prior to Pregnancy

Future mothers and fathers should make healthy diet and lifestyle choices prior to pregnancy. For healthier sperm, men should stop smoking, abstain from alcohol or drink only in moderation, strive for a healthy body weight, and consume a balanced diet. Prior to and during pregnancy, women should also abstain from alcohol, smoking, illicit drugs, and certain prescription and over-the-counter medications and supplements. They should also limit caffeine and, before conception, strive for a healthy weight on a balanced diet. In addition, women should consume adequate amounts of folic acid to reduce the risk of neural tube defects. Women in their childbearing years should avoid fish that contain high amounts of methylmercury but eat fish considered safe. Women with preexisting conditions should work closely with their health care professional to manage them prior to and during pregnancy.

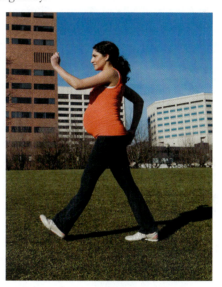

LO 17.3 A Nutritious Diet Is Critical during the First Trimester

A woman who starts her pregnancy at a healthy weight should gain 25–35 pounds during the course of her pregnancy. Women who are underweight or overweight prior to pregnancy, or who are carrying multiple fetuses, will have different weight gain goals. A woman's needs for many nutrients, including folate, iron, zinc, and copper, increase by up to 50 percent during pregnancy. With the exception of iron, for which a prenatal supplement is usually needed, most nutrient requirements can be met with a balanced diet. Care should be taken to avoid consuming too much preformed vitamin A (retinol), which can cause birth defects. Sufficient energy, carbohydrates, protein, alpha-linolenic acid, and choline are necessary throughout pregnancy. Awareness of food safety is also important, as bacteria such as *Listeria monocytogenes* may cause problems ranging from premature birth to infant death.

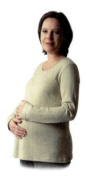

Third trimester

Total weight gain ~30 lbs

- Maternal fat stores (~7 lbs)
- Uterus and breast (4 lbs)
- Blood (3–4 lbs)
- Fetus (~7 lbs)
- Placenta, amniotic fluid, and other fluids (~8 lbs)

LO 17.4 Additional Energy Is Important during the Second and Third Trimesters

Many pregnant women find that the nausea and fatigue of the first trimester diminish during the second trimester and appetite begins to return. The mother's kilocalorie needs also increase. Women who begin pregnancy at a healthy weight need about 340 more kilocalories daily and should gain about a pound per week. Pregnant women need at least 175 grams of carbohydrate and 71 grams of protein. The risk of gestational diabetes and hypertension can be reduced during the second trimester with a healthy diet, daily exercise, and gaining the appropriate amount of weight.

During the last trimester of pregnancy, women who began pregnancy at a healthy weight should be consuming about 450 more kilocalories daily and continue to gain about 1 pound per week. Women who were underweight or overweight will need to eat more or less. The slower movement of food through the GI tract can contribute to heartburn and constipation. To minimize heartburn, pregnant women should eat frequent but smaller healthy meals, eliminate spicy foods, and avoid lying down immediately after meals. Exercise and consuming fiber-rich foods, along with plenty of fluids, can help prevent or alleviate constipation.

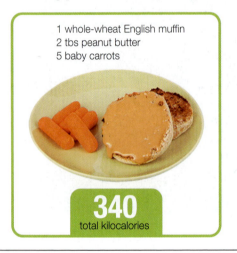

1 whole-wheat English muffin
2 tbs peanut butter
5 baby carrots

340 total kilocalories

LO 17.5 Younger, Older, or Low-Income Mothers-to-Be Face Special Challenges

Teenagers and women over age 35 may face additional challenges during pregnancy. Teenage mothers are at greater risk for pregnancy-induced hypertension, iron-deficiency anemia, premature birth, and low-birthweight babies. While many older women have healthy pregnancies, they are at increased risk for gestational diabetes and hypertension and for having a baby with Down syndrome or another birth defect. Low-income women, who may not have access to quality health care and a steady supply of healthy food, are at greater risk of iron-deficiency anemia and premature and low-birthweight infants.

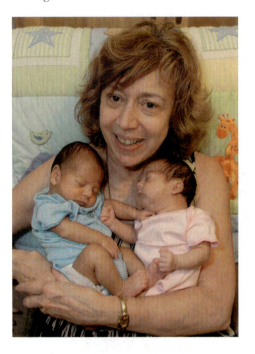

LO 17.6 Breastfeeding Benefits Both Mother and Child

Breastfeeding is the gold standard for feeding an infant. It provides physical, emotional, and financial benefits and convenience for the mother and nutritional and health benefits for the infant. Breast milk is rich in nutrients, antibodies, and other compounds that provide the infant with a disease-fighting boost until the baby's own immune system matures. Experts recommend that women exclusively breastfeed for the first 6 months of a baby's life, at which point they should add solid foods. Breastfeeding should continue to at least 12 months and for as long after that as baby and mother desire. Breastfeeding mothers should eat an additional 330–400 kilocalories daily as part of a balanced diet to produce adequate amounts of nutrient-rich breast milk.

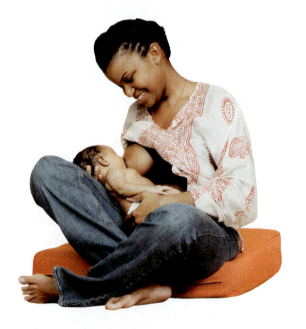

LO 17.7 Infant Formula Is the Only Healthy Alternative to Breast Milk

If an infant isn't breast-fed, the only healthy alternative is commercially made formula, which is modified from soy or cow's milk and patterned as much as possible after human breast milk. For some women, formula-feeding is a personal preference. For others, it is necessary, as breastfeeding may not be possible. To prevent tooth decay and ear infections, infants should never be put to sleep with a bottle of infant formula, breast milk, or juice.

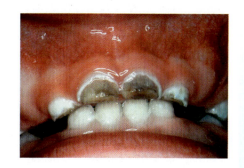

LO 17.8 Infants Have Specific Nutrient Needs

An infant typically doubles his or her birthweight by around 6 months of age and triples it by 12 months. Poor infant nutrition interferes with proper growth and a child's ability to meet developmental milestones. Infants need approximately 108 kilocalories per kilogram of body weight during the first 6 months of life. All infants should receive a vitamin K injection at birth, and breast-fed infants need vitamin D supplements. Infants older than 6 months, particularly those who are breast-fed, need to begin consuming iron through food sources, as their stored iron supply is depleted around this time.

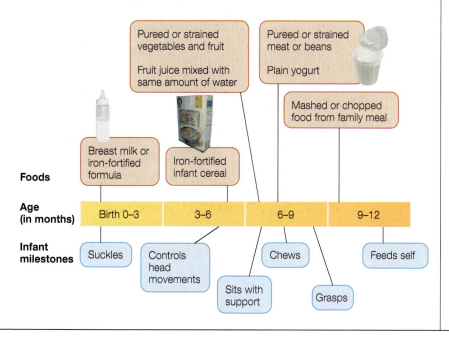

LO 17.9 Solid Foods Should Be Introduced Gradually

Infants are ready to begin eating solid foods if their birthweight has doubled, they can sit with support and control their head and neck, their tongue-thrust reflex has faded, and their swallowing skills are mature. Foods should be introduced gradually—one new food per week—to make sure the child isn't allergic or intolerant. Choking hazards should be avoided, and children should always be supervised while eating. Avoid excessive amounts of seasonings such as salt, sugar, and butter in the infant's diet.

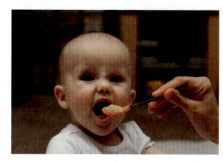

LO 17.10 A Food Allergy Is an Abnormal Immune Reaction

Food allergies are caused by specific proteins in foods that trigger an abnormal response by the immune system. The mast cells that respond to the allergen release heparin, histamine, and other chemicals that cause itching, swelling, hives, nausea and vomiting, constricted airways, and decreased blood pressure. A severe allergic reaction can lead to anaphylaxis and, potentially, unconsciousness and death. Epinephrine injections can counteract allergic reactions. Recent research suggests that delayed introduction of allergenic foods may have contributed to an increased prevalence of food allergies. Ninety percent of food allergies are caused by eight common foods: eggs, cow's milk, peanuts, soy, wheat, tree nuts, fish, and shellfish. The FDA requires labeling to indicate the presence of any of these ingredients. Many children outgrow food allergies.

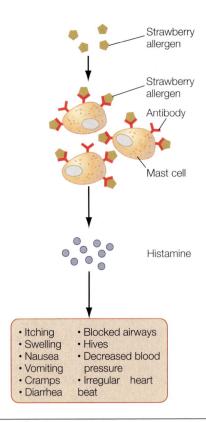

Strawberry allergen

Strawberry allergen

Antibody

Mast cell

Histamine

- Itching
- Swelling
- Nausea
- Vomiting
- Cramps
- Diarrhea
- Blocked airways
- Hives
- Decreased blood pressure
- Irregular heart beat

Terms To Know

- conception
- zygote
- embryo
- placenta
- fetus
- umbilical cord
- critical periods
- metabolic programming
- low birthweight
- small for gestational age (SGA)
- sudden infant death syndrome (SIDS)
- botanicals
- hyperemesis gravidarum
- pica
- gestational diabetes
- macrosomia
- jaundice
- pregnancy-induced hypertension
- gestational hypertension
- preeclampsia
- eclampsia
- lactation
- letdown response
- breastfeeding
- colostrum
- early-childhood caries
- infancy
- growth charts
- percentile
- milestones
- solid foods
- tongue-thrust reflex
- botulism
- food allergy
- food allergens
- mast cells
- anaphylaxis
- food intolerance

Mastering Nutrition

Visit the Study Area in Mastering Nutrition to hear an MP3 chapter summary.

Check Your Understanding

LO17.1 1. An embryo/fetus is most vulnerable to nutritional deficiencies, toxins, and other potentially harmful factors during the
    a. first trimester.
    b. second trimester.
    c. third trimester.
    d. second and third trimesters.

LO17.2 2. Sarah is trying to get pregnant. When should she start consuming 400 micrograms of folic acid every day to reduce the risk of neural tube defects?
    a. Immediately
    b. As soon as she finds out she is pregnant
    c. During the second trimester
    d. During the third trimester

LO17.3 3. A woman who began pregnancy at a healthy weight should gain _____ pounds during pregnancy.
    a. 15–25
    b. 20–30
    c. 25–35
    d. 30–40

LO17.4 4. During the second trimester of pregnancy, a woman who began her pregnancy at a healthy weight should increase her daily kilocalorie intake by
    a. 240 kilocalories.
    b. 340 kilocalories.
    c. 440 kilocalories.
    d. 540 kilocalories.

LO17.5 5. An adolescent mother is more likely than an adult mother to have which of the following pregnancy complications?
    a. Pregnancy-induced hypertension
    b. Iron-deficiency anemia
    c. A premature baby
    d. All of the above

LO17.6 6. Breastfeeding can have which of the following benefits for both mother *and* child?
   a. Relief of intestinal disorders
   b. Reduced risk of type 2 diabetes
   c. Fewer respiratory infections
   d. Reduced risk for ear infections

LO17.7 7. An HIV-positive mother living in an underdeveloped village in Kenya should do which of the following to feed her infant?
   a. Only provide formula to reduce the risk for transmitting HIV to the infant
   b. Breastfeed because the benefits outweigh the risks of transmitting HIV in regions that lack adequate sanitation
   c. Feed the baby cow's milk because it is highest in protein
   d. Feed the baby water and cereal

LO17.8 8. Which three nutrients are needed as supplements to an infant's diet?
   a. Folic acid, calcium, potassium
   b. Vitamin K, vitamin B$_{12}$, vitamin A
   c. Vitamin K, iron, and vitamin D
   d. Supplements are not needed in infancy

LO17.9 9. Solid foods should be introduced to an infant when which milestones have been reached?
   a. The infant turns 3 months and can roll over
   b. The infant can sit up with support and no longer thrusts the tongue
   c. The infant has reached 6 months and can crawl
   d. The infant no longer shows an interest in the breast or bottle

LO17.10 10. Which of the following statements about food allergies is true?
   a. Peanuts are responsible for about 90 percent of all allergic reactions to foods.
   b. Food allergies can be prevented by delaying introduction of allergenic foods until a child's 5th birthday.
   c. Food allergies are caused by allergenic proteins called antibodies present in certain foods.
   d. Breastfeeding offers some protection against food allergies.

Answers

1. (a) An embryo/fetus is most vulnerable to nutritional deficiencies, toxins, and other potentially harmful factors during the first trimester, when cell division and differentiation is rapid and tissues and organs are forming.
2. (a) Sarah should begin taking folic acid supplements immediately. Experts recommend that all women who are capable of becoming pregnant should consume 400 micrograms of folic acid daily to reduce the risk of neural tube defects, which occur during the first 30 days after conception. Folic acid is important throughout pregnancy, too.
3. (c) A woman who begins pregnancy at a healthy weight should gain 25–35 pounds by the time she gives birth.
4. (b) A pregnant woman needs 340 extra kilocalories daily during the second trimester to meet her needs. During the third trimester, she needs an extra 450 kilocalories every day. She doesn't need additional daily kilocalories during the first trimester, but does have additional nutrient needs, so she should be sure to eat nutrient-dense foods.
5. (d) all of the above. As compared to an adult mother, an adolescent mother is at increased risk for developing pregnancy-induced hypertension and iron-deficiency anemia as well as having a premature baby.
6. (b) Breastfeeding reduces the risk of type 2 diabetes in both the mother and child. The other benefits—fewer intestinal disorders and respiratory infections and lower risk of ear infections—affect the baby only.
7. (b) For HIV-infected women living in underdeveloped regions where there is an unsafe food and water supply and/or frequent incidences of infectious diseases, the benefits of breast milk often outweigh the risks of HIV infection for the baby.
8. (c) Infants are injected with vitamin K shortly after birth, and those who are breastfed, require supplementation of vitamin D and the introduction of an iron-fortified cereal when solids are started.
9. (b) An infant is ready for solid foods when the tongue-thrust reflex has gone away and when he or she can sit up with assistance. This usually occurs between 4 and 6 months of age.
10. (d) Breast milk contains components that offer some protection against food allergies. A total of eight common foods—not just peanuts—are together responsible for about 90 percent of allergic reactions to foods. Delaying introduction of allergenic foods into a child's diet has not been shown to be helpful in preventing food allergies. Antibodies are proteins produced during the immune response to foods. They do not trigger the response.

Answers to True or False?

1. **False.** A man's diet and other lifestyle habits, such as smoking and drinking alcohol, can affect his fertility.
2. **False.** Any type of alcohol, including red wine, can harm a growing fetus.
3. **False.** Though it's called morning sickness, nausea and vomiting can happen at any time of day and may last past the first trimester.
4. **False.** Physical activity is beneficial for most mothers-to-be, though certain potentially dangerous activities need to be avoided.
5. **False.** Formula is a healthy alternative, but breast milk is nearly always best for a baby.
6. **True.** Antibodies in breast milk are passed from the mother to the baby,

and support the infant's immune system.

7. **False.** Infants should never be put on a weight-loss diet. Babies need kilocalories and fat to support their rapid growth and development.

8. **False.** Most infants receive an injection of vitamin K at birth, and supplemental vitamin D is needed in an infant's diet.

9. **False.** Commercially prepared baby food can be as nutritious as home-made foods.

10. **False.** There is no evidence that restricting known allergens in an infant's diet reduces a child's food allergy risk; in fact, careful introduction of known allergens may be helpful.

Web Resources

- For more information on meal planning during pregnancy and lactation, visit ChooseMyPlate for pregnant and breastfeeding women at www.choosemyplate.gov/pregnancy-breastfeeding/pregnancy-nutritional-needs.html

- For more information on breastfeeding, visit the La Leche League International website at www.llli.org

- For more information on children and their dietary needs, visit the American Academy of Pediatrics at www.aap.org

- To obtain growth charts and guidelines for their use, visit www.cdc.gov/nchs/nhanes.htm

- For more information on food allergies, visit the Food Allergy and Anaphylaxis Network at www.foodallergy.org

References

1. American Congress of Obstetrians and Gynecologists, American College of Obstetricians and Gynecologists Committee on Obstetric Practice Society for Maternal-Fetal Medicine. 2013. Ob-Gyns Redefine Meaning of "Term Pregnancy." Available at http://www.acog.org/About-ACOG/News-Room/News-Releases/2013/Ob-Gyns-Redefine-Meaning-of-Term-Pregnancy. Accessed March 2017.

2. Stein, Z., and M. Susser. 1975. The Dutch Famine, 1944–1945, and the Reproductive Process. *Pediatric Research* 9:70–76.

3. Roseboom, T., de Rooij, S., and Painter, R. 2006. The Dutch Famine and Its Long-Term Consequences for Adult Health. *Early Human Development* 82(8):485–491.

4. Heindel, J. J., and Vandenberg, L. N. 2015. Developmental Origins of Health and Disease: A Paradigm for Understanding Disease Etiology and Prevention. *Current Opinion in Pediatrics* 27(2):248–253.

5. Radlowski, E. C., and Johnson, R. W. 2013. Perinatal Iron Deficiency and Neurocognitive Development. *Frontiers in Human Neuroscience* 7:585.

6. Block, S. R., Watkins, S. M., Salemi, J. L., Rutkowski, R., Tanner, J. P., Correia, J. A., and Kirby, R. S. 2013. Maternal Pre-Pregnancy Body Mass Index and Risk of Selected Birth Defects: Evidence of a Dose–Response Relationship. *Paediatric Perinatal Epidemiology* 27:521–531.

7. Bider-Canfield, Z., Martinez, M. P., Wang, X., Yu, W., Bautista, M. P., Brookey, J., Page, K. A., Buchanan, T. A., and Xiang, A. H. 2017. Maternal Obesity, Gestational Diabetes, Breastfeeding and Childhood Overweight at Age 2 years. *Pediatric Obesity* 12: 171–178.

8. Reynolds, R. M., Allan, K. M., Raja, E. A., Bhattacharya, S., McNeill, G., Hannaford, P. C., et al. 2013. Maternal Obesity During Pregnancy and Premature Mortality from Cardiovascular Event in Adult Offspring: Follow-up of 1,323,275 Person Years. *British Medical Journal* 347:4539.

9. Sharma, R., Harlev, A., Agarwal, A., and Esteves, S. C. 2016. Cigarette Smoking and Semen Quality: A New Meta-analysis Examining the Effect of the 2010 World Health Organization Laboratory Methods for the Examination of Human Semen. *European Urology* 70(4):635–645.

10. Dattilo, M., Cornet, D., Amar, E., Cohen, M., and Menezo, Y. 2014. The Importance of the One Carbon Cycle Nutritional Support in Human Male Fertility: A Preliminary Clinical Report. *Reproductive Biology and Endocrinology* 12:71.

11. Stuppia, L., Franzago, M., Ballerini, P., Gatta, V., and Antonucci, I. 2015. Epigenetics and Male Reproduction: The Consequences of Paternal Lifestyle on Fertility, Embryo Development, and Children Lifetime Health. *Clinical Epigenetics* 7:120.

12. Proctor, S. B., and C. G. Campbell. 2014. Position of the American Dietetic Association: Nutrition and Lifestyle for a Healthy Pregnancy Outcome. *Journal of the American Dietetic Association* 114:1099–1103.

13. Poston, L., Caleyachetty, R., Cnattingius, S., Corvalán, C., Uauy, R., Herring, S., and Gillman, M. W. 2016, Preconceptional and Maternal Obesity: Epidemiology and Health Consequences. *The Lancet Diabetes and Endocrinology* 4(12):1025–1036.

14. Bider-Canfield, Z., Martinez, M. P., Wang, X., Yu, W., Bautista, M. P., Brookey, J., Page, K. A., Buchanan, T. A., and Xiang, A. H. 2017 Maternal Obesity, Gestational Diabetes, Breastfeeding and Childhood Overweight at Age 2 Years. *Pediatric Obesity* 12:171–178.

15. Catalano, P. M., and S. Kartik. 2017. Obesity and Pregnancy: Mechanisms of Short Term and Long Term Adverse Consequences for Mother and Child. *British Medical Journal* 356:j1.

16. Poston, L., Caleyachetty, R., Cnattingius, S., Corvalán, C., Uauy, R., Herring, S., and Gillman, M. W. 2016, Preconceptional and Maternal Obesity: Epidemiology and Health Consequences. *The Lancet Diabetes and Endocrinology* 4(12):1025–1036.

17. Cnattingius, S., Villamor, E., Johansson, S., Bonamy, A. E., Persson, M., Wikström, A., and Granath, F. 2013. Maternal Obesity and Risk of Preterm Delivery. *Journal of the American Medical Association* 309(22):2362–2370.

18. Kaiser, et al. 2008. Position of the American Dietetic Association: Nutrition and Lifestyle for a Healthy Pregnancy Outcome.

19. Tam, W. H., R. C. Ma, X. Yang, A. M. Li, G. T. C. Ko, A. P. S. Kang, et al. 2010. Glucose Intolerance and Cardiometabolic Risk in Adolescents Exposed to Maternal Gestational Diabetes. *Diabetes Care* 122:1229–1234.

20. Hoellen, F., Hornemann, A., Haertel, C., Reh, A., Rody, A., Schneider, S., Tuschy, B., and Bohlmann, M. K. 2014. Does Maternal Underweight Prior to Conception Influence Pregnancy Risks and Outcome? *In Vivo* 28(6):1165–1170.

21. U.S. Department of Health and Human Services, Health Resources and Services Administration, Maternal and Child Health Bureau. *Child Health USA 2014*. Rockville, MD: U.S. Department of Health and Human Services, 2014.

22. U.S. Preventive Services Task Force. 2017. Folic Acid for the Prevention of Neural Tube Defects: Preventive Medication. Available at https://www.uspreventiveservicestaskforce.org/Page/Document/UpdateSummaryFinal/folic-acid-for-the-prevention-of-neural-tube-defects-preventive-medication. Accessed March 2017.

23. Viswanathan, M., Treiman, K. A., Kish Doto, J., Middleton, J. S., Coker-Schwimmer, E. J., and Nicholson, W. S. 2017. Folic Acid Supplementation: An Evidence Review for the US Preventive Services Task Force. *Journal of the American Medical Association* 317(2):190–203.

24. Ibid.

25. March of Dimes Foundation. 2012. *Caffeine in Pregnancy*. Available at www.marchofdimes.com/pregnancy/caffeine-in-pregnancy.aspx. Accessed March 2017.

26. American Society for Reproductive Medicine. Smoking and Infertility. Available at https://www.asrm.org/uploadedFiles/ASRM_Content/Resources/Patient_Resources/Fact_Sheets_and_Info_Booklets/smoking.pdf. Accessed March 2017.

27. U.S. Department of Health and Human Services. U.S. Surgeon General. 2014. *The Health Consequences of Smoking—50 Years of Progress: A Report of the Surgeon General, 2014*. Available at www.surgeongeneral.gov/library/

reports/50-years-of-progress. Accessed March 2017.

28. Been, J. V., Nurmatov, U. B., Cox, B., Nawrot, T. S., van Schayck, C. P., and Sheikh, A. Effect of Smoke-Free Legislation on Perinatal and Child Health: A Systematic Review and Meta-Analysis. *The Lancet* 383(9928):1549–1560.

29. Ibid.

30. U.S. Department of Health and Human Services. 2005. *U.S. Surgeon General Releases Advisory on Alcohol Use in Pregnancy.* Available at www.surgeongeneral.gov/news/2005/02/sg02222005.html. Accessed March 2017.

31. Varner, M. W., Silver, R. M., Hogue, C. J. R., et al. 2014. Association Between Stillbirth and Illicit Drug Use and Smoking During Pregnancy. *Obstetrics and Gynecology* 123(1):113–125.

32. Dante, G., Bellei, G., Neri, I., and Facchinetti, F. 2014. Herbal Therapies in Pregnancy: What Works? *Current Opinion in Obstetrics and Gynecology* 26(2):83–91.

33. Ibid.

34. Li, K., Wahlqvist, M., and Li, D. 2016. Nutrition, One-Carbon Metabolism and Neural Tube Defects: A Review. *Nutrients* 8(11):741.

35. Centers for Disease Control and Prevention. *National Diabetes Statistics Report: Estimates of Diabetes and Its Burden in the United States, 2014.* Atlanta, GA: U.S. Department of Health and Human Services; 2014.

36. American Diabetes Association. 2016. Management of Diabetes in Pregnancy. *Diabetes Care* 39(Suppl. 1):S94–S98.

37. National Heart, Lung, and Blood Institute. High Blood Pressure in Pregnancy. Available at https://www.nhlbi.nih.gov/health/resources/heart/hbp-pregnancy. Accessed March 2017.

38. Centers for Disease Control and Prevention. 2017. Weight Gain in Pregnancy. Available at https://www.cdc.gov/reproductivehealth/maternalinfanthealth/pregnancy-weight-gain.htm. Accessed March 2017.

39. Abdullah, A., Mamun, A. A., Kinarivala, M., O'Callaghan, M. J., Williams, G. M., Najman, J. M., and Callaway, L. K. 2010. Associations of Excess Weight Gain During Pregnancy with Long-Term Maternal Overweight and Obesity: Evidence from 21 y Postpartum Follow-Up. *American Journal of Clinical Nutrition* 91(5):1336–1341.

40. Institute of Medicine. 2009. *Weight Gain during Pregnancy: Reexamining the Guidelines.*

41. Bricker, L., Reed, K., Wood, L., and Neilson, J. P. 2015. Nutritional advice for improving outcomes in multiple pregnancies. *The Cochrane Library.*

42. Kaiser, L. L., and C. G. Campbell on behalf of the Academy Positions Committee Workgroup. 2014. Practice Paper of the Academy of Nutrition and Dietetics Abstract: Nutrition and Lifestyle for a Healthy Pregnancy Outcome. *Journal of the Academy of Nutrition and Dietetics* 114(9):1447.

43. Ibid.

44. Ibid.

45. Young, B. E., T. J. McNanley, E. M. Cooper, A. W. McIntyre, F. Witter, Z. L. Harris, and K. O. O'Brien. 2012. Maternal Vitamin D Status and Calcium Intake Interact to Affect Fetal Skeletal Growth in Utero in Pregnant Adolescents. *American Journal of Clinical Nutrition* 95:1103–1112.

46. World Health Organization. 2012. Guideline: Vitamin D supplementation in pregnant women. *The WHO Reproductive Health Library.* Geneva: World Health Organization. Available at http://apps.who.int/iris/bitstream/10665/85313/1/9789241504935_eng.pdf Accessed March 2017.

47. Yan, Y., Jiang, X., West, A. A., Perry, C. A., Malysheva, O. V., Brenna, J. T., Stabler, S. P., Allen, R. H., Gregory, J. F., and Caudill, M. A. 2013. Pregnancy Alters Choline Dynamics: Results of a Randomized Trial Using Stable Isotope Methodology in Pregnant and Nonpregnant Women. *American Journal of Clinical Nutrition* 98:1459–1467.

48. Lauritzen, L., Brambilla, P., Mazzocchi, A., Harsløf, L. B. S., Ciappolino, V., Agostoni, C. 2016. DHA Effects in Brain Development and Function. *Nutrients* 8(1):6.

49. Einarson, T. R., Piwko, C., and Koren, G. 2013. Prevalence of Nausea and Vomiting of Pregnancy in the USA: A Meta Analysis. *Journal of Population Therapeutics and Clinical Pharmacology* 20(2):e163–170.

50. Ibid.

51. Festin, M. 2014. Nausea and Vomiting in Early Pregnancy. *BMJ Clinical Evidence* 3:1405.

52. National Institutes of Health. U.S. National Library of Medicine. 2012. *Morning Sickness.* www.nlm.nih.gov/medlineplus/ency/patientinstructions/000604.htm. Accessed March 2017.

53. Festin, M. 2014. Nausea and Vomiting in Early Pregnancy.

54. Fawcett, E. J., Fawcett, J. M., and Mazmanian, D. 2016. A Meta-Analysis of the Worldwide Prevalence of Pica During Pregnancy and the Postpartum Period. *International Journal of Gynecology and Obstetrics* 133(3):277–283.

55. Miao, D., Young, S. L., and Golden, C. D. 2015. A Meta-Analysis of Pica and Micronutrient Status. *American Journal of Human Biology* 27(1):84–93.

56. Fawcett, E. J., Fawcett, J. M., and Mazmanian, D. 2016. A Meta-Analysis of the Worldwide Prevalence of Pica During Pregnancy and the Postpartum Period.

57. Kaiser, L. L., and C. G. Campbell on behalf of the Academy Positions Committee Workgroup. 2014. Practice Paper of the Academy of Nutrition and Dietetics Abstract: Nutrition and Lifestyle for a Healthy Pregnancy Outcome.

58. Pope, E., Koren, G., and Bozzo, P. 2014. Sugar Substitutes During Pregnancy. *Canadian Family Physician* 60(11):1003–1005.

59. Morisaki, N., Esplin, M. S., Varner, M. W., Henry, E., and Oken, E. 2013. Declines in Birth Weight and Fetal Growth Independent of Gestational Length. *Obstetrics and Gynecology* 121(1):51–58.

60. Centers for Disease Control and Prevention. 2017. Weight Gain in Pregnancy. Available at https://www.cdc.gov/reproductivehealth/maternalinfanthealth/pregnancy-weight-gain.htm. Accessed March 2017.

61. American College of Obstetricians and Gynecologists. 2015. Physical activity and exercise during pregnancy and the postpartum period. Committee Opinion No. 650. *Obstetrics and Gynecology* 126:e135–142.

62. Ibid.

63. Ibid.

64. Kaiser, L. L., and C. G. Campbell on behalf of the Academy Positions Committee Workgroup. 2014. Practice Paper of the Academy of Nutrition and Dietetics Abstract: Nutrition and Lifestyle for a Healthy Pregnancy Outcome.

65. DeSisto, C. L., Kim, S. Y., and Sharma, A. J. 2014. Prevalence Estimates of Gestational Diabetes Mellitus in the United States, Pregnancy Risk Assessment Monitoring System (PRAMS), 2007–2010. *Preventing Chronic Disease* 11:1304–1315.

66. American Diabetes Association. 2017. Gestational Diabetes. Available at www.diabetes.org/diabetes-basics/gestational. Accessed March 2017.

67. Mohammadbeigi, A., Farhadifar, F., Soufizadeh, N., Mohammadsalehi, N., Rezaiee, M., and Aghaei, M. 2013. Fetal Macrosomia: Risk Factors, Maternal, and Perinatal Outcome. *Annals of Medical and Health Sciences Research* 3(4):546–550.

68. Moore, T. R., Hauguel-De Mouzon, S., and Catalano, P. 2014. Diabetes in Pregnancy. In R. K. Creasy, R. Resnik, J. D. Iams, C. J. Lockwood, T. R. Moore, M. F. Greene, eds. *Creasy and Resnik's Maternal-Fetal Medicine: Principles and Practice.* 7th ed. Philadelphia, PA: Elsevier Saunders; chap. 59.

69. Ibid.

70. National Institute of Diabetes, Digestive and Kidney Diseases. Did you have gestational diabetes when you were pregnant? Available from: https://www.niddk.nih.gov/health-information/health-communication-programs/ndep/am-i-at-risk/gdm/gestational-diabetes-pregnancy/Pages/publicationdetail.aspx. Accessed March 2017.

71. Ibid.

72. Mayo Clinic. Gestational Diabetes: Risk Factors. 2017. Available from http://www.mayoclinic.org/diseases-conditions/gestational-diabetes/basics/risk-factors/con-20014854. Accessed March 2017.

73. Ibid.

74. National Heart, Lung, and Blood Institute. High Blood Pressure in Pregnancy. Available from https://www.nhlbi.nih.gov/health/resources/heart/hbp-pregnancy. Accessed March 2017.

75. Williams, D. 2011. Long-Term Complications of Preeclampsia. *Seminars in Nephrology* 31:111–122.

76. James, P. A., Oparil, S., Carter, B. L., Cushman, W. C., Dennison-Himmelfarb, C., Handler, J., et al. 2014. Evidence-Based Guideline for the Management of High Blood Pressure in Adults Report From the Panel Members Appointed to the Eighth Joint National Committee (JNC 8). *Journal of the American Medical Association* 311(5):507–520.

77. Ibid.

78. National Institutes of Health. U.S. National Library of Medicine. 2016. *Preeclampsia*. Available at www.nlm.nih.gov/medlineplus/ency/article/000898.htm. Accessed March 2017.

79. The American College of Obstetricians and Gynecologists. 2013. *Hypertension in Pregnancy*. Available at http://www.acog.org/Resources-And-Publications/Task-Force-and-Work-Group-Reports/Hypertension-in-Pregnancy. Accessed March 2017.

80. James, P. A., et al. 2014 Evidence-Based Guideline for the Management of High Blood Pressure in Adults. Report From the Panel Members Appointed to the Eighth Joint National Committee (JNC 8).

81. Kaiser, L. L., and C. G. Campbell on behalf of the Academy Positions Committee Workgroup. 2014. Practice Paper of the Academy of Nutrition and Dietetics Abstract: Nutrition and Lifestyle for a Healthy Pregnancy Outcome

82. Centers for Disease Control and Prevention. 2014. *Teen Pregnancy in the US*. Available at https://www.cdc.gov/teenpregnancy/about/. Accessed March 2017.

83. Cavazos-Rehg, P. A., Krauss, M. J., Spitznagel, E. L., Bommarito, K., Madden, T., Olsen, M. A., et al. 2015. Maternal Age and Risk of Labor and Delivery Complications. *Maternal and Child Health Journal* 19(6):1202–1211.

84. National Institutes of Health, U.S. National Library of Medicine. 2011. *Adolescent Pregnancy*. Available at https://www.hhs.gov/ash/oah/adolescent-health-topics/reproductive-health/teen-pregnancy/. Accessed May 2017.

85. Ibid.

86. Martin, J. A., Hamilton, B. E., Osterman, M. J., Driscoll, A. K., and Mathews, T. J. 2017. Births: Final Data for 2015. *National Vital Statistics Report* 66(1):1.

87. Mark V., and Sauer, M. V. 2015. Reproduction at an advanced maternal age and maternal health. *Fertility and Sterility* 103(5):1136–1143.

88. Food and Nutrition Service. 2013. *About WIC: WIC at a Glance*. Available at www.fns.usda.gov/wic/about-wic-wic-glance. Accessed March 2017.

89. United States Department of Agriculture. 2016. Women Infants and Children: Final Rule: Revisions in the WIC Food Packages. Available at https://www.fns.usda.gov/wic/final-rule-revisions-wic-food-packages. Accessed March 2017.

90. Thorn, B., Tadler, C., Huret, N., Trippe, C., Ayo, E., Mendelson, M., Patlan, K. L., Schwartz, G., & Tran, V. (2015). WIC Participant and Program Characteristics 2014. Prepared by Insight Policy Research under Contract No. AG-3198-C- 11-0010. Alexandria, VA: U.S. Department of Agriculture, Food and Nutrition Service.

91. Ibid

92. Ibid.

93. American Academy of Pediatrics, American College of Obstetricians and Gynecologists. 2013. Breastfeeding Handbook for Physicians, 2nd ed.

94. Carrothers, J. M., York, M. A., Brooker, S. L., Lackey, K. A., Williams, J. E., Shafii, B., Price, W. J., Settles, M. L., McGuire, M. A., and McGuire, M. K. 2015. Fecal Microbial Community Structure Is Stable Over Time and Related to Variation in Macronutrient and Micronutrient Intakes in Lactating Women. *Journal of Nutrition* 145(10):2379–2388.

95. Kornides, M., and Kitsantas, P. 2013. Evaluation of Breastfeeding Promotion, Support, and Knowledge of Benefits on Breastfeeding Outcomes. *Journal of Child Health Care* 17(3):264–273.

96. Ballard, O., and Morrow, A. L. 2013. Human Milk Composition: Nutrients and Bioactive Factors. *Pediatric Clinics of North America* 60(1):49–74.

97. Lessen, R., and Kavanagh, K. 2015. Position of the Academy of Nutrition and Dietetics: Promoting and Supporting Breastfeeding. *Journal of the Academy of Nutrition and Dietetics* 115(3):444–449.

98. Ibid.

99. Casey, C. F., D. Slawson, and L. R. Neal. 2010. Vitamin D Supplementation in Infants, Children, and Adolescents. *American Family Physician* 81:745–748.

100. Wagner, C. L., F. R. Greer, and the Section on Breast-Feeding and Committee on Nutrition. 2008. Prevention of Rickets and Vitamin D Deficiency in Infants, Children, and Adolescents. *Pediatrics* 122:1142–1152.

101. Lessen, R., and Kavanagh K. Position of the Academy of Nutrition and Dietetics: Promoting and Supporting Breastfeeding.

102. Breakey, A. A., Hinde, K., Valeggia, C. R., Sinofsky, A., and Ellison, P. T. 2015. Illness in Breastfeeding Infants Relates to Concentration of Lactoferrin and Secretory Immunoglobulin A in Mother's Milk. *Evolution, Medicine, and Public Health* 1:21–31.

103. Lessen, R., and Kavanagh, K. Position of the Academy of Nutrition and Dietetics: Promoting and Supporting Breastfeeding.

104. Ibid.

105. Woo Baidal, J. A., Locks, L. M., Cheng, E. R., Blake-Lamb, T. L., Perkins, M. E., Taveras, E. M. 2016. Risk Factors for Childhood Obesity in the First 1,000 Days: A Systematic Review. *American Journal of Preventive Medicine* 50(6):761–779.

106. Jasani, B., Simmer, K., Patole, S. K., and Rao, S. C. 2017. Long Chain Polyunsaturated Fatty Acid Supplementation in Infants Born at Term. *Cochrane Database of Systematic Reviews* Issue 3, Art. No.: CD000376.

107. Office on Women's Health, U.S. Department of Health and Human Services. 2017. Recovering from Birth. Available at https://www.womenshealth.gov/pregnancy/childbirth-and-beyond/recovering-birth. Accessed March 2017.

108. U.S. Department of Health and Human Services. Office on Women's Health. 2011. *Breast-Feeding: Why Breast-Feeding Is Important*. Available at www.womenshealth.gov/breastfeeding/why-breastfeeding-is-important/. Accessed March 2017.

109. U.S. Department of Health and Human Services. 2011. *The Surgeon General's Call to Action to Support Breast-Feeding*. Available at www.surgeongeneral.gov/library/calls/breastfeeding/factsheet.html. Accessed March 2017.

110. Batrick, M., and A. Reinhold. 2010. The Burden of Suboptimal Breast-Feeding in the United States. *Pediatrics* 125:e1048–e1056.

111. Ibid.

112. Dieterich, C. M., Felice, J. P., O'Sullivan, E., and Rasmussen, K. M. 2013. Breastfeeding and Health Outcomes for the Mother–Infant Dyad. *Pediatric Clinics of North America* 60(1):31 –48.

113. Ibid.

114. Centers for Disease Control and Prevention. 2014. Breast-Feeding Report Card—United States, 2014. Available at ttps://www.cdc.gov/breastfeeding/pdf/2014breastfeedingreportcard.pdf. Accessed March 2017.

115. Department of Health and Human Services. 2010. Healthy People 2020. *Maternal, Infant, and Child Health*. Available at www.healthypeople.gov/2020/topicsobjectives2020/over_view.aspx?topicid=26. Accessed March 2017.

116. Centers for Disease Control and Prevention. 2014. Breast-Feeding Report Card—United States, 2014. Available at ttps://www.cdc.gov/breastfeeding/pdf/2014breastfeedingreportcard.pdf. Accessed March 2017.

117. Institute of Medicine. Food and Nutrition Board. 2005. Dietary Reference Intakes for Energy, Carbohydrate, Fiber, Fat, Fatty Acids, Cholesterol, Protein, and Amino Acids. Washington, DC: The National Academies Press. Available at https://www.nap.edu/read/11537/chapter/8. Accessed March 2017.

118. Ibid.

119. Haastrup, M. B., Pottegård, A., and Damkier, P. (2014) Alcohol and Breastfeeding. *Basic and Clinical Pharmacology and Toxicology* 114(2):168–173.

120. Behnke, M., Smith, V. C., Behnke, M., Smith, V. C., Levy, S., Ammerman, S. D., et al. 2013. Prenatal Substance

Abuse: Short- and Long-term Effects on the Exposed Fetus. *Pediatrics* 131(3):e1009–e1024.

121. U.S. Department of Health and Human Services. *Let's Make the Next Generation Tobacco-Free: Your Guide to the 50th Anniversary Surgeon General's Report on Smoking and Health.* Atlanta: U.S. Department of Health and Human Services, Centers for Disease Control and Prevention, National Center for Chronic Disease Prevention and Health Promotion, Office on Smoking and Health, 2014.

122. Thygarajan, A., and A. Wesley Burks. 2008. American Academy of Pediatrics Recommendations on the Effects of Early Nutritional Interventions on the Development of Atopic Disease. *Current Opinions in Pediatrics* 20:698–702.

123. American Academy of Pediatrics. Section on Breast-Feeding. 2012. Breast-Feeding and the Use of Human Milk. *Pediatrics* 129:e827–e841. Available at www.pediatrics.aappublications.org/content/129/3/e827.full. Accessed March 2017.

124. Ibid.; Lawrence, et al. 2011. Breast-Feeding: More Than Just Good Nutrition.

125. Baker, R. D., F. R. Greer, and the Committee on Nutrition. 2010. Diagnosis and Prevention of Iron Deficiency and Iron-Deficiency Anemia in Infants and Young Children (0–3 Years of Age). *Pediatrics* 126:1040–1050.

126. American Academy of Pediatrics, Section on Breastfeeding. 2012. Breastfeeding and the use of human milk. *Pediatrics* 129:e827–841.

127. U.S. Department of Health and Human Services. U.S. Food and Drug Administration. 2013. *Food Safety for Moms-to-Be.* Available at www.fda.gov/food/resources-foryou/healtheducators/ucm089629.htm. Accessed March 2017.

128. American Dental Association. 2017. Statement on Early Childhood Caries. Available at http://www.ada.org/en/about-the-ada/ada-positions-policies-and-statements/statement-on-early-childhood-caries. Accessed March 2017.

129. Ibid

130. Kuczmarski, R. J., Ogden, C. L., Guo, S. S., et al. 2002. 2000 CDC growth charts for the United States: methods and development. National Center for Health Statistics. *Vital Health Statistics* 11(246).

131. Reynolds, G. D., and Romano, A. C. 2016. The Development of Attention Systems and Working Memory in Infancy. *Frontiers in Systems Neuroscience* 10:15.

132. U.S. National Library of Medicine. Failure to thrive. Available at https://medlineplus.gov/ency/article/000991.htm. Accessed March 2017.

133. Institute of Medicine. Food and Nutrition Board. 2005. Dietary Reference Intakes for Energy, Carbohydrate, Fiber, Fat, Fatty Acids, Cholesterol, Protein, and Amino Acids.

134. Lessen, R., and Kavanagh, K. 2015. Position of the Academy of Nutrition and Dietetics: Promoting and Supporting Breastfeeding.

135. Ibid.

136. Ibid.

137. Ibid.

138. Institute of Medicine. Food and Nutrition Board. 2005. Dietary Reference Intakes for Energy, Carbohydrate, Fiber, Fat, Fatty Acids, Cholesterol, Protein, and Amino Acids.

139. Reynolds, G. D., and Romano, A. C. 2016. The Development of Attention Systems and Working Memory in Infancy.

140. American Academy of Pediatrics. 2017. Infant Food and Feeding. Available at www.aap.org/en-us/advocacy-and-policy/aap-health-initiatives/HALF-Implementation-Guide/Age-Specific-Content/Pages/Infant-Food-and-Feeding.aspx#none. Accessed March 2017.

141. American Academy of Pediatrics. Infant Food and Feeding. Available from https://www.aap.org/en-us/advocacy-and-policy/aap-health-initiatives/HALF-Implementation-Guide/Age-Specific-Content/pages/infant-food-and-feeding.aspx. Accessed March 2017.

142. Reynolds, G. D., and Romano, A. C. 2016. The Development of Attention Systems and Working Memory in Infancy.

143. American Academy of Pediatrics. 2017. Infant Food and Feeding.

144. Ibid.

145. American Academy of Pediatrics. 2013. Switching to Solid Foods. Available at www.healthychildren.org/English/ages-stages/baby/feeding-nutrition/Pages/Switching-To-Solid-Foods.aspx. Accessed March 2017.

146. Ross, E. S. 2017. Flavor and Taste Development in the First Years of Life. *Nestle Nutrition Institute Workshop Series* 87:49–58.

147. Ibid.

148. Fleischer, D. M., J. M. Spergel, A. H. Assa'ad, and J. A. Pongracic. 2013. Primary Prevention of Allergic Disease through Nutrition Interventions. *Journal of Allergy and Clinical Immunology: In Practice* 1:29–36.

149. National Library of Medicine. 2017. Infant Botulism. Available from https://medlineplus.gov/ency/article/001384.htm. Accessed April 2017.

150. Birch L. 1979. Dimensions of Preschool Children's Food Preferences. *Journal of Nutrition Education* 11:77–80.

151. National Institute of Allergy and Infectious Diseases. 2012. Food Allergy: An Overview. Available at www.niaid.nih.gov/topics/foodallergy/documents/foodallergy.pdf. Accessed March 2017.

152. Food and Drug Administration. 2016. Frequently Asked Questions about Food Allergies. Available at https://www.fda.gov/Food/IngredientsPackagingLabeling/FoodAllergens/ucm530854.htm. Accessed March 2017.

153. Centers for Disease Control and Prevention. 2013. *NCHS Data Brief Number 121: Trends in Allergic Conditions among Children: United States, 1997–2011.* Available at www.cdc.gov. Accessed March 2017.

154. Du Toit, G., Roberts, G., Sayre, P. H., Bahnson, H. T., Radulovic, S., Santos, A. F., et al. 2015. Randomized Trial of Peanut Consumption in Infants at Risk for Peanut Allergy. *New England Journal of Medicine* 372(9):803–813.

155. Fleischer, D. M., Sicherer, S., Greenhawt, M., et al. 2017. Consensus Communication on Early Peanut Introduction and the Prevention of Peanut Allergy in High-risk Infants. *Pediatrics* 136;600.

156. American Academy of Pediatrics. 2013. Food Allergies in Children. Available at www.healthychildren.org/English/healthy-living/nutrition/Pages/Food-Allergies-in-Children.aspx. Accessed March 2017.

157. The Food Allergy and Anaphylaxis Network. 2014. About Food Allergens. Available at www.foodallergy.org. Accessed March 2017.

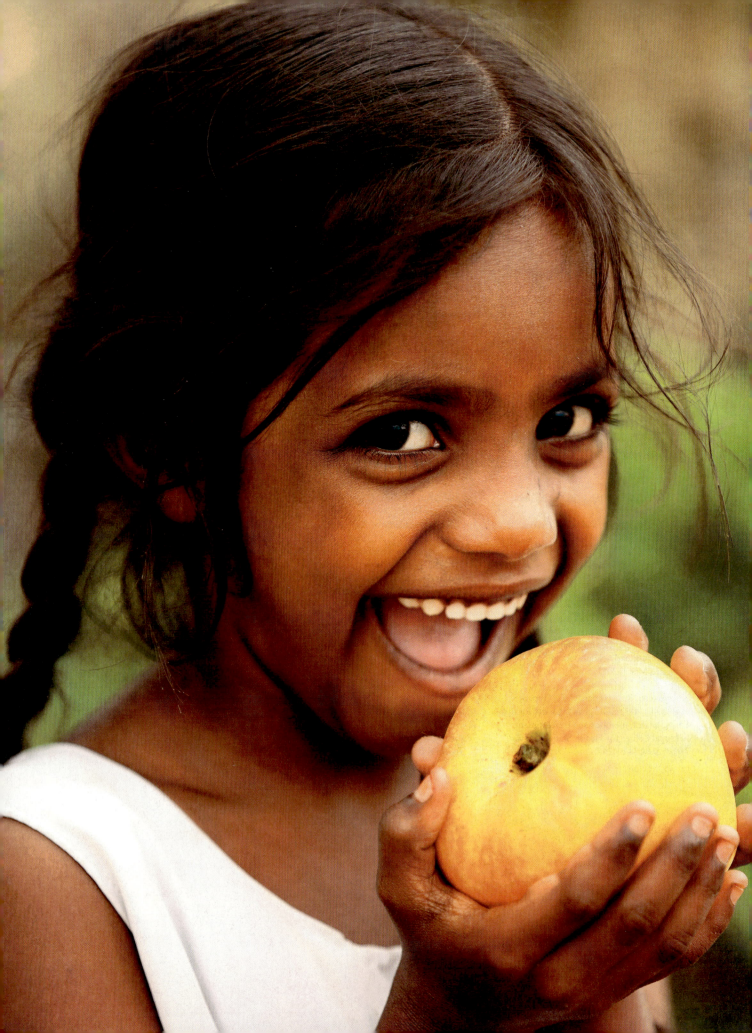

Life Cycle Nutrition

Toddlers through Adolescents

Learning Outcomes

After reading this chapter, you will be able to:

18.1 Describe the nutritional needs of toddlers and preschoolers.

18.2 Discuss how parents influence a child's food preferences.

18.3 Describe the effects of food choices, school lunches, food allergies, and poverty on the nutritional status of school-age children.

18.4 Explain why school-age children are experiencing high rates of obesity.

18.5 Describe the nutritional needs of adolescents.

18.6 Discuss the nutritional issues that affect adolescents, including disordered eating.

18.7 Identify the health risks of obesity in children and teens.

True or False?

1. Toddlers grow at the same rate as infants. **T**/**F**

2. Toddlers and preschoolers are often too busy exploring to eat. **T**/**F**

3. Children can receive all the nutrients they need by drinking milk. **T**/**F**

4. Iron deficiency in young children is caused by eating too much chicken. **T**/**F**

5. Once a child refuses a new food, there is no point in offering it again. **T**/**F**

6. Young children often go on food "jags." **T**/**F**

7. The rise in childhood obesity is due entirely to fast food. **T**/**F**

8. Lunches served under the National School Lunch Program have to follow certain nutritional regulations. **T**/**F**

9. As long as teens drink diet soda, they don't have to worry about negative health effects. **T**/**F**

10. Most teens consume adequate amounts of calcium and iron. **T**/**F**

See page 692 for the answers.

As children age, their nutritional needs and eating habits continually evolve. Whereas infants are relatively immobile much of the time, once children learn to stand and walk, they'd rather explore the world than sit quietly at the table for a meal or snack. Just when parents think they have a handle on toddler nutrition, they find they are parenting a preschooler who presents them with a new set of nutritional challenges. And so it goes through the school-age and teen years.

In this chapter, we explore the unique nutrition needs of toddlers, preschoolers, school-age children, and adolescents as they grow and change.

What Are the Nutritional Needs of Toddlers and Preschoolers?

LO 18.1 Describe the nutritional needs of toddlers and preschoolers.

Early childhood consists of two distinct age categories: **toddlers** (ages 1 and 2) and **preschoolers** (ages 3–5). Toddlers and preschoolers are still growing rapidly, but less rapidly than infants. During the second year of life the average weight gain is about 3 to 5 pounds, and the average height or length increase is about 3–5 inches.[1] As a result of their slowed growth, the appetites of toddlers diminish relative to infancy. This is normal. Children are likely eating enough as long as there are no prolonged dramatic changes in their health, including decreased energy level, diarrhea, nausea and vomiting, or changes in the child's hair, skin, or nails.

The growth chart shown in **Figure 18.1** is used to track the growth through childhood and to determine how an individual child's growth rate compares to other children of the same age and sex. Growth charts can be used to assess whether a child is growing at a consistent rate. In general, the growth of a healthy child should continue roughly along the same percentile for age and sex, and large increases or decreases should be evaluated by a health professional. See the Calculation Corner to practice reading a growth chart.

Young Children Need Frequent, Small, Nutrient-Dense Meals and Snacks

To fuel their activity, toddlers need between 1,000 and 1,400 kilocalories per day from nutrient-dense foods. Toddlers eat small amounts and may need several meals and snacks. Meals and snacks should consist of small portions of protein-rich foods, including lean meat, poultry, seafood, eggs, tofu, beans, fruits, vegetables, milk, and whole grains, instead of lower-nutrient fare such as fried chicken nuggets, French fries, sugary drinks, cookies, and crackers.[2] (The Daily Food Plans for Preschoolers and Kids, discussed later in this chapter, can be used to determine specific numbers of servings for young children.)

Parents must be mindful about portion sizes for young children and avoid encouraging them to eat more than they need. One way to help ensure proper portion sizes is to use child-sized plates and cups, which are more appropriate for the quantity of food a child can eat.

Children will eat different amounts at each meal. Parents should serve small portions, such as a few tablespoons of cooked whole-grain pasta or vegetables or an ounce or so of protein-rich foods, such as chicken, to start. If a child wants more food, then he or she should have it. Caregivers looking after a group of children with larger or smaller appetites should tailor portion sizes to each child's individual needs.

toddlers Children 1 or 2 years old.

preschoolers Children 3–5 years old.

Growth Chart

Birth to 36 months: Boys
Length-for-age and weight-for-age percentiles

Name _____

Record # _____

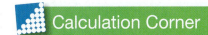
Calculation Corner

Interpreting a Growth Chart

Properly interpreting a CDC growth chart is essential for monitoring a child's growth patterns. Marcus is 21 months old, weighs 32 pounds, and is 35 inches tall. Follow the steps below to determine where he falls on the growth chart.

Step 1. Select the appropriate chart for age and gender.

Step 2. Locate Marcus's age at the top of the chart.

Step 3. Locate Marcus's weight along the side of the chart.

Step 4. Mark where Marcus's age and weight meet.

Step 5. Locate Marcus's height (length) in inches along the side of the chart.

Step 6. Mark where Marcus's age and height meet.

What is Marcus's percentile for weight? for height?

Answer:

Marcus is at the 90th percentile for weight. Ten percent of the population falls above Marcus's weight, and 90 percent below. He is also at the 90th percentile for height. Ten percent of the population falls above that, and 90 percent below.

Go to Mastering Nutrition and complete a Math Video activity similar to the problem in this Calculation Corner.

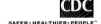

▲ **Figure 18.1 Growth Chart**
Growth charts can be used to assess whether a child is developing at a rate comparable to other children of the same age and gender.

Source: Developed by the National Center for Health Statistics in collaboration with the National Center for Chronic Disease Prevention and Health Promotion. 2000. Clinical Growth Charts. Available at www.cdc.gov/growthcharts/clinical/_charts.htm. Accessed May 2017.

To prevent choking in children under the age of 4, food should be cut into bite-sized pieces. Some foods are particularly problematic for very young children. The American Academy of Pediatrics (AAP) recommends keeping hot dogs, nuts and seeds, chunks of meat or cheese, whole grapes, hard candy, popcorn, chunks of peanut butter, raw vegetables, raisins, and chewing gum away from children younger than age 4.[3] Children should always sit when eating to reduce the likelihood of food entering the trachea during a stumble or fall. The Table Tips provide some ideas for healthy, toddler-friendly snacks.

Children who attend daycare may receive a substantial portion of their daily food in that setting. In some cases, daycare providers may offer menu items or snacks that are

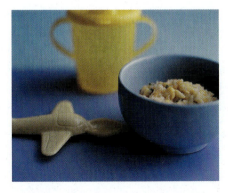

Using child-sized dishes at mealtimes can help caregivers monitor portion sizes.

Prepare Tasty Treats for Toddlers

Fresh pear, peach, or plum, peeled and cut into very small pieces

Whole-wheat English muffin with 1 tsp butter and cinnamon, cut into small pieces

Whole-grain pumpkin or bran muffin, cut into small pieces

Applesauce (no added sugar)

Yogurt with diced bananas

Remember: Young children should always be supervised while eating!

superior to what is given at home. Every state requires that licensed child-care centers meet minimum standards for nutrition. The National Resource Center for Health and Safety in Child Care and Early Education website (*http://nrckids.org*) posts all childcare regulations for each state.[4] Parents should know what is being offered at the daycare site and provide alternative foods for their child when necessary. This is particularly important for children with food allergies or food intolerances. Even if children do not have special dietary concerns, parents have the right to be firm about what their child eats in the daycare setting.

Young Children Need Adequate Carbohydrate, Fat, and Protein

The AMDR and RDA for carbohydrate—45–65 percent of daily kilocalories and 130 grams, respectively—do not change from toddlerhood through adulthood. Fruits, vegetables, and grains should provide the majority of carbohydrate for children. Added sugars—found in sugary drinks, candy, desserts, and many processed foods—should be strictly limited. Many parents blame high sugar consumption for **attention-deficit/hyperactivity disorder (ADHD)** in children. Does research support a link? Read the nearby Examining the Evidence box to find out.

At least half of the grains in a child's diet should be whole grains to help achieve the suggested intake for fiber and certain vitamins and minerals.[5] The recommended daily intake for fiber increases by age, as toddlers (1- to 3-year-olds) require 19 grams per day, whereas school-age children (age 4–8 years) need 25 grams per day. Like adults, toddlers need fiber to promote bowel regularity and prevent constipation.[6] A balanced diet with whole fruits, vegetables, and whole grains can easily meet a toddler's daily fiber needs.

The AMDR for protein is 5–20 percent of total energy needs for toddlers and increases to 10–30 percent for childhood and adolescence (4–18 years). The RDA for protein for toddlers is set at 1.1 grams per kilogram of body weight and decreases to 0.95 gram per kilogram of body weight in school-age children.[7] Consuming an adequate amount of carbohydrate has a protein-sparing effect, allowing protein to be used for growth and tissue repair rather than for energy.

The AMDR for total daily fat intake is 30–40 percent of total kilocalories for children 1 to 3 years old, and 25–35 percent for children age 4 through 18.[8] Dietary fat contributes to normal development of the brain and nerve cells and is a concentrated source of energy to fuel growth. Fat is used for the synthesis of the myelin sheath that insulates neurons and aids in nerve impulse conduction. Some neurons are fully myelinated at birth, such as those in the motor cortex that control the infant's ability to suckle. Intensive myelination continues as children fine-tune their vision, hearing, language, emotions, and physical capabilities during the first 2 years of life. Unsaturated fats, found in foods such as fish, nuts, and vegetable oils, should be the dominant fats in the diets of children ages 2 and older. It is also recommended that toddlers receive 0.7 grams of omega-3 fatty acids and that school-age children consume 0.9 grams per day. Solid fats, such as butter and lard, should be limited given their saturated fat content.

Young Children Need Adequate Iron, Calcium, and Vitamin D

Iron, calcium, and vitamin D are particularly important to a young child's development and growth. Iron is needed to prevent developmental delays, and calcium and vitamin D support rapid bone growth.

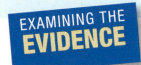

Can a Change in Diet Prevent or Treat ADHD in Children?

Parents often wonder if their child's diet is responsible for all or some of their children's behavior. Observing young children after they eat cake at a birthday party, for example, can lead one to wonder whether the sugar in the cake causes children to become hyperactive. In the United States, an estimated 3–5 percent of children (about 2 million) have been diagnosed with **attention-deficit/ hyperactivity disorder (ADHD)** (sometimes called attention-deficit disorder, or ADD).[1] ADHD is a condition—generally identified in early childhood—in which children are inattentive, hyperactive, and impulsive.[2] Children with ADHD have difficulty controlling their behavior, which can be disruptive in the home and classroom. The condition can be difficult and frustrating to manage for parents, caregivers, and teachers, and many people would like to believe that a solution—namely, changing their child's diet—could prevent or treat it. Is this true?

Dietary approaches proposed for the prevention and treatment of ADHD include sugar restriction, additive/ preservative-free diets, allergy elimination diets, and omega-3 fatty-acid supplementation. Whereas research consistently supports that sugar consumption does not cause ADHD, the research literature is equivocal regarding the other dietary approaches.[3–5] Moreover, some research suggests that children who consume a diet very different from the Mediterranean diet have a higher prevalence of ADHD.[6] Further research is needed to clarify the relationship between diet and ADHD.

With so many children and families affected by ADHD, research into

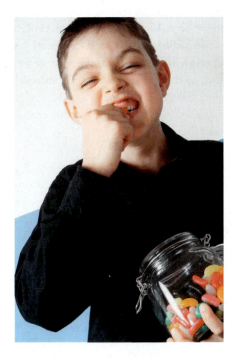

potential causes has increased in recent years. Attention disorders often run in families, so there may be genetic influences.[7]

Clinical treatments for ADHD include medications, psychotherapy, behavioral therapies, and dietary therapy. Parents of children with ADHD may want to consult with a registered dietitian nutritionist before making changes to their child's diet or to address any nutritional issues, such as underweight due to side effects of medications that decrease appetite. Disruptive mealtimes may also be a concern (if ADHD is not well managed). Organizations such as the National Institute of Mental Health (*www.nimh.nih.gov*) and the American Academy of Child and Adolescent Psychiatry (*www.aacap*

.org/index.ww) provide information for families of children with ADHD.

References

1. National Library of Medicine. 2016. Attention Deficit Hyperactivity Disorder. Available from https://medlineplus.gov/ attentiondeficithyperactivitydisorder.html. Accessed May, 2017.
2. National Institute of Mental Health. 2016. *Attention Deficit Hyperactivity Disorder.* Available at www.nimh.nih.gov/health/topics/ attention-deficit-hyperactivity-disorder-adhd/index.shtml. Accessed May 2017.
3. Pelsser, L.M., Frankena, K., Toorman, J., and Pereira, R.R. 2017. Diet and ADHD, Reviewing the Evidence: A Systematic Review of Meta-Analyses of Double-Blind Placebo-Controlled Trials Evaluating the Efficacy of Diet Interventions on the Behavior of Children with ADHD. *PloS One* 12(1).
4. Millichap, J. G., and Yee, M. M. 2012. The Diet Factor in Attention-Deficit/ Hyperactivity Disorder. *Pediatrics* 129(2):330–337.
5. Sonuga-Barke, E. J., Brandeis, D., Cortese, S., Daley, D., Ferrin, M., et al., 2013. Non-pharmacological Interventions for ADHD: Systematic Review and Meta-Analyses of Randomized Controlled Trials of Dietary and Psychological Treatments. *American Journal of Psychiatry* 170(3):275–289.
6. Ríos-Hernández, A., Alda, J. A., Farran-Codina, A., Ferreira-García, E., and Izquierdo-Pulido, M. 2017. The Mediterranean Diet and ADHD in Children and Adolecents. *Pediatrics* 139(2).
7. Larsson, H., Chang, Z., D'Onofrio, B. M., and Lichtenstein, P. 2014. The Heritability of Clinically Diagnosed Attention Deficit Hyperactivity Disorder across the Lifespan. *Psychological Medicine* 44(10):2223–2229.

attention-deficit/hyperactivity disorder (ADHD) Condition characterized by impulsivity, high distractibility, and hyperactivity; previously known as attention-deficit disorder, or ADD.

Iron Needs

Toddlers need 7 milligrams of iron daily and school-age children require 10 milligrams each day.[9] To help children meet their iron needs, parents and caregivers should offer iron-rich lean meats, poultry, and fish and fortified grains such as breakfast cereal on a daily basis. If children get too large a percentage of their kilocalories from iron-poor cow's milk, iron-rich foods may be displaced.[10] The Table Tips list kid-friendly ways to enjoy foods that have plenty of iron.

Create Kid-Friendly, Iron-Rich Foods

Serve iron-fortified cereal. (*Note:* No raisins under age 4.)

Add mashed, cooked chickpeas to tossed salads.

Serve tuna sandwiches on iron-enriched bread.

Tote iron-enriched ready-to-eat breakfast cereal on trips.

Serve iron-enriched pastas with meatballs or a meat sauce.

Mix enriched rice with dinnertime veggies for a nutrient-dense meal.

Iron needs are highest during periods of rapid growth, and young children are more prone to iron deficiency because they are growing so fast. Among children, iron deficiency is seen most often between 6 months and 3 years of age. It is the most common nutritional deficiency and the leading cause of anemia in the United States.[11] Among children living in the United States, an estimated 14 percent of 1- to 2-year-olds and 4 percent of 3- to 4-year-olds experience iron deficiency.[12] Worldwide, iron-deficiency anemia, the result of severe iron deficiency, affects an estimated 2 billion people, and young children and their mothers are the most often afflicted.[13] Iron-deficiency anemia during infancy and early childhood can impair a child's cognition, behavior, and overall neurodevelopment and leave lasting damage,[14] so it is crucial to ensure that children get sufficient iron in their diets.

Iron Toxicity

Although iron deficiency is a big concern in young children, it is possible to get too much iron, usually due to an overdose from iron-containing dietary supplements and medications. Children may be attracted to pills with iron because they can look like candy.[15] To prevent accidental iron poisoning, the FDA requires warning labels on iron-containing drugs and dietary supplements.[16] Parents and other caregivers should keep pills in containers with safety caps and out of reach of children.

Calcium Needs

Toddlers need calcium to develop healthy bones. Children between 1 and 3 years of age should consume 700 milligrams of calcium per day, and children age 4 and 5 should consume 1,000 milligrams.[17] Eight ounces of any type of cow's milk, 8 ounces of yogurt, and $1\frac{1}{2}$ ounces of hard cheese each provide about 300 milligrams of calcium. Children should drink cow's milk or soymilk that is fortified with both calcium and vitamin D.

Vitamin D Needs

The AAP recommends that all children over the age of 1 year consume 15 micrograms (600 IU) of vitamin D daily.[18] Vitamin D is found in fortified milk and soymilk and naturally in egg yolk and certain types of fish. Two eight-ounce cups of milk and a variety of fortified foods daily can help to satisfy a child's vitamin D needs. If the child does not consume adequate amounts of vitamin D from foods, the AAP recommends vitamin D supplements to fill the gap.[19]

Young Children Need Adequate Fluid

A child's daily fluid needs are based on age, body weight, and gender. Young children require 5 cups of fluid per day (1–8 years of age).[20] The best source of fluids is water, but drinking too much fluid of any kind may reduce a child's intake of nutrient-dense solid foods and important nutrients such as iron. Therefore, caregivers should encourage water intake, monitor a child's milk intake, limit juice to no more than 4–6 ounces of 100-percent fruit juice daily, and avoid offering soda and other sugary drinks. A child may require additional fluids on hot days and during vigorous activity. If a child is physically active, it is important to drink water every 15–20 minutes.

Young Children Can Grow Healthfully on Vegetarian Diets

Young children can grow and develop normally on a vegetarian diet, as long as it is balanced. Generally speaking, vegetarian diets are rich in whole grains, vegetables, and fruits—foods that experts encourage all children and adults to eat. Vegetarian diets may be high in fiber, which is helpful in promoting GI health and function; however, too much fiber may prevent children from getting all the nutrients they need by making them feel full too quickly. As with any eating plan, a vegetarian diet should include adequate kilocalories, protein, calcium, iron, vitamin B_{12}, and zinc.[21] Vegan children must be given vitamin B_{12}–fortified foods or supplements as their diets include no animal-based foods.[22] Vitamin B_{12} is available, for example, from fortified breakfast cereals and milk alternatives.

Added Sugars Should Be Limited in Young Children's Diets

As noted earlier, foods high in added sugars displace nutrient-dense foods and should be strictly limited in a child's diet. These foods also promote tooth decay, the potential for which begins as soon as teeth emerge from the gums. Prolonged contact with sugary drinks, candies, and other sweets encourages the growth of bacteria that contribute to the breakdown of tooth enamel. In addition to limiting added sugars, parents and caregivers should help young children practice tooth-friendly dental hygiene. Unfortunately, many children do not practice good dental hygiene, and the Centers for Disease Control and Prevention (CDC) reports that tooth decay affects more than one-fourth of U.S. children age 2–5 years.[23] Left untreated, dental caries can cause serious health problems in addition to pain and discomfort.[24]

LO 18.1: THE TAKE-HOME MESSAGE Toddlers grow more slowly than infants and have appetites that may fluctuate from day to day. Adults should offer children appropriate portion sizes. Toddlers need adequate amounts of kilocalories, carbohydrate, protein, fat, calcium, iron, vitamin D, and other nutrients and must avoid excess iron and too much dietary fiber. Caregivers also need to monitor a child's beverage intake and provide water, milk, and no more than 6 ounces of 100-percent juice daily while avoiding soda and other sugary drinks. Vegetarian toddlers need adequate calcium, iron, and zinc and a daily source of vitamin B_{12}. Caregivers should help young children practice tooth-friendly dental hygiene and limit their intake of added sugars.

How Can Adults Influence Young Children's Food Preferences?

LO 18.2 Discuss how parents influence a child's food preferences.

As toddlers grow and learn to eat independently (see **Table 18.1**), their variety of healthy food choices should increase, too. Eating habits form early in life, and parents and other caregivers can help children establish a lifelong appreciation for a variety of nutrient-dense foods.

According to Ellyn Satter, an expert on child feeding and nutrition, there is a "division of responsibility" when it comes to control of feeding.[25] The adult is responsible for what the child is offered to eat, as well as when and where the food is offered. The child, however, is responsible for how much he or she eats, if anything at all. Food issues and power struggles can occur when adults think that their job is not only to provide the food but also to make sure that the child eats it. Some parents encourage their children to "clean their plates," even when they have indicated that they are full. This is a risky habit

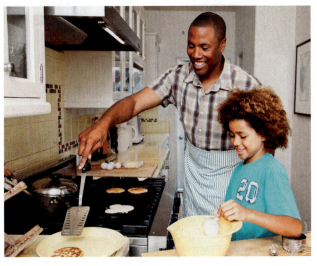

Encourage children to enjoy a variety of healthy foods by involving them in preparing the family meal.

TABLE 18.1 Food Skills of Young Children

Age	Developmental Feeding Skill
1–2	Child uses the big muscles of the arm and can tear and snap vegetables, help scrub, drink from a cup, and help feed self.
3	Child uses the medium muscles of the hand and can help pour, mix, shake, and spread foods. With supervision, child can feed self independently.
4	Child uses the small muscles of the fingers and can peel, juice, crack raw eggs, and use all utensils and napkins.
5	Child uses eye–hand coordination and can measure, cut with supervision, grind, and grate.

that encourages overconsumption and is associated with obesity in later childhood and adolescence.[26] Parents should allow children to stop eating once they are full.

Small children may seem to have very narrow food preferences. Parents may think, "My child only likes chicken nuggets and fries" or "She hates all vegetables." Though it's true that toddlers may be selective in their eating, parents should not give up on encouraging them to try and to accept new foods because it's likely that their food preferences will change with time. For example, they should not hesitate to offer healthy foods with strong tastes, such as broccoli or brussels sprouts, to their children. Some research suggests that it can take up to 14 introductions to a new food before the child both accepts it and enjoys it.[27]

Parents have tremendous influence on their child's food preferences and can act as positive role models for nutritious food choices.[28] Adults should load up their own plates with a variety of fruits and vegetables, lean protein sources, and whole grains and snack on items like carrot sticks and apple slices between meals so that children will be more likely to follow suit. On the other hand, children will also mimic adults' unhealthy behaviors. A mom who only drinks diet soda for dinner or a dad who fills his plate with French fries sends the child a message that these behaviors are appropriate. Involving children in food shopping, menu selection, and preparation of meals is another way to encourage them to enjoy a variety of foods.

Food jags occur when a child refuses anything but a limited selection of foods. This behavior of getting "stuck" on a small selection of foods is quite common and normal in young children. Luckily, food jags are usually temporary. A child who only wants to eat pretzels and oranges, or refuses to eat anything green, will likely emerge from the phase within a few days or weeks.

If a parent or caregiver senses that the food jag is not going away, then the situation might require the parent to pay more careful attention to what the child is eating as well as what he or she is avoiding. Is the child really "eating only crackers" or is the parent forgetting that the child is also drinking milk and eating green beans and orange slices when offered? A parent or caregiver can keep a food diary of everything the child eats and drinks for a few days to help identify any problems. Sharing concerns (and the food diary) with the child's health care provider or a registered dietitian nutritionist and asking for advice may prevent serious nutrient deficiencies in the long run.

In some cases, indulging the food jag may be the best option. If a child is stuck on something like pasta, a parent or caregiver can still offer a variety of foods within that category, such as whole-grain versions or those with added nutrients, such as omega-3 fats.

MyPlate for Preschoolers is a tool that can help adults plan a healthy diet for this age group (see the Web Resources section at the end of this chapter).

food jag Period of time in which a child will eat only one food or a few limited foods meal after meal.

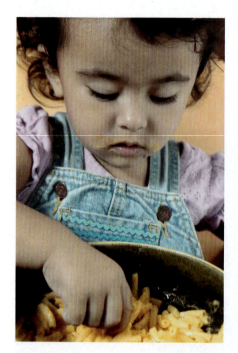

Food jags, such as wanting to only eat one food (like macaroni and cheese), or avoiding certain foods, are common among toddlers.

What Factors Affect School-Age Children's Nutrition?

LO 18.3 Describe the effects of food choices, school lunches, food allergies, and poverty on the nutritional status of school-age children.

School-age children, usually considered those between the ages of 6 and 12, still have plenty of growing to do, and the quality of their diet affects their growth. See **Table 18.2** for the range of energy needs for children in this age group. The table provides wide ranges for each age group. Children who are fairly sedentary have energy needs closer to the lower end of the range, whereas those who are active likely have needs at the higher end of each range. During the school years, gross- and fine-motor skills become more refined, and children's growth rates are steady until the adolescent growth spurt. While school-age children develop at different rates, they add, on average, 7 pounds and 2.5 inches per year.[29]

Because they're in class and away from home, school-age children do not eat as often throughout the day as toddlers and preschoolers. However, they can eat more at one meal, are better able to maintain their blood glucose longer, and tend to be less hungry between meals and snacks. Families, caregivers, and school staff members can help ensure that children make healthy food choices, get regular exercise, and maintain a healthy body weight.

MyPlate Can Help Guide Food Choices

Most parents are not nutrition experts, and the idea of trying to meet their child's entire nutrient needs can be overwhelming and confusing. Fortunately, user-friendly versions of

TABLE 18.2	Kilocalorie Needs for Children and Adolescents		
Age	**Life Stage**	**Gender**	**Energy Needs***
2–3 years	Toddlers	Female and male	1,000–1,400
4–8 years	Preschoolers and school age	Female	1,200–1,800
		Male	1,200–2,000
9–13 years	School age	Female	1,400–2,200
		Male	1,600–2,600
14–18 years	Adolescent	Female	1,800–2,400
		Male	2,000–3,200

Note: These levels are based on Estimated Energy Requirements (EER) from the Institute of Medicine (IOM) Dietary Reference Intakes macronutrients report, 2002, calculated by gender, age, and activity level for reference-sized individuals. "Reference size," as determined by the IOM, is based on median height and weight for ages up to 18 years. Sedentary children have needs at the lower end of each range, whereas those who are active have needs closer to the higher end of each range.

Source: HHS/USDA. 2015. Dietary Guidelines for Americans, 2015–2020 Available at https://health.gov/dietaryguidelines/2015/guidelines/. Accessed May 2017.

school-aged children Children between the ages of 6 and 12.

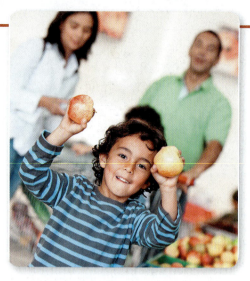

Cut back on kid's sweet treats

1 Serve small portions
2 Sip smarter
3 Use the check-out lane that does not display candy
4 Choose not to offer sweets as rewards
5 Make fruit the everyday dessert
6 Make food fun
7 Encourage kids to invent new snacks
8 Play detective in the cereal aisle
9 Make treats "treats," not everyday foods
10 If kids don't eat their meal, they don't need sweet "extras"

Be a healthy role model for children

1 Show by example
2 Go food shopping together
3 Get creative in the kitchen
4 Offer the same foods for everyone
5 Reward with attention, not food
6 Focus on each other at the table
7 Listen to your child
8 Limit screen time
9 Encourage physical activity
10 Be a good food role model

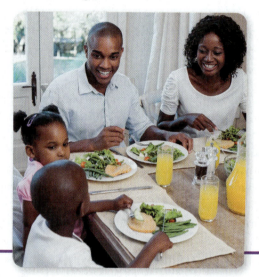

▲ **Figure 18.2** **Tips and Daily Food Plans from ChooseMyPlate.gov**
Source: Adapted from USDA. 2011. 10 Tips Nutrition Education Series. Available at www.choosemyplate.gov/healthy-eating-tips/ten-tips.html.

the Daily Food Plans and the extensive 10 Tips Nutrition Education System (**Figure 18.2**) available at ChooseMyPlate.gov can help parents guide their children's choices. The Super-Tracker creates a meal plan that shows what and how much the child should eat to meet his or her needs. It also provides ideas to help with meal planning (**Figure 18.3**) as well as tips for making healthy foods fun for children.

The portions of the ChooseMyPlate.gov website about children encourage kids to:

- **Be physically active every day.**
- **Choose healthier foods from each of the five food groups every day.** The different colors of the food groups shown in MyPlate represent the five different food groups (and don't forget healthy oils). Within each food group are healthier foods that should be eaten more often than others. Choices from the vegetables, fruits, grains, protein, and dairy groups should be varied.
- **Eat more of some food groups than others.** The sizes of the food groups as highlighted in MyPlate indicate suggested relative proportions.
- **Make the right choices for the whole family.** ChooseMyPlate.gov gives everyone in the family personal ideas on how to eat better and exercise more.
- **Take it one step at a time.** Start with one new, good thing a day and continue to add another new one every day.

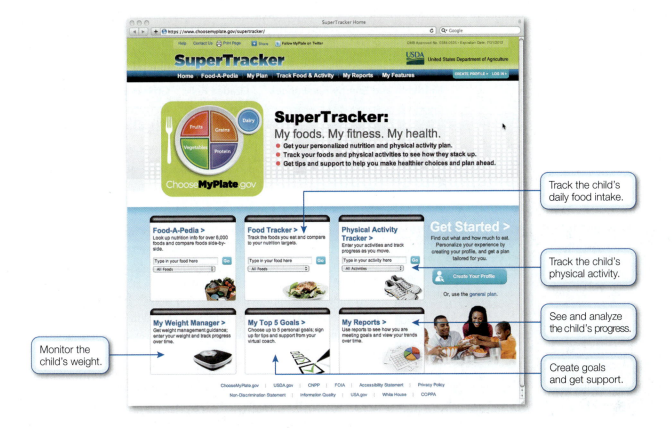

▲ **Figure 18.3 The USDA's SuperTracker Offers Personalized Plans and Food Trackers**
The USDA's SuperTracker is an online diet and physical activity tool that parents and caregivers can use to plan, assess, and analyze a child's daily food intake and activities.
Source: www.choosemyplate.gov.

Children with health-related issues or chronic diseases may not be able to follow the Daily Food Plans for Preschoolers and Kids. For example, children with autism may become especially fixated on specific foods or be reluctant to try new foods. Overcoming these issues generally requires intervention and support from professionals who work with children with special needs, such as registered dietitian nutritionists (RDNs).

School Lunches Contribute to Children's Nutritional Status

The National School Lunch Program (NSLP) provides nutritionally balanced lunches for school-age children throughout the United States. The NSLP serves more than 30 million lunches each day.[30] In 2014–2015, more than 21.5 million low-income children received free or reduced-price meals through the NSLP.[31] Providing healthy meals at school, particularly to children who may not be able to afford them without financial assistance, is one of the greatest successes of the NSLP. For some children, the food that they eat at school is the healthiest meal—perhaps the *only* meal—they eat all day.

Meals served as part of the NSLP are required to meet nutrition standards. As of 2010, NSLP nutrition standards have been updated to more closely match the Federal Dietary Guidelines for Americans.[32] For example, the percentage of total kilocalories from saturated fat is limited to 10 percent per meal for all age groups. **Table 18.3** presents recommended levels for other nutrients.

TABLE 18.3

TABLE 18.3 Minimum Nutrient and Kilocalorie Levels for School Lunches (School Week Averages)

Nutrients and Energy Allowances	Minimum Requirements*		
	Grades K–5	Grades 6–8	Grades 9–12
Energy allowances (kilocalories)	550–650	600–700	750–850
Saturated fat (% of kilocalories)	Less than 10	Less than 10	Less than 10
Sodium (mg)	640 or less	710 or less	740 or less

Source: USDA Food and Nutrition Service. Available at www.fns.usda.gov/sites/default/files/dietaryspecs.pdf. Accessed July 2014.

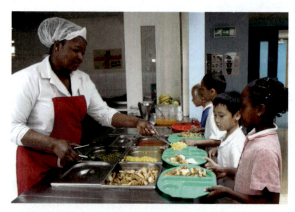

The National School Lunch Program provides lunch for millions of school-age children every day.

Tips for Packing School Lunches

Get children interested in packing their lunches by having them pick out a fun lunch box or decorate a brown paper bag with stickers.

Involve the child in planning lunches and then shopping for the items.

Make a lunch calendar and go over which days kids will eat a school lunch and which days they'll pack their lunch.

Invite children to pack their own lunch. Be sure to give them options, like leftovers or a choice of healthy ingredients.

Select new foods that kids will like and ask them if there are new items they want to try.

Ask children what they are actually eating and what they might be leaving behind or throwing away. If, for example, the apple keeps coming back day after day, it's time to try an orange.

Research suggests children who take part in the NSLP have lower intakes of sugar-sweetened beverages and a lower percentage of kilocalories from low-nutrient-density foods and beverages than nonparticipants. The recent changes in nutrition standards have led to increased vegetable consumption and improved overall diet quality in children who participate in the NSLP.[33] The challenge is to provide healthy options that consist of whole, unprocessed foods that kids will eat and enjoy, while staying within budget.

Children who are not taking part in the NSLP need a healthy substitute. Research shows that lunch meals from home contain more sodium and less fruit, vegetable, and milk servings as compared to those provided by the NSLP.[34] To improve both the quality of lunch and its acceptability, the parent *and* the child can use MyPlate as a guide to pack a mutually agreeable, healthy, and appealing lunch for the child to take to school. Children who plan and make their own lunch are more likely to eat it. The Table Tips can help provide some useful ideas to improve the likelihood that children actually eat the lunch that they pack.

Breakfast Is Important

Research suggests an association between eating breakfast regularly and both better diet quality and a healthier body weight in children and adolescents.[35,36] When children skip breakfast, they lose out on an opportunity for good nutrition. Traditional breakfast foods—such as milk, fortified whole-grain breads and whole-grain breakfast cereal, fruit, and eggs—are sources of important nutrients for kids. Breakfast-skippers may not make up for the nutrients they miss at breakfast during the rest of the day.

Over 90 percent of schools that participate in the NSLP also offer the School Breakfast Program (SBP). Eligible students receive nutritious free or reduced-price breakfasts. In 2015–2016, 12.1 million low-income children, representing 56 percent of all participants, received breakfast via the SBP.[37]

Hunger at any time of the school day can disrupt learning and behavior. Evidence suggests that habitual breakfast eating at home or in school breakfast programs has a positive effect on children's academic performance; the clearest effects of the lack of a morning meal are seen on mathematic and arithmetic grades in undernourished children.[38] Five states and the District of Columbia have passed legislation to fund breakfast in the classroom to ensure that all children eat breakfast regardless of financial need.[39]

If children don't have time to eat breakfast at home or don't receive breakfast at school, caregivers can provide nutritious morning meals for children to eat on the way to school or when they arrive. Another option is to offer a glass of milk or soymilk at home and send the rest of breakfast to school with the child to have as a mid-morning snack. See the Table Tips for some on-the-go breakfast ideas.

Most Children Need to Eat More Fruits and Vegetables

Healthy People 2020 encourages Americans to eat more fruits and vegetables.[40] Suggested fruit and vegetable intake for children is based on their daily energy needs, as produce is part of a balanced eating plan; however, many children, and their caregivers, do not consume the recommended amount of fruits and vegetables every day.[41] How do we get children to enjoy vegetables? In addition to providing well-prepared, fresh, and tasty vegetables, caregivers should give strong verbal encouragement—at school, at home, and in the community—to help children obtain their recommended servings.[42]

Parents can help establish healthy eating habits, such as filling their plate with vegetables at every meal or ending each meal with fruit. A little effort in planning meals that incorporate more produce in the family's diet can have big payoffs for the whole family. Parents can also substitute pureed vegetables in traditional dishes, like casseroles and breads, to increase vegetable intake and decrease energy density of foods. Other suggestions on increasing fruit and vegetable consumption are provided in **Table 18.4**.

Food Allergies Remain a Concern

The Health Connection in Chapter 17 explored the problem of food allergies in infants, but food allergies remain a concern throughout childhood. An estimated 8 percent of U.S. children under age 18 have one or more food allergies.[43] Whereas most children outgrow allergies to cow's milk, egg, soy, and wheat, they are less likely to outgrow allergies from peanuts, tree nuts, fish, and shellfish. Accordingly, most public schools are either entirely peanut-free or have peanut-free zones. The Food and Drug Administration (FDA) requires U.S. food manufacturers to use plain language to disclose whether their products contain (or may contain) any of the top eight allergenic foods: eggs, milk, peanuts, tree nuts, soy, wheat, shellfish, and fish.[44] An RDN with expertise in food allergies can provide guidance on how best to avoid allergenic foods and how to plan nutritious diets for children with one or more food allergies.

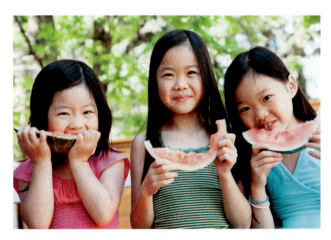

Children should be encouraged to eat fruits and vegetables every day.

TABLE TIPS
Breakfast on the Go

Mix dry, unsweetened, whole-grain cereal with an individual-sized container of low-fat yogurt. Throw in banana slices, berries, or dried fruit to make it even more nutritious.

Sprinkle reduced-fat cheese on a corn tortilla and melt it in the oven or microwave. Add some salsa and corn and roll it up into a portable tortilla tube.

Spread a thin layer of natural peanut butter or all-fruit preserves on a toasted whole-wheat waffle and pair it with a travel cup of skim milk.

TABLE 18.4	TASTE: Increasing Fruits and Vegetables in the Family Meal
T: Try something new at every eating occasion	• Add shredded carrots to casseroles, chili, lasagna, meatloaf, or soup. • Drop berries into cereal, pancakes, or yogurt. • Make fruit smoothies and veggie burritos. • Use leftover veggies for salad, or add them to a can of soup. • Keep grab-and-go snacks handy (e.g., apple slices with peanut butter or carrot sticks with hummus)
A: All forms of fruits and veggies count!	• Consider fresh, frozen, 100% juice, canned, and dried. • Cook fruits and veggies in different ways, including steamed, slow-cooked, sautéed, stir-fried, grilled, and microwaved.
S: Shop smart	• Fresh produce in season is more affordable. Look for specials. • Clean and cut up the produce so it is ready to use. • At a restaurant, substitute vegetables for high-fat side orders.
T: Turn it into a family activity	• Kids can skewer a shish-kabob or make pizza. • A trip to a farmers' market is fun for kids and gets them interested in trying new fruits and vegetables.
E: Explore the bountiful variety	• Use salad bars or buffets to try new types of produce. • When shopping, kids can pick out a new produce item for the family meal.

Source: Table adapted from Fruits & Veggies—More Matters website, September 6, 2012. T.A.S.T.E. Tips and Information for Moms. Copyright © 2012 by Produce for Better Health Foundation. Reprinted with permission.

Poverty Influences Children's Nutritional Status

In 2015, 19.7 percent of American children lived in poverty, and one in five American households with children could not afford to buy adequate food to feed their family.[45] Energy-dense, nutrient-poor foods cost less per kilocalorie than nutrient-dense foods, and an abundance of research evidence suggests that families living in poverty are more likely to purchase low-cost, low-quality food to prevent hunger.[46] Accordingly, children and adults living in poverty consume diets of lower quality than those from higher-income families. Their diets are often higher in calories, sugar, and fat and lower in vegetables,[47] and they are 1.7 times more likely to be obese as compared to their higher-income peers.[48] Their diets are improved, to an extent, by participation in the NSLP and SBP and by parents who do their best to shield their children from hunger.[49]

> **LO 18.3: THE TAKE-HOME MESSAGE**   MyPlate can help people of all ages make good food choices. School meals provide nourishment for many children at breakfast and lunch. Nutritious meals boost children's cognitive function, academic performance, school attendance rates, psychosocial function, and mood. Caregivers and other adults should be aware of the potential for a child's exposure to food allergens at home and at school. Children living in poverty consume lower-quality diets and are more likely to be obese; however, school-based meal programs have the potential to reduce these disparities.

Why Are School-Age Children Experiencing High Rates of Obesity?

LO 18.4 Explain why school-age children are experiencing high rates of obesity.

Childhood obesity is more than a matter of extra "baby fat." It has substantial short- and long-term health consequences. In the short term, it is a recognized risk factor for hypertension, type 2 diabetes, sleep apnea, and cardiovascular disease as well as poor self-esteem and depression. In the long term, obese children are more likely to become obese adults at greater risk for morbidity and premature death.[50] For more on the health risks of childhood obesity, see the Health Connection later in this chapter.

About 17 Percent of U.S. School-Age Children Are Obese

More than 17 percent of U.S. school-age children, age 6–11, are obese.[51] As shown in **Figure 18.4**, the prevalence of childhood obesity in this age group increased from 11.3 percent in 1988–1994 to 17.4 percent in 2013–2014. Although 9.4 percent of preschool age children in 2013–2014 were obese, 20.6 percent of adolescents were, suggesting that the prevalence of obesity steadily increases across the pediatric life course.[52]

Beginning at 2 years of age, body mass index (BMI) is used to identify overweight and obesity. CDC growth charts are used to determine the BMI-for-age and sex percentile in children. Because children's body composition varies as they age and between males and females, health professionals use an age- and sex-specific method to determine BMI in those age 2–19 years.[53]

In children and teens, overweight is defined as a BMI at or above the 85th percentile but lower than the 95th percentile, and obesity is defined as a BMI at or above the 95th percentile.[54] However, while BMI is a reasonable indicator of body fatness for most children and adolescents, it is not considered a diagnostic tool.[55] If a child has a high BMI

childhood obesity Condition of a child's having too much body weight for his or her height. Defined as a BMI at or above the 95th percentile.

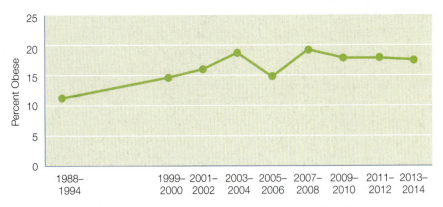

▲ **Figure 18.4 Increase in Obesity Among U.S. School-Age Children**
Note: Obesity is defined as a BMI greater than or equal to the sex- and age-specific 95th percentile from the CDC 2000 Growth Charts.

Source: Data from Ogden, C. L., Carroll, M. D., Lawman, H. G., et al. (2016). Trends in Obesity Prevalence among Children and Adolescents in the United States, 1988–1994 through 2013–2014. Journal of the American Medical Association 315(21):2292–2299..

for his age and sex, a health care provider should perform further assessments, including skinfold thickness measurements; evaluations of diet, physical activity, and family history; and other appropriate health screenings.

Multiple Factors Contribute to Childhood Obesity

Several factors can contribute to obesity among U.S. school-age children, including excessive energy consumption, genetics, a child's environment, a lack of physical activity, sedentary behavior, and outside influences such as peers and the media. No single food, nutrient, or behavior is to blame.

Overconsumption of Kilocalories

Childhood obesity results from consuming more energy than is expended.[56] Obviously, children and caregivers are making food choices that result in overconsumption of kilocalories. Today, for example, children consume 168 more kilocalories per day as snacks than they did in 1977.[57] Moreover, children's portion sizes have increased both inside and outside the home. But what factors are driving children's increased energy intake?

First, children eat fewer meals at home and more meals out, often at fast-food restaurants.[58] The relatively low levels of fiber and nutrients in foods eaten away from home, and the high levels of kilocalories, saturated fat, and added sugars, may contribute to excess energy intake in children.[59] Many children drink excess energy as well. From 1989 to 2008, the percentage of children drinking sugary beverages increased from 79 percent to 91 percent, and kilocalories from sugary beverages increased by 60 percent in children age 6–11, from 130 to 209 kilocalories per day.[60] While consumption of these drinks has been on the decline since 2007,[61] they remain one of the biggest culprits for excess weight gain in Americans of all ages.[62] Even drinking excessive amounts of milk or 100-percent juice may lead to a kilocalorie imbalance that contributes to obesity.

Genetics

A small percentage of overweight or obesity in children can be attributed to genetics; however, for the majority of children, obesity is not due to a single genetic defect. Although studies indicate a strong connection for BMI between identical twins,[63] during the past 30 years, while childhood obesity rates have increased, the human gene pool has stayed largely the same. Thus, it is likely that changes in nutrition and physical activity over these decades have influenced gene expression in ways that have contributed to the present childhood obesity epidemic.[64]

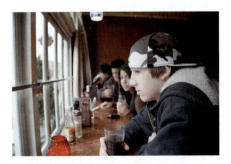

Increased consumption of sugary drinks is widely believed to have contributed to rising rates of obesity in children.

The Family

We noted earlier that parents and other caregivers are powerful role models for children. Among children under age 3, the strongest predictor of adulthood obesity is parental obesity, which, in part, may be due to genetics but is likely a by-product of learned personal health habits and the home environment. The risk of becoming an obese adult is 50 percent if one parent is obese and 80 percent if both parents are obese.[65]

Parents also exert their influence on a child's propensity for obesity well before birth. As discussed in Chapter 17, childhood obesity may have its origins in metabolic programming in the womb. Recall that if a pregnant woman experiences undernutrition, gains too much weight, or has uncontrolled gestational diabetes, the decreased or increased availability of energy may irreversibly alter appetite, endocrine function, and/or energy metabolism in her child.[66]

In older children, family habits—including watching TV while eating dinner, skipping breakfast, and consuming more food prepared outside of the home—are linked to higher BMI.[67] Parents may inadvertently reinforce a child's avoidance of unfamiliar foods if they try to avoid food-related conflicts by offering only the child's favorite foods.[68] Conversely, trying to control children's food intake by pressuring them to eat healthy food, usually fruits and vegetables, restricting access to sweets and fatty snacks, and using food as a reward may backfire.[69] Restriction is directly associated with children's BMI. The more restrictive parents are in what, and how much, food they offer children, the greater the risk for a child's overeating in the absence of parental oversight.[70]

Treatment for childhood obesity often takes the form of a family-based behavioral intervention in which parents are intricately involved.[71] Modeling healthy behaviors sends a strong message to children about what to value. When children see adults enjoying healthy foods and physical activity, they are more likely to do the same now and for the rest of their lives. Approaching healthy eating as a family fosters positive change in every member and helps to remove the stigma of overweight from the child. Parents and other caregivers play a crucial role in helping overweight children feel loved and accepted at any size and in control of their weight.

Most Children Don't Move Enough

Engaging in at least 1 hour of physical activity daily has many benefits for children, including helping them to attain and maintain a healthy weight as they grow and promoting lifelong health and well-being.[72] Despite these benefits, levels of physical activity among youth are insufficient.[73] Specifically, a recent assessment of physical activity in American youth showed that only 25 percent of children age 6–15 were moderately active on at least 5 days of the week.[74]

Children age 6–12 spend much of their day at school, and most of the time they are sitting in the classroom. Daily, quality physical education in schools can help students meet the 60-minutes-a-day guideline for exercise as outlined in the *2008 Physical Activity Guidelines for Americans*.[75] However, opportunities for regular physical activity are limited in many schools; daily physical education is provided in only 4 percent of elementary schools and 8 percent of middle schools in the United States.[76]

One major factor that affects activity levels in American youth is "screen time," or time spent in front of a television or on computers, tablets, or smartphones for entertainment purposes. Children in the United States spend 6 hours per day, on average, in front of screens for entertainment purposes.[77] While a certain amount of screen time is necessary for homework, especially in older school-age kids, excessive screen time, which is usually sedentary, is unhealthy. It may also result in increased energy intake, as children, and their parents, may snack and eat meals in front of the television or computer. In addition, TV food advertisements may influence families to purchase and eat kilocalorie-dense, low-nutrient foods.[78]

Striking a balance between the role of screens in school and homework with the harmful effects of screen time on sleep, physical activity, and diet, the AAP revised screen-time guidelines to recommend that parents address media use for each child or teenager and place consistent limits on hours per day of media use as well as types of media used.[79] To help families set and abide by screen-time limits, the AAP suggests that parents establish "screen-free" zones at home by allowing no televisions, computers, or video games in children's bedrooms and by turning off the TV during dinner.[80]

The AAP also recommends that children keep all screens out of their bedroom at night. The blue light emitted from television, computer/tablet, and cell-phone screens can disrupt melatonin release and affect a child's sleep duration and quality.[81] Disrupted sleep is associated with obesogenic behaviors as well as reduced academic performance.[82] Whereas more research is needed to understand the relationship between screen time, sleep, and obesity risk, having a TV in the bedroom continues to be associated with increased risk of obesity.[83]

The Environment Outside the Home

According to the socioecological model of childhood obesity, children's obesity risk depends not only on their behaviors and genetics, but also on the social, cultural, economic, and environmental influences to which they are exposed.[84] These influences include the staff, policies, and programs within schools, after-school and childcare settings, recreational facilities, faith-based institutions, and governmental agencies. They also include the influence of media and entertainment and the built environment, including community and transportation infrastructure. Promoting healthy lifestyle habits including healthy eating and regular physical activity on several fronts can reduce the risk of obesity.[85] Government policies not traditionally thought of as health policies, such as those involving transportation, land use, education, agriculture, and economics, affect health and obesity rates.[86] Federal agencies and nongovernmental health organizations are working together to develop healthy environments by improving access to healthy and fresh foods and by building walk paths, bike paths, and playgrounds in underserved communities.[87]

Media and Advertising Target Children

Food and beverage companies market extensively to children, even those as young as 2 years old.[88] A large meta-analysis of studies examining the influence of food and beverage marketing on children found that it affects not only what and how much they eat, but also what they want to buy and their overall diet.[89] Despite efforts of federal policymakers to impose nutrition guidelines asking companies to voluntarily limit the marketing of foods high in saturated fats, added sugars, and sodium to youth, evidence suggests that in 2015, children saw just 3 percent fewer food ads than they had in 2007, the year after the regulations were proposed.[90] Marketers are finding more ways to target children online and through smartphone applications, but television remains the top vehicle for food marketing to children. A recent study showed that from 2009 to 2014, 954 brands marketd to youth through product placement, or when a brand logo or product is featured in mass media, particularly TV shows. More specifically, four beverage brands—The Coca-Cola Company, Dr Pepper Snapple Group, PepsiCo, and Starbucks—were responsible for more than half of those appearances.[91]

Friends Can Negatively Influence Food Preferences

As children age, they spend more time interacting with peers and their peers' families. For children whose parents are inconsistent about offering healthy foods and getting regular exercise, peers can be positive role models. But peers may also negatively influence a child's food preferences. It's important for parents to lay a strong foundation of healthy habits at home so that kids know what's expected of them when they are away from the house. One of the best ways to establish expectations about behavior is to practice healthy eating and staying physically active as a family. Children need to know that each family conducts itself differently and that, for their family, healthy living is a priority.

> **LO 18.4: THE TAKE-HOME MESSAGE** The prevalence of childhood obesity increased from 11.3 percent in 1988–1994 to 17.4 percent in 2013–2014. Although genetics are thought to influence BMI, parents and other caregivers are strong models for food choices. A child's home environment exerts the most influence over health behaviors and obesity risk now and in the future. Social, cultural, economic, and environmental influences can also be modified to support healthy eating and adequate physical activity. Food and beverage marketing strongly influences children's diets. Peers may positively or negatively influence a child's food preferences and engagement in physical activity.

What Are the Nutritional Needs of Adolescents?

LO 18.5 Describe the nutritional needs of adolescents.

Adolescence is the stage of the life cycle between ages 9 and 19, which bridges the challenging transition from childhood to adulthood. It is characterized by two significant physical changes, a rapid **growth spurt** and the onset of **puberty**—the period during which an adolescent becomes sexually mature. Adolescents attain about 15 percent of their adult height and about 50 percent of their ideal adult weight during this stage. Bones grow significantly. Increases in lean muscle mass and body fat stores are also part of the adolescent growth spurt. For boys, the onset of puberty is marked by linear growth and maturation of the genitals. For girls, the onset of puberty is marked by the first menstrual period, or **menarche**.

The timing of the growth spurt and the onset of puberty depends on an interaction between the adolescent's genetics and environment, including nutritional status. Growth must be supported with adequate energy and nutrients; however, given the complex relationship between puberty and obesity, youth should take care to avoid excess weight gain. Research supports that excess adiposity may cause puberty to begin earlier in youth and it can limit peak height as well.[92] Currently, one in five American adolescents is obese.[93] This is especially problematic, as obese adolescents are 16 times more likely to become severely obese adults.[94] Therefore, children and adolescents should choose nutrient-dense foods to meet their increased nutrient needs and optimize their development without consuming excess kilocalories.

Adolescents Need Calcium and Vitamin D for Bone Development

Adolescents experience rapid bone growth. Most of the growth occurs in the **epiphyseal plate** (**Figure 18.5**), the area of tissue near the end of the long bones. The growth plate determines the future length and shape of the mature bone. At some point during adolescence, bone growth stops, the plates close, and they are replaced by solid bone.[95]

Almost half of peak bone mass is accumulated during adolescence. Thus, adequate calcium and vitamin D intake are critical during this life stage. Inadequate calcium intake during childhood and adolescence can lead to low peak bone mass and is considered a risk

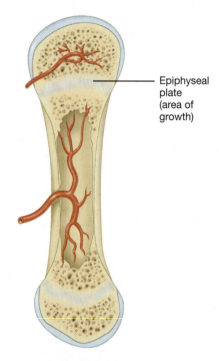

Epiphyseal plate (area of growth)

▲ **Figure 18.5 Epiphyseal Plate in Long Bone**
Adolescent bone growth takes place along the epiphyseal plate. Once the plate closes, lengthening of the bone stops.

adolescence Developmental transition between childhood and early adulthood (approximately ages 9–19).

growth spurt Rapid increase in height and weight.

puberty Period during which adolescents reach sexual maturity and become capable of reproduction.

menarche Onset of menstruation.

factor for osteoporosis.[96] The RDA for calcium is 1,300 milligrams for those age 9–18. The RDA for vitamin D is 600 IU for all children over 1 year old.[97]

Getting enough dietary calcium is a concern for adolescents, particularly for females.[98] Just 15 percent of girls age 9–13 years and about 10 percent of those age 14–19 meet the 1,300-milligram-a-day requirement.[99]

Teens don't take in enough calcium if they replace calcium-rich milk products with soft drinks, energy drinks, and juice drinks. Nearly all of the milk sold in the United States is fortified with vitamin D, so when teens don't drink milk, they miss out on a substantial source of this nutrient. For example, 8 ounces of fortified milk supplies 100 I.U. of vitamin D, or one-sixth of a teen's daily requirement.

The Calculation Corner shows how to determine how much of a teen's daily calcium requirement is fulfilled by a glass of milk.

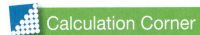

Calculation Corner

Adolescent Calcium Needs

Teens need an adequate intake of calcium to support bone growth and mass.

Approximately how much calcium is found in an 8-ounce serving of milk containing 30 percent of the Daily Value for calcium? Refer to the Daily Values for Food Labels in the inside back cover of the textbook.

$$\text{Daily Value of calcium} = 1{,}000 \text{ mg}$$
$$0.30 \times 1{,}000 \text{ mg} = 300 \text{ mg}$$

Answer: Eight ounces of milk contains 300 milligrams of calcium.

The Recommended Dietary Allowance (RDA) for calcium for teens is 1,300 milligrams per day. An 8-ounce serving of milk contributes what proportion of a teen's RDA?

$$8 \text{ ounces of milk contains } 300 \text{ milligrams of calcium.}$$
$$300 \text{ mg calcium} \div 1{,}300 \text{ mg calcium recommended} = 0.23 \times 100 = 23\%$$

Answer: One 8-ounce serving represents 23 percent of a teen's daily recommended intake for calcium.

Go to Mastering Nutrition and complete a Math Video activity similar to the problem in this Calculation Corner.

Adolescents Need Iron for Muscle Growth and Blood Volume

Iron needs are highest during growth spurts and after the onset of menstruation. Adolescents need more iron than younger children to support their rapid muscle growth and increased blood volume. Adolescent girls need additional iron to replace monthly losses due to menstruation. The RDA for iron for females age 14–18 years is 15 milligrams per day; males require 11 milligrams per day.[100] These recommendations are based on the amount of dietary iron needed to maintain adequate iron stores.

According to the USDA, the average daily iron intake from foods is about 15 milligrams per day in those age 12–19 years; however, among females it is only 12 milligrams per day.[101] Teens, particularly girls, may have inadequate iron intake if they restrict their overall food intake or avoid fortified grains, lean meats, seafood, nuts, and legumes. The symptoms and diagnosis of iron deficiency and iron-deficiency anemia are discussed in Chapter 13. In most cases, dietary iron supplements as part of a balanced diet are prescribed to replenish and maintain iron stores.[102]

What Nutritional Issues Affect Adolescents?

LO 18.6 Discuss the nutritional issues that affect adolescents, including disordered eating.

In addition to being a time of great physical change, adolescence is a time of significant social and emotional change. Because emotion centers in the brain mature faster than cognitive control regions, teens often experience intense emotions yet have difficulty controlling those emotions. They experience a strong desire for independence and individuality and want to make their own decisions, yet they have difficulty foreseeing the consequences of their decisions and inhibiting behaviors that put them at risk. During adolescence, teens establish patterns of behavior, including eating and exercise habits, that track into adulthood. Therefore, it is of utmost importance to support teens in developing healthy habits.

Social Factors Can Influence Teens' Health Habits

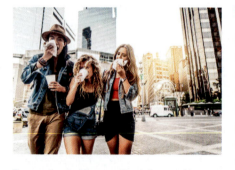
Teen eating habits are often influenced by peers and social settings.

Parents and siblings, peers, sports figures and other celebrities, and images in traditional and social media influence adolescents. Teens may adopt damaging health habits in order to emulate what they see in the media or to fit in with their peer group. Social media have transformed the teenage years. It used to be that the pressures of high school could be left at the front door and home was a safe haven from peer pressure. The advent of social media may increase pressure on teens to be thin or popular, or both. It's important for teenagers to feel that home is a safe, loving environment where they will be nurtured and won't be judged.

Strong family bonds promote healthier habits. Much has been made, for example, about the benefits of family meals for teen nutrition: Parents can model good behavior at the table and serve healthy foods at family meals, and mealtime is often the only time of the day when family members speak face to face. However, it's difficult to isolate family mealtime benefits: Families that dine together most nights may also have other healthy behaviors. The good news is that when parent–child bonds are strong, dining together may contribute to fewer depressive symptoms and less tobacco, drug, and alcohol use in teens.[103,104]

Diet May Play a Modest Role in Adolescent Acne

Whereas the relationship between adolescent acne and diet is not fully understood, evidence suggests that diet may play a role in its onset. It is well established that both vitamins A and D play a role in overall skin health.[105] There is also evidence that following a low-glycemic-index diet is associated with reduced acne,[106] while other studies have found that high consumption of chocolate, sweets, and dairy foods and low consumption of fish, fruits, and vegetables may also be related to acne.[107] While there are no definitive dietary guidelines for acne prevention, collective evidence indicates that teens who consume a balanced diet are less likely to suffer from acne than those who do not.

Adolescents Are at Risk for Disordered Eating

As discussed in Chapter 14, teenagers may experience poor body image that could result in disordered eating. Both anorexia nervosa and bulimia nervosa are more prevalent among adolescent females than adolescent males; however, recent evidence suggests that one-third of those suffering from eating disorders are male.[108] Moreover, transgender and LGBTQ youth are also at increased risk for eating disorders.[109] Preteens and younger teens seem to be at greatest risk: The median age for anorexia nervosa, bulimia nervosa, and binge eating disorder is about 12–13 years of age.[110]

Teens grapple with trying to fit in and must adjust to new bodies, new thoughts, new situations, and new experiences. As they do, several risk factors put them at risk for eating disorders, including perceived or real pressure to be thin; a distorted body image; low self-esteem; participation in activities such as figure skating, gymnastics, or wrestling, where body image and weight can be major issues; and personality traits such as perfectionism.[111] All of this, along with the typical adolescent feeling of immortality, may encourage an adolescent to engage in risky tactics to reach a desired weight. These risky tactics include eating very little food, skipping meals, smoking cigarettes, using diet pills, self-inducing vomiting, or abusing laxatives or diuretics.

It's not always possible, even for the most motivated and caring parents, to prevent disordered eating in teens. Experts recommend open communication about healthy eating. As a parent, concentrating on good health, not thinness, may promote the idea that health, not appearance, is the primary value.

Early intervention programs are crucial for those with disordered eating; thus, it's important that caregivers recognize the signs (see Chapter 14). As discussed in the nearby Nutrition in Practice, early intervention can increase the adaptability and coping skills of teens and family members and may be able to prevent disordered eating from developing into a clinical eating disorder.

LO 18.6: THE TAKE-HOME MESSAGE Adolescents want to have control over their food and lifestyle decisions. At the same time, their ability to control their emotions and to appreciate the consequences of their actions is not yet mature. Family, peers, and media all exert a strong influence on adolescents' eating, physical activity, and other health habits. Because adolescents often live in the present, they may not think about the long-term health consequences of poor diet and lifestyle habits they adopt during their teen years. Whereas the role of diet in acne is not well understood, following a healthy eating pattern may reduce the onset of adolescent acne. Adolescents are sometimes at risk of developing disordered eating patterns due to poor body image, emotional issues, or peer pressure. Early intervention is critical.

NUTRITION *in* PRACTICE:
Psychologist

Erinn is a 16-year-old high school student who has gained over 15 pounds in the last year. While she is active and walks to school daily, she has noticed that she can't fit into the jeans that she wore last summer and is not happy with her recent weight gain. During her annual physical at the pediatrician's office, Erinn admitted that she has been experiencing a huge amount of anxiety during the last year and found herself snacking every time she felt a wave of stress in her life. Concerned, the pediatrician asked her to explain her anxiety. After some tears, Erinn told the pediatrician that her mom and dad were filing for a divorce and that she didn't understand why this was happening. Erinn has found that they only way to ease her stress is to snack on sweet foods. She admits that she has consumed an entire pint of ice cream over the course of a day or will eat three to four chocolate bars on the way home from school when she is having a "bad day." Concerned, the pediatrician asked Erinn if she would like to get some support regarding her weight gain and anxiety. She agreed. The pediatrician spoke with Erinn's mom, and they both agreed that she would meet with a registered dietitian nutritionist (RDN) about her diet and a psychologist about her anxiety. Her mother was very supportive of any help that the RDN and psychologist could provide to Erinn during this stressful time.

Erinn's Stats
- ❏ Age: 16
- ❏ Height: 5 feet 4 inches
- ❏ Weight: 140 pounds

Critical Thinking Questions
1. Why is Erinn so hungry at lunch?
2. According to Erinn's food log, she isn't hungry in the afternoon and evening but appears to be snacking due to stress. What suggestions can the RDN provide her?

RDN's Observation and Plan for Erinn
- ❏ Discuss the importance of consuming a healthy breakfast in the morning so that

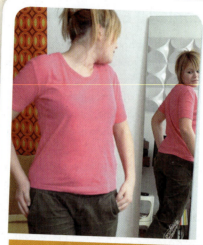

Erinn

ERINN'S FOOD LOG

Food/Beverage	Time Consumed	Hunger Rating*	Location
No breakfast		1	
Pizza and cola	12 NOON	5	High school cafeteria
Chocolate bars	3:30 P.M.	1	Walking home from school
Chicken, rice, and broccoli	6:00 P.M.	3	With her mom at the dining room table
Cookies	10:00 P.M.	1	In her bedroom while on Facebook

*Hunger Rating (1–5): 1 = not hungry; 5 = super hungry.

Erinn isn't so ravenous at lunch. Erinn agrees to have a Greek yogurt with fruit in the morning before walking to school.
- ❏ Discuss her snacking issue in the afternoon and evening. The RDN and Erinn discuss healthier options to release her stress, such as calling a friend, rather than snacking.

Psychologist Observation and Plan for Erinn
- ❏ Suggest Erin begin a course of cognitive-behavioral therapy (CBT). This type of therapy is a goal-oriented treatment that empowers a person with practical suggestions to reverse the negative pattern of behaviors and thoughts that may be occurring in his or her life.
- ❏ Using CBT, teach Erinn to identify the negative thoughts that she may be having, reflect on the actual evidence for feeling this way, and then find an alternative non-eating-related activity to challenge the negative thoughts and release her stress. Also

recommend that Erinn practice mindful breathing to calm her nerves when she is feeling anxious.
- ❏ Recommend that Erinn keep a journal of her daily thoughts to be discussed at the next session.

Erinn returns to the psychologist a week later and is feeling a little better. She is having difficulties initiating the mindful breathing exercises so the psychologist recommends a few mindful breathing apps that Erinn can download on her phone and listen to when she is feeling stressed.

The following week Erinn reports that she is enjoying her breakfast and is less hungry at lunch. She is still having some snacking issues in the evening. The RDN suggests some new strategies to help her in the evening such as going to sleep earlier. Together, they continue to work on making healthy improvements in her diet, such as adding more dairy, fruits, and vegetables.

What Are the Health Effects of Childhood Obesity?

LO 18.7 Identify the health risks of obesity in children and teens.

Childhood obesity can have multiple health consequences, including physical, mental, and even social problems. Generally speaking, the more obese the child is, the worse the potential health outcomes. Some effects of childhood overweight and obesity are apparent in youth, whereas many others may appear decades later.

Obese Children Are at Increased Risk for Type 2 Diabetes

The obesity epidemic has been accompanied by an associated increase in the rate of type 2 diabetes in youth. As you learned in Chapter 4, type 2 diabetes was previously an adult-onset disease, but is now common among U.S. children and adolescents, with a 30 percent increase over the last two decades.[112] Prevalence increased in both sexes, among all age groups, and in white, black, and Hispanic youth.[113] Moreover, an estimated 20–40 percent of teens age 12–19 years have prediabetes, which often goes undiagnosed because clinical symptoms are not apparent.[114] Increasing diabetes and prediabetes rates among U.S. youth is of great concern, as they are more likely to have diabetes in adulthood and struggle with diabetes-related complications, such as heart and kidney disease, nerve damage, and vision problems.

Childhood obesity and low levels of physical activity, as well as exposure to diabetes in utero, may contribute to this increased incidence. Children and teens diagnosed with prediabetes or type 2 diabetes are typically obese, have a strong family history of diabetes, and have insulin resistance. Among youth, Native Americans have the highest prevalence of type 2 diabetes.[115]

It's possible to delay and even prevent the onset of type 2 diabetes in at-risk obese youth. Eliminating from the diet sugary drinks, desserts, and snack foods; increasing nutrient-dense foods such as fruits, vegetables, whole grains, lean-protein foods, and low-fat dairy; and increasing physical activity can make a big difference in an obese child's chances for avoiding the disease.[116]

If a child has already been diagnosed with type 2 diabetes, early intervention and treatment are a must. The sooner the family learns the dietary and activity changes needed and how to manage all other aspects of the disease, the better off the child will be. The entire family should consider eating in the same healthy way as the child. All family members should take part in physical activity as well. Taking a family walk or bike ride after dinner or enjoying weekend games of basketball or tennis are excellent ways to teach the importance of exercise. The child is more likely to feel supported and succeed with keeping diabetes under control if everyone in the family is educated about what to do to help.

Other Risks Are Associated with Childhood Obesity

Obese children are more likely to have hypertension and high cholesterol, which are risk factors for cardiovascular disease (CVD). In a nationally representative survey of American adolescents, 37 percent, 49 percent, and 61 percent of the normal-weight, overweight, and obese adolescents, respectively, had at least one CVD risk factor.[117]

Children and adolescents with obesity also suffer emotional problems. Research shows that children with obesity tend to experience more depression and have lower self-esteem compared with their normal-weight peers.[118] Low self-esteem can create overwhelming feelings of hopelessness in some obese children.[119] In addition, some children overeat to cope with problems or deal with emotions, such as stress, or to fight boredom or loneliness, which may intensify their weight issues. It's important to support obese children in their daily lives and while they are in treatment. Research shows improved psychosocial functioning in children participating in weight-control treatments, and that these changes are typically independent of weight-loss outcomes.[120]

Perhaps one of the most obvious risks of childhood obesity is that it will continue into adulthood, bringing with it all of the obesity-related risks for chronic disease. Children and adolescents who are obese are likely to be obese as adults and therefore at increased risk for type 2 diabetes and CVD, as just mentioned, as well as several types of cancer, sleep apnea, asthma, nonalcoholic fatty liver disease, and osteoarthritis.[121]

Early Assessment and Treatment Can Help Address Childhood Obesity

Childhood obesity is a multifactorial public health problem with personal, psychosocial, and financial ramifications. Addressing the problem is crucial, however, because childhood obesity can lead to costly and life-threatening medical problems later in life.[122]

The U.S. Preventive Services Task Force (USPSTF) recommends that physicians screen for childhood obesity in children over 6 years of age.[123] However, childhood obesity often goes undiagnosed.

The USPSTF advises pediatricians to refer obese children to comprehensive, intensive behavioral intervention to promote improvement in weight status.[124] For younger children, family-based interventions are recommended, whereas with older children and adolescents, the evidence for family-based interventions is not as clear. Interventions should target diet, physical activity, and behavioral modification.

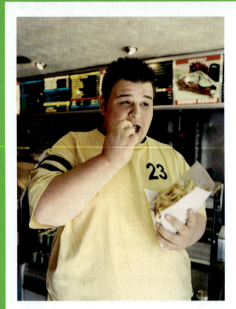

The first step in helping an overweight child is to get him or her evaluated by a health professional.

The most effective programs include more than 26 hours of contact with the child and/or the family over weeks or months.[125]

Parents who are concerned about their child's weight should first consult with the child's pediatrician. Putting a child on a restrictive diet, which may lack the essential nutrients children need to grow and develop properly, may encourage disordered eating in the long run. An RDN can provide dietary counseling and help families implement the eating plan.

The AAP is focused on preventing childhood obesity. Parental obesity and rapid infant weight gain increase a child's risk. Parents and caregivers of children with these risk factors should provide a healthy diet that includes adequate nutrients without excessive kilocalories, sugars, and saturated fats and support the child in participating in plenty of physical activity. The AAP recommends that parents and caregivers serve as role models when it comes to healthy eating and physical activity.

LO 18.7: THE TAKE-HOME MESSAGE

Obese children and adolescents are at greater risk for health problems. Increasing obesity rates are contributing to rising rates of prediabetes, type 2 diabetes, hypertension, and other health problems in children and teenagers. Early assessment and intervention, including changes in diet and exercise, can prevent or reverse obesity, and may delay or prevent the onset of type 2 diabetes and other health problems.

Visual Chapter Summary

LO 18.1 The Needs of Toddlers and Preschoolers Are Met with Small, Nutrient-Dense Meals

Toddlers and preschoolers need frequent, small, nutrient-dense meals and snacks to consume adequate amounts of kilocalories and nutrients to fuel their growth and development. The RDA for carbohydrate is the same for children and adults, but the RDA for protein is higher in children. Adequate fat intake supports the intensive myelination of the nervous system that continues through early childhood. Young children need enough iron, calcium, and vitamin D to ensure healthy growth and adequate fiber and fluid for bowel regularity. Milk, water, and diluted 100-percent juice are better beverage choices than sugary drinks.

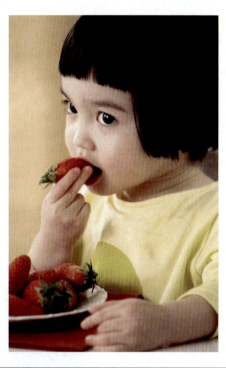

LO 18.2 Adults Influence Young Children's Eating Habits

Young children may be picky eaters and go on food jags, but these behaviors are normal and usually temporary. Caregivers should allow children to participate in food preparation and to choose the foods they eat from among several healthy options. New foods may need to be offered multiple times before the child accepts them. Caregivers should act as role models by adopting the lifelong healthy eating habits they want to see in their children.

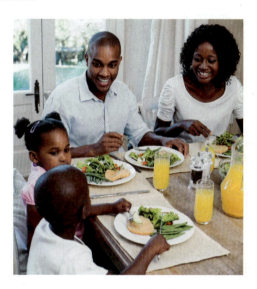

LO 18.3 MyPlate Helps School-Age Children to Meet Their Nutritional Needs

The quality of the diet influences growth and development of school-age children. School-age children have the capacity to eat more and maintain blood glucose levels longer and are less hungry between meals than younger children. Children who participate in the National School Lunch Program have higher-quality lunch meals as compared to those who bring lunch from home. Children who bring lunch from home should be involved in the planning and preparation of the lunch so they are more likely to consume it. Research shows that eating breakfast positively influences a child's energy levels, nutrient intake, and mental performance throughout the day. Most public schools participate in the School Breakfast Program and many provide free in-class breakfasts to all children regardless of need. Federal school meal programs can help to prevent hunger and improve diet quality for children who live in poverty.

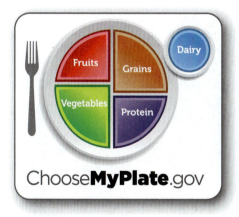

LO 18.4 Multiple Factors Contribute to Childhood Obesity

About 17 percent of U.S. school-age children, ages 6–11, are obese. Overconsumption of energy, inadequate physical activity, genetics, the home and community environment, and media and advertising contribute to this problem.

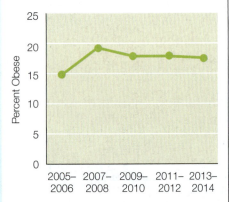

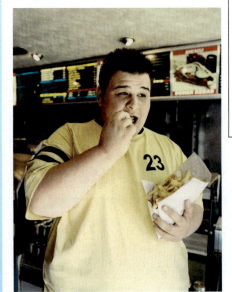

LO 18.5 Nutritional Needs of Adolescents Are Based on Characteristic Physical Changes

The transition from childhood to adolescence is marked by two key physical changes: the adolescent growth spurt and the onset of puberty. Adolescents require a nutrient-dense diet to meet their high nutrient needs. Because of rapid bone growth, adequate calcium and vitamin D intake are critical. Overconsumption of soda may interfere with calcium intake if it displaces milk in the diet. Adequate iron intake is important for growth of lean muscle and blood volume. Girls' need for dietary iron increases after the onset of menstruation. Dieting, or limiting enriched grains, lean meats, and legumes, may result in inadequate iron intake.

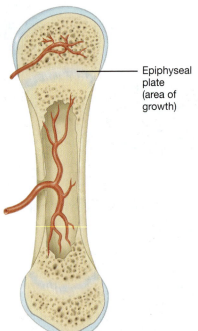

Epiphyseal plate (area of growth)

LO 18.6 Nutritional Issues That Affect Adolescents Are Due to Social and Emotional Changes

Adolescents are heavily influenced by peers, media, and other nonparental role models, which may lead them to adopt unhealthy eating and lifestyle habits, such as skipping meals, choosing unhealthy foods, excessive dieting, or smoking. However, strong family bonds promote healthier habits. Whereas the role of diet in acne is not fully understood, following a healthy eating pattern may help to reduce outbreaks. Adolescents are sometimes at risk of developing disordered eating patterns due to poor body image, emotional issues, or peer pressure.

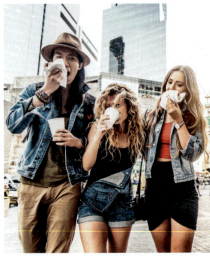

LO 18.7 Childhood Obesity Has Several Negative Health Effects

More children are obese than ever before. These children are likely to remain obese in adulthood, and have an increased risk for obesity-related chronic diseases. Type 2 diabetes resulting from obesity affects an increasing number of children in the United States, particularly teens. Type 2 diabetes can damage the heart, kidney, nerves, and vision. Obesity also increases the risk for hypertension and high cholesterol and a variety of psychosocial health challenges.

Terms to Know

- toddlers
- preschoolers
- attention-deficit/hyperactivity disorder (ADHD)
- food jags
- school-age children
- childhood obesity
- adolescence
- growth spurt
- puberty
- menarche
- epiphyseal plate

Mastering Nutrition
Visit the Study Area in Mastering Nutrition to hear an MP3 chapter summary.

Check Your Understanding

LO18.1 1. When feeding toddlers and preschoolers, what is a good rule to follow?
   a. Decide for the child how much to eat at each meal.
   b. Offer small portions of a variety of healthy foods at each meal.
   c. Offer three tablespoons of food per year of age.
   d. Don't offer a new food that the toddler has rejected previously.

LO18.1 2. During periods of rapid growth, young children are at a particular risk for developing
   a. iron deficiency.
   b. calcium toxicity.
   c. vitamin D toxicity.
   d. vitamin C deficiency.

LO18.2 3. In order to foster healthy eating habits in children, caregivers should
   a. serve them only the foods they like.
   b. offer them a limited variety of foods.
   c. insist that they eat everything on their plate.
   d. allow them to stop eating when they are full.

LO18.3 4. MyPlate illustrates the _____ food groups that are the building blocks of a healthy diet.
   a. four
   b. five
   c. seven
   d. 10

LO18.4 5. Children are considered obese if they have a BMI greater than or equal to the _____ percentile.
   a. 85th
   b. 90th
   c. 95th
   d. 99th

LO18.4 6. The American Academy of Pediatrics recommends that screen time should be
   a. limited to 2 hours per day in children of all ages.
   b. set by parents for each individual child.
   c. set by schools to accommodate the amount of homework they assign.
   d. used for both education and entertainment and limited to 4 hours per day.

LO18.5 7. Which mineral supports healthy bone development and is particularly important during adolescence?
   a. Calcium
   b. Iron
   c. Zinc
   d. Copper

LO18.5 8. The need for iron increases during adolescence to support muscle growth and _____.
   a. blood volume
   b. bone development
   c. heart health
   d. kidney function

LO18.6 9. Which of the following behaviors may play a protective role in reducing the risk of disordered eating in adolescents?
   a. Participation in competitive figure skating, gymnastics, or ballroom dancing
   b. Use of mild weight-loss supplements
   c. Parental emphasis on good health
   d. Peer emphasis on a slender appearance

LO18.7 10. The USPSTF recommends which treatment for childhood obesity?
   a. Monthly weight checks with the child's pediatrician
   b. Referral to an intensive behavioral intervention that targets diet and physical activity and promotes behavior change
   c. Diets that reduce energy intake by 500 kilocalories per day
   d. Weekly family-based therapy to support behavior modification

Answers

1. (b) A young child's appetite can fluctuate. Offer small portions of a variety of healthy foods at every meal and allow children to choose. A new food may need to be offered many times before a child accepts it.

2. (a) Iron deficiency is the most common nutrient deficiency among young children. This is often due to an overly heavy milk diet. Iron is critical to support children's rapid growth.

3. (d) Caregivers should allow young children to stop eating when they are full. Forcing children to clean their plate may result in food struggles or overeating. Offer children new foods, not just what they are accustomed to.

4. (b) MyPlate illustrates these five food groups: vegetables, fruits, grains, dairy, and protein foods. They are the building blocks for a healthy diet using a familiar image—a place setting for a meal.

5. (c) Children with a BMI greater than or equal to the 95th percentile are considered obese. They are considered overweight if their BMI is between the 85th and 94th percentile.

6. (b) The American Academy of Pediatrics recommends that parents set screen-time limits based on each individual child's relationship with digital media.

7. (a) Adolescents need adequate amounts of calcium to support their growing bones.

8. (a) The need for iron is increased in adolescents to support their growing muscles and blood volume. Adolescent girls also need to replace iron loss as part of the blood loss of menstruation.

9. (c) Parental emphasis on health rather than weight may play a protective role in preventing disordered eating.

10. (b) The USPSTF recommends that pediatricians screen for obesity in children ages 6 and older, and that those who are obese be referred to intensive behavioral intervention that targets diet and physical activity and promotes behavior change.

Answers to True or False?

1. **False.** After infancy, growth slows down significantly. During the second year of life, a toddler may gain 3–5 pounds.

2. **True.** Between the ages of 1 and 4, small children are extremely active and may not be as interested in eating.

3. **False.** Milk is a source of important nutrients; however, it doesn't provide all the nutrients that growing children need. A variety of other foods are also needed to provide key nutrients for proper growth and development.

4. **False.** Iron deficiency may be caused by a limited diet that relies too heavily on milk or other iron-poor food sources.

5. **False.** Parents and caregivers may need to offer foods numerous times before a child accepts them.

6. **True.** Young children often refuse foods of a certain color, texture, or taste. Alternatively, they may get hooked on a particular food and eat only that item for a while.

7. **False.** Though high-fat, high-sugar foods often found in fast-food restaurants are part of the problem, that's not the whole story. An overall poor diet with kilocalorie-dense foods and inadequate physical activity also contribute.

8. **True.** The school lunch and school breakfast programs must meet specific requirements in order to receive funding from the USDA.

9. **False.** Diet sodas provide nothing but fluid and may displace nutrient-dense foods and beverages.

10. **False.** Inadequate calcium and iron intakes are common among adolescents. Teens tend to prefer sugar-sweetened soft drinks to calcium-rich milk. Teens need iron to support muscle growth and increased blood volume. Adolescent females also need more iron than males to support the onset of menstruation.

Web Resources

- For more information on nutrition for preschoolers, visit www.ChooseMyPlate.gov/preschoolers.html
- For more information on nutrition during the younger years, visit www.cdc.gov/healthyyouth/nutrition/facts.htm
- For more information on children's and teens' health, visit http://kidshealth.org
- To learn about practical tools for keeping kids at a healthy weight, visit We Can! at www.nhlbi.nih.gov/health/public/heart/obesity/wecan/index.htm
- For more about the USDA's National School Lunch Program, visit www.fns.usda.gov/cnd/lunch
- For more information on increasing fruit and vegetable consumption, visit Fruits & Veggies—More Matters, at www.fruitsandveggiesmorematters.org

References

1 US National Library of Medicine. 2016. *Normal Growth and Development.* Available at https://medlineplus.gov/ency/article/002456.htm. Accessed March 2017.

2 Reidy, K. C., Deming, D. M., Briefel, R. R., Fox, M. K., Saavedra, J. M., and Eldridge, A. L. 2017. Early Development of Dietary Patterns: Transitions in the Contribution of Food Groups to Total Energy—Feeding Infants and Toddlers Study, 2008. *BMC Nutrition* 3:5.

3 American Academy of Pediatrics. 2012. *Age-Related Safety Sheets: 6–12 Months.* Available at www.healthychildren.org/English/tips-tools/Pages/Safety-for-Your-Child-6-to-12-Months.aspx. Accessed March 2017.

4 National Resource Center for Health and Safety in Child Care and Early Education. 2017. State Licensing and Regulation Information. Available at http://nrckids.org. Accessed March 2017.

5 Institute of Medicine. 2005. *Dietary Reference Intakes for Energy, Carbohydrate, Fiber, Fat, Fatty Acids, Cholesterol, Protein, and Amino Acids (Macronutrients).* Washington, DC: National Academies Press. Available at https://www.nal.usda.gov/sites/default/files/fnic_uploads//macronutrients.pdf. Accessed March 2017.

6 Ibid.

7 Ibid.

8 Ibid.

9 Institute of Medicine. 2001. *Dietary Reference Intakes for Vitamin A, Vitamin K, Arsenic, Boron, Chromium, Copper, Iodine, Iron, Manganese, Nickel, Silicon, Vanadium, and Zinc.* Washington, DC: National Academies Press.

10 Domellöf, M., Braegger, C., Campoy, C., Colomb, V., Decsi, T., Fewtrell, M., et al. 2014. Iron Requirements of Infants and Toddlers. *Journal of Pediatric Gastroenterology and Nutrition* 58(1):119–129.

11 National Library of Medicine. 2017. Anemia Caused by Low Iron - Infants and Toddlers. Available at https://medlineplus.gov/ency/article/007618.htm. Accessed March 2017.

12 Centers for Disease Control and Prevention. 2013. *FastStats.* Available at www.cdc.gov. Accessed May 2014.

13 World Health Organization. 2017. *Micronutrient Deficiencies.* Available at www.who.int/nutrition/topics/ida/en/. Accessed March 2017.

14 Domellöf, M., Braegger, C., Campoy, C., Colomb, V., Decsi, T., Fewtrell, M., et al. 2014. Iron Requirements of Infants and Toddlers.

15 National Institutes of Health. 2015. *Iron Overdose.* Available at www.nlm.nih.gov/medlineplus/ency/article/002659.htm. Accessed March 2017.

16 U.S. Food and Drug Administration. 2016. *Code of Federal Regulations Title 21. Sec. 101.17 Food Labeling Warning, Notice, and Safe Handling Statements.* Available at www.accessdata.fda.gov/scripts/cdrh/cfdocs/cfcfr/CFRSearch.cfm?fr=101.17. Accessed March 2017

17 Committee to Review Dietary Reference Intakes for Vitamin D and Calcium, Food and Nutrition Board, Institute of Medicine. Dietary Reference Intakes for Calcium and Vitamin D. Washington, DC: National Academy Press, 2010.

18 National Institutes of Health. Office of Dietary Supplements. 2016. Vitamin D: Fact Sheet for Health Professionals. Available

from https://ods.od.nih.gov/factsheets/ VitaminD-HealthProfessional/. Accessed March 2017.

19 Ibid.

20 Academy of Nutrition and Dietetics. 2016. Water: How Much Do Kids Need? Available from http://www.eatright.org/resource/ fitness/sports-and-performance/hydrate-right/water-go-with-the-flow. Accessed March 2017.

21 Schürmann, S., Kersting, M., and Alexy, U. 2017. Vegetarian Diets in Children: A Systematic Review. *European Journal of Nutrition* 1:21.

22 Craig, W. J., and A. R. Mangels. 2009. Position of the American Dietetic Association: Vegetarian Diets. *Journal of the American Dietetic Association* 109:1266–1282.

23 Centers for Disease Control and Prevention. 2014. Untreated Dental Caries (Cavities) in Children Ages 2–19, United States. Available at https://www.cdc.gov/Features/ dsUntreatedCavitiesKids/. Accessed March 2017.

24 Ibid.

25 Satter, E. 2015. *Ellyn Satter's Division of Responsibility in Feeding.* Available at http:// ellynsatterinstitute.org/cms-assets/ documents/203702-180136.dor-2015-2.pdf. Accessed March 2017.

26 Rollins, B., Savage, J., Fisher, J., and Birch, L. 2015. Alternatives to Restrictive Feeding Practices to Promote Self-Regulation in Childhood: A Developmental Perspective. *Pediatric Obesity* 11(5):326–332.

27 Fildes, A., van Jaarsveld, C., Wardle, J., and Cooke, L. 2014. Parent-Administered Exposure to Increase Children's Vegetable Acceptance: A Randomized Controlled Trial. *Journal of the Academy of Nutrition and Dietetics* 114(6):881–888.

28 Gibson, E. L., et al. 2012. A Narrative Review of Psychological and Educational Strategies Applied to Young Children's Eating Behaviours Aimed at Reducing Obesity Risk. *Obesity Review* Suppl. 1:85–95.

29 National Library of Medicine. 2017. Normal Growth and Development. Available from https://medlineplus.gov/ency/ article/002456.htm. Accessed April 2017.

30 U.S. Department of Agriculture. Economic Research Service. 2013. *National School Lunch Program.* Available at www.ers.usda.gov/ topics/food-nutrition-assistance/child-nutrition-programs/national-school-lunch-program.aspx/#.U5iYn8aEQ58. Accessed June 2014.

31 Food Research Action Center. The National School Lunch Program. Available at http:// frac.org/programs/national-school-lunch-program. Accessed March 2017.

32 Ibid.

33 Cohen, J. F. W., Richardson, S., Parker, E., Catalano, P. J., Rimm, E. B. 2014. Impact of the New U.S. Department of Agriculture School Meal Standards on Food Selection, Consumption, and Waste. *American Journal of Preventive Medicine* 46(4):388–394.

34 Caruso, M. L., and Cullen, K. W. 2015. Quality and Cost of Student Lunches Brought from Home. *JAMA Pediatrics* 169(1):86–90.

35 Affenito, S. G., Thompson, D., Dorazio, A., Albertson, A. M., Loew, A., and Holschuh, N. M. 2013. Ready-to-Eat Cereal Consumption and the School Breakfast Program: Relationship to Nutrient Intake and Weight. *Journal of School Health* 83:28–35.

36 Marlatt, K. L., Farbakhsh, K., Dengel, D. R., and Lytle, L. A. 2016. Breakfast and Fast Food Consumption Are Associated with Selected Biomarkers in Adolescents. *Preventive Medicine Reports* 3:49–52.

37 Food Research Action Council. 2017. School Breakfast Program. Available at http://frac .org/programs/school-breakfast-program. Accessed March 2017.

38 Adolphus, K., C. L. Lawton, and L. Dye. 2013. The Effects of Breakfast on Behavior and Academic Performance in Children and Adolescents. *Frontiers in Human Neuroscience.* Available at www.ncbi.nlm.nih.gov/pmc/ articles/PMC3737458/. Accessed June 2014.

39 Food Research Action Center. State School Breakfast Legislation. Available at http:// www.frac.org/state-school-breakfast-legislation. Accessed March 2017.

40 Healthy People 2020. 2012. *Nutrition and Weight Status Objectives.* Available at www. healthypeople.gov/2020/topicsobjec-tives2020/objectiveslist.aspx?topicid=29. Accessed April 2014.

41 Kim, S. A., Moore, L. V., Galuska, D., Wright, A. P., and Harris, D. 2014. Progress on Children Eating More Fruit, Not Vegetables. *Morbidity and Mortality Weekly Report* 63(31):671–676.

42 Natale, R. A., Messiah, S. E., Asfour, L., Uhlhorn, S. B., Delamater, A., Arheart, K. L. 2014. Role Modeling as an Early Childhood Obesity Prevention Strategy: Effect of Parents and Teachers on Preschool Children's Healthy Lifestyle Habits. *Journal of Developmental and Behavioral Pediatrics* 35(6):378–387.

43 Centers for Disease Control and Prevention. 2015. Food Allergies in School. Available from https://www.cdc.gov/healthyschools/ foodallergies/index.htm. Accessed April 2017.

44 Food and Drug Administration. 2014. *Guidance for Industry: Questions and Answers Regarding Food Allergens, Including the Food Allergen Labeling and Consumer Protection Act of 2004 (Edition 4); Final Guidance.* Available at www.fda.gov/food/guidanceregulation/ guidancedocumentsregulatoryinformation/ allergens/ucm059116.htm. Accessed June 2014.

45 Food Research Action Center. 2016. Food Hardship in America: Households with Children Especially Hard Hit. Available from www.frac.org/wp-content/uploads/food-hardship-report-households-with-children-sep-2016.pdf. Accessed March 2017.

46 Darmon, N., and Drewnowski, A. 2015. Contribution of Food Prices and Diet Cost to Socioeconomic Disparities in Diet Quality and Health: A Systematic Review and Analysis. *Nutrition Reviews* 73(10):643–660.

47 Fram, M. S., Ritchie, L. D., Rosen, N., and Frongillo, E. A. 2015. Child Experience of Food Insecurity Is Associated with Child Diet and Physical Activity. *Journal of Nutrition* 145(3):499–504.

48 Skelton, J., Cook, S., Auinger, P., Klein, J., and Barlow, S. 2009. Prevalence and Trends of Severe Obesity among US Children and Adolescents. *Academy of Pediatrics* 9(5):322–329.

49 Hanson, K. L., and Connor, L. M. 2014. Food Insecurity and Dietary Quality in US Adults and Children: A Systematic Review. *American Journal of Clinical Nutrition* 100(2):684–692.

50 Centers for Disease Control and Prevention. 2015. *Childhood Obesity Causes and Consequences.* Available at https://www.cdc.gov/ obesity/childhood/causes.html. Accessed March 2017.

51 Ogden, C. L., Carroll, M. D., Lawman, H. G., et al. 2016. Trends in Obesity Prevalence among Children and Adolescents in the United States, 1988–1994 through 2013–2014. *Journal of the American Medical Association* 315(21):2292–2299.

52 Ibid.

53 Centers for Disease Control and Prevention. 2015. *Defining Childhood Obesity.* Available at www.cdc.gov/obesity/childhood/defining .html. Accessed March 2017.

54 Ibid.

55 Centers for Disease Control and Prevention. 2015. *About BMI for Children and Teens.* Available at www.cdc.gov/healthyweight/ assessing/bmi/childrens/_bmi/about/ _childrens-_bmi.html. Accessed April 2017.

56 Daniels, S. R., D. K. Arnett, R. H. Eckel, S. S. Gidding, L. L. Hayman, S. Kumanyika, et al. 2005. Overweight in Children and Adolescents: Pathophysiology, Consequences, Prevention, and Treatment. *Circulation* 111:1999–2002. Available at www.circ .ahajournals.org/content/111/15/1999.full. Accessed June 2014.

57 Piernas, C., and Popkin, B. M. 2011. Food Portion Patterns and Trends among U.S. Children and the Relationship to Total Eating Occasion Size 1977–2006. *Journal of Nutrition.* 141:1159–1164.

58 Daniels, S. R., M. S. Jacobson, B. W. McCrindle, R. H. Eckel, and B. McHugh Sanner. 2009. American Heart Association Childhood Obesity Research Summit Report. *Circulation* 119:e489–e517. Available at http:// circ.ahajournals.org/content/119/15/e489 .full.pdf. Accessed June 2014.

59 Powell, L. M., and Nguyen, B. T. 2013. Fast-Food and Full-Service Restaurant Consumption Among Children and Adolescents: Effect on Energy, Beverage, and Nutrient Intake. *JAMA Pediatrics* 167(1):14–20.

60 HHS/USDA. 2011. *Dietary Guidelines for Americans, 2010.* Available at www.cnpp.usda. gov/publications/dietaryguidelines/2010/ policydoc/chapter3.pdf. Accessed June 2014

61 Miller, G., Merlo, C., Demissie, Z., Sliwa, S., and Park, S. 2017. Trends in Beverage Consumption Among High School Students — United States, 2007–2015. *Morbidity and Mortality Weekly Report*, 66(4):112–116.

62 Hu, F. B. 2013. Resolved: There is Sufficient Scientific Evidence That Decreasing Sugar-Sweetened Beverage Consumption Will Reduce the Prevalence of Obesity and Obesity-Related Diseases. *Obesity Reviews* 14:606–619.

63 Dubois, L., K. O. Kyvik, M. Girard, F. Tatone-Tokuda, D. Perusse, J. Hjelmborg, A. Skytthe, F. Rasmussen, M. J. Wright, P. Lichtenstein, and N. G. Martin. 2012. Genetic and Environmental Contributions to Weight, Height, and BMI from Birth to 19 Years of Age: An International Study of Over 12,000 Twin Pairs. Available at www .plosone.org/article/inf0/%3Adoi/%2F10 .1371/%2Fjournal.pone.0030153. Accessed June 2014.

64 van Dijk, S. J., Molloy, P. L., Varinli, H., Morrison, J. L., Muhlhausler, B. S., members of Epi S. 2015. Epigenetics and Human Obesity. *International Journal of Obesity* 39(1):85–97.

65 American Academy of Child and Adolescent Psychiatry. 2014. *Facts for Families: Obesity in Children and Teens*. Available at https://www .aacap.org/AACAP/Families_and_ Youth/Facts_for_Families/Facts_for_ families_Pages/Obesity_In_Children_And_ Teens_79.aspxf. Accessed April 2017.

66 Sridhar S. B., et al. 2014. Maternal Gestational Weight Gain and Offspring Risk for Childhood Overweight or Obesity. *American Journal of Obstetrics and Gynecology* 211(3):259. e1–8. Available at www.ncbi.nlm.nih.gov/ pubmed/24735804. Accessed June 2014.

67 Jerica, M., Bergel, J. M., Meyer, C., MacLehose, R. F., Crichlow, R., and Newmark-Sztainer, D. 2015. All in the Family: Correlations Between Parents' and Adolescent Siblings' Weight and Weight-Related Behaviors. *Obesity* 23:833–839.

68 Russell, C. G., Worsley, A., and Campbell, K. J. 2015. Strategies Used by Parents to Influence Their Children's Food Preferences. *Appetite* 90:123–130.

69 Liang, J., Matheson, B. E., Rhee, K. E., Peterson, C. B., Rydell, S., and Boutelle, K. N. 2016. Parental Control and Overconsumption of Snack Foods in Overweight and Obese Children. *Appetite* 100:181–188.

70 Lumeng, J. C., Ozbeki, T. N., Appugliese, D. P., Kaciroti, N., Corwyn, R. F., and Bradley, R. H. 2012. Observed Assertive and Intrusive Maternal Feeding Behaviors Increase Child Adiposity. *American Journal of Clinical Nutrition* 95:640–647.

71 Wilfley, D. E., Staiano, A. E., Altman, M., Lindros, J., Lima, A., Hassink, S. G., Dietz, W. H., Cook, S. and The Improving Access and Systems of Care for Evidence-Based Childhood Obesity Treatment Conference Workgroup. 2017. Improving access and systems of care for evidence-based childhood

obesity treatment: Conference key findings and next steps. *Obesity* 25:16–29.

72 U.S. Department of Health and Human Services. Subcommittee of the President's Council on Fitness, Sports & Nutrition. 2012. *Physical Activity Guidelines for Americans Midcourse Report. Strategies to Increase Physical Activity among Youth.* Available at www.health .gov/paguidelines/midcourse/pag-mid-course-report-final.pdf. Accessed March 2017.

73 Centers for Disease Control and Prevention. 2013. *A Growing Problem.*

74 Dentro, K., Beals, K., Crouter, S., Eisenmann, J., McKenzie, T., Pate, R., et al. 2014. Results from the United States' 2014 Report Card on Physical Activity for Children and Youth. *Journal of Physical Activity and Health* 11(1).

75 U.S. Department of Health and Human Services. 2008. *2008 Physical Activity Guidelines for Americans.* Available at www.health.gov/ paguidelines/pdf/paguide.pdf. Accessed June 2014.

76 U.S. Department of Health and Human Services. 2012. *Physical Activity Guidelines for Americans Midcourse Report. Strategies to Increase Physical Activity among Youth.*

77 Common Sense Media. The Common Sense Census: Media Use by Tweens and Teens. Available from https://www.commonsen-semedia.org/sites/default/files/uploads/ research/census_executivesummary.pdf. Accessed May 2017.

78 Tarabashkina, L., Quester, P., and Crouch, R. 2016. Food Advertising, Children's Food Choices and Obesity: Interplay of Cognitive Defences and Product Evaluation: An Experimental Study. *International Journal of Obesity* 40(4):581–586.

79 Hill, D., Ameenuddin, N., Chassiakos, Y. R., Cross, C., Radesky, J., Hutchinson, J., et al. 2016. Media Use in School-Aged Children and Adolescents. *Pediatrics* 138(5).

80 Ibid.

81 Buxton, O. M., Chang, A. M., Spilsbury, J. C., Bos, T., Emsellem, H., Knutson, K. L. 2015. Sleep in the Modern Family: Protective Family Routines for Child and Adolescent Sleep. *Sleep Health* 1(1):15–27.

82 Borghese, M. M., Tremblay, M. S., Katzmarzyk, P. T., et al. 2015. Mediating Role of Television Time, Diet Patterns, Physical Activity and Sleep Duration in the Association between Television in the Bedroom and Adiposity in 10 Year-Old Children. *International Journal of Behaviorial Nutrition and Physical Activity* 12:60–70.

83 Ibid.

84 Ohri-Vachaspati, P., DeLia, D., DeWeese, R. S., Crespo, N. C., Todd, M., and Yedidia, M. J. 2015. The Relative Contribution of Layers of the Social Ecological Model to Childhood Obesity. *Public Health Nutrition* 18(11):2055–2066.

85 Ibid.

86 Roberto, C. A., Swinburn, B., Hawkes, C., Huang, T. T. K., Costa, S. A., Ashe, M., et

al. 2015. Patchy Progress on Obesity Prevention: Emerging Examples, Entrenched Barriers, and New Thinking. *The Lancet* 385(9985):2400–2409.

87 Casey, R., Oppert, J.-M., Weber, C., et al. 2014. Determinants of Childhood Obesity: What Can We Learn from Built Environment Studies? *Food Quality and Preference* 31:164–172.

88 American Psychological Association. The Impact of Food Advertising on Childhood Obesity. Available from http://www.apa .org/topics/kids-media/food.aspx. Accessed March 2017.

89 Boyland, E. J., Nolan, S., Kelly, B., Tudur-Smith, C., Jones, A., Halford, J. C., et al. 2016. Advertising as a Cue to Consume: A Systematic Review and Meta-Analysis of the Effects of Acute Exposure to Unhealthy Food and Nonalcoholic Beverage Advertising on Intake in Children and Adults. *American Journal of Clinical Nutrition*. [Epub ahead of print]

90 Frazier, W. C., and Harris, J. L. 2016. Trends in Television Food Advertising to Young People: 2015 Update. Available at http://uconnruddcenter.org/files/ TVAdTrends2016.pdf. Accessed May 2017.

91 Elsey, J., and Harris, J. 2015. Trends in Food and Beverage Television Brand Appearances Viewed by Children and Adolescents from 2009 to 2014 in the USA. *Public Health Nutrition* 19(11):1928–1933.

92 De Leonibus, C., Marcovecchio, M., Chiavaroli, V., Giorgis, T., Chiarelli, F., and Mohn, A. 2014. Timing of Puberty and Physical Growth in Obese Children: A Longitudinal Study in Boys and Girls. *Pediatric Obesity* 9(4):292–299.

93 Ogden, C. L., Carroll, M. D., Lawman, H. G., et al. 2016. Trends in Obesity Prevalence among Children and Adolescents in the United States, 1988–1994 through 2013–2014.

94 Simmonds, M., Llewellyn, A., Owen, C.G. and Woolacott, N. 2016. Predicting adult obesity from childhood obesity: a systematic review and meta-analysis. *Obesity Reviews* 17(2):95–107.

95 Donaldson, A., and Gordon, C. 2013. Bone Health in Adolescents. *Contemporary Pediatrics*.

96 Institute of Medicine. 2011. *Dietary Reference Intakes for Calcium and Vitamin D.*

97 Institute of Medicine, Food and Nutrition Board. 1997. *Dietary Reference Intakes for Calcium, Phosphorus, Magnesium, Vitamin D, and Fluoride.* Available at http://fnic.nal.usda. gov/dietary-guidance/dri-reports/calcium-phosphorus-magnesium-vitamin-d-and-fluoride. Accessed June 2014.

98 Golden, N. H., and Abrams, S. A. 2014. Optimizing Bone Health in Children and Adolescents. *Pediatrics* 134(4):e1229–e1243.

99 Ibid.

100 Institute of Medicine. 2001. *Dietary Reference Intakes for Vitamin A, Vitamin K, Arsenic, Boron, Chromium, Copper, Iodine, Iron, Manganese, Nickel, Silicon, Vanadium, and Zinc.*

101 U.S. Department of Agriculture, Agricultural Research Service. 2016. Nutrient Intakes from Food and Beverages: Mean Amounts Consumed per Individual, by Gender and Age, What We Eat in America, NHANES 2013–2014.

102 U.S. Department of Health and Human Services. National Heart, Lung, and Blood Institute. 2014. *How Is Iron-Deficiency Anemia Treated?* Available at https://www.nhlbi.nih.gov/health/health-topics/topics/ida/treatment Accessed March 2017.

103 Meier, A., and K. Musick. 2014. Variation in Associations between Family Dinners and Adolescent Well-Being. *Journal of Marriage and Family* 76(1):13–23. Available at http://onlinelibrary.wiley.com/doi/10.1111/jomf.12079/abstract. Accessed June 2014.

104 CASAColumbia. 2012. *The Importance of Family Dinners VIII.* Available at www.casacolumbia.org/addiction-research/reports/importance-of-family-dinners-2012. Accessed July 2014.

105 Grossi, E., Cazzaniga, S., Crotti, S., Naldi, L., Di Landro, A., Ingordo, V., Cusano, F., Atzori, L., Tripodi Cutrì, F., Musumeci, M. L., and Pezzarossa, E. 2016. The Constellation of Dietary Factors in Adolescent Acne: A Semantic Connectivity Map Approach. *Journal of the European Academy of Dermatology and Venereology* 30(1):96–100.

106 Burris, J., Rietkerk, W., and Woolf, K., 2014. Relationships of Self-Reported Dietary Factors and Perceived Acne Severity in a Cohort of New York Young Adults. *Journal of the Academy of Nutrition and Dietetics* 114(3):384–392.

107 Grossi, E., Cazzaniga, S., Crotti, S., Naldi, L., Di Landro, A., Ingordo, V., Cusano, F., Atzori, L., Tripodi Cutrì, F., Musumeci, M.L., Pezzarossa, E., Bettoli, V., Caproni, M., Bonci, A., and the GISED Acne Study Group. 2016. The Constellation of Dietary Factors in Adolescent Acne: A Semantic Connectivity Map Approach.

108 National Eating Disorders Association. 2012. *Research on Males and Eating Disorders.* Available at https://www.nationaleating-disorders.org/research-males-and-eating-disorders. Accessed March 2017.

109 Diemer, E. W., Grant, J. D., Munn-Chernoff, M. A., Patterson, D. A., and Duncan, A. E. 2015. Gender Identity, Sexual Orientation, and Eating-related Pathology in a National Sample of College Students. *Journal of Adolescent Health: Official Publication of the Society for Adolescent Medicine* 57(2):144–149.

110 Herpertz-Dahlmann, B. 2015. Adolescent Eating Disorders: Update on Definitions, Symptomatology, Epidemiology, and Comorbidity. *Child and Adolescent Psychiatric Clinics of North America* 24(1):177–196.

111 Rohde, P., Stice, E., and Marti, C. N. 2015. Development and Predictive Effects of Eating Disorder Risk Factors During Adolescence: Implications for Prevention Efforts. *International Journal of Eating Disorders* 48:187–198.

112 Dabelea, D., Mayer-Davis, E. J., Saydah, S., Imperatore, G., Linder, B., Divers, J., Bell, R., Badaru, A., Talton, J. W., Crume, T., Liese, A. D., Merchant, A. T., Lawrence, J. M., Reynolds, K., Dolan, L., Liu, L. L., Hamman, R. F., for the SEARCH for Diabetes in Youth Study. 2014. Prevalence of Type 1 and Type 2 Diabetes Among Children and Adolescents From 2001 to 2009. *Journal of the American Medical Association* 311(17):1778–1786.

113 Ibid.

114 Dingle, E., and Brar, P. 2017. Prediabetes in Obese Adolescents: An Emerging Clinical Priority. *Clinical Pediatrics* 56(2):115–116.

115 Ibid.

116 American Diabetes Association. 2014. *Preventing Type 2 Diabetes in Children.* Available at www.diabetes.org/living-with-diabetes/parents-and-kids/children-and-type-2/preventing-type-2-in-children.html. Accessed March 2017.

117 May, A. L., Kuklina, E. V., and Yoon, P. W. 2012. Prevalence of Cardiovascular Disease Risk Factors Among US Adolescents, 1999–2008. *Pediatrics* 129(6):1035–1041.

118 Pulgarón, E. R. 2013. Childhood Obesity: A Review of Increased Risk for Physical and Psychological Comorbidities. *Clinical Therapeutics* 35(1):A18–A32.

119 Ibid.

120 Lloyd-Richardson, E. E., Jelalian, E., Sato, A. F., Hart, C. N., Mehlenbeck, R., Wing, R. R. 2012. Two-Year Follow-up of an Adolescent Behavioral Weight Control Intervention. *Pediatrics* 130(2):e281–e288.

121 Mayo Clinic. 2014. *Childhood Obesity Complications.* Available at http://www.mayoclinic.org/diseases-conditions/childhood-obesity/symptoms-causes/dxc-20268891. Accessed March 2017.

122 Finkelstein, E. A., Graham, W. C. K., and Malhotra, R. 2014. Lifetime Direct Medical Costs of Childhood Obesity. *Pediatrics* 133(5):854–862.

123 US Preventive Services Task Force. 2010. Screening for Obesity in Children and Adolescents: US Preventive Services Task Force Recommendation Statement. *Pediatrics* 125:361–367.

124 Ibid.

125 Ibid.

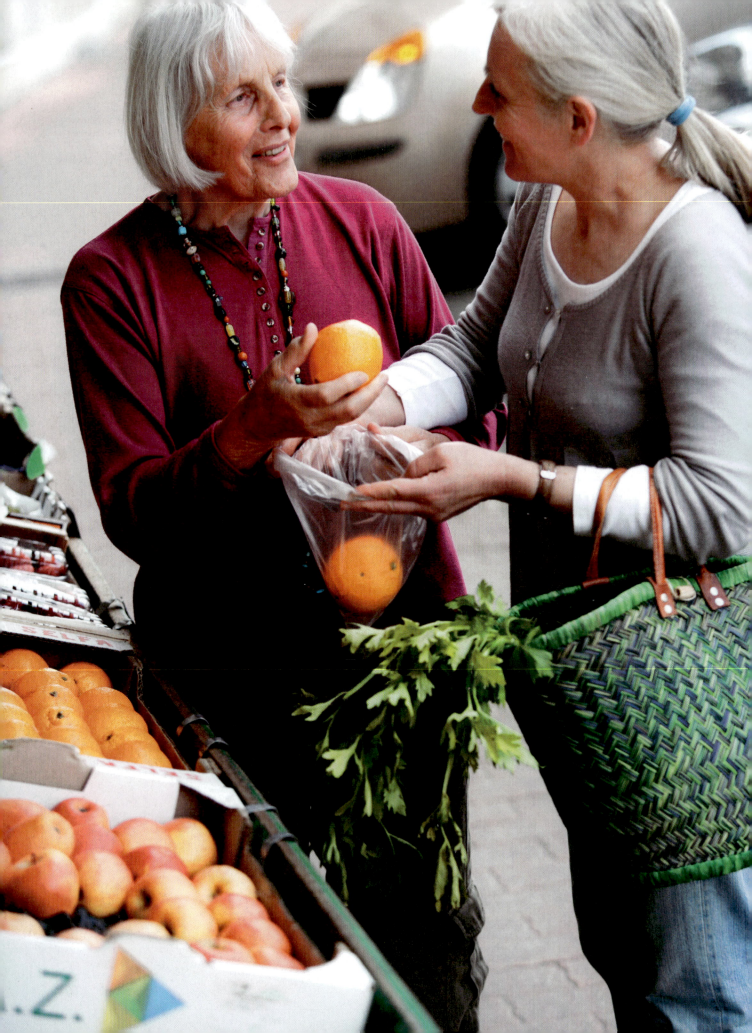

Life Cycle Nutrition
Older Adults

Learning Outcomes

After reading this chapter, you will be able to:

19.1 Discuss the demographics of aging in America and the links between health care, lifestyle choices, and longevity.

19.2 Describe common changes in bodily functions that occur as a result of the aging process.

19.3 Summarize the nutrient needs of older adults.

19.4 Discuss key nutrition-related health concerns common among older adults.

19.5 Describe several social, economic, and psychological factors that commonly affect the health of older Americans.

19.6 Identify the age-related risk factors for hypertension and the dietary interventions that help control it.

True or False?

1. Chronic disease is an inevitable part of aging. **T**/**F**

2. Heart disease is the number-one cause of death among older Americans. **T**/**F**

3. Inadequate dietary fiber leads many older adults to suffer from constipation. **T**/**F**

4. The percentage of the population age 65 years and older is declining in the United States. **T**/**F**

5. Older adults are more susceptible to osteoporosis in part because of low sun exposure and insufficient intake of vitamin D. **T**/**F**

6. Too much vitamin A can increase the risk of bone fractures. **T**/**F**

7. Older adults rarely use dietary supplements. **T**/**F**

8. On average, older adults need fewer daily kilocalories than younger adults. **T**/**F**

9. Food insecurity among elders is a nonissue in the United States. **T**/**F**

10. Alcohol abuse is extremely rare among older adults. **T**/**F**

See page 725–726 for the answers.

Aging is a natural, complex process that occurs at the cellular level and results in physical and psychological changes. It begins during early middle age, which may be considered the years from 35 to 50, when bodily functions begin to gradually decline. Age 65 is often designated as the beginning of old age, but there is no single age at which people become old.[1] **Senescence**, another term for growing old, is defined as a process that begins at conception and ends at death.

Each aging experience is unique, and changes in bodily functions do not occur at the same rate or to the same degree in any two people. Perhaps the reason 65 is considered old is that traditionally, that's when many people retired from full-time employment, although now people are working well into their later years and living longer in better health.

Although the older years are often seen as a positive time, aging can make people more vulnerable to disease and disability. It can also inflict heavy health and financial burdens on people and diminish their quality of life. While the risk of illness increases with age, poor health is not inevitable.

In this chapter we discuss the physical, economic, and emotional aspects of aging and the nutrient needs of older adults. We also examine the most common dietary challenges older adults face and ways to minimize health risks and promote a healthier older age.

What Are the Demographics of Aging in America?

LO 19.1 Discuss the demographics of aging in America and the links between health care, lifestyle choices, and longevity.

The potential **lifespan** of the human body—about 120 years—hasn't changed much during the last century. From the early 1900s, **life expectancy** has increased from 48 to 81.2 years for women and from 46 to 76.3 years for men.[2] Fewer deaths from infectious disease at an early age, better nutrition, and advances in medicine, including interventions to diagnose, manage, and treat chronic illness, have led to increased **longevity**, or duration of life.[3] Some researchers now make a distinction between lifespan and health span and between longevity and healthy longevity; that is, the number of years of good health and functioning is a different consideration from the total number of years lived.[4]

America's Population Is Getting Older and More Diverse

The United States' population is aging at a rapid rate. The large, so-called baby boomer generation—children born between 1946 and 1964—is expected to be the fastest-growing segment of the population over the next decade. About 14.5 percent of the U.S. population, or one in seven people, are over age 65. In 2014, there were 64.8 million people age 65 and older in the United States, up from 48.9 million in 2004.[5] By 2060, the number of Americans aged 65 and older is projected to be 98 million.[6] See **Figure 19.1**.

The 85-and-older population is also growing rapidly. The number of people in this oldest age group is projected to grow from 6 million in 2014 to 20 million by 2060.[7] Whereas the U.S. population is becoming more diverse, this diversity is less pronounced among older Americans. Specifically, among those age 65 and older, more than 75 percent were non-Hispanic white in 2014 compared to 50 percent of Americans age 18 and younger. It is expected, however, that by 2060, 45 percent of the older population will identify as belonging to a minority group: non-Hispanic black (12 percent), Asian (9 percent), Hispanic (22 percent), Other (3 percent).[8]

aging Declines in bodily functions that accumulate with time, ultimately leading to death.

senescence Another term for aging.

lifespan Maximum age to which members of a species can live.

life expectancy Average length of life for a population of individuals.

longevity Duration of an individual's life.

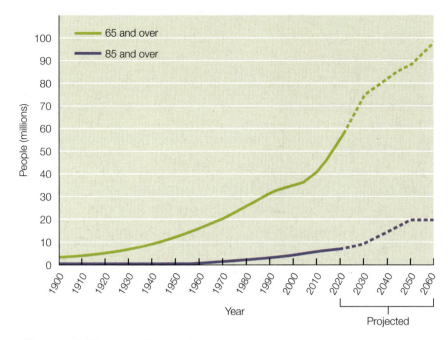

▲ **Figure 19.1 The Aging Population**
The number of older adults in the United States is projected to increase significantly during the next several decades.

Source: Data from Administration on Aging (AoA). 2014. Projected Future Growth of the Older Population. Available from https://aoa.acl.gov/Aging_Statistics/future_growth/future_growth.aspx. Accessed May 2017.

Improved Health Care Is Increasing Lifespan

Medical advances and public health campaigns have greatly contributed to Americans' longer lives. Since the 1900s, the incidence of potentially fatal infectious diseases, such as tuberculosis, pneumonia, polio, mumps, and measles, has been dramatically reduced by vaccination programs, antibiotics, and better medical care. In addition, modern medical technology contributes to earlier diagnosis and better management of chronic conditions such as cancer, cardiovascular disease, diabetes, and osteoporosis that could prove disabling or deadly.

For decades, public health campaigns have encouraged Americans to eat a balanced diet and get regular physical activity to help prevent obesity and reduce the risk for obesity-related conditions and chronic diseases. Moreover, people of all ages now have access to a vast amount of health information via the Internet and other media and may be using it to make healthier choices than previous generations. Whereas the overall age-adjusted death rate for the total population increased 1.2 percent from 2014 to 2015, much of this increase was due to a 6.7 percent increase in unintentional injuries and a 15.7% increase in Alzheimer's disease as opposed to a large increase in obesity-related diseases.[9]

Poor Lifestyle Choices Contribute to the Leading Causes of Death in Older Adults

Despite these advances in health care and subsequent increases in life expectancy, recent evidence suggests that poor lifestyle choices may be slowing this trend. These include poor nutrition and a sedentary lifestyle, both of which contribute to obesity, which greatly increases the risk for chronic disease, especially in adults over age 65. Since 1980, for example, the number of Americans diagnosed with diabetes, primarily type 2 diabetes, has more than tripled. This surge has been linked to our rising obesity rates, sedentary lifestyles, and advancing age. The Centers for Disease Control and Prevention (CDC) estimates that 29.1 million Americans have diabetes, and 8.1 million of them do not know it.[10]

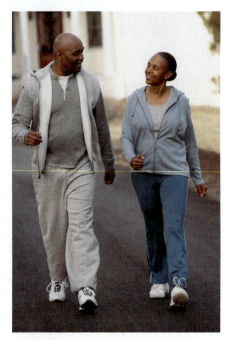

The number-one physical activity among older Americans is walking. Gardening is second most prevalent, followed by bicycling. Don't know what to get your grandparents for a birthday gift? Consider a pedometer.

Poor nutrition and inactivity are key risk factors not only for obesity and diabetes, but also for hypertension, high cholesterol, heart disease, stroke, and cancer.[11] Unfortunately, just 16 percent of Americans aged 65 and older meet the physical activity guidelines for their age group as suggested in the *Physical Activity Guidelines for Americans*.[12]

Even with the physical changes that accompany aging, many people can remain physically active in their later years. Routine exercise improves sleep, flexibility, and range of motion and can help postpone the decline in cognitive ability that naturally occurs in aging.[13] Working in the garden, mowing the lawn, walking the dog, and dancing provide health benefits. Older adults also benefit from strength-training activities such as lifting weights and calisthenics at least twice a week to help maintain muscle strength.[14] Physical fitness can enable older adults to live independently longer, reducing their need for assistance with activities of everyday living, preserving their quality of life, and reducing health care costs.

The CDC's *State of Aging and Health* report assesses the health status and health behaviors of adults aged 65 years and older in the United States. The most recent report encourages older adults to adopt healthier behaviors to reduce their risk for many chronic diseases.[15]

LO 19.1: THE TAKE-HOME MESSAGE Lifespan is the maximum age to which members of a species can live, and longevity is the duration of an individual's life. Life expectancy has increased markedly in the United States since the 1900s. There are more older Americans than ever, and that population is expected to grow further. The U.S. population is living longer due to improved health care, disease prevention, and, for some, because of healthier lifestyle choices. Some of the leading causes of death among older adults are related to nutrition and inactivity. These include heart disease, stroke, cancer, and type 2 diabetes.

What Changes Occur as Part of the Aging Process?

LO 19.2 Describe common changes in bodily functions that occur as a result of the aging process.

As we age, changes occurring at the cellular level cause changes in tissues and organs that affect a person's health, function, and appearance.[16] Aging and damaged cells undergo cell death, a normal process that makes room for new cells. However, in some organs, cells die and are not replaced. A reduced number of cells then affects organ function.

Most age-related changes are gradual and their effects accumulate with time. The rate at which individuals age depends on their genes, environment, and lifestyle choices:

- Genetics affect the rate at which cells are maintained and repaired and can influence development of a number of chronic diseases, such as cardiovascular disease and cancer.
- Environmental factors such as oxidative stress caused by excessive sun exposure or cigarette smoking can cause cell damage and lead to cell mutation or death. Poverty, discrimination, and many other factors can cause excessive, persistent stress, which in turn provokes higher levels of the hormone cortisol in the body. High cortisol levels can lead to increases in body weight, decreased immune function, and an increased inflammatory response.[17]

- Important lifestyle choices, including diet and exercise, affect the rate of aging. A diet high in saturated fat and low in antioxidants and fiber can accelerate the aging process. Regular aerobic activity and strength training help to control blood pressure, blood lipids, and blood glucose.

Because these three variables influence aging, the **physiologic age** of a person can vary greatly from that person's **chronologic age**. The following sections discuss the most important physiological changes that occur with age and their nutritional implications.

Muscle and Bone Mass Decline

Aging leads to changes in body composition that can affect overall health and nutrition status. Many adults lose between 10 and 15 percent of their peak muscle mass and strength during their lifetime[18] (**Figure 19.2**). As a result of this slowly declining muscle mass, basal metabolic rate (BMR) starts to slow around age 30.

Sarcopenia, or a loss of muscle mass and function, is caused by changes in muscle and nerve tissue that result from decreased physical activity. It is a common cause of disability in older adults, making day-to-day activities more difficult and increasing the risk for falls and fractures. Although everyone experiences muscle loss, regular physical activity and optimal nutrition can slow or minimize the effects.

As a result of a lower BMR, reduced physical activity, or both, it's common for older adults to gain weight, usually fat tissue. In the United States, 38 percent of males and 39 percent of females over age 60 are obese.[19] While many people in their 50s, 60s, and 70s grapple with excess body fat, those in their 80s and beyond may experience unintentional weight loss. Chronic inadequate food intake due to dental problems, difficulty preparing food, reduced appetite, and other causes, can lead to undernutrition, which in turn reduces resistance to infections and can lead to frailty, loss of independence, and functional decline.[20]

The aging process also affects bones and joints. With time, bones become less dense due to calcium loss. As a result, they are more prone to fracture. The significant estrogen losses caused by menopause accelerate bone loss in women. In addition, with age, the body becomes less efficient at absorbing calcium from foods and dietary supplements, so there is less available to bones. Older people lose height because spinal vertebrae lose density and the disks between them get thinner, shortening the spine.

Immune Function Decreases

As a person ages, the function of the immune system decreases, reducing the body's ability to protect itself against bacteria and viruses, cancer, and autoimmune diseases, such as lupus and autoimmune hepatitis.[21]

A decrease in immunity may be due in part to inadequate nutrient intake. The immune response depends on an adequate supply of protein and key vitamins and minerals. Older adults, especially those who have limited food intake, may not consume adequate amounts of vitamins A, C, B$_{12}$, and E, as well as iron and zinc. Deficiency of key nutrients such as these in conjunction with advanced age can decrease the body's ability to fight illness.

Sensory Abilities Decline

Aging brings a progressive decline in vision and hearing, although the extent of these impairments varies among individuals. This decline can result in decreased food intake. For example, poor vision can make shopping for food and preparing meals more difficult. Hearing loss can lead to social isolation, solitary eating, and depression, which in turn may limit a person's interest in food.

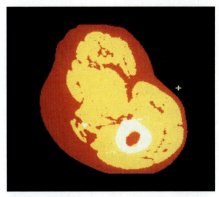

a Cross-section of a young adult's thigh

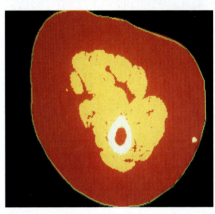

b Cross-section of an older adult's thigh

▲ **Figure 19.2 Aging Leads to Decrease in Muscle Mass**
Note the proportionally reduced muscle area (in yellow) of the older, sedentary adult in the bottom image compared with that of a younger, more active adult. Most people lose a significant amount of muscle as they age, some of which could be prevented by engaging in regular physical activity.

physiologic age Person's age estimated in terms of body health, function, and life expectancy.

chronologic age Person's age in number of years of life.

sarcopenia Age-related progressive loss of muscle mass, muscle strength, and function.

Aging also reduces sense of smell, as do certain medications and nutritional deficiencies. There is no treatment for age-related loss of smell.[22] Because the sense of smell contributes to our ability to taste, a decline in sense of smell may reduce an older adult's appetite and food intake. If a person's diet allows, they should flavor foods with some butter or olive oil, cheese, nuts, fresh herbs, mustard, hot pepper, spices, or lemon or lime juice to make them more appealing.[23] Assisting older adults to maintain an adequate and varied diet through the use of highly seasoned foods can help offset nutritional deficiencies and make meals more enjoyable.

Gastrointestinal Functions Change

As a person ages, a number of changes occur within the GI tract and its accessory organs that affect chewing, swallowing, digestion, and nutrient absorption. One of the most important is decreased saliva production, which is especially common in the very old and in those who take certain medications. Decreased saliva production increases the risk for oral health problems, makes swallowing more difficult (a condition known as *dysphagia*), and may reduce taste perception. It also increases the risk of tooth decay and gum disease. Moreover, some elderly people have missing teeth or wear ill-fitting dentures, which can make chewing difficult, limit food choices, and contribute to poor nutrition.

Dysphagia is another common age-related change in GI function. It currently affects up to 68 percent of nursing home residents, up to 64 percent of stroke patients, and between 13 and 38 percent of elderly who live independently.[24] Dysphagia is caused not only by decreased saliva production, but also by reduced muscle mass and a decrease in the elasticity of connective tissue that occurs with aging. Regardless of the cause, dysphagia increases the risk for nutrient deficiencies and aspiration-related pneumonia (which can occur when food or liquid enters the respiratory tract). Simple dietary modifications that can prevent these outcomes include thickening liquids and softening solid foods so that they are mashed, moist, semi-solid, or pureed.[25]

Aging also causes changes in gastric secretions. Decreased production of hydrochloric acid and pepsin can contribute to the development of atrophic gastritis, which affects protein digestion and can reduce the absorption of nutrients, notably vitamin B_{12}.[26] Vitamin B_{12} deficiency affects up to 15 percent of the elderly population; thus, older adults should consume vitamin B_{12} in fortified foods or supplements or have regular intramuscular injections of vitamin B_{12}.[27]

A decline in GI motility also occurs with aging. Stomach emptying may slow, reducing hunger and thus food and nutrient intake. Slowed peristalsis can lead to constipation, gas, and bloating. Consuming adequate fiber and fluid and remaining physically active can help to alleviate some of the consequences of reduced GI motility.

Brain Function Changes

Much of aging focuses on what people lose as they grow older. The brain, however, is one organ of the body that adapts well to aging. Improved technology such as functional magnetic resonance imaging (fMRI) has generated a wealth of information about the physical changes in the aging brain. This new research suggests that the aging brain is far more resilient than was previously believed, changing and reorganizing to maintain its functions.[28]

So why do older people become more forgetful or process new information more slowly? Experts cannot say for sure, but such changes might be due to an age-related decline in the levels of neurotransmitters, which allow for communication among brain cells, and reduced blood flow to the brain. Older people may therefore react more slowly and take more time to accomplish tasks, but when given plenty of time, they are successful.[29] Dementia—a form of cognitive impairment more common with age—is discussed later in this chapter.

The rate at which individuals age depends on their genes, environment, and lifestyle choices. Among the notable physiologic effects of aging are declines in muscle mass and bone density. Weight loss occurring among older adults may result in malnutrition, reducing the function of the immune system and increasing the risk for infection. Vision, hearing, taste, and smell are diminished with age, and these losses may in turn reduce appetite, food intake, and eating enjoyment. Older adults may also experience gastrointestinal difficulties, such as reduced saliva production, dysphagia, reduced gastric secretions, and slower GI motility. Brain function may slow because of an age-related decline in the levels of neurotransmitters and in blood flow. Optimal nutrition can help to prevent further declines in health and preserve bodily functions.

What Are the Nutrient Needs of Older Adults?

LO 19.3 Summarize the nutrient needs of older adults.

The Dietary Reference Intakes (DRIs) for a few nutrients differ for older adults, and several other dietary changes are recommended. These are summarized in **Table 19.1**. In addition, **Figure 19.3** shows the Tufts University *MyPlate for Older Adults*, which illustrates healthy food and beverage choices for this population. Like people of all ages, older adults should make half of their plate fruits and vegetables; 25 percent grains, most of which should be whole grains; and 25 percent lean proteins and dairy. Also, older adults should consume adequate low-kilocalorie fluids, include healthy plant oils, and use herbs and spices in place of table salt.[30]

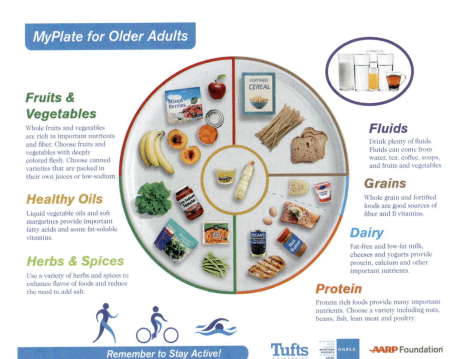

MyPlate for Older Adults

Fruits & Vegetables
Whole fruits and vegetables are rich in important nutrients and fiber. Choose fruits and vegetables with deeply colored flesh. Choose canned varieties that are packed in their own juices or low-sodium.

Healthy Oils
Liquid vegetable oils and soft margarines provide important fatty acids and some fat-soluble vitamins.

Herbs & Spices
Use a variety of herbs and spices to enhance flavor of foods and reduce the need to add salt.

Remember to Stay Active!

Fluids
Drink plenty of fluids. Fluids can come from water, tea, coffee, soups, and fruits and vegetables.

Grains
Whole grain and fortified foods are good sources of fiber and B vitamins.

Dairy
Fat-free and low-fat milk, cheeses and yogurts provide protein, calcium and other important nutrients.

Protein
Protein rich foods provide many important nutrients. Choose a variety including nuts, beans, fish, lean meat and poultry.

◀ **Figure 19.3 Older Adults Benefit from Good Nutrition and Physical Activity**
Older adults need to focus on nutrient-dense foods that contain adequate fiber, calcium, vitamin B12, vitamin D, and many other nutrients. With a declining metabolic rate, seniors require fewer kilocalories. Food choices should emphasize fresh and lightly processed foods rich in nutrient-dense carbohydrates, lean protein, and healthy fats. Older people also need to ensure adequate fluid intake and regularly engage in physical activity.
Source: Tufts University Jean Mayer USDA Human Nutrition Research Center on Aging. 2016. MyPlate for Older Adults. Available at http://hnrca.tufts.edu/myplate/. Accessed April 2017.

TABLE 19.1 Dietary Changes for Older Adults

Recommended Change	Rationale	Examples
Increase protein intake	Older people may need more protein to protect against lean tissue loss	Focus on lean sources of protein such as lean beef, skinless poultry, seafood, and legumes
Consume adequate amounts of nutrient-dense foods	Older adults continue to need vitamins, minerals, and phytonutrients	Choose foods in each food group that are low in added sugars and fats
Consume most carbohydrates in the complex form	Complex carbohydrate keeps blood glucose levels stable better than simple sugars	Eat whole grains, fruits, and vegetables, including legumes, daily; limit refined grains, sugary drinks, and desserts
Consume most fat as the unsaturated variety	Saturated fat increases heart disease risk; unsaturated fats help to reduce it	Include at least two seafood meals weekly; choose foods such as avocados, nuts, and olive and canola oils
Limit sodium intake to 1,500 milligrams daily	Decreases risk for high blood pressure	Eat more fresh and lightly processed foods; limit restaurant foods and packaged products
Consume adequate fiber	Helps prevent constipation and diverticulosis and type 2 diabetes	Choose at least three servings of whole grains, such as whole-wheat bread, whole-grain cereals, and brown rice, daily. Include whole fruits, and legumes and other vegetables in meals and snacks
Consume adequate fluid	Decreased ability of kidneys to concentrate urine and decreased thirst mechanism can both increase risk of dehydration	Drink 1% low-fat or fat-free milk and water with and between meals; limit sugary, low-nutrient soft drinks
Increase intake of foods high in beta-carotene to meet vitamin A needs and limit dietary supplements with high levels of retinol (preformed vitamin A)	Higher amounts of retinol in the body can increase fracture risk	Choose brightly colored fruits and vegetables, including carrots, cantaloupe, broccoli, spinach, kale, and winter squash for beta-carotene
Increase intake of vitamin D–fortified foods	Lower ability to make the active form of vitamin D in the body decreases the absorption of calcium and phosphorus and increases the risk of osteoporosis	Choose vitamin D–fortified milk, soymilk, yogurt, and breakfast cereals. Many older people will need a vitamin D supplement to satisfy suggested intakes
Increase intake of synthetic form of vitamin B_{12}	Decreased stomach acid reduces the absorption of naturally occuring vitamin B_{12} in foods	Choose vitamin B_{12}–fortified breakfast cereals and soy beverages. A daily multivitamin typically supplies the suggested amount of vitamin B_{12} for those age 51 and older
Choose adequate amounts of iron-rich foods	Prevents iron deficiency, which is more common in people who don't eat iron-rich foods	Choose lean meat, fish, and poultry; enjoy iron-fortified grains along with vitamin C–rich foods (such as citrus and tomatoes) to enhance iron absorption
Increase intake of zinc-rich foods	Zinc deficiency can suppress immune system and appetite	Choose zinc-fortified cereals, lean meats, poultry, legumes, and nuts
Increase intake of calcium-rich foods	Calcium needs increase with age; adequate calcium intake helps protect against osteoporosis	Consume at least three servings of dairy foods daily; older people may need a dietary supplement

Older Adults Have Lower Energy Needs

Given their previously discussed reductions in BMR, adults typically need fewer kilocalories as they age. The decline in metabolism is a result of the natural loss of muscle mass (recall that muscle mass requires more energy for maintenance than fat mass). A lower metabolic rate combined with less physical activity reduces energy needs. (See the Calculation Corner for one way of estimating energy expenditure.) For example, a 70-year-old moderately active man needs about 400 fewer kilocalories—about the amount in a turkey sandwich—than his 40-year-old counterpart. By the age of 80, a sedentary female requires only about 1,600 kilocalories a day, which are 600 fewer kilocalories than she needed when she was

Estimating Energy Expenditure Using the Harris-Benedict Equation

Sue, a 70-year-old retired nurse, walks 2 miles every day, as she has since she was 30. She is 5 feet 7 inches (170.2 cm) tall and maintains her weight at 154 pounds (70 kg). Use the Harris-Benedict equation below to determine her Estimated Energy Requirement (EER). How has Sue's EER changed from when she was 30 years old?

Answer

1. Use the Harris-Benedict equation for females to calculate Sue's RMR:

   $RMR = 655.1 + (9.6 \times \text{weight in kg}) + (1.8 \times \text{height in cm}) - (4.7 \times \text{age in years})$

   $655.1 + (9.6 \times 70 \text{ kg}) + (1.8 \times 170.2 \text{ cm}) - (4.7 \times 70) = 1{,}304.46 \text{ kcalories}$

   $655.1 + 672 + 306.36 - 329 = 1{,}304.46$

2. Next, apply the activity factor to determine total daily energy expenditure:

   Sedentary: 1.00; Low level of activity: 1.12; Active: 1.27; Very Active: 1.48

   $1{,}304.46 \times 1.12 = 1{,}461 \text{ kcalories}$

3. Now put the equations together to calculate her EER at age 30:

   $655.1 + (9.6 \times 70 \text{ kg}) + (1.8 \times 170.2 \text{ cm}) - (4.7 \times 30) = 1{,}492.46 \text{ kcalories}$

   $1{,}492.46 \times 1.27 \text{ activity factor} = 1{,}895 \text{ kcalories}$

Compared with her needs at age 30, Sue now requires 434 fewer daily kilocalories. Most vitamin and mineral requirements remain the same for her, and some, such as for calcium and vitamin D, have increased since she was 30. Lower energy requirements mean that Sue should select nutrient-dense foods with fewer kilocalories to maintain her body weight.

> Go to Mastering Nutrition and complete a Math Video activity similar to the problem in this Calculation Corner.

---

a moderately active 20-year-old.[31] Examining the Evidence: Does Kilocalorie Restriction Extend Life? explores the possible benefits of intentionally decreasing energy intake.

Though energy needs may be reduced, the need for most nutrients does not decline, and the need for certain nutrients increases. For many seniors it's challenging to get the nutrients they need on a more limited-kilocalorie budget, on a dietary plan designed to manage chronic conditions, or when they have a diminished appetite. Choosing nutrient-dense foods becomes even more important in aging because these foods supply the most nutrition for the lowest number of kilocalories.

Older Adults Need Ample Protein

Protein is essential for reducing the loss of lean tissue and bone mass and for tissue repair, wound healing, and immune function. According to the DRIs, protein requirements (expressed as grams per kilogram of body weight) do not change with age. However, because overall kilocalorie needs decline, individuals must obtain a relatively higher proportion of kilocalories from protein-rich foods. For healthy older people, the RDA is 0.8 grams per kilogram of body weight.[32] Although the role of dietary protein in the prevention of sarcopenia remains unclear, a protein intake greater than that suggested by the DRI may enhance muscle protein anabolism and reduce progressive loss of muscle mass with age. There is debate as to exactly how much protein older adults need, as some nutrition experts recommend protein intake of 1.0–1.6 g/kg daily for healthy older adults.[33]

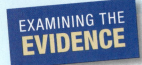

Does Kilocalorie Restriction Extend Life?

In the last several decades, the number of centenarians, or people who have reached the age of 100, has increased around the world. Researchers are actively gathering information about where these people live, how they live, and what they eat to gain a better understanding of the factors that contribute to longevity. Longevity tends to run in families.[1] However, research suggests that lifestyle influences longevity.

Epidemiologists have studied populations with large numbers of centenarians, with the most notable and longest-running study being conducted on the Japanese island of Okinawa, which has the greatest number of centenarians per capita worldwide. The Okinawa Centenarian Study examined over 900 Okinawan centenarians and numerous other adults in their 70s, 80s, and 90s to identify factors associated with their increased lifespan.[2] The findings suggested that genetics and lifestyle habits explain why Okinawans live so long and remain healthy well into their senior years. A lower kilocaloric intake, first reported in Okinawans in 1967, led researchers to hypothesize that kilocaloric restriction could partly explain their longevity. Okinawans have been shown to follow the "less is more"

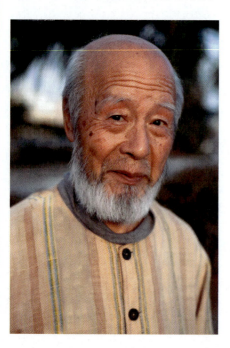

philosophy when it comes to eating, regularly eating only to the point at which they are 80 percent full.[3]

In animal studies, research about consuming significantly fewer kilocalories is mixed. Studies show that a kilocalorie-restricted diet can extend the lives of underfed rats up to 50 percent longer than those of rats given an unlimited supply of food.[4] However, another study on rhesus monkeys showed that those on restricted diets aged as quickly as their counterparts who were not restricted.[5] Human studies on kilocaloric restriction are limited, but recent studies suggest that restricting kilocalories may reduce risk factors for diabetes and cardiovascular disease.[6,7]

How might eating less lead to a longer life? Nobody yet knows exactly how calorie restriction works at the cellular level, but experts hypothesize that it reduces oxidative damage through lower metabolism. Free radicals damage cellular material, including DNA. Damage accumulates with time, accelerating the "aging process."[8]

It's worth noting that kilocalorie restriction is not the sole distinguishing factor in the Okinawan diet. It is also rich in green leafy and yellow root vegetables, sweet potatoes, and soy, and is supplemented with fish. This plant-based diet is high in nutrient-dense carbohydrates and antioxidants and lower in protein than the typical American diet.[9] The health benefits that have been linked to the Okinawan diet and lifestyle are numerous and include decreased mortality from diseases of the heart and cancer as well as increased functional and cognitive capacity at older ages versus Americans.[10]

It's not possible to say whether kilocalorie restriction is the key to a longer life, nor yet what the ideal BMI is for humans.[11] People who are interested in kilocalorie restriction should consult a registered dietitian nutritionist (RDN) to establish a meal plan that meets their health goals. We do know that eating the right number of kilocalories to achieve and maintain a healthy weight on a balanced diet can contribute to a

better quality of life by supporting good health and reducing the risk for chronic disease.

It's also important to consider lifestyle choices other than diet when it comes to longevity. Generally speaking, Okinawans are physically active into their later years, they have low rates of tobacco and alcohol use, a long tradition of caring for one another's welfare, and their lifestyle is less stressful than that of residents of mainland Japan,[12] factors that also contribute to well-being in older adults everywhere.

References

1. Beekman, M., H. Blanché, et al. 2013. Genome-wide linkage analysis for human longevity: Genetics of Healthy Aging Study. *Aging Cell* 12:184–193.
2. Willcox, D.C., B. J. Willcox, et al. 2006. Caloric Restriction and Human Longevity: What Can We Learn from the Okinawans? *Biogerontology* 7:173–177.
3. Ibid.
4. Omodei, D. and L. Fontana. 2011. Calorie Restriction and Prevention of Age-Associated Chronic Disease. *Federation of European Biochemical Societies Letters* 585:1537–1542.
5. Maxmen, A. 2012. Calorie Restriction Falters in the Long Run. *Nature: International Weekly Journal of Science* 488:569.
6. Ortiz-Bautista, R. J., et al. 2013. Caloric Restriction: About Its Positive Metabolic Effects and Cellular Impact [in Spanish]. *Cirugía y Cirujanos* 459–464.
7. Ravussin, E., L. M. Redman, et al. 2015. A 2-Year Randomized Controlled Trial of Human Caloric Restriction: Feasibility and Effects on Predictors of Health Span and Longevity. *Journals of Gerontology. Series A, Biological Sciences and Medical Sciences* 70(9):1097–1104.
8. Ibid.
9. Willcox, D. C. et al. 2006. Caloric Restriction and Human Longevity: What Can We Learn from the Okinawans?
10. Le Couteur, D. G., S. Solon-Biet, et al. 2016. New Horizons: Dietary Protein, Ageing and the Okinawan Ratio. *Age Ageing* 45(4):443–447
11. Willcox, D. C., G. Scapagnini, et al. 2014. Healthy Aging Diets Other Than the Mediterranean: A Focus on the Okinawan Diet. *Mechanisms of Ageing and Development*. 136–137:148–162.
12. Santrock, J. Physical Development and Biological Aging. In M. Ryan, et al., eds., *A Topical Approach to Life-Span Development* (New York: McGraw-Hill, 2008), 129–132.

Carbohydrates Should Be Nutrient Dense and High in Fiber

Older adults are encouraged to consume 45–65 percent of their total daily energy as carbohydrates, which is no change from their younger years. However, because kilocalorie requirements decrease with age, older adults on average need fewer carbohydrates. So, most of the carbohydrates they consume should come from foods that are nutrient dense and high in fiber, such as fruits, vegetables, and whole grains.

Dietary fiber can help to prevent constipation, diverticulosis, and type 2 diabetes. The AI for fiber is 14 grams per 1,000 kilocalories. While fiber intake is related to kilocalorie consumption, generally speaking, women age 51 and older need 21 grams of daily fiber and men of the same age require 30 grams.[34] Research suggests that most adults over the age of 51 do not meet the AI for fiber.[35]

The AMDR for Fat Does Not Change with Age

Fat provides kilocalories, supplies essential fatty acids, and is needed for the absorption of fat-soluble vitamins. Omega-3 fats are heart healthy, and the AHA recommends eating fish at least twice weekly.[36] However, a diet rich in saturated fat, *trans* fats, or both increases the risk for cardiovascular disease. In addition, because fat is kilocalorie-dense, eating too much fat may contribute excess kilocalories and lead to overweight and obesity. Healthy older adults without evidence of heart disease, or unless otherwise advised by their doctor, should aim to meet the AMDR of 20–35 percent of kilocalories from fat, with no more than 7 percent of kilocalories from saturated fat, and should consume as little *trans* fat as possible.[37]

Older Adults Need to Stay Hydrated

Several factors make older people more prone to dehydration: As we age, the body's ability to conserve water is decreased and changes in the central nervous system decrease thirst sensations, which leads to reduced fluid intake.[38] Kidney disease and other chronic conditions, such as uncontrolled diabetes, further increase dehydration risk.[39] Additionally, certain medications commonly prescribed to older adults, such as diuretics, cause their body to lose water. Thus, older adults who don't eat enough watery foods, such as fruits and vegetables, and who don't drink adequate fluid can quickly become mildly or severely dehydrated. Symptoms of dehydration, which include weakness, confusion, and fatigue, should not be dismissed as effects of aging. Constipation is another side effect of dehydration.

Older adults have the same fluid requirements as younger people—13 cups a day, most of it as plain water. *Urinary incontinence* (loss of bladder control) is more common with aging, and older adults often fail to meet their fluid requirements because they wish to avoid frequent trips to the bathroom. The incidence of urinary incontinence also increases with age because of prostate problems in men and weakened pelvic floor muscles in women after pregnancy. Foods such as fruits and vegetables provide fluid and adults of all ages should be encouraged to eat five servings daily. All beverages, including coffee and tea, are considered fluid sources. Drinking water or milk with meals is a productive way to take in adequate fluid.

Older Adults Need the Right Amounts of Vitamins A, D, and B$_{12}$

Though the recommended daily amount of vitamin A doesn't change for those over age 50, there is a concern that, because preformed vitamin A can accumulate to toxic amounts in the body, older adults consuming it in excess of the RDA may develop toxicity (see Chapter 9). When choosing dietary supplements, such as a multivitamin, it's wise

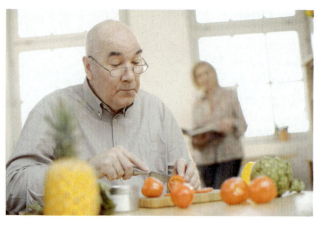

The beta-carotene found in many fruits and vegetables is a good source of vitamin A for seniors, as it won't contribute to vitamin A toxicity.

to choose products with the majority of vitamin A as beta-carotene rather than as retinol. The body will convert beta-carotene, which also acts on its own as an antioxidant, into vitamin A on an as-needed basis.

The skin's ability to use sunlight to initiate vitamin D production declines with age. Furthermore, vitamin D absorption declines and the kidneys lose some ability to convert vitamin D to its active form.[40] For all these reasons, the RDA for dietary vitamin D increases from 600 IU to 800 IU at age 71. Recall that vitamin D's main role is to help the body properly use calcium and phosphorus to strengthen bones and that inadequate amounts of this vitamin can increase the risk of osteoporosis. It's difficult for most older adults to get the recommended 600–800 IU of vitamin D from foods alone. Vitamin D supplements help to fill in gaps in the diet and are especially helpful for those who avoid vitamin D–fortified products, such as milk, soymilk, and some yogurts (review Table 19.1).

The RDA for vitamin B_{12} is the same for younger and older adults; however, because the stomach produces fewer acidic digestive juices as it ages, it's estimated that up to 30 percent of people over the age of 50 do not properly absorb the form of vitamin B_{12} that naturally occurs in foods. They can, however, absorb the synthetic variety found in fortified foods and supplements, and the majority of older people should add these sources.[41] Proper nervous system function requires vitamin B_{12}, and prolonged deficiencies can lead to permanent nerve damage. Vitamin B_{12}, along with adequate amounts of folate and vitamin B_6, may keep levels of homocysteine normal in the bloodstream, helping to reduce the risk for heart disease and stroke.

Older Adults Need the Right Amounts of Iron, Zinc, Calcium, and Sodium

Postmenopausal women, who are typically over age 50, need less dietary iron than they did in their younger years. Specifically, a menstruating woman needs 18 mg/day, whereas an older woman requires only 8 mg/day—the same requirement for an adult male.[42] While older people need only 8 mg/day, they are still at risk of iron deficiency if their diets do not supply adequate amounts of iron. Foods rich in iron, including meat, chicken, and seafood, are good choices for older people because they also supply protein, vitamins, and minerals to support good health. Older people are more prone to chronic conditions that can result in iron-deficiency anemia, such as an ongoing intestinal blood loss from an ulcer, cancer, and liver or kidney disease.[43] Iron deficiency can lead to fatigue, decreased physical activity, and impaired immunity.

Zinc is found in many of the same foods as iron, so if a person is iron deficient, he or she may also be zinc deficient. Zinc is necessary for many bodily functions including immunity, wound healing, and supporting a strong sense of taste and smell. Zinc deficiency may occur from inadequate zinc intake or absorption. Several chronic conditions, including diabetes, chronic liver disease, and chronic kidney disease, are associated with zinc deficiency. Research suggests many elderly people who live in food-insecure households are at risk for inadequate zinc intake.[44]

Calcium needs increase to 1,200 milligrams daily for women over the age of 50, whereas the requirement for men is 1,000 milligrams daily until age 71, when it increases to 1,200 milligrams daily.[45] Calcium absorption decreases by 10–15 percent in adulthood and continues to decrease with age, which is why recommended calcium intakes are higher for females older than 50 years and for both males and females older than 70 years. Surveys of calcium intake among people living in the United States suggest that women age 51–70 years and both men and women older than 70 years fail to consume adequate amounts of calcium from food. However, many people take calcium supplements, which may increase their intake to the recommended levels.[46]

Recall that the body breaks down bone tissue to maintain calcium concentrations in blood, muscle, and intercellular fluids. Thus, calcium must be replenished on a daily basis.[47] Inadequate calcium intake increases the risk for osteoporosis. Experts estimate that, by 2020, that more than half of all Americans over age 50 will have low bone mass or osteoporosis unless we make changes to our diet and lifestyle.[48] Older adults should consume at least three servings of dairy foods daily or the equivalent in calcium-fortified foods. They may need to take a calcium supplement if they don't meet these recommendations.

The 2015–2020 *Dietary Guidelines for Americans* recommends that everyone over the age of 50 limit their sodium intake to 2,300 milligrams a day to reduce their risk of hypertension, which is more common with advancing age. People who have hypertension, or who have diabetes or chronic kidney disease, may need to make further modifications to their sodium intake.[49]

Older Adults May Benefit from Vitamin and Mineral Supplements

As discussed, physiological alterations, medications, and changes in dietary intake patterns increase the risk for nutritional deficiencies with age. In the last decade, older adults have increased their intake of multivitamin-mineral supplements, and an estimated 35% of older adults now take a multivitamin-mineral supplement daily.[50,51]

Despite this frequent use, not all older adults need to take a multivitamin-mineral supplement. There are, however, three micronutrients that older adults may need to take as supplements: vitamin D, calcium, and vitamin B_{12}.[52] Moreover, older adults who take medications that deplete certain nutrients may require a supplement even if their appetite is adequate. For example, proton-pump inhibitors, which reduce stomach acidity, reduce iron absorption and blood levels of magnesium.[53] Therefore, a health care provider may prescribe both iron and magnesium supplements to patients taking proton-pump inhibitors.

Like anyone else, older adults should consult with their health care provider before they use nutritional supplements. They must read labels carefully to avoid exceeding the Tolerable Upper Intake Level for any micronutrient. They should also consult with their pharmacist to see if their supplements interact with any prescription or over-the-counter medication they consume. (Medication–supplement interactions are discussed in more detail shortly.) Using a checklist like the one in **Table 19.2** can help an individual have an effective conversation about nutritional supplements with a health care provider.

TABLE 19.2 Checklist for Talking about Nutritional Supplements
Questions about Nutritional Supplements to Ask a Health Care Provider
Can I obtain the same nutrients in adequate amounts from my diet?
Is taking a nutritional supplement an important part of my total diet, given my current intake?
Are there any precautions or warnings I should know about (e.g., is there an amount or "upper limit" I should not go above)?
Are there any known side effects (such as loss of appetite, nausea, or headaches)? Do they apply to me?
Are there any foods, medicines (prescription or over the counter), or other supplements I should avoid while taking this product?
If I am scheduled for surgery, should I be concerned about the nutritional supplements I am taking?

Source: Adapted from U.S. Food and Drug Administration. 2014. *Tips for Dietary Supplement Users.* Available at http://www.fda.gov/food/dietarysupplements/usingdietarysupplements/ucm110567.htm. Accessed April 2017.

Healthy Eating for Older Adults

Eat a fiber-rich diet by including 2 servings of fruits, 3 servings of vegetables, and 3 servings of whole grains daily.

Drink enough fluid by sipping six to eight (8-ounce) glasses of fluids every day, most of it as water.

Consume three servings of calcium- and vitamin D–rich foods, including fortified fat-free and 1% low-fat milk or soymilk, yogurt, greens, canned salmon with bones, legumes, and tofu processed with calcium sulfate.

Eat protein-rich foods including lean meats, seafood, poultry, eggs, legumes, seeds, nuts, and soy products.

Focus on a plant-based diet—research reveals that a variety of nutrient-dense fruits and vegetables provide antioxidants and phytochemicals that help protect cells against free radicals.

Older Adults Should Eat Right for Good Health and Disease Prevention

The best dietary strategy for aging adults to maintain good health and to prevent chronic diseases is to consume a varied, nutrient- and phytochemical-dense, heart-healthy diet.[54] The Table Tips give some guidelines for healthy eating for older adults.

Like their younger counterparts, many older Americans do not eat according to expert advice, and their diets may be too high in saturated fat, cholesterol, and sodium. Recent evidence suggests that those who consume a diet that adheres to the *Dietary Guidelines for Americans* reduce their risk for all-cause mortality as well as mortality from cancer and cardiovascular disease.[55] As adults age, a registered dietitian nutritionist (RDN) is uniquely equipped to help them adjust the content and/or texture of their diet to their needs without sacrificing diet quality. **Table 19.3** identifies some age-related disorders that a healthy diet may help prevent.

TABLE 19.3 Eating Right to Fight Age-Related Disorders

A varied, plant-based diet that supplies adequate nutrients, fiber, and phytochemicals is the best diet defense against age-related disorders.

Condition/Disease	Disease-Fighting Compounds That May Help to Prevent It
Alzheimer's disease, Parkinson's disease	Antioxidant, vitamins C and E and carotenoids
Anemia	Iron Folate Vitamin B_{12}
Cancer (colon, prostate, breast)	Fiber found in whole grains, fruits, vegetables Phytochemicals (phenols, indoles, lycopene, beta-carotene)
Cataracts, age-related macular degeneration	Vitamins C and E Phytochemicals (lutein and zeaxanthin) Zinc
Constipation, diverticulosis	Fiber Fluid
Heart disease	Vitamins B_6, B_{12}, and folate Omega-3 fatty acids Soluble fiber Phytochemicals in whole grains, fruits, vegetables
Hypertension	Calcium Magnesium Potassium
Impaired immune response	Iron Zinc Vitamin B_6 Protein
Obesity	Fiber as part of a balanced eating plan with the appropriate number of kilocalories to achieve and maintain a healthy weight
Osteoporosis	Calcium Vitamins D and K Protein
Type 2 diabetes	A healthy weight Chromium Fiber

Older adults typically require fewer kilo-calories but not less nutrition than they did when they were younger. Meals and snacks should be nutrient dense to maximize nutrient intake. Protein requirements may increase. Carbohydrates should be nutrient dense and high in fiber, and fat consumption should be moderate. Fruits and vegetables should be emphasized to ensure sufficient intake of antioxidant nutrients and phytochemicals, fluid, and fiber. Some vitamin and mineral consumption, including vitamins A, D, and B_{12} and the minerals iron, zinc, and calcium, should be particularly monitored to ensure adequate intake. Consuming adequate fluid is necessary to prevent dehydration and constipation. As much as possible, older adults should eat right to maintain their health.

What Nutrition-Related Health Concerns Affect Older Adults?

LO 19.4 Discuss key nutrition-related health concerns common among older adults.

Aging is often associated with significant health problems and a diminished quality of life, especially in the very old. Almost 80 percent of older adults have one chronic condition, and half of all older adults have two or more.[56] Dealing with one or more chronic conditions can affect a person's ability to perform activities of daily living, including shopping for food and preparing meals, managing money, and taking medications as prescribed. It can also increase the individual's risk for harmful medication interactions.

Medications, Foods, and Supplements Can Interact in Harmful Ways

We noted earlier that about 35 percent of older adults take a multivitamin-mineral supplement; moreover, almost 36 percent of older Americans take five or more prescription medications daily.[57] When considered together, these statistics help explain the increased risk among older Americans for harmful interactions. Moreover, both dietary supplements and medications can interact harmfully with foods and related metabolites.

Dietary supplements include not only micronutrient supplements, but also herbs and other botanicals, amino acids, enzymes, and animal extracts. Whereas the roles of most vitamins and minerals are well understood, little high-quality research has been done on these other types of supplements. Recall from Chapter 9 that the Food and Drug Administration does not have the authorization to review dietary supplements for safety, efficacy, or effectiveness claims before they come to market; thus, Americans of all ages should consult their health care provider before starting any dietary supplement.[58] **Table 19.4** provides key examples of the potential side effects of various supplements.

Food can also interact with medications in several ways. First, foods can affect the metabolism of drugs. For example, calcium can bind with tetracycline (an antibiotic), decreasing its absorption. For this reason, tetracycline shouldn't be taken with milk or calcium-fortified foods. In contrast, grapefruit juice alters the metabolism of several medications commonly prescribed to older adults. For example, it increases the absorption of statins, drugs used to improve blood lipids, and calcium channel blockers, which are used to treat heart disease. Drugs can also interfere with the metabolism of certain substances in foods. An enzyme called monoamine oxidase metabolizes the compound tyramine, which is abundant in aged cheese, smoked fish, yogurt, and red wine. Certain medications called *monoamine oxidase inhibitors (MAOIs)*, which may be prescribed to treat depression,

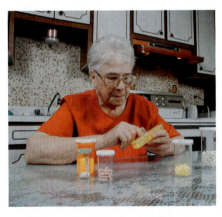

Older individuals who are taking multiple medications must regularly review potential drug interactions with their doctor or pharmacist.

Herb/Nutrient	Purported Use	Potential Side Effects	Drug Interactions
Coenzyme Q-10	Hypertension, diabetes mellitus, congestive heart failure, increased energy levels	Nausea and vomiting, appetite loss	Do not combine with chemotherapy, antihypertensive drugs, and warfarin and red yeast
DHEA	Slow aging process, improve cognition, increase muscle mass, and improve sexual function	High blood pressure, liver problems, lower blood glucose levels	Corticosteroids decrease DHEA production in body; soy may decrease DHEA effectiveness; DHEA may increase effectiveness of insulin
Dong Quai root	Relieve menopausal symptoms, manage hypertension	Excessive bleeding due to blood thinning	Enhances the effectiveness of blood-thinning drugs and aspirin as well as vitamin E, garlic, and ginkgo biloba
Echinacea	Treat upper respiratory conditions, including the common cold	Rash, increased asthma, allergic reactions in sensitive individuals	May decrease effectiveness of immune-suppressing drugs (cyclosporine, corticosteroids)
Evening primrose oil	Reduce eczema, inflammation, menopausal symptoms	Mild stomach and intestinal discomfort; headaches	May increase bleeding in people also taking blood thinners
Garlic, garlic supplements	Lower blood cholesterol levels, reduce heart disease risk, lower blood pressure	Possible stomach and intestinal discomfort, bad breath	Increases the blood-thinning actions of aspirin and prescription blood thinners and supplements such as vitamin E and ginkgo biloba
Ginkgo	Reduce memory loss, treat or prevent dementia	Possible stomach and intestinal discomfort, headache	Increases the risk of bleeding and should not be combined with aspirin or prescription blood thinners; enhances the blood-thinning actions of vitamin E and garlic
Ginseng, American	Reduce fatigue and stress, boost immune system, general stimulant	May lower blood glucose levels, insomnia	Enhances the action of medications to lower blood glucose levels; promotes blood thinning, so do not take with prescription blood thinners, aspirin, or vitamin E
Hawthorn	Hypertension, congestive heart failure	Upset stomach, dizziness, headache	May not be combined with certain heart medications
Kava	Reduce anxiety, stress, insomnia	Possible severe liver damage, drowsiness, scaly yellow skin in long-term use	The FDA has issued a warning that kava supplements increase liver damage; do not combine with drugs used for Parkinson's disease
St. John's wort	Reduce depression, anxiety, fatigue, menopausal symptoms	Insomnia, vivid dreams, restlessness, dizziness, headache, severe reactions to sun exposure	Interacts with several medications; may decrease effectiveness of anti-anxiety drugs, heart medications, and antidepressants

Sources: U.S. Food and Drug Administration. 2014. *Tips for Older Dietary Supplement Users.* Available at https://www.fda.gov/Food/DietarySupplements/UsingDietarySupplements/ucm110493.htm. Accessed April 2017; National Institutes of Health, Office of Dietary Supplements. 2016. *Calcium.* Available at www.ods.od.nih.gov/factsheets/Calcium-HealthProfessional/#h10. Accessed April 2017; U.S. National Library of Medicine. National Institutes of Health. 2017. *Herbs and Supplements.* Available at www.nlm.nih.gov/medlineplus/druginfo/herb_All.html. Accessed April 2017.

prevent tyramine from being properly metabolized. High levels of tyramine in the blood can result in dangerously high blood pressure.[59]

Decreased Mobility Affects Many Older Adults

About 36 percent of people age 65 and older in the United States report living with a disability, including vision and hearing impairments, chronic respiratory distress, and decreased mobility, such as difficulty carrying groceries, reaching overhead, climbing stairs, and rising from a chair. Living alone increases disability risk, and the risk increases further when that person living alone has no children or siblings nearby, a condition that is more common among those 85 years and older.[60]

The decline in mobility seen in some older adults can be attributed to sarcopenia. However, the more common causes are **arthritis** (*arthr* = joint, *itis* = inflammation), back or spine disorders, and heart problems, in that order.[61] Osteoporosis can also affect mobility in aging adults.

Arthritis can cause pain, stiffness, and swelling in joints, muscles, tendons, ligaments, and bones. Getting out of bed, trying to open a jar, or climbing stairs can be challenging for those with arthritis. Of the more than 100 types of arthritis, osteoarthritis, rheumatoid arthritis, and gout are the most common in older adults.

Osteoarthritis

Nearly half of Americans aged 65 and older report having received a diagnosis of osteoarthritis.[62] The disorder develops when the cartilage, which covers the ends of the bones at the joints, wears down, causing the bones to rub together. Repeated friction in the joint causes swelling, loss of motion, and pain. Osteoarthritis commonly occurs in the fingers, neck, lower back, knees, and hips (see **Figure 19.4**). Exercises that increase flexibility, keep joints limber, and improve the range of motion can help people with osteoarthritis stay mobile. Losing excess weight also helps relieve some of the stress at the weight-bearing hip and knee joints.[63]

Many older adults turn to the dietary supplements glucosamine and chondroitin sulfate, which are naturally found in cartilage, to reduce their symptoms of osteoarthritis. However, the research on these supplements is inconclusive. Some evidence supports their efficacy, particularly with high pain levels in the back and knee, but an equal amount of evidence suggests that they provide no improvement over a placebo.[64,65] Individuals with osteoarthritis should speak with their health care provider before using these supplements.

Rheumatoid Arthritis

Rheumatoid arthritis (RA), which occurs in at least 1.3 million U.S. adults, is an inflammatory disease of the joints that causes pain, swelling, and deformity.[66] The typical Western diet, which is high in fat, protein, sugar, salt, and energy-dense processed or convenience foods, may heighten the symptoms of RA.[67] Research suggests a link between diet and inflammation, and eating fish and foods rich in antioxidants may help ease the inflammation characteristic of RA. Fish supply omega-3 fatty acids, which play a role in modifying inflammation and pain; therefore, people with RA who don't eat fish at least twice weekly should consult with their health care provider about taking omega-3 supplements. Other potential anti-inflammatory foods include foods rich in the antioxidant vitamins C and E and the flavonoid group of phytochemicals, cooked vegetables, and olive oil.[68,69]

Routine physical activity can help those who suffer from RA. Swimming, aquatic exercises, and walking can all help reduce joint pain and stiffness, increase range of motion, build muscle, and increase flexibility.

Gout

Crystallization of excess uric acid within joints and soft tissues causes **gout**, an inflammatory arthritis. For many people, gout initially occurs as pain and swelling in the joints of the big toe. The needlelike uric acid crystals can also affect the insteps, ankles, heels, knees, wrists, fingers, and elbows.[70]

Gout is a growing health problem among older adults. Doctors may have difficulty diagnosing it because the symptoms can be vague, and gout often mimics other conditions.[71] An estimated 3 percent of American adults have gout; however, an additional 21 percent of Americans have hyperuricemia (elevated uric acid levels), a risk factor for

▲ **Figure 19.4 Effects of Osteoarthritis**
Osteoarthritis can affect any joint. When multiple hand joints become affected, pain, swelling, and stiffness make routine tasks difficult to accomplish. Studies show that people who actively manage their osteoarthritis have less pain and function better.

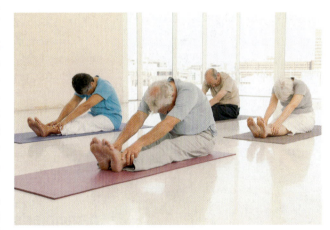

Routine physical activity can help with arthritis by building muscles and increasing flexibility.

arthritis Inflammation in the joints that can cause pain, stiffness, and swelling.

gout Disease in which high levels of uric acid build up in the blood and cause inflammation in the joints. Chronic gout causes episodes of acute arthritis pain, especially in the feet.

gout.[72,73] Other risk factors include obesity, hypertension, diabetes, kidney disease, excessive alcohol intake, and a family history of gout.[74] Consumption of sugar-sweetened soft drinks and meat is also associated with hyperuricemia and gout.[75] Managing gout means controlling weight; limiting purine-rich foods, such as meat, poultry, and fish; cutting back on saturated fat; limiting or avoiding alcohol, especially beer; limiting or avoiding foods with high-fructose corn syrup; eating more whole grains and fewer refined grains; choosing low-fat or fat-free dairy products; and drinking 8–16 glasses of fluid daily, mostly as water.[76] People with gout should consult with an RDN.

Osteoporosis

The bone disease osteoporosis was discussed in the Health Connection in Chapter 12. Recall that osteoporosis leads to thinning and hardening of the vertebrae, which reduce height and spine flexibility, making bending, reaching, and walking difficult.[77] Moreover, older adults who suffer falls and fractures can have limited mobility, as they have to walk with a walker for assistance or are confined to a wheelchair, making living independently and cooking and preparing healthy meals difficult. There is no cure for osteoporosis, but medications and a balanced diet, dietary supplements as necessary, and regular weight-bearing exercise can slow bone loss.

Eye Disease Is a Concern for Many Older Adults

Vision disorders are prevalent in older age. As described in Chapter 9, age-related macular degeneration (AMD) is the most common cause of blindness in older Americans. AMD results from oxidative damage to the macula, the area of the retina that distinguishes fine detail. It is the leading cause of blindness in older adults, with a two-fold increase in prevalence expected in the United States by 2020.[78] A combination of antioxidant vitamins C and E, zinc, and beta-carotene has been shown to slow the progression of AMD.[79] Moreover, consumption of the phytochemicals lutein and zeaxanthin, carotenoids found primarily in broccoli, corn, squash, and dark green, leafy vegetables such as spinach and kale, may also reduce the risk for AMD.[80,81]

Cataracts, cloudy spots on the lens of the eye, also cause loss of vision. The lens is made mostly of water and protein, which is arranged in a way that allows light to pass through. As a person ages, some of the protein may clump together and form a cataract, reducing the sharpness of the image reaching the retina.[82] Cataracts develop in more than half of all Americans by age 80.[83] A family history increases the risk, as do diabetes, excessive alcohol intake, hypertension, obesity, and smoking.[84] Research associates a diet rich in antioxidants as well as B-vitamins with reduced risk for cataracts. Accordingly, eating more green, leafy vegetables and fruits such as blueberries, cherries, and raspberries, as well as whole grains, may help reduce the risk.[85]

Alzheimer's Disease Is a Progressive, Irreversible Form of Dementia

Although cognitive changes, such as taking longer to learn new information, are a normal part of aging, more serious mental declines may be indicative of disease. **Dementia** is a group of symptoms that affect memory, thinking, and social function to the point that they interfere with daily functioning. Dementia is often characterized by memory loss, though the two are not synonymous.[86] **Alzheimer's disease** is the most common cause of progressive dementia. This irreversible disease slowly damages the brain tissues and can progress over the years to severe brain damage. An estimated 5 million Americans have Alzheimer's disease, with most showing signs of the condition in their 60s.[87]

Research, including through postmortem studies, indicates that Alzheimer's disease develops when plaques made of "sticky" amyloid proteins and tangles of a fibrous

dementia Disorder of the brain that interferes with a person's memory, learning, and mental stability.

Alzheimer's disease Progressive and irreversible type of dementia characterized by distinct changes in brain tissue.

protein called tau disrupt connections between nerve cells and cause nerve cell death and tissue loss throughout the brain. The brain shrinks and is less able to function. It appears likely that the toxic changes begin to damage the brain a decade or more before symptoms appear.[88] Whereas there appears to be a genetic component to Alzheimer's disease, chronic diseases and lifestyle choices may play a role. Physical and mental inactivity, smoking, obesity, diabetes, hypertension, and depression are linked to the development of Alzheimer's disease.[89] Evidence from a recent randomized controlled trial suggests that a multicomponent intervention including diet, exercise, and cognitive training may be effective in maintaining or improving cognition in older adults.[90]

Generally speaking, a lifestyle that supports heart health also supports brain health. A balanced diet with the recommended amounts of fruits, vegetables, and whole grains, as well as lean-protein foods and low-fat dairy, helps to prevent atherosclerosis in arteries that feed the heart and brain and provide the nutrients to support tissue health. Recently, a large trial studying the effect of the MIND diet, a hybrid of the Mediterranean and DASH diets, showed that adherence to the diet was associated with a reduced risk for Alzheimer's disease.[91]

Older adults with dementia may experience mental deterioration, but they should be encouraged to stay active as long as possible to prevent physical deterioration. Accompanying an elder on a walk or jog is a great way for two people to get some exercise.

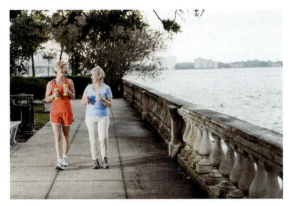

Accompanying an elder during a walk is a great way for two people to get some exercise and boost their physical and mental health.

LO 19.4: THE TAKE-HOME MESSAGE Older adults face various health concerns that can have an impact on nutrition needs or that can be affected by nutrition. Dietary supplements and medications can interact harmfully with each other or with foods and related metabolites. Decreased mobility is common in older age and is frequently due to osteoarthritis, rheumatoid arthritis, gout, or osteoporosis. Vision disorders, including macular degeneration and cataracts, are also common. Risk of developing eye disease may be reduced by a diet that includes foods rich in antioxidant nutrients and phytochemicals. Alzheimer's disease and other forms of dementia affect some older adults. Some evidence indicates that the MIND diet, a hybrid of the Mediterranean and DASH diets, may help reduce the risk of Alzheimer's disease.

What Socioeconomic and Psychological Issues Affect the Nutrition of Older Adults?

LO 19.5 Describe several social, economic, and psychological factors that commonly affect the health of older Americans.

In addition to physical ailments, as older adults retire and lose loved ones, they may have to deal with various social, psychological, and financial issues, any of which can affect their nutritional health.

Food Insecurity Has Nutritional Impacts

In 2014, 4.5 million Americans age 65 and older lived in poverty (defined as at or below $15,730 for a household of two or $11,170 for a person living alone).[92] Women and racial and ethnic minorities are more likely to experience poverty than white males.[93] In light of these numbers, it's not surprising that, in 2015, 8.1 percent of American households with elders experienced **food insecurity**, or limited or uncertain access to sufficient food to reliably feed those living there.[94]

Limited finances aren't always the cause of food insecurity. Some elders may be able to afford food but because of disability are unable to obtain it, prepare it, or eat it.[95] Whatever the reason, food-insecure older adults run the risk of lower intakes for kilocalories and essential nutrients and are more likely to be in poor or fair rather than good health.

Participation by older adults in food assistance programs can improve nutritional status and quality of life and in turn reduce health care expenses. To help community advocates identify older adults at risk for food insecurity, the American Academy of Family Physicians and other organizations created the Nutrition Screening Initiative (NSI). The NSI is designed to promote routine screening of older persons in both community and institutional settings through a network of clinical and public health RDNs, community workers, and physicians (see the Self-Assessment).[96]

Self-Assessment

DETERMINE Your Nutritional Health

The DETERMINE checklist was developed by the American Academy of Family Physicians, the National Council on Aging, and other partners as part of the Nutrition Screening Initiative. It is a tool that can be used with older adults to assess their risk for poor nutritional status or malnutrition or to understand how their risk changes over time. To complete the questionnaire, circle the number in the right-hand column for the statements that apply to you (or someone you know, if you are taking the assessment for a friend or relative).

YES

I have an illness or condition that has made me change the kind and/or amount of food I eat.	2
I eat fewer than two meals per day.	3
I eat few fruits or vegetables or milk products.	2
I have three or more drinks of beer, liquor, or wine almost every day.	2
I have tooth or mouth problems that make it hard for me to eat.	2
I don't always have enough money to buy food.	4
I eat alone most of the time.	1
I take three or more different prescribed or over-the-counter drugs a day.	1
Without wanting to, I have lost or gained 10 pounds in the last 6 months.	2
I am not always physically able to shop, cook, and/or feed myself.	2
Total	____

Once the checklist is completed, add up the circled number to calculate the score. Individuals who score a 6 or higher on the DETERMINE checklist are at "high nutritional risk." They should bring the checklist with them to their next appointment with a physician, RDN, or social worker to identify available social services and to review any existing problems. A score of 3–5 indicates "moderate nutritional risk." Individuals who are at moderate nutritional risk should determine what changes they can make to their diet and/or lifestyle to improve their status and repeat the checklist in 3 months.

Source: The Nutrition Screening Initiative. The DETERMINE Checklist. Available from http://nutritionandaging.org/wp-content/uploads/2017/01/DetermineNutritionChecklist.pdf. Accessed April 2017.

food insecurity Limited or uncertain access to adequate food within a household.

Community Resources Exist for Older Adults

Government-supported food assistance programs that are available to the larger population, such as food stamps, also serve older adults; however, there are also federally funded food assistance programs specifically for older adults. These programs are funded under the 1965 Older Americans Act, the goal of which is to provide support and services to help individuals age 60 and older maintain good health, an adequate quality of life, and an acceptable level of independence.[97] The Act brought federal support to **Meals on Wheels**, making it one of the most significant volunteer programs in the country. A large assessment study of Meals on Wheels found that, compared to those on the waiting list, daily participants reported improvements in mental health, anxiety, self-rated health, and feelings of isolation and loneliness as well as reductions in falls.[98]

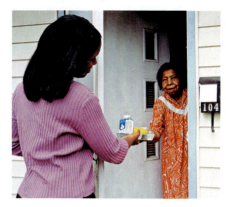

Programs such as Meals on Wheels provide hot meals to older adults who cannot leave their home.

In addition to Meals on Wheels, the Older Americans Act funds the Elderly Nutrition Program (ENP), which provides **congregate meals**—hot meals served at specified sites in the community, such as churches, synagogues, and senior centers. This guarantees that older adults receive a nutritious daily meal and provides an opportunity for them to socialize. Often, transportation to these meals is also available. The program brings consistency and quality to senior center programs.

Young people in the community can help make sure that older adults are familiar with and take advantage of the numerous services available to them. Consider "adopting" a senior neighbor or family member and, if necessary, help him or her locate these services.

Depression and Alcohol Abuse Can Affect Nutritional Health

Whereas many seniors live happy, fulfilled lives, some struggle with grief, isolation, loneliness, and a reduced sense of self-worth as they lose family or friends, retire, learn to live alone, or adjust to living with their grown children or in an assisted-living facility. These seniors are at increased risk for depression and alcohol abuse.

Depression

Depression affects 1–5 percent of older Americans living in the community.[99] The loss of friends and loved ones, as well as chronic pain and concerns about their own health, can add to feelings of grief, sadness, and isolation. Depression can interfere with an older adult's motivation to eat, be physically active, and socialize—all of which can reduce mental and physical health.

Depression in the elderly, especially the very old, may be difficult to detect. Characteristic symptoms such as fatigue, appetite loss, and trouble sleeping can be part of the aging process or a physical illness, so depression may be confused with other conditions common to older adults. Family and friends should be aware of the changes in elders' eating and lifestyle habits, and help them seek treatment for depression, if necessary. Younger adults need to help elders reconnect with their communities after a loss and adjust to a new lifestyle. As mentioned, neighbors can "adopt an elder" who may be living alone and coordinate regular visits and delivery of meals. A quick visit by several supportive friends over the course of a month can go a long way to help seniors stay healthy.

Alcohol Abuse

Chronic health problems, loss of friends and loved ones, or financial stress can make alcohol an appealing sedative to temporarily ease discomfort or depression. Yet heavy drinking can exacerbate depression, which can lead to more drinking.[100] Also, because alcohol impairs judgment and interferes with coordination and reaction time, older adults who have been drinking are at a higher risk for stumbling, falling, and fracturing bones.

Meals on Wheels Program that delivers nutritious meals to homebound older adults.

congregate meals Low- or no-cost meals served at churches, synagogues, or other community sites where older adults can receive a nutritious meal and socialize.

With age, adults become more sensitive to alcohol, in part because of a decline in body water. Individuals with a lower percentage of body water will have a higher blood alcohol concentration (BAC) and thus feel its effects sooner. In addition, many adults over age 65 take several medications daily, and numerous medications can be harmful if mixed with alcohol.[101] Moreover, alcohol intake is associated with a poorer diet quality, putting older adults at greater risk for micronutrient deficiencies and related comorbidities.

Health care providers and family members may not recognize alcohol abuse in older adults, mistaking it for the forgetfulness and disorientation of "normal aging."[102] The National Institute on Alcohol Abuse and Alcoholism recommends that those over age 65 who are healthy and do not take medications should limit alcohol consumption to seven drinks a week and no more than three drinks on a given day. People with health problems or who take certain medications may need to drink less or not at all.[103]

> **LO 19.5: THE TAKE-HOME MESSAGE** In 2015, 8.1 percent of American households with elders experienced food insecurity. Depression, social isolation, and other emotional and psychological conditions can impair the abilities of older adults to maintain healthy diets and lifestyles. Alcohol can reduce an older adult's nutritional health and interfere with the actions of prescription drugs. Many community resources exist to help elders cope with their life challenges. The Older Americans Act has been particularly effective at providing nutritional support to seniors.

HEALTHCONNECTION

Why Are Older Adults at Increased Risk for Hypertension?

LO 19.6 Identify the age-related risk factors for hypertension and the dietary interventions that help control it.

Blood pressure is a measure of the force that blood exerts against the walls of arteries. It is highest at the moment of the heartbeat (measured as **systolic**

systolic pressure Top number in a blood pressure reading that measures the pressure in the arteries when the heart muscle contracts.

diastolic pressure Bottom number in a blood pressure reading that measures the minimal arterial pressure during relaxation of the heart muscle when the ventricles fill with blood.

pressure) and lower when the heart is at rest between beats (measured as **diastolic pressure**). As discussed in Chapter 5, an individual's blood pressure is expressed as a reading of systolic over diastolic pressure. A blood pressure reading of less than 120/80 mm Hg (millimeters of mercury) is considered normal. A blood pressure that is consistently at or above 140/90 mm Hg is called *hypertension (HTN)*. Among Americans age 65 and older, 64 percent of men and 69 percent of women have HTN.[104]

Hypertension Develops Over Time

Although the condition can exist for decades without producing obvious symptoms, HTN is a serious disorder that increases the risk for a heart attack, sudden cardiac arrest, stroke, kidney failure, and peripheral artery disease.[105] Moreover, individuals with chronic HTN may develop an enlarged and weakened heart because it has to work harder to pump blood throughout the body. This can lead to fatigue, shortness of breath, and heart failure.[106] For these reasons, HTN is often referred to as the "silent killer." The only way to be sure that blood pressure levels are within normal range is to have regular blood pressure screenings.

In most cases, HTN develops over time. The first stage, prehypertension, occurs as blood pressure begins to rise above normal—that is, systolic blood pressure measures between 120 and 139 mm Hg or the diastolic reading reaches 80–89 mm Hg.[107] Untreated prehypertension can advance to Stage 1 hypertension, which is characterized by a systolic pressure between 140 and 159 mm Hg or a diastolic pressure of 90–99 mm Hg. The most severe hypertension is Stage 2,

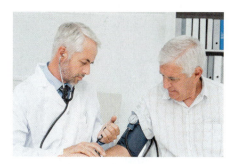

Having your blood pressure checked regularly is the only way to make sure you aren't developing hypertension.

which occurs when the systolic pressure is consistently 160 mm Hg or higher or the diastolic pressure is 100 mm Hg or higher. Both numbers are important, but after age 50 the most common form of hypertension is characterized by a high systolic blood pressure and a normal diastolic pressure.[108] **Table 19.5** summarizes the classifications of blood pressure.

As a group, older adults have a higher rate of HTN than younger adults.[109] Generally speaking, most people experience a moderate rise in blood pressure as they age for a variety of reasons, including that arteries, such as the aorta, become thicker and less flexible.[110] This stiffening of arterial walls is further complicated by atherosclerosis and inflammation, two common conditions associated with aging.

Some Risk Factors for Hypertension Are Not Controllable

Among the factors affecting the risk of developing HTN, age, gender, race/ethnicity, and family history are not controllable. Before age 55, men have a greater

prevalence of HTN, whereas women are more likely to develop the condition after menopause.[111] Also, HTN is more prevalent and tends to occur earlier in life and be more severe in African Americans.[112] People with a family history of HTN are also at increased risk.

Many Risk Factors for Hypertension Are Within Your Control

The good news is that many risk factors for HTN are controllable, including diet, alcohol intake, smoking, body weight, and level of physical activity.

Diet

Recall from Chapter 12 that the DASH diet, which is relatively low in sodium and rich in potassium and other nutrients, has been proven to help control blood pressure.[113] It emphasizes fruits, legumes and other vegetables, and low-fat dairy foods and includes whole grains, fish, poultry, nuts, and seeds, while limiting sodium, sugar, and red meat. You can find the DASH eating plan online at *www.nhlbi.nih.gov*.

The DASH diet is based on research studies sponsored by the National Heart, Lung, and Blood Institute (NHLBI). The initial DASH study found that subjects who followed the eating plan experienced a significant reduction in blood pressure compared with those who followed two other diets. Because all three diets in the study contained approximately 3,000 milligrams of sodium per day, researchers were unable to attribute the lowered blood pressure experienced by the DASH dieters

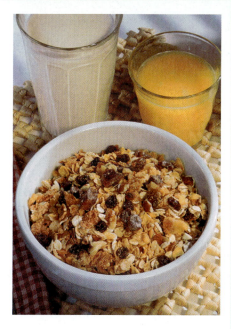

to a reduction in sodium intake. Rather, the researchers concluded that the blood pressure–lowering effect of the DASH diet was due to its abundance of fruits and vegetables, which provide healthy doses of potassium and magnesium, and because of its numerous servings of dairy foods, which are rich in calcium. The study concluded that dietary potassium, magnesium, and calcium could all play a role in lowering blood pressure.[114]

A follow-up to the DASH study, called the DASH-Sodium study, investigated whether reducing the amount of dietary sodium in each of the three diets could also help lower blood pressure. Not surprisingly, it did. While the result of this study showed that reducing dietary sodium from about 3,300 milligrams to 2,400 milligrams daily lowered blood pressure, the biggest blood pressure reduction occurred when sodium intake was limited to 1,500 milligrams daily.[115]

The DASH studies reinforced our understanding of sodium's role in blood pressure and showed that a largely plant-based diet with lean sources of protein significantly reduces HTN. The authors of the Optimal Macronutrient Intake Trial to Prevent Heart Disease (OMNIHeart Trial) compared the effects on blood pressure of

TABLE 19.5	Classification of Blood Pressure	
Category	Systolic Blood Pressure, mmHg	Diastolic Blood Pressure, mmHg
Normal	< 120 and	< 80
Prehypertension	120–139 or	80–89
Hypertension, Stage 1	140–159 or	90–99
Hypertension, Stage 2	≥ 160 or	≥ 100

Source: National Institute on Aging. 2016. *Health and Aging: High Blood Pressure.* Available at https://www.nia.nih.gov/health/publication/high-blood-pressure. Accessed April 2017.

substituting protein (about half as plant protein) or unsaturated fat (mostly monounsaturated) for some of the carbohydrate in healthy diets such as DASH. The results suggest that replacing 10 percent of kilocalories from carbohydrate with either protein or monounsaturated fat in isocaloric diets reduced systolic blood pressure by an additional 1.4 mm Hg over the DASH diet.[116] The researchers concluded that all three diets (the DASH diet, as well as the higher-protein eating plan and higher monounsaturated fat versions in the OMNI diet) lowered blood pressure and thus cardiovascular disease risk.

Alcohol Consumption and Smoking

Chronic heavy alcohol consumption can significantly increase blood pressure. Older people who drink should do so in moderation, especially if they have HTN. The American Heart Association recommends that men limit alcohol to no more than two drinks daily and women to one drink daily or less.[117]

Although the relationship between smoking and HTN is not entirely clear, both smoking and exposure to second-hand smoke are known to increase the risk of atherosclerosis.[118] As you learned in Chapter 5, chronic high blood pressure thickens and stiffens the arteries and may injure arterial walls and accelerate plaque buildup. Atherosclerosis in turn is a key risk factor for heart disease and stroke.

Body Weight

Achieving and maintaining a healthy body weight can also markedly reduce the risk for HTN. When you're overweight, your heart works harder to pump blood. Losing as few as 10 pounds can reduce blood pressure and/or prevent hypertension in many people with a body mass index of 25 or higher.[119]

Physical Activity

Regular physical activity—at least 30–60 minutes on most days of the week—can lower blood pressure by 4–9 millimeters of mercury (mm Hg). People with prehypertension can avoid developing HTN and bring their blood pressure down to safer levels with regular exercise.[120]

The research on HTN is clear: Diet and lifestyle changes help reduce blood pressure. Table 19.6 summarizes the steps that anyone of any age can take to reduce their risk of developing hypertension. See the Nutrition in Practice for an example of how these strategies can help an older adult with HTN.

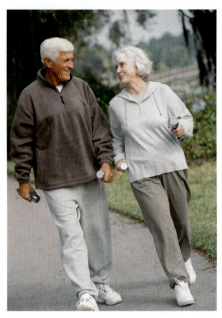

Regular physical activity can help older adults keep their blood pressure under control.

TABLE 19.6	Take Charge of Your Blood Pressure!	
If You	**By**	**Your Systolic Blood Pressure* May Be Reduced by**
Reduce your sodium intake	Limiting dietary sodium consumption to no more than 2,400 mg daily	2–8 mm Hg
Follow the DASH diet	Consuming a heart-healthy diet that is abundant in fruits, vegetables, and low-fat dairy products; 58% carbohydrate, 15% protein, and 27% fat	8–14 mm Hg
Achieve and maintain a healthy body weight	Consuming the right number of kilocalories that allows you to maintain a normal, healthy BMI	5–20 mm Hg for every 22 lbs of weight loss
Stay physically active	Participating in aerobic exercise (such as brisk walking) 30 minutes per day most days of the week	4–9 mm Hg
Drink alcohol only in moderation	Limiting consumption to no more than two drinks daily for men and one drink daily for women	2–4 mm Hg

*Controlling the systolic pressure is more difficult than controlling the diastolic pressure, especially for individuals 50 years of age and older. Therefore, lowering systolic pressure is the primary focus for lowering blood pressure. Typically, as systolic pressure goes down with diet and lifestyle changes, the diastolic pressure does, too.
Source: Data from A. V. Chobanian, et al. 2003. The Seventh Report of the Joint National Committee on Prevention, Detection, Evaluation, and Treatment of High Blood Pressure. *Journal of the American Medical Association* 289:2560–2572.

NUTRITION *in* PRACTICE:
Occupational Therapist

Craig and his wife have been married for more than 40 years and live in their original home in the suburbs of Chicago. At age 72, Craig experienced a stroke and was hospitalized. Luckily, the stroke was considered mild, but he lost some movement in his left arm and hand. Craig's wife mentioned to the doctor that she was concerned that he would not be able to feed himself or perform other activities of daily living once he was discharged from the hospital. The doctor asked for an occupational therapist (OT) consult to assess Craig's condition.

Because Craig has hypertension, a registered dietitian nutritionist (RDN) was also consulted to assess his diet. Craig admitted to the RDN that he is a meat and potatoes eater and doesn't care much for fruits or vegetables, other than mashed potatoes. He also admits that he has a "salt tooth" and shakes salt on almost everything he eats.

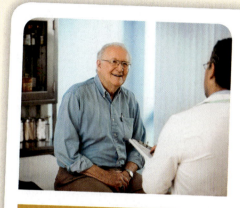

Craig

CRAIG'S FOOD LOG

Food/Beverage	Time Consumed	Hunger Rating*	Location
Scrambled eggs, bacon, and white toast	6:00 A.M.	4	In the kitchen
Ham and cheese sandwich, chips, and lemonade	12:00 P.M.	5	In the kitchen
Pretzel, lemonade	3:00 P.M.	2	Reading the newspaper on the porch
Grilled steak, mashed potatoes, lemonade	6:30 P.M.	3	In kitchen with wife

* Hunger Rating (1–5): 1 = not hungry; 5 = super hungry

Craig's Stats
- Age: 72
- Height: 5 feet 11 inches
- Weight: 210 pounds
- BMI: 29.3
- Blood Pressure: 150/90 mm Hg

Critical Thinking Questions
1. How does Craig's BMI influence his health?
2. What foods are missing from his diet that may help him lower his blood pressure?
3. What dietary changes can the RDN suggest to lower the sodium in this diet?

Occupational Therapist's Observation and Plan for Craig
- Ask if Craig is left-hand dominant.
- Evaluate Craig's ability to perform everyday living activities, such as feeding himself. Based on her observation, recommend that he use adapted utensils that have built-up handles to make dining easier.
- Instruct Craig and his wife on how to use these adapted utensils.

RDN's Observation and Plan for Craig
- Discuss the role of weight loss in helping Craig lower his blood pressure. Craig's BMI is 29.3, which means that he is not only overweight, but also close to being categorized as obese. Suggest that diet lemonade be substituted for regular lemonade.
- Explain that consuming adequate amounts of dietary potassium can help lower his blood pressure. Craig's diet is low in potassium-rich foods, such as fruits, vegetables, and dairy. Suggest adding a fruit or vegetable to every meal and a yogurt snack during the day.
- Increase amount of dairy in Craig's diet, such as whole-grain cereal with milk and fruit for breakfast. Decrease the amount of sodium-laden foods consumed daily by swapping the chips and pretzels for unsalted popcorn and low-sodium ham for deli ham at lunch.

❏ Recommend that Craig make an appointment in the outpatient nutrition clinic a month after his discharge to assess how Craig's diet is progressing.

The OT discusses Craig's limitations with the MD. The MD recommends nursing and OT home health care once Craig is discharged from the hospital. The OT will conduct a home assessment once Craig is discharged to make recommendations for any modifications to help him be as independent as possible in his activities of daily living.

A month later, Craig and his wife visit the RDN in the outpatient clinic.

He is trying to add more fruits and vegetables to his meals and snacks, and he has lost 2 pounds. He complains that his meals taste bland without shaking on some salt. The RDN recommends a no-salt seasoning blend that Craig can use to add some flavor to his meals.

LO 19.6: THE TAKE-HOME MESSAGE The risk for hypertension increases with age. Older Americans should attempt to prevent and control hypertension to reduce the risk for heart attack and stroke. Some risk factors for hypertension, including obesity, alcohol intake, diet, and physical activity, are under personal control. The DASH diet, a plant-based eating plan with lean sources of protein, has been proven to reduce blood pressure.

Visual Chapter Summary

LO 19.1 America Is Aging

Improved health care, public health initiatives, and widespread access to health information have helped lead to a longer life expectancy for Americans. The average life expectancy for men in the United States is 76 years and for women, 81 years. By 2060, the number of Americans aged 65 and older is projected to be 98 million. While heart disease and cancer remain the leading causes of death in older Americans, people are living longer and better lives, in large part because of better medical care. Despite these advances, poor nutrition and a sedentary lifestyle are increasing older Americans' risk for chronic disease and premature death.

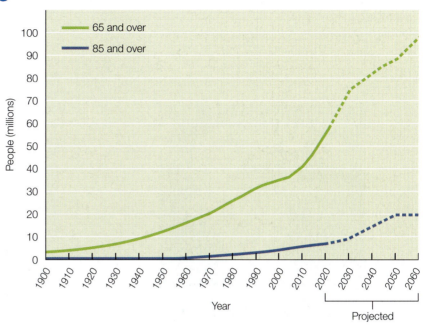

LO 19.2 Age-Related Changes Can Affect Nutrition

The majority of age-related changes are gradual and accumulate over time. Physiological effects of aging include changes in body composition, including reduced muscle mass (sarcopenia) and increased body fat; a decrease in immune function; declining sensory abilities; gastrointestinal changes such as slower digestion; and changes in brain function. These changes can have a negative influence on the desire to eat and on the body's ability to extract nutrients from food.

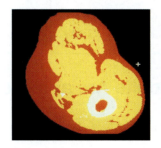

Young adult's thigh   Older adult's thigh

LO 19.3 The Nutrient Needs of Older Adults Reflect Their Changing Metabolism

Metabolism slows with age, so older adults need fewer kilocalories than their younger counterparts. Older adults should ensure that they get an adequate intake of high-quality lean protein, complex carbohydrates, and unsaturated fat, and that they consume enough fluid, vitamins D and B_{12}, and the minerals iron, calcium, and zinc, and decrease sodium intake. Vitamin D requirements increase from 600 IU to 800 IU at age 71.

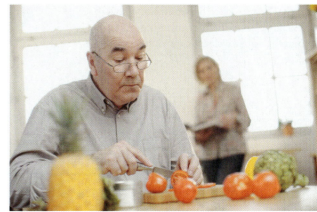

LO 19.4 Older Adults Have a Variety of Nutrition-Related Health Concerns

About 36 percent of people age 65 and older in the United States report living with a disability, such as trouble with mobility, vision, or hearing. Nearly half of Americans age 65 and older report having been diagnosed with arthritis; others are affected by rheumatoid arthritis and gout, which is on the rise. Other nutrition-related health issues include osteoporosis, eye problems such as macular degeneration and cataracts, and dementia, including Alzheimer's disease.

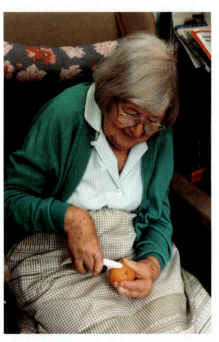

LO 19.5 Socioeconomic and Psychological Issues Affect the Nutrition of Older Adults

Older adults sometimes suffer from food insecurity because of financial hardship or physical disabilities. Federal food assistance programs specifically for older adults are funded under the 1965 Older Americans Act to provide support and services to individuals age 60 and older. Loss of loved ones coupled with social isolation can lead to depression and grief in older adults. This may lead to a decreased motivation to eat as well as an increased reliance on alcohol.

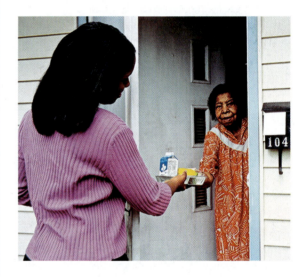

LO 19.6 Older Adults Are at Increased Risk for Hypertension

Hypertension is characterized by a systolic pressure at or above 140 mm Hg or a diastolic pressure at or above 90 mm Hg. Age increases the risk for hypertension, but several positive lifestyle choices, including eating a balanced diet, limiting alcohol intake, and achieving and maintaining a healthy weight, help to keep blood pressure within normal range. The DASH diet is a plant-based diet with lean sources of protein that helps reduce hypertension. Staying physically active can help lower the risk of hypertension, as well as many other chronic conditions.

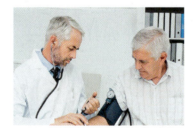

Terms to Know

- aging
- senescence
- lifespan
- life expectancy
- longevity
- physiologic age
- chronologic age
- sarcopenia
- arthritis
- gout
- dementia
- Alzheimer's disease
- food insecurity
- Meals on Wheels
- congregate meals
- systolic pressure
- diastolic pressure

Check Your Understanding

LO 19.1 1. Which of the following factors has contributed to the increased longevity of older Americans?
   a. Decrease in infant mortality
   b. Rising health care costs
   c. Advances in medical care
   d. Increase in incidence of dementia

LO 19.1 2. Since 1980 the prevalence of _____ has more than tripled among older Americans.
   a. lung cancer
   b. osteoporosis
   c. Alzheimer's disease
   d. diabetes

LO 19.2 3. Which of the following refers to the loss of muscle that occurs with aging?
   a. Senescence
   b. Sarcopenia
   c. Osteoarthritis
   d. Dysphagia

LO 19.2 4. Constipation in older adults can be caused by
   a. decreased GI motility.
   b. insufficient vitamin B_{12}.
   c. physical activity.
   d. excessive fluid intake.

LO 19.3 5. Older adults may benefit from adding zinc to their diet to
   a. help with weight loss.
   b. boost the immune system.
   c. promote bone growth.
   d. increase muscle mass.

LO 19.3 6. The DRI for both _____ increases with age.
   a. water and iron
   b. calcium and vitamin D
   c. protein and fat
   d. vitamin K and biotin

LO 19.4 7. Alzheimer's disease
   a. is an inevitable part of aging.
   b. is caused by a high-fat diet.
   c. leads to loss of memory.
   d. leads to thinning of the bones.

LO 19.4 8. The risk of developing osteoporosis can be reduced by
   a. eating a diet high in fat.
   b. drinking plenty of fluids.
   c. engaging in weight-bearing exercise.
   d. taking herbal supplements.

LO 19.5 9. Which of the following best describes food insecurity?
   a. Inability to afford the cost of high-quality food
   b. Inequitable food distribution
   c. Hunger
   d. Limited or uncertain access to adequate food

LO 19.6 10. Why are older adults at greater risk for hypertension?
   a. Arteries become thicker and less flexible with age
   b. Atherosclerosis is more common with age
   c. Inflammation is more common with age
   d. All of the above

Answers

1. (c) Advances in medical care are a key reason for increased longevity. Infant mortality rates, though relevant to overall life expectancy, are not a direct factor in the longevity of older adults. Rising health care costs and the incidence of dementia are also irrelevant.

2. (d) The prevalence of Americans with diabetes has tripled from the 1980s. An estimated 29.1 million Americans have diabetes.

3. (b) Sarcopenia refers to a loss of muscle mass that occurs with aging. Senescence is the scientific term for the physical changes that occur with age. Osteoarthritis is an inflammation of the joints, and dysphagia is difficulty swallowing.

4. (a) As people age, GI motility slows, leading to problems with constipation. Vitamin B_{12} absorption decreases with age, but this does not affect GI motility. A high-fiber, high-fluid diet helps relieve constipation; it doesn't cause it.

5. (b) Adequate zinc is needed for a healthy immune system. Zinc has nothing to do with losing weight, promoting bone growth, or increasing muscle mass.

6. (b) The need for both vitamin D and calcium is increased in older adults. Generally speaking, protein, fat, and water needs don't change with aging. Iron, vitamin K, and biotin are necessary for health, but are not needed in higher amounts by older adults.

7. (c) Alzheimer's disease leads to memory loss. It does not cause thinning of the bones and is not linked to a high-fat diet, nor is it inevitable.

8. (c) The risk of developing osteoporosis can be reduced by engaging in regular weight-bearing exercise. A diet rich in calcium and vitamin D can also slow its progression.

9. (d) Food insecurity refers to limited or uncertain access to adequate food. A person in a household that is food insecure may or may not be hungry. Moreover, affordability is the most common but not the only factor in food insecurity, as for example cognitive impairment or physical disability can contribute to food insecurity even in people with adequate financial means.

10. (d) Older adults are at increased risk for hypertension as their arteries, such as the aorta, become thicker and less flexible with age. This is further complicated by atherosclerosis and inflammation, two common conditions associated with aging.

Answers to True or False?

1. **False.** Chronic disease is not inevitable, although if you live to be very old, chances are you will develop at least one chronic condition. Healthy eating, physical activity, moderate alcohol intake, and not smoking are the best prevention for chronic conditions.

2. **True.** Heart disease remains the number-one cause of death in the United States among older adults.

3. **True.** A slowed gastrointestinal system in conjunction with low fluid and fiber intakes can lead to constipation in older adults.

4. **False.** The percentage of the population made up of adults over the age of 65 continues to rise.
5. **True.** Vitamin D helps the body absorb calcium from foods and dietary supplements. Calcium is necessary for strong bones.
6. **True.** Vitamin A is stored in the body and too much can increase the risk for osteoporosis and fractures.
7. **False.** The use of dietary supplements is common among older people.
8. **True.** Because a person's metabolism slows naturally with age, older adults need less energy (kilocalories) than younger adults.
9. **False.** Inadequate income and savings and/or reduced mobility can cause older adults to experience food insecurity, often for the first time in their lives.
10. **False.** Older adults sometimes turn to alcohol to deal with discomfort, loneliness, or boredom.

Web Resources

- For more general health information for older adults, visit www.cdc.gov/aging/aginginfo/index.htm
- For more information on herbs and interactions, visit the National Center for Complementary and Integrative Health, National Institutes of Health, at https://nccih.nih.gov
- For more information on Meals on Wheels, visit www.mowaa.org
- For information on legislative updates related to congregate meals and resources on diseases, elder rights, and nutrition, visit the Administration for Community Living, part of the Administration on Aging, at www.aoa.gov
- For information on good nutrition for all ages, visit the Academy of Nutrition and Dietetics (formerly the American Dietetic Association) at www.eatright.org

References

1. U.S. Department of Health and Human Services, Administration on Aging. 2016. *Statistics on Aging.* Available at https://aoa.acl.gov/Aging_Statistics/Index.aspx. Accessed April 2017.
2. Xu, J., S. L. Murphy, et al. 2016. Mortality in the United States, 2015 (NCHS Data Brief No. 267). Available at https://www.cdc.gov/nchs/products/databriefs/db267.htm. Accessed April 2017.
3. U.S. Department of Health and Human Services, Administration on Aging. 2016. A Profile of Older Americans: 2015. Available from https://aoa.acl.gov/Aging_Statistics/Profile/2015/docs/2015-Profile.pdf. Accessed April 2017.
4. National Institutes of Health. 2017. *Living Long and Well: Can We Do Both? Are They the Same?* Available from https://www.nia.nih.gov/health/publication/aging-under-microscope/living-long-and-well-can-we-do-both-are-they-same. Accessed April 2017.
5. U.S. Department of Health and Human Services, Administration on Aging. 2016. *A Profile of Older Americans: 2015.* Available from https://aoa.acl.gov/Aging_Statistics/Profile/2015/docs/2015-Profile.pdf. Accessed April 2017.
6. Ibid.
7. Population Reference Bureau. 2015. *Population Bulletin.* Available from http://www.prb.org/pdf16/aging-us-population-bulletin.pdf. Accessed April 2017.
8. Ibid
9. Xu, J., S. L. Murphy, et al. 2016. Mortality in the United States, 2015.
10. Centers for Disease Control and Prevention. 2015. *2014 National Diabetes Statistics Report.* Available from https://www.cdc.gov/diabetes/data/statistics/2014statisticsreport.html. Accessed April 2017.
11. Office of Disease Prevention and Health Promotion. 2017. *Healthy People 2020: Nutrition, Physical Activity and Obesity.* Available from https://www.healthypeople.gov/2020/leading-health-indicators/2020-lhi-topics/Nutrition-Physical-Activity-and-Obesity. Accessed April 2017.
12. Centers for Disease Control and Prevention. 2013. Adult Participation in Aerobic and Muscle-Strengthening Physical Activity—United States, 2011. *Morbidity and Mortality Weekly Report.* Available at www.cdc.gov/mmwr/preview/mmwrhtml/mm6217a2.htm?s_cid=mm6217a2_w. Accessed July 2014.
13. National Institutes of Health. 2017. *Exercise: Benefits of Exercise.* Available at https://nihseniorhealth.gov/exerciseforolderadults/healthbenefits/01.html. Accessed April 2017.
14. Ibid.
15. Centers for Disease Control and Prevention. 2013. *State of Aging and Health in America.* Available at https://www.cdc.gov/aging/pdf/State-Aging-Health-in-America-2013.pdf. Accessed April 2017.
16. National Institutes of Health. 2017. *What is Aging?* Available from https://www.nia.nih.gov/health/publication/aging-under-microscope/what-aging. Accessed April 2017.
17. Mayo Clinic. 2017. *Stress Management.* Available at www.mayoclinic.org/healthy-living/stress-management/in-depth/stress/art-20046037. Accessed April 2017.
18. The Merck Manual Home Health Book. 2013. *Overview of Aging.* Available at www.merckmanuals.com/home/older_peoples_health_issues/the_aging_body/changes_in_the_body_with_aging.html. Accessed July 2014.
19. National Center for Health Statistics. 2016. *Prevalence of Overweight, Obesity, and Extreme Obesity Among Adults: United States, Trends 1960–1962 Through 2013–2014.* Available at https://www.cdc.gov/nchs/data/hestat/obesity_adult_13_14/obesity_adult_13_14.pdf. Accessed April 2017.
20. Jahangir, E., A. De Schutter, et al. 2014. Low Weight and Overweightness in Older Adults: Risk and Clinical Management. *Progress in Cardiovascular Diseases* 57(2):127–133.
21. Castelo-Branco, C., and I. Soveral. 2014. The Immune System and Aging: A Review. *Gynecological Endocrinology* 30(1):16–22.
22. U.S. National Library of Medicine. National Institutes of Health. 2013. *Smell—Impaired.* Available at www.nlm.nih.gov/medlineplus/ency/article/003052.htm. Accessed August 2014.
23. National Institute of Aging, National Institutes of Health. 2017. *Smell and Taste: Spice of Life.* Available at www.nia.nih.gov/health/publication/smell-and-taste. Accessed April 2017.
24. Sura, L., A. Madhavan, et al. 2012. Dysphagia in the elderly: management and nutritional considerations. *Clinical Interventions in Aging* 7:287–298.
25. Ibid.
26. Rémond, D., D. R. Shahar, et al. 2015. Understanding the Gastrointestinal Tract of the Elderly to Develop Dietary Solutions That Prevent Malnutrition. *Oncotarget* 6(16):13858–13898.
27. Office of Dietary Supplements, National Institutes of Health. 2016, February. Vitamin B-12. Available from https://ods.od.nih.gov/factsheets/VitaminB12-HealthProfessional/. Accessed May 2017.
28. Gutchess, A. 2014. Review: Plasticity of the aging brain: New directions in cognitive neuroscience. *Science* 346(6209):579–582.
29. Ibid.
30. Tufts University, Jean Mayer USDA Human Nutrition Research Center on Aging. 2016. *MyPlate for Older Adults.* Available at http://hnrca.tufts.edu/myplate/. Accessed April 2017.
31. U.S. Department of Health and Human Services, U.S. Department of Agriculture. 2015, December. 2015–2020 Dietary Guidelines for Americans, 8th edition. Available at http://health.gov/dietaryguidelines/2015/guidelines/.
32. Institute of Medicine, Food and Nutrition Board. 2002. *Dietary Reference Intakes for Energy, Carbohydrate, Fiber, Fat, Fatty Acids,*

Cholesterol, Protein, and Amino Acids. Washington, DC: National Academies Press.

33. Paddon-Jones, D., W. W. Campbell, et al. 2015. Protein and Healthy Aging. *American Journal Clinical Nutrition* 101(6): 1339S–1345S.

34. Institute of Medicine, Food and Nutrition Board. 2002. *Dietary Reference Intakes for Energy, Carbohydrate, Fiber, Fat, Fatty Acids, Cholesterol, Protein, and Amino Acids.*

35. Deierlein, A. L., K. B. Morland, et al. 2014. Diet Quality of Urban Older Adults Age 60 to 99 Years: The Cardiovascular Health of Seniors and Built Environment Study. *Journal of Academy of Nutrition and Dietetics* 114(2):279–287.

36. American Heart Association. 2017. *Fish and Omega-3 Fatty Acids.* Available at www.heart. org/HEARTORG/HealthyLiving/Healthy-Eating/HealthyDietGoals/Fish-and-Omega-3-Fatty-Acids_UCM_303248_Article.jsp#. WOultkXyuig. Accessed April 2017.

37. American Heart Association. 2017. *Know Your Fats.* Available at www.heart.org/ HEARTORG/Conditions/Cholesterol/ PreventionTreatmentofHighCholesterol/ Know-Your-Fats_UCM_305628_Article.jsp. Accessed April 2017.

38. Begg, D. P. 2017. Disturbances of thirst and fluid balance associated with aging. *Physiology and Behavior.* Epub ahead of print.

39. Mayo Clinic. 2017. *Dehydration.* Available at www.mayoclinic.org/diseases-conditions/ dehydration/home/ovc-20261061. Accessed April 2017.

40. Bruyère, O., E. Cavalier, et al. 2014. Effects of Vitamin D in the Elderly Population: Current Status and Perspectives. *Archives of Public Health* 72(1):32.

41. National Institutes of Health. Office of Dietary Supplements. 2017. *Vitamin B12 Fact Sheet for Health Professionals.* Available at https://ods.od.nih.gov/factsheets/ VitaminB12-HealthProfessional/. Accessed April 2017.

42. National Institutes of Health, Office of Dietary Supplements. 2017. *Iron Fact Sheet for Health Professionals.* Available at https://ods. od.nih.gov/factsheets/Iron-HealthProfessional/. Accessed April 2017

43. Ibid.

44. National Institutes of Health. Office of Dietary Supplements. 2017. *Zinc Fact Sheet for Health Professionals.* Available at www.ods.od.nih.gov/ factsheets/Zinc-HealthProfessional/#en21. Accessed April 2017.

45. National Institutes of Health. Office of Dietary Supplements. 2017. *Calcium Fact Sheet for Health Professionals.* Available at https:// ods.od.nih.gov/factsheets/Calcium-Health-Professional/. Accessed April 2017.

46. Ibid.

47. Institute of Medicine. Food and Nutrition Board. 2010. *Dietary Reference Intakes for Calcium, Phosphorus, Magnesium, Vitamin D, and Fluoride.* Washington, DC: National Academies Press.

48. Wright, N. C., A. C. Looker, et al. 2014. The Recent Prevalence of Osteoporosis and Low Bone Mass in the United States Based on Bone Mineral Density at the Femoral Neck or Lumbar Spine. *Journal of Bone and Mineral Research* 29(11):2520–2526.

49. U.S. Department of Health and Human Services and U.S. Department of Agriculture. 2015, December. 2015–2020 Dietary Guidelines for Americans, 8th ed.

50. Qato, D. M., J. Wilder, et al. 2016. Changes in Prescription and Over-the-Counter Medication and Dietary Supplement Use Among Older Adults in the United States, 2005 vs 2011. *JAMA Internal Medicine* 176(4): 473–482.

51. Ibid.

52. National Institute on Aging. 2016. Dietary Supplements. Available from https://www .nia.nih.gov/health/publication/dietary-supplements. Accessed April 2017.

53. Nguyen, T., A. Cina, et al. 2016. The Effects of Concomitant Use of Proton Pump Inhibitors on Iron Supplements. *Journal for Nurse Practitioners* 13(2):e95–e97.

54. U.S. Department of Health and Human Services. 2015. *Dietary Guidelines for Americans, 2015–2020.*

55. Reedy, J., S. M. Krebs-Smith, et al. 2014. Higher Diet Quality Is Associated with Decreased Risk of All-Cause, Cardiovascular Disease, and Cancer Mortality among Older Adults. *Journal of Nutrition* 144(6):881–889.

56. Centers for Disease Control and Prevention. 2011. *Helping People to Live Long and Productive Lives and Enjoy a Good Quality of Life: At a Glance, 2015.* Available at https://stacks.cdc. gov/view/cdc/43961/Print. Accessed April 2017.

57. Qato, D. M., J. Wilder, et al. 2016. Changes in Prescription and Over-the-Counter Medication and Dietary Supplement Use Among Older Adults in the United States, 2005 vs 2011.

58. Food and Drug Administration. 2016. Information for Consumers on Using Dietary Supplements. Available from https://www. fda.gov/Food/DietarySupplements/Using-DietarySupplements/default.htm. Accessed April 2017.

59. Mayo Clinic. 2017. Monoamine Oxidase Inhibitors. Available from http://www. mayoclinic.org/diseases-conditions/ depression/in-depth/maois/art-20043992. Accessed April 2017.

60. US Department of Health and Human Services, Administration on Aging. 2016. A Profile of Older Americans: 2015. Available from https://aoa.acl.gov/Aging_Statistics/Profile/2015/docs/2015-Profile.pdf. Accessed April 2017.

61. Centers for Disease Control and Prevention. 2015. *Prevalence of Disability and Disability Type Among Adults—United States, 2013.* Available at https://www.cdc.gov/mmwr/preview/ mmwrhtml/mm6429a2.htm. Accessed April 2017.

62. Centers for Disease Control and Prevention. 2017. *Arthritis-Related Statistics.* Available at https://www.cdc.gov/arthritis/data_statistics/arthritis-related-stats.htm. Accessed April 2017.

63. Barbour, K. E., C. G. Helmick, et al. 2017. Vital Signs: Prevalence of Doctor-Diagnosed Arthritis and Arthritis-Attributable Activity Limitation–United States, 2013–2015. *Morbidity and Mortality Weekly Report.*

64. Hochberg, M. C., J. Martel-Pelletier, et al., on behalf of the MOVES Investigation Group. on behalf of the MOVES Investigation Group, et al. 2016. Combined Chondroitin Sulfate and Glucosamine for Painful Knee Osteoarthritis: A Multicentre, Randomised, Double-Blind, Non-Inferiority Trial versus Celecoxib *Annals of the Rheumatic Diseases* 75:37–44.

65. National Center for Complimentary and Integrative Health. 2016. Glucosamine and Chondroitin for Osteoarthritis Available from https://nccih.nih.gov/health/ glucosaminechondroitin#hed2. Accessed May 2017.

66. American College of Rheumatology. 2017. Prevalence Statistics. Available at http:// www.rheumatology.org/Learning-Center/ Statistics/Prevalence-Statistics. Accessed August 2017.

67. Manzel, A., D. N. Muller, et al. 2014. Role of "Western Diet" in Inflammatory Autoimmune Diseases. *Current Allergy and Asthma Reports* 14(1):404.

68. Marino, A., I. Paterniti, et al. 2015. Role of Natural Antioxidants and Potential Use of Bergamot in Treating Rheumatoid Arthritis. *PharmaNutrition* 3(2):53–59.

69. Lahiri, M., C. Morgan, et al. 2012. Modifiable Risk Factors for RA: Prevention Better than Cure? *Rheumatology* 51:499–512.

70. National Institutes of Health, National Institute of Arthritis and Musculoskeletal and Skin Diseases. 2016. *Questions and Answers about Gout.* Available at www.niams.nih.gov/ Health_Info/Gout/. Accessed April 2017.

71. Ibid.

72. Roddy, E., and H. K. Choi. 2014. Epidemiology of Gout. *Rheumatic Disease Clinics of North America* 40(2):155–175.

73. Zhu, Y., B. J. Pandya, et al. 2011. Prevalence of Gout and Hyperuricemia in the US General Population: The National Health and Nutrition Examination Survey 2007–2008. *Arthritis Rheumatology* 63:3136–3141.

74. Roddy, E., and H. K. Choi. 2014. Epidemiology of Gout.

75. Mayo Clinic. 2017. Gout: Risk Factors. Available at http://www.mayoclinic.org/diseases-conditions/gout/basics/risk-factors/ con-20019400. Accessed April 2017.

76. Mayo Clinic. 2017. *Gout Diet: What's Allowed, What's Not.* Available at http:// mayoclinic.org/healthy-lifestyle/nutrition-and-healthy-eating/in-depth/gout-diet/art-20048524. Accessed April 2017.

77. National Institutes of Health Osteoporosis and Related Bone Diseases, National

Resource Center. 2016. Osteoporosis Overview. Available at https://www.niams.nih.gov/Health_Info/Bone/Osteoporosis/overview.asp. Accessed April 2017.

78. Chew, E. Y., T. E. Clemons, et al., for the Age-Related Eye Disease Study Research Group. 2014. Ten-Year Follow-up of Age-Related Macular Degeneration in the Age-Related Eye Disease Study AREDS Report No. 36. *JAMA Ophthalmology* 132(3):272–277.

79. Chew, E. Y., T. E. Clemons, et al. 2013. Age-Related Eye Disease Study Research Group. Long-term effects of vitamins C, E, β-carotene and zinc on age-related macular degeneration in the Age-Related Eye Disease Study: AREDS Report No. 35. *Ophthalmology* 120(8):1604–1611.

80. Wang, J. J., G. H. S. Buitendijk, et al. 2014. Genetic Susceptibility, Dietary Antioxidants, and Long-Term Incidence of Age-Related Macular Degeneration in Two Populations. *Ophthalmology* 121(3):667.

81. American Macular Degeneration Foundation. 2016. *Nutrition and Macular Degeneration*. Available at www.macular.org/nutrition-macular-degeneration. Accessed April 2017.

82. National Eye Institute. 2015. *Cataracts*. Available at https://nei.nih.gov/health/cataract/cataract_facts. Accessed April 2017.

83. Ibid.

84. Ibid.

85. Rautiainen, S., B. E. Lindblad, et al. 2014. Total Antioxidant Capacity of the Diet and Risk of Age-Related Cataract A Population-Based Prospective Cohort of Women. *JAMA Ophthalmology* 132(3):247–252.

86. U.S. National Library of Medicine. 2017. Dementia. Available from https://medlineplus.gov/dementia.html. Accessed April 2017.

87. National Institutes of Health. National Institute on Aging. 2017. *Alzheimer's Disease Fact Sheet*. Available at www.nia.nih.gov/alzheimers/publication/alzheimers-disease-fact-sheet. Accessed April 2017.

88. U.S. Department of Health and Human Services, National Institute on Aging. 2014. *A Primer on Alzheimer's Disease and the Brain*. Available at www.nia.nih.gov/alzheimers/publication/2013-2014-alzheimers-disease-progress-report/primer-alzheimers-disease-and#characteristics. Accessed July 2014.

89. Hersi, M., B. Irvine, et al. 2017. Risk Factors Associated with the Onset and Progression of Alzheimer's Disease: A Systematic Review of the Evidence. *Neurotoxicology*. [Epub ahead of print]

90. Ngandu, T., J. Lehtisalo, et al. 2015. A 2 Year Multidomain Intervention of Diet, Exercise, Cognitive Training, and Vascular Risk Monitoring versus Control to Prevent Cognitive Decline in At-Risk Elderly People (FINGER): A Randomized Controlled Trial. *Lancet* 385(9984):2255–2263.

91. Morris, M. C., C. C. Tangney, et al. 2015. MIND Diet Associated with Reduced Incidence of Alzheimer's Disease. *Alzheimer's and Dementia* 11(9):1007–1014.

92. U.S. Department of Health and Human Services, Administration on Aging. 2016. A Profile of Older Americans: 2015. Available from https://aoa.acl.gov/Aging_Statistics/Profile/2015/docs/2015-Profile.pdf. Accessed April 2017.

93. Ibid

94. Coleman-Jensen, A., M. P. Rabbitt, et al. 2016, September. Household Food Security in the United States in 2015, ERR-215, U.S. Department of Agriculture, Economic Research Service.

95. Seligman, H. K., B. A. Laraia, et al. 2010. Food Insecurity Is Associated with Chronic Disease among Low-Income NHANES Participants. *Journal of Nutrition* 140:304–310.

96. Sinnett, S. S., R. Bengle, et al. 2010. The Validity of Nutrition Screening Initiative DETERMINE Checklist Responses in Older Georgians. *Journal of Nutrition for the Elderly* 29:393–409.

97. Administration on Aging. 2016. *Older Americans Act*. Available at https://aoa.acl.gov/aoa_programs/oaa/index.aspx Accessed May 2012.

98. Meals on Wheels of America. Results from a Pilot Randomized Control Trial of Home-Delivered Meal Programs. 2015. Available from: http://www.mealsonwheelsamerica.org/docs/default-source/News-Assets/mtam-full-report—march-2-2015.pdf?sfvrsn=6. Accessed April 2017.

99. Center for Disease Control. 2017. Depression Is Not a Normal Part of Growing Older. Available from https://www.cdc.

gov/aging/mentalhealth/depression.htm. Accessed April 2017.

100. National Institute on Aging. 2016. Alcohol Use in Older People. Available from https://www.nia.nih.gov/health/publication/alcohol-use-older-people. Accessed April 2017.

101. National Institutes of Health, National Institute on Alcohol Abuse and Alcoholism. 2014. *Harmful Interactions*. Available at www.pubs.niaaa.nih.gov/publications/Medicine/medicine.htm. Accessed August 2014.

102. Ibid.

103. National Institutes of Health, National Institute on Alcohol Abuse and Alcoholism. *Older Adults*. Available at http://www.niaaa.nih.gov/alcohol-health/special-populations-co-occurring-disorders/older-adults. Accessed April 2017.

104. Mozzafarian, E. J. Benjamin, et al. 2015. Heart Disease and Stroke Statistics-2015 Update: a report from the American Heart Association. *Circulation* e29–322.

105. National Institute on Aging. 2016. *Health and Aging: High Blood Pressure*. Available at https://www.nia.nih.gov/health/publication/high-blood-pressure. Accessed April 2017.

106. Ibid.

107. U.S. National Library of Medicine. 2017. *High Blood Pressure*. Available at www.nlm.nih.gov/medlineplus/highbloodpressure.html. Accessed April 2017

108. National Institute on Aging. 2016. *Health and Aging: High Blood Pressure*. Available at https://www.nia.nih.gov/health/publication/high-blood-pressure. Accessed April 2017.

109. Sun, Z. 2015. Aging, Arterial Stiffness, and Hypertension. *Hypertension* 65:252–256.

110. Ibid.

111. National Institute on Aging. 2016. Health and Aging: High Blood Pressure. Available at https://www.nia.nih.gov/health/publication/high-blood-pressure. Accessed April 2017.

112. Centers for Disease Control and Prevention. 2016. High Blood Pressure Facts. Available at https://www.cdc.gov/bloodpressure/facts.htm. Accessed April 2017.

113. National Institutes of Health, National Heart, Lung and Blood Institute. 2015. *What Is the DASH Eating Plan?* Available at www.nhlbi.nih.gov/health/health-topics/topics/dash/. Accessed April 2017.

114. Harsha, D. W., W. P. Lin, et al. 1999. Dietary Approaches to Stop Hypertension: A Summary of Study Results. *Journal of the American Dietetic Association* 99:S35–S39.

115. Sacks, F. M., L. P. Svetkey, et al. DASH-Sodium Collaborative Research Group. 2001. Effects on Blood Pressure of Reduced Dietary Sodium and the Dietary Approaches to Stop Hypertension (DASH) Diet. *New England Journal of Medicine* 344(1):3–10.

116. Appel, L. J., F. M. Sacks, et al. 2005. Effects of Protein, Monounsaturated Fat, and Carbohydrate Intake on Blood Pressure and Serum Lipids: Results of the OMNIHeart

Randomized Trial. *Journal of the American Medical Association* 294:2455–2464.

117. American Heart Association. 2016. *Limiting Alcohol to Manage High Blood Pressure*. Available at http://www.heart.org/HEARTORG/Conditions/HighBloodPressure/MakeChangesThatMatter/Limiting-Alcohol-to-Manage-High-Blood-Pressure_UCM_303244_Article.jsp#.WO4zqkUrKig. Accessed April 2017.

118. American Heart Association. 2016. Smoking, High Blood Pressure and Your Health, Available from www.heart.org/HEARTORG/Conditions/HighBloodPressure/MakeChangesThatMatter/Smoking-High-Blood-Pressure-and-Your-Health_UCM_301886_Article.jsp#.WQJF-VLMyu4. Accessed May 2017.

119. American Heart Association. 2016. *Weight Management and Blood Pressure*. Available at www.heart.org/HEARTORG/Conditions/HighBloodPressure/PreventionTreatmentofHighBloodPressure/Weight-Management-and-Blood-Pressure_UCM_301884_Article.jsp. Accessed April 2017.

120. American Heart Association. 2016. Getting Active to Control High Blood Pressure. Available from http://www.heart.org/HEARTORG/Conditions/HighBloodPressure/MakeChangesThatMatter/Getting-Active-to-Control-High-Blood-Pressure_UCM_301882_Article.jsp#.WO40O0UrKig. Accessed April 2017.

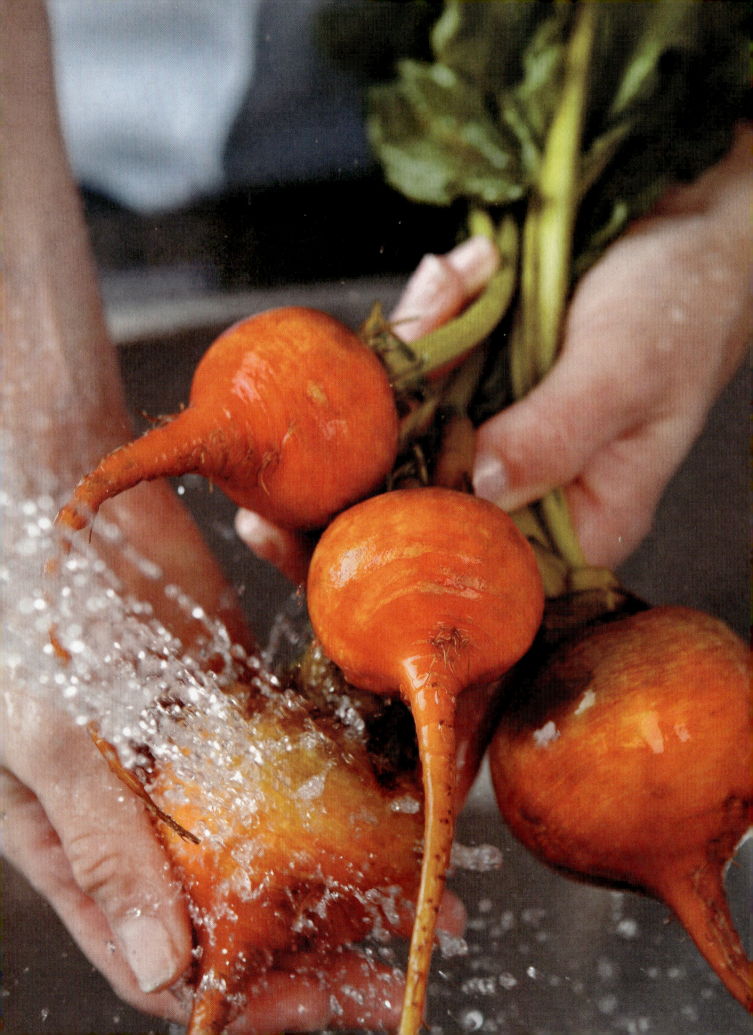

Food Safety, Technology, and Sustainability

Learning Outcomes

After reading this chapter, you will be able to:

20.1 Distinguish between foodborne infection and foodborne intoxication and provide an example of each.

20.2 Summarize strategies to prevent foodborne illness in the home and when traveling.

20.3 Describe how the food supply is protected in the United States.

20.4 Compare the risks and benefits of food additives and the use of hormones, antibiotics, and pesticides in both traditionally and organically grown food.

20.5 Explain what constitutes a sustainable food system.

20.6 Compare the benefits and risks of the use of biotechnology in our current food system.

True or False?

1. Foods that contain pathogens that cause foodborne illness always smell bad. **T/F**

2. Handwashing is more effective in preventing food contamination than using a hand sanitizer. **T/F**

3. A kitchen sponge is a prime environment for the breeding and spread of bacteria. **T/F**

4. Freezing foods kills the harmful bacteria. **T/F**

5. Leftovers that have been stored in the fridge for a week are safe to eat. **T/F**

6. As long as the expiration date hasn't passed, packaged food is always safe to eat. **T/F**

7. Food additives must demonstrate a "zero risk" of cancer to human beings in order to meet FDA approval. **T/F**

8. A diet consisting only of locally grown foods is a sustainable diet. **T/F**

9. Foods grown organically that carry the USDA organic seal are free of pesticides. **T/F**

10. Genetically engineered foods are plentiful in the United States. **T/F**

See page 773–774 for the answers.

Have you ever thought about where food comes from before it appears on the supermarket shelf or how safe that food is for you? No matter what you are eating, it likely started out on a farm. Getting food safely from farms to your plate requires several steps and a huge investment of human and natural resources.

Thanks to monitoring and regulation by the U.S. Food and Drug Administration (FDA), the U.S. Department of Agriculture (USDA), and other government agencies, consumers in the United States enjoy a relatively safe food supply. As we explain this chapter, however, foodborne illness continues to be a threat. Moreover, as the world's population continues to increase, the pressure to produce more food with limited natural resources has led to technological changes in the **food system** that have had environmental costs, including depletion of natural resources and pollution of air, soil, and water. In this chapter we discuss the causes of foodborne illnesses and strategies to prevent them. We also explore techniques of modern food production and their effects on our health and our environment.

What Causes Foodborne Illness?

LO 20.1 Distinguish between foodborne infection and foodborne intoxication and provide an example of each.

Foodborne illness is any disorder caused by consuming contaminated food. It is a major preventable public health threat worldwide. Every year in the United States, 1 in 6 Americans (or 48 million people) experience foodborne illness, and about 128,000 are hospitalized.[1] Foodborne illness most commonly results in gastrointestinal symptoms such as cramps, diarrhea, and nausea and vomiting, but in extreme circumstances it can result in death. Approximately 3,000 Americans die of foodborne illness every year.[2]

Pathogens and Their Toxins Cause Most Foodborne Illness

The two types of foodborne illness are infection and intoxication. Consuming foods or beverages that are contaminated with disease-causing organisms, known as **pathogens**, causes foodborne infection. Once ingested, the pathogens multiply in the GI tract and cause illness. Pathogens commonly implicated in foodborne infection include viruses, bacteria, molds, parasites, and prions (**Table 20.1**).

Eating foods contaminated with a **toxin** causes foodborne intoxication. Viruses and parasites do not cause foodborne intoxication. Certain species of bacteria, however, do secrete toxins. These include *Clostridium botulinum*, *Staphylococcus aureus*, *Bacillus cereus*, and *Escherichia coli*. Bacterial foodborne intoxication generally is caused by enterotoxins (*entero* = intestine, *toxin* = toxic), which quickly produce gastrointestinal symptoms such as nausea and vomiting—in some cases within 30 minutes of consuming the contaminated food.[3] Some bacteria, such as *C. botulinum*, secrete neurotoxins (*neuro* = nerve) that harm the nervous system. Toxins can also accumulate naturally in plants or seafood or result from chemical contamination. These types are discussed later in this chapter. Pathogens may be present in the raw ingredients of the food or may contaminate the food at any stage of the food system. For example, fruit flies have been shown to transfer toxin-producing *Escherichia coli* O157:H7 to apples under laboratory conditions.[4] *E. coli* as well as several other pathogens are found in the GI tract and fecal matter of humans or animals. Food may become contaminated with these pathogens if it comes into contact with fecal matter, and individuals can become infected by putting food or hands that have been in contact with fecal matter into their mouths. This is a common route of transmission of foodborne illness and is called the **fecal-to-oral transmission** route.

food system All processes and infrastructure involved in feeding a population: growing, harvesting, processing, packaging, transporting, marketing, and consuming food.

foodborne illness Sickness caused by consuming pathogen- or toxin-containing food or beverages. Also known as *foodborne disease* or *food poisoning*.

pathogens Collective term for disease-causing organisms. Pathogens include microorganisms (viruses, bacteria) and parasites and are the most common source of foodborne illness.

toxin Poison that can be produced by living organisms.

fecal-to-oral transmission Spread of pathogens by putting something in the mouth, such as hands or food, that has been in contact with infected stool.

TABLE 20.1 Pathogens That Commonly Cause Foodborne Illness

Microbe	Where You Find It	How You Can Get It	What You May Experience
Viruses			
Norovirus	In the stool or vomit of infected individuals	Fecal-to-oral transmission; eating ready-to-eat foods or drinking liquids contaminated by an infected person; eating contaminated shellfish; touching contaminated objects and then putting hands in mouth	Watery diarrhea, nausea and vomiting, flulike symptoms; possible fever. Symptoms can appear 24–48 hours after onset, last 24–60 hours, and are typically not serious.
Hepatitis A (HAV)	In the stool of infected individuals	Fecal-to-oral transmission; eating raw produce irrigated with contaminated water; eating raw or undercooked foods that have not been properly reheated; drinking contaminated water	Diarrhea, dark urine, jaundice, flulike symptoms that can appear 30 days after incubation and can last 2 weeks to 3 months.
Bacteria			
Campylobacter jejuni	GI tracts of animals and birds, unpasteurized milk, untreated water, and sewage	Drinking contaminated water or raw milk; eating raw or undercooked meat, poultry, or shellfish	Fever, headache, and muscle pain followed by diarrhea (sometimes bloody), abdominal pain, and nausea; appears 2–5 days after eating; may last 7–10 days; Guillain-Barré syndrome may occur.
Clostridium botulinum	Widely distributed in nature in soil, water, on plants, and in the GI tracts of animals and fish; grows only in environments with little or no oxygen	Eating improperly canned foods, garlic in oil, vacuum-packaged and tightly wrapped food	Bacteria produce a toxin that causes illness by affecting the nervous system. Symptoms usually appear after 18–36 hours. May experience double vision, droopy eyelids, trouble speaking and swallowing, and difficulty breathing. Fatal in 3–10 days if not treated.
Clostridium perfringens	Soil, dust, sewage, and GI tracts of animals and humans; grows only in little or no oxygen	Called "the cafeteria germ" because many outbreaks result from eating food left for long periods in steam tables or at room temperature; bacteria are destroyed by cooking, but some spores may survive	Bacteria produce toxin that causes illness. Diarrhea and gas pains may appear 8–24 hours after eating; usually last about 1 day, but less severe symptoms may persist for 1–2 weeks.
Escherichia coli O157:H7	GI tracts of some mammals, unpasteurized milk, unchlorinated water; one of several strains of *E. coli* that can cause human illness	Drinking contaminated water, unpasteurized apple juice or cider, or unpasteurized milk; eating raw or rare ground beef or uncooked fruits and vegetables	Diarrhea or bloody diarrhea, abdominal cramps, nausea, and weakness. Can begin 2 to 5 days after food is eaten, lasting about 8 days. Small children and older adults may develop hemolytic uremic syndrome (HUS), which causes acute kidney failure. A similar illness, thrombotic thrombocytopenic purpura (TTP), may occur in adults.
Enterotoxigenic *Escherichia coli* (major cause of traveler's diarrhea)	GI tracts of some mammals and unpasteurized dairy products; more common in developing countries	Fecal-to-oral transmission; consuming stool-contaminated water and foods from unsanitary water supplies and food establishments	Diarrhea, nausea and vomiting, stomach cramping, bloating, fever, and weakness
Listeria monocytogenes	GI tracts of humans and animals, milk, soil, leafy vegetables; can grow slowly at refrigerator temperatures	Eating ready-to-eat foods such as hot dogs, luncheon meats, cold cuts, fermented or dry sausage, other deli-style meat and poultry, or soft cheeses; drinking unpasteurized milk	Fever, chills, headache, backache, sometimes upset stomach, abdominal pain, and diarrhea; may take up to 3 weeks to become ill; may later develop more serious illness in high-risk individuals

(continued)

TABLE 20.1 Pathogens That Commonly Cause Foodborne Illness (*continued*)

Microbe	Where You Find It	How You Can Get It	What You May Experience
Salmonella (over 2,300 types)	GI tracts and feces of animals; *Salmonella enteritidis* in eggs	Eating raw or undercooked eggs, poultry, and meat, unpasteurized milk and dairy products, and seafood; can also be spread by infected food handlers	Stomach pain, diarrhea, nausea, chills, fever, and headache usually appear 8–72 hours after eating. May last 1–2 days.
Shigella (over 30 types)	Human GI tract; rarely found in other animals	Fecal-to-oral transmission by consuming contaminated food and water. Most outbreaks result from eating food, especially salads, prepared and handled by workers with poor personal hygiene	Disease referred to as "shigellosis" or bacillary dysentery. Diarrhea containing blood and mucus, fever, abdominal cramps, chills, and vomiting begin 12–50 hours from ingestion of bacteria; can last a few days to 2 weeks.
Staphylococcus aureus	On humans (skin, infected cuts, pimples, noses, and throats)	Consuming foods that were contaminated by being improperly handled; bacteria multiply rapidly at room temperature	Bacteria produce a toxin that causes illness. Severe nausea, abdominal cramps, vomiting, and diarrhea occur 1–6 hours after eating; recovery within 2–3 days.
Parasites			
Cryptosporidium parvum	In the intestines of humans and animals	Fecal-to-oral transmission; drinking contaminated water; eating contaminated produce	Stomach pains, diarrhea, cramps, fever, and vomiting
Cyclospora cayetanensis	Human stool	Fecal-to-oral transmission; drinking contaminated water; eating contaminated produce	Diarrhea, flatulence, stomach cramps, vomiting, fatigue
Giardia lamblia	In the intestines of humans and animals	Fecal-to-oral transmission; drinking contaminated water; eating contaminated produce	Diarrhea, stomach pains, flatulence
Trichinella spiralis	In undercooked or raw meats containing *Trichinella* worms	Raw or undercooked contaminated meat, usually pork or game meats	Nausea and vomiting, diarrhea, fever, aching joints and muscles

Sources: Data from Centers for Disease Control and Prevention (CDC). 2004. *Diagnosis and Management of Foodborne Illness: A Primer for Physicians*; CDC. 2012. *Norovirus*; CDC. 2014. *Hepatitis A Information for the Public*; CDC. 2006. *Traveler's Diarrhea*; Diagnosis and Management of Foodborne Illnesses: A Primer for Physicians. *MMWR Recommendations and Reports* 50 (January 2001):1–69; CDC. 2014. *Parasites: Food*. All available at www.cdc.gov. USDA Food Safety and Inspection Service. 2013. *Foodborne Illness: What Consumers Need to Know*. Available at https://www.fsis.usda.gov/wps/portal/fsis/topics/food-safety-education/get-answers/food-safety-fact-sheets/foodborne-illness-and-disease/foodborne-illness-what-consumers-need-to-know/CT_Index. Accessed April 2017; USDA Food Safety and Inspection Service. 2015. *Parasites and Foodborne Illness*. Available at https://www.cdc.gov/parasites/food.html. Accessed April 2017.

Eating contaminated food does not always result in foodborne illness. Many pathogens are killed in the mouth by antimicrobial enzymes and in the stomach by hydrochloric acid. In addition, the potential for a pathogen to cause illness depends on the amount that is consumed, the potency, and the nutritional and immune status of the person who consumes it. Pathogens that survive the natural defense systems of the body undergo an *incubation period* before the symptoms of illness begin. The delay in the time between when the pathogen is consumed and when it causes illness depends on the type and number of pathogens swallowed and can range from a few hours to a few weeks (refer to Table 20.1).

In the United States the majority of foodborne illness is caused by infection or intoxication from five pathogens: norovirus, *Salmonella* (bacterium), *Clostridium perfringens* (bacterium), *Campylobacter* (bacterium), and *Staphylococcus aureus* (bacterium that produces a toxin).[5] Together these pathogens are estimated to account for 91 percent of all domestically acquired cases of foodborne illness in the United States. The differences between the major pathogen groups are discussed next.

Viruses

The term **virus** denotes a microscopic infectious agent that contains genetic information (DNA or RNA) but must enter a living **host**, such as a plant or animal cell, to engage in metabolism and reproduction and thus survive. When an individual eats a food that is

virus Microscopic organism that carries genetic information for its own replication; can infect a host and cause illness.

host Living plant or animal (including a human) that a microbe infects for the sake of reproducing.

contaminated with a virus, the pathogen can invade the cells of the stomach and intestinal walls. The virus can then cause the cells' genetic material to start producing more viruses, ultimately leading to illness.[6] One virus species—**norovirus**—is currently responsible for more than half of all foodborne illness in the United States, making it the single most common cause of foodborne disease in this country.[7]

Bacteria

Bacteria are single-celled organisms that lack a nucleus. Thousands of types of bacteria are naturally present in our environment. If you were to swab your kitchen sink right now and look at the results under a microscope, you would find that there are about 16 million bacteria living on each square centimeter (less than half an inch) of the sink. Whereas viruses need a host to survive, bacteria can flourish on both living and nonliving surfaces and can multiply on sponges, dishtowels, cutting boards and countertops, and in sinks. Given the right conditions, a single bacterium can produce colonies of billions of bacteria over the course of just one day.

Not all bacteria cause disease in humans. Recall from Chapter 3 that the GI tract harbors in excess of 1,000 different types of bacteria, many of which are beneficial to health.[8] Some produce small amounts of vitamins or enhance GI functioning, whereas others may aid in weight regulation or maintenance of the lining of the GI tract.[9] Harmful bacteria that enter the GI tract compete for resources with the resident GI flora and, depending on the amount and species of invading bacteria and the condition of the human host, may cause illness.

Contamination of food by certain types of bacteria causes it to spoil; that is, the quality of the food deteriorates. The same bacterial species may or may not introduce pathogens that cause foodborne illness. Though most individuals do not become seriously ill after eating spoiled foods, these items can cause nausea and shouldn't be eaten. In contrast to spoiled foods, contaminated foods that contain bacterial pathogens may look and smell perfectly fine. It is not safe to eat food just because it "looks fine" or "smells OK."

Bacteria may contaminate raw meat, poultry, seafood, eggs, and produce. Lettuce, tomatoes, sprouts, and melons—which are eaten raw—frequently carry pathogenic bacteria. Although they can grow in just about any food, bacteria grow particularly well on foods high in protein, such as meat, dairy foods, and cooked beans. Even ready-to-eat foods that have been cooked may become contaminated with bacteria from raw products or poor personal hygiene of food handlers.

The foodborne bacterium that causes the largest number of illnesses in the United States is *Salmonella*. *Salmonella* is found in the GI tract and feces of animals and in eggs. Most people infected with *Salmonella* experience diarrhea, fever, and abdominal cramps within 12–72 hours after eating the infected food. The illness usually lasts 4–7 days. People in generally good health before becoming infected usually recover without treatment, but *Salmonella* infection is the most common cause of foodborne illness that results in hospitalization and death in the United States.[10]

One type of foodborne bacterium that is not as common, but is of particular concern, is *Escherichia coli* O157:H7. Although most strains of *E. coli* are benign, *E. coli* O157:H7 secretes a toxin that results in severe, even life-threatening illness for some individuals. *E. coli* O157:H7 intoxication can cause **hemolytic uremic syndrome** (*hemo* = blood, *lyti* = destroyed, *uremic* = too much urea in blood), which results in the destruction of red blood cells and damage to and eventual failure of the kidneys.[11] Contaminated ground beef has been the culprit behind most cases of foodborne illness caused by *E. coli* O157:H7. Because bacteria live in the GI tracts of healthy cattle, they can easily come into contact with the meat of the animal during slaughtering and then get mixed in when the beef is being ground. *E. coli* is destroyed by heat, and most outbreaks occur when people eat undercooked meat, unpasteurized milk, or raw produce contaminated with the bacterium.

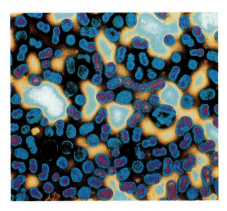

Viruses, such as the hepatitis A virus, need a host to survive and multiply.

norovirus Most common type of virus that causes foodborne illness; can cause gastroenteritis, or the "stomach flu."

bacteria Single-celled microorganisms without an organized nucleus. Some are benign or beneficial to humans, whereas others can cause disease.

hemolytic uremic syndrome Rare condition that can be caused by *E. coli* O157:H7 and results in the destruction of red blood cells and kidney failure. Very young children and older adults are at a higher risk of developing this syndrome.

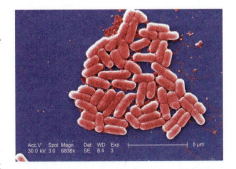

E. coli O157:H7 is a toxin-producing strain of *Escherichia coli* that can cause severe and even fatal foodborne illness. Most other forms of *E. coli* are harmless.

Molds

Molds are multicellular fungi that form a filamentous growth and thrive on damp surfaces. Spores give mold the color you see, and when airborne they spread very easily. Some molds cause allergic reactions and respiratory problems. A number of molds grow on foods such as breads, cheeses, and fruits, and not all of them are detrimental; some are used to make certain cheeses like Roquefort, blue, Gorgonzola, and Brie. Molds flourish in foods such as breads made without preservatives because they prefer warmer temperatures and thrive at room temperature. Molds also grow on fruits and vegetables and in the refrigerator on jams, jellies, and even cured, salty meats, given enough time.

Some molds in the right conditions produce mycotoxins that can lead to food intoxication if ingested. One example of this is aflatoxin, a carcinogen sometimes found on moldy peanuts. To avoid mold growth in peanuts and other legumes, store them in a dry environment; avoid eating any legumes that have an off color. Many countries, including the U.S., monitor foods for aflatoxin. Because of their visibility, molds are easy to identify and food that is moldy should be discarded. Cooking and freezing stop mold growth but do not kill the toxins present.[12]

Parasites

Parasites are small organisms, occasionally in the egg or larval phase, that take their nourishment from hosts. They can be found in food and water and are often transmitted through the fecal-to-oral route.[13] Foodborne illness caused by parasites is much less common in the United States than is illness caused by other types of pathogens.[14]

The most common parasitic illness outbreaks in the United States have been caused by just a few types: *Cryptosporidium parvum*, *Cyclospora cayetanensis*, *Giardia lamblia*, and *Trichinella spiralis*. Both *Cryptosporidium parvum* and *Cyclospora cayetanensis* can be found in contaminated water or food sources. *Giardia lamblia* is one of the most common sources of waterborne illness. Hikers who drink unfiltered water from streams or lakes often become infected with the *Giardia* parasite. *Trichinella spiralis* (see photo) is an intestinal worm whose larvae (hatched eggs) can travel from the digestive tract to the muscles of the body. See Table 20.1 for a summary of these parasites and the foodborne illnesses they cause.

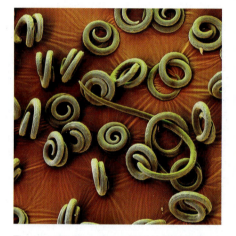

The parasitic roundworm *Trichinella spiralis*.

Prions

A **prion** is an infectious agent composed of an incorrectly folded protein particle. Prions are responsible for diseases known as spongiform encephalopathies, such as bovine spongiform encephalopathy (BSE, or mad cow disease) in cattle and variant Creutzfeldt-Jakob disease (vCJD) in humans. All known prion diseases affect the structure of neural tissue and are untreatable. Cattle and other ruminant animals develop the disease after consuming feed that contains prion-containing tissues of infected animals. Humans can be infected by consuming the meat or brain tissue of infected livestock.

Great Britain experienced an outbreak of BSE in the 1990s that resulted in vCJD in 150 people. Since that time, the United States has taken specific steps to protect its citizens against beef contaminated with BSE, such as limiting imported meat from countries at risk for BSE and banning ruminant feed containing mammalian protein.[15] BSE has not been eradicated, but the incidence of infection is sporadic and rare, and no one is known to have developed vCJD because of eating infected meat in the United States. Since 2003 there have been only four cases of BSE reported in the U.S. cattle supply, the most recent being in 2012.[16] In a press briefing, the USDA's chief veterinary officer said the cow's meat did not enter the food supply and the carcass was destroyed, so the risk to human health was minimal.[17] The World Organization for Animal Health (OIE) recently upgraded the United States' risk classification for BSE from controlled risk to negligible risk.[18]

molds Microscopic fungi that live on plant and animal matter; some can produce mycotoxins, which are harmful.

parasites Organisms that live on or in another organism; obtain their nourishment from their hosts.

prion Short for proteinaceous infectious particle; self-reproducing protein particles that cause degenerative brain diseases.

Some Illnesses Are Caused by Natural Toxins

Many toxins that occur in plants and animals function as natural pesticides and assist in fending off predators. In many cases, these natural toxins are present in amounts too small to harm humans, but there are instances in which these naturally occurring toxins can make a person seriously ill.

Marine Toxins

Cooking fish thoroughly may or may not destroy naturally occurring **marine toxins**. Eating spoiled finfish, such as tuna and mackerel, can cause **scombrotoxic fish poisoning**, in which the spoilage bacteria break down proteins in the fish and secrete histamine, a toxin that can accumulate to harmful levels. Consuming fish that contain large amounts of histamine can cause symptoms such as diarrhea, flushing, sweating, and vomiting within 2 minutes to 2 hours.[19]

Large, predatory reef fish, such as barracuda and grouper, can sometimes be contaminated with ciguatoxins, which when eaten can cause **ciguatera poisoning**. In this case, toxins travel through the food chain and **bioaccumulate** in larger species (see **Figure 20.1**). Ciguatoxins originate in microscopic sea organisms called *dinoflagellates*, which are eaten by small tropical fish, which in turn are eaten by larger fish. When people consume the larger fish, the consumption of the accumulated concentrations of toxin can result in illness.[20] In addition to experiencing various gastrointestinal discomforts, individuals infected with ciguatera may have temperature sensation reversal in their mouth when they eat.[21] For example, hot liquids and hot foods feel cold, and vice versa.

Marine neurotoxins can contaminate certain shellfish, such as mussels, clams, scallops, oysters, crabs, and lobsters, that typically live in the coastal waters of New England and the Pacific states. Neurotoxins are also produced by a particular reddish-brown-colored dinoflagellate. These reddish-brown dinoflagellates can become so abundant that the ocean appears to have red streaks, also known as red tides. Eating shellfish contaminated with neurotoxins can lead to **paralytic shellfish poisoning**. Symptoms include mild numbness or tingling in the face, arms, and legs, as well as headaches and dizziness. In severe cases muscle paralysis, the inability to breathe, and death could result.[22]

Toxins in Other Foods

Many plant foods naturally contain toxins in small amounts and don't generally present problems when eaten in reasonable portions; however, consuming them in large amounts could be harmful. For example, potatoes that have been exposed to light can

marine toxins Chemicals that occur naturally and contaminate some fish.

scombrotoxic fish poisoning Condition caused by consuming spoiled fish that contain large amounts of histamines; also referred to as *histamine fish poisoning*.

ciguatera poisoning Condition caused by marine toxins that are produced by dinoflagellates and have bioaccumulated in fish that the affected person consumes.

bioaccumulate To build up the levels of a substance or chemical in an organism over time, so that the concentration of the chemical is higher than would be found naturally in the environment.

paralytic shellfish poisoning Condition caused by a reddish-brown-colored dinoflagellate that contains neurotoxins.

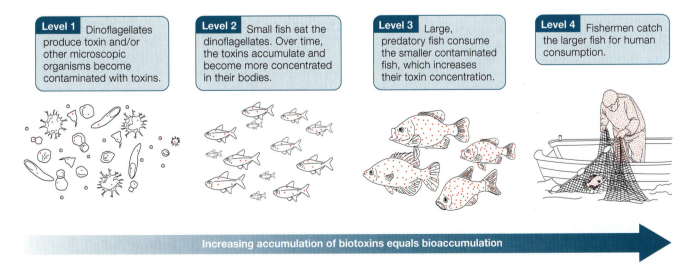

Level 1 Dinoflagellates produce toxin and/or other microscopic organisms become contaminated with toxins.

Level 2 Small fish eat the dinoflagellates. Over time, the toxins accumulate and become more concentrated in their bodies.

Level 3 Large, predatory fish consume the smaller contaminated fish, which increases their toxin concentration.

Level 4 Fishermen catch the larger fish for human consumption.

Increasing accumulation of biotoxins equals bioaccumulation

▲ Figure 20.1 **Bioaccumulation of Toxins**

develop a green tinge on the surface, which indicates that they contain increased amounts of **solanine**, a toxin that can cause fever, diarrhea, paralysis, and shock. Peeling potatoes and removing the green layer ensures that the potato can be safely eaten. Eating 2–5 milligrams of solanine per kilogram of body weight results in symptoms and eating 3–6 milligrams of solanine per kilogram of body weight may result in death.[23] The amount of solanine in potatoes is very small, on the order of about 0.2 milligrams per gram of potato. Eating approximately 1 pound of green potatoes would likely make a 100-pound person ill.

However, other foods contain toxins that are harmful even in trace amounts, and so should be avoided altogether. Certain wild mushrooms, for example, are poisonous; they contain toxins that can cause nausea and vomiting, liver damage, and death.

Chemical Agents Sometimes Cause Foodborne Illness

Consumers are becoming increasingly concerned about environmental damage caused by industrial and household chemicals. Traces of these substances can travel through the food chain and be ingested by people, posing numerous risks to health. Awareness of the potential environmental and health risks caused by these chemicals has led to a search for safer alternatives.

Polychlorinated Biphenyls

Polychlorinated biphenyls (PCBs) are industrial pollutants that occur in the food supply. These chemicals were used as coolants and insulating fluids for transformers and capacitors, as flame-retardants, and in the manufacture of plasticizers, waxes, and paper. Production of PCBs was banned in 1979 due to their high toxicity and persistence—resistance to being broken down—in the environment.[24]

PCB exposure in adults can cause skin conditions such as acne and rashes as well as liver damage. It is of particular concern for pregnant and lactating women because prenatal exposure and consumption of contaminated breast milk can damage a child's nervous system and cause learning defects. Also, because young children are smaller, exposure to PCBs has a proportionately greater effect on them than would the same level of exposure in adults. Moreover, exposure to PCBs can cause cancer in animals and may be carcinogenic in humans.[25]

Although PCBs are no longer manufactured in the United States, they do not degrade and can therefore still make their way into the environment through releases from hazardous waste sites, the burning of commercial or municipal waste, and the improper disposal of consumer products, such as old television sets and electrical fixtures and devices.[26] PCBs in the air eventually return to our land and water by runoff in snow and rain and may bioaccumulate in larger predatory fish that live in polluted waters (see Figure 20.1).[27]

The EPA began regulating PCBs in drinking water in 1992, and the agency is working to lower the amount of PCBs in the environment.[28] Although the FDA routinely monitors PCB levels in the food supply, the toxin can be found in nonregulated food sources, such as locally caught fish. Consumers should therefore research and adhere to local fish consumption advisories. See the Table Tips for the EPA website that lists current advisories, as well as tips to minimize exposure to toxins and chemical agents in fish and seafood.

Methylmercury

Mercury occurs naturally, but is also produced as an industrial by-product or pollutant. An airborne form of mercury can accumulate on the surface of streams and oceans and be transformed by the bacteria in the water into the toxic form of methylmercury. Methylmercury toxicity is associated with nervous system damage in adults and impaired neurological development in infants and children.[29] Methylmercury may bioaccumulate in

---

TABLE TIPS

Avoid Toxins and Chemical Agents in Seafood

Keep fish, especially finfish—such as fresh tuna, mackerel, grouper, and mahi mahi—chilled in the refrigerator to prevent spoilage and the formation of histamine toxins.

Never consume finfish or shellfish that is sold as bait, as these do not meet food safety regulations.

Observe all fish consumption advisories. To learn if an advisory is in place for the fish in your area, search for "Fish Consumption Advisories" at *www.epa.gov*.

If you fish recreationally, always check with the local or state health department for specific advice based on the local waters to avoid eating PCB-containing fish.

Eat a variety of types of fish to minimize the exposure to a particular toxin.

Source: Adapted from Centers for Disease Control and Prevention. 2016. *Harmful Algal Bloom (HAB)-Associated Illness*. Available at https://www.cdc.gov/habs/illness-symptoms-marine.html; Agency for Toxic Substances and Disease Registry. Updated 2014. *ToxFAQ for Polychlorinated Biphenyls (PCBs)*. Available at https://www.atsdr.cdc.gov/toxfaqs/tf.asp?id=140&tid=26.

solanine Toxin found in potato surfaces exposed to light that can cause fever, diarrhea, and shock if consumed in large amounts.

polychlorinated biphenyls (PCBs) Synthetic chemicals that have been shown to cause cancer and other adverse effects on the immune, reproductive, nervous, and endocrine systems in animals; may cause cancer in humans.

fish, seafood, and other wildlife and cause toxicity to humans if consumed in sufficient quantities. Larger fish—including shark, swordfish, king mackerel, and tilefish—contain high levels of mercury, so the FDA and EPA recommend that women who are or may become pregnant, women who are nursing, and young children should avoid consuming these fish.[30]

Some People Are at Higher Risk for Foodborne Illness

Older adults, young children, pregnant women, and people with certain disorders have compromised immunity. They are therefore more susceptible to contracting foodborne illness and suffering complications than the rest of the population.

Age-related deterioration of the immune system increases the risk for foodborne illness. In addition, because the level of acidic gastric juice produced by the stomach declines with age, fewer foodborne pathogens are destroyed in the stomach. This puts older adults at higher risk of serious disease and death from foodborne illness.[31] As the percentage of Americans 65 years of age and older increases—it is projected to reach 21.7 percent by the year 2040—more Americans will be at higher risk for severe foodborne illness.[32]

In addition to age, any condition that weakens a person's immune system, such as HIV, AIDS, cancer, or diabetes, can increase the risk of serious foodborne illness.[33] Also, the hormonal shifts that occur during pregnancy can weaken a pregnant woman's immune system, making her more vulnerable to a potentially life-threatening illness caused by the bacterium *Listeria monocytogenes*. (See Spotlight: The Lowdown on *Listeria*.)

Individuals in institutional settings (such as nursing homes, hospitals, schools, and on cruise ships), where groups of people eat foods from the same source, are also at higher risk of foodborne illness. Improper food handling and poor hygiene practices of foodservice workers are often the causes of foodborne disease outbreaks in institutional settings.

LO 20.1: THE TAKE-HOME MESSAGE Foodborne illness is a serious public health problem. Consuming pathogens in contaminated food or drinks causes foodborne infection, whereas consuming toxins causes foodborne intoxication. Viruses and bacteria are the most common causes of foodborne infection in the United States, although parasites and prions can also cause foodborne illness. Toxins can be released into foods by bacteria or can occur naturally in foods such as mushrooms or as the result of bioaccumulation of industrial chemicals such as polychlorinated biphenyls (PCBs) and methylmercury. Certain populations, including older adults, children, pregnant women, and those with compromised immune systems, are at higher risk of contracting foodborne illness and suffering complications.

What Strategies Can Prevent Foodborne Illness?

LO 20.2 Summarize strategies to prevent foodborne illness in the home and when traveling.

One of the best ways to prevent foodborne illness is to keep the pathogens that cause it from flourishing in foods. For example, in order for bacteria to thrive and multiply, they must have the proper conditions. These include (1) a source of nutrients (including glucose, amino acids, or vitamins and/or minerals), (2) moisture, (3) a pH above 4.6 (considered low acidity), (4) temperatures in the range of 40–140°F (4.4–60°C), and (5) time (at least 20 minutes) to multiply.[34] Protein- and nutrient-rich animal-based foods, such as

The Lowdown on *Listeria*

Listeriosis, the illness caused by the bacterium *Listeria monocytogenes*, seriously affects approximately 1,600 individuals in the United Sates annually, with pregnant women being 10 times more likely than other people to become infected.[1] *Listeria* can reach the fetus through the placenta, be transmitted to the developing fetus, and lead to severe illness, premature birth, miscarriage, and stillbirth. Older adults and those with a weakened immune system are also at risk for becoming very sick or even dying.

Animals can harbor *Listeria*, which leads to contamination of meat and dairy foods. Pasteurization kills *Listeria*, so unpasteurized soft cheeses, such as Camembert, Brie, and blue cheeses, carry a higher risk of contamination. Compared with hard cheeses such as Parmesan, these soft cheeses are less acidic and contain more moisture, two conditions that enhance bacterial growth. Even though cooking can also destroy *Listeria*, the lower cooking temperature used during the processing of soft cheeses isn't high enough to destroy this bacterium. Because contamination can also occur after processing, many outbreaks have been associated with other foods such as hot dogs, deli-style luncheon meats, salami, and paté. *Listeria* can also

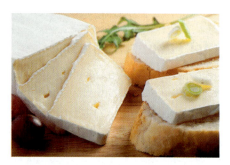

Unpasteurized soft cheese can be contaminated with *Listeria*.

continue to multiply at refrigerated temperatures.

The following tips can help pregnant women and other higher-risk individuals reduce their likelihood of contracting *Listeria*:[2,3]

- Heat ready-to-eat luncheon meats, cold cuts, fermented and dry sausage, deli-style meat and poultry products, and hot dogs until they are steamy hot to kill any existing bacteria before serving.
- Wash your hands with hot, soapy water after touching these types of ready-to-eat foods, or any foods for that matter. Also thoroughly wash cutting boards, dishes, and utensils.
- Avoid soft cheeses such as feta, Brie, Camembert, blue-veined (blue) cheese, and Mexican-style cheeses unless they are made with pasteurized

milk. (Read the ingredients list to see if pasteurized milk was used.) You can safely eat hard cheeses, semi-soft cheese such as mozzarella, pasteurized processed cheeses, cream cheese, and cottage cheese.
- Avoid unpasteurized milk and foods made from unpasteurized milk.
- Avoid refrigerated smoked seafood such as smoked salmon (lox or nova style), trout, whitefish, cod, tuna, or mackerel unless they are used in an entrée such as a heated casserole. You can safely eat canned fish and shelf-stable smoked seafood.
- Avoid refrigerated paté or meat spreads. You can safely eat canned or shelf-stable varieties.
- Eat precooked or ready-to-eat perishable items before the expiration date on the food label.

References

1. Centers for Disease Control and Prevention. 2016. Listeria *(Listeriosis)*. Available at www.cdc.gov/listeria. Accessed April 2017.
2. Ibid.
3. USDA. 2016. *Fact Sheets: Protect Your Baby and Yourself from Listeriosis.* Available at https://www.fsis.usda.gov/wps/portal/fsis/topics/food-safety-education/get-answers/food-safety-fact-sheets/foodborne-illness-and-disease/protect-your-baby-and-yourself-from-listeriosis/CT_Index. Accessed April 2017.

raw and undercooked meat, poultry, seafood, eggs, and unpasteurized milk, are the most common types of foods that provide conditions for rapid bacterial growth.

Bacteria thrive in moist environments, such as in raw chicken that is sitting in its juices. Dry foods, such as uncooked rice, sugar, flour, and cereals, do not usually support bacterial growth until they are hydrated with a liquid. However, infected utensils or hands can contaminate these foods. For example, a person with infected hands who takes a handful of cereal directly out of the box transfers bacteria onto the cereal. Although the bacteria may not multiply, they survive and, once eaten, will grow in the moist environment of the GI tract, possibly resulting in foodborne illness.

Bacteria don't thrive in acidic foods (pH less than 4.6) such as vinegar and citrus fruits, so these foods seldom provide the conditions necessary for growth. However, animal-based foods have a higher pH and provide the right conditions for bacteria to flourish.

Bacteria multiply most abundantly between the temperatures of about 40°F and 140°F. At body temperature, or 98.6°F (37°C), bacteria can divide and double within

20 minutes and multiply to millions in about 12 hours.[35] Because bacteria need such a short time period to multiply, it is important to realize that perishable food, such as raw meat, left at room temperature for an extended period can become a feast for bacterial growth.

Consumers can take various measures when consuming and handling food to reduce the risk of foodborne illness. These include preventing the growth of bacteria and destroying any pathogens that may be present. This can be done through the consistent practice of proper food consumption, handling, and storage strategies at home and while traveling.

Practice Food Safety at Home

An easy way to remember the important points of home food safety is by focusing on the "Core Four" of the Fight BAC! campaign of the nonprofit Partnership for Food Safety Education: Cleaning, Combating cross-contamination (or separating), Cooking, and Chilling (**Figure 20.2**).[36]

Clean Hands and Produce

Cleaning is one of the simplest ways to reduce the chances of microbial contamination, and proper handwashing is one of the most important overall strategies for preventing foodborne illness. If everyone practiced proper handwashing techniques, the incidences of foodborne illness could decrease by about half.[37] The Table Tips summarize proper handwashing techniques.

Proper handwashing refers to washing hands *thoroughly*, as well as washing hands *regularly*. This last part, regular washing, is where many people fall short. Germs accumulate on hands from a variety of sources throughout the day, and if hands are not regularly washed, these germs can infect the body after being passed into the mouth, nose, and eyes. Individuals also spread the germs to others by touching surfaces such as doorknobs.[38]

In instances where handwashing is not an option, such as when traveling or eating on the run, using disposable wipes or hand gel sanitizers can be an excellent

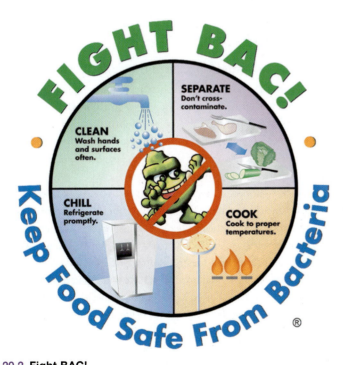

▲ **Figure 20.2 Fight BAC!**
The Fight BAC!® symbol sums up the "Core Four" of keeping food safe in the kitchen: clean, combat cross-contamination (separate meats from ready-to-eat foods), cook thoroughly, and chill to a cold enough temperature.
Source: www.fightbac.org/food-safety-basics/the-core-four-practices/

TABLE TIPS
Wash Your Hands!
After using the toilet
After changing a diaper
After touching animals
Before and after food preparation, especially when handling raw meat or poultry
After blowing your nose
After coughing or sneezing into your hands
Before and after treating wounds
After handling garbage
Before inserting or removing contact lenses
Proper handwashing:
Wet hands with warm, running water and apply liquid soap or use clean bar soap. Lather well.
Rub hands together vigorously for at least 20 seconds (recite the alphabet twice or sing "Happy Birthday" twice).
Scrub all surfaces, including the backs of hands, wrists, between fingers, and under fingernails.
Rinse well.
Dry hands with a clean cloth towel or disposable towel.
Use a towel to turn off the faucet and, if in a public restroom, use a clean towel to open the door as well.

Source: Adapted from Mayo Clinic. 2016. *Hand Washing: Do's and Don'ts*. Available at www.mayoclinic.org/healthy-lifestyle/adult-health/in-depth/hand-washing/art-20046253. Accessed April 2017.

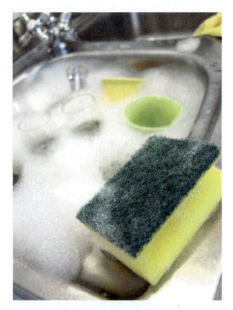

The countertop sponge may very well be the most contaminated item in your kitchen. Food scraps, moisture, and room temperature can lead to a thriving bacterial colony on this common cleaning item.

alternative. Only the alcohol-based products are effective in killing germs. The Centers for Disease Control and Prevention (CDC) recommends choosing products that contain at least 60 percent alcohol.[39] Individuals should keep hand sanitizers in the car, purse, desk drawer, and backpack so that proper hand hygiene can be practiced at all times.[40]

In addition to hands, anything that touches food, such as knives, utensils, and countertops, should be thoroughly cleaned between each use. Cutting boards should be placed in the dishwasher or scrubbed with hot, soapy water and rinsed after each use. Nonporous cutting boards made of plastic, marble, and tempered glass are easier to keep clean than the more porous wooden cutting boards or wooden surfaces. Cracked cutting boards should be discarded, as they can harbor pathogenic microbes. Kitchen sinks and cutting boards should be regularly sanitized by filling the sink with hot water and adding one teaspoon of bleach per quart of water. Let the board sit in the sanitizing liquid for a few minutes to kill the microbes, then rinse it thoroughly.

A kitchen sponge is an ideal environment for bacteria because it provides the ideal temperature, moisture, and nutrients (food particles). Household kitchen sponges and dishcloths have been shown to harbor more bacteria than toilet seats.[41] Consequently, sponges and dishcloths need to be replaced often and between replacements washed after each use in the hot cycle of the washing machine, preferably with bleach in addition to soap. They can also be soaked in a bleach solution along with the cutting boards, run through the dishwasher (including the dry cycle), or placed in the microwave for 1 minute at its highest setting.[42] To avoid fire hazards, be sure to use the microwave method only with damp sponges and those without metal.

All fruits and vegetables should be thoroughly washed under running tap water before eating. Even foods like cantaloupe, which doesn't have an edible peel or rind, have been known to carry *Salmonella* and *E. coli*, and the microbe can be transferred from the peel or rind to the fruit by the knife used to cut it open. Washing firm fruit with a vegetable brush helps remove any dirt or microbes on its surface. Fruit should be cut only on a clean cutting board. Washing fruits and vegetables offers the additional advantage of removing most of the pesticide residue that may be present. Pesticides are discussed in more detail later in this chapter.

Combat Cross-Contamination

Cross-contamination is the spread of microbes from one item to another. It can occur, for example, when washed lettuce—which is going to be eaten raw—comes into contact with raw meat, poultry, or fish during food preparation. To avoid cross-contamination between animal-based foods and fresh bread or raw fruits and vegetables, maintain separate cutting boards for meat and nonmeat foods. If you have just one cutting board, wash it thoroughly in hot, soapy water immediately after use.

Also, when grocery shopping, raw meats, fish, and poultry should be bagged separately from produce. Once home, these foods should either be frozen or stored in airtight containers on the bottom shelf of the refrigerator. This prevents contaminated drippings from coming in contact with cooked foods or raw fruits and vegetables. Marinades that are used to tenderize and flavor raw meats, poultry, or fish should never be reused as a basting or serving sauce. All plates and bowls that have contained raw meats, poultry, and fish should be thoroughly washed before reuse. For example, at a barbecue, the plate that held the raw hamburgers should *never* be used to serve the cooked burgers unless it has been thoroughly washed.

Another common source of cross-contamination occurs when soiled dishtowels are used to dry clean hands, dishes, or utensils. A towel that was used to wipe up raw meat juices or your hands can transfer those microbes to your clean dishes or utensils. You could easily coat those clean surfaces with a layer of germs. **Figure 20.3** summarizes some of the ways to combat cross-contamination in the kitchen.

cross-contaminate Transfer of pathogens from a food, utensil, cutting board, kitchen surface, and/or hands to another food or object.

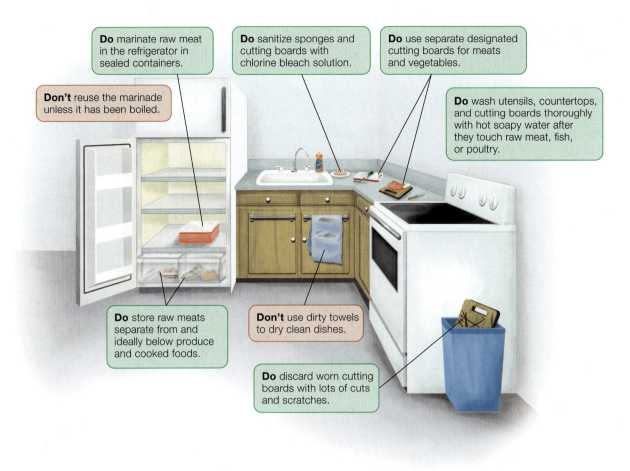

▲ Figure 20.3 **The Do's and Don'ts of Avoiding Cross-Contamination**

Cook Foods Thoroughly

A common food safety misconception is that meat that looks brown is fully cooked. Look at the two hamburger patties in **Figure 20.4**. The brown patty on the bottom might look more thoroughly cooked than the pinker patty above, but it's not. The color of beef is largely determined by **myoglobin**, the iron-containing protein that provides the purplish-red pigment in meat (and in human muscle tissue). The denaturing of this protein is what causes meat to turn from pink to brown during cooking. However, if the meat starts out brown, this color change won't occur. Thus, a burger could look "done" when it may still be raw in places. Research has shown that hamburgers can look "well done" while only having reached an internal temperature of approximately 135°F (57.2°C).[43] Ground meat (beef, pork, veal, and lamb) must reach an internal temperature of 160°F (71.1°C) to kill pathogens known to cause illness. In contrast, some lean or treated varieties of beef can remain pink even though they have reached an internal temperature of 160°F.

Poultry color can also be misleading because it can remain pink after thorough cooking. This is caused by a chemical reaction that occurs in the poultry from gases in the oven that give the meat a pink tinge. Because younger birds have thin skins, the gases can react with their flesh more easily and make the meat look pinker than that of older birds. Also, nitrates and nitrites added to some poultry as a preservative can give poultry a pink tinge (see the discussion of food additives later in the chapter).[44]

The only way to determine if food has reached an internal temperature high enough to kill pathogens is to use a food thermometer. **Figure 20.5** shows several types of food thermometers available for use when cooking. **Table 20.2** provides a list of the internal temperatures that foods should reach to ensure that they are safe to eat.

myoglobin Protein that provides the purplish-red color in meat and poultry.

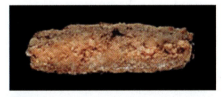

a Cooked to internal temperature of 160°F

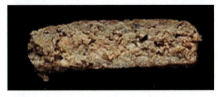

b Cooked to internal temperature of 135°F

▲ Figure 20.4 **Cook Meats Thoroughly to Kill Pathogens**
A hamburger needs to reach an internal temperature of 160°F to ensure that all foodborne pathogens are killed. Color is not an indication of "doneness."

If You Are Cooking This Food	The Food Thermometer Should Reach (°F)*
TABLE 20.2 Safe Food Temperatures	
Ground Meat and Meat Mixtures	
Beef, pork, veal, lamb	160
Turkey, chicken	165
Fresh Beef, Veal, Lamb	145**
Poultry	
Chicken, turkey, whole or parts	165
Duck and goose	165
Fresh Pork	
Ham, raw	145**
Ham, precooked (to reheat)	140
Fish and Shellfish	145
Eggs and Egg Dishes	
Eggs	Cook until yolk and white are firm
Egg dishes	160
Leftovers and Casseroles	165

*The thermometer should be placed in the thickest part of the food item.
**Meat should rest for 3 minutes before consumption to ensure that pathogens are destroyed.

Sources: Adapted from USDA Food Safety and Inspection Service. 2015. *Kitchen Thermometers*. Available at https://www.fsis.usda.gov/wps/portal/fsis/topics/food-safety-education/get-answers/food-safety-fact-sheets/appliances-and-thermometers/kitchen-thermometers/ct_index. Accessed April 2017; USDA Food Safety and Inspection Service. 2016. Keep Food Safe! Food Safety Basics. Available at https://www.fsis.usda.gov/wps/portal/fsis/topics/food-safety-education/get-answers/food-safety-fact-sheets/safe-food-handling/keep-food-safe-food-safety-basics/ct_index. Accessed April 2017.

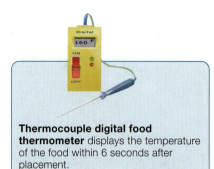

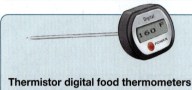

Thermocouple digital food thermometer displays the temperature of the food within 6 seconds after placement.

Thermistor digital food thermometers take approximately 10 seconds to display the temperature of the food on the dial.

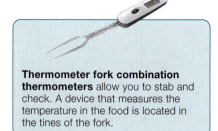

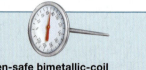

Thermometer fork combination thermometers allow you to stab and check. A device that measures the temperature in the food is located in the tines of the fork.

Oven-safe bimetallic-coil thermometers are most useful when cooking thick foods such as roasts and turkeys. They are unique, as they can stay in the food during cooking.

▲ **Figure 20.5 Food Thermometers**
There are several types of food thermometers available for measuring the internal temperature of cooked foods. The thermometer should be inserted at least one-half-inch deep into the food and should be washed thoroughly after each use and before insertion into any food.

Chill Foods at a Low Enough Temperature

Proper chilling and refrigeration of foods is essential to inhibit the growth of pathogens. But just how low must the temperature be? Foodborne bacteria multiply most rapidly in temperatures between 40° and 140°F (or 4.4–60°C), a range known as the "**danger zone**." To keep foods out of the danger zone, hot foods must be kept *hot*, above 140°F, and cold foods kept *cold*, below 40°F, or even lower (see **Figure 20.6**). This means that when cooked foods like lasagna are on a buffet table, they should be sitting on a hot plate or other heat source that keeps their temperature above 140°F, while cold prepared foods such as potato salad should be kept at 40°F or below at all times.[45]

Refrigerating foods for storage is another key aspect of keeping them chilled and inhibiting the growth and reproduction of pathogenic microbes. With the exception of the *Listeria* bacterium, cold temperatures *slow down* microbes' ability to multiply to dangerous levels; note that chilling does not kill them or completely stop their growth. To ensure that the growth of microbes on foods is controlled, refrigerator temperatures should be set at or below 40°F (4.4°C). The temperature for the freezer should be set at 0°F (−17.7°C) or below. Food stays safe in the freezer indefinitely, though its quality may deteriorate. "Freezer burn" may occur if frozen food is not tightly wrapped and gets exposed to air. Freezer burn causes the texture of food to change, as it dries out and accumulates ice crystals. This results in a less pleasant taste and appearance, but it isn't harmful. Most microbes become dormant and are unable to multiply when they are frozen, but they aren't destroyed. When food is defrosted the microbes can multiply again under the right conditions.

Two hours is the critical time to remember. Perishables such as raw meat and poultry left out at room temperature (a temperature within the danger zone) for more than 2 hours may not be safe to eat. In temperatures above 90°F (32.2°C), such as in the kitchen in the summertime, foods shouldn't be left out at room temperature for more than 1 hour.[46] Leftovers should be refrigerated within 2 hours of being prepared. Large roasts and pots of soup or stews should be divided into smaller batches and placed in shallow containers in order to cool more quickly in the refrigerator. If these items have been left in the danger zone for too long, bacteria can grow and may also produce toxins that are heat resistant.

danger zone Range of temperatures between 40° and 140°F at which foodborne bacteria multiply most rapidly; room temperature falls within the danger zone.

These toxins are not destroyed even if the food is cooked to a proper internal temperature and could cause illness if consumed.[47]

Once food is refrigerated it shouldn't be held for more than a few days, even when kept at the proper temperature. A good rule of thumb is that leftovers can be in the refrigerator at 40°F or below for no more than 4 days. Remember, after *4* days in the refrigerator, leftovers are ready *for* disposal. Raw meats, poultry, and seafood can be safely kept in the refrigerator for a maximum of 2 days. A good food safety strategy is the acronym FIFO, which means "first in, first out." In other words, use food that has been in the refrigerator the longest first. **Table 20.3** lists the storage times for various foods. Don't eat food that you suspect may not be safe. If you are unsure about the safety of a food, remember this rhyme: *When in doubt, throw it out.*

Minimizing the risk for developing a foodborne illness requires a conscious effort to clean, avoid cross-contamination, cook, and chill to keep foods safe. Think about how many of these strategies you use in your own kitchen and use the Self-Assessment to help identify areas in which you may need to improve your food safety habits.

TABLE 20.3 Safe Storage of Perishable Foods

Product	Storage Time after Purchase*	
For Raw Foods		
Poultry	1 or 2 days	
Beef, veal, pork, and lamb	3–5 days	
Ground meat and ground poultry	1 or 2 days	
Fresh variety meats (liver, tongue, brain, kidneys, heart, intestines)	1 or 2 days	
Cured ham, cook-before-eating	5–7 days	
Sausage from pork, beef, or turkey, uncooked	1 or 2 days	
Fish	1 or 2 days	
Eggs	3–5 weeks	
	Unopened, after Purchase*	**After Opening***
For Processed Product Sealed at Plant		
Cooked poultry	3–4 days	3–4 days
Cooked sausage	3–4 days	3–4 days
Sausage, hard/dry, shelf-stable	6 weeks/pantry	3 weeks
Corned beef, uncooked, in pouch with pickling juices	5–7 days	3–4 days
Vacuum-packed dinners, commercial brand with USDA seal	2 weeks	3–4 days
Bacon	2 weeks	1 week
Hot dogs	2 weeks	1 week
Luncheon meat	2 weeks	3–5 days
Ham, fully cooked, whole	7 days	3 days
Ham, canned, labeled "keep refrigerated"	9 months	3–4 days
Ham, canned, shelf-stable	2 years/pantry	3–5 days
Canned meat and poultry, shelf-stable	2–5 years/pantry	3–4 days
Leftovers		3–4 days

*Based on refrigerator home storage (at 41°F [5°C] or below) unless otherwise stated.
Source: Adapted from USDA Food Safety and Inspection Service. 2016. *Keep Foods Safe! Food Safety Basics.* Available at https://www.fsis.usda.gov/wps/portal/fsis/topics/food-safety-education/get-answers/food-safety-fact-sheets/safe-food-handling/keep-food-safe-food-safety-basics/ct_index. Accessed April 2017.

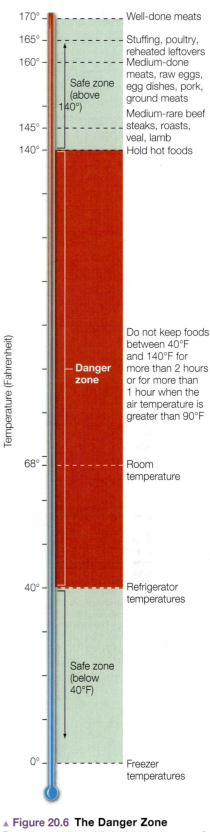

▲ **Figure 20.6 The Danger Zone**
Bacteria multiply rapidly in the "danger zone," between temperatures of 40° and 140°F.

Avoiding Foodborne Illness While Traveling

If you are traveling abroad, look up the country you're visiting on the Centers for Disease Control's National Center for Infectious Diseases Travelers' Health Destination website at www.cdc.gov/travel/destinat.htm to find out about any specific health advisories for that area.

Do not eat raw or undercooked meat or seafood.

Do not consume raw fruits and vegetables unless you wash and peel them. Thoroughly cooked fruits and vegetables should be safe to eat.

Do not consume foods from street vendors or other vendors who appear to leave food at room temperature for extended periods of time.

Do not consume food or beverages from vendors who appear unclean or have unclean establishments. A clean environment is no guarantee against foodborne illness, but unclean environments are more likely to spread foodborne illness.

Do not drink tap water or use ice made from tap water unless it has been boiled first or treated with iodine or chlorine. Bottled water should be safe.

Do not consume unpasteurized milk or other unpasteurized dairy foods.

Source: Adapted from Centers for Disease Control and Prevention, Division of Bacterial and Mycotic Diseases. 2013. *Travelers' Diarrhea*. Available at https://wwwnc.cdc.gov/travel/page/travelers-diarrhea. Accessed April 2017.

traveler's diarrhea Common pathogen-induced intestinal disorder experienced by some travelers who visit areas with unsanitary conditions.

How Do Your Food Safety Habits Stack Up?

Take the following quiz to find out.

How Often Do You	Always	Sometimes	Never
Wash your hands before preparing food?			
Scrub your fruits and vegetables under cold, running water before eating them?			
Use an insulated pouch with an ice pack to carry your perishable lunches and snacks, such as meat-filled sandwiches and/or yogurt and cheese?			
Wash your hands after using the bathroom?			
Throw out refrigerated leftovers after 4 days?			
Chop raw vegetables on a clean chopping board rather than the one you just used for raw meat, fish, or poultry?			
Use a thermometer to determine if the meat or poultry you are cooking is done?			

Answer

If you answered "Always" to all of the above you are practicing superior food safety skills. If you didn't, there's more you can do to reduce your chances of contracting a foodborne illness.

Practice Food Safety While Traveling

Travelers should follow food safety procedures to reduce the risk of illness while traveling abroad. Each year, up to 50 percent of international travelers are estimated to have their trips interrupted by foodborne illness.[48] One type of *E. coli*, enterotoxigenic (*entero* = intestines, *toxi* = toxin, *genic* = forming) *E. coli*, is a common cause of **traveler's diarrhea**. Traveler's diarrhea causes watery diarrhea and gastrointestinal cramps and is primarily caused by consuming contaminated food, water, or ice. People visiting countries where sanitation is poor, including some developing countries in Latin America, Africa, the Middle East, and Asia, are at a higher risk of contracting it.[49] See the Table Tips for suggestions on how to avoid traveler's diarrhea and other forms of foodborne disease while traveling.

LO 20.2: THE TAKE-HOME MESSAGE Proper food handling and storage strategies—particularly cleaning, preventing cross-contamination, cooking to recommended temperatures—and chilling at recommended temperatures, can help reduce the risk of foodborne illness. Anything that comes in contact with foods, including hands, should be thoroughly washed, and produce should always be washed before eating it. Fresh bread, fruits, and vegetables need to be kept separate from raw meats, poultry, and fish and from any utensils that touch them. Checking the internal temperature of cooked food with a food thermometer is the only accurate way to tell if it is safe to eat. Perishables should be properly and promptly chilled to minimize the growth of bacteria. Raw meat, poultry, and seafood should be used within 2 days. Leftovers that are refrigerated should be discarded after 4 days. Extra caution is needed when traveling abroad to avoid foodborne illness.

How Is the Food Supply Protected?

LO 20.3 Describe how the food supply is protected in the United States.

The food system includes the techniques and resources involved in growing, harvesting, processing, packaging, transporting, selling, and consuming food. Risks to both food safety and availability occur at each point in the food system. The **farm-to-table continuum** is a visual tool that shows how farmers, food manufacturers, transporters, retailers, and you, the consumer—following regulations and guidelines from the U.S. government—can help ensure a safe food supply. **Figure 20.7** shows the steps in this continuum.

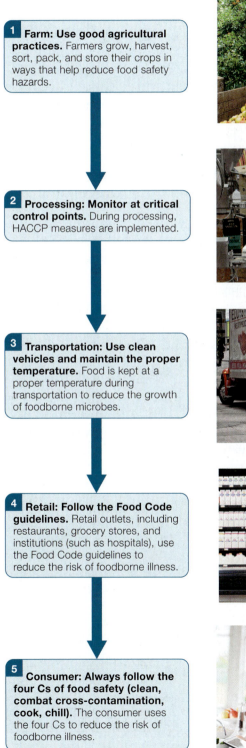

1 Farm: Use good agricultural practices. Farmers grow, harvest, sort, pack, and store their crops in ways that help reduce food safety hazards.

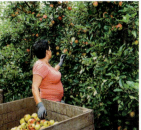

2 Processing: Monitor at critical control points. During processing, HACCP measures are implemented.

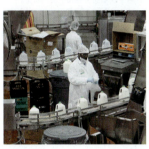

3 Transportation: Use clean vehicles and maintain the proper temperature. Food is kept at a proper temperature during transportation to reduce the growth of foodborne microbes.

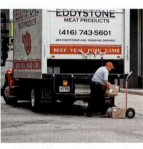

4 Retail: Follow the Food Code guidelines. Retail outlets, including restaurants, grocery stores, and institutions (such as hospitals), use the Food Code guidelines to reduce the risk of foodborne illness.

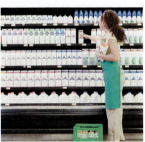

5 Consumer: Always follow the four Cs of food safety (clean, combat cross-contamination, cook, chill). The consumer uses the four Cs to reduce the risk of foodborne illness.

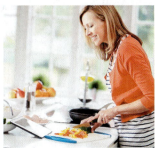

◀ **Figure 20.7 The Farm-to-Table Continuum**
Every step in the farm-to-table continuum plays an important role in reducing microbes and the spread of foodborne illness.

farm-to-table continuum Illustrates the roles that farmers, food manufacturers, food transporters, retailers, and consumers play in ensuring that the food supply, from the farm to the plate, remains safe.

Several Government Agencies and Programs Protect the Food Supply

In 1906 Congress charged the USDA with the responsibility for monitoring the safety of our nation's food. Today, several federal agencies share the responsibility for food safety in the United States.[50] **Table 20.4** lists these agencies and summarizes the roles they each play in safeguarding foods. The **Food Safety Initiative (FSI)**, begun in 1997, coordinates the research, inspection, outbreak response, and educational activities of the various government agencies.

An example of collaboration among these government agencies is FoodNet (*www.cdc. gov/foodnet*), which is a combined effort of the CDC, the USDA's Food Safety Inspection Service (FSIS), the FDA, and 10 state health departments. The program consists of active surveillance for foodborne diseases and related studies designed to help public health officials understand the cause and effect of foodborne diseases in the United States. The objectives of the program include determining the burden of foodborne illness in the United States, monitoring trends over time, assessing the incidence of foodborne illness and its relation to specific foods and settings, and developing interventions to reduce the overall burden of foodborne illness.

The CDC coordinates another program called PulseNet (*www.cdc.gov/pulsenet*), which is a national network of public health and food regulatory agency laboratories—including those at the CDC, USDA/FSIS, and FDA—designed to identify and contain foodborne illness outbreaks. PulseNet participants perform **DNA fingerprinting**, a sort of molecular identification, on pathogenic bacteria. DNA fingerprinting uses the bacteria's unique genetic code to identify different strains of pathogens. These "fingerprints" are submitted electronically to a database at the CDC and the information is available on demand to public health and food regulatory agencies. Finding similar strains of a bacterium in both a person and a food suggests a common source and potential connection. If similar patterns emerge at the same time in different states, this could indicate a potential outbreak. Once a suspicious foodborne illness outbreak is reported and a source is identified, several government agencies then work together to contain the disease.

The *E. coli* outbreak in spinach that occurred in the fall of 2006 is one example of how multiple government agencies work together to identify and contain an outbreak. The CDC, through its monitoring and surveillance programs, detected an outbreak of illness due to *E. coli* O157:H7 and immediately alerted the FDA. DNA fingerprinting was used by PulseNet to determine that all infected individuals had consumed the same strain of *E. coli* and to trace the strain to bagged raw spinach grown in California. The fingerprinting also allowed the agencies to link the tainted food to reported illnesses in 26 states. Once the source of the outbreak was confirmed, the CDC issued an official health alert about the outbreak, and the FDA advised consumers to stop eating raw spinach. Before the outbreak was over, more than 200 people had been infected, and more than half of them

Food Safety Initiative (FSI) Coordinates the research, surveillance, inspection, outbreak response, and educational activities of the various government agencies that work together to safeguard food.

DNA fingerprinting Technique in which bacterial DNA "gene patterns" (or "fingerprints") are detected and analyzed to distinguish between different strains of a bacterium.

TABLE 20.4	Agencies that Oversee the Food Supply
Agency	**Responsible for**
USDA Food Safety and Inspection Service (FSIS)	Ensuring safe and accurately labeled meat, poultry, and eggs
Food and Drug Administration (FDA)	Ensuring the safety of all other foods besides meat, poultry, and eggs
Environmental Protection Agency (EPA)	Protecting you and the environment from harmful pesticides
Animal and Plant Health Inspection Service (APHIS)	Protecting against plant and animal pests and disease
Centers for Disease Control and Prevention	Surveillance of foodborne disease

had been hospitalized.[51,52] Three individuals died and 31 developed hemolytic uremic syndrome from the outbreak. However, through the collaborative efforts and swift action of these federal and state agencies, the outbreak was contained in a short period of time and its impact was minimized.

Hazard Analysis and Critical Control Points (HACCP) is a program used to identify and control foodborne hazards that may occur in all stages of the food production process.[53] The HACCP approach was first conceived in the 1960s when the U.S. National Aeronautics and Space Administration (NASA) asked a private food manufacturer to design the foods for space flights. Since then, the FDA and USDA have mandated HACCP programs for seafood, juice, and meat processing in the United States. The use of HACCP is recommended, but not mandated, for other food industries as well. HACCP includes seven principles that focus on the analysis of potential hazards associated with foods and the identification of critical control points in the production of a food so that preventative measures can be put in place to minimize risks. For example, procedures for monitoring temperatures throughout a food's production need to be in place. Manufacturers also apply food preservation techniques to some foods to make them safer for consumers. We discuss these techniques later in the chapter.

Issues regarding food safety are also important at retail establishments. Grocery stores and restaurants must comply with FDA regulations. The Food Code is a reference document published by the FDA that local, state, and federal regulators use as a model for the development of their own food safety rules and to be consistent with national food regulatory policy. The Food Code provides practical, science-based guidance, including HACCP guidelines, and provisions to help purveyors minimize foodborne illness.[54]

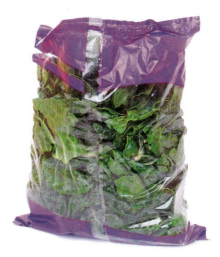

The FDA, CDC, and USDA worked together to combat an outbreak of *E. coli* O157:H7 in 2006 that was traced to bagged prewashed spinach.

Food Manufacturers Use Preservation Techniques to Destroy Contaminants

In addition to government efforts to help prevent foodborne illness, food manufacturers also work to safeguard food. **Food preservation** methods, some of which have been in use for thousands of years, include heating, canning, pickling, salting, drying, and freezing, all of which help to keep foods safe. At the same time, manufacturers' use of newer techniques such as irradiation and chemical additives has expanded as consumers demand fast and convenient foods, new flavors, increased shelf-life, and improved textures.

Pasteurization and Canning

Pasteurization is a process for destroying pathogenic bacteria in which liquid foods are heated to a prescribed temperature for a specified time. The process kills *E. coli* O157:H7, *Salmonella*, and *Listeria monocytogenes*, all of which can be present in raw milk. Pasteurization improves the quality of dairy products and keeps all products fresh for a longer period of time. In addition to dairy products, pasteurization is required for some juices like fresh apple juice and other foods. Unpasteurized juices must display a warning on the label to alert consumers.[55]

Canning is a process in which foods are packed into airtight containers and then heated to temperatures of 240–250°F (115.5–121.1°C) to kill microorganisms. The amount of exposure time to heat varies by the type of food, its acidity, and its density. Processing conditions are chosen to ensure that the foods are sterile while retaining the most nutrients.[56]

Commercial canning is regulated by the FDA and HACCP procedures, which virtually eliminates foodborne illness. However, improperly home-canned products can be the source of *Clostridium botulinum*, one of the toxin-producing foodborne bacterial species mentioned earlier in this chapter. *C. botulinum* can survive in airless environments and create **spores** that are not destroyed at normal cooking temperatures (refer to Table 20.2 on page 744). A temperature higher than boiling water (212°F [100°C]) is needed to kill

food preservation Treatment of foods to reduce deterioration and spoilage and help prevent the multiplication of pathogens that can cause foodborne illness.

pasteurization Process of heating liquids or food at high temperatures to destroy foodborne pathogens.

canning Process of packing food in airtight containers and heating them to a temperature high enough to kill bacteria.

spores Hardy reproductive structures that are produced by certain bacteria and fungi.

these spores.[57] Botulism, the foodborne illness caused by consumption of the botulism neurotoxin produced by *Clostridium botulinum*, can be deadly, as it can cause paralysis of respiratory and other muscles.[58]

Two newer preservation methods used to keep foods fresh are **modified atmosphere packing (MAP)** and **high-pressure processing (HPP)**. MAP is a process during which the manufacturer modifies the composition of the air surrounding the food in a package, thereby extending shelf-life and preserving the quality of packaged fruits and vegetables.[59] HPP is a method in which foods are exposed to pulses of high pressure that destroy microorganisms. Foods such as jams, fruit juices, fish, vacuum-packed meat products, fruits, and vegetables can be treated with HPP.[60]

Irradiation

Foods can also be treated with ionizing radiation to kill pathogenic bacteria and parasites. During the process of **irradiation**, foods are subjected to a radiant energy source within a protective, shielded chamber called an *irradiator*. The energy from the radiant waves damages the DNA of the pathogens, causing defects in their genetic instructions. Unless the microbes can repair the damage, they die. Because pathogens differ in their sensitivity to irradiation, the process either kills all of them or greatly reduces their numbers, thus reducing the risk of foodborne illness.[61] Unfortunately, irradiation can cause mutations in some bacteria and viruses and may lead to the development of irradiation-resistant strains of these pathogens.[62]

Irradiation is a cold process and does not significantly increase the temperature or change the physical characteristics of most foods, which helps prevent nutrient loss. Also, just as foods cooked in a microwave do not retain microwaves, irradiated foods do not retain the energy waves used during the irradiation process.[63] Most of the irradiating energy passes through the food and the packaging without leaving any residue behind.[64]

Irradiation destroys bacteria such as *Campylobacter*, *E. coli* O157:H7, and *Salmonella* and helps control insects and parasites.[65] It does not destroy viruses, such as norovirus and hepatitis A, or the prions associated with mad cow disease (BSE). The nucleic acid of viruses is too small to be destroyed, and prions—which are protein particles—do not have nucleic acids.

Irradiation can also stop the ripening process in some fruits and vegetables and reduce the number of food spoilage bacteria. Irradiated strawberries can last up to 3 weeks in the refrigerator, compared with only a few days for untreated berries.

Irradiated food has been evaluated for safety by the FDA for more than 30 years.[66] Irradiation has been used for years to sterilize surgical instruments and implants and to destroy disease-promoting microbes in foods served to hospital patients who have weakened immune systems. However, the use of irradiation in foods is not widespread due to consumer concerns and the expense of building the facilities.

Since 1986, all irradiated products must carry the international "radura" symbol, along with the phrase "treated by irradiation" or "treated with radiation" on the package (**Figure 20.8**). If a product such as sausage contains irradiated meat or poultry, these items must be listed as "irradiated pork" or "irradiated chicken" on the food label.[67] A label is not required if a minor ingredient, such as a spice, has been irradiated and used in the product.

Irradiation cannot be used with all foods. It causes undesirable flavor changes in dairy products, egg whites tend to become milky and liquid, fatty meats may develop an odor, and it causes tissue softening in some fruits such as peaches, nectarines, and grapefruits. Foods that are currently approved for irradiation in the United States include fruits and vegetables; herbs and spices; fresh meat, pork, and poultry; wheat flour; and white potatoes.[68]

Although irradiation has many advantages, it doesn't guarantee that a food is free from all pathogens, and some foods such as steak tartare (a dish that contains raw ground

modified atmosphere packaging (MAP) Food preservation technique that changes the composition of the air surrounding the food in a package to extend its shelf-life.

high-pressure processing (HPP) Method used to pasteurize foods by exposing the items to pulses of high pressure, which destroys the microorganisms that are present.

irradiation Process in which foods are placed in a shielded chamber, called an *irradiator*, and subjected to a radiant energy source; kills specific pathogens in food by breaking up the cells' DNA.

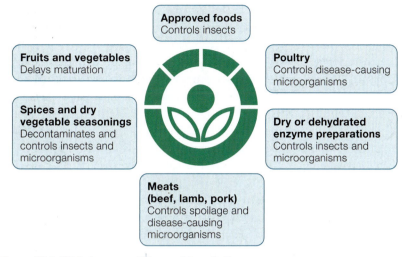

Approved foods
Controls insects

Fruits and vegetables
Delays maturation

Poultry
Controls disease-causing
microorganisms

**Spices and dry
vegetable seasonings**
Decontaminates and
controls insects and
microorganisms

**Dry or dehydrated
enzyme preparations**
Controls insects and
microorganisms

**Meats
(beef, lamb, pork)**
Controls spoilage and
disease-causing
microorganisms

▲ **Figure 20.8 FDA-Approved Uses of Irradiation**
The international radura symbol must appear on all irradiated foods.

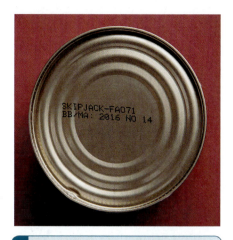

a Closed food product dating refers to the coded packing numbers that you often see on nonperishable foods such as canned soups.

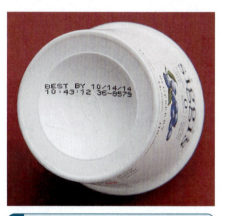

b Open food product dating must contain a calendar date and is used on perishable food items along with information on how to use the date.

▲ **Figure 20.9 Closed and Open Food Product Dating**

beef) should still not be eaten raw, even if they have been irradiated. Irradiation complements but does not replace the need for proper food-handling practices by food growers, processors, and consumers.

Product Dating Identifies Peak Quality

Expiration dates on almost all food products, with the exception of certain poultry, baby food products, and infant formulas, are provided voluntarily by food manufacturers and are not required by federal law. However, currently more than 20 states require some form of mandatory food product dating.

There are two types of food product dating: closed dating and open dating. **Closed (or coded) dating** refers to the packing numbers used by manufacturers that are often found on nonperishable, shelf-stable foods, such as cans of soup and fruit (**Figure 20.9a**). The manufacturer uses this type of dating to keep track of date and time of production, product inventory, and the location of products in the event of a recall.[69]

Open dating is more useful for the consumer and is typically found on perishable items such as meat, poultry, eggs, and dairy foods. Open dating must include at least a month and a day, and if the product is shelf-stable or frozen, the year must also be included (see **Figure 20.9b**). Open dating can help consumers determine if a product is at its peak quality but not if it is safe to eat. For example, a carton of yogurt that has been mishandled and not refrigerated for several hours may be unsafe to eat even though the date on the container hasn't passed.

Open-dated products must also contain a phrase next to the date that tells the consumer how to interpret it. If there is "Sell By" next to the date, the product should be purchased on or before that date. This date takes into consideration additional time for storage and use at home, so if the food is bought by the "Sell By" date it can still be eaten at a later date. If there is "Best if Used By" or "Use By" next to it, the date shows how long the manufacturer thinks a food will be of optimal quality. This does not necessarily mean that the product should not be used after the suggested date, as these dates refer to product quality, not safety.[70]

The Safety of the Water Supply Is Regulated

The Environmental Protection Agency (EPA) is the government body responsible for ensuring that consumers have a safe water supply; the Safe Drinking Water Act (SDWA) is the principal federal statute that affords that protection. Health-based standards are

closed or "coded" dating Refers to the packing numbers that are decodable only by manufacturers and are often found on nonperishable, shelf-stable foods.

open dating Typically found on perishable items such as meat, poultry, eggs, and dairy foods; must contain a calendar date.

set by the EPA to protect the drinking water in the United States from unsafe levels of contaminants. In most cases the EPA delegates to the states responsibility for ensuring that the health standards are met. The EPA collects and stores annual reports of each state's drinking water in a database called the Safe Drinking Water Information System (SDWIS). If there is an immediate threat to consumer health due to violation of a drinking water standard, the SDWA requires that public water systems notify consumers through the media or mail.[71]

Lead is a naturally occurring element found in the soil, air, and water around our homes. Lead exposure from paint and pipes made with lead can be harmful. In children, even low levels of lead in the blood can impair cognitive development. Pregnant women exposed to lead are at risk of premature birth and reduced growth of the fetus, while other adults can experience cardiovascular and kidney dysfunction.[72]

Whereas a small amount of lead in public water is normal, the EPA declared a federal state of emergency when Flint, Michigan, residents were exposed to water containing high levels of lead. The exposure occurred when the city switched to the Flint River as its source for public drinking water. This water's high acidity caused lead in the outdated municipal pipes to leach into the water. Residents were warned to use bottled water for drinking and bathing until the pipes could be replaced in 2020. The city's slow response to the crisis contributed to the residents' contamination and became the subject of national news.

LO 20.3: THE TAKE-HOME MESSAGE Several government agencies, including the FDA and USDA, share responsibility for food safety in the United States. HACCP is a food safety program used by the FDA, the USDA, and the food industry to identify and control hazards that may occur in any part of the food system. Manufacturers may use techniques such as pasteurization, canning, and irradiation to preserve food and destroy contaminants. The FDA has approved the use of irradiation in the U.S. food supply even though some consumers have concerns about the safety of irradiated foods. Most food product dating is provided voluntarily and can help determine peak quality but not food safety. The EPA is responsible for ensuring the safety of our water supply.

What Role Do Food Additives and Other Chemicals Play in Food Production and Safety?

LO 20.4 Compare the risks and benefits of food additives and the use of hormones, antibiotics, and pesticides in both traditionally and organically grown food.

Food manufacturers use various types of **food additives** for many different reasons. Commonly used additives include preservatives (such as antioxidants and sulfites), nutrients, and flavor enhancers (such as MSG). Food producers also give food-producing animals hormones and antibiotics to improve the health and food yield of these animals, but they may cause unintentional side effects in consumers.[73] Other food producers use pesticides on plants to protect them and boost production.

Some Additives Are Used to Preserve Foods

Most food additives are **preservatives** that are added to foods to prevent spoilage (usually by destroying microbes) and increase shelf-life. The most common antimicrobial preservatives are salt and sugar. Salt has been used for centuries, particularly in meat and fish, to

food additives Substances added to food that affect its quality, flavor, freshness, and/or safety.

preservatives Substances that extend the shelf-life of a product by retarding chemical, physical, or microbiological changes.

create a dry environment in which bacteria cannot multiply. Most (65 percent) of the salt consumed in the United States comes from processed and prepared foods that you find in grocery and convenience stores.[74] Sugar is used for the same preserving effect in products such as canned and frozen fruits and condiments.

Nitrites and nitrates are ionic salts, chemical compounds that result from the bonding of a positively charged ion to a negatively charged ion, that are added to foods to prevent microbial growth. They are used in cured meats such as hot dogs and hams to prevent the growth of *Clostridium botulinum*. These chemicals give processed meats their pink color. The use of these salts has been controversial because they form carcinogenic nitrosamines in the GI tract of animals.[75]

The addition of antioxidants to foods can prevent an off taste or off color in a product that's vulnerable to damage by oxidation. Currently the antioxidant vitamins E and C are approved for use as food additives. Fat-soluble vitamin E is often added to oils and cereals to prevent rancidity. Water-soluble vitamin C is often added to cut fruit to prevent premature browning. Butylated hydroxyanisole (BHA) and butylated hydroxytoluene (BHT) are chemical antioxidants that are also used as preservatives. Although some studies into BHT and BHA have linked high amounts to cancer, the current body of research evidence suggests that their use in foods is safe.[76]

Sulfites are a group of antioxidants that are used as preservatives to help prevent the oxidation and browning of some foods and to inhibit the growth of microbes.[77] Sulfites are often found in dried fruits and vegetables, packaged and prepared potatoes, wine, beer, bottled lemon and lime juice, and pickled foods. For most people sulfites pose no risk, but sulfur dioxide causes adverse reactions in some people.[78] The FDA has prohibited the use of sulfites on fruits and vegetables that are served raw, and foods containing sulfite additives or ingredients treated with sulfites must declare "added sulfites" in the ingredients list on the label. Food sold in bulk, such as dried fruit treated with sulfites, must display the ingredients on a sign near the food. Because sulfites destroy the B vitamin thiamin, the FDA prohibits their use in enriched grain products and other foods that are good sources of this vitamin.[79]

Some Additives Enhance Food Quality and Appeal

Food manufacturers also use additives to increase the quality or appeal of their products. Some additives improve food texture and consistency. Others enhance the nutrient content, color, or flavor of food. **Table 20.5** lists some commonly used nonpreservative additives and their functions in foods.

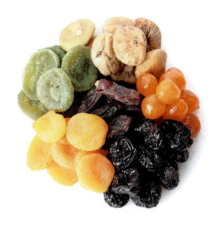

Dried fruits often have sulfur dioxide or other sulfites added to them to preserve color and flavor. People with sulfite sensitivity should avoid products containing these additives.

nitrites and nitrates Substances that can be added to foods to function as a preservative and to give meats such as hot dogs and luncheon meats a pink color.

sulfites Preservatives used to help prevent foods from turning brown and to inhibit the growth of microbes; often used in wine and dried fruit products.

TABLE 20.5	Commonly Used Food Additives	
Additive(s)	**Function(s)**	**Found in**
Alginates, carrageenan, glyceride, guar gum, lecithin, mono- and diglycerides, methyl cellulose, pectin, sodium aluminosilicate	Impart/maintain desired consistency	Baked goods, cake mixes, coconut, ice cream, processed cheese, salad dressings, table salt
Ascorbic acid (vitamin C), calcium carbonate, folic acid, thiamine (B_1), iron, niacin, pyridoxine (B_6), riboflavin (B_2), vitamins A and D, zinc oxide	Improve/maintain nutritive value	Biscuits, bread, breakfast cereals, desserts, flour, gelatin, iodized margarine, milk, pasta, salt
Ascorbic acid, benzoates, butylated hydroxyanisole (BHA), butylated hydroxytoluene (BHT), citric acid, propionic acid and its salts, sodium nitrite	Maintain palatability and wholesomeness	Bread, cake mixes, cheese, crackers, frozen and dried fruit, lard, margarine, meat, potato chips
Citric acid, fumaric acid, lactic acid, phosphoric acid, sodium bicarbonate, tartrates, yeast	Produce light texture and control acidity/alkalinity	Butter, cakes, cookies, chocolates, crackers, quick breads, soft drinks
Annatto, aspartame, caramel, cloves, FD&C Red No. 40, FD&C Blue No. 1, fructose, ginger, limonene, MSG, saccharin, turmeric	Enhance flavor or provide desired color	Baked goods, cheeses, confections, gum, spice cake, gingerbread, jams, soft drinks, soup, yogurt

Source: Adapted from FDA. 2014. *Food Additives Status List*. Available at https://www.fda.gov/food/ingredientspackaginglabeling/foodadditivesingredients/ucm091048.htm. Accessed April 2017.

Additives to Enhance Texture and Consistency

Food additives can enhance the texture and consistency of food in a number of ways. Gums and pectins are often added to thicken yogurts and puddings. Emulsifiers improve the stability, consistency, and homogeneity of high-fat products like mayonnaise and ice cream. Lecithin is an example of an emulsifier that is often added to salad dressings. Leavening agents such as yeast or baking powder cause dough to rise before it's baked. Anticaking agents such as sodium aluminosilicate and calcium carbonate prevent products like powdered sugar that are crystalline in nature from absorbing moisture and lumping. Humectants such as propylene glycol increase moisture in products so that they stay fresh.

Additives to Improve Nutrient Content

Additives can be used to enhance a product's nutritional content, such as when refined grains are enriched and fortified with added B vitamins (folic acid, thiamin, niacin, and riboflavin) and iron. In some cases, the federal government mandates such additions. This was the case in 1996, when the FDA published regulations requiring the addition of folic acid to enriched breads, cereal, and other grain products in order to help decrease the risk of neural tube defects in newborns.

Additives to Improve Color

Additives can also enhance the color of foods. There are two main categories that make up the FDA's list of permitted colors. "Certifiable" color additives are man-made and are derived primarily from petroleum and coal. You can recognize these types of additives by the following prefixes: FD&C, D&C, or Ext. An example is FD&C Yellow, which is often found in cereals and baked goods. The second main category of color additives is obtained largely from plants, animals, or minerals. Examples include caramel and grape color extract.

Adverse physical or allergic reactions to color additives are rare, although FD&C Yellow No. 5 may cause itching and hives in some people. This additive is found in beverages, desserts, and processed vegetables and must be listed as an ingredient on food labels.

MSG to Enhance Flavor

Monosodium glutamate (MSG) is the sodium salt of glutamic acid, a nonessential amino acid, and is often used as a flavor enhancer in Asian foods, canned vegetables and soups, and processed meats. Consumers can buy it in a form that is similar in texture to salt. Although it doesn't have a strong taste of its own, it enhances sweet, salty, sour, and bitter tastes.

After an extensive review, the FDA confirmed that MSG is safe to consume in the amounts typically used in processed foods and cooking (a typical meal that contains MSG has less than 0.5 gram). However, when consumed in large quantities such as 3 or more grams at a time, it may cause short-term reactions in people who are sensitive to it.[80] These reactions, which are called the MSG symptom complex, can include numbness, a burning sensation, facial pressure or tightness, chest pain, rapid heartbeat, and drowsiness. In addition, people with asthma may have difficulty breathing after consuming MSG. For these reasons, the FDA requires that all foods containing MSG declare this ingredient on the food label.

Food Additives Are Regulated by the FDA

Food additives are strictly regulated by the FDA, with consumer safety a top priority. The Federal Food, Drug, and Cosmetic Act of 1938 gave the FDA authority to regulate food and food ingredients, including the use of food additives. The 1958 Food Additives Amendment further mandated that manufacturers document a food additive's safety and obtain FDA approval before using it in a food.[81]

monosodium glutamate (MSG) Sodium salt of glutamic acid, used as a flavor enhancer.

Two categories of food additives were exempted from this amendment. The first category includes substances that were known to be safe before 1958 and were given **prior-sanctioned** status.[82] For example, because nitrates were used to preserve meats before 1958, they have prior-sanctioned status, but *only* for their use in meats. They can't be used in other foods, such as vegetables, without FDA approval. The second category includes substances that have a long history of being safe for consumption, such as salt, sugar, and spices, or have extensive research documenting that they are safe to consume, such as vitamins and MSG. These additives are categorized as **generally recognized as safe (GRAS)** and are exempt from FDA approval.[83]

The FDA continually monitors both prior-sanctioned additives and those with GRAS status to ensure that current research continues to support their safety. To remain on the GRAS list, an additive must not have been found to be carcinogenic in animals or humans and must be safe for human consumption. The 1958 Food Additives Amendment also included the **DeLaney Clause**, which states that no substances that have been shown to cause cancer in animals or humans at any dosage may be added to foods. However, with the present increases in technology and the ability to detect substances at very low levels, the clause is considered outdated. To address this issue the FDA deems additives safe if lifetime use presents no more than a one-in-a-million risk of cancer in human beings. If an additive is suddenly called into question, the FDA can prohibit its use or require that the food manufacturer conduct additional studies to ensure its safety.

The food additives discussed in the preceding sections are all **intentional food additives** used to improve the quality of food products. However, the FDA also regulates **unintentional food additives**, very small amounts of substances that enter foods during packaging or processing. For example, dioxins used during the manufacture of bleached paper such as coffee filters may end up in coffee and other foods and beverages. Dioxins can accumulate in the food chain and are carcinogenic to animals. The FDA requires that dioxin levels in products be so low as to present no health risks to people.[84]

Hormones and Antibiotics Are Provided to Food-Producing Animals

Hormones and antibiotics are two classes of compounds that are sometimes used to improve the health or output of food-producing animals. While the use of these substances is intentional, the resulting changes in the final food product are not, and these changes are a subject of controversy and consumer concern.

Bovine Growth Hormone

Cows naturally produce **bovine growth hormone (BGH)**, also known as bovine somatotropin. Some dairy farmers and ranchers treat their cattle with the naturally occurring form of BGH in order to produce animals that are leaner and produce more milk. Scientists can also produce a synthetic version of the hormone, **recombinant bovine somatotropin (rBST)**, and cows injected with this form can produce up to 25 percent more milk than untreated cows.[85]

Consumer groups and Health Canada (the FDA equivalent in Canada) have questioned the long-term safety of rBST. Traces of both the synthetic and natural form of BGH remain in the meat and milk of cows, and milk from rBST-treated cows has higher levels of IGF-1, a hormone that normally helps some types of cells to grow.[86] The FDA's extensive review of the safety of the use of rBST has found no evidence that it poses any long-term health threat to humans.[87] However, consumer concerns over the long-term safety

prior-sanctioned Substances that the FDA had determined were safe for use in foods prior to the 1958 Food Additives Amendment.

generally recognized as safe (GRAS) Designation given by the FDA to substances intentionally added to food, indicating that the substance is considered safe by experts and is exempted from further testing.

DeLaney Clause Clause in the Food Additives Amendment mandating that additives shown to cause cancer at any level must be removed from the marketplace.

intentional food additives Substances added intentionally to foods to improve food quality.

unintentional food additives Substances that enter into foods unintentionally during manufacturing or processing.

bovine growth hormone (BGH) Hormone that is essential for normal growth and development in cattle.

recombinant bovine somatotropin (rBST) Synthetically made hormone identical to a cow's natural growth hormone, somatotropin, that stimulates milk production; also known as *rBGH (recombinant bovine growth hormone)*.

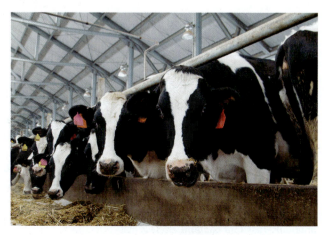

Natural bovine growth hormone, or its synthetic version, are sometimes injected into cows to increase milk production.

of rBST has led to a decrease in the percent of milk produced in the United States from cows treated with rBST.

Other steroid hormones are sometimes used to increase the amount of weight that cattle gain and the amount of meat they produce and to increase milk production in dairy cows. The FDA has approved the use of these hormones in cattle, as they have been shown to be safe at their approved level of use and not a health concern to consumers.[88] However, meat and milk that carry the USDA Organic seal cannot come from cows that were treated with these hormones.

Antibiotics

Antibiotics are sometimes given to livestock for three purposes: (1) to treat animals that are sick, (2) to prevent disease, and (3) to promote growth. When antibiotics are used properly in the treatment of sick animals and to prevent the spread of disease, they are used for a relatively short period of time. However, when used to promote growth and increase the amount of meat and milk produced, they are used over a long period of time.

Pathogenic bacteria such as *Campylobacter*, *E. coli* O157:H7, and *Salmonella* are commonly found in the GI tracts of animals without making them sick. The long-term use of antibiotics in animals can, however, promote the growth of strains of these bacteria that are **antibiotic-resistant**; that is, the bacteria develop features that make them unaffected by the administration of conventional antibiotic medications.[89] This practice poses a risk to anyone who contracts a foodborne infection from the resistant bacteria and is treated with the same antibiotic used to treat the animals. The antibiotic will not destroy the "super bug" because it has developed resistance to the antibiotic during its chronic use in the animals. For example, an outbreak of *Campylobacter*-induced foodborne illness in humans was found to involve a "super-bug" strain of *Campylobacter* that was resistant to treatment with fluoroquinolone, a conventional antibiotic that had been regularly added to animal feed.[90] Health care providers treating infections caused by resistant bacteria must use more powerful antibiotics and/or a longer treatment period.[91]

In 2015 the FDA implemented an update to the veterinary feed directive (VFD), which allows caregivers to use animal feed containing drugs. The new rule requires use of prescription drugs with the oversight of a veterinarian. It thereby helps ensure the judicious use of antibiotics in animals used for food.

Label Terms Indicate How Foods from Animals Are Produced

Both the FDA and USDA are the consumer watchdogs for food labeling, and labeling of foods from animals is essential when it comes to determining how the animals were fed, housed, and treated. The label terms for meat and poultry are determined and defined by the USDA. The following list includes terms often found on prepackaged meat products:[92]

- **No Hormones (pork or poultry).** Hormones are not allowed in raising hogs or poultry. Therefore, the claim "no hormones added" cannot be used on the labels of pork or poultry unless followed by the statement, "Federal regulations prohibit the use of hormones."
- **No Hormones (beef).** The phrase "no hormones administered" may be approved for use on the label of beef products if no hormones have been used in raising the animals.
- **No Antibiotics.** May be used on labels for meat or poultry products if the animals were raised without antibiotics.
- **Certified.** Indicates that the USDA has evaluated a meat product for class, grade, or other quality characteristics (e.g., "Certified Angus Beef").
- **Fresh Poultry.** Poultry that has never had an internal temperature below 26°F (−3.3°C).

antibiotics Drugs that kill or slow the growth of bacteria.

antibiotic-resistant bacteria Bacteria that have developed a resistance to an antibiotic such that they are no longer affected by it.

- **Free Range.** Producers must demonstrate that the animal has been allowed access to the outdoors.
- **Kosher.** Meat and poultry products that were prepared under the supervision of a rabbi.
- **Natural.** The food contains no artificial ingredient or added color and is only minimally processed; that is, using processes that do not fundamentally alter the raw product. The label must explain the use of the term *natural* (such as "no added colorings or artificial ingredients").

Pesticides Are Widely Used in Agriculture

Pesticides are used to prevent plant disease and insect infestations and can be applied to crops in the fields or after harvest. These chemicals increase crop yield by controlling threats to the food supply. Despite the beneficial role that they play in ensuring consumers a wide variety of foods, concerns about pesticides in food persist. The EPA continues to evaluate the safety of each pesticide used on food every 15 years. The Food Quality Protection Act (FQPA) ensures that all pesticides meet strict safety standards.[93]

Types of Pesticides

Several different types of pests can diminish or destroy crop yields, including weeds, insects, microorganisms (bacteria, viruses), fungi (mold), and rodents (rats and mice). **Herbicides** are a type of pesticide used to kill weeds, **insecticides** kill insects, **antimicrobials** are used on microorganisms, **fungicides** are used to destroy mold, and **rodenticides** poison and kill rodents.

Pesticides can be biologically or chemically based. Biologically based pesticides, such as biopesticides and sex pheromones, use material from animals, plants, bacteria, and some minerals and are typically less toxic than chemical pesticides.[94] Unlike chemical pesticides, biopesticides only harm a specific pest, and thus are not harmful to birds and other animals that may come into contact with them. For example, baking soda can be diluted with water and sprayed on plants to inhibit the growth of fungi without risk to animals or humans. Insect sex pheromones can be used to interfere with the reproduction of insects known to harm plants.

Chemically based **organophosphates** make up about half of all insecticides in the United States and are used on fruits, nuts, vegetables, corn, wheat, and other crops, as well as on commercial and residential lawns and plants. They are also used to help control mosquitoes and termites.[95] These pesticides kill pests by affecting their nervous systems, and exposure to humans may have effects on our nervous systems as well.

Antimicrobials, a special type of chemical pesticide that includes disinfectants and sanitizers, are used to destroy and control the spread of microorganisms on surfaces or objects, such as walls, countertops, and floors.[96] Sanitizers are often used in addition to washing with soap and water in food processing plants and in restaurants. Waterless, alcohol-based hand gels that are useful against pathogens are approved by the FDA for use in health care settings but are not approved for use in foodservice and retail establishments. Alcohol-based hand gels do not kill all types of pathogens, though using an antimicrobial hand gel is better than nothing when water and soap are not available for handwashing.[97]

Risks of Pesticides

Chemically based pesticides are not without risks to animals, the environment, and even humans. Residues of these chemicals remain on fruits and vegetables that reach consumers, and infants and young children are particularly susceptible to their hazards. Although a recent EPA review concluded that exposure to organophosphates in food and water to people in the United States likely causes no harm,[98] the EPA has also found that certain pesticides, depending on their level of toxicity and how much is consumed, may cause serious health problems, such as cancer, birth defects, and nerve damage.[99]

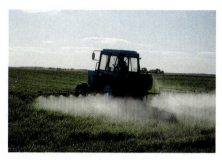

Farmers use pesticides on food crops to diminish the damage from pests such as weeds or insects.

pesticides Substances that kill or repel pests such as insects, weeds, microorganisms, rodents, or fungi.

herbicides Substances that are used to kill and control weeds.

insecticides Pesticides used to kill insects.

antimicrobials Substances or a combination of substances, such as disinfectants and sanitizers, that kill or inhibit the growth of microorganisms.

fungicides Chemicals used to kill mold.

rodenticides Poisons used to kill rats, mice, and other rodents.

organophosphates Group of synthetic pesticides that adversely affect the nervous systems of pests.

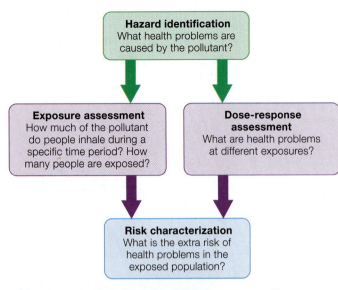

▲ Figure 20.10 EPA's Four-Step Risk Assessment Process
This four-step process is used by the EPA to assess risk of pesticides to humans.

Source: Adapted from Environmental Protection Agency. 1991. *Risk Assessment for Toxic Air Pollutants: A Citizen's Guide.* Available at https://www3.epa.gov/airtoxics/3_90_024.html. Accessed April 2017.

risk assessment Process of determining the potential human health risks posed by exposure to substances such as pesticides.

acceptable tolerance levels Maximum amount of pesticide residue that is allowed in or on foods.

To address these issues, *Healthy People 2020* includes an objective focused on reducing the number of health care visits related to pesticide exposure per year and advocates a reduction in the use of certain potentially dangerous pesticides.[100] In addition, the American Academy of Pediatrics has urged the U.S. government to improve public education, workplace training, science-based research, and the ongoing surveillance of pesticide usage.[101] In order to protect public health and the environment, the types of pesticides and how often they can be used, as well as the amount of residue that can remain on foods when they reach consumers, are heavily regulated in the United States.

Regulation of Pesticides

The EPA requires extensive test data from pesticide producers demonstrating that pesticide products can be used with "a reasonable certainty of no harm." To determine this, the EPA uses a four-step human health **risk assessment** that includes hazard identification, dose–response assessment, exposure assessment, and risk characterization (**Figure 20.10**).

The first step, hazard identification, identifies the potential hazards or ill effects that may develop after exposure to a specific pesticide. Tests looking at a wide range of side effects, from eye and skin irritations to more serious health effects such as cancer, are often performed on laboratory animals.

Because "the dose makes the poison," the second step, dose–response assessment, determines the dose levels at which adverse effects occur in animals and then uses this information to calculate a potentially equal dose in humans.

The third step, exposure assessment, determines all the ways that a person could typically be exposed to that specific pesticide. Most foods are grown with the use of pesticides, so one route of exposure is through eating food. Some pesticides applied to farmland make their way into drinking water supplies, which is another route of exposure. Exposure could also occur through inhalation or absorption through the skin when using household disinfectants or gardening pesticides around the home. The EPA has a separate program for assessing occupational risk and the level of exposure that pesticide applicators and vegetable and fruit pickers face due to the nature of their jobs.

The fourth and last step, risk characterization, is the process of combining the hazard, dose–response, and exposure assessments to determine the pesticide's overall risk. Using the conclusions of a risk assessment, the EPA can make an informed decision regarding whether to approve a pesticide or chemical for use freely or with restrictions.[102]

Acceptable tolerance levels are set using a margin of safety due to the potential differences that exist between the effects of a pesticide on animals and its effect on humans, as well as differences among humans. A safety factor of tenfold or less, depending on the evidence, is added to protect the most vulnerable groups, such as infants and children, for whom the same amount of pesticide provides a larger dose per unit of body weight than for adults.[103] Thus, much effort goes into ensuring that the food supply is safe, yet affordable, so that consumers obtain foods that are nutrient dense while being exposed to a minimum amount of pesticide.

In addition to the EPA, the USDA and the FDA are also involved in regulating pesticides. The EPA is charged with approving pesticides for their specific usages, regulating how much of the pesticide can be used, and establishing acceptable tolerance levels. The USDA enforces the tolerance levels for meat, poultry, and eggs, and the FDA enforces tolerance levels for all other foods.[104]

Alternatives to Pesticides

One method that some growers use to manage pests in their crops is **integrated pest management (IPM)**, which emphasizes the use of the most economical methods to control pests while causing the least risk of harm to the consumer, the crops, or the environment. Growers using the IPM approach use preventative measures, such as rotating crops, choosing pest-resistant strains of plants, and planting nonfood crops nearby to lure away pests.[105] When an infestation occurs, IPM programs are allowed to use targeted spraying of chemical pesticides as a last resort. Most crops in the United States are grown using at least a minimal form of IPM in which farmers identify pests and use a targeted pesticide to treat them.[106]

Minimizing Pesticides in the Diet

More than 80 percent of the pesticide residue remaining on the skins of fruits and vegetables can be removed simply by washing them with clean, running water and scrubbing them with a vegetable brush.[107] Peeling the skin from fruits and vegetables can help reduce pesticide residues and harmful microbes, but it also eliminates some of the fiber and micronutrients. For leafy vegetables such as cabbage and lettuce, the outer leaves can be removed and discarded to minimize risk. Consumers should also be aware that because of the strict pesticide guidelines in place in the United States, the amount of pesticide residue on fruits and vegetables should be below the EPA acceptable tolerance levels even *before* they reach the market.

Eating a variety of produce from a variety of locations also minimizes the consumption of any one type of pesticide. Although people who eat more fruits and vegetables potentially increase their exposure to pesticides, they still typically have a lower risk of cancer than those who eat fewer fruits and vegetables.[108] Locally grown produce may contain fewer pesticides than shipped produce because it does not contain pesticides applied to extend shelf-life. See **Figure 20.11** for a summary of strategies to minimize pesticides in the diet.

Organic Foods Meet USDA National Organic Standards

Organic food production involves growing food using approved methods that integrate cultural, biological, and mechanical practices that conserve resources, promote ecological balance, and conserve biodiversity.[109] Organically grown foods are grown without

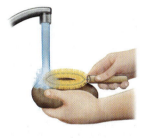
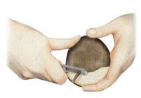
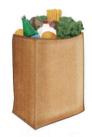
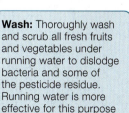

Wash: Thoroughly wash and scrub all fresh fruits and vegetables under running water to dislodge bacteria and some of the pesticide residue. Running water is more effective for this purpose than soaking the fruit and vegetables.

Peel and trim: Peeling fruits and vegetables and discarding the outer leaves of leafy vegetables helps reduce pesticides. Trimming the visible fat from meat and the fatty skin from poultry and fish helps reduce some of the pesticide residue that remains in the fatty tissue of the animal.

Eat a variety of foods: Eating a variety of foods reduces the chance of being overexposed to any particular pesticide.

▲ Figure 20.11 **Reducing Pesticides in Foods**

integrated pest management (IPM) Agricultural technique that uses the most economical and the least harmful methods of pest control to minimize risk to consumers, crops, and the environment.

organic Being free of chemical-based pesticides, synthetic fertilizers, irradiation, and bioengineering; a USDA-accredited certifying inspector must certify organic foods.

the use of most synthetic pesticides, synthetic fertilizers, bioengineering, or irradiation. Only antibiotic-free or growth hormone–free animals can be used to produce organic meat, poultry, eggs, and dairy foods.[110] Many consumers choose organically grown foods over traditionally grown foods because they are concerned about exposure to pesticides and other chemicals or perceive organic foods to be healthier. Consequently, consumer demand for organically grown products continues to increase. The annual growth rate of organically grown foods was 11 percent in 2015.[111] Organically grown foods are big business and annual sales of organically grown products topped $43.3 billion in 2015, according to a survey on the organic food industry from the Organic Trade Association.[112]

The Organic Foods Production Act and the National Organic Standards (NOS) developed in 2002 by the USDA are intended to ensure that the organic foods consumers purchase are produced, processed, and certified consistent with national standards.[113] The NOS provide specific criteria that food producers must meet during production, handling, and processing in order to label their products USDA *organic*. These standards define substances both approved for use and prohibited from use in organic food production. For example, organically grown foods cannot be grown using sewage sludge, and a USDA-accredited inspector must certify the farming and processing operations that produce and handle foods labeled as organic.[114]

Consumers who purchase organically grown and processed foods should not assume that they are pesticide free. Organically grown crops may come into contact with chemicals due to drift from wind and rainwater. Also, though organic farmers use IPM, and grow more disease- and pest-resistant plants, they can also use synthetic pesticides and biopesticides to control weeds and insects. Allowed synthetic pesticides include certain insecticidal soaps, microbials, botanicals, and minerals, whereas some natural substances, such as ash from the burning of manure, are prohibited from use in organic farming.[115]

There is no conclusive evidence that organically grown foods are nutritionally superior to foods grown using conventional methods.[116,117] Although organically grown foods differ in the ways they are grown, handled, and processed, and these differences do reduce exposures to pesticide residues, growth hormones, and antibiotic-resistant strains of bacteria, they do not appear to result in significant differences to the nutrient content of food.[118] A balanced and varied diet can support health regardless of whether the foods were grown organically or conventionally.

The USDA strictly regulates labeling of organic foods. Foods that display the USDA Organic Seal (**Figure 20.12**) or otherwise state that they are organic must contain at least 95 percent organic ingredients. A food label can state, "Made with Organic Ingredients" if it contains at least 70 percent organic ingredients. Labels of foods with less than 70 percent organic ingredients can make no organic claims.

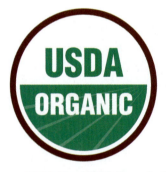

▲ **Figure 20.12 The USDA Organic Seal** Foods that are labeled or advertised with the USDA Organic Seal must contain at least 95 percent organic ingredients.

LO 20.4: THE TAKE-HOME MESSAGE The FDA strictly regulates all compounds intentionally added to foods or provided to food-producing animals. Food additives have long been used for food preservation and are often used by modern manufacturers to enhance texture, color, flavor, or nutrient content. Growth hormone is often given to dairy cows to increase milk production. Animal feed containing low doses of antibiotics has been used to increase the growth of cattle, poultry, and pigs, but can lead to the development of antibiotic-resistant strains of bacteria. All intentional food additives must be listed on food labels. Pesticides are used to destroy or mitigate pests and increase crop yield. Consumers can minimize exposure to plant pesticides by washing and trimming foods during preparation and by eating a wide variety of foods. The USDA developed National Organic Standards (NOS) that help to assure consumers that foods labeled as USDA organic are grown without the use of most synthetic pesticides, synthetic fertilizers, bioengineering, or irradiation.

What Is a Sustainable Food System?

LO 20.5 Explain what constitutes a sustainable food system.

There are currently more than 7 billion people in the world and that number is expected to increase by 2 billion people by 2050.[119] How will we provide safe and nutritious food for the growing number of people, given the limited resources available? This question deserves our attention and will require changes at all levels of our current food system.

A **sustainable** food system is one that can be maintained indefinitely without depleting or polluting natural resources. According to the position of the Academy of Nutrition and Dietetics, sustainable food systems conserve, renew, and protect natural resources; empower social responsibility to uphold the system; and are economically viable because they build community wealth (**Figure 20.13**).[120] All food systems are affected by social, political, economic, and environmental factors and depend on both human and natural resources. Sustainable food systems produce food using minimal natural resources, such as soil and water, and transport food using minimal energy. Thus, a sustainable diet contains foods that are produced in ways that are ecologically neutral.

Numerous natural resources, of two types, are used when growing crops and raising animals for food. *Internal natural resources* are used to produce foods. *External natural resources* are used to move food products from the farm to the consumer. Both internal and external resources generate natural and man-made by-products that affect the environment.

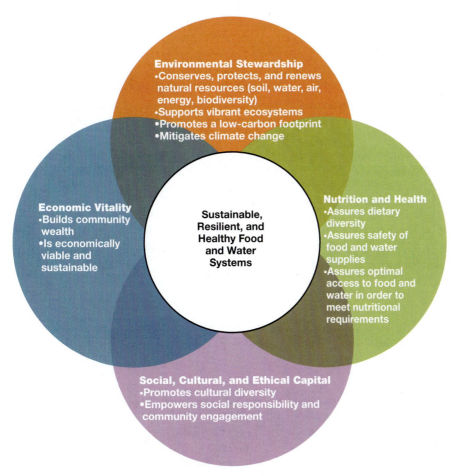

▲ **Figure 20.13 Sustainable, Resilient, and Healthy Food and Water Systems Framework**

Source: A. Tagtow, K. Robien, E. Bergquist, M. Mruening, L. Dierks, B. E. Hartman, et al. 2014. Academy of Nutrition and Dietetics: Standards of Professional Performance for Registered Dietitian Nutritionists (Competent, Proficient, and Expert) in Sustainable, Resilient, and Healthy Food and Water Systems. *Journal of the Academy of Nutrition and Dietetics* 114(3):475–488.

sustainable Referring to a method of resource use that can be maintained indefinitely because it does not deplete or permanently damage the resource.

Preserving Internal Natural Resources Is the First Step toward Sustainability

Abuse of any of the natural resources required to grow foods can prevent sustainability. Soil, biodiversity, energy, and water are the key internal natural resources that must be preserved in a sustainable food system. **Table 20.6** describes several of the challenges associated with using internal resources, including land and water, to produce food, and various strategies that can be employed to protect the environment.

Soil

More than a billion tons of topsoil, the layer of soil that sits atop the earth's crust, is lost each year from erosion.[121] It's not surprising, then, that numerous experts are concerned about soil degradation. All land organisms ultimately depend on the earth's soil. Organisms within the soil, such as bacteria and other microorganisms, feed on the nutrients provided by animal waste products and decaying plant and animal matter. Plants use nutrients in the soil to grow and to produce fruits, vegetables, nuts, and seeds. Humans and animals later obtain these same nutrients when they eat the plants and plant products.

Just as all organisms depend on healthy soil for survival, healthy soil depends on the organisms to anchor it in place and to keep it well oxygenated. Plant roots help hold soil in place, which protects it from water and wind erosion, and they also break up the soil to allow the dispersal of oxygen. As topsoil is formed and regenerated from decaying plants, organisms, animals, and rocks, a perpetual web of dependency is formed.

TABLE 20.6 Environmental Effects of Food Production

The Effect	The Challenge	How Can We Minimize the Environmental Impact?
Land overuse	Excessive use of farming equipment, overtilling, and livestock overgrazing can all damage soil.	Proper land management and conservation methods of tilling can help preserve the land and replenish soil nutrients.
Soil erosion	Wind and rain can cause more than 1.5 billion tons of nutrient-rich topsoil to be blown and washed away each year. When fertile topsoil is lost, crop yield declines.	Proper crop covering and shielding from wind as well as proper tillage of the soil can dramatically reduce erosion.
Water depletion	Irrigation accounts for 80 percent of water consumption in the United States; hence, excessive irrigation can deplete naturally occurring groundwater.	Precision farming and the conscious reduction of overwatering can help preserve water.
Water runoff	After a rainfall (or watering of crops), the water runoff from farms can spread pesticides from crops and pathogens in animal manure to other fields, surface water, and downfield rivers and streams, contaminating these ecosystems.	Basins can be installed to collect the runoff water to prevent contamination prior to discharge to streams and rivers.
Airborne emissions	Emissions of ammonia and nitrogen in manure are released into the air. The ammonia released from these airborne emissions can settle on water surfaces, killing fish and encouraging the growth of toxic algae, both of which disrupt the natural ecosystem.	The proper handling of manure (see below) mitigates this problem.
Nitrate production	The production of nitrates from the nitrogen in manure can pollute surface water and groundwater that is used as drinking water.	Proper collection, stockpiling, and disposal of manure to minimize the leaching of nitrates into runoff and groundwater, as proposed in the latest EPA regulations, helps concentrated animal feeding operations (CAFOs) to safely manage manure.

Sources: Data from A. H. Harmon and B. L. Gerald. 2007. Position of the American Dietetic Association: Food and Nutrition Professionals Can Implement Practices to Conserve Natural Resources and Support Ecological Sustainability. *Journal of the American Dietetic Association* 107:1033–1043; US Department of Agriculture, Economic Research Service. 2016. *Irrigation and Water Use*. Available at https://www.ers.usda.gov/topics/farm-practices-management/irrigation-water-use.aspx Accessed April 2017; U.S. Environmental Protection Agency. 2015. *Ag 101: Beef Production*. Available at https://www.epa.gov/sites/production/files/2015-07/documents/ag_101_agriculture_us_epa_0.pdf. Accessed April 2017.

Problems arise when the topsoil can't be regenerated and/or is less fertile. When this happens plants cannot grow, the web is severed, and nourishment for the local microorganisms, plants, animals, and humans is reduced. The natural process of regenerating one inch of nutrient-rich topsoil takes more than 500 years.[122] Improper agricultural practices that facilitate erosion of soil faster than it can be regenerated disrupt the entire web and food system.[123] However, research shows that crop rotation and other aspects of organic farming result in less soil erosion than conventional farming methods.[124]

Biodiversity

Achieving and maintaining biodiversity is an important part of a sustainable food system, and the extinction of even one member of the web can have dramatic consequences. Since 2006 the United States has seen the rapid decline in the honeybee population, termed *colony collapse disorder*, which has reduced the pollination, and therefore availability, of fruits, vegetables, and tree nuts (an estimated 30 percent of the foods that you eat need pollination to flourish).[125] Lack of biodiversity among aquatic systems is also a potential problem. More than 60 percent of commercial fisheries are overharvested, endangering the existence of more than 30 percent of native fish in North America.[126] As biodiversity is reduced, the variety and nutritional quality of foods available may also be reduced.

Plants draw nutrients from the soil through their roots, which in turn help anchor the soil in place, preventing erosion.

Energy

Research suggests that around 15 percent of the total energy consumption in the United States is used in the production, processing, transport, and preparation of our food.[127] Much of this is consumed as an external resource during processing and transport; however, some is used as an internal resource during the growth and production of food. For example, more energy (as well as land and water) is required to produce a meat-based diet than to produce a plant-based diet.[128] In order to produce every pound of animal protein in the form of edible beef, 10.6 pounds of plant food and 8 gallons of water in the form of feed are required.[129] Allowing livestock to graze on pasture rather than feeding them a grain diet would cut the amount of fuel needed to produce and transport feed grain in half. Producing chemical fertilizers and pesticides for crops also requires large amounts of fossil fuels.[130] Avoiding these chemicals and using natural fertilizers, such as animal manure, not only cuts the use of fossil fuel, but also can make soil more fertile.[131]

Water

According to the EPA, since the 1950s, the population in America has nearly doubled and our water consumption has more than tripled.[132] This heightened demand for water is a danger not only to the environment but also to your health. You need water to survive; therefore, conserving water now to ensure a healthy supply in the future makes sense.

In 2016 more than 40 percent of America's total water use went to toilets and showers.[133] In order to reduce this water waste, the EPA sponsors Water Sense, which is a voluntary label that manufacturers, retailers, and distributors can use to indicate that their models use at least 20 percent less water than regular product models.[134] If all households installed water-efficient fixtures, the United States would save more than 3 trillion gallons of water annually.[135] Other steps you can take to reduce water waste include using water-saving washing machines and dishwashers, taking short showers, and turning off the tap while washing dishes or brushing your teeth.

Locally Grown Food Requires Fewer External Natural Resources

External natural resources used to move food products from the farm to the consumer can contribute greatly to the environmental costs of food production. For example, the use of fossil fuels to grow, process, and transport food contributes to the release of carbon dioxide gas emissions. The carbon dioxide and other gases released when fossil fuels are burned for energy are referred to as *greenhouse gases*, as these gases absorb and trap heat in the air and re-radiate that heat downward. Global temperature has increased by 1.4°F since the 20th century and continues to increase because of the release of these greenhouse gases.[136] Carbon emissions associated with the transport of food from farm to supermarket are substantial, and consumers use additional fuel to drive to the supermarket and to prepare food at home. The amount of fossil fuel used to transport that produce all those miles, coupled with the increase in carbon dioxide gas emissions into the air from burning that fuel, has enormous environmental costs.

Natural resources aside, these fuel costs are factored into the price of the food, so they affect consumers' financial resources. A percentage of your food dollars goes toward the cost of getting food from the farm to your plate, though fuel is used in other aspects of food production as well.[137] And as the price of fuel increases, the price that you pay for food increases. Thus, the farther your food has to travel, the more resources it uses, which not only has a negative effect on the environment, but also is a drain on your wallet.

Because of the environmental and financial costs of shipping foods over long distances, some people are becoming **locavores**. Locavores try to buy from local farms, farmers markets, and roadside stands rather than supermarkets. They may have difficulty consuming 100 percent of their diet from local sources year round. For example, although Vermonters have access to fresh dairy foods 365 days a year, robust fruit and vegetable crops are hard to find under a foot of snow in the winter. Depending on where they live, locavores may have to supplement with foods from the supermarket. Farmers markets are an important resource for people who value food grown locally. See the Spotlight on page 765.

Many large supermarkets now sell locally grown produce. This combining of locally grown foods with conventionally grown foods allows consumers to do "one-stop shopping" rather than have to drive to farmers markets, farm stands, or **community-supported agriculture (CSA)** pickups in addition to the supermarket. Corporate America is also making it easier to eat locally. Some large corporations and industrial complexes have weekly farmers markets on their premises. Employees can shop for locally grown foods during the day and head home with the fixings for dinner.[138] The USDA recently awarded more than $5 million in grants to support local food connections between farmers and consumers, even in large cities, with its "Know Your Farmer, Know Your Food" initiative.[139]

Some individuals wrongfully assume that locally grown food is the same as sustainably grown food. A *sustainable diet* contains foods that meet your nutrient and health needs but can be produced for a long time without negatively affecting the environment.[140] Buying food from small local farms doesn't guarantee that the foods were grown in a sustainable way, nor does being from a distant farm mean that those farmers didn't practice sustainable agriculture.

> **LO 20.5: THE TAKE-HOME MESSAGE** A sustainable food system is one that will survive over the long term. To maintain a sustainable food system, the natural resources used to produce, transport, and distribute the food are conserved instead of being destroyed or depleted. Minimal natural resources such as soil and water and energy are depleted to grow, harvest, and transport the food. A sustainable diet contains foods that are produced in a way that is ecologically neutral. Natural resources are used internally to produce foods and externally to move foods from producers to consumers. Buying locally grown food decreases the amount of fuel needed to transport food and is one way to reduce the use of external natural resources in food systems.

locavore Person who eats locally grown food whenever possible.

community-supported agriculture (CSA) Arrangement where individuals pay a fee to support a local farm, and in exchange receive a weekly or biweekly box of fresh produce from the farm.

Farmers Markets

According to the USDA, farmers markets are an integral part of the urban–farm linkage and their growth has continued to rise. The number of farmers markets nationwide has increased 2.3 percent, from 1,755 in 1994 to 8,669 in 2016.[1] The USDA estimates that these markets generate approximately $1 billion in consumer spending each year. Most of this growth, a boon to local communities' economies, can be attributed to consumer interest in obtaining fresh products directly from the farm. In many cases consumers have the opportunity to personally interact with the farmer who grows the produce.

The USDA, in conjunction with the Agricultural Marketing Service (AMS), provides technical support to managers of farmers markets by hosting conferences and training sessions throughout the country to present research findings and information on marketing strategies with agricultural producers, economists, state Department of Agriculture personnel,

and other parties interested in supporting direct farm marketing venues. Many farmers markets accept WIC (Women, Infants, and Children) vouchers and SNAP (Supplemental Nutrition Assistance Program) vouchers and provide nutrition education and food preparation demonstrations in conjunction with local and state health departments.

The USDA's AMS has also formed the Farmers Market Consortium, which is a public-/private-sector partnership dedicated to helping farmers markets by sharing information about funding and resources available to them. The consortium publishes the *Farmers Market Resource Guide* that provides a centralized repository of information about federal and private resources that support farmers markets. The USDA also publishes the *National Farmers Market Directory* that organizes farmers markets by state and includes contact information, dates, and times of operation.

Produce sold at farmers markets is available according to the season;

although adapting to eating seasonally can be an adjustment, it is more environmentally friendly because produce is not transported long distances for sale.

Farmers markets vary by what can be sold but generally a product must be grown or raised or made (baked, canned, and so on) by the farm selling it. "Local" is also usually understood to mean food that comes from independent farmers and producers rather than from large corporations.

Costs at farmers markets vary and sometimes produce may be more expensive than at a grocery store. Food bought in the conventional system where pesticides are used and the food is transported thousands of miles and stored in warehouses is heavily subsidized at all stages of production and incurs costs not reflected in the purchase price. These costs include depleted fossil fuel reserves for fertilizer, cultivation, and transportation; water pollution from pesticide runoff; and the contribution of emissions to global warming.

Some products sold at farmers markets are certified organic, whereas others use integrated pest management (IPM) or use organic methods but are not USDA certified. Farmers sell directly to consumers for a number of reasons and those who do generally care for their land and use sustainable growing practices to keep it healthy.

Farmers markets are good for the local economy, the health of the land, and the health of the people. The USDA's farmers market locator tells you where to find a farmers market near you: *http://search. ams.usda.gov/farmersmarkets*.

Reference

1. USDA. Agricultural Marketing Service. n.d. *Farmers Markets and Direct-to-Consumer Marketing.* Available at https://www.ams.usda.gov/services/local-regional/farmers-markets-and-direct-consumer-marketing. Accessed April 2017.

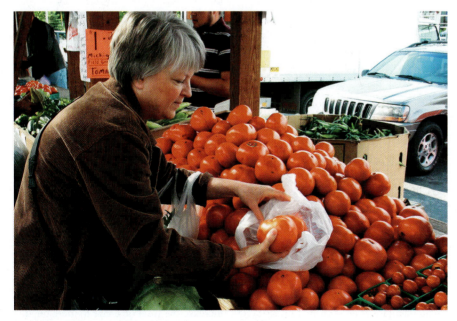

Farmers markets provide fresh produce to the consumer.

Is Genetically Engineered Food Safe?

LO 20.6 Compare the benefits and risks of the use of biotechnology in our current food system.

Historically, farmers have crossbred plants by trial and error, crossing two plants to produce a hybrid offspring with the desired combination of characteristics. For example, if one tree produced large apples with thinner skins and another produced smaller, sour apples with thicker skins, an ancient apple farmer might have bred the two in the hope of producing a tree with large, fleshy, hardy fruit. This process is called **cross-breeding**. Today's apples are an example of a plant food that has resulted from generations of deliberate cross-breeding.

For thousands of years, humans have cross-bred different versions of plants and animals to produce more desirable offspring. The offspring contain qualities from both parents, and it usually takes dozens of additional crosses and many years to separate the desirable traits from the less desirable ones.

In the last century, as scientists have come to understand more about the workings of DNA and how to manipulate it, the process of cross-breeding for particular

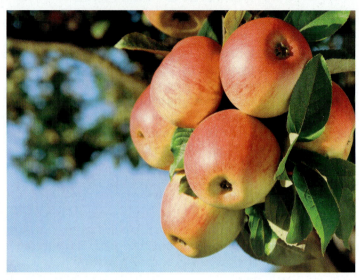

The apples of today are larger and sweeter than their ancestors, thanks to hundreds of years of selective breeding.

characteristics has become faster and more controlled. Today, scientists use **biotechnology** to modify the **genomes** of plants and animals to create desired characteristics with great precision. American farmers routinely use selectively bred, genetically modified plants to create disease-resistant crops that produce larger, hardier fruits and vegetables and increase overall crop yields. The production of foods using plant or animal products that have been modified genetically helps to keep food costs low and availability high. In fact, the majority of fruits and vegetables on the market today are a product of genetic modification.[141]

Genetic Engineering Is the Latest Form of Biotechnology

Genetic engineering (GE) allows scientists to alter the genetic makeup of an organism by manipulating DNA sequences. In genetic engineering, or bio-engineering, an exact gene or genes from the DNA sequence of an organism are isolated and inserted into the DNA of another species to create the genetically modified product (**Figure 20.14**).

This cutting and splicing of genes into the genome of another cell is called *recombinant DNA technology*. Organisms that have

been genetically engineered to contain both original and foreign genes are called **genetically modified organisms (GMOs)**. These GMOs are used to grow genetically engineered (GE) plants that produce GE foods.

Farmers in the United States have adopted GE crops widely since their introduction in 1996. Soybeans and cotton genetically engineered with herbicide-resistant traits have been the most widely accepted crops. According to the USDA's National Agricultural Statistics Service (NASS), in 2013, 90 percent of the corn, 93 percent of the soybeans, and 90 percent of the cotton planted in the United States were genetically engineered varieties.[142]

Proponents Believe GMOs Can Increase the World's Food Supply

Many experts believe that GMOs are part of the solution to the problem of meeting the world population's need for food with limited resources. GMOs have helped to increase the yield of crops in the United States and can do the same for developing countries that struggle to produce food.[143] Genetic engineering may also create new uses for plants in industries such as pharmaceuticals and manufacturing.

cross-breeding Type of biotechnology in which two plants or two animals with different qualities are bred to produce offspring with desired traits from both.

biotechnology Manipulation of living organisms or their components to develop or manufacture useful products.

genome Total genetic information of an organism stored in the DNA of its chromosomes.

genetic engineering (GE) Biological technique that isolates and manipulates the genes of organisms to produce a targeted, modified product.

genetically modified organisms (GMOs) Organisms that have been genetically engineered to contain both original and foreign genes.

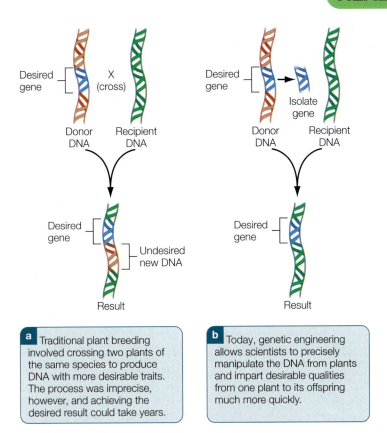

a Traditional plant breeding involved crossing two plants of the same species to produce DNA with more desirable traits. The process was imprecise, however, and achieving the desired result could take years.

b Today, genetic engineering allows scientists to precisely manipulate the DNA from plants and impart desirable qualities from one plant to its offspring much more quickly.

▲ **Figure 20.14 Traditional Cross-Breeding versus Genetic Engineering**

The original purpose of GE plants was to reduce the amount of pesticides used on food crops by engineering the plants themselves to be more resistant to pests. This would benefit both the health of consumers and the environment.[144] For example, the bacterium *Bacillus thuringiensis (Bt)*, which is found naturally in soil, produces a toxin that is poisonous to certain pests but not to humans or animals. When the gene for this toxin is inserted into a crop plant, the plant becomes resistant to these pests.[145] Some corn crops in the United States contain the *Bt* gene, which makes them resistant to some insect pests (**Figure 20.15**). Because chemical insecticides are not necessary, many benign insects are spared, and insect **biodiversity** is retained. Almost 15 percent of corn and cotton harvested in the United States in 2012 were varieties genetically engineered to contain the *Bt* gene.[146]

Another goal of the first-generation GE products was to use this technology to improve a crop's tolerance to herbicides. With an herbicide-resistant version of a desired crop, a farmer can spray herbicide over a field to kill a variety of weeds without harming the crop. Unfortunately, this liberal application of herbicide has led to the development of herbicide-resistant "super-weeds," as discussed shortly. According to the USDA, approximately 93 percent of soybeans planted in 2013 were genetically modified to be herbicide resistant.[147]

The second generation of GE products to hit the market was designed for increased shelf-life and improved nutrient composition.[148] Tomatoes that stay firm and ripe longer were among the first genetically engineered foods to be sold to consumers. An example of a genetically altered plant with an improved nutrient profile is "golden rice." In countries like Southeast Asia, India, and Africa rice is a staple of the diet. Golden rice has gene segments from a bacterium and a daffodil that instruct the rice plant cells to synthesize beta-carotene and to concentrate the levels of iron (**Figure 20.16**). If successfully cultivated by farmers and accepted

biodiversity Variability among living organisms on the earth, including the variability within and between species and within and between ecosystems.

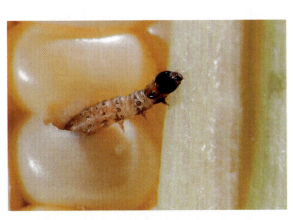

▲ **Figure 20.15 European Corn Borer Caterpillar**
Bt corn has been genetically engineered to produce a protein that is toxic to the larvae of the European corn borer, the most damaging insect pest of corn in North America.

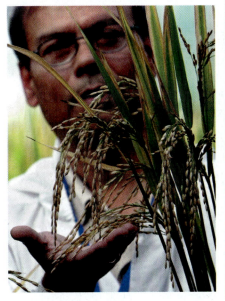

▲ **Figure 20.16 Genetically Engineered Golden Rice**
"Golden rice" is rich in both beta-carotene and iron and is a product of genetic engineering. Because of agricultural and political challenges, golden rice is not yet commercially available.

by consumers, golden rice could help eliminate the epidemic of vitamin A and iron deficiency in Asia and worldwide.[149] Although the beta-carotene from golden rice has been found to be bioavailable[150] and despite decades of development, golden rice has yet to be distributed, as finding a strain productive enough for farms to grow successfully and gaining consumer acceptance have been challenges. Another example of a genetically modified food with an improved nutrient profile is high-oleic-acid soybeans, which produce oil that is less prone to becoming rancid and thus is more stable when used for frying foods.

Genetic research has progressed to third-generation GE products that hold promise in the pharmaceutical, environmental, and industrial arenas. In fact, the first GE product created for commercial use was human insulin (needed by diabetics) produced by genetically engineered *E. coli* bacteria. Geneticists are currently exploring techniques for genetically engineering GI tract cells to produce insulin for patients with diabetes.[151] Plants can also be genetically modified to create substances with numerous medical uses, such as vaccines, antibiotics, anticlotting drugs, hormones, and substitutes for certain blood substances.[152] Scientists are currently experimenting with the concept of "growing" vaccines for measles, hepatitis B, and norovirus in produce.[153]

Some Consumers and Environmentalists Have Concerns about GMOs

Some consumers and environmentalists have concerns about the long-term effects of GMOs on human health and on the environment. These include the unintentional introduction of genes and proteins into non-GM foods, disruption of ecosystems, and introduction of herbicide-resistant superweeds, as mentioned earlier.[154]

Unintentional Transfer of Genes and Proteins

Proteins from GM crops have been found in wild, non-GM crops several miles distant. Wind pollination and seed dispersal are mechanisms that can lead to this unintentional cross-breeding. Some of the proteins transferred to non-GM foods could be allergens.[155] Under the FDA's biotech policy, food companies must declare on food labels when a product includes a gene from one of the common allergy-causing foods, unless the company can show that the protein produced by the added gene does not cause allergies.[156] The following eight foods account for 90 percent of all food allergies: milk, eggs, peanuts, tree nuts, fish, shellfish, soy, and wheat.[157] The effects of introducing genes from allergenic foods into other products must be carefully assessed before these GM products are released for human consumption. Recently, GE salmon was approved by the FDA. This salmon grows twice as fast as wild salmon, and therefore has the potential to supply an increasingly demanding food market. The salmon are sterile and are confined to enclosures; however, if only a small percentage of the fish were not sterile and escaped into the wild, genes could be transferred from GE salmon to wild salmon.[158]

Disruption of Ecosystems and Development of Superweeds

We noted above concerns that GMOs could lead to the disruption of ecosystems. A common example is the recent and dramatic decline (by about 80 percent between 2005 and 2015) in the population of monarch butterflies. Although climate change is almost certainly a factor, depletion of milkweed (the monarch caterpillar's food source) due to heavy application of powerful herbicides on herbicide-resistant GM crops is also thought to play a key role.[159]

Similarly, liberal application of herbicides on genetically engineered herbicide-resistant crops has fostered the development of superweeds throughout the United States and in 18 countries worldwide.[160] Some experts predict that, as a direct result of the use of herbicide-resistant GM crops, the use of herbicides will more than double between 2013 and 2025.[161]

Other concerns have arisen about GMOs leading to the unintentional production of plant toxins, changes in the nutrient content and substances in foods, and the production of unsafe animal feed. **Table 20.7** lists the regulations the FDA has put in place to address these issues.

GE Foods Are Highly Regulated in the United States

Genetic engineering is tightly regulated in the United States. GE foods are regulated by the same three government agencies that regulate pesticides: the FDA, USDA, and EPA. The FDA ensures that GE foods are safe to eat and labeled if they contain a suspected allergen. The USDA ensures that the plants are safe to grow, while the EPA makes certain that the gene for any pesticide, such as that for *Bt* toxin, inserted into a plant is safe and won't have adverse environmental effects. Though these agencies work together to ensure the safety of GE foods, the FDA has the overall authority to remove any GE food that doesn't meet the same high safety standards that are set for its conventionally grown equivalent.[162]

The FDA must review and approve all GE products before they are allowed on the market. As part of this process, the FDA mandates that the developers of GE foods conduct extensive tests to ensure their safety, then send the FDA a report of the findings. The FDA reviews the documentation and seeks additional information as warranted. Once all

TABLE 20.7	Concerns and Regulations for GE Foods
Concern	**FDA Regulation**
Undesirable genetic modification	To avoid the creation of undesirable products, all genes used must not have prior evidence of encoding any harmful substances. The genes must also be stably inserted into the plant in order to avoid any rearranging of genetic information that would produce an undesirable substance.
Introduction of allergens	GE foods must be monitored for food allergens. Protein encoded from common allergen food sources (such as milk, eggs, fish, tree nuts, and legumes) should be presumed to be allergens and should be labeled as such on the GE food.
Excessive level of toxins	GE foods should not contain natural toxins at levels that are higher than those found naturally in plants.
Changes in nutrients	All GE foods should be monitored to assess unintentional changes in the nutrient levels in the plants and their ability to be utilized in the human body as compared with their conventional counterparts.
Creation of new substances	If the genes that are introduced into plants encode substances that are different in structure and function than those normally found in foods, these substances would need to be approved by the FDA, as would any other food additive. However, if these substances are GRAS or "substantially equivalent" to substances that already exist in foods, they do not need the FDA's premarket approval.
Unsafe animal feeds	Because a single plant type may be the predominant food source in an animal feed, all GE animal feeds must meet the same strict safety standards that are in place for food that is grown for humans.

Source: U.S. FDA. 2017. *How FDA Regulates Food from Genetically Engineered Plants*. Available at https://www.fda.gov/Food/IngredientsPackagingLabeling/GEPlants/ucm461831.htmhtm. Accessed April 2017.

FDA guidelines are satisfied, the food is considered safe and is allowed to enter the market. More than 50 GE foods, including canola oil, corn, cottonseed oil, potatoes, soybeans, squash, and tomatoes, have been evaluated by the FDA and are considered as safe as their conventional counterparts.[163] The FDA has yet to approve any GE meat for human consumption, but as noted earlier has approved a GE salmon that grows faster than normal.[164]

Most consumers want genetically engineered foods to be labeled; however, the FDA has concluded that because there isn't any scientific evidence that GE foods differ from their conventionally grown counterparts, labeling isn't warranted.[165] The American Medical Association and the Society of Toxicology share this position.[166,167] Canada follows the United States in this regard. If a manufacturer chooses to voluntarily label a product, it may state that the product has been "genetically engineered." Mandatory labeling of GE foods is required in other countries across the world, including in the European Union, Japan, Australia, and New Zealand.[168]

Consumer acceptance of GE foods is increasing as a result of such foods becoming more common, their putative health benefits, and improved quality, but many consumers remain skeptical. In a recent survey, 88 percent of scientists but only 37 percent of the general public agreed that it is generally safe to eat GE foods.[169] Though many questions remain as to the long-term safety and impact of introducing GE foods into the world's food supply, GMOs offer attractive options for feeding the world's population now and in the future. An advanced technology of direct genome editing may permit modification without the use of recombinant DNA. This may increase the acceptance of GE foods in countries where they are poorly accepted.[170]

LO 20.6: THE TAKE-HOME MESSAGE Traditional cross-breeding and modern genetic engineering are types of biotechnology that alter an organism's genetic makeup to create a new plant or animal with more desirable traits. Many GM crops, including corn, soybeans, and potatoes, are currently available in the United States and are commonly used as ingredients in processed foods. Genetically engineered crops can be developed to be pest resistant, to provide additional nutrients, and to enhance flavor and quality. GE products are heavily regulated to minimize undesirable genetic modifications, the introduction of potential allergens, and unfavorable nutrient changes in food. However, health and environmental concerns remain. Labeling is not currently mandatory for GE foods in the United States.

Visual Chapter Summary

LO 20.1 Foodborne Illness Is Caused by Pathogens and Toxins

Pathogens (viruses, bacteria, molds, parasites, and prions) cause foodborne infection. Toxins produced by bacteria or present in food, either naturally or through chemical contamination, can cause foodborne intoxication. Norovirus is the single greatest cause of foodborne illness in the United States. The most common bacteria that cause foodborne illness are *Salmonella*, *Clostridium perfringens*, *Campylobacter*, and *Staphylococcus aureus*. Marine toxins and chemical contaminants, such as PCBs and methylmercury, can bioaccumulate to toxic levels in large fish. Older adults, children, pregnant women, and people with certain disorders have compromised immunity and are at higher risk of contracting foodborne illness and suffering complications.

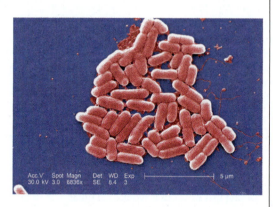

LO 20.2 Proper Food Handling Can Prevent Foodborne Illness

Proper food-handling techniques during four critical steps—cleaning, combating cross-contamination, cooking, and chilling—can help reduce the risk of foodborne illness. Handwashing is the first step in avoiding foodborne illness. Foodborne bacteria multiply most rapidly in temperatures between 40° and 140°F (4.4–60°C), a range known as the danger zone. Cold foods should be stored and served below 40°F, and hot foods must be kept above 140°F. The only sure way to tell if a food has reached a safe temperature is to measure it using a kitchen thermometer. Extra caution is needed when traveling abroad, particularly in developing countries, to avoid foodborne illness. As a general guideline to avoid foodborne illness while traveling, do not eat raw produce unless you wash and peel it first, and avoid drinking tap water or using ice made from tap water unless the water is boiled or treated with iodine or chlorine first.

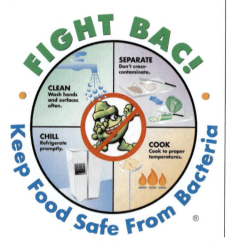

LO 20.3 Everyone Plays a Role in Protecting Our Food Supply

Everyone, from the farmer to the consumer, plays an important role in food safety. Through the coordinated effort of the Food Safety Initiative, numerous U.S. government agencies work together to safeguard America's food supply against foodborne illness. Hazard Analysis and Critical Control Point (HACCP) procedures are used by both the FDA and USDA to identify and control foodborne hazards that occur in all stages of the food system. Food manufacturers use techniques such as pasteurization, canning, and irradiation to help keep food safe for extended periods of time. Food irradiation exposes a food item to a radiant energy source that kills or greatly reduces some pathogens. Food product dating is not a measure of food safety, but can be used to determine peak quality. The EPA monitors and regulates the safety of the water supply.

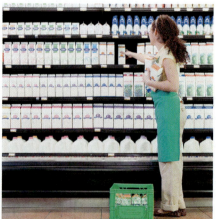

LO 20.4 Food Additives and Other Chemicals Play a Role in Food Production and Safety

Food additives are used as preservatives, antioxidants, flavoring, coloring, and leavening agents; to maintain a food's consistency; and to add nutrients. Pesticides are substances that allow crops to flourish by killing or repelling damaging pests. Natural biopesticides and antimicrobials are less toxic than chemical pesticides such as organophosphates. Integrated pest management (IPM) is used by many farmers and is designed to use the most economical methods to control pests with the least risk of harm to the consumer, the crops, and the environment. The FDA regulates the use of additives and, along with the EPA and USDA, regulates the use of pesticides. Growth hormones are sometimes provided to food-producing animals to increase the yield of product. The FDA regulates the administration of antibiotics to food animals. Foods with the USDA organic seal are grown without the use of most synthetic pesticides, synthetic fertilizers, bioengineering, or irradiation. Only antibiotic-free or growth hormone–free animals can be used to produce organic meat, poultry, eggs, and dairy foods.

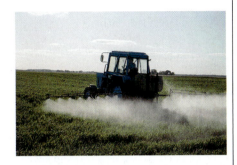

LO 20.5 A Sustainable Food System Conserves Natural Resources

A sustainable food system is one that can be maintained indefinitely because it conserves and protects natural resources, empowers social responsibility, and is economically viable. Food systems are impacted by social, political, economic, and environmental factors and depend on human and natural resources. Soil, biodiversity, energy, and water are key natural resources that must be preserved. Buying locally grown food decreases the amount of fuel needed to transport food and is one way to reduce the use of external natural resources in food systems.

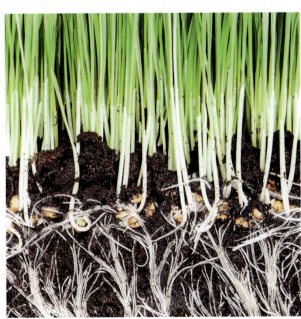

LO 20.6 Biotechnology Is Used to Alter the Genetic Makeup of Foods

Biotechnology, such as traditional cross-breeding and genetic engineering, is the application of biological techniques to alter the genetic makeup of living cells in order to produce organisms with a desired trait. Genetic engineering uses recombinant DNA technology to insert a gene or genes into the DNA of another cell to create a genetically modified product. Genetic engineering is conducted to improve crop yields, reduce the use of pesticides, and in some cases enhance the nutritional value of foods. Genetically engineered foods are heavily regulated in the United States, but some consumers and environmentalists are concerned about the long-term effects of these products. More and longer-term studies examining the effects of genetically engineered foods are needed.

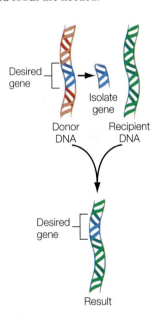

Desired gene → Isolate gene

Donor DNA | Recipient DNA

Desired gene

Result

Terms to Know

- food system
- foodborne illness
- pathogens
- toxin
- fecal-to-oral transmission
- virus
- host
- norovirus
- bacteria
- hemolytic uremic syndrome
- molds
- parasites
- prion
- marine toxins
- scombrotoxic fish poisoning
- ciguatera poisoning
- bioaccumulate
- paralytic shellfish poisoning
- solanine
- polychlorinated biphenyls (PCBs)
- cross-contaminate
- myoglobin
- danger zone
- traveler's diarrhea
- farm-to-table continuum
- Food Safety Initiative (FSI)
- DNA fingerprinting
- food preservation
- pasteurization
- canning
- spores
- modified atmosphere packaging (MAP)
- high-pressure processing (HPP)
- irradiation
- closed (or coded) dating
- open dating
- food additives
- preservatives
- nitrites and nitrates
- sulfites
- monosodium glutamate (MSG)
- prior-sanctioned
- generally recognized as safe (GRAS)
- DeLaney Clause
- intentional food additives
- unintentional food additives
- bovine growth hormone (BGH)
- recombinant bovine somatotropin (rBST)
- antibiotics
- antibiotic-resistant bacteria
- pesticides
- herbicides
- insecticides
- antimicrobials
- fungicides
- rodenticides
- organophosphates
- risk assessment
- acceptable tolerance levels
- integrated pest management (IPM)
- organic
- sustainable
- locavore
- community-supported agriculture (CSA)
- cross-breeding
- biotechnology
- genome
- genetic engineering
- genetically modified organisms (GMOs)
- biodiversity

Mastering Nutrition
Visit the Study Area in Mastering Nutrition to hear an MP3 chapter summary.

Check Your Understanding

LO 20.1 1. Which of the following produce toxins that may cause foodborne illness?
   a. Parasites
   b. Viruses
   c. Bacteria
   d. Food additives

LO 20.1 2. Which of the following pathogens is the most common cause of foodborne infection in the United States?
   a. *Clostridium botulinum*
   b. norovirus
   c. *Trichinella spiralis*
   d. *Escherichia coli* O157:H7

LO 20.2 3. Which of the following sets of four steps is recommended by the Fight BAC! campaign?
   a. Cutting, cleaning, chopping, and chilling
   b. Cleaning, combating cross-contamination, cutting, and chilling
   c. Clearing, combating cross-contamination, cutting, and chilling
   d. Cleaning, combating cross-contamination, cooking, and chilling

LO 20.2 4. At what temperature, known as the danger zone, do bacteria readily thrive and multiply?
   a. Any temperature above 40°F
   b. Between 20° and 120°F
   c. Between 40° and 140°F
   d. Any temperature below 140°F

LO 20.3 5. Which two government agencies oversee the safety of the majority of foods in the United States?
   a. United States Department of Agriculture (USDA) and Environmental Protection Agency (EPA)
   b. Centers for Disease Control and Prevention (CDC) and USDA
   c. USDA and Food and Drug Administration (FDA)
   d. FDA and EPA

LO 20.3 6. Which of the following preservation techniques destroys specific foodborne pathogens by breaking up the cells' DNA?
   a. Irradiation
   b. Pasteurization
   c. Canning
   d. High-pressure processing

LO 20.4 7. Which of the following food additives is on the FDA's GRAS list, is often added to enhance the flavor of savory foods, and causes adverse reactions among some individuals?

   a. Nitrites
   b. Sulfites
   c. Monosodium glutamate
   d. Vitamin E

LO 20.4 8. A frozen chicken enchilada that has the USDA Organic seal on its label means which of the following?

   a. One hundred percent of the ingredients in the product are organic.
   b. No pesticides were used to grow the corn from which the tortillas were made.
   c. The chickens in the enchilada were grown without using antibiotics or growth hormones.
   d. The organic enchilada is better for you because it is indisputably more nutrient-dense than a nonorganic chicken enchilada.

LO 20.5 9. Which of the following is a justified reason for buying food grown and produced locally?

   a. Locally grown food is more nutrient dense than non–locally grown food.
   b. Locally grown foods are organic foods.
   c. Locally grown foods are free from pesticides.
   d. Locally grown foods use fewer external natural resources than do non–locally grown foods.

LO 20.6 10. Which of the following is a key reason that consumers want genetically engineered (GE) foods labeled?

   a. GE foods can cause cancer.
   b. GE foods are linked to impaired cognitive growth in children.
   c. GE foods are not regulated by the FDA.
   d. GE foods may contain allergens.

Answers

1. (c) Bacteria are the only pathogens that produce toxins and cause illness due to foodborne intoxication. Some but not all parasites, viruses, and bacteria cause illness due to foodborne infection. Food additives are common in food and should not cause illness. Food additives are either approved by the FDA prior to their use or have GRAS or prior-sanctioned status based on a history of safe consumption.

2. (b) Half of all foodborne illness is caused by infection due to the noro-virus. Illnesses due to *Clostridium botulinum*, *Trichinella spiralis*, and *Escherichia coli* O157:H7 are much less common. *Clostridium botulinum* and *Escherichia coli* O157:H7 are species of bacteria that produce toxins. *Trichinella spiralis* is a parasite.

3. (d) To prevent foodborne illness, clean, combat cross-contamination, cook, and chill.

4. (c) Bacteria thrive and multiply best between the temperatures of 40° and 140°F. Below 40°F, bacterial replication slows. Temperatures above 140°F destroy bacteria involved in foodborne illness.

5. (c) The USDA and FDA oversee the safety of most foods in the United States. Neither the CDC nor the EPA has direct regulatory oversight of the food supply.

6. (a) Irradiation involves using radiation to damage the DNA of pathogens. Pasteurization and canning both use high temperatures to kill pathogens, while high-pressure processing employs pulses of high pressure.

7. (c) Monosodium glutamate is a flavor enhancer and has GRAS status, but some people may experience symptoms such as numbness, a burning sensation, facial pressure or tightness, chest pain, and rapid heartbeat after consuming MSG. Nitrites and sulfites and vitamin E are additives that help preserve food.

8. (c) The USDA Organic seal indicates that 95 percent of the ingredients in a food are grown organically and that food-producing animals used in the product were grown without the use of hormones or antibiotics. Some, but not all, pesticides may be used by organic farmers. There is little evidence that organically grown foods are more nutritious or safer for you than foods grown using conventional methods.

9. (d) Locally grown food requires fewer external natural resources in the form of fossil fuels from farm to your fork. However, just because a food is grown locally does not necessarily mean that it is grown organically, free from pesticides, or more nutrient dense than foods that are grown further from your home.

10. (d) Many consumers are concerned that GE foods may contain unintentional allergens. No evidence suggests that consumption of GE foods causes cancer. Lead exposure causes impaired cognitive growth in children. The USDA, EPA, and FDA regulate all GE foods.

Answers to True or False?

1. **False.** A food may contain disease-causing bacteria or other contaminants, yet look and smell perfectly fine.

2. **False.** Hand sanitizer kills most disease-causing pathogens, as do soap and water. It is not necessary to wash your hands with soap and water if you use hand sanitizer.

3. **True.** A kitchen sponge provides the perfect medium for bacterial growth: moisture, nutrients, and room temperature.

4. **False.** Freezing doesn't kill bacteria but puts them in a dormant state. Once thawed, some bacteria can continue to grow and reproduce.

5. **False.** Leftovers should be thrown out if they're not consumed within 3–5 days.

6. **False.** Package dates refer to food quality, not safety.

7. **False.** The FDA deems food additives safe if they present a "negligible risk" of cancer to human beings with lifetime use.

8. **False.** A diet consisting only of locally grown foods might or might not be a sustainable diet because not all local farms guarantee that the foods were grown in a sustainable way. A sustainable diet contains foods that meet your nutrient and health needs but can be produced for a long time without negatively affecting the environment.

9. **False.** Some synthetic pesticides have been approved for use on organic crops.

10. **True.** Corn, potatoes, and soybeans have been genetically modified to include a bacterial gene that makes them more resistant to insects since the 1990s. Labeling of genetically engineered foods is not mandatory in the United States, but many products contain genetically modified ingredients.

Web Resources

- For food safety education, visit www.fightbac.org
- For foodborne illness fact sheets, visit https://www.fsis.usda.gov/wps/portal/fsis/topics/food-safety-education/get-answers/food-safety-fact-sheets
- For more information on organic foods, visit https://www.ams.usda.gov/about-ams/programs-offices/national-organic-program
- For information on biotechnology, visit https://www.fda.gov/food/guidanceregulation/guidancedocumentsregulatoryinformation/biotechnology/default.htm

References

1. Centers for Disease Control and Prevention. 2016. *CDC Estimates of Foodborne Illness in the United States.* Available at https://www.cdc.gov/foodborneburden/2011-foodborne-estimates.html. Accessed April 2017.

2. Ibid.

3. Centers for Disease Control and Prevention. 2016. *Botulism.* Available at https://www.cdc.gov/botulism/. Accessed April 2017.

4. U.S. Food and Drug Administration. 2015. *Preventive Control Measures for Fresh & Fresh-Cut Produce: Chapter IV: Outbreaks Associated with Fresh and Fresh-Cut Produce. Incidence, Growth, and Survival of Pathogens in Fresh and Fresh-Cut Produce.* Available at https://www.fda.gov/Food/FoodScienceResearch/ucm090977.htm. Accessed April 2017.

5. Centers for Disease Control and Prevention. 2016. *Burden of Foodborne Illness: Findings.* Available at https://www.cdc.gov/foodborneburden/2011-foodborne-estimates.html. Accessed April 2017.

6. US Food and Drug Administration. 2016. *Food Safety A to Z Reference Guide: Virus.* Available at https://www.fda.gov/food/foodscienceresearch/toolsmaterials/ucm216150.htm. Accessed April 2017.

7. Ibid.

8. Shreiner, A. B., Kao, J. Y., and Young, V. B. 2015. The Gut Microbiome in Health and in Disease. *Current Opinion in Gastroenterology* 31(1):69–75.

9. DiBaise, J. K., Frank, D. N., and Mathur, R. 2012. Impact of the Gut Microbiota on the Development of Obesity: Current Concepts. *American Journal of Gastroenterology Supplement* 1:22–27.

10. Centers for Disease Control and Prevention. 2016. *Burden of Foodborne Illness: Findings.* Available at https://www.cdc.gov/foodborneburden/2011-foodborne-estimates.html. Accessed April 2017.

11. Centers for Disease Control and Prevention. 2017. *E. coli (Escherichia coli).* Available at https://www.cdc.gov/ecoli/index.html. Accessed April 2017.

12. United States Department of Agriculture. 2013. *Molds on Foods: Are They Dangerous?* Available at https://www.fsis.usda.gov/wps/portal/fsis/topics/food-safety-education/get-answers/food-safety-fact-sheets/safe-food-handling/molds-on-food-are-they-dangerous_/ct_index. Accessed April 2017.

13. Food Safety and Inspection Service. 2013. *Fact Sheet: Parasites and Foodborne Illness.* Available at https://www.fsis.usda.gov/wps/portal/fsis/topics/food-safety-education/get-answers/food-safety-fact-sheets/foodborne-illness-and-disease/parasites-and-foodborne-illness/ct_index. Accessed April 2017.

14. Cody, M.M. and Stretch, T. 2014 Position of the Academy of Nutrition and Dietetics: Food and Water Safety. *Journal of the Academy of Nutrition and Dietetics* 114(11):1819–1829.

15. U.S. Department of Agriculture. 2016. *About BSE.* Available at https://www.aphis.usda.gov/aphis/ourfocus/animalhealth/animal-disease-information/cattle-disease-information/sa_bse/ct_about_bse. Accessed April 2017.

16. Centers for Disease Control and Prevention. 2015. *BSE (Bovine Spongiform Encephalopathy, or Mad Cow Disease): News and Highlights.* Available at https://www.cdc.gov/prions/bse/news.html. Accessed April 2017.

17. USDA. 2012. *Statement by USDA Chief Veterinary Officer John Clifford Regarding a Detection of Bovine Spongiform Encephalopathy (BSE) in the United States.* Release No. 0132.12, April 24, 2012. Available at https://www.usda.gov/media/press-releases/2012/04/24/statement-usda-chief-veterinary-officer-john-clifford-regarding. Accessed April 2017.

18. United States Department of Agriculture. 2013. Statement from Agriculture Secretary Tom Vilsack Regarding World Organization for Animal Health (OIE) Upgrade of United States' BSE Risk Status. Statement Release no. 0106.13. Available at https://www.usda.gov/media/press-releases/2013/05/29/statement-agriculture-secretary-tom-vilsack-regarding-world. Accessed April 2017.

19. Centers for Disease Control and Prevention. 2016. *Harmful Algal Bloom (HAB)-Associated Illness.* Available at https://www.cdc.gov/habs/illness-symptoms-marine.html. Accessed April 2017.

20. Ibid.

21. Ibid.

22. Ibid.

23. Dolan, L. C., Matulka, R. A., Burdock, G. A. 2010. Naturally Occurring Food Toxins. *Toxins (Basel)* 2(9):2289–2332. doi: 10.3390/toxins2092289.

24. U.S. Environmental Protection Agency. 2017. *Polychlorinated Biphenyls (PCBs).* Available at https://www.epa.gov/pcbs/learn-about-polychlorinated-biphenyls-pcbs. Accessed April 2017.

25. Agency for Toxic Substances and Disease Registry. 2014. *ToxFAQs™ for Polychlorinated Biphenyls (PCBs).* Available at https://www.atsdr.cdc.gov/toxfaqs/tf.asp?id=140&tid=26 Accessed April 2017

26. U.S. Environmental Protection Agency. 2017. *Polychlorinated Biphenyls (PCBs).* Available at https://www.epa.gov/pcbs/learn-about-polychlorinated-biphenyls-pcbs. Accessed April 2017.

27. Ibid.

28. Environmental Protection Agency. 2017. *Consumer Fact Sheet on PCBs.* Available at https://www.epa.gov/environmental-topics/water-topics Accessed July 2017.

29. Rice, K. M., E. M. Walker, Jr., M. Wu, C. Gillette, and E. R. Blough. 2014. Environmental Mercury and Its Toxic Effects. *Journal of Preventive Medicine and Public Health* 47(2):74–83.

30. Environmental Protection Agency. 2017. *Guidelines for Eating Fish that Contain Mercury.* Available at https://www.epa.gov/mercury/guidelines-eating-fish-contain-mercury Accessed April 2017.

31. Food Safety.gov. 2017. *Food Safety for Older Adults.* Available at https://www.foodsafety.gov/risk/olderadults/. Accessed April 2017.

32. U.S. Department of Health and Human Services, Administration on Aging. 2016. *A Profile of Older Americans 2016.* Available at https://aoa.acl.gov/aging_statistics/profile/index.aspx Accessed April 2017.

33. Cody, M. M., and Stretch, T. 2014. Position of the Academy of Nutrition and Dietetics: Food and Water Safety.

34. United States Department of Agriculture Food Safety and Inspection Service. 2017. *Fact Sheets: Safe Food Handling.* Available at https://www.fsis.usda.gov/wps/portal/fsis/topics/food-safety-education/get-answers/food-safety-fact-sheets/safe-food-handling. Accessed April 2017.

35. US Food and Drug Administration. 2016. *Science and Our Food Supply: Free Supplementary Curriculum for Middle Level and High School Classrooms.* Available at https://www.fda.gov/food/foodscienceresearch/toolsmaterials/scienceandthefoodsupply/default.htm. Accessed April 2017.

36. Partnership for Food Safety Education. 2017. *Food Safety Basics: The Core Four Practices.* Available at http://www.fightbac.org/food-safety-basics/the-core-four-practices/ Accessed April 2017.

37. US Food and Drug Administration. 2016. *Food Safety A to Z Reference Guide: Handwashing.* Available at https://www.fda.gov/food/foodscienceresearch/toolsmaterials/ucm216150.htm. Accessed April 2017.

38. CDC. 2016. *Handwashing: Clean Hands Save Lives.* Available at www.cdc.gov/handwashing. Accessed May 2017.

39. Ibid

40. Ibid

41. Academy of Nutrition and Dietetics. 2015. *The Do's and Don'ts of Kitchen Sponge Safety.* Available at http://www.eatright.org/resource/homefoodsafety/four-steps/wash/dos-and-donts-of-kitchen-sponge-safety Accessed May 2017.

42. Ibid.

43. Sorheim O., Hoy, M. 2013. Effects of food ingredients and oxygen exposure on premature browning in cooked beef. *Meat Science* 93(1):105–110.

44. US Department of Agriculture. Food Safety and Inspection Service. Modified August 2013. *The Color of Meat and Poultry.* Available at https://www.fsis.usda.gov/wps/portal/fsis/topics/food-safety-education/get-answers/food-safety-fact-sheets/meat-preparation/the-color-of-meat-and-poultry/the-color-of-meat-and-poultry/ct_index. Accessed April 2017.

45. Food and Drug Administration. 2013. *Food Code 2013.* Available at https://www.fda.gov/Food/GuidanceRegulation/RetailFoodProtection/FoodCode/ucm374275.htmww.fda.gov/Food/FoodSafety/RetailFoodProtection/FoodCode/default.htm. Accessed April 2017.

46. Food Safety and Inspection Service. Modified June 2013. *How Temperatures Affect Food.* Available at https://www.fsis.usda.gov/wps/portal/fsis/topics/food-safety-education/get-answers/food-safety-fact-sheets/safe-food-handling/how-temperatures-affect-food/ct_indexAccessed April 2017.

47. Ibid.

48. Centers for Disease Control and Prevention. 2013 *Travelers' Diarrhea.* https://wwwnc.cdc.gov/travel/page/travelers-diarrhea. Accessed April 2017.

49. Centers for Disease Control and Prevention. 2015. *Travelers' Health: Food and Water Safety.* Available at https://wwwnc.cdc.gov/travel/page/food-water-safety. Accessed April 2017.

50. Food and Drug Administration and U.S. Department of Agriculture. 2000. *A Description of the U.S. Food Safety System.* Available at www.fsis.usda.gov/OA/codex/system.htm. Accessed April 2017.

51. U.S. Food and Drug Administration. 2014. *Congressional Testimony: Ensuring Food Safety: Tracking and Resolving the E.coli Spinach Outbreak.* Available at https://www.fda.gov/NewsEvents/Testimony/ucm110926.htm. Accessed April 2017.

52. Centers for Disease Control and Prevention. 2006. *Press Release: Multistate Outbreak of E. coli O157:H7 Infections Linked to Fresh Spinach.* Available at https://www.cdc.gov/ecoli/2006/spinach-10-2006.html. Accessed April 2017.

53. US Food and Drug Administration. 2017. Hazard Analysis Critical Control Point (HACCP). Available at https://www.fda.gov/food/guidanceregulation/haccp/. Accessed April 2017.

54. Food and Drug Administration. 2013. *Food Code 2013.* Available at https://www.fda.gov/Food/GuidanceRegulation/RetailFoodProtection/FoodCode/ucm374275.htmww.fda.gov/Food/FoodSafety/RetailFoodProtection/FoodCode/default.htm. Accessed April 2017.

55. US Food and Drug Administration. 2015. *Talking about Juice Safety: What You Need to Know.* Available at https://www.fda.gov/food/resourcesforyou/consumers/ucm110526.htm. Accessed April 2017.

56. FoodReference.com. n.d. *The History of Food Canning: About Canned Food and Whence It Came.* Available at www.foodreference.com/html/artcanninghistory.html. Accessed April 2017.

57. Centers for Disease Control and Prevention. 2016. *Botulism.* Available at https://www.cdc.gov/botulism/. Accessed April 2017.

58. Ibid.

59. Center for Food Safety and Applied Nutrition. 2015. *Analysis and Evaluation of Preventive Control Measures for the Control and Reduction/Elimination of Microbial Hazards on Fresh and Fresh-Cut Produce.* Available at https://www.fda.gov/Food/FoodScienceResearch/ucm090977.htm. Accessed April 2017.

60. Finley, J., D. Deming, and R. Smith. 2006. Food Processing: Nutrition, Safety, and Quality. In Shils, M., M. Shike, A. Ross, B. Caballero, and R. Cousins, eds. *Modern Nutrition in Health and Disease.* 10th ed. Philadelphia: Lippincott Williams & Wilkins.

61. Food and Drug Administration. 2016. *Food Irradiation: What You Need to Know.* Available at https://www.fda.gov/food/resourcesforyou/consumers/ucm261680.htm. Accessed April 2017.

62. Kindu, D., A. Gill, and R. Holley. 2013. Use of Low-Dose Irradiation to Evaluate the Radiation Sensitivity of *Escherichia coli* O157:H7, non-O157 Verotoxigenic *Escherichia coli,* and Salmonella in Phosphate-Buffered Saline. *Journal of Food Protection* 76(8):1438–1442.

63. Food and Drug Administration. 2016. *Food Irradiation: What You Need to Know.*

64. Ibid.

65. Ibid.

66. Ibid.

67. Ibid.

68. Ibid.

69. Food Safety and Inspection Service. 2016. Food Product Dating. U.S. Department of Agriculture. www.fsis.usda.gov. Accessed May 2017.

70. Ibid.

71. Environmental Protection Agency. 2017. *Safe Drinking Water Act: Consumer Confidence Reports (CCR).* Available at https://www.epa.gov/ccr Accessed April 2017.

72. Environmental Protection Agency. 2017. *Learn About Lead.* Available at https://www.epa.gov/lead/learn-about-lead#lead. Accessed April 2017.

73. Cody, M. M., and Stretch, T. 2014. Position of the Academy of Nutrition and Dietetics: Food and Water Safety.

74. Centers for Disease Control and Prevention (CDC). 2012. Vital Signs: Food Categories Contributing the Most to Sodium Consumption' United States, 2007–2008. *Morbidity and Mortality Weekly Report* 6:62–98.

75. Bouvard, V., Loomis, D., Guyton, K. Z., Grosse, Y., Ghissassi, F. E., Benbrahim-Tallaa, L. Guha, N., Mattock, H., Straif, K., on behalf of the International Agency for Research on Cancer Monograph Working Group. 2015. Carcinogenicity of consumption of red and processed meat. *Lancet Oncology* 16(16):1599–1600.

76. National Toxicology Program. 2011. NTP 12th Report on Carcinogens. *Report on Carcinogens: Carcinogen Profiles* iii–449.

77. FDA. 2014. *Food Additives Status List.* Available at https://www.fda.gov/food/ingredientspackaginglabeling/foodadditivesingredients/ucm091048.htm. Accessed April 2017.

78. Ibid.

79. Ibid.

80. FDA. 2014. *Questions and Answers on Monosodium Glutamate (MSG).* Available at https://www.fda.gov/food/ingredientspackaginglabeling/foodadditivesingredients/ucm328728.htm Accessed April 2017.

81. FDA. 2014. *Food Additives Status List.* Available at https://www.fda.gov/food/ingredientspackaginglabeling/foodadditivesingredients/ucm091048.htm Accessed April 2017.

82. FDA. 2017. *Generally Recognized as Safe (GRAS).* Available at https://www.fda.gov/food/ingredientspackaginglabeling/gras/ Accessed April 2017.

83. FDA. 2014. *Food Additives Status List.*

84. Food and Drug Administration. Modified 2017. *Questions and Answers about Dioxins and Food Safety.* Available at https://www.fsis.usda.gov/wps/wcm/connect/fsis-content/internet/main/topics/data-collection-and-reports/chemistry/dioxin-related-activites Accessed April 2017.

85. Food and Drug Administration. Modified 2014. *Report on the Food and Drug Administration's Review of the Safety of Recombinant Bovine Somatotropin.* Available at

https://www.fda.gov/animalveterinary/safetyhealth/productsafetyinformation/ucm130321.htm. Accessed April 2017.

86. American Cancer Society. 2014. *Learn About Cancer: Recombinant Bovine Growth Hormone.* Available at https://www.cancer.org/cancer/cancer-causes/recombinant-bovine-growth-hormone.html. Accessed April 2017.

87. Food and Drug Administration. 2015. *Steroid Hormone Implants Used for Growth in Food-Producing Animals.* Available at https://www.fda.gov/animalveterinary/safetyhealth/productsafetyinformation/ucm055436.htm Accessed April 2017.

88. Ibid.

89. Centers for Disease Control and Prevention, National Antimicrobial Resistance Monitoring System. Updated 2016. *Antibiotic Use in Food-Producing Animals: Tracking and Reducing the Public Health Impact.* Available at https://www.cdc.gov/narms/faq.html. Accessed April 2017.

90. Iovine, N. M., and M. J. Blaser. 2004. Antibiotics in Animal Feed and Spread of Resistant *Campylobacter* from Poultry to Humans. *Emerging Infectious Diseases* 10(6):1158–1189. doi: 10.3201/eid1006.040403.

91. U.S. FDA. 2015. *Veterinary Feed Directive.* Available at https://www.federalregister.gov/documents/2015/06/03/2015-13393/veterinary-feed-directive. Accessed April 2017.

92. USDA. Modified 2015. *Meat and Poultry Labeling Terms.* https://www.fsis.usda.gov/wps/portal/fsis/topics/food-safety-education/get-answers/food-safety-fact-sheets/food-labeling/meat-and-poultry-labeling-terms. Accessed April 2017.

93. U.S. Environmental Protection Agency. 2017. *Food and Pesticides.* Available at https://www.epa.gov/safepestcontrol/food-and-pesticides. Accessed May 2017.

94. U.S. Environmental Protection Agency. n.d. *Pesticides.* Available at https://www.epa.gov/pesticides. Accessed April 2017

95. Ibid.

96. U.S. Environmental Protection Agency. 2017. *What are Antimicrobial Pesticides.* Available at https://www.epa.gov/pesticide-registration/what-are-antimicrobial-pesticides. Accessed April 2017

97. Food and Drug Administration. 2014. *FDA Fact Sheet on Hand Hygiene in Retail and Food Service Establishments.* Available at https://www.fda.gov/food/guidanceregulation/retailfoodprotection/industryandregulatoryassistanceandtrainingresources/ucm135577.htm. Accessed April 2017.

98. U.S. Environmental Protection Agency. 2017. *Cumulative Assessment from Risk of Pesticides.* Available at https://www.epa.gov/pesticide-science-and-assessing-pesticide-risks/cumulative-assessment-risk-pesticides. Accessed May 2017.

99. U.S. Environmental Protection Agency. 2017. *Pesticides* Available at https://www.epa.gov/pesticides. Accessed April 2017.

100. Office of Disease Prevention and Health Promotion. U.S. Department of Health and Human Services. 2017. *Healthy People 2020: Environmental Health Objectives.* Available at https://www.healthypeople.gov/2020/topics-objectives/topic/environmental-health/objectives. Accessed April 2017.

101. American Academy of Pediatrics. 2012. Policy Statement on Pesticide Exposure in Children. *Pediatrics* 130(6):e1757–e1763.

102. U.S. Environmental Protection Agency. 2017. *Pesticides: Risk Assessment.* Available at https://www.epa.gov/pesticide-science-and-assessing-pesticide-risks/overview-risk-assessment-pesticide-program. Accessed April 2017.

103. U.S. Environmental Protection Agency. 2017. *Pesticides: Pesticide Registration.* Available at https://www.epa.gov/pesticide-registration/about-pesticide-registration. Accessed April 2017.

104. U.S. Environmental Protection Agency. 2012. *Pesticides and Food: How the Government*

105. U.S. Environmental Protection Agency. 2016. *Pesticides: Topical and Chemical Fact Sheets' Integrated Pest Management (IPM) Principles.* Available at https://www.epa.gov/safepestcontrol/integrated-pest-management-ipm-principles. Accessed April 2017.

106. Ibid.

107. Food and Drug Administration. 2017. *Pesticides.* Available at https://www.fda.gov/food/foodborneillnesscontaminants/pesticides/. Accessed April 2017.

108. American Cancer Society. 2016. *Common Questions About Diet and Cancer.* Available at www.cancer.org. Accessed May 2017.

109. United States Department of Agriculture. 2017. *National Organic Program.* Available at www.ams.usda.gov/AMSv1.0/nop. Accessed April 2017.

110. Ibid.

111. Organic Trade Association. 2016. *U.S. Organic Industry Survey.* Available at https://www.ota.com/news/press-releases/19031. Accessed May 2017.

112. Ibid.

113. International Food Information Council. 2003. *USDA Launches Organic Standards.* Available at http://www.foodinsight.org/Portals/0/pdf/May-June-2003-PDF.pdf. Accessed April 2017.

114. Agricultural Marketing Service, National Organic Program. Revised 2016. *National Organic Program Handbook: Guidance and Instructions for Accredited Certifying Agents and Certified Operations.* https://www.ams.usda.gov/rules-regulations/organic/handbook/. Accessed April 2017.

115. Electronic Code of Federal Regulations. 2014. *Title 7: Agriculture, Part 205' National Organic Program, Subpart G' Administrative: National List of Allowed and Prohibited Substances.* Available at https://www.federalregister.gov/documents/2014/09/30/2014-23135/national-organic-program-nop-amendments-to-the-national-list-of-allowed-and-prohibited-substances. Accessed April 2017.

116. Bara?ski, M., Srednicka-Tober, D., Volakakis, N., Seal, C., Sanderson, R., Stewart G. B., Benbrook, C., Biavati, B., Markellou, E., Giotis, C., Gromadzka-Ostrowska, J., Rembia?kowska, E., Skwar?o-So?ta, K., Tahvonen, R., Janovská, D., Niggli, U., Nicot, P., and Leifert, C. 2014. Higher Antioxidant and Lower Cadmium Concentrations and Lower Incidence of Pesticide Residues in Organically Grown Crops: A Systematic Literature Review and Meta-analyses. *British Journal of Nutrition* 112(15):794–811. doi: 10.1017/S0007114514001366.

117. Smith-Spangler, C., M. L. Brandeau, G. E. Hunter, J. C. Bavinger, M. Pearson, P. J. Eschbach, V. Sundaram, et al. 2012. Are Organic Foods Safer or Healthier than Conventional Alternatives?: A Systematic Review. *Annals of Internal Medicine* 157(5):348–366.

118. Ibid.

119. United Nations, Department of Economic and Social Affairs, Population Division. 2015. *Population Trends.* Available at http://www.un.org/en/development/desa/population/theme/trends/. Accessed April 2017.

120. Tagtow, A., K. Robien, E. Bergquist, M. Mruening, L. Dierks, B. E. Hartman, et al. 2014. Academy of Nutrition and Dietetics: Standards of Professional Performance for Registered Dietitian Nutritionists (Competent, Proficient, and Expert) in Sustainable, Resilient, and Healthy Food and Water Systems. *Journal of the Academy of Nutrition and Dietetics* 114(3):475–488.

121. Center for Sustainable Food Systems, University of Michigan. 2016. U.S. Food System Factsheet. Pub. No. CSS01-06. Available at http://css.snre.umich.edu/sites/default/files/U.S._Food_System_Factsheet_CSS01-06.pdf. Accessed May 2017.

122. USDA National Resources Conservation Service. 2017. *Soil Health.* Available at https://www.nrcs.usda.gov/wps/portal/nrcs/main/national/soils/health/. Accessed April 2017.

123. Tagtow, A., and Harmon A. 2009. *Healthy Land, Healthy Food and Healthy Eaters. Dieticians Cultivating Sustainable Food Systems.* Available at www.uwyo.edu/winwyoming/pubs/healthyland%20healthyfood%20healthyeaters.pdf. Accessed April 2017.

124. USDA Economic Research Service. 2017. Soil Tillage and Crop Rotation. Available at https://www.ers.usda.gov/topics/farm-practices-management/crop-livestock-practices/soil-tillage-and-crop-rotation/. Accessed May 2017.

125. United States Department of Agriculture. 2012. *Colony Collapse Disorder Progress Report.* Available at https://www.ars.usda.gov/is/br/ccd/ccdprogressreport2012.pdf. Accessed April 2017.

126. Allendorf, F. W., O. Berry, and N. Ryman. 2014. So Long to Genetic Diversity, and Thanks For All the Fish. *Molecular Ecology* 23(1):23–25. doi: 10.1111/mec.12574.

127. Center for Sustainable Food Systems, University of Michigan. 2016. U.S. Food System Factsheet. Pub. No. CSS01-06. Available at http://css.snre.umich.edu/sites/default/files/U.S._Food_System_Factsheet_CSS01-06.pdf Accessed May 2017.

128. Herrero, M., Havlik, P., Valin, H., Notenbaert, A., Rufino, M.C., Thornton, P.K., Blummel, M., Weiss, F., Grace, D., and Obersteiner, M. 2013. Biomass Use, Production, Feed Efficiencies, and Greenhouse Gas Emissions from Global Livestock Systems. *Proceedings of the National Academy of Sciences of the United States of America* 110(52):20888–20893. doi: 10.1073/pnas.1308149110.

129. Beef Cattle Research Council. 2014. How Much Feed and Water are Used to Make a Pound of Beef? Available at www.beefresearch.ca/blog/cattle-feed-water-use/. Accessed May 2017.

130. Center for Sustainable Food Systems, University of Michigan. 2016. U.S. Food System Factsheet. Pub. No. CSS01-06. Available at http://css.snre.umich.edu/sites/default/files/U.S._Food_System_Factsheet_CSS01-06.pdf. Accessed May 2017.

131. Harmon, A. H., and B. L. Gerald. 2007. Position of the American Dietetic Association: Food and Nutrition Professionals Can Implement Practices to Conserve Natural Resources and Support Ecological Sustainability. *Journal of the American Dietetic Association* 107(6):1033–1043.

132. Environmental Protection Agency. 2017. *Watersense*. Available at https://www.epa.gov/watersense/about-watersense Accessed April 2017.

133. Ibid.

134. Ibid.

135. Ibid.

136. National Oceanic and Atmospheric Administration, National Centers for Environmental Information. *Global Climate Change Indicators*. Available at https://www.ncdc.noaa.gov/monitoring-references/faq/indicators.php. Accessed May 2017.

137. USDA Economic Research Service. ERS Report Summary. 2016. *Food Prices and Spending*. Available at https://www.ers.usda.gov/data-products/ag-and-food-statistics-charting-the-essentials/food-prices-and-spending/. Accessed April 2017.

138. Harmon, A. H., and B. L. Gerald. 2007. Position of the American Dietetic Association: Food and Nutrition Professionals Can Implement Practices to Conserve Natural Resources and Support Ecological Sustainability. *Journal of the American Dietetic Association* 107(6):1033–1043.

139. United States Department of Agriculture. 2017. *Know Your Farmer, Know Your Food*. Available at https://www.cnpp.usda.gov/KnowYourFarmer. Accessed April 2017.

140. Tagtow, A., et al. 2014. Academy of Nutrition and Dietetics: Standards of Professional Performance for Registered Dietitian Nutritionists (Competent, Proficient, and Expert) in Sustainable, Resilient, and Healthy Food and Water Systems.

141. United States Department of Agriculture. Modified 2013. *Biotechnology Frequently Asked Questions (FAQs)*. Available at https://www.usda.gov/topics/biotechnology/biotechnology-frequently-asked-questions-faqs. Accessed April 2017.

142. Economic Research Service. 2016. *Adoption of Genetically Engineered Crops in the U.S.* Available at https://www.ers.usda.gov/data-products/adoption-of-genetically-engineered-crops-in-the-us.aspx. Accessed April 2017.

143. Quaim, M., Kouser, S. 2013. Genetically Modified Crops and Food Security. *PLoS One* 8(6):e64879. doi: 10.1371/journal.pone.0064879

144. USDA Economic Research Service. 2016. Adoption of Genetically Engineered Crops in the U.S. Available at https://www.ers.usda.gov/data-products/adoption-of-genetically-engineered-crops-in-the-us.aspx Accessed May 2017.

145. Ibid.

146. Economic Research Service. 2016. *Adoption of Genetically Engineered Crops in the U.S.* Available at https://www.ers.usda.gov/data-products/adoption-of-genetically-engineered-crops-in-the-us.aspx.

147. Economic Research Service. Updated 2016. *Adoption of Genetically Engineered Crops in the U.S.* Available at https://www.ers.usda.gov/data-products/adoption-of-genetically-engineered-crops-in-the-us.aspx. Accessed April 2017.

148. Ibid.

149. Bren, L. 2003. Genetic Engineering: The Future of Foods. *FDA Consumer* 37:28–34.

150. Tang, G., Hu Y., Yin, S., Wang, Y., Dallal, G. E., Grusak, M. A., and Russel, R. M. 2012. Beta Carotene in Golden Rice is as good as Beta carotene in oil at providing vitamin A to children. Golden Rice. *American Journal of Clinical Nutrition* 96:658–664.

151. Kieffer, T. J., and Seino, Y. 2016. Engineering the gut for insulin replacement to treat diabetes. *Journal of Diabetes Investigation* 7(Suppl. 1): 87–93. doi: 10.1111/jdi.12479.

152. Peplow, M. 2016. Synthetic Biology's First Malaria Drug Meets Market Resistance. *Nature*. Available at www.nature.com/news/synthetic-biology-s-first-malaria-drug-meets-market-resistance-1.19426. Accessed May 2017.

153. Ibid.

154. Kramkowska, M., T. Grzelak, and K. Czy?ewska. 2013. Benefits and Risks Associated with Genetically Modified Food Products. *Annals of Agricultural and Environmental Medicine* 20(3):413–419.

155. Buiatti, M, Christou, P., and Pastore, G. 2012. The Application of GMOs in Agriculture and in Food Production for a Better Nutrition: Two Different Scientific Points of View. *Genes and Nutrition* 8(3):255–270. doi: 10.1007/s12263-012-0316-4

156. Food and Drug Administration. 2017. *Biotechnology: Genetically Engineered Plants for Food and Feed*. Available at https://www.fda.gov/Food/IngredientsPackagingLabeling/GEPlants/default.htm. Accessed April 2017.

157. U.S. Food and Drug Administration. 2012. *Have Food Allergies? Read the Label*. Available at https://www.fda.gov/forconsumers/consumerupdates/ucm254504.htm. Accessed April 2017.

158. Ledford, H. 2016. Transgenic Salmon Nears Approval. *Nature*. Available at https://www.nature.com/news/transgenic-salmon-nears-approval-1.12903. Accessed May 2017.

159. Semmens, B. X, et al. 2016. Quasi-Extinction Risk and Population Targets for the Eastern, Migratory Population of Monarch Butterflies. *Scientific Reports* 6, Article No. 23264. doi: 10.1038/srep23265.

160. Gilbert, G. 2013. A Hard Look at GM Crops. *Nature* 497:24–26.

161. Ibid.

162. Food and Drug Administration. 2015. *Questions and Answers on Food from Genetically Engineered Plants*. Available at www.fda.gov/food/ingredientspackaginglabeling/geplants/ucm346030.htm. Accessed April 2017.

163. U.S. Food and Drug Administration. 2017. *Food from Genetically Engineered Plants*. Available at https://www.fda.gov/Food/IngredientsPackagingLabeling/GEPlants/default.htm. Accessed April 2017.

164. Reuters. 2014. *USDA Is Still Weighing If Genetically Modified Salmon Is Safe to Eat*. Available at www.reuters.com/article/2014/03/13/us-usa-health-salmon-fda-idUSBREA2C23L20140313. Accessed April 2017.

165. Food and Drug Administration. 2015. *Questions and Answers on Food from Genetically Engineered Plants*.

166. American Medical Association. 2012. *Policy H-480.958 Bioengineered (Genetically Engineered)Crops and Foods*. Available at https://searchpf.ama-assn.org/SearchML/searchDetails.action?uri=%2FAMADoc%2FHOD.xml-0-4359.xml. Accessed April 2017.

167. Society of Toxicology. 2003. The Safety of Genetically Modified Foods Produced through Biotechnology. *Toxicological Sciences* 71:2–8.

168. Center for Food Safety. 2014. *Genetically Engineered Foods Labeling Laws*. Available at www.centerforfoodsafety.org/ge-map. Accessed April 2017.

169. Pew Research Center. 2015. Chapter 3: Attitudes and Beliefs on Science and Technology Topics. Available at www.pewinternet.org/2015/01/29/chapter-3-attitudes-and-beliefs-on-science-and-technology-topics/. Accessed May 2017.

170. Kamthan, A., Chaudhuri, A., Kamthan, M., and Datta, A. 2016. Genetically Modified (GM) Crops: Milestones and New Advances in Crop Improvement. *Theoretical and Applied Genetics* 129(9):1639–1655. doi: 10.1007/s00122-016-2747-6.

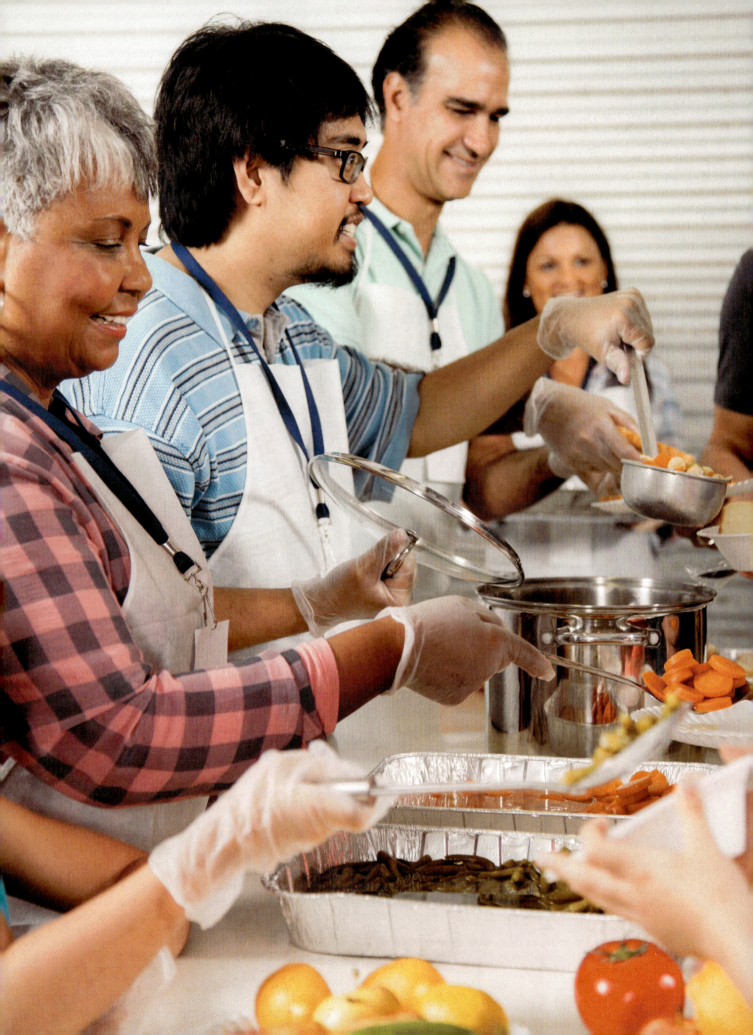

Global Nutrition and Malnutrition

21

Learning Outcomes

After reading this chapter, you will be able to:

21.1 Discuss the extent of food insecurity in the United States and the contributing factors.

21.2 Describe the causes of malnutrition worldwide.

21.3 Identify populations that are at greatest risk for malnutrition.

21.4 Explain several ways to reduce hunger.

21.5 Describe the health consequences of undernutrition.

True or False?

1. Malnutrition exists in every country in the world—including the United States. **T/F**

2. More than one-tenth of the world's population does not have enough to eat. **T/F**

3. If you have a job, you will never experience food insecurity. **T/F**

4. Depression among mothers has been associated with food insecurity. **T/F**

5. Farmers grow enough food to feed everyone on the planet today. **T/F**

6. Earthquakes can cause food shortages. **T/F**

7. Once you reach a certain age, you don't need to worry about malnutrition. **T/F**

8. Fortifying foods is a good idea, but it doesn't really affect malnutrition. **T/F**

9. You can't be obese and food insecure at the same time. **T/F**

10. Iodine deficiency is the world's most prevalent, yet easily preventable, cause of brain damage in children. **T/F**

See page 798 for the answers.

We all know what hunger feels like. After a long day, a grumbling or gnawing in the stomach or feelings of fatigue or lightheadedness are signs that tell us we need to eat. However, how many of us know what it is like to be hungry day in and day out, never to feel truly full, or to lose weight even though we don't want to?

Conversely, how many of us, though we satisfy our hunger, are malnourished without realizing it? As you learned in Chapter 2, malnutrition is a lack of proper nutrition. It may appear as undernutrition. Typically, undernutrition is caused by not having enough to eat, not eating enough of the right things, or being unable to use the food that one does eat, either because of repeated infections or poor nutrient absorption.[1] Children who are undernourished can't grow properly and have an increased risk for a variety of diseases and death. Inadequate intake of vitamin A, for example, is a leading cause of blindness. According to the World Health Organization (WHO), "an estimated 250,000 to 500,000 vitamin A–deficient children become blind every year, half of them dying within 12 months of losing their sight."[2] Women who are undernourished during pregnancy risk giving birth to low-birthweight babies.[3] The health effects of undernutrition are discussed in detail later in this chapter.

Malnutrition may also appear as overnutrition, which can lead to overweight or obesity or a specific micronutrient toxicity. Overnutrition and undernutrition may coexist, as when an individual consumes a diet high in refined carbohydrates and low in micronutrients. Even people at a healthy weight may be malnourished if they, like many Americans, are deficient in calcium, iron, or another micronutrient.

Who are the malnourished people in the United States and the rest of the world? What factors contribute to this problem, and what can we do about it? Can one person's actions really help people who are hungry? In this chapter, we explore malnutrition, its causes and effects, and potential solutions in the United States and around the world.

What Factors Contribute to Malnutrition in the United States?

LO 21.1 Discuss the extent of food insecurity in the United States and the contributing factors.

The United States is a **developed country**, one of the wealthiest in the world,[4] yet many Americans cannot afford to buy adequate amounts of nourishing foods at a grocery store or dine out at a local restaurant. Hunger and malnutrition are very real problems across the United States, in inner cities, the suburbs, and in rural areas, and food insecurity is a large part of the problem.

Food Insecurity in the United States Is Significant

developed country Country that is advanced in multiple areas, such as income per capita, life expectancy, rate of literacy, industrial capability, technological sophistication, and economic productivity.

food security Household-level economic and social condition characterized by reliable access to adequate amounts of healthy foods.

food insecurity Household-level economic and social condition characterized by uncertain access to adequate food.

The Economic Research Service (ERS) of the United States Department of Agriculture (USDA) uses four categories to identify different levels of **food security** in the United States (**Table 21.1**).[5] **Food insecurity** describes "limited or uncertain availability of nutritionally adequate and safe foods or limited or uncertain ability to acquire acceptable foods in socially acceptable ways."[6] The ERS reports that 12.7 percent (15.8 million) of U.S. households were food insecure at some time during 2013, including 5.0 percent (6.3 million) with very low food security.[7] About 42.2 million people in the United States lived in food-insecure households in 2015; 6.4 million of those households include children. About 5 percent of households were in the lowest-level category, classified as "very low food security."[8]

TABLE 21.1	Ranges of Food Security	
General Category	**Level of Food Security**	**Description of Conditions in the Household**
Food Security	High food security	No reported indications of food-access problems or limitations.
	Marginal food security	One or two reported indications—typically of anxiety over food sufficiency or shortage of food in the house. Little or no indication of changes in diets or food intake.
Food Insecurity	Low food security	Reports of reduced quality, variety, or desirability of diet. Little or no indication of reduced food intake.
	Very low food security	Reports of multiple indications of disrupted eating patterns and reduced food intake.

Source: Adapted from USDA Economic Research Service. 2016. *Definitions of Food Security.* Available at https://www.ers.usda.gov/topics/food-nutrition-assistance/food-security-in-the-us/definitions-of-food-security.aspx. Accessed February 2017.

Food Insecurity Is More Likely Among Certain Population Groups

According to the ERS, Americans most likely to be very food insecure live in households with one or more of these life situations:[9]

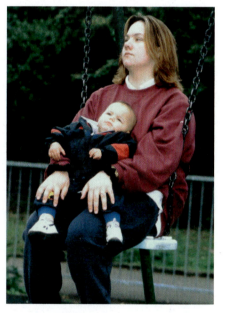

In the United States, poor single parents and their children can experience food insecurity due to unemployment, low wages, or other circumstances that lead to financial hardship.

- Households with children headed by a single parent
- Single people living alone
- Households with incomes below the poverty line
- Black, non-Hispanic households or Hispanic households
- Households located outside metropolitan areas (or rural)

For single parents heading a household, a lack of childcare may mean they can't work enough hours, and expensive childcare arrangements can drain an already-tight budget. Single parents may feel stuck in low-wage jobs, unable to explore more lucrative career paths requiring training or higher education because of their obligations to their children. In 2015, about 30.3 percent of single women heading up a household with children experienced food insecurity.[10]

Single people living alone include seniors, and 9 percent of all seniors were food insecure in 2014.[11] Seniors may be living on a fixed income and are less likely than other groups to enroll themselves in food-assistance programs.[12] They may also be disabled or have chronic conditions that decrease their ability to shop for themselves.

People living in households with incomes below the poverty line are at greater risk of being food insecure. Poverty is the primary factor in food insecurity and is discussed separately in the next section.

Because they experience disproportionate levels of poverty, it is not surprising that African Americans and Hispanics also experience higher rates of food insecurity than the national average, with 21.5 percent and 19.1 percent experiencing food insecurity, respectively, in 2015.[13] A number of factors may contribute to these statistics: African Americans experience unemployment at twice the rate of Caucasian Americans[14] and Hispanics tend to have larger family sizes and lower household incomes, which can make feeding the whole family difficult.[15]

Those living in households outside metropolitan areas struggle with multiple challenges to food security, including higher unemployment and lower wages, lower education levels, and lower access to affordable childcare and public transportation. Of rural households in the United States, 16.7 percent live below the poverty line and 15 percent are food insecure, with the South having the highest poverty rate.[16] Between 2013 and

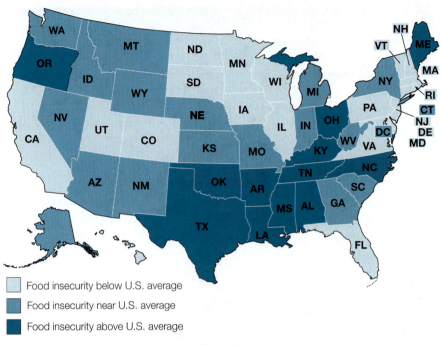

Food insecurity below U.S. average

Food insecurity near U.S. average

Food insecurity above U.S. average

▲ **Figure 21.1 Food Insecurity in the United States**
Though some areas of the United States have higher rates of food insecurity and/or hunger, these conditions can happen anywhere. In this map, data for 3 years, 2013–2015, were combined to provide more reliable statistics at the state level.
Source: United States Department of Agriculture, Economic Research Service. Updated 2015. *Food Security in the U.S.: Key Statistics & Graphics.* Available at www.ers.usda.gov. Accessed April 2017.

2015, the six states with the highest food-insecurity rates were Mississippi, Louisiana, Arkansas tied with Maine, and Kentucky tied with Alabama.[17] **Figure 21.1** shows levels of food insecurity in all U.S. states.

College students, too, experience food insecurity. Recent studies found that 21 percent of students at the University of Hawaii, 39 percent of students at the City University of New York (CUNY), and more than half of the students attending certain colleges in Oregon, Maryland, and Alaska were food insecure.[18,19,20,21,22] Some colleges are starting to offer campus food banks to support students who are food insecure. Does that include you? Take the Self-Assessment and find out.

Poverty Contributes to Food Insecurity

Poverty is the principal cause of food insecurity in the United States. The U.S. Census Bureau estimated that for 2015, the poverty rate was about 13.5 percent of the United States population. The poverty rate in 2015 for children under age 18 was 19.7 percent.[23] As of 2015, for a married couple or a single mother plus a child, poverty means a household income below $15,391 per year. A family of four would be impoverished with an income below $24,036.[24]

In 2012, about 9.5 million adults were classified among the **working poor**.[25] Though these people had jobs, they still had incomes below the poverty line. High housing and utility costs can consume most of the household budget and leave little money for food. Individuals in these households may be living "paycheck to paycheck." An unexpected expense, such as an illness or a costly auto repair, can force the working poor to choose between paying the bills and consuming a healthy, adequate diet.

People living in poverty often reside in rural regions or inner-city neighborhoods lacking healthy food stores. These regions are technically known as **food deserts**.[26] The U.S. Centers for Disease Control and Prevention (CDC) defines food deserts as areas

poverty Lacking the means to provide for material or comfort needs.

working poor Individuals or families who are steadily employed but still experience poverty due to low wages or high dependent expenses.

food deserts Parts of the country, usually impoverished areas, where fresh fruits, vegetables, and other healthful whole foods are scarce, largely due to a lack of grocery stores, farmers markets, and healthy-food providers.

without ready access to affordable fruits, vegetables, whole grains, lowfat milk, and other foods that make up the full range of a healthy diet.[27] Food deserts exist all over the United States. You can look for your community in the USDA Food Desert Locator by going to www.ers.usda.gov and searching for food desert locator.

Illness and Disability Can Lead to Food Insecurity

Adults who are chronically ill or disabled are less likely to earn a steady income and are therefore at increased risk of food insecurity. Even when they are employed, disease symptoms and health care appointments may cause them to miss work frequently. These absences can significantly reduce a paycheck, and thus available funds for food. Chronic illness and disability may also be accompanied by high out-of-pocket costs for medications, which can deplete income that would otherwise be available for food.

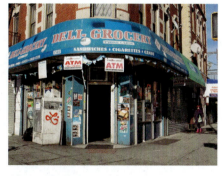

People in poor urban neighborhoods often find themselves in "food deserts," with little access to fresh, healthy food found in supermarkets.

Mental illness, including substance abuse disorders, can also contribute to food insecurity. People who suffer from anxiety disorders, depression, schizophrenia, alcoholism, or drug abuse may lose interest in eating. These individuals may also find it difficult to get and keep steady employment, may have decreased access to cooking facilities, and may have difficulty shopping for and preparing nutritious food. In a vicious cycle, mental health problems among mothers and their children increase when mothers are food insecure.[28]

According to the National Coalition for the Homeless, some 20–25 percent of individuals who are homeless are also mentally ill.[29] People who are homeless can be difficult to reach, counsel, or help. They may be forced to rely on charity, church meals, or public assistance programs for most of their food.

What Factors Contribute to Malnutrition around the World?

LO 21.2 Describe the causes of malnutrition worldwide.

Of a global population now exceeding 7.5 billion people, a minority—about 1.2 billion—live in developed countries.[30] The other 6 billion live in **developing** and **least developed** countries—collectively referred to as the developing world—where many lack full access to goods and services. The Food and Agriculture Organization (FAO) of the United Nations estimates that there were 795 million undernourished people in the world in 2014–2016.[31] **Figure 21.2** shows levels of undernourishment across the globe.

Malnutrition in the developing world is caused by a complex set of factors. Once again, poverty lies at the heart of the problem; however, discrimination, war and political unrest, agricultural challenges and food waste, climate change, natural disasters, resource depletion, and overpopulation all contribute to food insecurity for large numbers of people, particularly in Asia and Africa.

Discrimination Contributes to Malnutrition

In many poor countries, discrimination at both the national and local levels contributes to malnutrition. For example, at the national level, control over land and other assets is often unequal, so that even increased crop yields do not decrease food insecurity.

developing country Country that is growing in multiple areas, such as income per capita, life expectancy, rate of literacy, industrial capability, technological sophistication, and economic productivity.

least developed country Country that shows little growth in multiple areas, such as income per capita, life expectancy, rate of literacy, industrial capability, technological sophistication, and economic productivity.

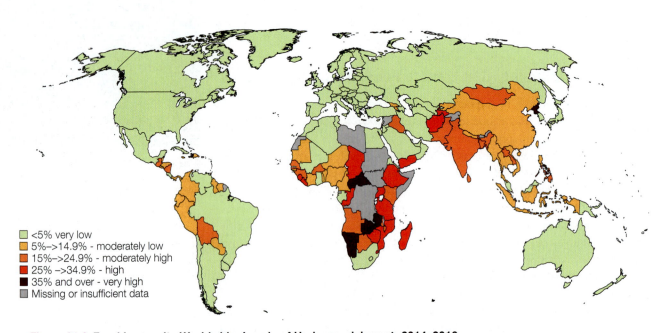

- <5% very low
- 5%–>14.9% - moderately low
- 15%–>24.9% - moderately high
- 25% –>34.9% - high
- 35% and over - very high
- Missing or insufficient data

▲ **Figure 21.2 Food Insecurity Worldwide, Levels of Undernourishment, 2014–2016**
Food insecurity is a global problem. This map shows which areas of the globe are most profoundly affected.
Source: FAO, IFAD, and WFP. 2015. *The State of Food Insecurity in the World 2015.* Available at www.fao.org. Accessed April 2017.

Very few people in certain developing countries own their own land, and a plentiful crop primarily benefits the landowner, not the farm laborer. Women, especially, suffer from discrimination.[32]

Cultural practices may also compromise access to food at the local or household level. In some cultures and within some families, the amount of food available to an individual is influenced by gender, control of income, education, birth order, and age. A study in Nigeria, for example, found that men controlled the household income and had preference in household food sharing.[33] Gender inequity is a serious problem worldwide. In many cultures women and girls are viewed as less valuable than men and boys, and they therefore receive less food and education. Of the 17 percent of the world population that is illiterate, two-thirds are women.[34] Young women are also disproportionately affected by lack of employment opportunities.[35]

Political Sanctions and Armed Conflicts Disrupt the Food Supply

Political sanctions can create or intensify food shortages by decreasing a population's access to agricultural supplies, fuel, or food imports. They can also result in higher local prices for fuel, food, and other essentials. Sanctions that block exports to other countries can also contribute indirectly to a failing economy by decreasing household income when workers in businesses that rely on this trade lose their jobs. All of these factors can lead to widespread food shortages that may cause a collapse in food production and distribution and, ultimately, widespread malnutrition.[36]

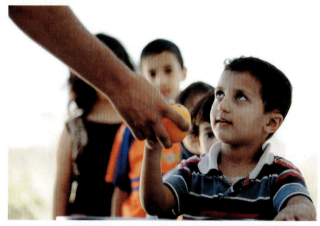

Many hunger relief programs work to provide food aid to nations in conflict. However, successfully delivering the food to those who need it is often challenging.

According to the World Food Programme, armed conflicts are another major cause of world malnutrition.[37] War and civil and political unrest lead to malnutrition by disrupting agriculture, food distribution, and normal community activities. During the past two decades, the world has experienced terrorism, tribal and religious warfare, and civil war in countries such as Somalia, the Democratic Republic of Congo, and Syria. During wars and regional conflicts, government money is often diverted from nutrition and food distribution programs and redirected toward weapons and military support. Moreover, political turbulence can compromise humanitarian food distribution efforts, making it difficult for food aid to reach the people in need. In some cases, assistance programs and aid workers have to abandon war-torn areas and curtail their relief efforts.

Agricultural Challenges and Food Waste Limit the Food Supply

Because of advances in agricultural technologies, including the introduction and widespread adoption of genetically modified high-yield crops, world agriculture produces 17 percent more kilocalories per person today than it did 30 years ago, which is enough to provide everyone in the world with at least 2,700 kilocalories per day.[38] Unfortunately, these advances are leading to the loss of genetic diversity of plants, damaging use of pesticides, evolution of pesticide-resistant pests, pollution by run-off of fertilizers, and depletion of water reservoirs. While these practices may increase crop yield in the short term, they are unsustainable in the long term.[39]

Moreover, agricultural challenges still persist in many regions, contributing to global food insecurity. A lack of access to information about modern farming practices, seeds, and equipment can keep farmers from reaching the land's full potential. Establishing efficient irrigation systems is another major challenge. Underground drip systems allow farmers to water crops accurately, without wasting water, and yet such systems are expensive

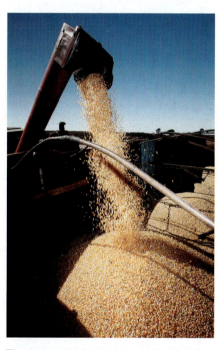

Thanks to agricultural advances, the world's farmers can grow plenty of food. However, distribution problems and other factors keep some people from getting enough to stave off hunger.

Reducing Food Waste

Shopping tips:

Plan out meals for a week at a time.

Check your fridge and cabinets before you shop.

Buy only foods you really need.

When you shop, stick to the list!

Cooking and storage tips:

Understand and use expiration dates properly.

Use up older foods in the fridge first.

Have "leftover night" once a week.

Compost!

Serve yourself only what you can eat.

Cook meals in large batches; freeze portions for later.

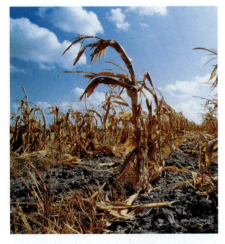

Shortsighted farming techniques can deplete natural resources and take a heavy toll on crops and farmland.

famine Severe shortage of food caused by weather-related crop destruction, poor agricultural practices, pestilence, war, or other factors.

overpopulation Condition in which a region has more people than its natural resources can support.

to buy and require some knowledge to install and maintain. Furrow irrigation systems, which are inexpensive and simple, can get water where it needs to go, but water is lost in transit, and these systems cause soil erosion.[40]

Finally, an astonishing one-third of all food produced is never consumed.[41] According to the FAO, tons of food is wasted all along the food chain from farm to table, with larger losses occurring during agricultural production in developing countries, and at the consumer level in wealthier regions—like the overripe bananas no one purchases at the grocery store.[42] Tackling the food waste problem involves reducing production to meet actual demand, directing surplus to regions in need, and responsibly recycling what can't be reused. For ideas on how you can reduce food waste, see the Table Tips.

Climate Change, Natural Disasters, and Depleted Resources Limit Food Production

Climate change is affecting Earth's ability to produce food. We see evidence of this in droughts, floods, record-breaking heat waves, and emerging crop diseases and infestations around the world, all of which ruin crops. In the United States, technological advances can help farmers cope with the effects of climate change, and relief programs can help affected communities. Nevertheless, devastating weather events can still wipe out crops.[43] In contrast, in the developing world, the effects of climate change and natural disasters can completely devastate communities. In just one example, entire villages in southern Madagascar are in the midst of **famine** as a result of a persistent drought attributed to climate change. Lack of communication and transportation systems, inadequate funding for relief programs, an inability to relocate populations from disaster-prone areas, and the incapacity to make homes and farms less vulnerable to destructive weather forces can all contribute to the problem.

Drought is the leading cause of severe food shortages not only in Madagascar but throughout the developing world. When drought conditions exist, crops cannot be adequately irrigated. In addition, access to safe and clean drinking water becomes limited, increasing a population's risk for infectious disease and dehydration. Undernutrition results, particularly in people who depend on agriculture for both food and income. Lack of water can even force livestock owners to slaughter part of their herd or sell animals at "distress sales."[44]

Floods and excessive rain can also destroy food crops and are major causes of food shortage. For example, in India, more than 70 percent of the annual rainfall occurs during the 3 months of monsoon season. Farmers must contend with water scarcity for 9 months of the year only to be faced with crop failure later if monsoon rains are overly heavy.

Depletion of natural resources also threatens the world's food supply. Water is one example; this natural resource is not infinite. About 3 percent of the water on Earth is fresh water, and most of that is locked up in ice or inaccessible underground.[45] Industrial waste, pesticides, and untreated human wastewater pollute the fresh water supply and make it unusable for drinking water.[46] Agriculture uses about 70 percent of the available fresh water, and yet wastes about 60 percent of this water through leaky irrigation systems, inefficient watering systems, and poor choice of crops for the land.[47] Without better management, a lack of water will reduce the food supply.

Overpopulation Leads to Food Scarcity

The world population is projected to reach 8.5 billion people by 2030, and 9.7 billion by 2050.[48] Much of this growth is taking place in the least developed regions, where the population is expected to increase from about 900 million people currently to 1.8 billion in 2050, as shown in **Figure 21.3**.[49] Whenever rapid population growth occurs in areas that are strained for food production, the resulting **overpopulation** can take a toll on the local people's nutritional status.

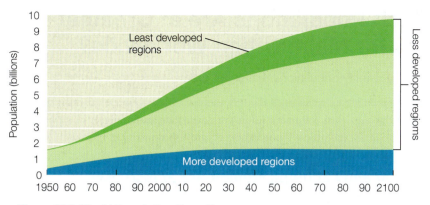

▲ **Figure 21.3 World Population Growth**
The majority of people in the world live in developing countries, and this number is expected to grow.

Source: United Nations Population Division. 2015. *World Population Prospects: The 2015 Revision, medium variant.* Available at http://esa.un.org. Accessed April 2017.

People in the developing world tend to have more children than people in developed regions for a variety of reasons. The infant and child mortality rate is high, so parents have more children to ensure that some of their offspring survive into adulthood. Large families are also needed to work on farms to help generate income and to support older family members later in life. Additionally, women in developing regions have reduced access to reliable methods of contraception, higher education, and career opportunities, all of which work to limit family size in developed nations. The World Bank promotes gender equality and development to break this cycle and ensure that girls and women receive a basic education.[50]

The Nutrition Transition Can Contribute to Malnutrition

Ironically, malnutrition is not confined to those who are food insecure or even hungry. In countries that are becoming more prosperous, while people are getting more food to eat, they are not necessarily eating high-quality food. As nations get richer, people who formerly ate meals full of vegetables and grains may shift over to diets higher in saturated fats and sugars. And as workers move from rural locations to cities, and from agricultural jobs to sedentary jobs, they get less exercise. These factors contribute to a so-called **nutrition transition** that leads to overweight, obesity, and potentially malnutrition.[51]

One of the hallmarks of populations in nutrition transition is the coexistence of undernutrition and overnutrition in the same community, as some community members thrive while others remain in desperate poverty. This coexistence of under- and over-nutrition can also be seen within a single family or even in individuals. The boys in a family may be overweight, for example, while the girls are underweight, or an individual may be obese but deficient in certain micronutrients.[52] This phenomenon is called the *double burden of malnutrition.*

LO 21.2: THE TAKE-HOME MESSAGE Factors that give rise to malnutrition around the world include poverty, discrimination, political sanctions and armed conflicts, poor agricultural practices and food waste, climate change, natural disasters, resource depletion, overpopulation, and the nutrition transition.

nutrition transition Shift in dietary consumption and energy expenditure that may occur as people in developing countries shift from their traditional diet to diets higher in sugar, fat, and animal-based foods.

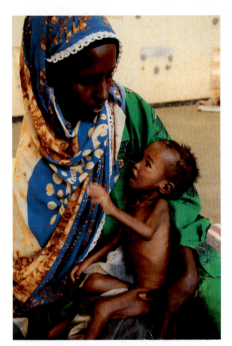

Because of the increased nutrient needs associated with pregnancy, lactation, and early childhood growth, mothers and their young children are at particular risk for malnutrition.

Which Populations Are at Greatest Risk for Malnutrition Worldwide?

LO 21.3 Identify populations that are at greatest risk for malnutrition.

Because of their increased nutritional needs, infants, children, and pregnant and lactating women are at higher risk for malnutrition worldwide than are other groups. Older adults, people who are ill, and people living in poverty are also at increased risk.

Pregnant and Lactating Women Are at Increased Risk for Malnutrition

As discussed in Chapter 17, nutrient requirements increase during pregnancy and lactation. Pregnant women need extra kilocalories and nutrients—in particular, protein, vitamins, and minerals—to support a healthy pregnancy. In general, during the first 6 months of a pregnancy, the majority of the additional kilocalories are used to nourish the mother as her body undergoes the changes necessary to support a pregnancy. During the last 3 months of a pregnancy, the majority of extra kilocalories are needed by the growing fetus to increase fetal reserves of protein, fat, and various micronutrients.[53] Improperly nourished pregnant women often give birth to malnourished infants.

Because human breast milk is the ideal nourishment for infants, women throughout the world are encouraged to breastfeed their babies. The global recommendation is for women to nurse their babies for the first 6 months and to continue nursing with supplemental foods into the child's second year of life.[54] Ideally, a woman of average weight who is breastfeeding would eat about 500 extra kilocalories per day to stay properly nourished. If this doesn't happen, the mother, and possibly the baby, will lose weight.[55]

One qualification to the breastfeeding recommendation applies to women who are HIV positive. Mothers with HIV risk passing the virus to their infants through breast milk, and therefore should be encouraged to use formula that is either canned or made from powder mixed with boiled, cool water, or to employ a noninfected wet nurse to feed their babies. However, HIV-positive women who can't afford these alternatives are advised to breastfeed their children. In these cases, the benefits of providing the nutrients in the breast milk, coupled with the risks of infection from making formula from contaminated water, outweigh the risks of passing the HIV infection on to the baby.

Infants and Children Are Highly Susceptible to Malnutrition

Infants are particularly susceptible to malnutrition because they are growing rapidly and have high nutrient requirements (per unit of body weight). Infants whose mothers are malnourished themselves are at particularly high risk for malnutrition because their mothers' supply of breast milk will be reduced.

After 6 months of age infants require solid food in addition to breast milk, which puts them at increased risk for malnutrition if food supplies are limited. As an infant transitions from an all–breast milk diet to a diet of breast milk plus solid foods, she or he is also at risk for improper weaning, which can lead to diminished growth during the first year of life and the potential for severe malnutrition during the second year of life.[56] Babies may be given foods that are inappropriate—too high in dietary fiber, for example, or too low in protein. During the sixth to twelfth months of life, children may be more likely to be exposed to contaminated food and water, which may cause diarrhea and dehydration. When infants begin to crawl and walk, their risk of exposure to and thus infection by bacteria and parasites increases. Some parasitic infestations cause nutritional deficiencies directly. For example, hookworms suck blood from the lining of the gut, causing iron-deficiency anemia.

The risk of malnutrition continues from infancy into early childhood and may result from food shortages within the family or chronic disease. If there is a severe lack of protein in the diet, for example, children may develop kwashiorkor (see Chapter 6). Malnourishment also builds on itself: Children who are ill or malnourished have poor appetites—their normal hunger sensations are diminished. In some children maldigestion and malabsorption exacerbate the problem by increasing the loss of nutrients.

The loss of one or both parents from disease may also lead to decreased family income and a greater risk of malnourishment. For example, about 17 million children in the world have lost one or both parents to HIV/AIDS in the last 30 years, increasing their risk of malnutrition.[57] An estimated 36.7 million people in the world had HIV/AIDS in 2015, including 1.8 million children under age 15.[58] Most of these children were born to mothers with HIV or obtained the virus during infancy (via childbirth or breastfeeding).

The Ill and the Elderly Are Also at High Risk for Malnutrition

People who are chronically ill may have malabsorption problems that reduce their nutritional status. Liver and kidney disease can impair the body's ability to process and use some nutrients. Some cancer patients and many people with AIDS experience loss of appetite, which reduces their kilocalorie intake and further complicates their treatment.

Although older adults need fewer kilocalories due to a decrease in their metabolic rate and lower levels of physical activity, they have higher requirements for vitamin D, vitamin B_6, and calcium, and are thought to need more protein per kilogram of body weight, as compared to younger adults. Older people may be at risk for nutrient deficiencies because of a decreased sense of taste and smell, immobility, malabsorption, or chronic illnesses. Loneliness, isolation, poverty, missing teeth, confusion, or disinterest in cooking and eating also contribute to malnutrition. In addition, most elderly people, whether in the United States or in other countries, live on a fixed income or have no income at all and must depend on family members to provide for them. In such cases, food is often stretched, and meals are smaller or are skipped altogether. All of these factors contribute to an increased rate of food insecurity and malnutrition in the older adult population.

People Living in Poverty Have Unique Risk Factors for Overnutrition

Unfortunately, overweight among those who are food insecure is common. High-fat, high-kilocalorie diets are more affordable than diets based on lean meats, fish, vegetables, and fruits. There is a clear link in women between food insecurity and overweight and obesity. Research suggests that mothers often restrict their food intake during periods of food insufficiency to protect their children from malnutrition, and then overcompensate when food is available. These chronic ups and downs of food intake can contribute to obesity.[59]

For those living on a limited budget, filling their cupboards with food, even if that food is low in nutrients, takes precedence over choosing foods with nutritional value. If they live in a food desert, people who are poor may not even have access to nutritious foods.

Living in poverty increases stress,[60] but sugar consumption has been shown to reduce secretion of the stress hormone cortisol.[61] This may make foods high in added sugars particularly appealing as a way to manage the chronic stresses of poverty.

Finally, cheaper foods tend to be low in protein and high in kilocalories. To get the same level of satiety, you would have to eat more kilocalories from chips and candy than you would from a high-protein snack like a hard-boiled egg. As you have learned from previous chapters, a diet high in empty kilocalories and low in nutrient-dense kilocalories can increase the risk of overnutrition.

How Can We Reduce Hunger?

LO 21.4 Explain several ways to reduce hunger.

In the United States, hunger relief efforts exist at many levels. At the local level, individuals, families, churches, and community relief agencies seek out and assist people who have insufficient resources. Examples of assistance include hot meals and free food provided by local shelters and food banks, as well as education and job training provided by local and state governments, nonprofit organizations, and faith-based organizations. See the Spotlight on America's Second Harvest for more information about food banks and how you can help.

The U.S. government also engages in hunger relief efforts, providing food aid and creating economic opportunities for people who want to improve their lives. The USDA, for example, spent over $104 billion in 2015 on numerous food assistance programs to feed Americans in need.[64] **Table 21.2** identifies some of the main USDA food assistance programs.

TABLE 21.2 Food Assistance Programs in the United States

Program	Eligibility	Description	Prevalence
Supplemental Nutrition Assistance Program (SNAP; formerly the Food Stamp Program)	Low income (for a family of four in 2016, the net monthly income could not exceed $2,025)	Eligible individuals are issued a debit card to purchase food at their local authorized supermarket. (Items such as alcohol, tobacco, nonfood items, vitamins and medicines, and hot foods are not covered.)	In 2016, more than 44.2 million people per month in the United States
Special Supplemental Nutrition Program for Women, Infants and Children (WIC)	At-risk low-income pregnant and lactating women, infants, and children less than 5 years old	The program provides nutritious, culturally appropriate foods to supplement the diet. The program also emphasizes nutrition education and offers referrals to health care providers	About 8 million women, infants, and children per month in 2015
National School Lunch Program; School Breakfast Program	Children with families with incomes at or below 130% of the poverty level are eligible for free meals and those with incomes between 130% and 185% of the poverty level are eligible for reduced-price meals	Eligible children receive free or reduced-price lunches and/or breakfasts at school each day.	More than 30 million American children joined the lunch program in 2016, and almost 14.5 million children participated in the breakfast program
Summer Food Service Program	Available to communities based on income data	Federal program that combines a meal or feeding program with a summer activity program for children	During 2016, more than 2.8 million children daily at 42,654 sites
Child and Adult Care Food Program	Available to communities based on income data	Program provides nutritious meals to low-income children and older adults who receive daycare or adult care outside the home. There are income guidelines for program participation	More than 4.4 million children and adults receive meals and snacks each day as part of this program
Congregate Meals for the Elderly and Meals on Wheels	Age 60 or over	The programs provide meals at a community site or delivered to the home	More than 1 million meals per day served at sites across the country

Sources: Data from USDA, Food and Nutrition Service. 2017. *Supplemental Nutrition Assistance Program (SNAP), WIC Program, National School Lunch Program (NSLP), Summer Food Service Program, Child/Adult Care Food Program,* www.fns.usda.gov. Meals on Wheels Association of America. 2017. www.mowaa.org.

Hunger Among Us (and How You Can Help!)

Food insecurity may be closer than you think. In fact, you may have friends, relatives, or neighbors who've experienced hunger sometime in their lives, or perhaps you've been hungry yourself.

America's Second Harvest, the largest hunger relief organization in the United States, was started to help individuals who are routinely without food. The mission of this organization is to eradicate hunger and ensure that no American goes to bed hungry. They redistribute excess and donated food and grocery items, work to increase public awareness of hunger, and advocate for those who are hungry. America's Second Harvest distributed more than 52 million pounds of food from July 2015 through June 2016, through partnerships with over 320 nonprofit agencies.[62]

America's Second Harvest stores surplus food from national food companies and other large donors in a centralized location. Volunteers travel to these

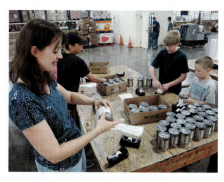

Everyone—from children to adults—can help eradicate hunger.

centers and gather and transport the donated foods to local **food pantries** or **emergency kitchens**. Volunteers and workers also staff food rescue organizations that "rescue" prepared foods, such as ready-to-eat surplus items from banquets, company and college cafeterias, and restaurants, that would otherwise go to waste.[63] Sometimes food rescue centers are located in the same building as food banks.

When it comes to fighting hunger in America, everyone needs to pitch in. You can help your needy neighbors in three ways: give funds, give food, and give time. Funds can be donated online at www.secondharvest.org. You can donate food by hosting a food drive. Finally, you can volunteer your time by helping out in your local community, perhaps by tutoring children on healthy eating practices, repackaging donated food, stocking shelves at a local food pantry, or transporting food to the hungry.

To find out where you can help, visit the America's Second Harvest website (www.secondharvest.org) and click on the volunteer link.

food pantry Community food assistance location where food is provided to needy individuals and families.

emergency kitchen Kitchen or a commercial food service that prepares for natural disasters, emergencies, or terrorist attacks.

In addition to the human (person-to-person) help provided by people and organizations, technology also plays a role in alleviating malnutrition by improving agricultural techniques, land management, water use, and sanitation and by fortifying common foods with iodine and other micronutrients of concern. The following discussion looks at a number of these solutions.

Improve Agriculture

The long-term solution to malnutrition in any given region requires balancing the number of people in that region with the amount of food that can be locally produced. Even where poverty is widespread, the region's capacity to feed its population can be increased by developing manageable systems for producing food.[65] Crop sales generate income that not only benefits the landowners and workers, but travels throughout the community to significantly decrease poverty and help reduce malnutrition.

Biotechnology, specifically the production of genetically modified foods, can create crops with increased yields and pest resistance. Some staple crops, such as corn and rice, can be bioengineered to contain an increased level of nutrients. Biotechnology can also be used to improve the taste or shelf-life of fruits and vegetables.

On the other end of the spectrum, many farmers are turning to organic farming. In organic farming, as defined by the USDA,

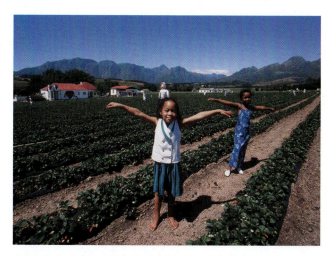

Better land management, appropriate crop selection, and biotechnology can all help eliminate malnutrition.

farmers do not use genetically modified organisms or toxic or persistent pesticides or fertilizers. They do support animal health and welfare, provide outdoor access for animals, use only approved materials, receive annual onsite inspections, and separate organic from nonorganic food. They thus preserve natural resources and biodiversity and reduce pollution.[66] As the soil on organic farms becomes balanced, the crops growing there tend to become healthier, and more disease resistant. While the yield from an organic farm may be lower than that of an industrial farm, organically grown plants tend to be more drought resistant.

In areas of Africa, farmers have had success leveraging the natural qualities of local plants as protection, where pests, climate change, and soil degradation have caused chronic food insecurity. For example, the local cereal crop, grown for its nutritional value, is planted with companion plants chosen specifically for their value in discouraging pests and nourishing the soil by capturing nitrogen. The whole field is then surrounded by a border of a third plant that attracts pests away from the main crop. Plants are chosen for their drought-resistant qualities as well. With better soil and fewer pests, the cereal crop can thrive and grain yields are higher.[67]

If farmers raised more crops for human consumption rather than for food-animal consumption, they could, generally speaking, feed more people. Right now, only a little over half of the world's crop kilocalories—kilocalories available from crops grown—actually feeds humans. About 36 percent goes to feed animals that are raised for human consumption. If we grew a greater percentage of crops for human consumption, rather than for raising meat, we could increase available kilocalories by as much as 70 percent.[68]

Increasing farmers' land ownership can also increase food security. Farmers who own their land are motivated to make better decisions regarding irrigation, crop rotation, land fallowing (leaving land plowed but unplanted), and appropriate soil management.[69] Unfortunately, land ownership is not evenly distributed across most populations. This situation is unlikely to change without *land reform*, in which governments create rules to reallocate land to landless people. In some countries, grassroots programs are providing access to land for women and their families for the purpose of growing food.

Improve Water and Sanitation

At least 1.8 billion people worldwide lack access to safe drinking water.[70] Providing safe water is critical in reducing malnutrition. The CDC stated in 2015 that 88 percent of all diarrheal illnesses in the world are attributable to unsafe water or inadequate sanitation.[71] Because diarrhea reduces nutrient absorption, a person who has diarrhea is at increased risk for malnutrition.[72]

Some innovative solutions are being proposed to alleviate the world's safe water problems. In some communities in Asia, Africa, and Latin America, for example, solar energy is used to thermally purify the water supply.[73] Water is poured into plastic PET jugs that are placed on black-covered roofs and allowed to heat for several hours. Once the temperature of the water exceeds 50°C (122°F), it becomes safe to drink. The heat and UV radiation effectively destroy common waterborne bacteria, viruses, and pathogens such as those that cause cholera, typhoid, dysentery, polio, and diarrhea.

About 2.4 billion people (36 percent of the developing world's population) lack basic sanitation facilities like flush toilets or covered latrines. They still use open-pit toilets or simply defecate on the ground.[74] Lack of proper toilets and sewage systems can lead to the contamination of rivers and groundwater. Poor sanitation is linked to the spread of diseases such as cholera, diarrhea, hepatitis A, and other communicable diseases.

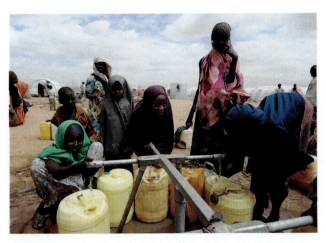

Access to clean drinking water is just as important as adequate nutrition for human health.

One initiative to improve sanitation in developing countries comes from the Gates Foundation, which has challenged engineers to create a toilet that would be cost effective, that would operate in conditions that mimic those in developing countries—without electricity, sewer lines, or water lines—and that would recapture energy, clean water, and nutrients from human waste. Developers are testing such toilets in India and China.[75]

Fortify Foods to Raise Nutrient Levels

Globally the most common micronutrient deficiencies include iodine, iron, and vitamin A. The fortification of staple foods with nutrients can help to alleviate these deficiencies. For food fortification to work, the staple foods must be shelf-stable, affordable, and consistently available in the food supply. Rice, cereals, flours, salt, and even sugar are examples of foods that can be successfully fortified.

Because food fortification is inexpensive, as well as enormously beneficial, fortification programs are being developed and implemented worldwide. Countries all across the globe fortify foods such as flour, salt, oil, sugar, and soy sauce with iron, iodine, and vitamin A.[76]

Promote Education

Education plays a critical role in improving food security, both directly and indirectly. Educating farmers on best agricultural practices—including crop rotation, irrigation, and fertilization—for sustainable farming can directly improve agricultural productivity, which in turns improves the chances of achieving food security.[77]

Education indirectly affects food security by reducing population growth. Educating girls and women is of particular importance: as noted earlier, population growth slows and children are healthier when women are educated.[78] Education must also focus on developing literacy, technical knowledge, agricultural skills, horticulture, human health and reproduction, and the preservation of natural resources.[79]

Assistance Programs Are Working to End Hunger Around the World

Across the globe many large and small international organizations are working to end hunger. The World Food Programme, which has the goal of getting to "Zero Hunger," provides hundreds of thousands of tons of food per year to people in need, and this is only one of its programs—it also provides cash and vouchers to people who have access to food but not enough money to buy it, and it has programs to put people to work to improve their community and get paid in food.[80] Another large organization, UNICEF, channels money for humanitarian aid from people in developed countries to help feed children in need in developing countries. UNICEF was founded after World War II to help children in war-torn countries, and it continues to help children worldwide today.[81]

The group Heifer International has the goal of ending poverty by providing families with animals such as sheep, goats, cows, or ducks.[82] The idea is that families can become self-sufficient and also sell surplus milk, eggs, and wool. The group also provides tools and training. Making families self-sufficient can help to lift them out of poverty.

The Peace Corps is another organization that helps reduce malnutrition by giving people the training and support they need to change their own situation. In one initiative, volunteers are helping to make sure girls get a chance to go to school. In another, they are helping local people establish sustainable methods to feed themselves, not just by growing more food, but by learning about health and nutrition.[83]

HEALTH**CONNECTION**

What Are the Effects of Chronic Undernutrition?

LO 21.5 Describe the health consequences of undernutrition.

The detrimental health effects of acute undernutrition can be reversible. In contrast, persistent undernutrition can prompt a downward health spiral that is hard to reverse (**Figure 21.4**).[84]

In times of reduced kilocalorie intake, such as when dieting to lose weight, fasting, ill, or experiencing famine, the body attempts to conserve energy and preserve body tissues by lowering basal metabolism. As the kilocalorie deficit continues, the body begins to break down its own tissues for energy. This results in the reduction of stored fat and ultimately the deterioration of internal organs and muscle mass. In prolonged starvation, adults can lose up to 50 percent of their body weight. The greatest amount of deterioration occurs in the GI tract and the liver; the loss is moderate in the heart and kidneys; and the least damage occurs in the brain and other parts of the nervous system.

Let's look at some individual effects of malnutrition.

growth stunting Impaired growth and development caused by undernutrition primarily in childhood. Once growth stunting occurs, it is usually permanent.

wasting Diminishment of muscle and fat tissue caused by extremely low energy intake.

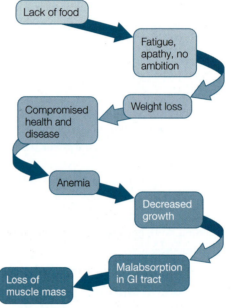

▲ **Figure 21.4 Downward Spiral of Hunger and Malnutrition**
Lack of food can lead to numerous other symptoms that compound the problem of hunger.

Children Suffer Impaired Growth and Development

The bodies of children who are undernourished compensate for a lack of food by decreasing physical and mental growth. An undernourished child is therefore likely to experience both physical and mental problems, including insufficient weight gain and reduced height, inadequate muscle development, lowered resistance to infection, and impaired brain development (**Figure 21.5**).[85]

Malnourished children experience **growth stunting** (lower than expected height for age). Globally, an estimated

156 million children experienced stunting in 2015, and about 145 million of these children lived in Africa and Asia.[86] Deficiencies of energy, protein, iron, and zinc, as well as prolonged infection, have been implicated as causes. In 2015, about 50 million children under 5 years old in the developing world suffered from **wasting** (decreased weight for age).[87]

If malnutrition occurs at early, crucial times of brain development, cognitive development is impaired.[88] Reduced cognitive development can in turn result in permanent lower intelligence and impaired learning. As a result, malnourished children may be unable to complete an elementary education and therefore have a reduced income-earning ability later in life. For example, iodine deficiency in a pregnant woman's diet can result in *congenital hypothyroidism*, also known as *cretinism*, in her child. In severe cases, the child may have brain damage, deaf-mutism, squinting, and difficulty walking.[89] The condition may be prevented by providing enough iodine in the mother's diet—typically via the use of iodized salt. According to the WHO, iodine deficiency is the most preventable cause of brain damage, and salt fortification programs are "spectacularly simple [and] universally effective."[90]

During their school years, children are more likely to show behavioral, emotional, and academic problems if they come from families that experience food insecurity. In particular, long-term undernutrition is associated with increased anxiety, irritability, attention problems, and school absence and tardiness rates.[91] Even if malnourished

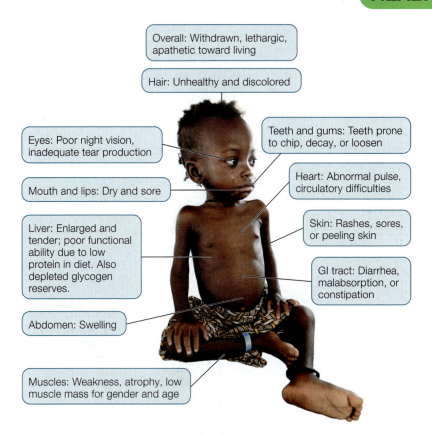

Overall: Withdrawn, lethargic, apathetic toward living

Hair: Unhealthy and discolored

Eyes: Poor night vision, inadequate tear production

Mouth and lips: Dry and sore

Liver: Enlarged and tender; poor functional ability due to low protein in diet. Also depleted glycogen reserves.

Abdomen: Swelling

Muscles: Weakness, atrophy, low muscle mass for gender and age

Teeth and gums: Teeth prone to chip, decay, or loosen

Heart: Abnormal pulse, circulatory difficulties

Skin: Rashes, sores, or peeling skin

GI tract: Diarrhea, malabsorption, or constipation

▲ **Figure 21.5 Symptoms of Starvation**
As hunger persists, physical symptoms set in and lead to further complications.

children are healthy enough to regularly attend school, they tend to be fatigued, inattentive, and unresponsive to their learning environment. Peers, teachers, and adult caregivers may neglect a child who does not respond to or interact with others.

Weakened Immunity Results in Disease

A malnourished individual has a weakened immune system, which increases his or her vulnerability to various infections. Fever, parasitic disease, pneumonia, measles, typhoid, cholera, diarrhea, and malaria are examples of conditions that can occur because of weakened immune systems and chronic malnutrition. Diarrhea alone kills an estimated 2.2 million people globally each year.[92]

The WHO estimates that about 45 percent of all childhood deaths in developing countries are associated with malnutrition.[93] The diseases that most commonly cause death in postneonatal children (i.e., those

who survive birth and the first 28 days of life) are pneumonia, diarrhea, and malaria (**Table 21.3**), and malnutrition—by impairing the immune system—makes children more vulnerable to these diseases.[94]

A deficiency of certain micronutrients contributes to weakened immunity. Vitamins A, C, and E, for example, are critical to a healthy immune response, as are copper, iron, selenium, and zinc. In addition to promoting a healthy immune response, supplemental use of zinc can reduce the severity and duration of diarrhea.[95]

Infant and Child Mortality Rates Increase

Malnutrition is part of a vicious cycle that passes hunger and illness from one generation to the next. Unfortunately, many young women experience undernutrition during their own infancy and childhood. About half of all pregnant women and about 40 percent of preschool children in the developing world are thought to be anemic.[96] In many developing countries the rate of low birth weight is as high as 30 percent.[97] Girls who were low birth weight babies or were undernourished and ill during the first 5 years of life may be physically stunted and less able to support a healthy pregnancy when they become adults. As we've seen, infants born to malnourished women are more likely to be malnourished themselves, to experience chronic illness, and to have an increased risk of premature death.[98]

LO 21.5: THE TAKE-HOME MESSAGE
The effects of chronic undernutrition can be severe and irreversible, depending on the stage of life. If undernutrition occurs during adulthood, the body first attempts to conserve energy by slowing basal metabolism, and then breaks down tissues for energy. The physical effects of undernutrition in infants and children include stunted growth, wasting, impaired cognitive development and academic performance, reduced immunity and higher likelihood of infectious disease, and increased infant and child mortality.

TABLE 21.3	Common Causes of Death in Malnourished Children	
Disease/Condition	**Cause**	**Effect**
Diarrhea	Pathogenic infections	Severe dehydration
Acute respiratory illness	Virus or bacteria	Pneumonia, bronchitis, colds, fast breathing, coughing, and fever
Malaria	Parasite (transmitted by a mosquito)	Flu, weakness, sweating, shivering, shaking, nausea, liver failure, infected red blood cells, and kidney failure or bleeding in the kidneys

Source: World Health Organization. Media Centre. 2017. *Children: Reducing Mortality.* Available at www.who.int. Accessed May 2017.

Visual Chapter Summary

LO 21.1 Several Factors Contribute to Malnutrition in the United States

Hunger and malnutrition are health conditions that can result from food insecurity. In the United States, food insecurity and malnutrition can occur anywhere, including in rural areas, inner cities, and suburbs. People may get too few nutrients and suffer from undernutrition, or they may eat too many or the wrong kind of nutrients, as in overnutrition. Causes include poverty, disease or disability, lack of education, and inadequate wages. People living in food deserts are at risk of malnutrition. Disease, disability, mental illness, and/or drug and alcohol abuse can lead to food insecurity, and sometimes contribute to homelessness, which in turn often results in hunger.

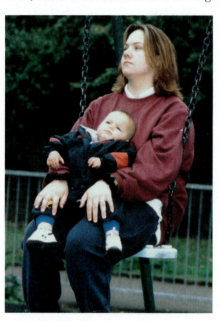

LO 21.2 Multiple Factors Contribute to Malnutrition Worldwide

Despite abundant food production, many people around the world suffer from chronic hunger, food insecurity, and malnutrition. The majority of the world's people live in developing countries where access to resources may be limited. Discrimination, political sanctions, armed conflicts, agricultural challenges, food waste, climate change, natural disasters, resource depletion, and overpopulation contribute to malnutrition in many countries. As a country becomes more prosperous, it may undergo a nutrition transition in which the population has access to more, but not necessarily better, food.

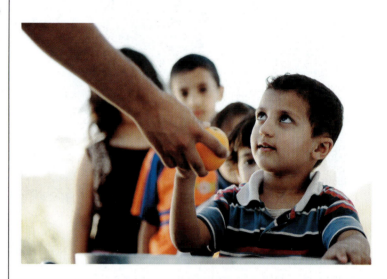

LO 21.3 Pregnant and Lactating Women, Children, the Ill, and Older Adults Are at Greatest Risk for Malnutrition

Pregnant and lactating women have higher kilocalorie and nutrient needs. If they are improperly nourished, their infants may be, too. Infants and children in general have high nutrient needs because they are growing rapidly. They are dependent on their caregivers for food, making them more susceptible to food insecurity. Chronically ill people may have malabsorption or metabolic problems or a reduced appetite. Older adults may be at risk for malnutrition because of higher needs for certain micronutrients, decreased senses of smell and taste, chronic illness, compromised immunity, and lack of mobility. People who are poor have unique risk factors for overnutrition, which is a form of malnutrition.

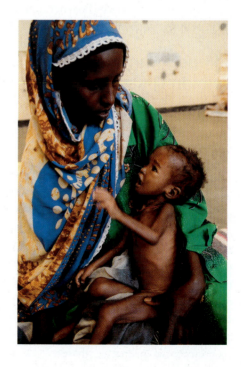

LO 21.4 Agricultural and Organizational Efforts Can Reduce Malnutrition

Agricultural practices such as using genetically modified high-yield crops and organic farming can help to reduce malnutrition, and safe water and sanitation practices are crucial to reducing illness. Because deficiencies of iron, iodine, and vitamin A are most common, these are the nutrients most often used to fortify foods.

Community organizations can help ease malnutrition by providing free food and meals and assistance programs to help people overcome poverty and food insecurity. Corporations and governments can invest in biotechnologies and education programs that provide more nutrient-dense foods and increase economic opportunity. The USDA funds multiple food assistance programs throughout the United States.

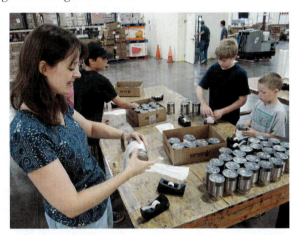

LO 21.5 Chronic Undernutrition Results in Disease and Death

Effects of undernutrition include stunted growth, wasting, and impaired cognitive development and academic performance. Reduced immune function increases vulnerability to infections. Infants and children who are malnourished are at increased risk for early death.

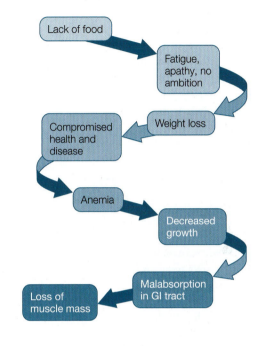

Terms to Know

- developed country
- food security
- food insecurity
- poverty
- working poor
- food deserts
- developing country
- least developed country
- famine
- overpopulation
- nutrition transition
- food pantry
- emergency kitchen
- growth stunting
- wasting

Mastering Nutrition
Visit the Study Area in Mastering Nutrition to hear an MP3 chapter summary.

Check Your Understanding

LO 21.1 1. Approximately how many people in the United States are food insecure?
   a. 11.3 million
   b. 14.8 million
   c. 42.2 million
   d. 16.2 million

LO 21.1 2. Which of the following states in the United States had one of the highest food insecurity rates between 2013 and 2015?
   a. Missouri
   b. Michigan
   c. North Dakota
   d. Mississippi

LO 21.2 3. What is the projected world population for 2050?
   a. 7.8 billion
   b. 9.7 billion
   c. 6 billion
   d. 6.2 billion

LO 21.2 4. Who are the "working poor"?
   a. Workers classified as low income by the United States Department of Labor
   b. Workers who have no steady employment
   c. Workers who are employed but have incomes that fall below the poverty line
   d. Workers who earn minimum wage

LO 21.3 5. The stress of poverty can contribute to overweight and obesity because
   a. people who are stressed cut down on exercise in order to get more work done.
   b. people who are dealing with stress feel some relief when they eat sugary foods, which are high in kilocalories.
   c. when a person is stressed, they don't have the time to choose a healthy snack over a sugary snack.
   d. stress reduces the body's ability to absorb protein.

LO 21.3 6. Infants and children are at higher risk of malnutrition than adults because
   a. they don't tend to wash their hands very often.
   b. they have a lower body mass index.
   c. they have higher nutrient requirements per unit bodyweight.
   d. they tend to prefer foods high in added sugar.

LO 21.4 7. Which nutrients are most likely to be used to fortify food?
   a. Vitamins D, E, and K
   b. Sodium, potassium, and chloride
   c. Magnesium, phosphorus, and sulfur
   d. Iron, iodine, and vitamin A

LO 21.4 8. Growing crops for human consumption, rather than to raise meat, could increase kilocalories available to humans by
   a. 36 percent.
   b. 70 percent.
   c. 25 percent.
   d. 60 percent.

LO 21.5 9. Which of the following conditions is usually permanent once it occurs?
   a. Hidden hunger
   b. Kwashiorkor
   c. Wasting
   d. Stunting

LO 21.5 10. Undernutrition increases deaths from pneumonia, diarrhea, and malaria by
   a. delaying cognitive development.
   b. impairing absorption of nutrients.
   c. impairing the immune system.
   d. contributing to overweight and obesity.

Answers

1. (c) About 42.2 million people in the United States lived in food-insecure households in 2015.
2. (d) Between 2013 and 2015, the six states with the highest food-insecurity rates were Mississippi, Louisiana, Arkansas tied with Maine, and Kentucky tied with Alabama.
3. (b) The projected world population for 2050 is 9.7 billion.
4. (c) The working poor include individuals who are employed yet still have incomes below the official poverty line.
5. (b) The stress of poverty can contribute to overweight and obesity because sugar consumption reduces release of the stress hormone cortisol, thereby helping reduce feelings of stress, yet foods high in added sugars are typically also high in kilocalories.
6. (c) Infants and children are at higher risk of malnutrition than adults because they have higher nutrient requirements per unit bodyweight.
7. (d) Iron, iodine, and vitamin A are the nutrients most commonly added to fortified foods worldwide.
8. (b) Growing crops for human consumption, rather than to raise meat, could increase calories available to humans by 70 percent.
9. (d) Growth stunting is usually permanent once it occurs.
10. (c) Undernutrition increases deaths from pneumonia, diarrhea, and malaria by impairing the immune system.

Answers to True or False?

1. **True.** While malnutrition may be more severe in developing countries, it occurs all over the globe.
2. **True.** An estimated 795 million people worldwide—more than one in 10—are hungry.
3. **False.** Even those who have jobs sometimes experience food insecurity.
4. **True.** Depression among mothers, particularly those in low-income families, has been associated with food insecurity in households.
5. **True.** The world's agricultural producers grow enough food to nourish every man, woman, and child on the planet. The challenge is distributing their products equitably.
6. **True.** Natural disasters such as droughts, floods, storms, earthquakes, crop diseases, and insect plagues can create food and water shortages in any country.
7. **False.** Malnutrition can occur in anyone. Those at greatest risk include pregnant and lactating women, infants and children, and the ill and elderly.
8. **False.** Fortifying foods can provide numerous nutrients that some populations wouldn't otherwise obtain.
9. **False.** There is a clear link in women between food insecurity and overweight and obesity.
10. **True.** The number-one cause of brain damage in children is iodine deficiency during pregnancy. Fortification of salt with iodine reduces the incidence of iodine-deficiency disorders.

Web Resources

- To learn more about one organization that is fighting global poverty, visit CARE at www.care.org
- To find out how the Food and Agriculture Organization of the United Nations leads international efforts to defeat hunger, visit www.fao.org

- To learn more about an international children's group, visit the UNICEF website at www.unicef.org
- For more about the World Health Organization, visit www.who.org
- To learn more about how biotechnology affects food production in developing countries, visit www.sustaintech.org
- To find out more about fighting hunger and reducing food waste in the United States, visit Feeding America at www.feedingamerica.org

References

1. Food and Agriculture Organization of the United Nations. 2017. *The State of Food Insecurity in the World 2015*. Available at www.fao.org. Accessed May 2017.
2. World Health Organization. 2017. *Micronutrient Deficiencies: Vitamin A Deficiency*. Available at www.who.int. Accessed March 2017.
3. World Health Organization. *Nutrition. Challenges*. Available at www.who.int/nutrition/challenges/en/. Accessed April 2017.
4. The World Bank. 2014. *Data. GDP Per Capita ($US)*. Available at http://data.worldbank.org. Accessed February 2017.
5. USDA. Economic Research Service. 2016. *Definitions of Food Security*. Available at www.ers.usda.gov. Accessed February 2017.
6. USDA. Economic Research Service. 2016. *Food Security in the U.S.* Available at www.ers.usda.gov. Accessed February 2017.
7. USDA. Economic Research Service. 2016. *Food Security Status of U.S. Households in 2015*. Available at www.ers.usda.gov. Accessed February 2017.
8. USDA. Economic Research Service. 2016. *How Many People Lived in Food-Insecure Households?* Available at www.ers.usda.gov. Accessed February 2017.
9. USDA. 2015. United States Department of Agriculture, Economic Research Service. *Key Statistics & Graphics*. www.ers.usda.gov. Accessed March 2017.
10. USDA. Economic Research Service. 2016. *Very Low Food Security by Household Characteristics*. Available at www.ers.usda.gov. Accessed February 2017.
11. Feeding America. 2017. Hunger and Poverty Facts and Statistics. *Poverty Statistics in the United States*. Available at www.feedingamerica.org/hunger-in-america/impact-of-hunger/hunger-and-poverty/hunger-and-poverty-fact-sheet.html. Accessed May 2017.
12. National Council on Aging. 2017. *SNAP and Senior Hunger Facts*. Available at https://www.ncoa.org/news/resources-for-reporters/get-the-facts/senior-hunger-facts/. Accessed May 2017.
13. USDA. Economic Research Service. 2016. *Food Security Status of U.S. Households in 2015*.
14. Feeding America. 2017. *African American Hunger Facts*. Available at www.feedingamerica.org/hunger-in-america/impact-of-hunger/african-american-hunger/african-american-hunger-fact-sheet.html. Accessed May 2017.
15. Feeding America. 2017. *Latino Hunger Facts*. Available at www.feedingamerica.org/hunger-in-america/impact-of-hunger/latino-hunger/latino-hunger-fact-sheet.html. Accessed May 2017.
16. Feeding America. 2017. *Rural Hunger Facts*. Available at www.feedingamerica.org/hunger-in-america/impact-of-hunger/rural-hunger/rural-hunger-fact-sheet.html. Accessed May 2017.
17. USDA. Economic Research Service. 2016. *State-Level Prevalence of Food Insecurity*. Available at www.ers.usda.gov. Accessed February 2017.
18. Chaparro, M. P., S. S. Zaghloul, et al. 2009. Food Insecurity Prevalence Among College Students at the University of Hawai'i at Mānoa. *Public Health Nutrition* 12(11):2097–2103. Available at http://scholarspace.manoa.hawaii.edu/handle/10125/20775. Accessed April 2017.
19. Freudenberg, N., L. Manzo, et al. 2011. *Food Insecurity at CUNY: Results from a Survey of CUNY Undergraduate Students*. New York, NY: Healthy CUNY Initiative, City University of New York. Available at https://www.gc.cuny.edu/CUNY_GC/media/CUNY-Graduate-Center/PDF/Centers/Center%20for%20Human%20Environments/cunyfoodinsecurity.pdf. Accessed April 2017.
20. Lindsley, K., and C. King. 2014. Food Insecurity of Campus-Residing Alaskan College Students. *Journal of the Academy of Nutrition and Dietetics* 9(114):A94.
21. Maroto, M. E., A. Snelling, et al. (2015). Food Insecurity Among Community College Students: Prevalence and Association with GRADE POINT AVERAGE. *Community College Journal of Research and Practice* 39(6):515–526. Available at www.tandfonline.com/doi/abs/10.1080/10668926.2013.850758. Accessed April 2017.
22. Patton-López, M. M., Daniel F. Lopezcevallos et al. 2014. Prevalence and Correlates of Food Insecurity Among Students Attending a Midsize Rural University in Oregon. *Journal of Nutrition Education and Behavior* 46(3):209–214. Available at www.jneb.org/article/S1499-4046(13)00707-0/abstract?cc=y=. Accessed April 2017.
23. U.S. Census Bureau. 2016. *Income and Poverty in the United States: 2015*. Available at https://www.census.gov/library/publications/2016/demo/p60-256.html. Accessed March 2017.
24. United States Census Bureau. 2015. *Poverty Thresholds*. Available at https://www.census.gov/data/tables/time-series/demo/income-poverty/historical-poverty-thresholds.html. Accessed March 2017.
25. U.S. Department of Labor, Bureau of Labor Statistics. 2016. *A Profile of the Working Poor, 2014*. Available at www.bls.gov. Accessed March 2017.
26. USDA. 2014. *Food Deserts*. Available at http://apps.ams.usda.gov. Accessed June 2014.
27. CDC Features. 2012. *A Look Inside Food Deserts*. Available at https://www.cdc.gov/features/FoodDeserts/index.html. Accessed March 2017.
28. Whitaker, R. C., S. M. Phillips, et al. 2006. Food Insecurity and the Risks of Depression and Anxiety in Mothers and Behavior Problems in their Preschool-Aged Children. *PEDIATRICS* 118:e859–e868. Available at http://pediatrics.aappublications.org/. Accessed April 2017.
29. National Coalition for the Homeless. 2009. *Mental Illness and Homelessness*. Available at www.nationalhomeless.org. Accessed March 2017.
30. Population Reference Bureau. 2016. *2016 World Population Data Sheet*. Available at www.prb.org. Accessed March 2017.
31. Food and Agriculture Organization. 2015. *The State of Food Insecurity in the World. Undernourishment around the world in 2015*. Available at www.fao.org. Accessed March 2017.
32. Doss, C., Chiara Kovarik et al. 2013. *Gender Inequalities in Ownership and Control of Land in Africa*. Washington, DC: International Food Policy Research Institute. Available at www.ifpri.org. Accessed March 2017.
33. Agada, M., and E. Igbokwe. 2016. Influence of Food Culture and Practices on Household Food Security in North Central Nigeria. *Journal of Food Security* 4(2):36–41. http://pubs.sciepub.com/jfs/4/2/2. Accessed May 2017.
34. Ibid.
35. United Nations. 2015. *Millenium Development Goals Report*. Available at http://www.un.org/millenniumgoals/reports.shtml. Accessed March 2017.
36. Petrescu, Ioana M. 2010. *The Humanitarian Impact of Economic Sanctions*. Available at www.essex.ac.uk. Accessed April 2017.
37. World Food Programme. 2013. *Hunger. What Causes Hunger?* Available at www.wfp.org. Accessed March 2017.
38. World Hunger Education Service. 2013. *2013 World Hunger and Poverty Facts and Statistics*. Available at www.worldhunger.org. Accessed March 2017.
39. Mission 2014: Feeding the World. 2014. *Ineffective/Inadequate Agricultural Practices*. Available at www.mit.edu. Accessed March 2017.
40. Dibal, J. M., H. E. Igbadun et al. 2014. *Modelling Furrow Irrigation-Induced Erosion on a Sandy Loam Soil in Samaru, Northern Nigeria*. International Scholarly Research Notices. Available at https://www.ncbi.nlm.nih.gov/pmc/articles/PMC4897171/. Accessed May 2017.

41. Mission 2014: Feeding the World. 2014. *Inadequate Food Distribution Systems*. Available at www.mit.edu. Accessed May 2017.

42. United Nations Environment. 2013. *Minimizing Food Waste*. Available at www.unep.org. Accessed March 2017.

43. Physicians for Social Responsibility. 2017. *Climate Change and Famine*. http://www.psr.org/resources/climate-change-and-famine.html. Accessed March 2017.

44. World Food Programme. 2013. *Hunger. What Causes Hunger?*

45. United States Geological Survey. 2016. *USGS Water Science School*. Available at https://water.usgs.gov/edu/earthhowmuch.html. Accessed May 2017.

46. CNN. 2017. *Flint Water Crisis Fast Facts*. Available at http://www.cnn.com/2016/03/04/us/flint-water-crisis-fast-facts/. Accessed May 2017.

47. Guarino, Arthur. 2017. The Economic Implications of Global Water Scarcity. *Research in Economics and Management* 2(1). Available at http://www.scholink.org/ojs/index.php/rem/article/view/799.

48. United Nations Department of Economic and Social Affairs. 2015. *World Population Projected to Reach 9.7 billion by 2050*. Available at www.un.org/en/development/desa/news/population/2015-report.html. Accessed March 2017.

49. Ibid.

50. The World Bank. 2017. *#BoldForChange: World Bank Group Helps Advance Education for Girls and Women*. Available at www.worldbank.org. Accessed March 2017.

51. Popkin, B. M., L. S. Adair, et al. 2012. NOW AND THEN: The Global Nutrition Transition: The Pandemic of Obesity in Developing Countries. *Nutrition Reviews*. Available at https://www.ncbi.nlm.nih.gov/pmc/articles/PMC3257829/. Accessed May 2017.

52. WHO. 2017. Nutrition. *Double Burden of Malnutrition*. Available at www.who.int/nutrition/double-burden-malnutrition/en/. Accessed May 2017.

53. FAO. 2004. Human Energy Requirements. Report of a Joint FAO/WHO/UNU Expert Consultation. *6. Energy Requirements of Pregnancy*. http://www.fao.org/docrep/007/y5686e/y5686e0a.htm. Accessed March 2017.

54. World Health Organization. 2016. *Infant and young child feeding*. Fact Sheet. Available at www.who.int/mediacentre/factsheets/fs342/en/. Accessed May 2017.

55. Mayo Clinic. 2017. *Infant and Toddler Health*. Available at www.mayoclinic.org/healthy-lifestyle/infant-and-toddler-health/in-depth/breastfeeding-nutrition/art-20046912. Accessed May 2017.

56. Shamim S,. F. Naz et al. 2006. Effect of Weaning Period on Nutritional Status of Children. *Journal of the College of Physicians and Surgeons (Pakistan)* 8:529–531.

57. USAID. 2016. *Orphans and Vulnerable Children Affected by HIV and AIDS*. Available at https://www.usaid.gov/what-we-do/global-health/hiv-and-aids/technical-areas/orphans-and-vulnerable-children-affected-hiv. Accessed March 2017.

58. AIDS.gov. 2016. *Global HIV/AIDS Overview*. Available at https://www.aids.gov/federal-resources/around-the-world/global-aids-overview/. Accessed March 2017.

59. Food Research and Action Center. 2017. *Why Low-Income and Food-Insecure People Are Vulnerable to Overweight and Obesity*. Available at http://frac.org. Accessed March 2017.

60. Haushofer, J., and E. Fehr, 2014. On the Psychology of Poverty. *Science* 344(6186):862–867. doi: 10.1126/science.1232491.

61. Tryon, Matthew, Kimber Stanhope et al. 2015. Excessive Sugar Consumption May Be a Difficult Habit to Break: A View From the Brain and Body. *Journal of Clinical Endocrinology and Metabolism*. doi: 10.1210/jc.2014-4353.

62. Second Harvest Food Bank. 2014. *How We Work*. Available at www.shfb.org. Accessed April 2017.

63. Ibid.

64. USDA. 2016. *The Food Assistance Landscape: FY 2015 Annual Report*. Available at www.ers.usda.gov. Accessed March 2017.

65. Food and Agriculture Organization of the United Nations. 2015. *The State of Food Insecurity in the World*. www.fao.org. Accessed March 2017.

66. Food and Agriculture Organization of the United Nations. 2017. Available at www.fao.org/organicag/oa-faq/oa-faq6/en/. Accessed April 2017.

67. Khan, Z., C. Midega et al. 2014. *Achieving Food Security for One Million Sub-Saharan African Poor Through Push–Pull Innovation by 2020*. Available at http://rstb.royalsocietypublishing.org/content/369/1639/20120284.short. Accessed May 2017.

68. Cassidy, E. S., P. C. West et al. 2013. *Redefining agricultural yields: from tonnes to people nourished per hectare*. Available at http://iopscience.iop.org/article/10.1088/1748-9326/8/3/034015/meta. Accessed May 2017.

69. Landesa Rural Development Institute. 2012. *Land Rights and Agricultural Activity*. Available at www.landesa.org. Accessed April 2017.

70. WHO. Media Centre (HELI). 2016. *Drinking-water*. Available at www.who.int. Accessed March 2017.

71. CDC. 2015. *Global Water, Sanitation, & Hygiene (WASH)*. Available at https://www.cdc.gov/healthywater/global/diarrhea-burden.html#five. Accessed April 2017.

72. WHO. Media Centre. 2013. *Diarrhoeal Disease. Fact Sheet no. 330*. Available at www.who.int. Accessed April 2017.

73. SODIS. 2017. *SODIS Method*. Available at www.sodis.ch/methode/index_EN. Accessed April 2017.

74. WHO. 2017. Media Centre. *Sanitation*. Available at www.who.int/mediacentre/factsheets/fs392/en/. Accessed May 2017.

75. Bill and Melinda Gates Foundation. 2014. *Reinvent the Toilet Challenge*. www.gatesfoundation.org/What-We-Do/Global-Development/Reinvent-the-Toilet-Challenge

76. CDC Food Fortification Initiative. 2017. *Global Progress*. Available at www.ffinetwork.org/global_progress/index.php. Accessed April 2017.

77. United Nations Educational, Scientific and Cultural Organization. 2016. *Global Education Monitoring Report. Education for People and Planet*. Available at http://en.unesco.org/gem-report/. Accessed May 2017.

78. Earth Policy Institute. 2011. *Education Leads to Lower Fertility and Increased Prosperity*. Available at www.earth-policy.org/data_highlights/2011/highlights13. Accessed April 2017.

79. United Nations Educational, Scientific and Cultural Organization. 2016. *Global Education Monitoring Report. Education for People and Planet*.

80. World Food Programme. 2017. *Overview*. Available at www.wfp.org. Accessed April 2017.

81. UNICEF. 2013. UNICEF in Emergencies and Humanitarian Action. *UNICEF's Role in Humanitarian Action*. Available at www.unicef.org. Accessed April 2017.

82. Heifer International. 2014. *About Heifer International*. Available at www.heifer.org. Accessed April 2017.

83. Peace Corps. 2016. *Global Initiatives*. Available at https://www.peacecorps.gov/about/global-initiatives/. Accessed April 2017.

84. Morley, J.E. 2016. *Merck Manual Professional Version. Overview of Undernutrition*. Available at www.merckmanuals.com/professional/nutritional-disorders/undernutrition/overview-of-undernutrition#v882492. Accessed April 2017.

85. American Psychological Association. Effects of Poverty, Hunger and Homelessness on Children and Youth. 2017. *What are the effects of hunger and undernutrition on child development?* Available at www.apa.org/pi/families/poverty.aspx. Accessed April 2017.

86. World Health Organization. 2016. Global Database on Child Growth and Malnutrition Joint Child Malnutrition Estimates–Levels and trends (2016 edition) UNICEF/WHO/World Bank Group. Available at www.who.int/

nutgrowthdb/estimates2015/en/. Accessed April 2017.

87. Ibid.

88. Ibid.

89. Chen, Z. P., and B. S. Hetzel. 2017. Cretinism Revisited. *Clinical Endocrinology and Metabolism* doi: http://dx.doi.org/10.1016/j.beem.2009.08.014.

90. World Health Organization. 2017. *Micronutrient Deficiencies: Iodine deficiency disorders.* Available at www.who.int. Accessed May 2017.

91. World Health Organization. 2016. *Global Database on Child Growth and Malnutrition* Joint Child Malnutrition Estimates–Levels and trends (2016 edition). UNICEF / WHO / World Bank Group.

92. World Health Organization. 2017. *Water Sanitation Health. Water-Related Diseases. Diarrhoea.* Available at www.who.int. Accessed April 2017.

93. World Health Organization. Media Centre. 2017. *Children: Reducing Mortality.* Available at www.who.int. Accessed April 2017.

94. Ibid.

95. Wessells, K. R. and Kenneth H. Brown. 2012. *Estimating the Global Prevalence of Zinc Deficiency: Results Based on Zinc Availability in National Food Supplies and the Prevalence of Stunting.* Public Library of Science. Available at https://doi.org/10.1371/journal.pone.0050568. Accessed May 2017.

96. World Health Organization. 2017. *Micronutrient Deficiencies: Iron-Deficiency Anaemia.* Available at www.who.int. Accessed March 2017.

97. World Health Organization. 2017. *Feto-Maternal Nutrition and Low Birth Weight.* Available at www.who.int. Accessed March 2017.

98. The Mother and Child Health and Education Trust. 2017. *Impact of Malnutrition.* Available at http://motherchildnutrition.org/malnutrition/about-malnutrition/impact-of-malnutrition.html.

Appendices

Appendix A Metabolism Pathways and Biochemical Structures

When learning about the science of nutrition, it is important to understand basic principles of metabolism and to know the molecular structures of important nutrients and molecules. Chapter 8 of the text provides a detailed discussion of the major metabolic processes that occur within the body. This appendix gives additional information and detail on several metabolism pathways and biochemical structures of importance.

Metabolism Pathways

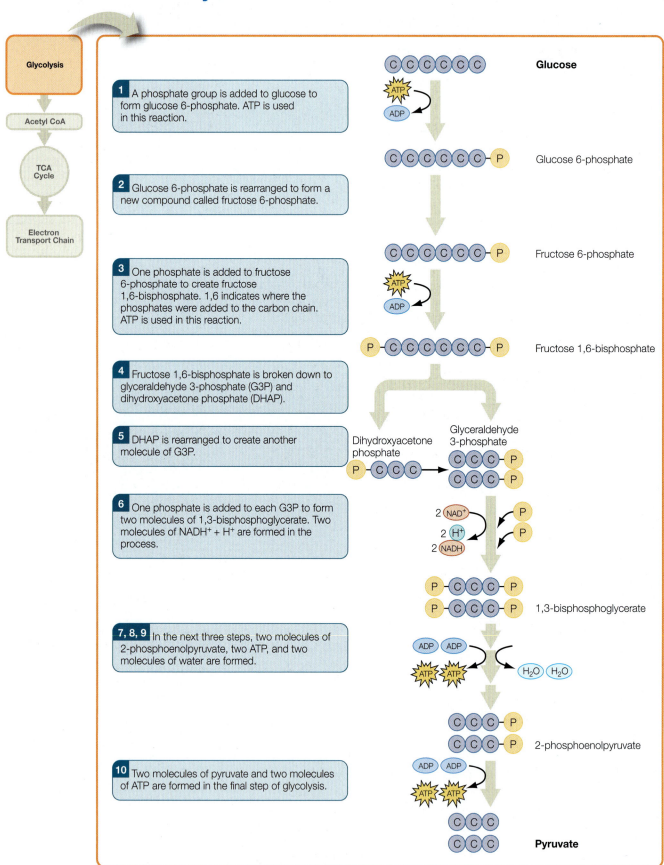

Glycolysis

Acetyl CoA

TCA Cycle

Electron Transport Chain

1 A phosphate group is added to glucose to form glucose 6-phosphate. ATP is used in this reaction.

2 Glucose 6-phosphate is rearranged to form a new compound called fructose 6-phosphate.

3 One phosphate is added to fructose 6-phosphate to create fructose 1,6-bisphosphate. 1,6 indicates where the phosphates were added to the carbon chain. ATP is used in this reaction.

4 Fructose 1,6-bisphosphate is broken down to glyceraldehyde 3-phosphate (G3P) and dihydroxyacetone phosphate (DHAP).

5 DHAP is rearranged to create another molecule of G3P.

6 One phosphate is added to each G3P to form two molecules of 1,3-bisphosphoglycerate. Two molecules of NADH + H+ are formed in the process.

7, 8, 9 In the next three steps, two molecules of 2-phosphoenolpyruvate, two ATP, and two molecules of water are formed.

10 Two molecules of pyruvate and two molecules of ATP are formed in the final step of glycolysis.

Glucose

Glucose 6-phosphate

Fructose 6-phosphate

Fructose 1,6-bisphosphate

Dihydroxyacetone phosphate

Glyceraldehyde 3-phosphate

1,3-bisphosphoglycerate

2-phosphoenolpyruvate

Pyruvate

▲ **Figure A.1 Glycolysis Pathway.**

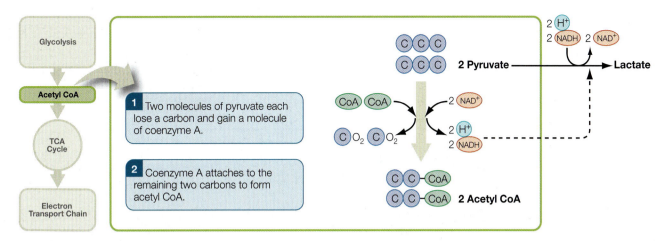

▲ Figure A.2 Acetyl CoA Pathway.

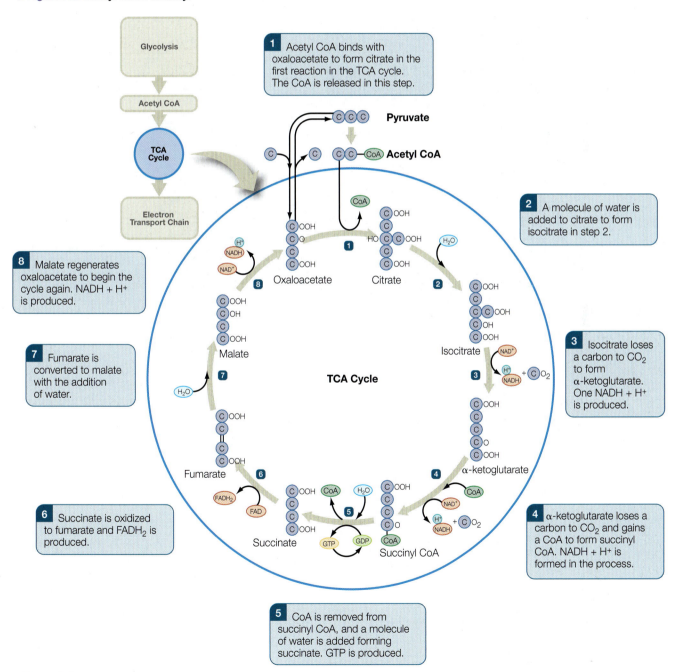

▲ Figure A.3 TCA Cycle.

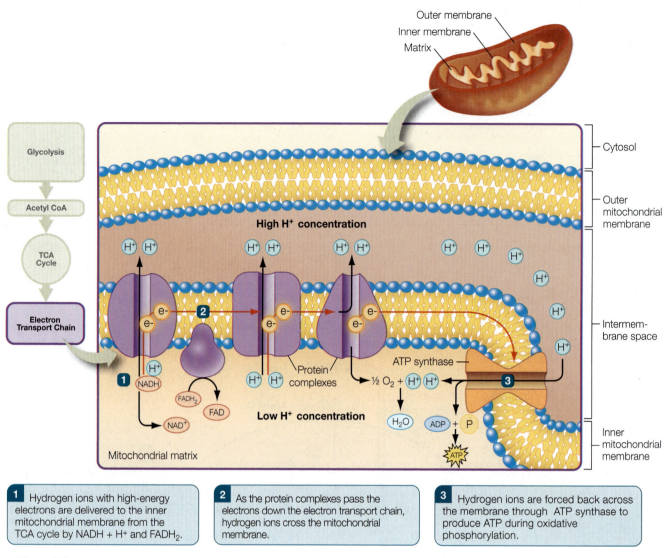

Figure A.4 Electron Transport Chain.

Glycolysis

Acetyl CoA

TCA Cycle

Electron Transport Chain

Outer membrane
Inner membrane
Matrix

Cytosol

Outer mitochondrial membrane

Intermembrane space

Inner mitochondrial membrane

High H$^+$ concentration

Low H$^+$ concentration

Mitochondrial matrix

Protein complexes

ATP synthase

$\frac{1}{2}$ O$_2$ + H$^+$ H$^+$

H$_2$O

ADP + P

ATP

NADH

NAD$^+$

FADH$_2$

FAD

1 Hydrogen ions with high-energy electrons are delivered to the inner mitochondrial membrane from the TCA cycle by NADH + H$^+$ and FADH$_2$.

2 As the protein complexes pass the electrons down the electron transport chain, hydrogen ions cross the mitochondrial membrane.

3 Hydrogen ions are forced back across the membrane through ATP synthase to produce ATP during oxidative phosphorylation.

a Sources of energy use and production in the different metabolic pathways

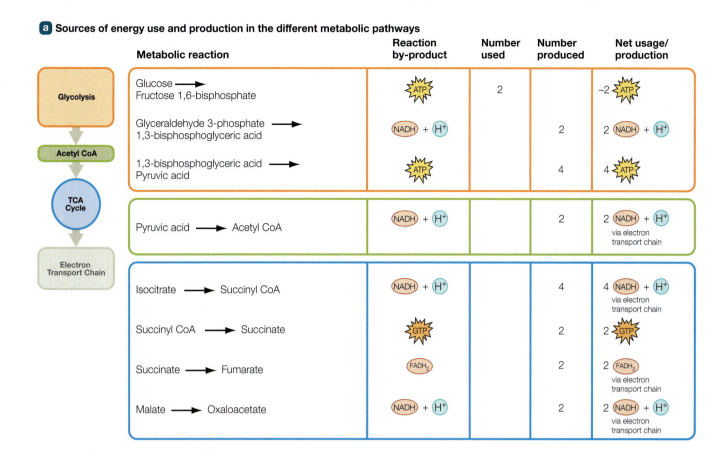

Metabolic reaction	Reaction by-product	Number used	Number produced	Net usage/ production
Glycolysis — Glucose → Fructose 1,6-bisphosphate	ATP	2		−2 ATP
Glyceraldehyde 3-phosphate → 1,3-bisphosphoglyceric acid	NADH + H⁺		2	2 NADH + H⁺
1,3-bisphosphoglyceric acid → Pyruvic acid	ATP		4	4 ATP
Acetyl CoA — Pyruvic acid → Acetyl CoA	NADH + H⁺		2	2 NADH + H⁺ via electron transport chain
TCA Cycle — Isocitrate → Succinyl CoA	NADH + H⁺		4	4 NADH + H⁺ via electron transport chain
Succinyl CoA → Succinate	GTP		2	2 GTP
Succinate → Fumarate	FADH₂		2	2 FADH₂ via electron transport chain
Malate → Oxaloacetate	NADH + H⁺		2	2 NADH + H⁺ via electron transport chain

(Left-side flow diagram: Glycolysis → Acetyl CoA → TCA Cycle → Electron Transport Chain)

b Energy balance sheet for glucose oxidation

Reaction by-product	Number produced	Number of ATP produced per product	Net usage/ production
ATP	4 − 2 = 2	1	2 × 1 = 2 ATP
NADH + H⁺ from glycolysis	2	2 to 3	2 × 2 = 4 or 2 × 3 = 6 ATP
NADH + H⁺ from TCA cycle	8	3	8 × 3 = 24 ATP
GTP	2	1	2 × 1 = 2 ATP
FADH₂ via electron transport chain	2	2	2 × 2 = 4 ATP
Balance of energy from the oxidation of one unit of glucose: 36 to 38 ATP			

▲ **Figure A.5 Products of Metabolic Pathways.**

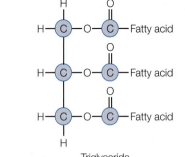
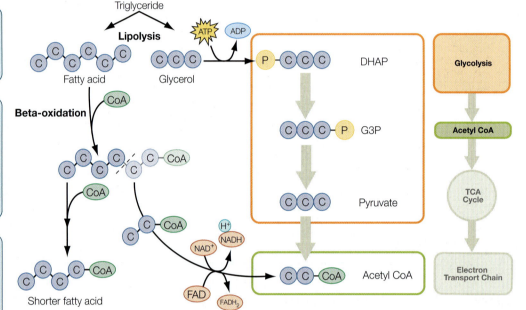

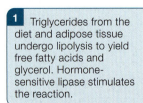
1 Triglycerides from the diet and adipose tissue undergo lipolysis to yield free fatty acids and glycerol. Hormone-sensitive lipase stimulates the reaction.

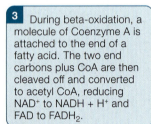
2 Glycerol is first converted to DHAP before it can enter anaerobic glycolysis to be converted to pyruvate. The first step requires ATP.

3 During beta-oxidation, a molecule of Coenzyme A is attached to the end of a fatty acid. The two end carbons plus CoA are then cleaved off and converted to acetyl CoA, reducing NAD$^+$ to NADH + H$^+$ and FAD to FADH$_2$.

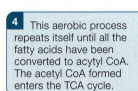
4 This aerobic process repeats itself until all the fatty acids have been converted to acytyl CoA. The acetyl CoA formed enters the TCA cycle.

▲ **Figure A.6** **Using Fat for Energy.**

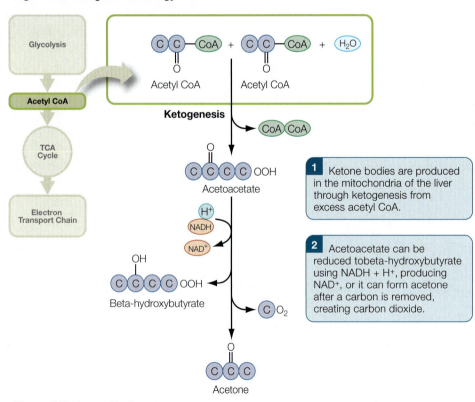

1 Ketone bodies are produced in the mitochondria of the liver through ketogenesis from excess acetyl CoA.

2 Acetoacetate can be reduced tobeta-hydroxybutyrate using NADH + H$^+$, producing NAD$^+$, or it can form acetone after a carbon is removed, creating carbon dioxide.

▲ **Figure A.7** **Ketone Bodies.**

Biochemical Structures

Amino Acid Structures

Amino acids all have the same basic core but differ in their side chains. The following amino acids have been classified according to their specific type of side chain.

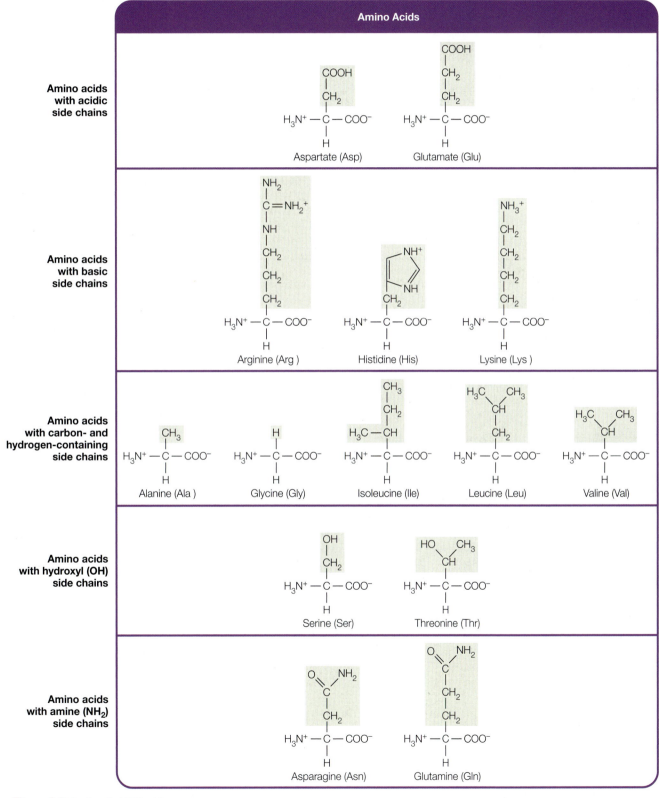

▲ **Figure A.8 Amino Acid Structures.**

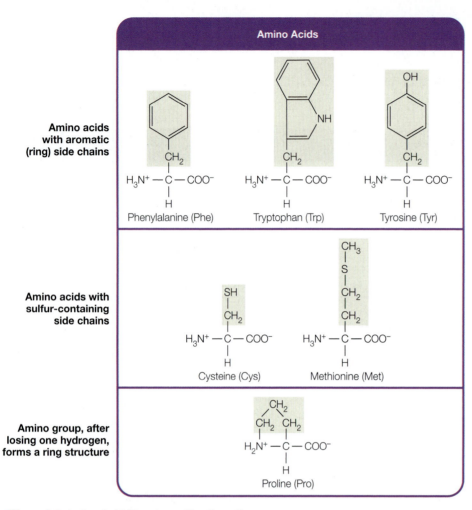

▲ **Figure A.8** Amino Acid Structures (Continued).

Vitamin Structures and Coenzyme Derivatives

Many vitamins have common names (e.g., vitamin C, vitamin E) as well as scientific designations (e.g., ascorbic acid and α-tocopherol). Most vitamins are found in more than one chemical form. Many of the vitamins illustrated here have an active coenzyme form; review both the vitamin and coenzyme structures and see if you can locate the "core vitamin" structure within each of the coenzymes. The vitamins found in food or supplements are not always in the precise chemical form needed for metabolic activity, and therefore the body often has to modify the vitamin in one way or another. For example, many of the B vitamins are phosphorylated, meaning that they have a phosphate group attached.

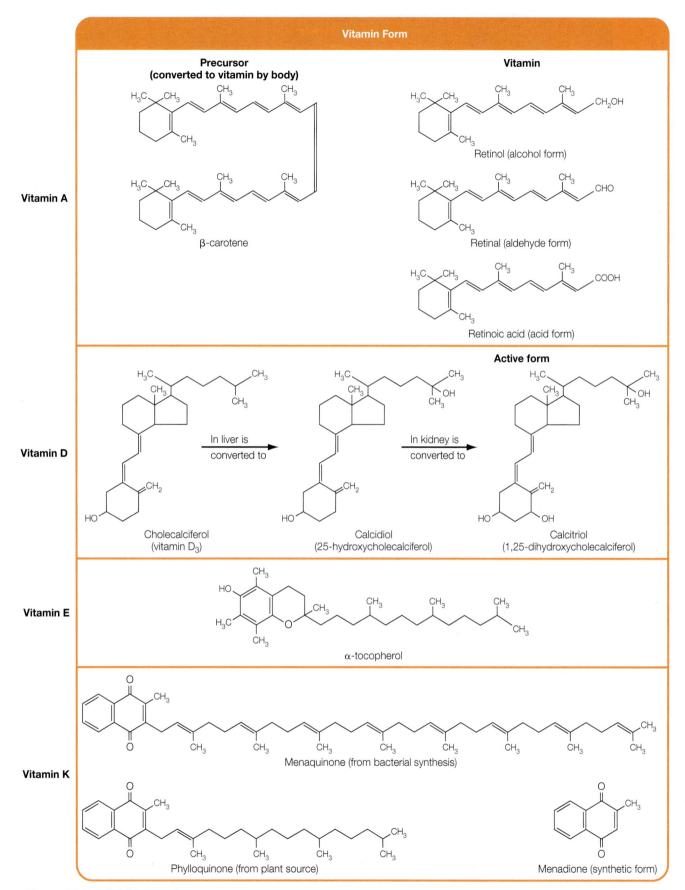

Vitamin Form

Vitamin A

Precursor (converted to vitamin by body)

β-carotene

Vitamin

Retinol (alcohol form)

Retinal (aldehyde form)

Retinoic acid (acid form)

Vitamin D

Cholecalciferol (vitamin D₃)

In liver is converted to

Calcidiol (25-hydroxycholecalciferol)

In kidney is converted to

Active form

Calcitriol (1,25-dihydroxycholecalciferol)

Vitamin E

α-tocopherol

Vitamin K

Menaquinone (from bacterial synthesis)

Phylloquinone (from plant source)

Menadione (synthetic form)

▲ **Figure A.9 Fat-Soluble Vitamins.**

Thiamin

Vitamin Form

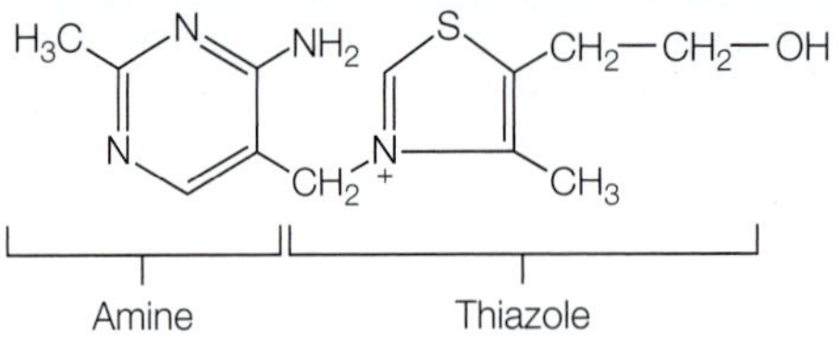

Coenzyme Form

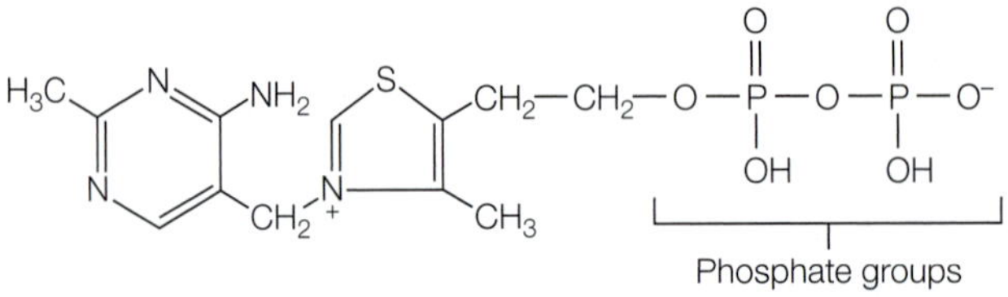

Thiamin pyrophosphate

Riboflavin

Vitamin Form

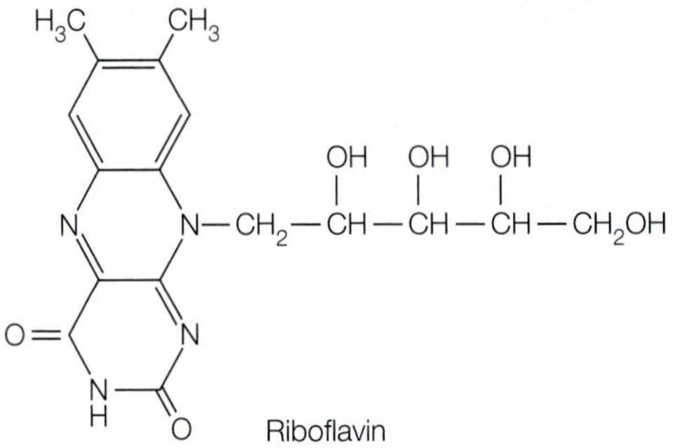

Riboflavin

Coenzyme Form

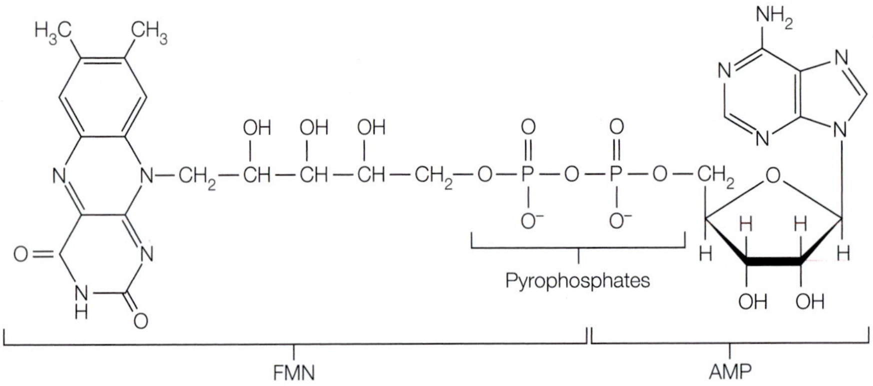

Flavin adenine dinucleotide (FAD)

▲ **Figure A.10 Water-Soluble Vitamins and Their Coenzymes.**

Niacin

Vitamin Form

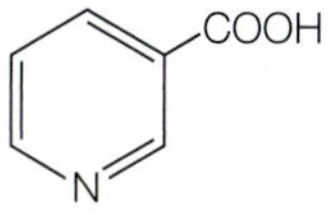

Nicotinic acid

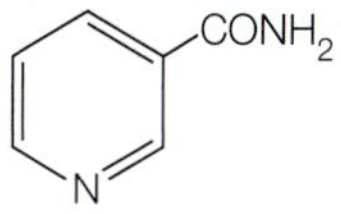

Nicotinamide

Coenzyme Form

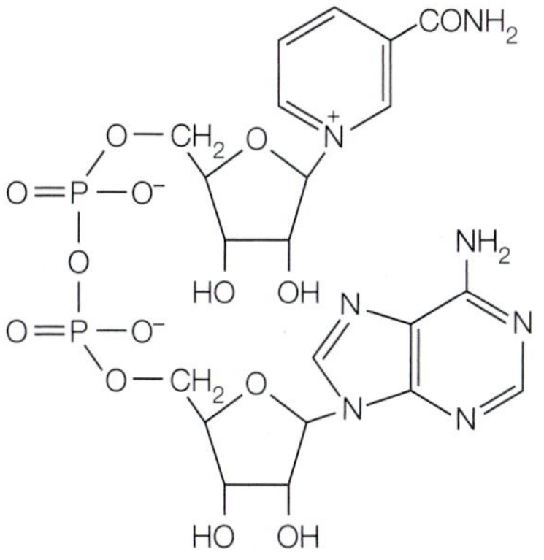

Nicotinamide adenine dinucleotide (NAD$^+$)

or

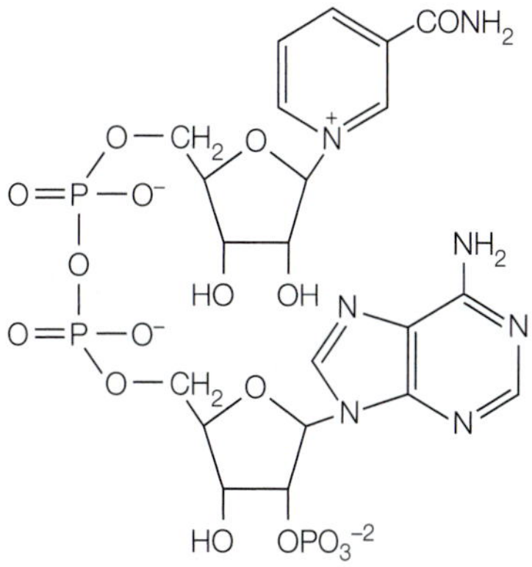

Nicotinamide adenine dinucleotide phosphate (NADP$^+$)

Pantothenic acid

Vitamin Form

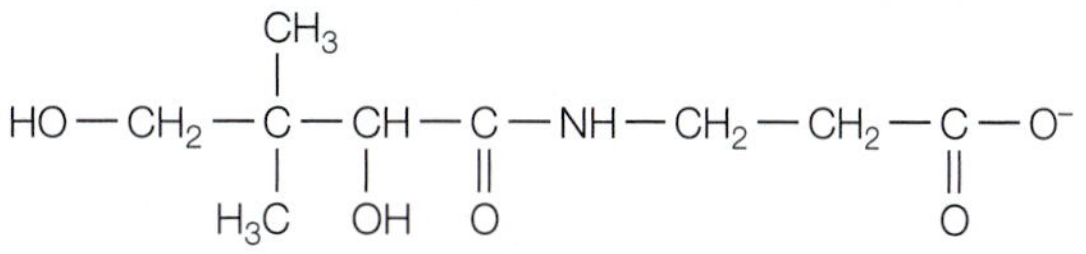

Pantothenic acid

Coenzyme Form

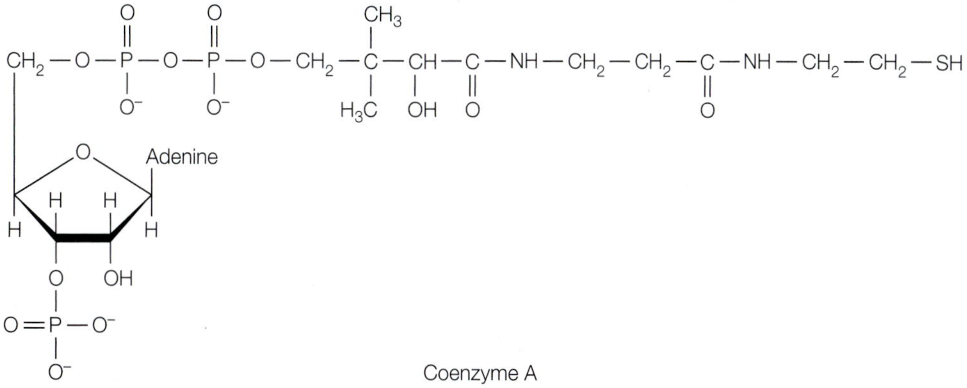

Coenzyme A

▲ Figure A.10 **Water-Soluble Vitamins and Their Coenzymes. (Continued)**

Biotin

Vitamin Form

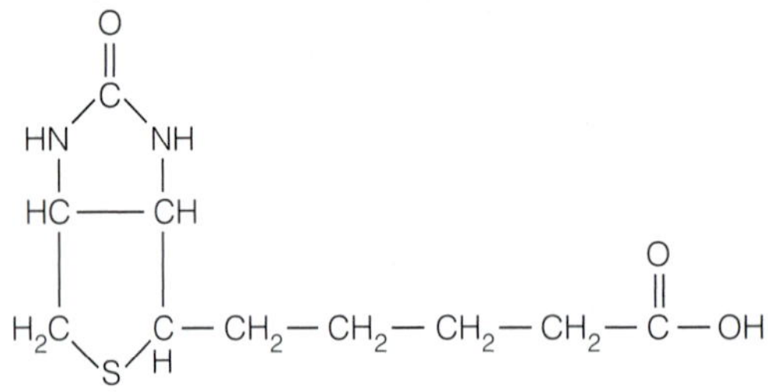

Vitamin B₆

Vitamin Form

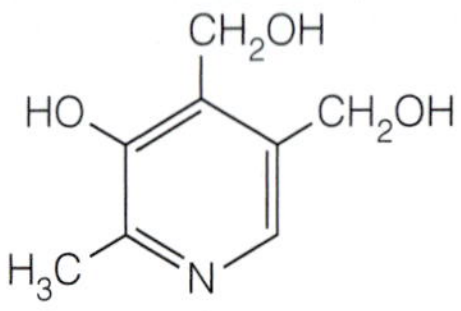

Pyridoxine (PN) 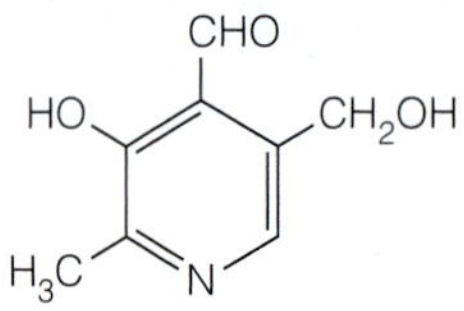 Pyridoxal (PL) 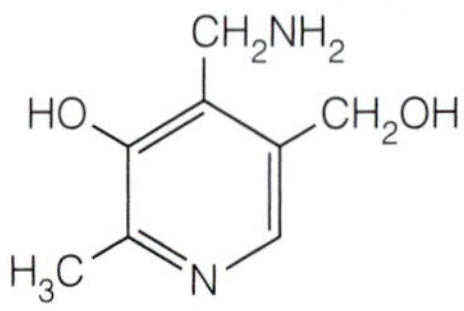 Pyridoxamine (PM)

Coenzyme Form

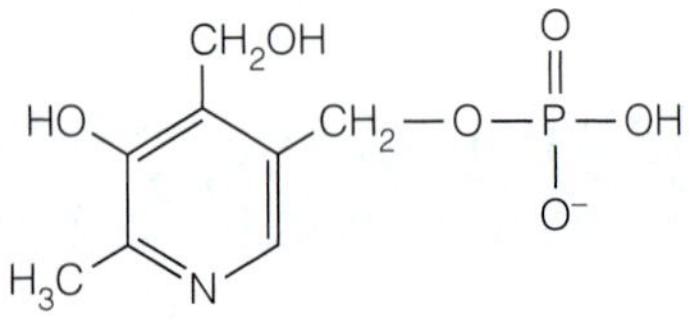

Pyridoxine 5′ phosphate (PNP) 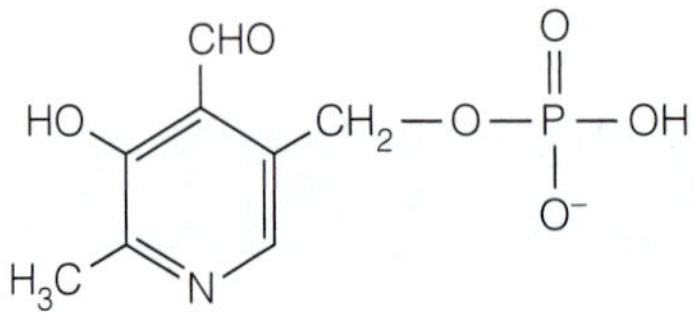 Pyridoxal 5′ phosphate (PLP) 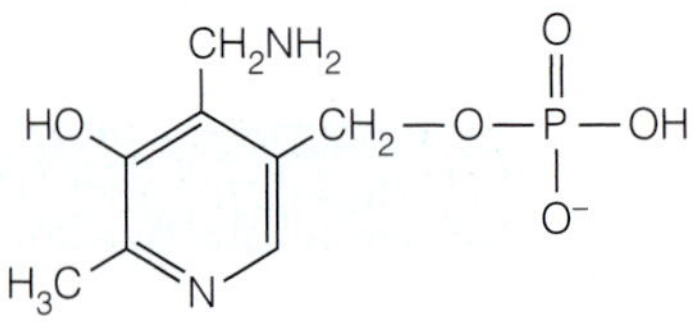 Pyridoxamine 5′ phosphate (PMP)

Folate

Vitamin Form

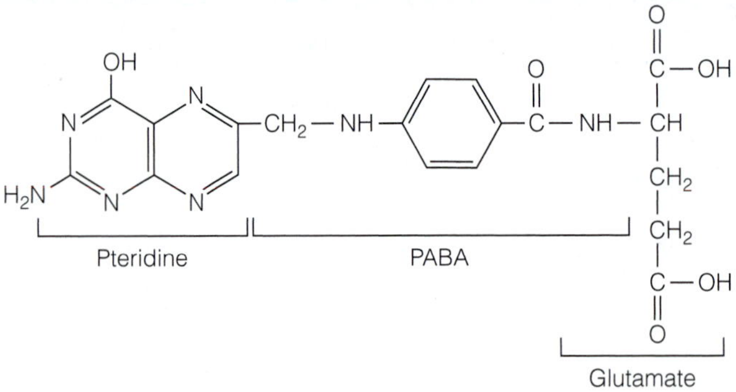

Pteridine PABA Glutamate

Coenzyme Form

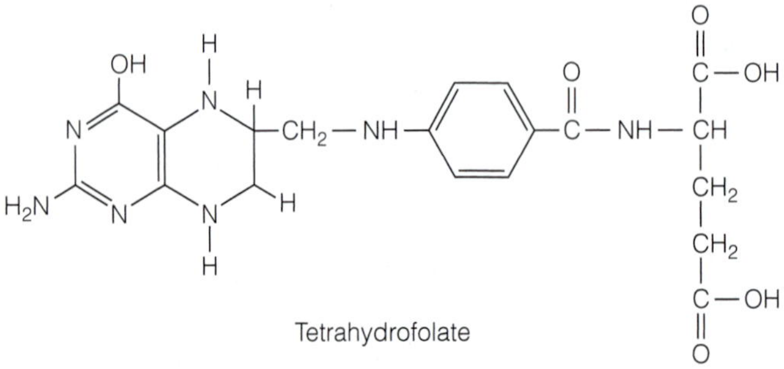

Tetrahydrofolate

▲ Figure A.10 Water-Soluble Vitamins and Their Coenzymes. (Continued)

Vitamin B₁₂

Vitamin Form

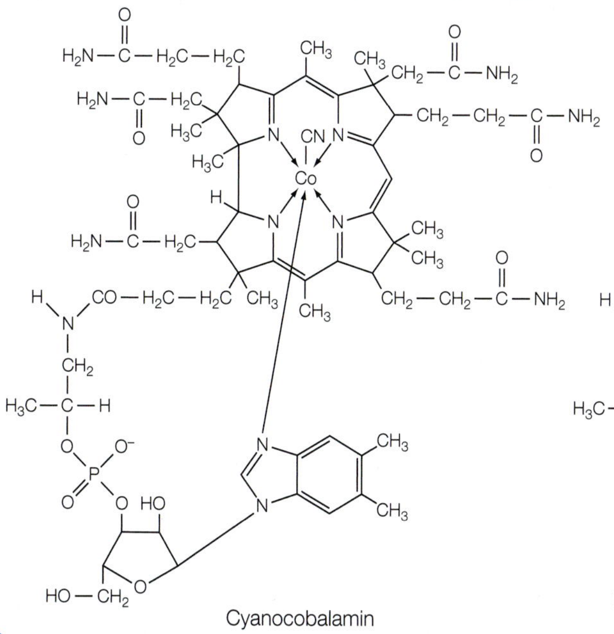

Cyanocobalamin

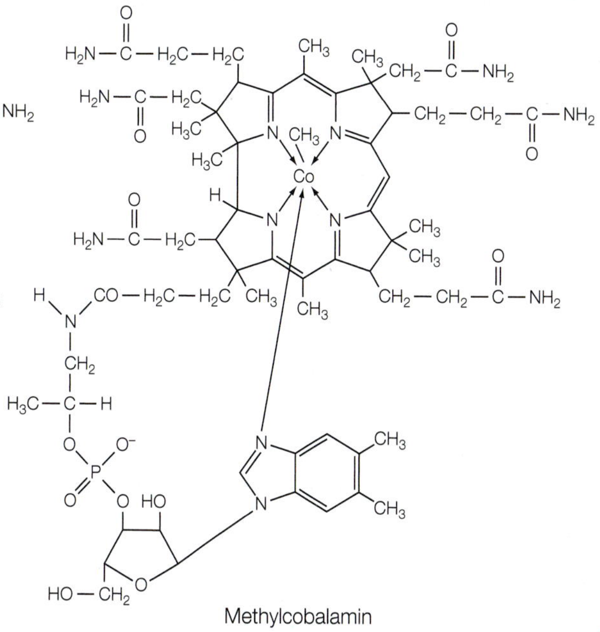

Methylcobalamin

Vitamin C

Vitamin Form

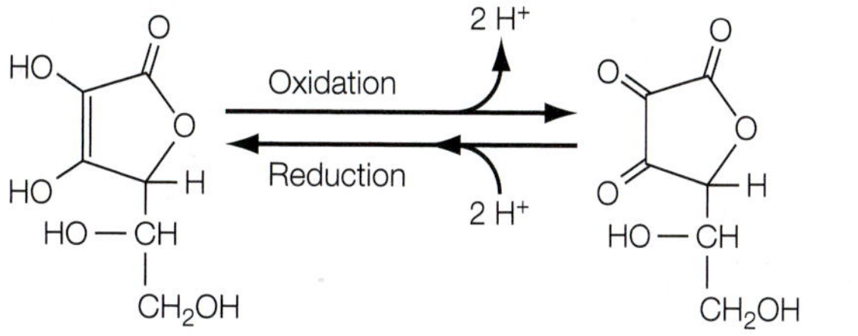

Oxidation

Reduction

$2 H^+$

$2 H^+$

Ascorbic acid

Dehydroascorbic acid

Choline

Vitamin Form

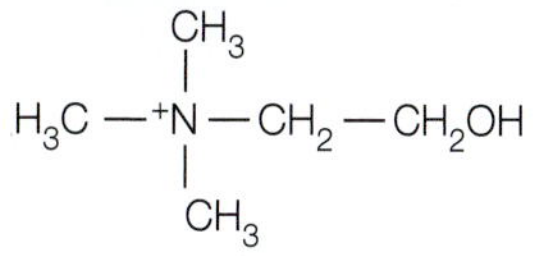

$H_3C - {}^+N - CH_2 - CH_2OH$

▲ **Figure A.10** **Water-Soluble Vitamins and Their Coenzymes. (Continued)**

Appendix B Calculations and Conversions

Calculation and Conversion Aids

Commonly Used Metric Units

millimeter (mm) : one-thousandth of a meter (0.001)

centimeter (cm) : one-hundredth of a meter (0.01)

kilometer (km) : one-thousand times a meter (1,000)

kilogram (kg) : one-thousand times a gram (1,000)

milligram (mg) : one-thousandth of a gram (0.001)

microgram (μg) : one-millionth of a gram (0.000001)

milliliter (ml) : one-thousandth of a liter (0.001)

Conversion Factors

Use the following table to convert U.S. measurements to metric equivalents:

Original Unit	Multiply By	To Get
ounces (avdp)	28.3495	grams
ounces	0.0625	pounds
pounds	0.4536	kilograms
pounds	16	ounces
grams	0.0353	ounces
grams	0.0022	pounds
kilograms	2.2046	pounds
liters	1.8162	pints (dry)
liters	2.1134	pints (liquid)
liters	0.9081	quarts (dry)
liters	1.0567	quarts (liquid)
liters	0.2642	gallons (U.S.)
pints (dry)	0.5506	liters
pints (liquid)	0.4732	liters
quarts (dry)	1.1012	liters
quarts (liquid)	0.9463	liters
gallons (U.S.)	3.7854	liters
millimeters	0.0394	inches
centimeters	0.3937	inches
centimeters	0.0328	feet
inches	25.4000	millimeters
inches	2.5400	centimeters
inches	0.0254	meters
feet	0.3048	meters
meters	3.2808	feet
meters	1.0936	yards
cubic feet	0.0283	cubic meters
cubic meters	35.3147	cubic feet
cubic meters	1.3079	cubic yards
cubic yards	0.7646	cubic meters

International Units

Some vitamin supplements may report vitamin content as International Units (IU).

To convert IU to:

› Micrograms of vitamin D (cholecalciferol), multiply the IU value by 0.025.

› Milligrams of vitamin E (alpha-tocopherol), multiply the IU value by 0.67 if vitamin E is from natural sources. Multiply the IU value by 0.45 if vitamin E is from synthetic sources.

› Vitamin A: 1 IU = 0.3 μg retinol or 0.3 μg RAE or 0.6 μg beta-carotene

Retinol Activity Equivalents

Retinol activity equivalents (RAE) are a standardized unit of measure for vitamin A. RAE account for the various differences in bioavailability from sources of vitamin A. Many supplements will report vitamin A content in IU, as shown above, or in retinol equivalents (RE).

$$1 \; \mu\text{g RAE} = 1 \; \mu\text{g retinol}$$
$$12 \; \mu\text{g beta-carotene}$$

To calculate RAE from the RE value of vitamin carotenoids in foods, divide RE by 2. Divide the amount of beta-carotene by 12 to convert to RAE.

For vitamin A supplements and foods fortified with vitamin A, 1 RE = 1 RAE.

Folate

Folate is measured as dietary folate equivalents (DFE). DFE accounts for the different factors affecting bioavailability of folate sources.

1 μg DFE = 1 μg food folate

0.6 μg folate from fortified foods

0.5 μg folate supplement taken on an empty stomach

0.6 μg folate as a supplement consumed with a meal

To convert micrograms of synthetic folate, such as that found in supplements or fortified foods, to DFE:

$$\mu\text{g synthetic folate} \times 1.7 = \mu\text{g DFE}$$

For naturally occurring food folate, such as spinach, each microgram of folate equals 1 microgram DFE:

$$\mu\text{g folate} = \mu\text{g DFE}$$

Niacin

Niacin is measured as niacin equivalents (mg NE). NE reflects the amount of preformed niacin in foods or the amount that can be formed from a food's content of the amino acid niacin.

To calculate mg NE from a meal:

If you know the tryptophan and preformed niacin in a meal: (tryptophan $\times$ 1,000 $\div$ 60) + preformed niacin = mg NE

If you know the total amount of protein in a meal but not the tryptophan content: (0.011 $\times$ g of protein) $\times$ 1,000 $\div$ 60 + preformed niacin = mg NE

Length: U.S. and Metric Equivalents

$\frac{1}{4}$ inch =	0.6 centimeters
1 inch =	2.5 centimeters
1 foot =	0.3048 meter
	30.48 centimeters
1 yard =	0.9144 meter
1 millimeter =	0.03937 inch
1 centimeter =	0.3937 inch
1 decimeter =	3.937 inches
1 meter =	39.37 inches
	1.094 yards
1 micrometer =	0.00003937 inch

Weights and Measures

Food Measurement Equivalencies from U.S. to Metric

Capacity

$\frac{1}{5}$ teaspoon =	1 milliliter
$\frac{1}{4}$ teaspoon =	1.23 milliliters
$\frac{1}{2}$ teaspoon =	2.5 milliliters
1 teaspoon =	5 milliliters
1 tablespoon =	15 milliliters
1 fluid ounce =	30 milliliters
$\frac{1}{4}$ cup =	59 milliliters
$\frac{1}{3}$ cup =	79 milliliters
$\frac{1}{2}$ cup =	118 milliliters
1 cup =	237 milliliters
1 pint (2 cups) =	473 milliliters
1 quart (4 cups) =	0.95 liter
1 liter (1.06 quarts) =	1,000 milliliters
1 gallon (4 quarts) =	3.79 liters

Weight

0.035 ounce =	1 gram
1 ounce =	28 grams
$\frac{1}{4}$ pound (4 ounces) =	113 grams
1 pound (16 ounces) =	454 grams
2.2 pounds (35 ounces) =	1 kilogram

U.S. Food Measurement Equivalents

3 teaspoons =	1 tablespoon
$\frac{1}{2}$ tablespoon =	$1\frac{1}{2}$ teaspoons
2 tablespoons =	$\frac{1}{8}$ cup
4 tablespoons =	$\frac{1}{4}$ cup
5 tablespoons + 1 teaspoon =	$\frac{1}{3}$ cup
8 tablespoons =	$\frac{1}{2}$ cup
10 tablespoons + 2 teaspoons =	$\frac{2}{3}$ cup
12 tablespoons =	$\frac{3}{4}$ cup
16 tablespoons =	1 cup
2 cups =	1 pint
4 cups =	1 quart
2 pints =	1 quart
4 quarts =	1 gallon

Volumes and Capacities

1 cup =	8 fluid ounces
	$\frac{1}{2}$ liquid pint
1 milliliter =	0.061 cubic inch
1 liter =	1.057 liquid quarts
	0.908 dry quart
	61.024 cubic inches
1 U.S. gallon =	231 cubic inches
	3.785 liters
	0.833 British gallon
	128 U.S. fluid ounces
1 British Imperial gallon =	277.42 cubic inches
	1.201 U.S. gallons
	4.546 liters
	160 British fluid ounces
1 U.S. ounce, liquid or fluid =	1.805 cubic inches
	29.574 milliliters
	1.041 British fluid ounces
1 pint, dry =	33.600 cubic inches
	0.551 liter
1 pint, liquid =	28.875 cubic inches
	0.473 liter
1 U.S. quart, dry =	67.201 cubic inches
	1.101 liters
1 U.S. quart, liquid =	57.75 cubic inches
	0.946 liter
1 British quart =	69.355 cubic inches
	1.032 U.S. quarts, dry
	1.201 U.S. quarts, liquid

Energy Units

$$1 \text{ kilocalorie (kcal)} = 4.2 \text{ kilojoules}$$
$$1 \text{ megajoule (MJ)} = 239 \text{ kilocalories}$$
$$1 \text{ kilojoule (kJ)} = 0.24 \text{ kcal}$$
$$1 \text{ gram carbohydrate} = 4 \text{ kcals}$$
$$1 \text{ gram fat} = 9 \text{ kcals}$$
$$1 \text{ gram protein} = 4 \text{ kcals}$$

Temperature Standards

	°Fahrenheit	°Celsius
Body temperature	98.6°	37°
Comfortable room temperature	65–75°	18–24°
Boiling point of water	212°	100°
Freezing point of water	32°	0°

Temperature Scales

To Convert Fahrenheit to Celsius

$[(°F − 32) \times 5]/9$

1. Subtract 32 from °F
2. Multiply (°F − 32) by 5, then divide by 9

To Convert Celsius to Fahrenheit

$[(°C \times 9)/5] + 32$

1. Multiply °C by 9, then divide by 5
2. Add 32 to (°C × 9/5)

Appendix C U.S. Exchange Lists for Meal Planning

Starch

One starch choice has 15 grams of carbohydrate, 3 grams of protein, 1 gram of fat, and 80 calories.

Icon Key

✔ = Good source of fiber

! = Extra fat

🧂 = High in sodium

Food	Serving Size
Bread	
Bagel	¼ large bagel (1 oz)
! Biscuit	1 biscuit (2½ inches across)
Breads, loaf-type	
white, whole-grain, French, Italian, pumpernickel, rye, sourdough, unfrosted raisin or cinnamon	1 slice (1 oz)
✔ reduced-calorie, light	2 slices (1½ oz)
Breads, flat-type (flatbreads)	
chapatti	1 oz
ciabatta	1 oz
naan	3¼ inch square (1 oz)
pita (6 inches across)	½ pita
roti	1 oz
✔ sandwich flat buns, whole-wheat	1 bun, including top and bottom 1½ oz)
! taco shell	2 taco shells (each 5 inches across)
tortilla, corn	1 small tortilla (6 inches across)
tortilla, flour (white or whole-wheat)	1 small tortilla (6 inches across) or ⅓ large tortilla (10 inches across)
Cornbread	1¾-inch cube (1½ oz)
English muffin	½ muffin
Hot dog bun or hamburger bun	½ bun (¾ oz)
Pancake	1 pancake (4 inches across, ¼ inch thick)
Roll, plain	1 small roll (1 oz)
! Stuffing, bread	⅓ cup
Waffle	1 waffle (4-inch square or 4 inches across)
Cereals	
✔ Bran cereal (twigs, buds, or flakes)	½ cup
Cooked cereals (oats, oatmeal)	½ cup
Granola cereal	¼ cup
Grits, cooked	½ cup
Muesli	¼ cup
Puffed cereal	1½ cups
Shredded wheat, plain	½ cup

Food	Serving Size
Sugar-coated cereal	½ cup
Unsweetened, ready-to-eat cereal	¾ cup
Grains (Including Pasta and Rice)	
Unless otherwise indicated, serving sizes listed are for cooked grains.	
Barley	⅓ cup
Bran, dry	
✔ oat	¼ cup
✔ wheat	½ cup
✔ Bulgur	½ cup
Couscous	⅓ cup
Kasha	½ cup
Millet	⅓ cup
Pasta, white or whole-wheat (all shapes and sizes)	⅓ cup
Polenta	⅓ cup
Quinoa, all colors	⅓ cup
Rice, white, brown, and other colors and types	⅓ cup
Tabbouleh (tabouli), prepared	½ cup
Wheat germ, dry	3 Tbsp
Wild rice	½ cup
Starchy Vegetables	
All of the serving sizes for starchy vegetables on this list are for cooked vegetables.	
Breadfruit	¼ cup
Cassava or dasheen	⅓ cup
Corn	½ cup
on cob	4- to 4½-inch piece (½ large cob)
✔ Hominy	¾ cup
✔ Mixed vegetables with corn or peas	1 cup
Marinara, pasta, or spaghetti sauce	½ cup
✔ Parsnips	½ cup
✔ Peas, green	½ cup
Plantain	⅓ cup
Potato	
baked with skin	¼ large potato (3 oz)
boiled, all kinds	½ cup or ½ medium potato (3 oz)
! mashed, with milk and fat	½ cup

Source: From *Choose Your Foods: Exchange Lists for Diabetes.* © Academy of Nutrition and Dietetics. Adapted and reprinted with permission.

Food	Serving Size
French-fried (oven-baked)*	1 cup (2 oz)
✔ Pumpkin puree, canned, no sugar added	¾ cup
✔ Squash, winter (acorn, butternut)	1 cup
✔ Succotash	½ cup
Yam or sweet potato, plain	½ cup (3½ oz)

Crackers and Snacks

Note: Some snacks are high in fat. Always check food labels.

Crackers

Food	Serving Size
animal	8 crackers
✔ crispbread	2–5 pieces ¾ oz
graham, 2½-inch square	3 squares
nut and rice	10 crackers
oyster	20 crackers
! round, butter-type	6 crackers
saltine-type	6 crackers
! sandwich-style, cheese or peanut butter filling	3 crackers
whole-wheat, baked	5 regular 1½-inch squares or 10 thins (¾ oz)
Granola or snack bar	1 bar (¾ oz)
Matzoh, all shapes and sizes	(¾ oz)
Melba toast	4 pieces (each about 2 by 4 inches)

Popcorn

Food	Serving Size
✔ no fat added	3 cups
‼ with butter added	3 cups
Pretzels	¾ oz
Rice cakes	2 cakes (4 inches across)

Snack chips

Food	Serving Size
baked (potato, pita)	about 8 chips (¾ oz)
‼ regular (tortilla, potato)	about 13 chips (1 oz)

! count as 1 starch choice + 1 fat choice
(1 starch choice plus 5 grams of fat)

‼ count as 1 starch choice + 2 fat choices
(1 starch choice plus 10 grams of fat)

Note: For other snacks, see the **Sweets, Desserts, and Other Carbohydrates** list, **page C-4**.

Beans, Peas, and Lentils

The choices on this list count as 1 starch choice + 1 lean protein choice.

Food	Serving Size
✔ Baked beans, canned	⅓ cup
✔ Beans (black, garbanzo, kidney, lima, navy, pinto, white), cooked or canned, drained and rinsed	½ cup
✔ Lentils (any color), cooked	½ cup
✔ Peas (black-eyed and split), cooked or canned, drained and rinsed	½ cup
🧂 ✔ Refried beans, canned	½ cup

Note: Beans, lentils, and peas are also found on the **Protein** list, **page C-6**.

Note: Restaurant-style French fries are on the **Fast Foods** list, **page C-11**.

Fruits

One fruit choice has 15 grams of carbohydrate and 60 calories.

Icon Key

✔	=	Good source of fiber
!	=	Extra fat
🧂	=	High in sodium

Food	Serving Size
Fruits	
The weights listed include skin, core, seeds, and rind.	
Apple, unpeeled	1 small apple (4 oz)
Apples, dried	4 rings
Applesauce, unsweetened	½ cup
Apricots	
canned	½ cup
dried	8 apricot halves
fresh	4 apricots (5½ oz total)
Banana	1 extra-small banana, about 4 inches long (4 oz)
✔ Blackberries	1 cup
Blueberries	¾ cup
Cantaloupe	1 cup diced
Cherries	
sweet, canned	½ cup
sweet, fresh	12 cherries (3½ oz)
Dates	3 small (deglet noor) dates or 1 large (medjool) date

Food	Serving Size
Dried fruits (blueberries, cherries, cranberries, mixed fruit, raisins)	2 Tbsp
Figs	
dried	3 small figs
✔ fresh	1½ large or 2 medium figs (3½ oz total)
Fruit cocktail	½ cup
Grapefruit	
fresh	½ large grapefruit (5½ oz)
sections, canned	¾ cup
Grapes	17 small grapes (3 oz total)
✔ Guava	2 small guava (2½ oz total)
Honeydew melon	1 cup diced
Kiwi	½ cup sliced
Loquat	¾ cup cubed
Mandarin oranges, canned	¾ cup

Food	Serving Size	Food	Serving Size
Mango	½ small mango (5½ oz) or ½ cup	dried (prunes)	3 prunes
Nectarine	1 medium nectarine (5½ oz)	fresh	2 small plums (5 oz total)
✓ Orange	1 medium orange (6½ oz)	Pomegranate seeds (arils)	½ cup
Papaya	½ papaya (8 oz) or 1 cup cubed	✓ Raspberries	1 cup
		✓ Strawberries	1¼ cup whole berries
Peaches		Tangerine	1 large tangerine (6 oz)
canned	½ cup	Watermelon	1¼ cup diced

Fruit Juice

Food	Serving Size
Peaches	
canned	½ cup
fresh	1 medium peach (6 oz)
Pears	
canned	½ cup
✓ fresh	½ large pear (4 oz)
Pineapple	
canned	½ cup
fresh	¾ cup
Plantain, extra-ripe (black), raw	¼ plantain (2¼ oz)
Plums	
canned	½ cup

Food	Serving Size
Apple juice/cider	½ cup
Fruit juice blends, 100% juice	⅓ cup
Grape juice	⅓ cup
Grapefruit juice	½ cup
Orange juice	½ cup
Pineapple juice	½ cup
Pomegranate juice	½ cup
Prune juice	⅓ cup

Milk and Milk Substitutes

One carbohydrate choice has 15 grams of carbohydrate and about 70 calories. One fat choice has 5 grams of fat and 45 calories.

Food	Serving Size	Choices per Serving
Milk and Yogurts		
Fat-Free (Skim) or Low-Fat (1%)		
milk, buttermilk, acidophilus milk, lactose-free milk	1 cup	1 fat-free milk
evaporated milk	½ cup	1 fat-free milk
yogurt, plain or Greek; may be sweetened with an artificial sweetener	⅔ cup (6 oz)	1 fat-free milk
Chocolate milk	1 cup	1 fat-free milk + 1 carbohydrate
Reduced-Fat (2%)		
milk, acidophilus milk, kefir, lactose-free milk	1 cup	1 reduced-fat milk
yogurt, plain	⅔ cup (6 oz)	1 reduced-fat milk
Whole		
milk, buttermilk, goat's milk	1 cup	1 whole milk
evaporated milk	½ cup	1 whole milk
yogurt, plain	1 cup (8 oz)	1 whole milk
chocolate milk	1 cup	1 whole milk + 1 carbohydrate
Other Milk Foods and Milk Substitutes		
Eggnog		
fat-free	⅓ cup	1 carbohydrate
low-fat	⅓ cup	1 carbohydrate ½ fat
whole milk	⅓ cup	1 carbohydrate + 1 fat
Rice drink		
plain, fat-free	1 cup	1 carbohydrate
flavored, low-fat	1 cup	2 carbohydrates
Soy milk		
light or low-fat, plain	1 cup	½ carbohydrate + ½ fat
regular, plain	1 cup	½ carbohydrate + 1 fat
Yogurt with fruit, low-fat	⅔ cup (6 oz)	1 fat-free milk + 1 carbohydrate

Note: Unsweetened nut milks (such as almond milk and coconut milk) are on the **Fats** list, **page C-8**.

Nonstarchy Vegetables

One nonstarchy vegetable choice (½ cup cooked or 1 cup raw) has 5 grams of carbohydrate, 2 grams of protein, 0 grams of fat, and 25 calories.

Icon Key

✓ = Good source of fiber

! = Extra fat

[s] = High in sodium

Nonstarchy Vegetables

Amaranth leaves (Chinese spinach)
Artichoke
Artichoke hearts (no oil)
Asparagus
Baby corn
Bamboo shoots
Bean sprouts (alfalfa, mung, soybean)
Beans (green, wax, Italian, yard-long beans)
Beets
Broccoli
Broccoli slaw, packaged, no dressing
✓ Brussels sprouts
Cabbage (green, red, bok choy, Chinese)
✓ Carrots
Cauliflower
Celery
Chayote
Coleslaw, packaged, no dressing
Cucumber
Daikon
Eggplant
Fennel
Gourds (bitter, bottle, luffa, bitter melon)
Green onions or scallions
Greens (collard, dandelion, mustard, purslane, turnip)

Hearts of palm
✓ Jicama
Kale
Kohlrabi
Leeks
Mixed vegetables (without starchy vegetables, legumes, or pasta)
Mushrooms, all kinds, fresh
Okra
Onions
Pea pods
Peppers (all varieties)
Radishes
Rutabaga
[s] Sauerkraut, drained and rinsed
Spinach
Squash, summer varieties (yellow, pattypan, crookneck, zucchini)
Sugar snap peas
Swiss chard
Tomato
Tomatoes, canned
[s] Tomato sauce (unsweetened)
Tomato/vegetable juice
Turnips
Water chestnuts

Note: Salad greens (like arugula, chicory, endive, escarole, lettuce, radicchio, romaine, and watercress) are on the **Free Foods** list, **page C-9**.

Sweets, Desserts, and Other Carbohydrates

One carbohydrate choice has 15 grams of carbohydrate and about 70 calories. One fat choice has 5 grams of fat and 45 calories.

Icon Key

✓ = Good source of fiber

! = Extra fat

[s] = High in sodium

Food	Serving Size	Choices per Serving
Beverages, Soda, and Sports Drinks		
Cranberry juice cocktail	½ cup	1 carbohydrate
Fruit drink or lemonade	1 cup (8 oz)	2 carbohydrates
Hot chocolate, regular	1 envelope (2 Tbsp or ¾ oz) added to 8 oz water	1 carbohydrate
Soft drink (soda), regular	1 can (12 oz)	2½ carbohydrates
Sports drink (fluid replacement type)	1 cup (8 oz)	1 carbohydrate
Brownies, Cake, Cookies, Gelatin, Pie, and Pudding		
Biscotti	1 oz	1 carbohydrate + 1 fat
Brownie, small, unfrosted	1¼-inch square, ⅞-inch high (about 1 oz)	1 carbohydrate + 1 fat

Food	Serving Size	Choices per Serving
Cake		
angel food, unfrosted	¹⁄₁₂ of cake (about 2 oz)	2 carbohydrates
frosted	2-inch square (about 2 oz)	2 carbohydrates + 1 fat
unfrosted	2-inch square (about 1 oz)	1 carbohydrate + 1 fat
Cookies		
100-calorie pack	1 oz	1 carbohydrate + ½ fat
chocolate chip cookies	2 cookies, 2¼ inches across	1 carbohydrate + 2 fats
gingersnaps	3 small cookies, 1½ inches across	1 carbohydrate
large cookie	1 cookie, 6 inches across (about 3 oz)	4 carbohydrates + 3 fats
sandwich cookies with crème filling	2 small cookies (about ⅔ oz)	1 carbohydrate + 1 fat
sugar-free cookies	1 large or 3 small cookies (¾ to 1 oz)	1 carbohydrate + 1 to 2 fats
vanilla wafer	5 cookies	1 carbohydrate + 1 fat
Cupcake, frosted	1 small cupcake (about 1¾ oz)	2 carbohydrates + 1 to 1½ fats
Flan	½ cup	2½ carbohydrates + 1 fat
Fruit cobbler	½ cup (3½ oz)	3 carbohydrates + 1 fat
Gelatin, regular	½ cup	1 carbohydrate
Pie		
commercially prepared fruit, 2 crusts	⅙ of 8-inch pie	3 carbohydrates + 2 fats
pumpkin or custard	⅛ of 8-inch pie	1½ carbohydrates + 1½ fats
Pudding		
regular (made with reduced-fat milk)	½ cup	2 carbohydrates
sugar-free or sugar- and fat-free (made with fat-free milk)	½ cup	1 carbohydrate

Candy, Spreads, Sweets, Sweeteners, Syrups, and Toppings

Food	Serving Size	Choices per Serving
Blended sweeteners (mixtures of artificial sweeteners and sugar)	1½ Tbsp	1 carbohydrate
Candy		
chocolate, dark or milk type	1 oz	1 carbohydrate + 2 fats
chocolate "kisses"	5 pieces	1 carbohydrate + 1 fat
hard	3 pieces	1 carbohydrate
Coffee creamer, nondairy type		
powdered, flavored	4 tsp	½ carbohydrate + ½ fat
liquid, flavored	2 Tbsp	1 carbohydrate
Fruit snacks, chewy (pureed fruit concentrate)	1 roll (¾ oz)	1 carbohydrate
Fruit spreads, 100% fruit	1½ Tbsp	1 carbohydrate
Honey	1 Tbsp	1 carbohydrate
Jam or jelly, regular	1 Tbsp	1 carbohydrate
Sugar	1 Tbsp	1 carbohydrate
Syrup		
chocolate	2 Tbsp	2 carbohydrates
light (pancake-type)	2 Tbsp	1 carbohydrate
regular (pancake-type)	1 Tbsp	1 carbohydrate

Condiments and Sauces

Food	Serving Size	Choices per Serving
Barbecue sauce	3 Tbsp	1 carbohydrate
Cranberry sauce, jellied	¼ cup	1½ carbohydrates
[s] Curry sauce	1 oz	1 carbohydrate + 1 fat
[s] Gravy, canned or bottled	½ cup	½ carbohydrate + ½ fat
Hoisin sauce	1 Tbsp	½ carbohydrate
Marinade	1 Tbsp	½ carbohydrate
Plum sauce	1 Tbsp	½ carbohydrate
Salad dressing, fat-free, cream-based	3 Tbsp	1 carbohydrate
Sweet-and-sour sauce	3 Tbsp	1 carbohydrate

Doughnuts, Muffins, Pastries, and Sweet Breads

Food	Serving Size	Choices per Serving
Banana nut bread	1-inch slice (2 oz)	2 carbohydrates + 1 fat
Doughnut		
cake, plain	1 medium doughnut (1½ oz)	1½ carbohydrates + 2 fats
hole	2 holes (1 oz)	1 carbohydrate + 1 fat

Food	Serving Size	Choices per Serving
yeast-type, glazed	1 doughnut, 3¾ inches across (2 oz)	2 carbohydrates + 2 fats
Muffin		
regular	1 muffin (4 oz)................................	4 carbohydrates + 2½ fats
lower-fat	1 muffin (4 oz)................................	4 carbohydrates + ½ fat
Scone...	1 scone (4 oz).................................	4 carbohydrates + 3 fats
Sweet roll or Danish...	1 pastry (2½ oz).............................	2½ carbohydrates + 2 fats

Frozen Bars, Frozen Dessert, Frozen Yogurt, and Ice Cream

Food	Serving Size	Choices per Serving
Frozen pops	1	½ carbohydrate
Fruit juice bars, frozen, 100% juice..	1 bar (3 oz)......................................	1 carbohydrate
Ice cream		
fat-free..	½ cup	1½ carbohydrates
light	½ cup...	1 carbohydrate + 1 fat
no-sugar-added	½ cup...	1 carbohydrate + 1 fat
regular	½ cup...	1 carbohydrate + 2 fats
Sherbet, sorbet	½ cup...	2 carbohydrates
Yogurt, frozen		
fat-free..	⅓ cup	1 carbohydrate
regular	½ cup...	1 carbohydrate + 0–1 fat
Greek, low-fat or fat-free..	½ cup...	1½ carbohydrates

Note: You can also check the **Fats** list and **Free Foods** list for other condiments.

Protein

One lean protein choice has 0 grams of carbohydrate, 7 grams of protein, 2 grams of fat, and 45 calories.

Icon Key

✔ = Good source of fiber

! = Extra fat

(S) = High in sodium (based on the sodium content of a typical 3-oz serving of meat, unless 1 oz or 2 oz is the normal serving size)

Food	Serving Size
Lean Protein	
Note: 1 oz is usually the serving size for meat, fish, poultry, or hard cheeses.	
Beef: ground (90% or higher lean/10% or lower fat); select or choice grades trimmed of fat: roast (chuck, round, rump, sirloin), steak (cubed, flank, porterhouse, T-bone), tenderloin	1 oz
(S) Beef jerky	½ oz
Cheeses with 3 grams of fat or less per oz	1 oz
Curd-style cheeses: cottage-type (all kinds); ricotta (fat-free or light)	¼ cup (2 oz)
Egg substitutes, plain	½ cup
Egg whites...	2
Fish	
fresh or frozen, such as catfish, cod, flounder, haddock, halibut, orange roughy, tilapia, trout...	1 oz
salmon, fresh or canned	1 oz
sardines, canned	2 small sardines

Food	Serving Size
tuna, fresh or canned in water or .... oil and drained	1 oz
(S) smoked: herring or salmon (lox)	1 oz
Game: buffalo, ostrich, rabbit, venison....................	1 oz
(S) Hot dog with 3 grams of fat or less per oz .... (*Note*: May contain carbohydrate.)	1 hot dog (1¾ oz)
Lamb: chop, leg, or roast	1 oz
Organ meats: heart, kidney, liver .... (*Note*: May be high in cholesterol.)	1 oz
Oysters, fresh or frozen..	6 medium oysters
Pork, lean	
(S) Canadian bacon	1 oz
(S) ham..	1 oz
rib or loin chop/roast, tenderloin	1 oz
Poultry, without skin: chicken; Cornish hen; domestic duck or goose (well drained of fat); turkey; lean ground turkey or chicken................	1 oz

Food	Serving Size	Food	Serving Size

Processed sandwich meats with 3 grams of fat or less per oz: chipped beef, thin-sliced deli meats, turkey ham, turkey pastrami .... 1 oz

Sausage with 3 grams of fat or less per oz .... 1 oz

Shellfish: clams, crab, imitation shellfish, lobster, scallops, shrimp.. 1 oz

Veal: cutlet (no breading), loin chop, roast .... 1 oz

Medium-Fat Protein

One medium-fat protein choice has 0 grams of carbohydrate, 7 grams of protein, 5 grams of fat, and 75 calories.

Note: 1 oz is usually the serving size for meat, fish, poultry, or hard cheeses.

Beef trimmed of visible fat: ground beef (85% or lower lean/15% or higher fat), corned beef, meatloaf, prime cuts of beef (rib roast), short ribs, tongue .... 1 oz

Cheeses with 4–7 grams of fat per oz: feta, mozzarella, pasteurized processed cheese spread, reduced-fat cheeses .... 1 oz

Cheese, ricotta (regular or part-skim) .... ¼ cup (2 oz)

Egg .... 1 egg

Fish: any fried .... 1 oz

Lamb: ground, rib roast .... 1 oz

Pork: cutlet, ground, shoulder roast .... 1 oz

Poultry with skin: chicken, dove, pheasant, turkey, wild duck, or goose; fried chicken..................... 1 oz

Sausage with 4–7 grams of fat per oz..................... 1 oz

High-Fat Protein

These foods are high in saturated fat, cholesterol, and calories and may raise blood cholesterol levels if eaten on a regular basis. Try to eat 3 or fewer choices from this group per week.

Note: 1 oz is usually the serving size for meat, fish, poultry, or hard cheeses.

Bacon, pork.. 2 slices (1 oz each before cooking)

Bacon, turkey .... 3 slices (½ oz each before cooking)

Cheese, regular: American, blue-veined, brie, cheddar, hard goat, Monterey jack, Parmesan, queso, and Swiss .... 1 oz

! Hot dog: beef, pork, or combination...................... 1 hot dog (10 hot dogs per 1 lb-sized package)

Hot dog: turkey or chicken .... 1 hot dog (10 hot dogs per 1 lb-sized package)

Pork: sausage, spareribs .... 1 oz

Processed sandwich meats with 8 grams of .... 1 oz fat or more per oz: bologna, hard salami, pastrami

Sausage with 8 grams fat or more per oz: .... 1 oz bratwurst, chorizo, Italian, knockwurst, Polish, smoked, summer

---

Protein

Icon Key

✓ = Good source of fiber

! = Extra fat

🧂 = High in sodium (based on the sodium content of a typical 3-oz serving of meat, unless 1 oz or 2 oz is the normal serving size)

Food	Serving Size	Choices per Serving
Plant-Based Protein		
Because carbohydrate and fat content varies among plant-based proteins, you should read the food labels.		
"Bacon" strips, soy-based	2 strips (½ oz)	1 lean protein
✓ Baked beans, canned	⅓ cup	1 starch + 1 lean protein
✓ Beans (black, garbanzo, kidney, lima, navy, pinto, white), cooked or canned, drained and rinsed....................	½ cup	1 starch + 1 lean protein
"Beef" or "sausage" crumbles, meatless	1 oz	1 lean protein
"Chicken" nuggets, soy-based...................................	2 nuggets (1½ oz)	½ carbohydrate + 1 medium-fat protein
✓ Edamame, shelled...	½ cup	½ carbohydrate + 1 lean protein
Falafel (spiced chickpea and wheat patties)	3 patties (about 2 inches across)	1 carbohydrate + 1 high-fat protein
Hot dog, meatless, soy-based..................................	1 hot dog (1½ oz)	1 lean protein
✓ Hummus	⅓ cup	1 carbohydrate + 1 medium-fat protein
✓ Lentils, any color, cooked or canned, drained and rinsed.........	½ cup	1 starch + 1 lean protein
Meatless burger, soy-based......................................	3 oz	½ carbohydrate + 2 lean proteins
✓ Meatless burger, vegetable and starch-based	1 patty (about 2½ oz)................	½ carbohydrate + 1 lean protein
Meatless deli slices..	1 oz	1 lean protein
Mycoprotein ("chicken" tenders or crumbles), meatless	2 oz	½ carbohydrate + 1 lean protein
Nut spreads: almond butter, cashew butter, peanut butter, soy nut butter	1 Tbsp.......................................	1 high-fat protein
✓ Peas (black-eyed and split peas), cooked or canned, drained and rinsed	½ cup	1 starch + 1 lean protein
🧂✓ Refried beans, canned..	½ cup	1 starch + 1 lean protein
"Sausage" breakfast-type patties, meatless	1 (1½ oz)....................................	1 medium-fat protein
Soy nuts, unsalted...	¾ oz	½ carbohydrate + 1 medium-fat protein
Tempeh, plain, unflavored	¼ cup (1½ oz)	1 medium-fat protein
Tofu	½ cup (4 oz)..............................	1 medium-fat protein
Tofu, light...	½ cup (4 oz)..............................	1 lean protein

Fats

One fat choice has 5 grams of fat and 45 calories.

Food	Serving Size
Unsaturated Fats—Monounsaturated Fats	
Almond milk (unsweetened)	1 cup
Avocado, medium	2 Tbsp (1 oz)
Nut butters (*trans* fat-free): almond butter, cashew butter, peanut butter (smooth or crunchy)	1½ tsp
Nuts	
almonds	6 nuts
Brazil	2 nuts
cashews	6 nuts
filberts (hazelnuts)	5 nuts
macadamia	3 nuts
mixed (50% peanuts)	6 nuts
peanuts	10 nuts
pecans	4 halves
pistachios	16 nuts
Oil: canola, olive, peanut	1 tsp
Olives	
black (ripe)	8
green, stuffed	10 large
Spread, plant stanol ester-type	
light	1 Tbsp
regular	2 tsp
Unsaturated Fats—Polyunsaturated Fats	
Margarine	
lower-fat spread (30–50% vegetable oil, *trans* fat-free)	1 Tbsp
stick, tub (*trans* fat-free), or squeeze (*trans* fat-free)	1 tsp
Mayonnaise	
reduced-fat	1 Tbsp
regular	1 tsp
Mayonnaise-style salad dressing	
reduced-fat	1 Tbsp
regular	2 tsp
Nuts	
pignolia (pine nuts)	1 Tbsp
walnuts, English	4 halves
Oil: corn, cottonseed, flaxseed, grapeseed, safflower, soybean, sunflower	1 tsp

Food	Serving Size
Salad dressing	
reduced-fat (*Note:* May contain carbohydrate.)	2 Tbsp
regular	1 Tbsp
Seeds	
flaxseed, ground	1½ Tbsp
pumpkin, sesame, sunflower	1 Tbsp
Tahini or sesame paste	2 tsp
Saturated Fats	
Bacon, cooked, regular or turkey	1 slice
Butter	
reduced-fat	1 Tbsp
stick	1 tsp
whipped	2 tsp
Butter blends made with oil	
reduced-fat or light	1 Tbsp
regular	1½ tsp
Chitterlings, boiled	2 Tbsp (½ oz)
Coconut, sweetened, shredded	2 Tbsp
Coconut milk, canned, thick	
light	⅓ cup
regular	1½ Tbsp
Coconut milk beverage (thin), unsweetened	1 cup
Cream	
half-and-half	2 Tbsp
heavy	1 Tbsp
light	1½ Tbsp
whipped	2 Tbsp
Cream cheese	
reduced-fat	1½ Tbsp (¾ oz)
regular	1 Tbsp (½ oz)
Lard	1 tsp
Oil: coconut, palm, palm kernel	1 tsp
Salt pork	¼ oz
Shortening, solid	1 tsp
Sour cream	
reduced-fat or light	3 Tbsp
regular	2 Tbsp

Free Foods

A "free" food is any food or drink choice that has less than 20 calories and 5 grams or less of carbohydrate per serving.

Icon Key

✔ = Good source of fiber

! = Extra fat

🧂 = High in sodium

Food	Serving Size	Food	Serving Size
Low-Carbohydrate Foods		*Salad dressing*	
Candy, hard (regular or sugar-free)	1 piece	fat-free	1 Tbsp
Fruits		fat-free, Italian	2 Tbsp
Cranberries or rhubarb, sweetened with sugar substitute	½ cup	Sour cream, fat-free or reduced-fat	1 Tbsp
Gelatin dessert, sugar-free, any flavor		*Whipped topping*	
Gum, sugar-free		light or fat-free	2 Tbsp
Jam or jelly, light or no-sugar-added	2 tsp	regular	1 Tbsp
Salad greens (such as arugula, chicory, endive, escarole, leaf or iceberg lettuce, purslane, romaine, radicchio, spinach, watercress)		**Condiments**	
		Barbecue sauce	2 tsp
		Catsup (ketchup)	1 Tbsp
Sugar substitutes (artificial sweeteners)		Chili sauce, sweet, tomato-type	2 tsp
Syrup, sugar-free	2 Tbsp	Horseradish	
Vegetables: any **raw** nonstarchy vegetables (such as broccoli, cabbage, carrots, cucumber, tomato)	½ cup	Hot pepper sauce	
		Lemon juice	
		Miso	1½ tsp
Vegetables: any **cooked** nonstarchy vegetables (such as carrots, cauliflower, green beans)	¼ cup	*Mustard*	
		honey	1 Tbsp
Reduced-Fat or Fat-Free Foods		brown, Dijon, horseradish-flavored, wasabi-flavored, or yellow	
Cream cheese, fat-free	1 Tbsp (½ oz)	Parmesan cheese, grated	1 Tbsp
Coffee creamers, nondairy		Pickle relish (dill or sweet)	1 Tbsp
liquid, flavored	1½ tsp	*Pickles*	
liquid, sugar-free, flavored	4 tsp	🧂 dill	1½ medium pickles
powdered, flavored	1 tsp	sweet, bread and butter	2 slices
powdered, sugar-free, flavored	2 tsp	sweet, gherkin	¾ oz
Margarine spread		Pimento	
fat-free	1 Tbsp	Salsa	¼ cup
reduced-fat	1 tsp	🧂 Soy sauce, light or regular	1 Tbsp
Mayonnaise		Sweet-and-sour sauce	2 tsp
fat-free	1 Tbsp	Taco sauce	1 Tbsp
reduced-fat	1 tsp	Vinegar	
Mayonnaise-style salad dressing		Worcestershire sauce	
fat-free	1 Tbsp	Yogurt, any type	2 Tbsp
reduced-fat	2 tsp		

Free Foods

Drinks/Mixes

🧂 Bouillon, broth, consommé
Bouillon or broth, low sodium
Carbonated or mineral water
Club soda
Cocoa powder, unsweetened (1 Tbsp)
Coffee, unsweetened or with sugar substitute
Diet soft drinks, sugar-free
Drink mixes (powder or liquid drops), sugar-free
Tea, unsweetened or with sugar substitute
Tonic water, sugar-free

Water
Water, flavored, sugar-free

Seasonings

Flavoring extracts (e.g., vanilla, almond, or peppermint)
Garlic, fresh or powder
Herbs, fresh or dried
Kelp
Nonstick cooking spray
Spices
Wine, used in cooking

Combination Foods

One carbohydrate choice has 15 grams of carbohydrate and about 70 calories.

Icon Key

✓ = Good source of fiber

! = Extra fat

(S) = High in sodium

Food	Serving Size	Choices per Serving
Entrees		
(S) Casserole-type entrees (tuna noodle, lasagna, spaghetti with meatballs, chili with beans, macaroni and cheese)	1 cup (8 oz)	2 carbohydrates + 2 medium-fat proteins
(S) Stews (beef/other meats and vegetables)	1 cup (8 oz)	1 carbohydrate + 1 medium-fat protein + 0–3 fats
Frozen Meals/Entrees		
(S) Burrito (beef and bean)	1 burrito (5 oz)	3 carbohydrates + 1 lean protein + 2 fats
Dinner-type healthy meal (includes dessert and is usually less than 400 calories)	about 9–12 oz	2–3 carbohydrates + 1–2 lean proteins + 1 fat
"Healthy"-type entree (usually less than 300 calories)	about 7–10 oz	2 carbohydrates + 2 lean proteins
Pizza		
(S) cheese/vegetarian, thin crust	¼ of a 12-inch pizza (4½–5 oz)	2 carbohydrates + 2 medium-fat proteins
(S) meat topping, thin crust	¼ of a 12-inch pizza (5 oz)	2 carbohydrates + 2 medium-fat proteins + 1½ fats
(S) cheese/vegetarian or meat topping, rising crust	⅙ of 12-inch pizza (4 oz)	2½ carbohydrates + 2 medium-fat proteins
(S) Pocket sandwich	1 sandwich (4½ oz)	3 carbohydrates + 1 lean protein + 1 to 2 fats
(S) Pot pie	1 pot pie (7 oz)	3 carbohydrates + 1 medium-fat protein + 3 fats
Salads (Deli-Style)		
Coleslaw	½ cup	1 carbohydrate + 1½ fats
Macaroni/pasta salad	½ cup	2 carbohydrates + 3 fats
(S) Potato salad	½ cup	1½–2 carbohydrates + 1–2 fats
Tuna salad or chicken salad	½ cup (3½ oz)	½ carbohydrate + 2 lean proteins + 1 fat
Soups		
✓ Bean, lentil, or split pea soup	1 cup (8 oz)	1½ carbohydrates + 1 lean protein
(S) Chowder (made with milk)	1 cup (8 oz)	1 carbohydrate + 1 lean protein + 1½ fats
(S) Cream soup (made with water)	1 cup (8 oz)	1 carbohydrate + 1 fat
(S) Miso soup	1 cup (8 oz)	½ carbohydrate + 1 lean protein
(S) Ramen noodle soup	1 cup (8 oz)	2 carbohydrates + 2 fats
(S) Rice soup/porridge (congee)	1 cup (8 oz)	1 carbohydrate
(S) Tomato soup (made with water), borscht	1 cup (8 oz)	1 carbohydrate
(S) Vegetable beef, chicken noodle, or other broth-type soup (including "healthy"-type soups, such as those lower in sodium and/or fat)	1 cup (8 oz)	1 carbohydrate + 1 lean protein

Fast Foods

One carbohydrate choice has 15 grams of carbohydrate and about 70 calories.

Icon Key

✓ = Good source of fiber

! = Extra fat

⬛ = High in sodium

Food	Serving Size	Choices per Serving
Main Dishes/Entrees		
Chicken		
⬛ breast, breaded and fried*	1 (about 7 oz)	1 carbohydrate + 6 medium-fat proteins
breast, meat only**	1	4 lean proteins
drumstick, breaded and fried*	1 (about 2½ oz)	$\frac{1}{2}$ carbohydrate + 2 medium-fat proteins
drumstick, meat only**	1	1 lean protein + ½ fat
⬛ nuggets or tenders	6 (about 3½ oz)	1 carbohydrate + 2 medium-fat proteins + 1 fat
thigh, breaded and fried*	1 (about 5 oz)	1 carbohydrate + 3 medium-fat proteins + 2 fats
thigh, meat only**	1	2 lean proteins + ½ fat
wing, breaded and fried*	1 wing (about 2 oz)	½ carbohydrate + 2 medium-fat proteins
wing, meat only**	1 wing	1 lean protein
⬛ ✓ Main dish salad (grilled chicken type, no dressing or croutons)	1 salad (about 1½ oz)	1 carbohydrate + 4 lean proteins
Pizza		
⬛ cheese, pepperoni, or sausage, regular or thick crust	⅛ of a 14-inch pizza (about 4 oz)	2½ carbohydrates + 1 high-fat protein + 1 fat
⬛ cheese, pepperoni, or sausage, thin crust	⅛ of a 14-inch pizza (about 2¾ oz)	1½ carbohydrates + 1 high-fat protein + 1 fat
⬛ cheese, meat, and vegetable, regular crust	⅛ of a 14-inch pizza (about 5 oz)	2½ carbohydrates + 2 high-fat proteins
Asian		
⬛ Beef/chicken/shrimp with vegetables in sauce	1 cup (about 6 oz)	1 carbohydrate + 2 lean proteins + 1 fat
Egg roll, meat	1 egg roll (about 3 oz)	1½ carbohydrates + 1 lean protein + 1½ fats
Fried rice, meatless	1 cup	2½ carbohydrates + 2 fats
Fortune cookie	1 cookie	½ carbohydrate
⬛ Hot-and-sour soup	1 cup	½ carbohydrate + ½ fat
⬛ Meat with sweet sauce	1 cup (about 6 oz)	3½ carbohydrates + 3 medium-fat proteins + 3 fats
⬛ Noodles and vegetables in sauce (chow mein, lo mein)	1 cup	2 carbohydrates + 2 fats
Mexican		
⬛ ✓ Burrito with beans and cheese	1 small burrito (about 6 oz)	3½ carbohydrates + 1 medium-fat protein + 1 fat
⬛ Nachos with cheese	1 small order (about 8 nachos)	2½ carbohydrates + 1 high-fat protein + 2 fats
⬛ Quesadilla, cheese only	1 small order (about 5 oz)	2½ carbohydrates + 3 high-fat proteins
Taco, crisp, with meat and cheese	1 small taco (about 3 oz)	1 carbohydrate + 1 medium-fat protein + ½ fat
⬛ ✓ Taco salad with chicken and tortilla bowl	1 salad (1 lb, including tortilla bowl)	3½ carbohydrates + 4 medium-fat proteins + 3 fats
⬛ Tostada with beans and cheese	1 small tostada (about 5 oz)	2 carbohydrates + 1 high-fat protein
Sandwiches		
Breakfast Sandwiches		
⬛ Breakfast burrito with sausage, egg, cheese	1 burrito (about 4 oz)	1½ carbohydrates + 2 high-fat proteins
⬛ Egg, cheese, meat on an English muffin	1 sandwich	2 carbohydrates + 3 medium-fat proteins + ½ fat

*Definition and weight refer to food **with** bone, skin, and breading.
Definition refers to above food **without bone, skin, and breading.

Food	Serving Size	Choices per Serving
Egg, cheese, meat on a biscuit	1 sandwich	2 carbohydrates + 3 medium-fat proteins + 2 fats
Sausage biscuit sandwich...	1 sandwich	2 carbohydrates + 1 high-fat protein + 4 fats
Chicken Sandwiches		
grilled with bun, lettuce, tomatoes, spread	1 sandwich (about 7½ oz).............	3 carbohydrates + 4 lean proteins
crispy, with bun, lettuce, tomatoes, spread	1 sandwich (about 6 oz)................	3 carbohydrates + 2 lean proteins + 3½ fats
Fish sandwich with tartar sauce and cheese............................	1 sandwich (5 oz)	2½ carbohydrates + 2 medium-fat proteins + 1½ fats
Hamburger		
regular with bun and condiments (catsup, mustard, onion, pickle)	1 burger (about 3½ oz)	2 carbohydrates + 1 medium-fat protein + 1 fat
4 oz meat with cheese, bun, and condiments (catsup, mustard, onion, pickle).........................	1 burger (about 8½ oz)	3 carbohydrates + 4 medium-fat proteins + 2½ fats
Hot dog with bun, plain..	1 hot dog (about 3½ oz)................	1½ carbohydrates + 1 high-fat protein + 2 fats
Submarine sandwich (no cheese or sauce)		
less than 6 grams fat	1 6-inch sub	3 carbohydrates + 2 lean proteins
regular..	1 6-inch sub	3 carbohydrates + 2 lean proteins + 1 fat
Wrap, grilled chicken, vegetables, cheese, and spread..........	1 small wrap (about 4–5 oz)............	2 carbohydrates + 2 lean proteins + 1½ fats

Sides/Appetizers

Food	Serving Size	Choices per Serving
French fries...	1 small order (about 3½ oz)	2½ carbohydrates + 2 fats
	1 medium order (about 5 oz)...........	3½ carbohydrates + 3 fats
	1 large order (about 6 oz)...............	4½ carbohydrates + 4 fats
Hashbrowns...	1 cup/medium order (about 5 oz)....	3 carbohydrates + 6 fats
Onion rings	1 serving (8–9 rings, about 4 oz).....	3½ carbohydrates + 4 fats
Salad, side (no dressing, croutons, or cheese)	1 small salad	1 nonstarchy vegetable

Beverages and Desserts

Food	Serving Size	Choices per Serving
Coffee, latte (fat-free milk)	1 small order (about 12 oz)	1 fat-free milk
Coffee, mocha (fat-free milk, no whipped cream)	1 small order (about 12 oz)	1 fat-free milk + 1 carbohydrate
Milkshake, any flavor...	1 small shake (about 12 oz)	5½ carbohydrates + 3 fats
	1 medium shake (about 16 oz)........	7 carbohydrates + 4 fats
	1 large shake (about 22 oz)............	10 carbohydrates + 5 fats
Soft-serve ice cream cone	1 small..	2 carbohydrates + ½ fat

Alcohol

One alcohol equivalent or choice (½ oz absolute alcohol) has about 100 calories. One carbohydrate choice has 15 grams of carbohydrate and about 70 calories.

Alcoholic Beverage	Serving Size	Choices per Serving
Beer		
light (less than 4.5% abv)......................................	12 fl oz	1 alcohol equivalent + ½ carbohydrate
regular (about 5% abv)...	12 fl oz	1 alcohol equivalent + 1 carbohydrate
dark (more than 5.7% abv)	12 fl oz	1 alcohol equivalent + 1 to 1½ carbohydrates
Distilled spirits: (80 or 86 proof): vodka, rum, gin, whiskey, tequila	1½ fl oz	1 alcohol equivalent
Liqueur, coffee (53 proof)..	1 fl oz	1 alcohol equivalent + 1 carbohydrate
Sake..	1 fl oz	½ alcohol equivalent
Wine		
champagne/sparkling	5 fl oz	1 alcohol equivalent
dessert (sherry)	3½ fl oz	1 alcohol equivalent + 1 carbohydrate
dry, red or white (10% abv)	5 fl oz	1 alcohol equivalent

Note: The abbreviation "% abv" refers to the percentage of alcohol by volume.

Appendix D Organizations and Resources

Academic Journals

International Journal of Sport Nutrition and Exercise Metabolism
www.humankinetics.com/IJSNEM

Journal of Nutrition
www.jn.nutrition.org

Nutrition Research
www.journals.elsevierhealth.com/periodicals/NTR

Nutrition
www.nutritionjrnl.com

Nutrition Reviews
http://onlinelibrary.wiley.com/journal/10.1111/%28ISSN%291753-4887

Obesity
http://onlinelibrary.wiley.com/journal/10.1111/%28ISSN%291753-4887

International Journal of Obesity
www.nature.com/ijo

Journal of the American Medical Association
http://jama.ama-assn.org

New England Journal of Medicine
www.nejm.org

American Journal of Clinical Nutrition
www.ajcn.org

Journal of the Academy of Nutrition and Dietetics
www.adajournal.org

Aging

Administration on Aging
www.aoa.gov

American Association of Retired Persons (AARP)
www.aarp.org

Health and Age
Sponsored by the Novartis Foundation for Gerontology and the Web-Based Health Education Foundation
www.healthandage.com

National Council on Aging
www.ncoa.org

International Osteoporosis Foundation
www.iofbonehealth.org

National Institute on Aging
www.nia.nih.gov

NIH Osteoporosis and Related Bone Diseases National Resource Center
www.niams.nih.gov

American Geriatrics Society
www.americangeriatrics.org

National Osteoporosis Foundation
www.nof.org

Alcohol and Drug Abuse

National Institute on Drug Abuse
www.nida.nih.gov

National Institute on Alcohol Abuse and Alcoholism
www.niaaa.nih.gov

Alcoholics Anonymous
www.alcoholics-anonymous.org

Narcotics Anonymous
www.na.org

National Council on Alcoholism and Drug Dependence
www.ncadd.org

National Clearinghouse for Alcohol and Drug Information
http://ncadi.samhsa.gov

Canadian Government

Health Canada
www.hc-sc.gc.ca

Canadian Council of Food and Nutrition
www.nin.ca

Agricultural and Agri-Food Canada
www.arg.gc.ca

Canadian Food Inspection Agency
www.inspection.gc.ca/english/toce.shtml

Canadian Institute for Health Information
www.cihi.ca

Canadian Public Health Association
www.cpha.ca

Canadian Nutrition and Professional Organizations

Dietitians of Canada, Canadian Dietetic Association
www.dietitians.ca

Canadian Diabetes Association
www.diabetes.ca

National Eating Disorder Information Centre
www.nedic.ca

Canadian Paediatric Society
www.cps.ca

Disordered Eating/Eating Disorders

American Psychiatric Association
www.psych.org

Harvard Eating Disorders Center
www.mcleanhospital.org/programs/klarman-eating-disorders-center

National Institute of Mental Health
www.nimh.nih.gov

National Association of Anorexia Nervosa and Associated Disorders (ANAD)
www.anad.org

National Eating Disorders Association
www.nationaleatingdisorders.org

Eating Disorder Referral and Information Center
www.edreferral.com

Overeaters Anonymous
www.oa.org

Weight Management
http://wmdpg.org

Exercise, Physical Activity, and Sports

American College of Sports Medicine (ACSM)
www.acsm.org

American Physical Therapy Association (APTA)
www.apta.org

Gatorade Sports Science Institute (GSSI)
www.gssiweb.com

National Coalition for Promoting Physical Activity (NCPPA)
www.ncppa.org

Sports, Cardiovascular, and Wellness Nutrition (SCAN)
www.scandpg.org

President's Council on Physical Fitness and Sports
www.fitness.gov

American Council on Exercise
www.acefitness.org

IDEA Health & Fitness Association
www.ideafit.com

Food Safety

Food Marketing Institute
www.fmi.org

Agency for Toxic Substances and Disease Registry (ATSDR)
www.atsdr.cdc.gov

Food Allergy and Anaphylaxis Network
www.foodallergy.org

Foodsafety.gov
www.foodsafety.gov

USDA Food Safety and Inspection Service
www.fsis.usda.gov

Consumer Reports
www.consumerreports.org

Center for Science in the Public Interest: Food Safety
www.cspinet.org/foodsafety/index.html

Center for Food Safety and Applied Nutrition
www.fda.gov/Food/FoodSafety

Food Safety Project
www.extension.iastate.edu/foodsafety

Organic Consumers Association
www.organicconsumers.org

Infancy and Childhood

Administration for Children and Families
www.acf.hhs.gov

American Academy of Pediatrics
www.aap.org

Kidshealth: The Nemours Foundation
www.kidshealth.org

National Center for Education in Maternal and Child Health
www.ncemch.org

Birth Defects Research for Children, Inc.
www.birthdefects.org

USDA/ARS Children's Nutrition Research Center at Baylor College of Medicine
www.kidsnutrition.org

Centers for Disease Control and Prevention—Healthy Youth
www.cdc.gov/healthyyouth

International Agencies

UNICEF
www.unicef.org

World Health Organization
www.who.int/en

Stockholm Convention on Persistent Organic Pollutants
www.pops.int

Food and Agricultural Organization of the United Nations
www.fao.org

International Food Information Council
www.ific.org

Pregnancy and Lactation

San Diego County Breastfeeding Coalition
www.breastfeeding.org

National Alliance for Breastfeeding Advocacy
www.naba-breastfeeding.org

American College of Obstetricians and Gynecologists
www.acog.org

La Leche League
www.lalecheleague.org

National Organization on Fetal Alcohol Syndrome
www.nofas.org

March of Dimes Birth Defects Foundation
http://modimes.org

Professional Nutrition Organizations

Academy of Nutrition and Dietetics (AND)
www.eatright.org

American Cancer Society
www.cancer.org

American Dental Association
www.ada.org

American Heart Association
www.americanheart.org

American Medical Association
www.ama-assn.org

Center for Science in the Public Interest
www.cspinet.org

American Society for Nutrition (ASN)
www.nutrition.org

Dietitians in Integrative and Functional Medicine
www.complementarynutrition.org

Institute for Functional Medicine
www.functionalmedicine.org

North American Association for the Study of Obesity (NAASO)
www.naaso.org

Society for Nutrition Education
www.sne.org

American College of Nutrition
www.americancollegeofnutrition.org

American Obesity Association
www.obesity.org

American Council on Science and Health
www.acsh.org

American Diabetes Association
www.diabetes.org

Institute of Food Technologists
www.ift.org

ILSI Human Nutrition Institute
www.ilsi.org

Trade Organizations

American Meat Institute
www.meatami.com

National Dairy Council
www.nationaldairycouncil.org

United Fresh Fruit and Vegetable Association
www.uffva.org

U.S.A. Rice Federation
www.usarice.com

U.S. Government

Agricultural Research Service
www.ars.usda.gov

USDA National Organic Program
Agricultural Marketing Service
www.ams.usda.gov

U.S. Department of Health and Human Services
www.hhs.gov

Food and Drug Administration (FDA)
www.fda.gov

Environmental Protection Agency
www.epa.gov

Federal Trade Commission
www.ftc.gov

Office of Dietary Supplements
National Institutes of Health
http://dietary-supplements.info.nih.gov

Nutrient Data Laboratory
Beltsville Human Nutrition Research Center, Agricultural
Research Service
www.ars.usda.gov/nutrientdata

National Digestive Diseases Information Clearinghouse
http://digestive.niddk.nih.gov

National Cancer Institute
www.cancer.gov

National Eye Institute
www.nei.nih.gov

National Heart, Lung, and Blood Institute
www.nhlbi.nih.gov/index.htm

National Institute of Diabetes and Digestive and Kidney
Diseases
www.niddk.nih.gov

National Center for Complementary and Alternative Medicine
http://nccam.nih.gov

U.S. Department of Agriculture (USDA)
www.usda.gov

Centers for Disease Control and Prevention (CDC)
www.cdc.gov

National Institutes of Health (NIH)
www.nih.gov

Food and Nutrition Information Center
Agricultural Research Service, USDA
www.nal.usda.gov/fnic

National Institute of Allergy and Infectious Diseases
www.niaid.nih.gov

Weight and Health Management

North American Association for the Study of Obesity (NAASO)
www.obesityresearch.org

Vegetarian Resource Group
www.vrg.org

American Obesity Association
www.obesity.org

Anemia Lifeline
www.anemia.com

The Arc
www.thearc.org

Bottled Water Web
www.bottledwaterweb.com

Food and Nutrition
Institute of Medicine
www.iom.edu/Global/Topics/Food-Nutrition.aspx

Calorie Control Council
www.caloriecontrol.org

TOPS (Take Off Pounds Sensibly)
www.tops.org

Shape Up America!
www.shapeup.org

World Hunger

Center on Hunger, Poverty, and Nutrition Policy
http://nutrition.tufts.edu

Freedom from Hunger
www.freefromhunger.org

Oxfam International
www.oxfam.org

WorldWatch Institute
www.worldwatch.org

The Hunger Project
www.thp.org

U.S. Agency for International Development
www.usaid.gov

Feeding America
www.feedingamerica.org

Food First
www.foodfirst.org

Glossary

1,25-dihydroxycholecalciferol (calcitriol) Active form of vitamin D.

5-methyltetrahydrofolate (5-methyl THF) Most active form of folate.

A

absorption Process of moving nutrients from the GI tract into the circulatory system.

absorptive state Period after you eat when the stomach and small intestine are full and anabolic reactions exceed catabolic reactions.

Acceptable Macronutrient Distribution Ranges (AMDRs) Healthy range of intakes for the energy-containing nutrients—carbohydrates, proteins, and fats—expressed as a percentage of total daily energy. The AMDRs for adults are 45–65 percent carbohydrates, 10–35 percent protein, and 20–35 percent fat.

acceptable tolerance levels Maximum amount of pesticide residue that is allowed in or on foods.

acetaldehyde dehydrogenase (ALDH) Alcohol-metabolizing enzyme found in the liver that converts acetaldehyde to acetate.

acetaldehyde One of the first compounds produced in the metabolism of ethanol. Eventually, acetaldehyde is converted to carbon dioxide and water and excreted.

acetyl CoA Two-carbon compound formed when pantothenic acid combines with acetate.

acid–base balance Mechanisms used to maintain body fluids close to a neutral pH so the body can function properly.

acidosis Condition in which the blood pH is too low, generally due to excessive hydrogen ions.

active transport Movement of substances across a cell membrane against their concentration gradient with the help of a carrier protein and energy expenditure.

acute dehydration Dehydration that sets in after a short period of time.

acute Characterized by a sudden onset and rapid progression of symptoms.

added sugars Sugars added to foods during processing and/or packaging.

adenosine diphosphate (ADP) Nucleotide composed of adenine, ribose, and two phosphate molecules; formed when one phosphate molecule is removed from ATP.

adenosine triphosphate (ATP) High-energy molecule composed of adenine, ribose, and three phosphate molecules; used by cells to fuel all biological processes.

Adequate Intake (AI) *Approximate* daily amount of a nutrient that is sufficient to meet the needs of similar individuals within a population group. The Food and Nutrition Board uses AIs for nutrients that do not have enough scientific evidence to calculate an RDA.

adipocytes Cells in adipose tissue that store fat; also known as *fat cells*.

adiponectin Hormone produced in the adipocytes that controls the body's response to insulin and may be involved in reducing the risk of obesity and type 2 diabetes.

adolescence Developmental transition between childhood and early adulthood (approximately ages 9–19).

aerobic Reaction that requires oxygen.

age-related macular degeneration (AMD) Disease that affects the macula of the retina, causing blurry vision and, potentially, blindness.

aging Declines in bodily functions that accumulate with time, ultimately leading to death.

air-displacement plethysmography Procedure used to estimate body volume based on the amount of air displaced.

albumin Protein produced in the liver and found in the blood that helps maintain fluid balance.

alcohol dehydrogenase (ADH) One of the alcohol-metabolizing enzymes, found in the stomach and the liver, that converts ethanol to acetaldehyde.

alcohol poisoning State in which the BAC rises to the point that a person's central nervous system is affected and his or her breathing and heart rate are interrupted.

alcohol tolerance State in which the body has adjusted to long-term alcohol use by becoming less sensitive to the alcohol. More alcohol needs to be consumed in order to get the same euphoric effect.

alcohol use disorder (AUD) Pattern of alcohol intake characterized by lack of control over drinking; preoccupation with drinking; continuation of drinking despite negative consequences; tolerance; or withdrawal symptoms when drinking is discontinued.

alcohol Class of organic compounds that contain one or more hydroxyl groups attached to carbons. Examples include ethanol, glycerol, and methanol. Ethanol is often referred to as "alcohol."

alcoholic hepatitis Stage 2 of alcoholic liver disease, in which the liver becomes inflamed.

alcoholic liver disease Degenerative liver condition that occurs in three stages: (1) fatty liver, (2) alcoholic hepatitis, and (3) cirrhosis.

alcoholism Chronic disease influenced by genetic, psychosocial, and environmental factors and characterized by a level of alcohol intake that causes physical, mental, social, and sometimes legal problems.

aldosterone Hormone secreted from the adrenal glands in response to reduced blood volume; signals the kidneys to reabsorb sodium, which increases blood volume and blood pressure.

alkalosis Condition in which the blood pH is too low due to a low concentration of hydrogen ions.

allergen Substance, such as wheat protein, that causes an allergic reaction.

alpha-ketoglutarate Compound that participates in the formation of nonessential amino acids during transamination.

alpha-linolenic acid Polyunsaturated essential fatty acid; part of the omega-3 fatty acid family.

alpha-tocopherol (α-tocopherol) Most active form of vitamin E in the body.

Alzheimer's disease Progressive and irreversible type of dementia characterized by distinct changes in brain tissue.

amenorrhea Absence of menstruation for at least three consecutive cycles.

amine group Nitrogen-containing compound (NH_2) connected to the central carbon of an amino acid.

amino acid pools Limited supplies of amino acids that accumulate in the blood and cells; amino acids are pulled from the pools and used to build new proteins.

amino acid score Composition of essential amino acids in a protein compared with a standard, usually egg protein.

amino acids Fundamental units of proteins; composed of carbon, hydrogen, oxygen, and nitrogen.

amylopectin Branched chain of polysaccharides found in starch.

amylose Straight chain of polysaccharides found in starch.

anabolic Energy-requiring process in which smaller molecules are combined to form larger molecules.

anaerobic Reaction that does not require oxygen.

anaphylaxis Severe, life-threatening allergic reaction involving a sudden drop in blood pressure and constriction of the airways in the lungs, which inhibits the ability to breathe.

anencephaly Neural tube defect that results in the absence of major parts of the brain.

angiotensin II Blood protein that causes vasoconstriction and triggers the release of aldosterone from the adrenal glands, which raises blood pressure.

anions Negatively charged ions.

anorexia nervosa Eating disorder in which people intentionally starve themselves, causing extreme weight loss.

antibiotic-resistant bacteria Bacteria that have developed a resistance to an antibiotic such that they are no longer affected by antibiotic medication.

antibiotics Drugs that kill or slow the growth of bacteria.

antibodies Proteins that identify and participate in the destruction of pathogens as part of the body's immune response.

antidiuretic hormone (ADH) Pituitary hormone secreted in response to low blood volume; acts to reduce renal excretion of water, constrict blood vessels, and raise blood pressure; also known as *vasopressin*.

antimicrobials Substances or a combination of substances, such as disinfectants and sanitizers, that kill or inhibit the growth of microorganisms.

antioxidants Nutrients and phytochemicals that act to neutralize free radicals.

anus Opening of the rectum, or end of the GI tract.

appetite Desire to eat food whether or not there is hunger; a taste for particular foods and cravings in reaction to cues such as the sight, smell, or thought of food.

arachidonic acid Omega-6 fatty acid formed from linoleic acid; used to synthesize the eicosanoids, including leukotrienes, prostaglandins, and thromboxanes.

ariboflavinosis Deficiency of riboflavin characterized by stomatitis, glossitis, and cheilosis.

ascorbic acid Active form of vitamin C.

atherosclerosis Narrowing of the coronary arteries due to buildup of debris along the artery walls.

atrophic gastritis Chronic inflammation of the stomach.

atrophy To shrink in size.

attention-deficit/hyperactivity disorder (ADHD) Condition characterized by impulsivity, high distractibility, and hyperactivity; previously known as attention-deficit disorder, or ADD.

avidin Protein in raw egg whites that binds biotin.

B

bacteria Single-celled microorganisms without an organized nucleus. Some are benign or beneficial to humans, whereas others can cause disease.

balance Diet principle of providing the correct proportion of nutrients to maintain health and prevent disease.

bariatric surgery Surgical procedure that promotes weight loss by limiting the amount of food that can be eaten or absorbed.

basal metabolic rate (BMR) Measure of basal metabolism taken when the body is at rest in a warm, quiet environment after a 12-hour fast; expressed as kilocalories per kilogram of body weight per hour.

basal metabolism Amount of energy expended by the body to meet its basic physiological needs, including muscle tone and heart and brain function.

behavior modification Changing behaviors to improve health outcomes. In the case of weight management, it involves identifying and altering eating patterns that contribute to weight gain or impede weight loss.

beriberi Thiamin deficiency that results in weakness; the name translates to "I can not."

beta-carotene One of the provitamin A carotenoids.

beta-oxidation Series of metabolic reactions in which fatty acids are oxidized to acetyl CoA; also called *fatty acid oxidation*.

bicarbonate Negatively charged alkali ion produced from bicarbonate salts; during digestion, bicarbonate ions released from the pancreas neutralize HCl in the duodenum.

bile Secretion produced by the liver, stored in the gallbladder, and released into the duodenum to emulsify dietary fat.

binders Compounds such as oxalates and phytates that bind to minerals in foods and reduce their bioavailability.

binge drinking Pattern of consuming five or more alcoholic drinks by men or four or more drinks by women in about 2 hours that raises BAC to 0.08 g/dl or more.

binge eating disorder Eating disorder characterized by recurrent episodes of binge eating without purging.

bioaccumulate To build up the levels of a substance or chemical in an organism over time, so that the concentration of the chemical is higher than would be found naturally in the environment.

bioavailability Degree to which a nutrient is absorbed from foods and used in the body.

biodiversity Variability among living organisms on the earth, including the variability within and between species and within and between ecosystems.

bioelectrical impedance analysis (BIA) Method used to assess the percentage of body fat by using a low-level electrical current; body fat resists or impedes the current, whereas water and muscle mass conduct electricity.

biotechnology Manipulation of living organisms or their components to develop or manufacture useful products.

biotinidase Enzyme in the small intestine that releases biotin from food to allow it to be absorbed.

blackout Amnesia for events that occurred while a person was intoxicated.

bleaching Reaction occurring when light enters the eye and interacts with rhodopsin, splitting it into *trans*-retinal and opsin.

blood alcohol concentration (BAC) Amount of alcohol in the blood. BAC is measured in grams of alcohol per deciliter of blood, usually expressed as a percentage.

blood lipid profile Measurement of blood lipids used to assess cardiovascular risk.

body composition Ratio of fat to lean tissue (muscle, bone, and organs) in the body; usually expressed as percent body fat.

body image How you perceive your physical appearance.

body mass index (BMI) Calculation of body weight in relationship to height.

body mass index (BMI) Measurement calculated using the metric formula of weight in kilograms divided by height in meters squared; used to determine whether an individual is underweight, at a healthy weight, overweight, or obese.

bolus Soft mass of chewed food.

bomb calorimeter Instrument used to measure the amount of heat released from food during combustion; the amount of heat produced is directly related to the number of kilocalories in a given food.

bone mineral density (BMD) Amount of minerals, in particular calcium, per volume in an individual's bone.

botanicals Part of a plant, such as its root, that is believed to have medicinal or therapeutic attributes.

botulism A rare but serious paralytic illness caused by a toxin secreted by the bacterium *Clostridium botulinum*.

bovine growth hormone (BGH) Hormone that is essential for normal growth and development in cattle.

bran Indigestible outer shell of the grain kernel.

breastfeeding Act of feeding an infant milk from a woman's breast.

brown adipose tissue (BAT) Type of adipose tissue, found primarily in infants, that produces body heat; gets its name from the large number of mitochondria and capillaries responsible for the brown color.

buffers Substances that help maintain the proper pH in a solution by accepting or donating hydrogen ions.

bulimia nervosa Eating disorder characterized by binging (consuming large quantities of food in a short period of time) and then purging through vomiting or other means.

C

calciferol Family of vitamin D compounds.

calcitonin Hormone secreted by the thyroid gland that lowers blood calcium levels.

calcium (Ca^{2+}) One of the most abundant divalent cations found in nature and in the body.

cancer General term for a large group of diseases characterized by uncontrolled growth of abnormal cells.

canning Process of packing food in airtight containers and heating them to a temperature high enough to kill bacteria.

carbohydrate loading Diet and training strategy that maximizes glycogen stores in the body before an endurance event.

carbohydrate-based fat substitutes Substances that use polysaccharides to retain moisture and provide a fatlike texture.

carboxylation Chemical reaction in which a carboxyl group is added to a molecule.

carcinogen Cancer-causing substance, including tobacco smoke, air and water pollution, ultraviolet radiation, and various chemicals.

carcinogenesis Process of cancer development.

cardiac arrhythmia Disturbance in the beating and rhythm of the heart; can be caused by excessive alcohol consumption.

cardiac myopathy Condition in which the heart becomes thin and weak and is unable to pump blood throughout the body; also called *disease of the heart muscle.*

cardiorespiratory conditioning Improvements in the delivery of oxygen to working muscles as a result of aerobic activity.

cardiorespiratory endurance Body's ability to sustain cardiorespiratory exercise for a prolonged period of time.

cardiovascular disease (CVD) General term for diseases of the heart and blood vessels.

carnitine Vitamin-like substance used to transport fatty acids across the mitochondrial membrane to properly utilize fat.

carotenodermia Presence of excess carotene in the blood, resulting in an orange color to the skin due to excessive intake of carrots or other carotene-rich vegetables.

catabolic Energy-releasing process that breaks larger molecules into smaller parts.

cataract Common eye disorder that occurs when the lens of the eye becomes cloudy.

cations Positively charged ions.

cecum Pouch at the beginning of the large intestine that receives waste from the small intestine.

celiac disease Genetic disease in which a hyperimmune response damages the villi of the small intestine when gluten is consumed.

cell differentiation Process of a less specialized immature cell becoming a specialized mature cell.

cell division Process of dividing one cell into two separate cells with the same genetic material.

cellulose Nondigestible polysaccharide found in plant cell walls.

central or android obesity Excess storage of visceral fat in the abdominal area, indicated by a waist circumference greater than 40 inches in males and 35 inches in females; central obesity increases the risk of heart disease, diabetes, and hypertension.

ceruloplasmin Protein found in the blood that transports copper.

cheilosis Noninflammatory condition of the lips characterized by chapping and fissuring.

chemical digestion Breaking down food through enzymatic reactions.

chief cells Specialized cells in the stomach that secrete pepsinogen, an inactive form of the protein-digesting enzyme pepsin.

childhood obesity Condition of a child's having too much body weight for his or her height. Defined as a BMI at or above the 95th percentile.

chloride (Cl⁻) Major anion in the extracellular fluid.

chlorophyll Green pigment in plants that absorbs energy from sunlight to begin the process of photosynthesis.

cholecalciferol (vitamin D₃) Form of vitamin D found in animal foods, supplements, and formed from precalciferol in the skin; absorbed from the skin into the blood.

cholecystokinin (CCK) Hormone released by the duodenum that stimulates the gallbladder to release bile.

cholesterol Common sterol found only in animal products and made in the liver from saturated fatty acids.

choline Member of the B vitamin family that is a component of the phospholipid lecithin.

choline Vitamin-like substance that is a precursor for the neurotransmitter acetylcholine, which is essential for healthy nerves.

chronic dehydration Dehydration over a long period of time.

chronic disease Noncommunicable disease characterized by a slow onset, long duration, and gradual progression.

chronologic age Person's age in number of years of life.

chylomicron Type of lipoprotein that carries digested fat and other lipids through the lymph system into the blood.

chyme Semiliquid, partially digested food mass that leaves the stomach and enters the small intestine.

ciguatera poisoning Condition caused by marine toxins that are produced by dinoflagellates and have bioaccumulated in fish that the affected person consumes.

cirrhosis Stage 3 of alcoholic liver disease, in which liver cells die and are replaced by scar tissue.

cis Configuration of a fatty acid in which the carbon atoms on each side of the double bond are on the same side.

closed or "coded" dating Refers to the packing numbers that are decodable only by manufacturers and are often found on non-perishable, shelf-stable foods.

clotting factors Substances involved in the process of blood clotting, such as prothrombin and fibrinogen.

coagulation The process of blood clotting.

cobalamin Vitamin involved in energy metabolism and the conversion of homocysteine to methionine; another name for vitamin vitamin B₁₂.

coenzymes Organic substances, often vitamins, that bind to an enzyme to facilitate enzyme activity; unlike enzymes, coenzymes can be altered by the chemical reaction.

coenzymes Substances, such as vitamins or minerals, that facilitate the activity of enzymes.

cofactor Substance that binds to an enzyme to help catalyze a reaction; generally refers to a metal ion, whereas a coenzyme is usually an organic compound such as a vitamin.

collagen Protein found in connective tissue, including bones, teeth, skin, cartilage, and tendons.

colon Another name for the large intestine.

colostrum Fluid that is expressed from the mother's breast after birth and before the development of breast milk.

community-supported agriculture (CSA) Arrangement where individuals pay a fee to support a local farm, and in exchange receive a weekly or biweekly box of fresh produce from the farm.

complete protein Protein that provides all the essential amino acids, along with some nonessential amino acids. Soy protein and protein from animal sources are complete proteins.

complex carbohydrates Category of carbohydrates that contain many sugar units combined. Oligosaccharides and polysaccharides are complex carbohydrates.

conception Moment when a sperm fertilizes an egg.

condensation Chemical reaction in which two molecules combine to form a larger molecule, and water is released.

conditionally essential amino acids Nonessential amino acids that become essential (and must be consumed in the diet) when the body cannot make them.

conditioning Process of improving physical fitness through repeated activity.

cones Light-absorbing cells responsible for color vision.

congeners Fermentation by-products in alcoholic beverages that may contribute to hangover symptoms.

congregate meals Low- or no-cost meals served at churches, synagogues, or other community sites where older adults can receive a nutritious meal and socialize.

consensus Agreed-upon conclusion of a group of experts based on a collection of information.

constipation Infrequent passage of dry, hardened stools.

control group In experimental research, the group that does not receive the treatment but may be given a placebo instead; used as a standard for comparison.

Cori cycle Metabolic pathway in the liver that regenerates glucose from lactate released from the muscle.

cortical bone Hard outer layer of bone.

cortisol Hormone produced by the adrenal cortex that stimulates gluconeogenesis and lipolysis.

C-reactive protein (CRP) Protein found in the blood that is released from the cells during inflammation; used as a marker for the presence of atherosclerosis.

creatine phosphate (PCr) Compound that provides a reserve of phosphate to regenerate ADP to ATP.

cretinism Condition caused by a deficiency of thyroid hormone during prenatal development, resulting in abnormal mental and physical development in children.

critical periods Developmental stages during which cells and tissues rapidly grow and differentiate to form body structures.

Crohn's disease Form of ulcerative colitis in which ulcers form throughout the GI tract and not just in the colon.

cross-breeding Type of biotechnology in which two plants or two animals with different qualities are bred to produce offspring with desired traits from both.

cross-contaminate Transfer of pathogens from a food, utensil, cutting board, kitchen surface, and/or hands to another food or object.

crypts Glands at the base of the villi; they contain stem cells that manufacture young cells to replace the cells of the villi when they die.

cupric copper Oxidized form of copper (Cu^{+2})

cuprous copper Reduced form of copper (Cu^+)

cytochromes Protein complexes that move electrons down the electron transport chain; contain the minerals iron and copper.

D

danger zone Range of temperatures between 40° and 140°F at which foodborne bacteria multiplies most rapidly; room temperature falls within the danger zone.

deamination Removal of the amine group from an amino acid.

dehydration Excessive loss of body fluids; usually caused by inadequate fluid intake, diarrhea, vomiting, or excessive sweating.

DeLaney Clause Clause in the Food Additives Amendment mandating that additives shown to cause cancer at any level must be removed from the marketplace.

dementia Disorder of the brain that interferes with a person's memory, learning, and mental stability.

denature To alter a protein's secondary, tertiary, or quaternary structure, thereby disabling its function; the amino acids of the primary structure remain linked together by peptide bonds.

dental caries Tooth decay.

deoxyadenosylcobalamin Coenzyme form of vitamin vitamin B_{12} that converts intermediate substances in the TCA cycle.

developed country Country that is advanced in multiple areas, such as income per capita, life expectancy, rate of literacy, industrial capability, technological sophistication, and economic productivity.

developing country Country that is growing in multiple areas, such as income per capita, life expectancy, rate of literacy, industrial capability, technological sophistication, and economic productivity.

diabetes mellitus Medical condition whereby an individual either doesn't have enough insulin or is resistant to the insulin available, resulting in a rise in blood glucose levels. Diabetes mellitus is often called diabetes.

diarrhea Abnormally frequent passage of watery stools.

diastolic pressure Bottom number in a blood pressure reading that measures the minimal arterial pressure during relaxation of the heart muscle when the ventricles fill with blood.

dietary fiber Food components that humans cannot digest; most are carbohydrates.

dietary folate equivalents (DFE) Measurement used to express the amount of folate in a food or supplement.

Dietary Guidelines for Americans Guidelines published every 5 years by the Department of Health and Human Services and the United States Department of Agriculture that provide dietary and lifestyle advice to healthy individuals age 2 and older to maintain good health and prevent chronic diseases. They are the basis for the federal food and nutrition education programs.

Dietary Reference Intakes (DRIs) Reference values for nutrients developed by the Food and Nutrition Board of the National Academy of Medicine, used to plan and evaluate the diets of healthy people in the United States and Canada. It includes the Estimated Average Requirement (EAR), the Recommended Dietary Allowance (RDA), the Adequate Intake (AI), and the Tolerable Upper Intake Level (UL).

digestion Process that breaks down food into individual molecules small enough to be absorbed through the intestinal wall.

diglyceride Remnant of fat digestion that consists of a glycerol with two attached fatty acids; also the form of fat used as an emulsifier in food production.

dipeptide Chain of two amino acids joined together by a peptide bond.

direct calorimetry Direct measurement of the energy expended by the body obtained by assessing heat loss;

disaccharide Simple sugar that consists of two sugar units combined. The three most common disaccharides are sucrose, lactose, and maltose.

disordered eating Abnormal and potentially harmful eating behaviors that do not meet specific criteria for a clinical eating disorder.

distillation Evaporation and then collection of a liquid by condensation. Liquors are made using distillation.

diuretics Substances that increase the production of urine; often used as antihypertensive drugs.

diverticula Small bulges at weak spots in the colon wall.

diverticulitis Infection of the diverticula.

diverticulosis Existence of diverticula in the lining of the large intestine or colon.

DNA fingerprinting Technique in which bacterial DNA "gene patterns" (or "fingerprints") are detected and analyzed to distinguish between different strains of a bacterium.

double-blind placebo-controlled study Experimental study in which neither the researchers nor the subjects in the study are aware of who is receiving the treatment or the placebo.

dual-energy X-ray absorptiometry (DEXA) Method that uses two low-energy X-rays to measure body density and bone mass.

E

Early-childhood caries Tooth decay from prolonged tooth contact with formula, milk, fruit juice, or other sugar-rich liquid offered to an infant in a bottle.

eating disorders Psychiatric illnesses that involve specific abnormal eating behaviors.

eclampsia Seizures or coma in a woman with preeclampsia.

edema Accumulation of excess water in the spaces surrounding the cells, which causes swelling of the body tissue.

eicosanoids Hormonelike substances in the body. Prostaglandins, thromboxanes, and leukotrienes are all eicosanoids.

eicosapentaenoic acid (EPA) and docosahexaenoic acid (DHA) EPA (C20:5n–3) and DHA (C22:6n–3) are omega-3 fatty acids that are synthesized in the body and found in cold-water fish. These compounds may be beneficial in reducing heart disease.

electrolytes Ions such as sodium, potassium, chloride, and calcium that are able to conduct electrical current when they are dissolved in body water.

electron transport chain Final stage of energy metabolism in which NADH and $FADH_2$ transport high-energy electrons to the protein complexes in the electron transport chain, resulting in the formation of ATP and water.

elimination Excretion of undigested and unabsorbed food through the feces.

elongation Phase of protein synthesis in which the polypeptide chain grows longer by adding amino acids.

embryo Fertilized egg during the third through the eighth week of pregnancy.

emergency kitchen Kitchen or a commercial food service that prepares for natural disasters, emergencies, or terrorist attacks.

emulsifier Compound that keeps two incompatible substances, such as oil and water, mixed together.

emulsify To break large fat globules into smaller droplets.

endocytosis Type of active transport in which the cell membrane forms an indentation, engulfs the substance to be absorbed, and releases it into the interior of the cell.

endosperm Starchy inner portion of a cereal grain.

endotoxins Damaging products released from the cell wall of dead bacteria, such as those in the GI tract. They can travel in the blood to the liver and initiate liver damage.

energy balance State at which energy (kilocalorie) intake from food and beverages is equal to energy (kilocalorie) output for basal metabolism, the thermic effect of exercise, and the thermic effect of food.

energy density Measurement of the kilocalories in a food compared with the weight (grams) of the food.

energy gap Difference between the numbers of kilocalories needed to maintain weight before and after weight loss.

energy Capacity to do work.

energy-yielding nutrients Three nutrients that provide energy to the body to fuel physiological functions: carbohydrates, lipids, and protein.

enriched grains Refined grain foods that have folic acid, thiamin, niacin, riboflavin, and iron added.

enteric nervous system Section of the peripheral nervous system that directly controls the gastrointestinal system.

enterocytes Absorptive epithelial cells that line the lumen of the small intestine.

enterogastrones Group of GI tract hormones, produced in the stomach and small intestine, that controls gastric motility and secretions.

enterohepatic circulation Process of recycling bile from the large intestine back to the liver to be reused during fat digestion.

enzymes Proteins in living cells that act as catalysts and control chemical reactions.

enzymes Substances, mostly proteins, that increase the rate of chemical reactions; also called *biological catalysts*.

epidemiological research Research that studies the variables that influence health in a population; it is often observational.

epigenetics Study of the variety of environmental factors and other mechanisms influencing gene expression.

epiglottis Cartilage at the back of the tongue that closes off the trachea during swallowing.

epinephrine Hormone produced by the adrenal glands that signals the liver cells to release glucose; also referred to as the "fight-or-flight" hormone.

epiphyseal plate Growth plate of the bone; in puberty, growth in this area leads to increases in height.

epithelial tissues Tissues that line body cavities or cover body surfaces.

ergocalciferol (vitamin D_2) Form of vitamin D found in plants and dietary supplements.

ergogenic aid Substance, such as a dietary supplement, used to enhance athletic performance.

esophagus Tube that connects the mouth to the stomach.

essential amino acids Nine amino acids that the body cannot synthesize; they must be obtained through dietary sources.

essential fat Component of body fat that is necessary for health and normal body functions; includes the fat stored in the bone marrow, heart, lungs, liver, spleen, kidneys, intestines, muscles, and the lipid-rich tissues of the central nervous system.

essential fatty acids Two polyunsaturated fatty acids that the body cannot make and that therefore must be eaten in foods: linoleic acid and alpha-linolenic acid.

essential nutrients Nutrients that must be consumed from foods because they cannot be made in the body in sufficient quantities to meet its needs and support health.

Estimated Average Requirement (EAR) Average daily amount of a nutrient needed by 50 percent of the individuals in a similar age and gender group.

Estimated Energy Requirement (EER) Amount of daily energy to maintain a healthy body weight and meet energy needs based on age, gender, height, weight, and activity level.

estimated energy requirement (EER) Average kilocalorie intake that is estimated to maintain energy balance based on a person's gender, age, height, body weight, and level of physical activity.

ethanol Type of alcohol, specifically ethyl alcohol (C_2H_5OH), found in alcoholic beverages such as wine, beer, and liquor.

exchange lists Diet-planning tool that groups foods together based on their carbohydrate, protein, and fat content. One food on the list can be exchanged for another food on the same list.

exercise Any type of structured or planned physical activity.

experimental group In experimental research, the group of participants given a specific treatment, such as a drug, as part of the study.

experimental research Research involving at least two groups of subjects receiving different treatments.

extracellular fluid (ECF) Water found outside the cell, including the intravascular fluid and the interstitial fluid.

F

facilitated diffusion Movement of substances across a cell membrane with the help of a carrier protein along their concentration gradient.

fad diet Diet that promises rapid weight loss via a method that is typically unproven and unhealthy.

famine Severe shortage of food caused by weather-related crop destruction, poor agricultural practices, pestilence, war, or other factors.

farm-to-table continuum Illustrates the roles that farmers, food manufacturers, food transporters, retailers, and consumers play in ensuring that the food supply, from the farm to the plate, remains safe.

fat substitutes Substances that replace added fat in foods; provide the creamy properties of fat for fewer kilocalories and total fat grams.

fat-based substitutes Substances that resemble triglycerides and are either chemically synthesized or derived from conventional fats and oils by enzymatic modification.

fat-soluble vitamins Vitamins that dissolve in fat and can be stored in the body.

fatty acid Most basic unit of triglycerides and phospholipids; fatty acids consist of carbon chains ranging from 2 to 80 carbons in length.

fatty liver Stage 1 of alcoholic liver disease, in which fat begins to build up in the liver cells.

fecal-to-oral transmission Spread of pathogens by putting something in the mouth, such as hands or food, that has been in contact with infected stool.

ferment (fermentation) Process by which yeast converts sugars in grains or fruits into ethanol and carbon dioxide.

ferment To metabolize sugar into carbon dioxide and other gases.

ferric iron Oxidized form of iron (Fe^{+3})

ferritin Protein that stores iron in the intestine.

ferroportin Protein found on the basolateral surface of the enterocyte that transports iron out of the enterocyte into the portal vein.

ferrous iron Reduced form of iron (Fe^{+2})

fetal alcohol spectrum disorders (FASDs) Range of conditions that can occur in children who are exposed to alcohol in utero.

fetal alcohol syndrome (FAS) Most severe of the fetal alcohol spectrum disorders (FASDs); children with FAS display physical, mental, and behavioral abnormalities.

fetus Developing embryo that is at least 8 weeks old.

flatulence Production of excessive gas in the stomach or the intestines.

flavin adenine dinucleotide (FAD) Electron carrier similar to NAD that picks up a hydrogen ion from the TCA cycle and carries it to the electron transport chain.

flavin mononucleotide (FMN) Coenzyme form of riboflavin, which functions in the electron transport chain.

flavonoids Phytochemicals found in fruits, vegetables, tea, nuts, and seeds that have antioxidant properties and neutralize free radicals.

flavoproteins Protein complexes that move electrons down the electron transport chain; contain the B vitamin riboflavin.

flexibility Ability to move joints freely through a full and normal range of motion.

fluoroapatite Crystalline structure that results when hydroxyapatite has been changed by exposure of the tooth to fluoride.

fluorosis Condition caused by excess amounts of fluoride, resulting in mottling of the teeth.

folate The B vitamin that functions as a coenzyme in cell growth and reproduction.

folic acid Form of folate often used in vitamin supplements and fortification of foods.

food additives Substances added to food that affect its quality, flavor, freshness, and/or safety.

food allergens Proteins that are not broken down by cooking or digestion and enter the body intact, causing an adverse reaction by the immune system of a susceptible individual.

food allergy Abnormal reaction by the immune system that occurs reproducibly in response to consumption of a particular food.

food deserts Parts of the country, usually impoverished areas, where fresh fruits, vegetables, and other healthful whole foods are scarce, largely due to a lack of grocery stores, farmers' markets, and healthy-food providers.

food insecurity Limited or uncertain access to adequate food within a household.

food intolerance Adverse reaction to a food that does not involve an immune response.

food jag Period of time in which a child will eat only one food or a few limited foods meal after meal.

food pantry Community food assistance location where food is provided to needy individuals and families.

food preservation Treatment of foods to reduce deterioration and spoilage and help prevent the multiplication of pathogens that can cause foodborne illness.

Food Safety Initiative (FSI) Coordinates the research, surveillance, inspection, outbreak response, and educational activities of the various government agencies that work together to safeguard food.

food security Household-level economic and social condition characterized by reliable access to adequate amounts of healthy foods.

food system All processes and infrastructure involved in feeding a population: growing, harvesting, processing, packaging, transporting, marketing, and consuming food.

foodborne illness Sickness caused by consuming pathogen- or toxin-containing food or beverages. Also known as *foodborne disease* or *food poisoning*.

fortified foods Foods with added vitamins and minerals; fortified foods often contain nutrients that are not naturally present in the food or that are in higher amounts than the food contains naturally.

free radicals Atoms or molecules that have an unpaired electron and are thus chemically unstable and destabilizing.

fructose Sweetest of all the monosaccharides; also known as *fruit sugar* or *levulose*.

functional fiber Nondigestible polysaccharides that are added to foods because of a specific desired effect on human health.

functional foods Foods that may provide additional health benefits beyond their basic nutrient value.

fungicides Chemicals used to kill mold.

G

galactose Monosaccharide that links with glucose to create the disaccharide found in dairy foods.

galactosemia Genetic disorder characterized by high levels of galactose in the blood; due to the inability to convert galactose to glucose.

gallbladder Pear-shaped organ that stores and concentrates bile produced by the liver and secretes it through the common bile duct into the small intestine.

gallstones Stones formed from cholesterol in the gallbladder or bile duct.

gastric bypass surgery Type of bariatric surgery that reduces the functional volume of the stomach to minimize the amount of food eaten. Such surgeries are sometimes used to treat extreme obesity.

gastric inhibitory peptide (GIP) Hormone produced by the small intestine that slows the release of chyme from the stomach.

gastric pits Indentations or small pits in the stomach lining where the gastric glands are located; gastric glands produce gastric juices.

gastrin Hormone released from the stomach that stimulates the release of acid.

gastritis Inflammation of the lining in the stomach.

gastroenteritis Inflammation of the lining of the stomach and intestines; also known as *stomach flu*.

gastroesophageal reflux disease (GERD) Chronic condition characterized by the backward flow of stomach contents into the esophagus, resulting in heartburn.

gastrointestinal (GI) tract Tubular organ system including the mouth, pharynx, esophagus, stomach, and small and large intestines, by means of which food is digested, nutrients absorbed, and wastes expelled.

gene expression Processing of genetic information to create a specific protein.

gene–environment interaction Interaction of genetics and environmental factors that increases the risk of obesity in susceptible individuals.

generally recognized as safe (GRAS) Designation given by the FDA to substances intentionally added to food, indicating that the substance is considered safe by experts and is exempted from further testing.

genes A segment of DNA that codes for a protein; genes are inherited from our parents and determines a variety of characteristics.

genetic engineering (GE) Biological technique that isolates and manipulates the genes of organisms to produce a targeted, modified product.

genetically modified organisms (GMOs) Organisms that have been genetically engineered to contain both original and foreign genes.

genome Total genetic information of an organism stored in the DNA of its chromosomes.

germ Vitamin-rich embryo, or seed, of a grain.

gestational diabetes Form of diabetes that may develop during pregnancy in women who were not previously diagnosed with diabetes.

gestational hypertension Hypertension occurring during pregnancy in a woman without prior history of high blood pressure.

ghrelin Hormone produced in the stomach that stimulates hunger.

GI flora Microorganisms that live in the GI tract of humans and animals.

glossitis Inflammation of the tongue.

glucagon Hormone secreted from the alpha cells of the pancreas that stimulates glycogenolysis and gluconeogenesis to increase blood levels of glucose.

glucogenic amino acids Amino acids that can be used to form glucose through gluconeogenesis.

gluconeogenesis Creation of glucose from noncarbohydrate sources, predominantly protein.

glucose Primary monosaccharide and primary energy source for the body.

glycemic index (GI) Rating scale of the likelihood of foods to increase the levels of blood glucose and insulin.

glycemic load (GL) Amount of carbohydrate in a food multiplied by the amount of the glycemic index of that food.

glycerol Three-carbon backbone of a triglyceride.

glycogen storage disease Genetic disorder characterized by a lack of glucose 6-phosphatase, which impairs the body's ability to break down glycogen.

glycogen Storage form of glucose in animals, including humans.

glycogenesis Process of assembling excess glucose into glycogen in the liver and muscle cells.

glycogenolysis Hydrolysis of glycogen to release glucose.

glycolysis Breakdown of glucose; for each molecule of glucose, two molecules of pyruvate and two ATP molecules are produced.

glycosidic bond Bond that forms when two sugar molecules are joined together during condensation.

goblet cells Cells throughout the GI tract that secrete mucus.

goiter Enlargement of the thyroid gland, mostly due to iodine deficiency.

goitrogens Substances in food that reduce the utilization of iodine by the thyroid gland, resulting in goiter.

growth charts Series of percentile curves that illustrate the distribution of selected body measurements in U.S. children.

growth hormone Hormone that regulates glucose metabolism by increasing glycogenolysis and lipolysis.

growth spurt Rapid increase in height and weight.

growth stunting Impaired growth and development caused by undernutrition primarily in childhood. Once growth stunting occurs, it is usually permanent.

gynoid obesity Excessive storage of body fat in the thighs and hips of the lower body.

H

hangover Collective term for the unpleasant symptoms, such as a headache and dizziness, that occur after drinking an excessive amount of alcohol; many of the symptoms are caused by high levels of acetaldehyde in the blood.

healthy weight Body weight in relationship to height that doesn't increase the risk of developing any weight-related health problems or diseases. A BMI between 18.5 and 24.9 is considered healthy.

heart attack Permanent damage to the heart muscle that results from a sudden lack of oxygen-rich blood; also called a *myocardial infarction (MI)*.

heme iron Iron that is part of a heme group found in hemoglobin in the blood, myoglobin in muscles, and in the mitochondria as part of the cytochromes.

hemochromatosis Blood disorder characterized by the retention of an excessive amount of iron.

hemochromatosis Genetic disorder that causes the body to store excessive amounts of iron.

hemoglobin Oxygen-carrying, heme-containing protein found in red blood cells.

hemolytic uremic syndrome Rare condition that can be caused by *E. coli* O157:H7 and results in the destruction of red blood cells and kidney failure. Very young children and older adults are at a higher risk of developing this syndrome.

hemopoiesis Formation of red blood cells.

hemorrhage Excessive bleeding or loss of blood.

hemorrhoid Swelling in the veins of the rectum and anus.

hemosiderin Protein that stores iron in the body.

hepatic portal vein Large vein that connects the GI tract to the liver and transports newly absorbed water-soluble nutrients.

hepatic vein Vein that carries the blood received from the hepatic portal vein away from the liver.

hepcidin Hormone produced in the liver that regulates the absorption and transport of iron.

hephaestin Copper-containing enzyme that catalyzes the conversion of ferrous to ferric iron before attaching to transferrin for transport.

herbicides Substances that are used to kill and control weeds.

hexose Sugar that contains six carbons; glucose, galactose, and fructose are all hexoses.

high-density lipoproteins (HDLs) Lipoproteins that remove cholesterol from the tissues and deliver it to the liver to be used as part of bile and/or to be excreted from the body. Because of this, HDL is known as the "good" cholesterol.

High-intensity interval training (HIIT) Interval training that includes short periods of intense anaerobic exercise alternating with less intense recovery periods.

high-pressure processing (HPP) Method used to pasteurize foods by exposing the items to pulses of high pressure, which destroys the microorganisms that are present.

homocystinuria Genetic disorder characterized by the inability to metabolize the essential amino acid methionine.

hormone-sensitive lipase Enzyme that catalyzes lipolysis of triglycerides.

host Living plant or animal (including a human) that a virus infects for the sake of reproducing.

hunger Strong sensation indicating a physiological need for food.

hydrochloric acid (HCl) Strong acid produced in the stomach that aids in digestion.

hydrogenation Adding hydrogen to an unsaturated fatty acid to make it more saturated and solid at room temperature.

hydrolysis Chemical reaction that breaks the bond between two molecules with water. A hydroxyl group is added to one molecule and a hydrogen ion is added to the other molecule.

hydrophobic "Water fearing." In nutrition, the term refers to compounds that are not soluble in water.

hydrostatic weighing Method used to assess body volume by underwater weighing.

hydroxyapatite Crystalline salt structure that provides strength in bones and teeth. Calcium and phosphorus are the main minerals found in the structure.

hypercalcemia Abnormally high levels of calcium in the blood.

hypercalcemia Chronically high amount of calcium in the blood.

hyperchloremia Abnormally high level of chloride in the blood.

hyperemesis gravidarum Excessive vomiting during pregnancy that can lead to dehydration and loss of electrolytes.

hyperkalemia Abnormally high levels of potassium in the blood.

hypernatremia Excessive amounts of sodium in the blood.

hyperphenylalanemia Elevated levels of blood phenylalanine due to a lack of the enzyme phenylalanine hydroxylase.

hyperphosphatemia Abnormally high level of phosphorus in the blood.

hyperplasia Increase in the number of cells due to cell division.

hypertension High blood pressure; defined as a systolic blood pressure higher than 140 mm Hg and/or a diastolic blood pressure greater than 90 mm Hg.

hyperthermia Rise in body temperature above normal.

hypertonic Having a high solute concentration.

hypertriglyceridemia Presence of high concentrations of triglycerides in the blood. Defined as triglyceride concentrations between 400 and 1,000 milligrams per deciliter.

hypertrophy Increase in size; in adipocytes, hypertrophy refers to the increase in size of the cells.

hypervitaminosis Condition resulting from the presence of excessive amounts of vitamins in the body; also referred to as *vitamin toxicity*.

hypervitaminosis A Serious condition in which the liver accumulates toxic levels of vitamin A.

hypervitaminosis D Condition resulting from excessive amounts of vitamin D in the body.

hypocalcemia Abnormally low levels of calcium in the blood.

hypochloremia Abnormally low level of chloride in the blood.

hypoglycemia Blood glucose level that drops to lower than 70 mg/dl.

hypokalemia Dangerously low level of blood potassium.

hyponatremia Dangerously low level of sodium in the blood that can result from dilution or depletion of sodium.

hypophosphatemia Abnormally low level of phosphorus in the blood.

hypothermia Drop in body temperature to below normal.

hypothesis Idea or explanation proposed by scientists based on observations or known facts.

hypotonic Having a low solute concentration.

hypovolemia Low blood volume.

I

ileocecal valve Sphincter that separates the small intestine from the large intestine.

immunity State of having built up memory immune cells that target a particular pathogen so that any subsequent encounter with that pathogen prompts rapid production of specific antibodies.

impaired glucose tolerance Condition whereby a fasting blood glucose level is higher than normal, but not high enough to be classified as having diabetes mellitus. Also called *prediabetes.*

incomplete protein Protein that is low in one or more of the essential amino acids. Proteins from plant sources tend to be incomplete.

indirect calorimetry Indirect measurement of energy expenditure obtained by measuring the amount of oxygen consumed and carbon dioxide produced.

infancy Age range from birth to 12 months.

inflammatory bowel disease (IBD) Chronic inflammation throughout the GI tract.

inorganic Describing elements or compounds that do not contain carbon.

inositol Water-soluble compound synthesized in the body that maintains healthy cell membranes.

insecticides Pesticides used to kill insects.

insensible water loss Loss of body water that goes unnoticed, such as by exhalation during breathing and the evaporation of water through the skin.

insoluble fiber Type of fiber that isn't dissolved in water or fermented by intestinal bacteria.

insulin Hormone secreted from the beta cells of the pancreas that stimulates the uptake of glucose from the blood into the cells.

insulin resistance Inability of the cells to respond to insulin.

integrated pest management (IPM) Agricultural technique that uses the most economical and the least harmful methods of pest control to minimize risk to consumers, crops, and the environment.

intensity Level of difficulty of an activity.

intentional food additives Substances added intentionally to foods to improve food quality.

international units (IU) System of measurement of a biologically active ingredient such as a vitamin that produces a certain effect.

interstitial fluid Tissue fluid; the fluid that surrounds cells.

intestinal permeability Condition in which the junctions between enterocytes allow large molecules to enter the bloodstream; also called *leaky gut syndrome.*

intracellular fluid (ICF) Fluid found in the cytoplasm within cells.

intravascular fluid Fluid found inside the blood and lymphatic vessels.

intrinsic factor (IF) Glycoprotein secreted by the stomach that facilitates the absorption of vitamin vitamin B_{12}

iodide Ionized form of iodine in the body (I^-)

iodopsin Compound found in the cones of the eye that is needed for color vision.

iron-deficiency anemia Type of anemia due to a lack of dietary iron or excessive loss of blood.

irradiation Process in which foods are placed in a shielded chamber, called an *irradiator,* and subjected to a radiant energy source; kills specific pathogens in food by breaking up the cells' DNA.

irritable bowel syndrome (IBS) Intestinal disorder resulting in abdominal discomfort, pain, diarrhea, constipation, and bloating; the cause is unknown.

isoflavones Naturally occurring phytoestrogens, or weak plant estrogens, that function in a similar fashion to the hormone estrogen in the human body.

J

jaundice Yellowish coloring of the skin due to the presence of bile pigments in the blood.

K

keratinization Accumulation of the protein keratin in epithelial cells, forming hard, dry cells unable to secrete mucus; due to vitamin A deficiency.

Keshan disease Disease related to a deficiency of selenium.

ketoacidosis Form of metabolic acidosis, or pH imbalance due to excess acid, that occurs when excess ketone bodies are present in the blood; most often seen in individuals with untreated type I diabetes.

ketogenesis Formation of ketone bodies from excess acetyl CoA.

ketogenic Describing molecules that can be transformed into ketone bodies.

ketone bodies By-products of the incomplete breakdown of fat.

ketosis Condition of increased ketone bodies in the blood.

kilocalorie Amount of energy required to raise the temperature of 1 kilogram of water 1 degree centigrade; used to express the measurement of energy in foods; 1 kilocalorie is equal to 1,000 calories.

kwashiorkor State of PEM in which there is a severe deficiency of dietary protein.

L

laboratory experiment Scientific experiment conducted in a laboratory; some involve animals.

lactate Three-carbon compound generated from pyruvate when mitochondria lack sufficient oxygen.

lactation Production of milk in a woman's body after childbirth and the period during which it occurs.

lactose intolerance When maldigestion of lactose results in symptoms such as nausea, cramps, bloating, flatulence, and diarrhea.

lactose maldigestion Inability to digest lactose due to low levels of the enzyme lactase.

lactose Disaccharide composed of glucose and galactose; also known as *milk sugar*.

lanugo Very fine, soft hair typically found on a newborn or a person who is malnourished.

large intestine Lowest portion of the GI tract, where water and electrolytes are absorbed and waste is eliminated.

lean body mass (LBM) Total body weight minus the fat mass; consists of water, bones, vital organs, and muscle; metabolically active tissue in the body.

least developed country Country that shows little growth in multiple areas, such as income per capita, life expectancy, rate of literacy, industrial capability, technological sophistication, and economic productivity.

lecithin Phospholipid made in the body that is integral in the structure of cell membranes; also known as *phosphatidylcholine*.

letdown response Release of milk from the mother's breast to feed a nursing baby.

licensed dietitian nutritionist (LDN) Individual who has met specified educational and experience criteria deemed by a state licensing board necessary to be considered an expert in the field of nutrition. An RDN would meet all the qualifications to be an LDN.

life expectancy Average length of life for a population of individuals.

lifespan Maximum age to which members of a species can live.

lignin Noncarbohydrate form of dietary fiber that binds to cellulose fibers to harden and strengthen the cell walls of plants.

limiting amino acid Essential amino acid that is in the shortest supply, relative to the body's needs, in an incomplete protein

linoleic acid Polyunsaturated essential fatty acid; part of the omega-6 fatty acid family.

lipases Group of lipid-digesting enzymes.

lipid Category of carbon, hydrogen, and oxygen compounds that are insoluble in water.

lipogenesis Process that converts excess glucose into fat for storage.

lipoic acid Vitamin-like substance used in energy production; may also act as an antioxidant.

lipoprotein lipase (LPL) Enzyme that hydrolyzes triglycerides in lipoproteins into three fatty acids and glycerol.

lipoprotein Capsule-shaped transport carrier that enables fat and cholesterol to travel through the lymph and blood.

liver Accessory organ of digestion located in the upper abdomen and responsible for the synthesis of bile, the processing of nutrients, the metabolism of alcohol, and other functions.

locavore Person who eats locally grown food whenever possible.

long-chain fatty acids Fatty acids with a chain of more than 12 carbons.

longevity Duration of an individual's life.

low birthweight Describes a baby weighing less than $5\frac{1}{2}$ pounds at birth.

low-density lipoproteins (LDLs) Lipoproteins that deposit cholesterol in the walls of the arteries. Because this can lead to heart disease, LDL is referred to as the "bad" cholesterol.

lower esophageal sphincter (LES) Muscular ring located between the base of the esophagus and the stomach.

Lp(a) protein Lipoprotein containing LDL cholesterol found in the blood; has been correlated to increased risk of heart disease.

lumen Channel or inside space of a vessel such as the intestine or artery.

lymphatic system System of interconnected vessels that contains lymph fluid in which fat-soluble nutrients are carried; also includes bone marrow, lymph nodes, and other tissues and organs that produce and store defensive cells.

M

macrocytic anemia Condition that results in abnormally large, pale, and fewer than normal red blood cells.

macronutrients Essential nutrients, including water and the energy-containing carbohydrates, lipids, and proteins that the body needs in large amounts.

macrosomia Term for a large newborn, weighing more than 8 pounds, 13 ounces.

magnesium (Mg^{+2}) Major divalent cation in the body.

major minerals Minerals found in the body in amounts greater than 5 grams; also referred to as *macrominerals*.

major minerals Minerals needed in amounts greater than 100 milligrams per day. These include sodium, chloride, potassium, calcium, phosphorus, magnesium, and sulfur.

malabsorption Condition characterized by impaired absorption of nutrients through the gastrointestinal tract.

malnourished Characterized by an inappropriate level of essential nutrients to maintain health; overnourishment and undernourishment are forms of malnutrition.

maltose Disaccharide composed of two glucose units joined together.

maple syrup urine disease (MSUD) Genetic disorder characterized by the inability to metabolize branched-chain amino acids; symptoms include a maple syrup smell in the urine.

marasmus State of PEM in which there is a severe deficiency of kilocalories, which perpetuates wasting; also called *starvation*.

marine toxins Chemicals that occur naturally and contaminate some fish.

mass movement (mass peristalsis) Strong, slow peristaltic movements, occurring only three or four times a day within the colon, that force waste toward the rectum.

mast cells Cells in connective tissue to which antibodies attach, setting the stage for potential future allergic reactions.

mastication Chewing food.

Meals on Wheels Program that delivers nutritious meals to homebound older adults.

mechanical digestion Breaking down food by chewing, grinding, squeezing, and moving it through the GI tract by peristalsis and segmentation.

medical nutrition therapy Integration of nutrition counseling and dietary changes, based on individual medical and health needs, to treat a patient's medical condition.

medium-chain fatty acids Fatty acids with a chain of 8–12 carbons.

megadose Amount of a vitamin or mineral that's at least 10 times the amount recommended in the DRI.

menaquinone (vitamin K$_2$) The form of vitamin K produced by bacteria in the colon.

menarche Onset of menstruation.

Menkes' disease Genetic disorder that interferes with copper absorption.

messenger RNA (mRNA) Type of RNA that copies the genetic information from the DNA and carries it from the nucleus to the ribosomes in the cell.

metabolic pathway Sequence of reactions that convert compounds from one form to another.

metabolic programming Process by which the prenatal environment interacts with genetic and other factors to produce permanent change; also called *fetal programming*.

metabolic water Water that is formed in the body as a result of metabolic reactions. Condensation reactions are an example of a chemical reaction that results in the production of water.

metabolism Sum of all chemical reactions in the body.

metalloenzymes Active enzymes that contain one or more metal ions that are essential for their biological activity.

metallothionine Metal-binding protein rich in sulfur-containing amino acids that transports ions.

methylcobalamin Coenzyme form of vitamin vitamin B$_{12}$ that converts homocysteine to methionine.

micelle Transport carrier in the small intestine that enables fatty acids and other compounds to be absorbed.

microcytic hypochromic anemia Form of anemia in which red blood cells are small and pale in color due to lack of hemoglobin synthesis.

micronutrients Essential nutrients the body needs in smaller amounts: vitamins and minerals.

microsomal ethanol oxidizing system (MEOS) Second major enzyme system in the liver that metabolizes alcohol.

microsomes Small vesicles in the cytoplasm of liver cells where oxidative metabolism of alcohol takes place.

microvilli Tiny projections on the villi in the small intestine.

milestones Objectives or significant events that occur during development.

mineralization Process of adding minerals, including calcium and phosphorus, to the collagen matrix in the bone, which makes the bone strong and rigid.

minerals Inorganic elements essential to the nutrition of humans.

mitochondrion Cellular organelle that releases energy from carbohydrates, proteins, and fats to make ATP; *pl.* mitochondria.

moderate drinking According to the *Dietary Guidelines for Americans,* up to one drink per day for women and up to two drinks a day for men.

moderate Diet principle of providing reasonable but not excessive amounts of foods and nutrients.

modified atmosphere packaging (MAP) Food preservation technique that changes the composition of the air surrounding the food in a package to extend its shelf-life.

molds Microscopic fungi that live on plant and animal matter; some can produce mycotoxins, which are harmful.

monoglyceride Remnant of fat digestion that consists of a glycerol with only one fatty acid attached to one of the three carbons.

monosaccharide Simple sugar that consists of a single sugar unit. The three most common monosaccharides are glucose, fructose, and galactose.

monosodium glutamate (MSG) Sodium salt of glutamic acid, used as a flavor enhancer.

monounsaturated fatty acid (MUFA) Fatty acid that has one double bond.

mucus Secretion produced throughout the GI tract that moistens and lubricates food and protects membranes.

muscular endurance Ability of the muscle to produce prolonged effort.

muscular strength Greatest amount of force exerted by the muscle at one time.

myelin sheath Tissue that surrounds nerves and speeds the transmission of nerve impulses.

myoglobin Oxygen-carrying, heme-containing protein found in muscle cells.

MyPlate Icon that serves as a reminder for healthy eating and a website providing nutritional information and educational tools based on the *Dietary Guidelines for Americans* and the Dietary Reference Intakes (DRIs).

N

negative energy balance State in which energy intake is less than energy expenditure; over time, this results in weight loss.

neural tube defects Any major birth defect of the central nervous system, including the brain, caused by failure of the neural tube to properly close during embryonic development.

niacin equivalents (NE) Measurement that reflects the amount of niacin and tryptophan in foods that can be used to synthesize niacin.

nicotinamide adenine dinucleotide (NAD⁺) Coenzyme form of niacin that functions as an electron carrier and can be reduced to NADH during metabolism.

nicotinamide adenine dinucleotide phosphate (NADP⁺) Coenzyme form of niacin that functions as an electron carrier and can be reduced to NADPH during metabolism.

night blindness Inability to see in dim light or at night due to a deficiency of retinal in the retina.

nitrites and nitrates Substances that can be added to foods to function as a preservative and to give meats such as hot dogs and luncheon meats a pink color.

nitrogen balance Difference between nitrogen intake and nitrogen excretion.

non-celiac gluten sensitivity (NCGS) Reaction to eating foods that contain gluten when celiac disease has been ruled out. Symptoms vary widely but may include abdominal pain, fatigue, headaches, rashes, or mental confusion.

nonessential amino acids Eleven amino acids the body can synthesize and that therefore do not need to be consumed in the diet.

nonessential nutrients Nutrients that can be made in sufficient quantities in the body to meet the body's requirements and support health.

nonexercise activity thermogenesis (NEAT) Energy expended for all activities not related to sleeping, eating, or exercise, including fidgeting, performing work-related activities, and playing.

nonheme iron Iron that is not attached to heme.

norepinephrine Hormone produced by the adrenal glands that stimulates glycogenolysis and gluconeogenesis.

normal blood pressure Systolic blood pressure less than 120 mm Hg (the top number) and a diastolic blood pressure less than 80 mm Hg (the bottom number); referred to as 120/80.

norovirus Most common type of virus that causes foodborne illness; can cause gastroenteritis, or the "stomach flu."

nutrient density Measurement of the nutrients in a food compared with the kilocalorie content; nutrient-dense foods are high in nutrients and low in kilocalories.

nutrient requirements Amounts of specific nutrients needed to prevent malnutrition or deficiency; reflected in the DRIs.

nutrients Compounds in foods that sustain body processes. There are six classes of nutrients: carbohydrates, fats (lipids), proteins, vitamins, minerals, and water.

nutrition Science that studies how nutrients and other components of foods nourish the body and affect body functions and overall health.

Nutrition Facts panel Area on the food label that provides a list of specific nutrients obtained in one serving of the food.

nutrition transition Shift in dietary consumption and energy expenditure that may occur as people in developing countries shift from their traditional diet to diets higher in sugar, fat, and animal-based foods.

nutritional genomics Study of the relationship between genes, gene expression, and nutrition.

nutritionist Generic term with no recognized legal or professional meaning. Some people may call themselves a nutritionist without having any credible training in nutrition.

O

obese Condition of excess body weight due to an abnormal accumulation of stored body fat; a BMI of 30 or more is considered obese.

observational research Research that involves systematically observing subjects to see if there is a relationship to certain outcomes.

oils Lipids that are liquid at room temperature.

oligosaccharides Three to 10 units of monosaccharides combined.

omega-3 fatty acid Family of polyunsaturated fatty acids with the first double bond located at the third carbon from the omega end.

omega-6 fatty acid Family of polyunsaturated fatty acids with the first double bond located at the sixth carbon from the omega end.

open dating Typically found on perishable items such as meat, poultry, eggs, and dairy foods; must contain a calendar date.

organic Being free of chemical-based pesticides, synthetic fertilizers, irradiation, and bioengineering; a USDA-accredited certifying inspector must certify organic foods.

organic Describing compounds that contain carbon or carbon–carbon bonds.

organophosphates Group of synthetic pesticides that adversely affect the nervous systems of pests.

osmolality Measurement of the concentration of solutes per kilogram of solvent in a solution.

osmosis Diffusion of water or any solvent across a semipermeable membrane from an area of lower solute concentration to an area of higher solute concentration.

osmotic gradient Difference in concentration between two solutions on either side of the cell membrane.

osmotic pressure Pressure that prevents the solutes in a solution from drawing water across a semipermeable membrane.

osteomalacia Adult equivalent of rickets, causing muscle and bone weakness and pain.

osteopenia Condition in which the bone mineral density is lower than normal but not low enough to be classified as osteoporosis.

osteoporosis Disorder characterized by low bone mineral density, which increases the individual's risk of fractures.

overexercise Excessive physical activity without adequate rest periods for proper recovery.

overnourished Characterized by an excessive intake of energy or one or more individual nutrients.

overpopulation Condition in which a region has more people than its natural resources can support.

overweight Body weight that increases risk of developing weight-related health problems; defined as having a BMI between 25 and 29.9.

oxaloacetate Starting molecule for the TCA cycle.

oxidative phosphorylation Metabolic pathway in the mitochondria in which ATP is formed using energy from the oxidation-reduction reactions in the electron transport chain.

oxidative stress Condition whereby free radicals are being produced in the body faster than they are neutralized.

P

pancreas Large gland located behind the stomach that releases digestive enzymes and bicarbonate after a meal. Also secretes the hormones insulin and glucagon, which control blood glucose.

paralytic shellfish poisoning Condition caused by a reddish-brown-colored dinoflagellate that contains neurotoxins.

parasites Organisms that live on or in another organism; obtain their nourishment from their hosts.

parathyroid hormone (PTH) Hormone secreted from the parathyroid glands that activates vitamin D formation in the kidney.

parietal cells Specialized cells in the stomach that secrete the gastric juices hydrochloric acid and intrinsic factor.

passive diffusion Movement of substances across a cell membrane along their concentration gradient.

pasteurization Process of heating liquids or food at high temperatures to destroy foodborne pathogens.

pathogens Collective term for disease-causing organisms. Pathogens include microorganisms (viruses, bacteria) and parasites and are the most common source of foodborne illness.

peak bone mass Genetically determined maximum amount of bone mass an individual can build up.

peer-reviewed journal Journal in which scientists publish research findings, after the findings have gone through a rigorous review process by other scientists.

pellagra Disease resulting from a deficiency of niacin or tryptophan.

pepsin Active protease that begins the digestion of proteins in the stomach.

pepsinogen Inactive protease secreted by the chief cells in the stomach; it is converted to the active enzyme pepsin in the presence of HCl.

peptide bonds Bonds that connect amino acids; created when the acid group of one amino acid is joined with the amine group of another through condensation.

peptide YY Hormone produced in the small intestine that reduces hunger.

peptide Chain of amino acids.

percent Daily Values (%DVs) Reference values developed by the Food and Drug Administration and used on the Nutrition Facts panel to describe the percentage of a daily nutrient intake provided in one serving of the food.

percentile Most commonly used clinical indicator to assess the size and growth patterns of children in the United States. An individual child is ranked according to the percentage of the reference population he or she equals or exceeds.

peripheral neuropathy Damage to the peripheral nerves causing pain, numbness, and tingling in the feet and hands and muscle weakness.

peristalsis Forward, rhythmic muscular contractions that move food through the GI tract.

pernicious anemia Form of anemia caused by a lack of intrinsic factor needed for absorption of vitamin vitamin B_{12} forming large, immature red blood cells.

pernicious anemia Form of macrocytic anemia caused by a lack of intrinsic factor due to either gastritis or an autoimmune disorder.

pesticides Substances that kill or repel pests such as insects, weeds, microorganisms, rodents, or fungi.

pH Measure of the acidity or alkalinity of a solution.

pharynx Area of the GI tract between the mouth and the esophagus; also called the *throat*.

phenylketonuria (PKU) Genetic disorder characterized by the inability to metabolize the essential amino acid phenylalanine.

phospholipids Category of lipids that consists of two fatty acids and a phosphate group attached to a glycerol backbone. Lecithin is an example of a phospholipid found in food and in the body.

phosphorus (P) Second most abundant mineral in the body.

photosynthesis Process by which plants create carbohydrates using the energy from sunlight.

phylloquinone (vitamin K_1) The form of vitamin K found in plants.

physical activity Voluntary movement that results in energy expenditure.

physical fitness Ability to perform physical activities requiring cardiorespiratory endurance, muscle endurance, strength, and/or flexibility, typically acquired through exercise and adequate nutrition.

physiologic age Person's age estimated in terms of body health, function, and life expectancy.

physiological fuel values Real energy value of foods that are digested and absorbed; adjusted from the results of bomb calorimetry because of the inefficiency of the body.

phytochemicals Non-nutritive plant compounds, found in fruits and vegetables, that may play a role in fighting chronic diseases.

phytostanols Type of plant sterol similar in structure to cholesterol.

phytosterols Naturally occurring sterols found in plants.

pica Eating nonfood substances such as dirt and clay.

placebo Inactive substance, such as a sugar pill, administered to a control group during an experiment.

placenta Organ that allows nutrients, oxygen, and waste products to be exchanged between a mother and fetus.

plaque Hardened buildup of cholesterol-laden foam cells, platelets, cellular waste products, and calcium in the arteries that results in atherosclerosis.

polychlorinated biphenyls (PCBs) Synthetic chemicals that have been shown to cause cancer and other adverse effects on the immune, reproductive, nervous, and endocrine systems in animals; may cause cancer in humans.

polypeptide Chain consisting of 10 or more amino acids joined together by peptide bonds.

polysaccharides Many sugar units combined. Starch, glycogen, and fiber are all polysaccharides.

polyunsaturated fatty acid (PUFA) Fatty acid with two or more double bonds.

portion Quantity of a food usually eaten at one sitting.

positive energy balance State in which energy intake is greater than energy expenditure; over time, this results in weight gain.

postabsorptive state Period when you haven't eaten for more than 4 hours and the stomach and intestines are empty. Energy needs are met by the breakdown of stores.

potassium (K$^+$) Main cation in the intracellular fluid.

poverty Lacking the means to provide for material or comfort needs.

prebiotics Nondigestible starch found in plant foods that promotes the growth and health of your GI flora.

preeclampsia Serious medical condition developed late in pregnancy in which hypertension, severe edema, and protein loss occur.

preformed vitamins Vitamins found in food.

pregnancy-induced hypertension High blood pressure resulting from pregnancy; includes gestational hypertension, preeclampsia, and eclampsia.

preschoolers Children 3–5 years old.

preservatives Substances that extend the shelf-life of a product by retarding chemical, physical, or microbiological changes.

primary malnutrition State of being malnourished due to poor diet, consuming either too much or too little of a nutrient or energy.

primary structure First stage of protein synthesis after transcription when the amino acids have been linked together with peptide bonds to form a simple linear chain.

prion Short for proteinaceous infectious particle; self-reproducing protein particles that cause degenerative brain diseases.

prior-sanctioned Substances that the FDA had determined were safe for use in foods prior to the 1958 Food Additives Amendment.

probiotics Live microorganisms that, when consumed in adequate amounts, confer a health benefit on the host.

progressive overload principle Gradual increase in exercise demands resulting from modifications to the frequency, intensity, time, or type of activity.

prohormone Physiologically inactive precursor to a hormone.

proof Measure of the amount of ethanol contained in alcoholic beverages.

proportionality Relationship of one entity to another. Vegetables and fruits should be consumed in a higher proportion than dairy and protein foods in the diet.

propulsion Process that moves food along the gastrointestinal tract during digestion.

proteases Classification of enzymes that catalyze the hydrolysis of proteins.

protein digestibility corrected amino acid score (PDCAAS) Score measured as a percentage that takes into account both digestibility and amino acid score and provides a good indication of the quality of a protein.

protein turnover Continual process of degrading and synthesizing protein.

protein-based fat substitutes Substances created from the protein in eggs and milk.

protein-energy malnutrition (PEM) Lack of sufficient dietary protein and/or kilocalories.

proteins Large molecules, made up of chains of amino acids, found in all living cells.

provitamin Vitamin precursor that is converted to a vitamin in the body.

provitamin-A carotenoids Group of yellow, red, and orange plant pigments that act as precursors to vitamin A.

puberty Period during which adolescents reach sexual maturity and become capable of reproduction.

public health nutritionists Individuals who may have an undergraduate degree in nutrition but who are not registered dietitian nutritionists.

pyridoxal phosphate (PLP) Active coenzyme form of vitamin vitamin B$_6$

pyruvate Three-carbon molecule formed from the oxidation of glucose during glycolysis.

Q

quackery Promotion and selling of health products and services of questionable validity. A quack is a person who promotes these products and services in order to make money.

quaternary structure Rod-like or globular structure of a protein formed when two or more polypeptide chains cluster together.

R

R protein Protein secreted from the salivary glands that binds vitamin vitamin B_{12} in the stomach and transports it into the small intestine during digestion.

rancidity Spoiling of lipids through oxidation.

rating of perceived exertion (RPE) Subjective measure of the intensity level of an activity using a numerical scale.

recombinant bovine somatotropin (rbST) Synthetically made hormone identical to a cow's natural growth hormone, somatotropin, that stimulates milk production; also known as *rbGH (recombinant bovine growth hormone)*.

Recommended Dietary Allowance (RDA) Recommended daily amount of a nutrient that meets the needs of nearly all individuals (97–98 percent) in a similar age and gender group. The RDA is set higher than the EAR.

rectum Final 8-inch portion of the large intestine.

refined grains Grain foods that are made with only the endosperm of the kernel. The bran and germ have been removed during milling.

registered dietitian nutritionist (RDN) Health professional who is a food and nutrition expert; RDNs obtain a college degree in nutrition from an Academy of Nutrition and Dietetics–accredited program and pass a national exam.

relative energy deficiency in sport (RED-S) Syndrome of low energy availability based on the balance between energy intake through food and energy expenditure for daily activities, growth, and training and competition.

renin Enzyme secreted by the kidneys that increases blood volume, vasoconstriction, and blood pressure.

repetition maximum (RM) Maximum amount of weight that can be lifted for a specified number of repetitions.

resistance training Exercising with weights to build, strengthen, and tone muscle to improve or maintain overall fitness; also called *strength training*.

resistant starch Type of starch that is not digested in the GI tract but has important health benefits in the large intestine.

resting metabolic rate (RMR) Measure of the amount of energy expended by the body at rest and after approximately a 3- to 4-hour fasting period; about 6 percent higher than BMR.

retinal Aldehyde form of preformed vitamin A.

retinoic acid Acid form of preformed vitamin A.

retinoids Term used to describe the family of preformed vitamin A compounds.

retinol activity equivalents (RAE) Unit of measure used to describe the total amount of all forms of preformed vitamin A and provitamin A carotenoids in food.

retinol Alcohol form of preformed vitamin A.

retinyl ester Ester form of preformed vitamin A found in foods and stored in the body.

rhodopsin Compound found in the rods of the eye that is needed for night vision; composed of *cis*-retinal and the protein opsin.

ribosomes Organelles found in the cytoplasm that read the mRNA and build the protein in the proper sequence during elongation.

rickets Vitamin D deficiency in children resulting in soft bones.

risk assessment Process of determining the potential human health risks posed by exposure to substances such as pesticides.

rodenticides Poisons used to kill rats, mice, and other rodents.

rods Light-absorbing cells responsible for black-and-white vision and night vision.

S

saliva Secretion from the salivary glands that softens and lubricates food and begins the chemical breakdown of starch.

salivary amylase Digestive enzyme that begins breaking down carbohydrate (starch) in the mouth; other important enzymes during carbohydrate digestion include pancreatic amylase, maltase, sucrase, and lactase.

salivary glands Cluster of glands located underneath and behind the tongue that release saliva in response to the sight, smell, and taste of food.

sarcopenia Age-related progressive loss of muscle mass, muscle strength, and function.

satiation State of being satisfactorily full during a meal, which inhibits the ability to eat more food.

satiety Feeling of satiation, or "fullness," after a meal before hunger sets in again.

saturated fatty acid Fatty acid in which all of the carbons are bound with hydrogen.

school-aged children Children between the ages of 6 and 12.

scientific method Process used by scientists to gather and test information for the sake of generating sound research findings.

scombrotoxic fish poisoning Condition caused by consuming spoiled fish that contain large amounts of histamines; also referred to as *histamine fish poisoning*.

scurvy Disease caused by a deficiency of vitamin C and characterized by bleeding gums and a skin rash.

secondary malnutrition State of being malnourished due to interference with nutrient absorption or metabolism.

secondary structure Shape of a protein in which hydrogen bonding between carboxyl and amine groups has caused the straight chain to fold and twist.

secretin A hormone secreted from the duodenum that stimulates the stomach to release pepsin, the liver to make bile, and the pancreas to release digestive juices.

segmentation Muscular contractions of the small intestine that move food back and forth, breaking the mixture into smaller and smaller pieces and combining it with digestive juices.

selectively permeable Characteristic of cell membranes that allows some substances to cross more easily than others.

selenomethionine Amino acid that contains selenium rather than sulfur.

selenoproteins Proteins that contain selenomethionine.

selenosis Presence of toxic levels of selenium.

senescence Another term for aging.

serving size Recommended portion of food that is used as a standard reference on food labels.

set point Weight-control theory proposing that each individual has a genetically established body weight and that significant deviation from this point stimulates changes in body metabolism to reestablish the normal weight.

severe obesity Defined as a BMI greater than 40 or more than 100 pounds over ideal body weight.

short-chain fatty acid Fatty acid with a chain of less than eight carbons.

sickle cell anemia Blood disorder caused by a genetic defect that results in the synthesis of hemoglobin S, which makes the red blood cells likely to distort into a sickle shape.

side chain Part of an amino acid that provides its unique qualities; also referred to as the R group.

simple carbohydrates Carbohydrates that consist of one sugar unit (monosaccharides) or two sugar units (disaccharides).

skinfold caliper Tool used to measure the thickness of subcutaneous fat.

small for gestational age (SGA) Term for babies who weigh less than the 10th percentile of weight for gestational age.

small intestine Long coiled chamber that is the major site of food digestion and nutrient absorption.

social drinking Moderate drinking of alcoholic beverages in social settings within safe limits.

sodium (Na$^+$) Major cation in the extracellular fluid.

sodium-potassium pump Protein located in the cell membrane that actively transports sodium ions out of the cell and potassium ions into the cell.

solanine Toxin found in potato surfaces exposed to light that can cause fever, diarrhea, and shock if consumed in large amounts.

solid foods Foods other than breast milk or formula given to an infant, usually around 4–6 months of age.

solubility Ability to dissolve into another substance.

soluble fiber Type of fiber that dissolves in water and is fermented by intestinal bacteria. Many soluble fibers are viscous and have thickening properties.

solvent Liquid in which substances dissolve to form a new solution. Water is called the universal solvent because it can dissolve a variety of substances, including minerals and glucose.

specific heat Measurement of the energy required to raise a gram of a substance, such as water, 1 degree Celsius.

sphincters Circular rings of muscle that open and close in response to nerve input.

spina bifida Serious birth defect in which a portion of the spinal cord and its protective membranes (meninges) protrude from the vertebral column.

spores Hardy reproductive structures that are produced by certain bacteria and fungi.

sports anemia Low concentrations of hemoglobin in the blood; results from an increase in blood volume during strenuous exercise.

starch Storage form of glucose in plants.

sterols Category of lipids that contains four connecting rings of carbon and hydrogen. Cholesterol is the most common sterol.

stomach J-shaped muscular organ that mixes and churns food with digestive juices and acid to form chyme.

stomatitis Inflammation of the mucous lining of the mouth.

stool Waste produced in the large intestine; also called *feces*.

stroke volume Amount of blood pumped by the heart with each heartbeat.

stroke Interruption or cessation of circulation to a region of the brain that deprives the area of oxygen and nutrients and can result in paralysis and possibly death.

subcutaneous fat Fat located under the skin and between the muscles.

substrate Substance or compound that is altered by an enzyme.

sucrose Disaccharide composed of glucose and fructose; also known as *table sugar*.

sudden infant death syndrome (SIDS) Unexplained death of an infant at less than 1 year of age.

sugar alcohols Type of sweetener often used in sugar-free foods. Includes xylitol, mannitol, and sorbitol. Also known as *polyols*.

sugar substitutes Alternatives to table sugar that sweeten foods for fewer kilocalories.

sulfate (SO$_4$) Oxidized form of the mineral sulfur.

sulfites Preservatives used to help prevent foods from turning brown and to inhibit the growth of microbes; often used in wine and dried fruit products.

sustainable Referring to a method of resource use that can be maintained indefinitely because it does not deplete or permanently damage the resource.

systolic pressure Top number in a blood pressure reading that measures the pressure in the arteries when the heart muscle contracts.

T

target heart rate Heart rate in beats per minute (expressed as a percentage of maximum heart rate) achieved during exercise that indicates the level of intensity at which fitness levels can increase.

tertiary structure Protein structure that occurs when the side chains of the amino acids, most often containing sulfur, form bonds resulting in loops, bends, and folds in the molecule.

thermic effect of exercise (TEE) Increase in muscle contraction that occurs during physical activity, which produces heat and contributes to the total daily energy expenditure.

thermic effect of food (TEF) Amount of energy expended by the body to digest, absorb, transport, metabolize, and store energy-yielding nutrients from foods.

thermogenesis Generation of heat from the basal metabolism, digestion of food, and all forms of physical activity.

thiamin pyrophosphate (TPP) Coenzyme form of thiamin with two phosphate groups as part of the molecule.

thirst mechanism Complex interaction between the brain and the hypothalamus triggered by a depletion of body water; the interaction leads to a feeling of thirst.

thyroxine Less active form of thyroid hormone; also known as *tetraiodothyronine* (T_4)

thyroxine-releasing hormone (TRH) Hormone secreted by the hypothalamus that stimulates the pituitary gland to release thyroxine-stimulating hormone (TSH).

thyroxine-stimulating hormone (TSH) Hormone released by the pituitary that stimulates the thyroid gland to trap more iodine to produce more thyroid hormone (T_4 and T_3).

toddlers Children 1 or 2 years old.

Tolerable Upper Intake Level (UL) Maximum daily amount of a nutrient considered safe in a group of similar individuals.

tongue-thrust reflex Forceful protrusion of the tongue in response to an oral stimulus, such as a spoon.

total daily energy expenditure (TDEE) Total kilocalories needed to meet daily energy requirements.

total iron-binding capacity (TIBC) Blood test that measures the amount of iron that transferrin can bind; a higher TIBC indicates iron-deficiency anemia.

toxicity Level of nutrient intake at which exposure to a substance becomes harmful.

toxin Poison that can be produced by living organisms.

trabecular bone Inner structure of bone, also known as *spongy bone* because of its appearance. This portion of bone is often lost in osteoporosis.

trace minerals Minerals needed in amounts less than 20 milligrams daily. These include iron, zinc, selenium, fluoride, chromium, copper, manganese, and molybdenum.

trans fats An unsaturated fatty acid formed as the result of hydrogenation. This type of fatty acid causes a reconfiguring of some of its double bonds. A small amount of *trans* fats occur naturally in foods from animal sources.

trans Configuration of a fatty acid in which the carbon atoms are on opposite sides of the double bond.

transamination Transfer of an amino group from one amino acid to a keto acid to form a new nonessential amino acid.

transcription First stage in protein synthesis, in which the DNA sequence is copied from the gene and transferred to messenger RNA.

transfer RNA (tRNA) Type of RNA that transfers a specific amino acid to a growing polypeptide chain in the ribosomes during protein synthesis.

transferrin Iron-transporting protein.

translation Second phase of protein synthesis; the process of converting the information in mRNA to an amino acid sequence in the ribosomes.

transport proteins Proteins that carry other substances, mainly nutrients, through the blood to various organs and tissues. Proteins can also act as channels through which some substances enter your cells.

traveler's diarrhea Common pathogen-induced intestinal disorder experienced by some travelers who visit areas with unsanitary conditions.

tricarboxylic acid (TCA) cycle Cycle of aerobic chemical reactions in the mitochondria that oxidize glucose, amino acids, and fatty acids, producing hydrogen ions to be used in the electron transport chain, some ATP, and by-products carbon dioxide and water.

triglycerides Type of lipid commonly found in foods and the body; also known as *fat*. Triglycerides consist of three fatty acids attached to a glycerol backbone.

tripeptide Chain of three amino acids joined together by peptide bonds.

trivalent chromium Oxidized form of chromium (Cr^{+3}) found in food.

type 1 diabetes Autoimmune form of diabetes in which the pancreas does not produce insulin.

type 2 diabetes Form of diabetes characterized by insulin resistance.

Type I osteoporosis Form of osteoporosis that results from reduced estrogen levels and is characterized by rapid loss of bone mass.

Type II osteoporosis Form of osteoporosis that results from aging and is characterized by the slow loss of bone mass over time.

U

ulcer Sore or erosion of the stomach or intestinal lining.

ulcerative colitis Chronic inflammation of the colon that results in ulcers forming in the lining.

umbilical cord Cord connecting the fetus to the placenta.

undernourished Characterized by an inadequate energy intake or a deficiency in quality or quantity of one or more individual nutrients.

underweight Weighing too little for your height; defined as a BMI less than 18.5.

unintentional food additives Substances that enter into foods unintentionally during manufacturing or processing.

United States Pharmacopeial Convention (USP) Nonprofit organization that sets quality standards for dietary supplements.

unsaturated fatty acid Fatty acid in which there are one or more double bonds between carbons.

upper esophageal sphincter Muscular ring located at the top of the esophagus.

urea Nitrogen-containing waste product of protein metabolism that is mainly excreted through the urine via the kidneys.

V

vary Diet principle of consuming a mixture of different food groups and foods within each group.

vegetarian Person who avoids eating animal foods. Some vegetarians only avoid meat, fish, and poultry, while others (vegans) avoid all animal products, including eggs and dairy.

very low-density lipoproteins (VLDLs) Lipoproteins that deliver fat made in the liver to the tissues. VLDL remnants are converted into LDLs.

villi Small, fingerlike projections that line the lumen of the small intestine.

virus Microscopic organism that carries genetic information for its own replication; can infect a host and cause illness.

visceral fat Body fat associated with the internal organs and stored in the abdominal area.

vitamins Thirteen essential, organic micronutrients that are needed by the body for normal functions.

VO$_2$ max Maximum amount of oxygen (ml) a person uses in 1 minute per kilogram of body weight.

W

waist circumference Measurement taken at the top of the iliac crest or hip bone; used to determine the pattern of obesity.

wasting Diminishment of muscle and fat tissue caused by extremely low energy intake.

water balance State of equilibrium when the intake of water equals the amount of water excreted.

water intoxication Potentially dangerous medical condition that results from drinking too much water too quickly, also known as *hyperhydration*; can lead to hyponatremia and possible death.

water-soluble vitamins Vitamins that dissolve in water; they generally cannot be stored in the body and must be consumed daily.

weight management Maintaining a healthy body weight; defined as having a BMI of 18.5–24.9.

Wernicke-Korsakoff syndrome Severe brain disorder associated with chronic excessive alcohol consumption; symptoms include vision changes, loss of muscle coordination, and loss of memory; the cause is a thiamin deficiency.

whole grains Grain foods that are made with the entire edible grain kernel: the bran, the endosperm, and the germ.

Wilson's disease Rare genetic disorder that results in accumulation of copper in the body.

working poor Individuals or families who are steadily employed but still experience poverty due to low wages or high dependent expenses.

X

xerophthalmia Permanent damage to the cornea causing blindness; due to a prolonged vitamin A deficiency.

Z

zoochemicals Non-nutritive animal compounds that play a role in fighting chronic diseases.

zygote Fertilized egg prior to the first cleavage (which occurs at approximately 72 hours).

Index

Credits

Photo Credits

Chapter 1   Chapter Opener: Darren Kemper/Corbis/Getty Images; **p. 4:** Karen Dreyer/Blend Images/Getty images; **p. 5:** Clive Streeter/Dorling Kindersley, Ltd.; Foodfolio/Alamy Stock Photo; Don Mason/Corbis Super/Alamy Stock Photo; **p. 6:** Singkham/Shutterstock; Taylor S. Kennedy/National Geographic/Getty Images; **p. 7:** Mars Incorporated; **p. 8:** Michael Jung/Shutterstock; A9photo/Shutterstock; Motorolka/Shutterstock; **p. 10:** Peter Bernik/Shutterstock; **p. 12:** Darqué/Photocuisine/AGE Fotostock; **p. 13:** D. Hurst/Alamy Stock Photo; **p. 14:** Purestock/Getty Images; **p. 15:** Don Smetzer/Alamy Stock Photo; **p. 18:** Tim Evans/Science Source; **p. 20:** Skynesher/E+/Getty Images; **p. 24:** Buena Vista Images/Digital Vision/Getty Images; Bill Aron/PhotoEdit, Inc.; **p. 25:** Biophoto Associates/Science Source; **p. 28:** US Food and Drug Administration FDA; **p. 29:** Kristen Piljay/Pearson Education, Inc.; **p. 31:** Karen Dreyer/Blend Images/Getty images; **p. 32:** Don Smetzer/Alamy Stock Photo; Peter Bernik/Shutterstock; **p. 33:** Skynesher/E+/Getty Images; **p. 34:** US Food and Drug Administration FDA

Chapter 2   Chapter Opener: Agencja Free/Alamy Stock Photo; **p. 40:** William Shaw/Dorling Kindersley, Ltd.; **p. 41:** Jiri Hera/Fotolia; Jupiterimages/Creatas/Getty Images; **p. 42:** Joe Gough/Shutterstock; **p. 46:** Samuel Borges/Shutterstock; **p. 50:** Peter Cavanagh/Alamy Stock Photo; **p. 55:** Richard Megna/Fundamental Photographs: NYC; **p. 56:** Radius Images/Alamy Stock Photo; Halfpoint/Shutterstock; **p. 59:** Guiding Stars Licensing Company; Pearson Education, Inc.; **p. 60:** B.A.E. Inc/Alamy Stock Photo; **p. 62:** Pearson Education, Inc.; **p. 63:** Sky Bonillo/PhotoEdit; **p. 65:** Kristen Piljay/Pearson Education, Inc.; **p. 66:** Kristen Piljay/Pearson Education, Inc.; **p. 68:** Radius Images/Alamy Stock Photo; **p. 69:** William Shaw/Dorling Kindersley, Ltd.; **p. 70:** Kristen Piljay/Pearson Education, Inc.

Chapter 3   Chapter Opener: Robert Deutschman/Palladium/AGE Fotostock; **p. 76:** Japack/AGE Fotostock; **p. 77:** Tom Grill/Corbis; **p. 78:** Wavebreakmedia/Shutterstock; **p. 80:** Maridav/Shutterstock; David Musher/Science Source; Steve Gschmeissner/Science Source; Don W Fawcett/Science Source; **p. 82:** Kristen Piljay/Pearson Education, Inc.; **p. 84:** Tom Grill/Corbis; **p. 85:** Tom Grill/Corbis; **p. 86:** Red Chopsticks/AGE Fotostock; **p. 95:** John Lund/Blend Images/Corbis; **p. 96:** Joana Lopes/Shutterstock; **p. 98:** Images USA/Alamy Stock Photo; **p. 99:** Dr. E. Walker/Science Source; Southern Illinois University/Science Source; **p. 101:** Koki Lino/Getty Images; **p. 102:** Cristovao/Shutterstock; **p. 103:** Wavebreakmedia/Shutterstock; **p. 104:** David Musher/Science Source; **p. 105:** Tom Grill/Corbis; **p. 106:** John Lund/Blend Images/Corbis

Chapter 4   Chapter Opener: Newpi/E+/Getty Images; **p. 115:** Kristen Piljay/Pearson Education, Inc.; **p. 117:** Kristen Piljay/Pearson Education, Inc.; **p. 118:** Barbro Bergfeldt/Fotolia; **p. 119:** Food Collection/Getty Images; **p. 121:** Kostudio/Shutterstock; **p. 123:** Hongqi Zhang/123RF; **p. 125:** Yuri Acurs/Shutterstock; Flashon Studio/Shutterstock; **p. 127:** Comstock/Stockbyte/Getty Images; Dragon Fang/Shutterstock; **p. 128:** Elenathewise/Fotolia; **p. 131:** Zstock/Fotolia; **p. 135:** Pearson Education, Inc.; Ingram Publishing/Alamy Stock Photo; James Benet/Getty Images; **p. 136:** Kristen Piljay/Pearson Education, Inc.; **p. 137:** Petro Perutsky/123RF; Rangizzz/123RF; **p. 141:** Pearson Education, Inc.; **p. 145:** Dragon Images/Shutterstock; **p. 146:** Arka38/Shutterstock; **p. 147:** Arek Malang/Shutterstock; **p. 149:** Yuri Acurs/Shutterstock; **p. 150:** Zstock/Fotolia; Pearson Education, Inc.; **p. 151:** Arka38/Shutterstock

Chapter 5   Chapter Opener: Creativ Studio Heinemann/Getty Images; **p. 158:** Ryan McVay/Photodisc/Getty Images; **p. 162:** Gemenacom/Fotolia;

p. 165: Charles Brutlag/Shutterstock; **p. 166:** Comstock Images/Stockbyte/Getty Images; **p. 172:** Jose Luis Calvo/Shutterstock; **p. 179:** Shebeko/Shutterstock; **p. 183:** Geo Grafika/Alamy Stock Photo; **p. 186:** Brand X Pictures/AGE Fotostock; **p. 187:** Dianne McFadden/Shutterstock; **p. 188:** Pearson Education, Inc.; **p. 191:** Eric Cohen/Biophoto Associates/Science Source; Pearson Education, Inc.; **p. 193:** Ligia Botero/Photodisc/Getty Images; NF-05-12: Luchschen/123RF; **p. 194:** Pearson Education, Inc.; **p. 195:** Comstock/Stockbyte/Getty Images; **p. 197:** Wavebreak Media ltd/Alamy Stock Photo; **p. 199:** Shebeko/Shutterstock; **p. 200:** Mariano Heluani/Shutterstock; Eric Cohen/Biophoto Associates/Science Source

Chapter 6   Chapter Opener: Love_Life/E+/Getty Images; **p. 206:** Pidjoe/E+/Getty Images; **p. 210:** Riou/Photo Cuisine/Alamy Stock Photo; **p. 214:** Frederic Cirou/PhotoAlto/Alamy Stock Photo; **p. 216:** Pearson Education, Inc.; **p. 219:** Dr P. Marazzi/Science Source; **p. 220:** Juergen Berger/Science Source; **p. 212:** John Lund/Tiffany Schoepp/Corbis; **p. 222:** Ruth Jenkinson/Dorling Kindersley, Ltd.; Monkey Business Images/Shutterstock; Pearson Education, Inc.; **p. 226:** Macdaddy/Pearson Education, Inc.; **p. 227:** Dustin Dennis/Shutterstock; **p. 228:** Stockstudios/Shutterstock; **p. 229:** Elena Elisseeva/Shutterstock; **p. 231:** Dolgachov/123RF; Svitlana Symonova/123RF; Maridav/123RF; **p. 235:** Dai Kurokawa/EPA/Newscom; Farah Abdi Warsameh/AP Images; **p. 236:** Elenathewise/Fotolia; **p. 237:** Cathy Yeulet/123RF; **p. 239:** Gun/Shutterstock; **p. 241:** Frederic Cirou/PhotoAlto/Alamy Stock Photo; Monkey Business Images/Shutterstock; Elena Elisseeva/Shutterstock; **p. 242:** Farah Abdi Warsameh/AP Images

Chapter 7   Chapter Opener: Shyripa Alexandr/Shutterstock; **p. 250:** Syracuse Newspapers/Jim Commentucci/The Image Works; **p. 251:** Pearson Education, Inc.; Yukata/Fotolia; **p. 252:** Foodcollection/Getty Images; Johnfoto18/Shutterstock; Pearson Education, Inc.; Rawpixel/Shutterstock; **p. 253:** Digital Vision/Getty Images; **p. 254:** Jim Varney/Science source; **p. 257:** Wavebreakmedia/Shutterstock; **p. 258:** Jack Dagley Photography/Shutterstock; **p. 259:** NF-07-06: Corbis/VCG/Getty Images; **p. 260:** Image Source/Corbis; **p. 261:** Richard Megna/Fundamental Photographs: NYC; **p. 262:** Antonio MP/Getty Images; Peepo/Vetta/Getty Images; OlegSam/Shutterstock; Iofoto/Shutterstock; Joy Brown/Shutterstock; npict/Fotolia; Danny Hooks/Fotolia; AmpFotoStudio.com/Fotolia; **p. 264:** Arthur Glauberman/Science Source; **p. 265:** Nd3000/Shutterstock; **p. 266:** Pearson Education, Inc.; **p. 267:** Ol_vic/Shutterstock; **p. 268:** Pearson Education, Inc.; **p. 271:** Joe Koshellek/MCT/Newscom; **p. 273:** Rawpixel/Shutterstock; Digital Vision/Getty Images; **p. 274:** Wavebreakmedia/Shutterstock; Image Source/Corbis; **p. 275:** Joe Koshellek/MCT/Newscom

Chapter 8   Chapter Opener: Tom Grill/JGI/AGE Fotostock; **p. 283:** Bloomimage/Corbis; **p. 290:** Don Mason/Blend Images/Alamy Stock Photo; **p. 295:** ESB Professional/Shutterstock; **p. 301:** Rudchenko Liliia/Shutterstock; **p. 303:** Sniegirova Mariia/Shutterstock; April_89/Fotolia; **p. 308:** Chris Rout/Alamy Stock Photo; **p. 309:** D.Hurst/Alamy Stock Photo; **p. 310:** Andy Dean Photography/Shutterstock; **p. 312:** Rudchenko Liliia/Shutterstock; **p. 313:** Andy Dean Photography/Shutterstock

Chapter 9   Chapter Opener: Burke's Backyard/Alamy Stock Photo; **p. 319:** Mtsyri/Shutterstock; Stockbyte/Getty Images; **p. 321:** Best View Stock/Alamy Stock Photo; **p. 322:** Dmytro Nikitin/123RF; **p. 323:** National Eye Institute; **p. 326:** A-plus image bank/Alamy Stock Photo; Pearson Education, Inc.; **p. 328:** Elena Schweitzer/Shutterstock; Sarsmis/Shutterstock; **p. 329:** Timmary/Shutterstock; **p. 331:** Siri Stafford/Digital Vision/Getty Images; **p. 332:** Suzanne Tucker/Shutterstock; **p. 334:** 09-11: James Stevenson/Science

Source, **p. 336:** Gustoimages/Science Source, **p. 337:** Seth Joel/Photographer's Choice/Getty Images, **p. 338:** John Smith/Photolibrary/Getty Images, **p. 340:** Pearson Education, Inc.; Jacek Chabraszewski/Fotolia; Biophoto Associates/Science Source; **p. 341:** Arek Malang/Shutterstock; **p. 342:** Ian O'Leary/Dorling Kindersley, Ltd.; M.pilot/Shutterstock; **p. 346:** Scott Camazine/Alamy Stock Photo; **p. 346:** SPL/Science Source; **p. 347** Suzifoo/Getty Images; **p. 348:** Kristin Piljay/Pearson Education, Inc.; Jupiterimages/Getty Images; **p. 349:** Registered trademark of The United States Pharmacopeial Convention. Used with Permission; **p. 351:** Mtsyri/Shutterstock, Stockbyte/Getty Images; **p. 353:** Kristin Piljay/Pearson Education, Inc.

Chapter 10 **Chapter Opener:** Lubos Chlubny/123RF; **p. 364:** Joe Gough/Fotolia; **p. 367:** Ralph Morse//Time Life Pictures/Getty Images; Jjava/Fotolia; **p. 369:** Biophoto Associates/Science Source; SPL/Science Source; **p. 370:** D.Hurst/Alamy Stock Photo; **p. 372:** Dr. M.A. Ansary/Science Source; **p. 373:** Smileus/Shutterstock; Justin Lightley/Photographer's Choice/Getty Images; **p. 374:** Richard Semik/Shutterstock; **p. 375:** MaxPhotographer/Shutterstock; **p. 376:** FoodCollection/Photolibrary/Getty Images; Brand X Pictures/AGE Fotostock; **p. 378:** Tim Ridley/Dorling Kindersley, Ltd.; **p. 380:** Biophoto Associates/Science Source/Getty Images; **p. 382:** Olga Miltsova/Shutterstock; AmpFotoStudio/Shutterstock; **p. 383:** Pearson Education, Inc.; **p. 384:** Wavebreakmedia/Shutterstock; **p. 386:** Syda Productions/Shutterstock; **p. 387:** Pikselstock/Shutterstock; Brand X Pictures/AGE Fotostock; **p. 388:** SPL/Science Source; **p. 389:** Pantakan Sakda/Shutterstock; **p. 390:** Jason Stitt/Shutterstock; Antagain/E+/Getty Images; **p. 394:** Brand X Pictures/AGE Fotostock; **p. 395:** Brand X Pictures/AGE Fotostock; **p. 400:** AmpFotoStudio/Shutterstock

Chapter 11 **Chapter Opener:** Westend61/Getty Images; **p. 406:** Orange Line Media/Shutterstock; **p. 407:** Steve HIx/Fuse/Getty Images; **p. 408:** Dea/L Ricciarini/De Agostini Editore/AGE Fotostock; Radius Images/Alamy Stock Photo; **p. 410:** Bit24/Fotolia; Odua Images/Fotolia; **p. 412:** TerryJ/E+/Getty Images; **p. 416:** Dave & Les Jacobs/Blend Images/Getty Images; **p. 417:** Wave Royalty Free/Design Pics Inc/Alamy Stock Photo; Dynamic Graphics Group/Getty Images; **p. 418:** Pearson Education, Inc.; **p. 420:** Lucianne Pashley/Age Fotostock; **p. 422:** Sergey Peterman/Shutterstock; **p. 422:** George Dolgikh/Shutterstock; Peter Bernik/Shutterstock; Jeremy Pembrey/Alamy Stock Photo; **p. 424:** Monika Wisniewska/Shutterstock; **p. 427:** Lucianne Pashley/Age Fotostock

Chapter 12 **Chapter Opener:** PhotoCuisine/Alamy Stock Photo; **p. 435:** Keko64/Shutterstock; **p. 436:** Eye of Science/Science Source; **p. 440:** Richard Megna/Fundamental Photographs, NYC; **p. 442:** Scott Thomas/Getty Images; **p. 443:** Nick Emm/Alamy Stock Photo; Joe Gough/Shutterstock; **p. 444:** Steve Sant/Alamy Stock Photo; **p. 446:** Smit/Shutterstock; Elena Schweitzer/Shutterstock; Motorlka/Fotolia; **p. 447:** Buena Vista Images/Stone/Getty Images; **p. 448:** Lehner/E+/Getty Images; D.Hurst/Alamy Stock Photo; **p. 449:** Brand X Pictures/AGE Fotostock; **p. 450:** Nitr/Shutterstock; Michael Klein/Photolibrary/Getty Images; **p. 451:** Vaivirga/Fotolia; **p. 452:** Ian O'Leary/Dorling Kindersley, Ltd.; **p. 453:** Dustin Dennis/Shutterstock; **p. 454:** Brand X Pictures/Getty Images; **p. 455:** Larry Korb/Shutterstock; **p. 456:** United States Department of Health and Human Services; **p. 457:** Catherine Ursillo/Science Source; **p. 458:** Stockbyte/Getty Images; **p. 460:** Monkey Business Images/Shutterstock; **p. 462:** Steve Sant/Alamy Stock Photo; Smit/Shutterstock; Elena Schweitzer/Shutterstock; Motorlka/Fotolia; Stockbyte/Getty Images; **p. 463:** Michael Klein/Photolibrary/Getty Images

Chapter 13 **Chapter Opener:** Elena Elisseeva/Alamy Stock Photo; **p. 472:** Olga Nayashkova/Shutterstock; **p. 473:** Steve Moss/Alamy Stock Photo; **p. 476:** C Squared Studios/Photodisc/Getty Images; **p. 477:** Dehooks/Getty Images; **p. 478:** Mimagephotography/Shutterstock; **p. 479:** Anna Sedneva/Getty Images; Foodcollection/Getty Images; **p. 483:** Jon Edwards Photography/Bon Appetit/Alamy Stock Photo; **p. 483:** Medical-on-Line/Alamy Stock Photo; **p. 484:** Olga Popova/Shutterstock; **p. 486:** Don Farrall/Getty Images; **p. 487:** 13-11: National Institute of Dental Research; John A Rizzo/Age Fotostock; **p. 488:** Hong Vo/Shutterstock; **p. 490:** Chatuphot/Shutterstock; Wavebreakmedia/Shutterstock; **p. 492:** Marco Mayer/Shutterstock; Anna Hoychuk/Shutterstock; Foodcollection/Getty Images; **p. 493:** Viktor/Fotolia; **p. 495:** Eric Grave/Science Source; Joaquin Carrillo Farga/Science Source; Ed Reschke/Photolibrary/Getty Images; **p. 496:** Lostinbids/Getty Images; **p. 497:** Dani

Vincek/Fotolia; **p. 498:** FoodCollection/SuperStock; **p. 500:** National Institute of Dental Research; Foodcollection/StockFood GmbH/Alamy Stock Photo; Mike Goldwater/Alamy Stock Photo; Marco Mayer/Shutterstock; **p. 501:** Foodcollection/Getty Images; **p. 501:** Anna Hoychuk/Shutterstock; Eric Grave/Science Source; Joaquin Carrillo Farga/Science Source

Chapter 14 **Chapter Opener:** Erik Isakson/Tetra Images/Alamy Stock Photo; **p. 509:** Helder Almeida/Shutterstock; Kenneth Man/Shutterstock; Maga/Shutterstock; Light poet/Shutterstock; Zurijeta/Shutterstock; Brian A Jackson/Shutterstock; **p. 513:** NF-14-01: 2/Jack Hollingsworth/Ocean/Corbis; **p. 514:** Cultura Limited/SuperStock; **p. 515:** Timothy A. Clary/AFP/Getty Images/Newscom; **p. 517:** St Bartholomew's Hospital/Science Source; Philippe Psaila/Science Source; **p. 522:** David Madison/Photographer's Choice/Getty Images; Joe Traver/The LIFE Images Collection/Getty Images; Mauro Fermariello/Science Source; Pearson Education, Inc.; **p. 523:** Inmagine/Alamy Stock Photo; **p. 526:** Julien Warnand/EPA/Newscom; **p. 527:** Michaela Begsteiger/Getty Images; **p. 528:** Barcroft Media/Getty Images; **p. 529:** Corbis/VCG/Getty Images; **p. 530:** D. Hurst/Alamy Stock Photo; **p. 532:** St Bartholomew's Hospital/Science Source; Mauro Fermariello/Science Source; **p. 533:** Corbis/VCG/Getty Images

Chapter 15 **Chapter Opener:** JGI/Jamie Grill/Blend Images/Getty Images; **p. 538:** Bill Aron/PhotoEdit: Inc; **p. 540:** SilviaJansen/Vetta/Getty Images; **p. 541:** Laurence Mouton/PhotoAlto Sas/Alamy Stock Photo; **p. 542:** Dmitri Maruta/Alamy Stock Photo; **p. 545:** Ilene MacDonald/Alamy Stock Photo; **p. 548:** Inmagine Asia/AGE Fotostock; **p. 549:** Catalin Petolea/Shutterstock; **p. 551:** ZUMA Press: Inc/Alamy Stock Photo; GlowImages/Alamy Stock Photo; **p. 554:** Department of Health and Human Services; **p. 555:** Bogdan Wankowicz/Shutterstock; Photolibrary/Alamy Stock Photo; Foodcollection RF/Getty Images; **p. 556:** James Benet/Getty Images; **p. 557:** Ruth Jenkinson/Dorling Kindersley, Ltd.; **p. 558:** William87/Fotolia; **p. 562:** Hoozone/Getty Images; **p. 563:** JGI/Blend Images/Getty Images; **p. 566:** Phanie/Alamy Stock Photo; **p. 567:** Peter Kramer/AP Images; **p. 568:** William87/Fotolia; Dmitri Maruta/Alamy Stock Photo; **p. 569:** Ilene MacDonald/Alamy Stock Photo; **p. 570:** Inmagine Asia/AGE Fotostock; Richard Megna/Fundamental Photographs, NYC; Ruth Jenkinson/Dorling Kindersley, Ltd.

Chapter 16 **Chapter Opener:** Stock4B-RF/Getty Images; **p. 578:** Dan Dalton/Digital Vision/Getty Images; **p. 580:** BananaStock/Getty Images; Tamara Lackey/Getty Images; Arpad/Fotolia; Dex Image/Alamy Stock Photo; **p. 581:** Tetra Images/Getty Images; Ryan McVay/Photodisc/Getty Images; Stockbyte/Getty Images; Stockbyte/Getty Images; **p. 582:** Aletia2011/Fotolia; Sirtravelalot/Shutterstock; **p. 589:** Webphotographeer/Getty Images; **p. 594:** Peter Bernik/Shutterstock; Nigel Roddis/EPA/Newscom; Koji Aoki/Getty Images; Maho/Fotolia; Piluhin/Alamy Stock Photo; Maridav/Shutterstock; **p. 596:** Stockbroker/MBI/Alamy Stock Photo; **p. 597:** Elena Gaak/Shutterstock; **p. 598:** Kristin Piljay/Pearson Education, Inc.; Kayte Deioma/PhotoEdit; **p. 600:** Skynesher/E+/Getty Images; **p. 601:** Duncan Selby/Alamy Stock Photo; **p. 602:** 101dalmatians/Getty Images; **p. 604:** John Giustina/SuperStock/Corbis; **p. 606:** Siegi/Fotolia; **p. 609:** Kristin Piljay/Pearson Education, Inc.; **p. 610:** Kristin Piljay/Pearson Education, Inc.; **p. 612:** Dan Dalton/Digital Vision/Getty Images; **p. 613:** Elena Gaak/Shutterstock; Stockbroker/MBI/Alamy Stock Photo; **p. 614:** Kristin Piljay/Pearson Education, Inc.

Chapter 17 **Chapter Opener:** Tetra Images/Brand X Pictures/Getty Images; **p. 624:** PictureIndia/Asia Images Group Pte Ltd/Alamy Stock Photo; **p. 626:** Dalaprod/Fotolia; **p. 628:** Andy Crawford/Dorling Kindersley, Ltd.; **p. 632:** Amarita/Shutterstock; **p. 633:** Shutterdandan/Shutterstock; **p. 634:** Freemixer/Getty Images; **p. 635:** Kristin Piljay/Pearson Education, Inc.; **p. 636:** Blend Images/SuperStock; **p. 639:** Erik Freeland/Corbis Historical/Getty Images; **p. 641:** Stewart Cohen/Blend Images/Getty Images; **p. 643:** It Stock Free/AGE Fotostock; **p. 645:** Sally and Richard Greenhill/Alamy Stock Photo; **p. 647:** Ted Croll/Science Source; **p. 651:** Mariusz S. Jurgielewicz/Shutterstock; **p. 653:** Serhiy Kobyakov/Shutterstock; **p. 654:** Kristin Piljay/Pearson Education, Inc.; **p. 655:** Blend Images/SuperStock; **p. 656:** Kristin Piljay/Pearson Education, Inc.; Erik Freeland/Corbis Historical/Getty Images; Andy Crawford/Dorling Kindersley, Ltd.; **p. 657:** Stewart Cohen/Blend Images/Getty Images; Mariusz S. Jurgielewicz/Shutterstock

Chapter 18 **Chapter Opener:** Werli Francois/Alamy Stock Images; **p. 667:** Simon Brown/Dorling Kindersley, Ltd.; **p. 669:** TF2/Picturesbyrob/Alamy Stock Photo; **p. 671:** Ronnie Kaufman/Larry Hirshowitz/Blend Images/Alamy Stock Photo; **p. 672:** Skip Nall/Alamy Stock Photo; **p. 674:** SB Professional/Shutterstock; Wavebreak Media Ltd/123 RF; **p. 677:** Marnie Burkhart/Fancy/Alamy Stock Photo; **p. 679:** Alin Dragulin/FogStock/Getty Images; Mike Booth/Alamy Stock Photo; **p. 684:** Oneinchpunch/Shutterstock; **p. 686:** Beyond/Kalle Singer/Micheko Productions Inh. Michele Vitucci/Alamy Stock Photo; **p. 688:** Digital Vision/Getty Images; **p. 689:** N. Aubrier/AGE Fotostock; Wavebreak Media Ltd/123 RF; **p. 690:** Oneinchpunch/Shutterstock; TF2/Picturesbyrob/Alamy Stock Photo; Digital Vision/Getty Images

Chapter 19 **Chapter Opener:** Phanie/Alamy Stock Photo; **p. 700:** Blend Images/Ariel Skelley/Brand X Pictures/Getty Images; **p. 701:** SDA Ag. Research Center; SDA Ag. Research Center; **p. 706:** Chris Willson/Alamy Stock Photo; **p. 708:** Altrendo images/Getty Images; **p. 711:** Pinkcandy/Shutterstock; **p. 713:** Sally and Richard Greenhill/Alamy Stock Photo; Fancy/Alamy Stock Photo; **p. 715:** Susan Chiang/Getty Images; **p. 717:** Tina Manley/Alamy Stock Photo; **p. 719:** WavebreakmediaMicro/Fotolia; Comstock/Getty Images; **p. 720:** Stockbyte/Getty Images; **p. 721:** Stevecoleimages/Getty Images; **p. 723:** SDA Ag. Research Center; Altrendo images/Getty Images; **p. 724:** Sally and Richard Greenhill/Alamy Stock Photo, Tina Manley/Alamy Stock Photo, WavebreakmediaMicro/Fotolia

Chapter 20 **Chapter Opener:** Lew Robertson/Corbis/Getty Images; **p. 735:** Phanie/Science Source; Cultura/REX/Shutterstock; **p. 736:** Eye of Science/Science Source; **p. 740:** Jacek Chabraszewski/Shutterstock; **p. 742:** Piga&catalano/Marka/AGE Fotostock; **p. 743:** United States Department of Agriculture; **p. 747:** Ruud Morijn/Fotolia; George Skene/MCT/Newscom; Andrew Rubtsov/Alamy Stock Photo; Paul Burns/Blend Images/Alamy Stock Photo; Monkey Business Images/Shutterstock; **p. 749:** Anke van Wyk/Shutterstock; **p. 751:** Pearson Education, Inc.; **p. 753:** Africa Studio/Fotolia; **p. 755:** Grigorenko/Getty Images; **p. 757:** Sauletas/iStock/Getty Images; **p. 763:** Vovan/Fotolia; **p. 765:** Dembinsky Photo Associates/Alamy Stock Photo; **p. 766:** Smileus/Shutterstock; **p. 767:** Michael Siluk/Alamy Stock Photo; Joel Nito/AFP/Getty Images; **p. 770:** Cultura/REX/Shutterstock; Paul Burns/Blend Images/Alamy Stock Photo; **p. 771:** Sauletas/iStock/Getty Images; Vovan/Fotolia

Chapter 21 **Chapter Opener:** Fstop123/Getty Images; **p. 781:** Jane Alexander/Photofusion Picture Library/Alamy Stock Photo; **p. 783:** David Grossman/Alamy Stock Photo; **p. 785:** ESB Professional/Shutterstock; Lulu/Fotolia; **p. 786:** Mike Boyatt/Agstockusa/AGE Fotostock; **p. 788:** Mike Goldwater/Alamy Stock Photo; **p. 791:** Susan Montoya Bryan/AP Images; Alain Evrard/Robert Harding; **p. 792:** Boris Roessler/DPA/Picture-alliance/Newscom; **p. 795:** Jean-Marc Giboux/Getty Images; **p. 796:** Jane Alexander/Photofusion Picture Library/Alamy Stock Photo; ESB Professional/Shutterstock; Mike Goldwater/Alamy Stock Photo; **p. 797:** Susan Montoya Bryan/AP Images

Tolerable Upper Intake Levels (ULs)

Life Stage Group	Vitamin A (µg/d)[a]	Vitamin C (mg/d)	Vitamin D (µg/d)	Vitamin E (mg/d)[b, c]	Niacin (mg/d)[c]	Vitamin B6 (mg/d)	Folate (µg/d)[c]	Choline (g/d)
Vitamins								
Infants								
0–6 mo	600	ND[d]	25	ND	ND	ND	ND	ND
6–12 mo	600	ND	38	ND	ND	ND	ND	ND
Children								
1–3 y	600	400	63	200	10	30	300	1.0
4–8 y	900	650	75	300	15	40	400	1.0
Males								
9–13 y	1,700	1,200	100	600	20	60	600	2.0
14–18 y	2,800	1,800	100	800	30	80	800	3.0
19–30 y	3,000	2,000	100	1,000	35	100	1,000	3.5
31–50 y	3,000	2,000	100	1,000	35	100	1,000	3.5
51–70 y	3,000	2,000	100	1,000	35	100	1,000	3.5
>70 y	3,000	2,000	100	1,000	35	100	1,000	3.5
Females								
9–13 y	1,700	1,200	100	600	20	60	600	2.0
14–18 y	2,800	1,800	100	800	30	80	800	3.0
19–30 y	3,000	2,000	100	1,000	35	100	1,000	3.5
31–50 y	3,000	2,000	100	1,000	35	100	1,000	3.5
51–70 y	3,000	2,000	100	1,000	35	100	1,000	3.5
>70 y	3,000	2,000	100	1,000	35	100	1,000	3.5
Pregnancy								
14–18 y	2,800	1,800	100	800	30	80	800	3.0
19–50 y	3,000	2,000	100	1,000	35	100	1,000	3.5
Lactation								
14–18 y	2,800	1,800	100	800	30	80	800	3.0
19–50 y	3,000	2,000	100	1,000	35	100	1,000	3.5

Note: A Tolerable Upper Intake Level (UL) is the highest level of daily nutrient intake that is likely to pose no risk of adverse health effects to almost all individuals in the general population. Unless otherwise specified, the UL represents total intake from food, water, and supplements. Due to a lack of suitable data, ULs could not be established for vitamin K, thiamin, riboflavin, vitamin B₁₂, pantothenic acid, biotin, and carotenoids. In the absence of a UL, extra caution may be warranted in consuming levels above recommended intakes. Members of the general population should be advised not to routinely exceed the UL. The UL is not meant to apply to individuals who are treated with the nutrient under medical supervision or to individuals with predisposing conditions that modify their sensitivity to the nutrient.

[a] As preformed vitamin A only.

[b] As α-tocopherol; applies to any form of supplemental α-tocopherol.

[c] The ULs for vitamin E, niacin, and folate apply to synthetic forms obtained from supplements, fortified foods, or a combination of the two.

[d] ND = Not determinable due to lack of data of adverse effects in this age group and concern with regard to lack of ability to handle excess amounts. Source of intake should be from food only to prevent high levels of intake.

Data from: DIETARY REFERENCE INTAKES series, National Academies Press. Copyright ©1997, 1998, 2000, 2001, and 2011, by the National Academy of Sciences. These reports may be accessed via www.nap.edu. Courtesy of the National Academies Press, Washington, DC. Reprinted with permission.

Tolerable Upper Intake Levels (ULs)

Elements

Life Stage Group	Boron (mg/d)	Calcium (mg/d)	Copper (µg/d)	Fluoride (mg/d)	Iodine (µg/d)	Iron (mg/d)	Magnesium (mg/d)[e]	Manganese (mg/d)	Molybdenum (µg/d)	Nickel (mg/d)	Phosphorus (g/d)	Selenium (µg/d)	Vanadium (mg/d)[f]	Zinc (mg/d)	Sodium (g/d)	Chloride (g/d)
Infants																
0–6 mo	ND[d]	1,000	ND	0.7	ND	40	ND	ND	ND	ND	ND	45	ND	4	ND	ND
6–12 mo	ND	1,500	ND	0.9	ND	40	ND	ND	ND	ND	ND	60	ND	5	ND	ND
Children																
1–3 y	3	2,500	1,000	1.3	200	40	65	2	300	0.2	3	90	ND	7	1.5	2.3
4–8 y	6	2,500	3,000	2.2	300	40	110	3	600	0.3	3	150	ND	12	1.9	2.9
Males																
9–13 y	11	3,000	5,000	10	600	40	350	6	1,100	0.6	4	280	ND	23	2.2	3.4
14–18 y	17	3,000	8,000	10	900	45	350	9	1,700	1.0	4	400	ND	34	2.3	3.6
19–30 y	20	2,500	10,000	10	1,100	45	350	11	2,000	1.0	4	400	1.8	40	2.3	3.6
31–50 y	20	2,500	10,000	10	1,100	45	350	11	2,000	1.0	4	400	1.8	40	2.3	3.6
51–70 y	20	2,000	10,000	10	1,100	45	350	11	2,000	1.0	4	400	1.8	40	2.3	3.6
>70 y	20	2,000	10,000	10	1,100	45	350	11	2,000	1.0	3	400	1.8	40	2.3	3.6
Females																
9–13 y	11	3,000	5,000	10	600	40	350	6	1,100	0.6	4	280	ND	23	2.2	3.4
14–18 y	17	3,000	8,000	10	900	45	350	9	1,700	1.0	4	400	ND	34	2.3	3.6
19–30 y	20	2,500	10,000	10	1,100	45	350	11	2,000	1.0	4	400	1.8	40	2.3	3.6
31–50 y	20	2,500	10,000	10	1,100	45	350	11	2,000	1.0	4	400	1.8	40	2.3	3.6
51–70 y	20	2,000	10,000	10	1,100	45	350	11	2,000	1.0	4	400	1.8	40	2.3	3.6
>70 y	20	2,000	10,000	10	1,100	45	350	11	2,000	1.0	3	400	1.8	40	2.3	3.6
Pregnancy																
14–18 y	17	3,000	8,000	10	900	45	350	9	1,700	1.0	3.5	400	ND	34	2.3	3.6
19–50 y	20	2,500	10,000	10	1,100	45	350	11	2,000	1.0	3.5	400	ND	40	2.3	3.6
Lactation																
14–18 y	17	3,000	8,000	10	900	45	350	9	1,700	1.0	4	400	ND	34	2.3	3.6
19–50 y	20	2,500	10,000	10	1,100	45	350	11	2,000	1.0	4	400	ND	40	2.3	3.6

Note: A Tolerable Upper Intake Level (UL) is the highest level of daily nutrient intake that is likely to pose no risk of adverse health effects to almost all individuals in the general population. Unless otherwise specified, the UL represents total intake from food, water, and supplements. Due to a lack of suitable data, ULs could not be established for vitamin K, thiamin, riboflavin, vitamin B_{12}, pantothenic acid, biotin, and carotenoids. In the absence of a UL, extra caution may be warranted in consuming levels above recommended intakes. Members of the general population should be advised not to routinely exceed the UL. The UL is not meant to apply to individuals who are treated with the nutrient under medical supervision or to individuals with predisposing conditions that modify their sensitivity to the nutrient.

[d] ND = Not determinable due to lack of data of adverse effects in this age group and concern with regard to lack of ability to handle excess amounts. Source of intake should be from food only to prevent high levels of intake.

[e] The ULs for magnesium represent intake from a pharmacological agent only and do not include intake from food and water.

[f] Although vanadium in food has not been shown to cause adverse effects in humans, there is no justification for adding vanadium to food, and vanadium supplements should be used with caution. The UL is based on adverse effects in laboratory animals, and this data could be used to set a UL for adults but not children and adolescents.